REHABILITATION
NURSING

PROCESS AND APPLICATION

REHABILITATION NURSING

PROCESS AND APPLICATION

SHIRLEY P. HOEMAN, PhD, RN, CRRN, CNAA, CCM

Health System Consultations
Long Valley, New Jersey

SECOND EDITION

with 190 illustrations

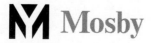 Mosby

St. Louis Baltimore Boston Carlsbad Chicago Naples New York Philadelphia Portland
London Madrid Mexico City Singapore Sydney Tokyo Toronto Wiesbaden

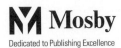

Mosby
Dedicated to Publishing Excellence

A Times Mirror Company

Publisher: Nancy Coon
Acquisitions Editor: Barry Bowlus
Developmental Editor: Nancy Baker
Senior Project Manager: Linda Clarke
Senior Production Editor: Vicki Hoenigke
Manufacturing Supervisor: David Graybill
Design Manager: Nancy McDonald
Cover illustration: David Noyes
Cover design: Sheriff Krebs Design

A NOTE TO THE READER

The author and publisher have made every attempt to check dosages and nursing content for accuracy. Because the science of pharmacology is continually advancing, our knowledge base continues to expand. Therefore we recommend that the reader always check product information for changes in dosage or administration before administering any medication. This is particularly important with new or rarely used drugs.

SECOND EDITION

Printed in the United States of America
Composition by The Clarinda Company
Printing/binding by Maple Vail

Mosby–Year Book, Inc.
11830 Westline Industrial Drive
St. Louis, Missouri 63146

Library of Congress Cataloging in Publication Data

Rehabilitation nursing : process and application/ [edited by] Shirley
  P. Hoeman. — 2nd ed.
       p.   cm.
    Includes bibliographical references and index.
    ISBN 0-8016-7766-1
    1. Rehabilitation nursing.   I. Hoeman, Shirley P.
    [DNLM: 1. Nursing Care.   2. Rehabilitation—nursing.   WY 150 R345
1996]
    RT120.R4R423   1996
    610.73′6—dc20
    DNLM/DLC   94-49100
    for Library of Congress   CIP

96 97 98 99 00 / 9 8 7 6 5 4 3 2

To Christopher, Timothy, and Jonathan

"They that wait upon the Lord shall renew their strength;
they shall mount up with wings as eagles;
they shall run, and not be weary;
and they shall walk, and not faint."
Isaiah 40:31

CONTRIBUTORS

Denise B. Angst, DNSc, RN
Clinical Research Associate
Department of Pediatrics
Lutheran General Hospital
Park Ridge, IL
Chapter 18

Judith A. Behm, MSN, RN, CRRN
Nursing Education Coordinator
Department of Nursing Education
Marianjoy Rehabilitation Hospital and Clinic
Wheaton, Illinois
Chapter 30

Jean M. Benjamin, MSN, RN, CRRN
Assistant Administrator-Rehabilitation Nursing
Southeastern Regional Rehabilitation Center
Cape Fear Valley Medical Center
Fayetteville, North Carolina
Chapter 6

Mary Frances Borgman-Gainer, EdD, RN
Nurse Consultant
Neuroscience Institute of Santa Fe
Gainesville, Florida
Chapter 14

Barbara J. Boss, PhD, RN, CS
Professor of Nursing
School of Nursing
University of Mississippi Medical Center
Jackson, Mississippi
Chapter 25

Linda Brewer, RN, MSN, ANP
Adult Nurse Practitioner
Scott Regional Hospital
Morton, Mississippi
Chapter 19

Lisa Cyr Buchanan, MS, RNC, CRRN
Rehabilitation Clinical Nurse Specialist
Lisa B. Cyr & Associates
Charleston, Maine
Chapter 9

Marci Catanzaro, RN, CS, PhD
Nurse Practitioner
Private Practice
Seattle, Washington
Chapter 4

Gloria T. Aubert Craven MSN, RN, CRRN
Director
Department of Legislation and Government Affairs
Massachusetts Nurses Association
Canton, Massachusetts

Editor/Publisher
Pertinent Legislation Affecting Nurses
Medford, Massachusetts
Chapter 5

Susan L. Dean-Baar, PhD, RN, CRRN, FAAN
Assistant Professor
Department of Health Restoration
University of Wisconsin-Milwaukee
Milwaukee, Wisconsin
Chapter 10

Pamela Muhm Duchene, DNSc, RN, CRRN
Vice President
Nursing and Clinical Services
New England Rehabilitation Hospital
Woburn, Massachusetts
Chapters 7 and 24

Elizabeth Forbes, RN, MSN, EdD, FAAN
Professor
Department of Nursing
College of Allied Health Science
Thomas Jefferson University
Philadelphia, Pennsylvania
Chapter 16

Cindy Gatens, MN, RN, CRRN
Clinical Nurse Specialist
Rehabilitation Nursing
Dodd Hall
The Ohio State University Medical Center
Columbus, Ohio
Chapter 26

Aloma R. Gender, MSN, RN, CRRN
Assistant Administrator/Director of Nursing
San Diego Rehabilitation Institute
San Diego, California
Chapter 21

Carol A. Gleason, RN, CRRN, CCM, LRC
Rehabilitation Consultant
Marblehead, Massachusetts
Chapter 5

Nancy H. Glenn, MSN, RN, CRRN
Rehabilitation Clinical Nurse Specialist
Education and Staff Development
Charlotte Mecklenburg Hospital Authority
Charlotte, North Carolina
Chapter 17

Cheryl Graham-Eason, MS, RN, CRRN
Professor
Nursing and Anthropology
Community College Allegheny County
Pittsburgh, Pennsylvania
Chapter 3

Susan B. Greco, MSN, RN, CRRN
Administrative Director of Patient Care Services
Relife, North Alabama Rehabilitation Hospital
Huntsville, Alabama
Chapter 27

Margaret J. Griffiths, MSN, RN
Associate Professor
Department of Nursing
College of Allied Health Sciences
Thomas Jefferson University
Philadelphia, Pennsylvania
Chapter 22

Maureen Habel, MA, RN, CRRN
Director, Nursing Staff Development
Department of Nursing
Rancho Los Amigos Medical Center
Downey, California
Chapter 23

A. René Hébert, MS, RN, CRRN
Clinical Nurse Specialist
Dodd Hall
The Ohio State University Medical Center
Columbus, Ohio

Staff Registered Nurse
Rehabilitation Department
Mt. Carmel Medical Center
Columbus, Ohio
Chapter 26

Joyce H. Johnson, PhD, RN
Associate Professor
Medical-Surgical Nursing Department
University of Illinois at Chicago
Chicago, Illinois
Chapter 18

Margaret Kelly-Hayes, EdD, RN, CRRN
Associate Clinical Professor of Neurology
Neurological Nursing
Department of Neurology
Boston University School of Medicine
Boston, Massachusetts
Chapter 11

Janet G. LaMantia, MA, RN, CRRN
Rehabilitation Clinical Specialist
Pain Management Associates
Jamestown, Rhode Island
Chapter 15

Janet L. Larson, PhD, RN
Associate Professor
Medical-Surgical Nursing Department
University of Illinois at Chicago
Chicago, Illinois
Chapter 18

Kay Lewis Abney, PhD, RN, CPNP
Department of Pediatrics
University of Mississippi Medical Center
Jackson, Mississippi
Chapter 25

Patricia L. McCollom, RN, MS, CRRN, CIRS, CCM
President/Nurse Consultant
Management Consulting & Rehabilitation Services, Inc.
LifeCare Economics, Ltd.
Ankeny, Iowa
Chapter 8

Angela Moy, MSN, RN, CRRN
Rehabilitation Admissions Coordinator
Rehabilitation Department
Rehabilitation Institute of Chicago
at Alexian Brothers Hospital
Elk Grove Village, Illinois
Chapter 29

Christina M. Mumma, PhD, RN, CRRN
Associate Professor
School of Nursing and Health Sciences
University of Alaska Anchorage
Anchorage, Alaska
Chapter 2

Audrey Nelson, PhD, RN
Associate Chief, Nursing Service for Research
James A. Henry Veterans' Hospital
Tampa, Florida
Chapter 2

Marilyn Pires, MS, RN, CRRN
Clinical Nurse Specialist-Spinal Cord Injury
Nursing
Rancho Los Amigos Medical Center
Downey, California
Chapter 20

Maria Brighton Radwanski, RN, MSN, CS, CRRN
Gerontological Clinical Nurse Specialist
Department of Nursing
Reading Rehabilitation Hospital
Reading, Pennsylvania
Chapter 31

Josephine Ricci-Balich, MSN, RNC, CRRN
Clinical Nurse Educator
(formerly: Clinical Nursing Director, Pediatric Program)
Division of Nursing
Rehabilitation Institute of Chicago
Chicago, Illinois
Chapter 30

Dorothy Sager, RN, CRRN, CIRS, CCM
President
Rehabilitation Network Corporation
Paoli, Pennsylvania
Chapter 8

Mary Ann E. Solimine, MLS, RN*
Eucharistic Minister: Medical Librarian
Kessler Institute for Rehabilitation, Inc.
West Orange, New Jersey
Chapter 28

Anaise (Sis) Theuerkauf, BS, MEd, RN, CRRN, CCM
President
ESCI
Shreveport, Louisiana
Chapter 12

Barbara H. Warner, MS, RN
Director Neuroscience/Psychiatric/Rehabilitation Nursing
Rehabilitation Nursing Department
The Ohio State University Hospitals
Columbus, Ohio
Chapter 6

*Research Assistant

ACKNOWLEDGMENTS FOR PREVIOUS CONTRIBUTORS

Mila A. Aroskar, RN, EdD

Rita J. Boucher, RN, EdD

Dorothy P. Byers, RN, MS

Sandra Chenelly, RN, MS

Sharon S. Dittmar, RN, PhD

Theresa P. Dulski, RN, C, MS

Susan M. Evans, RN, MS

Kathy M. Graham, RN, MS

Denise Hanlon, RN, MS

Brenda P. Haughey, RN, PhD

Margaret M. Hens, RN, MS

Linda M. Janelli, RN, C, MS, EdD

Judith A. Laughlin, RN, PhD

Martha F. Markarian, RN, MS

Elizabeth A. Moody-Szymanski, RN, MS

Mary Sue Niederpruem, RN, MS

Elizabeth C. Phelps, RN, MS

Joyce Santora, RN, MS

Yvonne Krall Scherer, RN, EdD

Jill A. Scott, RN, MS

Margie L. Scott, RN, EdD

Elizabeth L. Sharkey, RN, MS

Margaret A. Umhauer, RN, MS

Barbara G. White, RN, EdD

Barbara Wisnom, RN, MS

REVIEWERS

Judith L. Albers, RN
Acute Rehabilitation Staff Nurse
Deconess Hospital
St. Louis, Missouri

Jane Backer, DNS, RN
Assistant Professor
Indiana University School of Nursing
Indianapolis, Indiana

Susan Baltrus, BS, MSN
Senior Co-Coordinator Nursing Education
Central Maine Medical Center School of Nursing
Lewiston, Maine

Barbara Brillhart, RN, PhD, CRRN
Associate Professor
University of Colorado Health Sciences Center
Denver, Colorado

Barbara Brown, BSN, MN
Professor of Nursing
Community College of Allegheny County
Pittsburgh, Pennsylvania

Karen Anne Budenholzer, BSN, CRRN
Registered Nurse
Oakland Children's Hospital
Oakland, California

Sharon Burk, MBA, CRRN, CCM
National Director of Managed Care
The Hillhaven Corporation
Tacoma, Washington

Karen DeWitt, BSN, MA, EdD
Vice President of Nursing
Children's Specialized Hospital
Mountainside, New Jersey

Shirley Drayton-Hargrove, PhD, RN, CRRN
Assistant Professor of Nursing
Temple University College of Allied Health Professions
Philadelphia, Pennsylvania

Sharon A. Duncan, BSN, MSAC, MSN
Instructor
Indiana Vocational Technical College
Evansville, Indiana

Kristen L. Easton, MS, RN, CRRN
Assistant Professor of Nursing
Valparaiso University
Valparaiso, Indiana

Janet M. Farahmand, CGN, MSN, EdD
Associate Professor of Nursing
Neumann College Division of Nursing
Aston, Pennsylvania

Mary Anne Gaynor, MS, CRRN
Associate Professor of Nursing
Saint Xavier University
Chicago, Illinois

Susan Girvin-Quirk, MSN, RN
Clinical Nurse Specialist
Community Hospitals Indianapolis
Indianapolis, Indiana

Gail Goetz, BSN, MSN
Confidence Program Nurse Practitioner
Magee Rehabilitation Hospital
Philadelphia, Pennsylvania

Cynthia S. Jacelon, MS, RN, CRRN
Rehabilitation Clinical Nurse Specialist
Berkshire Medical Center
Pittsfield, Massachusetts

Mary Ann Jacobs, MSN, RN, CRRN
Physical Rehabilitation Clinician
Jewish Hospital of St. Louis
St. Louis, Missouri

Kara B. Jaffe, MA, RN
Vice President
Assisted Home Recovery
Los Angeles, California

Patricia A. Knecht, RN, BSN
Practical Nursing Instructor
Center for Arts and Technology/Brandywine Campus
Coatesville, Pennsylvania

Patricia A. Lockhart-Pretti, ADN, BSN
Practical Nursing Instructor
Center for Arts and Technology-Brandywine Campus
Coatesville, Pennsylvania

Joan E. Miller, BSN, MAM, CRRN
Rehabilitation Consultant
Miller Medical Consulting Services
Phoenix, Arizona

Myra E. Neal, MSN, RN, CRRN
Clinical Nurse Specialist, Retired
Community Hospitals Indianapolis
Indianapolis, Indiana

Terri Sue Patterson, BSN, MSN, CRRN
Consultant
Nursing Consultation Services, Ltd.
Norristown, Pennsylvania

Mary L. Pickerell, BA, RN, CCM, CIRS
Rehabilitation Nurse Consultant
Bethesda, Maryland

PREFACE

This edition of *Rehabilitation Nursing* is a work of caring about clients and of commitment to the nurses who practice the professional specialty of rehabilitation nursing. This book is intended to be another step in the growth and development of rehabilitation nursing theory, practice, education, and administration. From the beginning of this project, the rehabilitation nurses who contributed to this book joined in a conceptual contract about how we envisioned this book would improve outcome for clients, as well as guide and inspire rehabilitation nurses in their growing areas of practice.

This book is written by nurse experts from across the nation, who serve in a variety of rehabilitation settings. One goal is to translate theoretical concepts and findings from nursing and interdisciplinary health research into meaningful interventions in practice. The contributors, library research consultant, and editorial staff of Mosby Year Book have joined me in producing a scholarly work that is relevant and usable in education and practice. To this end, every chapter has been peer reviewed, every reference has been verified, primary resources and classic references have been included with current references, and the literature has been researched to determine the best practices.

Using the nursing process as a foundation, the conceptual framework for the book is expanded upon and adapted from Roper's activities of daily living and Gordon's functional health patterns. Certain themes are threaded throughout the book because I believed them to be appropriate and essential to all areas. These are professional practice that is both community-based and institutional; interdisciplinary collaboration and evaluation; family and community influences; managing care across the lifespan, even lifelong care; attaining cultural relevance and sensitivity; improving clients' quality of life, dignity, and self-determination; promoting clients' wellness while preventing further disability or complications; and achieving clients' maximum potential in functional and lifestyle independence in their self-care or self-directed care. Throughout, the focus is on the whole person, apart from the chronic, disabling, or developmental condition. In reality, some aspect of rehabilitation will touch all of us, whether individually or through family and friends, in the human experience.

The second edition is organized within the framework of five sections. Section I contains chapters that address concepts and principles basic to rehabilitation nursing and is supplemented by Section II, in which content basic to understanding the foundations of rehabilitation nursing is addressed. Many of the chapters in these two sections, such as Case Management and Total Quality Management/Outcome Evaluation, appear for the first time in a rehabilitation nursing book and are further evidence of the significant changes that continue to occur within this specialty. Sections III and IV contain chapters about functional health patterns and sensory and psychosocial patterns, including Cardiac Rehabilitation as well as new chapters on cognition and spirituality. All of the functional health pattern chapters have been fully revised and draw upon an extensive collection of current clinical information available on each topic. Section V provides essential chapters on three emerging specialty practice areas: burn, pediatric, and geriatric rehabilitation.

Two additional features found in this book are individualized assessments and nursing processes organized by topic or specialty area. Individualized assessment can be incorporated into existing assessments and nursing processes, as well as the unique case studies that appear at the end of most chapters. Each case study resembles a synthesis of care plan and case study, and is designed to illustrate how to apply rehabilitation nursing concepts and process with the client.

Shirley P. Hoeman PhD, RN, CRRN, CNAA, CCM

FOREWORD

Rehabilitation nursing is an excellent example of what holistic nursing is all about. In rehabilitation nursing, the client's physical, psychological, cognitive, social, and financial aspects and interactions are assessed and addressed. In addition to the usual client/nurse relationship, rehabilitation nursing involves the client's family and community in the treatment process. While some situations may require a large interdisciplinary team of knowledgeable health care professionals, others may be well served by a rehabilitation nurse practitioner who works with the desciplines that are selected on the basis of an individual patient's requirements.

Just how specialized is rehabilitation nursing? It can be very specialized, but the nurse in general practice needs to know its goals and capabilities, as well as the relationship between sound general practice and rehabilitation. There is a crying need for basic nursing programs to include the rudiments of the rehabilitation process in their curricula. By not understanding the intricacies of rehabilitation, nurses can actually limit a patient's opportunity for positive outcome.

The clientele who can benefit from rehabilitation is increasing rapidly. Some of these individuals are true pioneers. For example, adults with spina bifida were unheard of 15 years ago. Very small premature infants are surviving at weights that once, no one ever envisioned. Who would have thought that increasing numbers of octogenarians would be living in their own homes, and out volunteering their services?

These *new* clients will need assistance in maintaining their independence at the highest levels possible for as long as possible. Nurses play a key role in helping the client to accomplish these goals. The rehabilitation process may begin with specialists in an institution, but it continues in the home and the community, often for a lifetime.

In 406 B.C., Hippocrates said in his book *On Surgery,* "It should be kept in mind that exercise stengthens and inactivity wastes." Here we are 2,500 years later, and the dynamics of our society have changed dramatically. The scope of nursing practice has expanded and changed drastically in just the past few decades. We should no longer find elderly hospitalized persons restrained, as in years past, nor should we allow older persons who live in nursing homes, assistive living apartments, and at home, to remain sitting around in chairs, rarely moving and with minimal social, cognitive, or psychological stimulation.

Community accessibility is also critical to the rehabilitation process. Although there has been recent federal and state legislation requiring architectural accessibility for persons with disabilities, unfortunately in many circumstances the application of these laws ignores the obstacles that existed before the legislation. For example, one may find the wheelchair-accessible toilet the last on a line of toilets, making wheelchair access difficult, if not impossible. Another example of unthinking adherence to building codes is the addition of Braille signage in parking ramp elevators. Those who implement our laws and codes certainly need greater input from people who understand the immediate problems that face individuals involved in both short- and long-term rehabilitation care.

Shirley Hoeman, the editor of this book, and I met 25 years ago when we both worked at Sister Kenny Institute in Minneapolis, which was, at the time, one of only a dozen or so rehabilitation centers in the United States. We not only saw first hand the exciting results of a multidisciplinary rehabilitation team, but we also saw what one rehabilitation nurse could do in our outreach program to nursing homes and public institutions for children. At that time, I wrote what may have been the first rehabilitation nursing text. It went into two editions and was translated into both Spanish and Japanese. Since then, greater international interest, changes in technology and pharmaceuticals, altered life expectancy, community awareness, the expansion of nursing knowledge, and an emphasis on home care have expanded the scope of rehabilitation nursing application.

As new research-based resources are becoming available every day, it is a delight to be a part of this book, which encompasses the advances in both nursing and rehabilitation nursing. Rehabilitation nurses are indeed fortunate to have such a comprehensive text available.

Ruth Stryker, RN, MA
Associate Professor Emerita
Formerly Assistant Coordinator of Center for Long Term Care Education
School of Public Health
University of Minnesota

ACKNOWLEDGEMENTS

This book was written because of the encouragement and support of my family, friends, and professional colleagues around the world. I value my husband, Denny for his patience while living in a "paper blizzard"; I thank my sons, Chris, Tim, and Jon for their encouragement and humor; I thank Jean Lundy for notions of "possibilities," and I appreciate Mary Ann Solimine for her unconditional friendship and professional support, and my mother for a lifetime of support. I acknowledge the contributions of numerous Mosby–Year Book editors, particularly Brian Morovitz and Nancy Baker, and Vicki Hoenigke and members of the production staff toward completion of this book. Furthermore, it has been rewarding to warmly initiate or regenerate acquaintances with Ruth Stryker and other colleagues across the nation. And, as I think back over my more than 25 years in rehabilitation nursing, I often wonder about those who are somewhat unaccounted for in my address book . . . Alan Borgen, where are you?

CONTENTS

I

CONCEPTS AND PRINCIPLES

1

Conceptual Bases for Rehabilitation Nursing

Shirley P. Hoeman, PhD, RN, CRRN, CNAA, CCM

INTRODUCTION

This chapter presents theories, models, concepts, and principles important for understanding content in this book and to clarify their value and utility for rehabilitation nurses. The discussion of theories in this chapter is intended to assist rehabilitation nurses to

+ Define roles and practice
+ Assess and plan with a client to meet unique, complex, and multidimensional needs
+ Build interventions on a client's strengths and resources
+ Integrate theoretical concepts from multiple disciplines with practice, education, research, or administration
+ Employ concepts and principles from a comprehensive repertoire of models or theories
+ Envision rehabilitation as a logical and essential component in the health process across the life span

The scope of rehabilitation nursing practice extends from primary prevention through acute and subacute levels; beyond tertiary intervention into community and lifelong care transactions. Early on, Stryker defined rehabilitation for nursing as "a creative process that begins with immediate preventive care in the first stage of accident or illness. It is continued through the restorative phase of care and involves adaptation of the whole being to a new life" (Stryker, 1977, p. 15).

CHANGING HEALTHCARE AND REHABILITATION NURSING

Rehabilitation nurses rely on sound theoretic foundations and scientific knowledge as they work with clients and their families to

+ Set goals for maximum levels of interdependent functioning and activities of daily living
+ Promote self-care, prevent complications or further disability
+ Reinforce positive coping behaviors
+ Ensure access with continuity of services and care
+ Advocate for optimal quality of life
+ Improve outcome for clients
+ Contribute to reforms in the character, structure, and delivery of healthcare in the United States

Healthcare leaders predict healthcare services will center on needs, preferences, and informed consent of individuals and families in our society, as opposed to being system driven. Ideally less emphasis will be focused on medical cure, illness, paternalism, and prescribed activities and more attention paid to values for self-care and client participation, ecologic approaches, holistic wellness, primary care and prevention, and quality attributes of care.

These changes in healthcare offer opportunities for rehabilitation nurses to activate theories and models; to construct, replicate, or validate instruments; to test concepts and principles; and then to use research findings as guides in education, administration, and practice.

THEORIES AND REHABILITATION NURSING

From the beginning, nurse theorists have attempted to question and explain phenomena related to Nightingale's "grand theory" of nursing by formulating assumptions based on metaparadigms of person, health, environment, and nursing (McCourt, 1993) (Table 1-1).

Ideally a nurse theorist offers explanations about how a theory is actualized in practice, beginning with the nursing process. Nursing theories and models both provide key links for demonstrating relationships among practice, education, research, and administration. As an example, theories can provide explanations about the possible relationships between or among observed phenomena, which may be used to predict events or control expected outcomes (Dubin, 1978).

Although theories themselves are too abstract to be proven directly, concepts, frameworks, models, and principles are components of theories that are available for testing through research (Fawcett, 1989). Findings from research on theory components eventually may form the basis for decision-making in nursing (Grant, Kinney, & Davis, 1993). Often researchers do not illustrate how theory was used in research or its implications for practice. Unfortunately only a few concepts have been discussed, and not examined by research, for rehabilitation nursing.

For instance, self-care and wellness are two concepts relevant to rehabilitation nursing (Orem 1971/1985) that have been suggested as content for rehabilitation programs (Nadolsky, 1987) and rehabilitation nursing curricula (Derstine & O'Toole, 1987). Orem's model was found to be useful clinically when nurses implemented and evaluated care plans for pediatric clients in multidisciplinary pediatric residential treatment centers (Titus & Porter, 1989).

Although relationships between quality-of-life factors and assumptions from Neuman's systems model were found relevant for practice (Hinds, 1990), little is known about how models and concepts apply to the practice of rehabilitation nursing or influence client outcomes.

Table 1-1 Comparison of four nursing models

	King open systems model	Neuman healthcare systems model	Orem self-care model	Roy adaptation model
Major Focus	Goal attainment through interaction	Relationship and reaction to stressors and regenerative factors	Self-care Dependence Independence	Holistic, biopsychosocial adaptation
Pragmatic use for rehabilitation nursing	Strong interactive basis with a goal-setting emphasis	Strong intervention based on primary, secondary, and tertiary prevention activities	Individual and/or family self-care abilities; emphasizes independence	Strong nursing process base with heavy assessment
Client involvement	Unique open system (personal, interpersonal, social) interacting with the environment	Unique, holistic open system composed of physiologic, sociocultural, psychological, developmental, and spiritual variables	System that involves the client when self-care needs exceed capabilities	Holistic level-of-adaptation system (regulator and cognator mechanisms function as internal control processes)
Nursing involvement	Process of action, reaction, and interaction with the client	Concern for the total person and all the variables affecting the response to stressors	Helping the client and/or family to become capable of meeting self-care needs	Managing stimuli to promote adaptation
Goals for health and well-being	Attain, maintain, or restore health to function in life roles	Maintain adaptation after reconstitution and stability occur	A whole, sound state of being	Promote integrity and positive adaptation
Environment	Personal set of systems interacting with other personal systems in the environment	Reciprocal: Prevention-limitation of stressors and effects (flexible, internal, and adaptive lines of defense)	External surroundings, including biologic and psychosocial	Internal and external stimuli (focal, contextual, and residual)
Limitations	Interaction of clients with cognitive and/or communication deficits may be limited. Implies compliance as a result of interaction. Minimal guidelines for assessment, diagnosis, and intervention	Can apply to all healthcare disciplines (a two-edged sword, as it can be challenging and problematic to define each discipline's unique contribution)	Focus is on individual self-care deficits rather than biopsychosocial aspects; illness/acute care focus of philosophy may be a barrier to rehabilitation nursing practice. Assumes that independence is of value in self-care	Boundaries between psychosocial modes are blurred. Assessment and diagnoses focus on nursing, which may interfere with an interdisciplinary approach

From *The Specialty Practice of Rehabilitation Nursing: A Core Curriculum* (3rd ed.) (p. 15), by A.E. McCourt, 1993, Skokie, IL: Rehabilitation Nursing Foundation. Copyright 1993 by the Rehabilitation Nursing Foundation. Reprinted with permission.

Domains of Knowledge

Another view of theoretical constructs uses nursing knowledge in separate but combinable domains of client, client-nurse, practice, and environment (Kim, 1987). Others envision an eclectic menu from which nurses may "mix and match" theorists and concepts to achieve versatility in a scientific basis for practice (Moccia, 1986). Nurses do agree that theory development contributes to the unified body of scientific knowledge, enhances professional autonomy, and promotes collegiality and communication among colleagues. Combining models with different ways of organizing and thinking may be necessary to address the variety of nursing process activities and practice options for

rehabilitation nurses, as well as to meet the complex needs of clients. Correctly speaking, most nursing frameworks are conceptual models rather than theories. At the present level of theory development and concept testing, no one unified model or combination of theories is adequate or elegant enough to serve as the sole paradigm for professional nursing.

For example, clients participating in rehabilitation often enter the health system at an acute or trauma level, then move to other levels of care in an effort to attain maximum independent functioning. This involves a series of transitions seldom addressed by one model (Derstine, 1992). Clients and rehabilitation nurses will benefit as more is learned about how to validate instruments and reach similar conclusions, outcomes, and implications when different or multiple concepts and models are used as a basis for practice.

In the same manner the healthcare system will demand precision when evaluating practice and programs. We need to understand how nurses, clients, and members of the healthcare team communicate; how the development of critical thinking impacts research, education, and practice (Hickman, 1993); and how therapeutic plans are implemented in practice to improve outcomes for and with clients. Chapter 7 describes best practices and processes for total quality management in rehabilitation nursing.

HISTORICAL PERSPECTIVE ON NURSING FRAMEWORKS

Members of a profession cannot realize issues concerning what they know—or how they have come to think, or about what they think, or what and how they do things—without understanding the history of their profession within a societal context of change. We nurses need to tell our stories to one another about who we are, what we value, where we've been, and where we want to go. Ideally rehabilitation nurses are making a commitment to know, practice, and refine their shared values. Thus our history becomes a part of our present and shapes our future.

Nursing knowledge, values, and beliefs have not evolved in isolation from changes in the rest of the world. Wars, disasters, and social movements all influence ways of thinking for leaders in any era. Nursing is no exception. For example, Nightingale's work began as a result of her efforts during the Crimean War. Wald's work in the New York slums mirrored a social consciousness at the turn of the nineteenth century (Backer, 1993). Increasing numbers of men in nursing will impact directions of knowledge formerly framed by feminism (Perkins, Bennett, & Dorman, 1993). Today the social construction of health has expanded to encompass outcome in terms of quality of life, as well as by mortality and morbidity of life (Hoeman & Winters, 1988).

Although a history of nursing conceptual frameworks began with Florence Nightingale's *Notes on Nursing,* many years passed until an expansion of knowledge yielded formal frameworks by early American nursing leaders (Nightingale, 1860).

Martha Rogers

Rogers was one of the first nurse theorists, beginning her work in the 1930s. This surprises many because she did not begin to publish her work until 1970. Nurses who study Rogers's ideas may relate readily to notions about persons as energy fields, open systems constantly exchanging with the environment; or alternate patterns of healing such as therapeutic touch. Rogers, trained in physics, defined three principles of homeodynamics that influenced the evolution of unitary human beings: resonancy, helicy, and integrality. These principles dealt specifically with rhythmic, unpredictable, constant, and increasingly diverse field patterns of change, which are discussed further in this chapter. Although visionary, her theory is complex, containing terminology that must be comprehended before one can apply her theoretical concepts (Rogers, 1970).

Rosemary Parse

Ultimately Rogers influenced other nursing theorists, notably Parse. Parse continues to develop her man-living-health model, building on Rogers's existential and phenomenologic tenets, as well as integrating concepts from philosophy. Parse melds the interaction of environment and person as she stresses the importance of cultural and family values in determining health and health actions. Assisting clients to accept responsibility for their own health is an example of a nursing role function fostered by Parse (Parse, 1981; Heine, 1991).

Virginia Henderson

The earliest definitions of nursing roles and functions identified by Henderson have permeated the thinking of nursing theorists for more than three decades. Beginning in the 1960s Henderson laid groundwork for future nursing theorists with her definitions of the uniqueness of nursing. Primarily focused on institutional nursing practice, Henderson described health as basic to a person's independent function within her now familiar 14 components of basic nursing care (Henderson, 1966). As an educator Henderson also contributed to appreciation of a professional level of nursing practice requiring university education, research action, and collegial interaction with other health professions.

Ida Orlando

During the same period as Henderson, Orlando wrote about changing concepts in nurse-patient relationships. She introduced nurse-patient relationships, patient feedback and participation in care, and promoted nursing as a distinct health profession capable of delivering an optimal level of care. In turn, much of Orlando's and Henderson's work was influenced by Peplau (Orlando, 1961).

Hildegaarde Peplau

Peplau was a psychiatric nurse who promoted graduate education in nursing and recognized the importance of a strong definition of clinical nursing therapeutics in practice. She conceptualized a nurse moving through a progression of therapeutic roles when working with a client and family: A nurse enters a therapeutic relationship in the role of stranger, then progresses through roles of resource person, teacher, leader, surrogate, and eventually, counselor. According to Peplau's interpersonal process, a nurse, especially in the counselor role, facilitates behaviors that enable a client to advance toward health. By using available energy for problem-solving, a client logically would reduce energy devoted to unhealthful anxiety.

A nurse's changing role is complemented by the nurse and client moving together through four distinct but interlocking phases of interpersonal relationship: orientation, identification, exploitation, and resolution. These role relationships and processes were influenced and moderated by cultural, social, and environmental factors (Peplau, 1952).

Imogene King

About the time these early theorists began publishing their work, the federal government became interested in providing funds for expanding the scientific knowledge base for nursing. A number of nurse theorists accepted the support and challenge to propose a definition for professional nursing. King was one of the nurse theorists whose work originated under governmental funding in the 1960s. Notably, she continued to refine her theory of goal attainment and systems models over the next 20 years (King, 1981).

King viewed three interacting systems: personal, interpersonal, and social systems. Systems and nurse-patient relationships at the transactional level are viewed as essential means to achieve goal attainment. Many concepts from her theory are highly related to practices in rehabilitation nursing. Certainly transaction, role, body image, perception, time, space, stress, growth and development, and communication have become familiar terms in practice and research (King, 1968, 1971).

In practice a rehabilitation nurse may use King's intrapersonal system to assess how a client with a disability adopts and performs roles as a member of a family and in a society. When a client has impaired communication or altered cognitive states, rehabilitation nurses may find limited application for King's theory unless a client is able to value goals and actively participate in goal setting, or alternatively unless theoretical concepts are extended to family goal setting (Mumma, 1987).

King's Open Systems Model concepts are social systems, perception, health, and interpersonal relations. These concepts may be used in rehabilitation nursing for
+ Setting mutual and realistic goals
+ Identifying short-term, long-term, or lifelong goals
+ Attaining or revising goals
+ Participating with clients and families
+ Interfacing with components of King's intrapersonal system such as communication, stress, interactions, and transactions, to define the client's social system (King, 1968, 1971).

In the social system a person forms concepts of power and authority, decision-making, status, and organizing behaviors. Within these systems nurses interact with clients toward attaining mutually held goals using agreed-upon means. King's theory stresses the importance of assuring client rights, and values are respected as goals are set. When a client is unable to cope with changes in daily activities or to maintain life, the nurse intervenes to help a client attain, preserve, and restore health; or if this is not possible, to die with comfort and dignity (King, 1971).

Transaction between client and nurse occurs when mutual goals are accomplished as indicated by client satisfaction, improved learning, decreased stress and anxiety, and using role behaviors that meet goals. As an illustration, a client and nurse strive for mutual agreement about the specific content of goal objectives. This is necessary so resources can be used for maximum independent function in activities of daily living, considering the person's roles and lifestyle. For this reason, mutual agreement may involve a contractual arrangement with clients and families, as mentioned later with Neuman's model.

Sister Calista Roy

Roy's Adaptation Model was another valuable theoretic product of the 1960s. Like King, she was knowledgeable about theories from other disciplines and worked within these theories to clarify a science of nursing. Rehabilitation nurses know about systems and adaptation from other frameworks; they have been "borrowed" from other disciplines. Roy placed these concepts within sets of assumptions embedded in a nursing context, which are useful to rehabilitation nurses who often work with clients who are adapting or adjusting to loss and change (Roy, 1970).

Roy identified the following four modes of adaptation:
+ Physiologic needs
+ Self-concept
+ Role mastery
+ Interdependence

These modes are discussed in more detail with role theories later in this chapter.

Roy envisioned a person as an adaptive system. Thus the person who is disabled experiences both overt and covert physiologic changes that may affect self-concept negatively and hinder successful adaptation to a disability (Trieschman, 1987). The role of the nurse is to assist clients and families with a positive response to environmental stimuli (i.e., adaptation).

Myrna Levine

Nearly 10 years later, Levine, another nurse theorist, began to raise questions. Levine wondered about a nurse's understanding of an individual within the context of a particular time or in a certain situation and how understanding connected with reasons for nursing interventions. In the 1980s Levine expanded her model to a less institutional model that contributes to setting community-based rehabilitation goals. A primary reason for nursing intervention, according to Levine, was to assist a client to conserve energy as well as structural, personal, and social integrity. Optimal health would use principles of conservation to maintain function, balance, self-identity, and socialization (Levine, 1967). In rehabilitation nursing efficient energy conservation is an essential consideration when planning care with a client who must deal with fatigue, such as discussed in Chapter 23.

Dorothea Orem

Orem is another theorist whose work is applied frequently in rehabilitation nursing. She began presenting her ideas in 1958, formalized her model in the 1970s, and remained active into the 1980s (Orem, 1971/1980). Orem's definition of the nursing role is closely aligned with Henderson's concept of assisting a patient toward maximum independence or dignified death.

Rehabilitation nurses recognize the usefulness of Orem's multiple levels of a patient's self-care capabilities, attention to wholeness, and important contributions to patient education (Orem, 1985). Knust and Quarn suggest that "the key to utilizing self-care theory in rehabilitative nursing is a thorough assessment of each category of self-care (universal, developmental, and health deviation). The interrelationships among areas of the assessment indicate the uniqueness of the individual client and ultimately direct interventions that are holistic" (Knust & Quarn, 1983).

Thus a person may be dependent in certain areas of self-care but responsible for self-directing care. In this scenario all three of Orem's nursing systems operate simultaneously with the same person. Since rehabilitation is an active process, nursing systems are dynamic (Knust & Quarn, 1983). However, Orem's application to practice may be less effective with a client who has cognitive impairment.

On an individual client basis, Orem's Self-Care Model is widely used in institutional settings for determining activities that clients are able "to initiate and perform on their own behalf in maintaining life, health, and well-being" (Orem, 1971/1980). Rehabilitation nurses find Orem's model useful when assessing a client's functional status as "wholly compensatory, partially-compensatory, or supportive of educational needs" in order to guide nursing interventions.

Orem's model may be useful in community-based settings to assess a client's ability to live independently, the level of services needed, or to monitor progress. The model is not particularly useful for a pediatric population. Family members are included in care, but Orem's model is limited to self-care deficits, may be culture bound, and does not deal with either outcome or uncontrolled biopsychosocial issues such as those encountered with community-based programs.

Dorothy Johnson

The next nursing theorist in historical sequence is Johnson. Like Orem and King, Johnson's work evolved over several decades, beginning in the 1960s. Her behavioral systems model interrelated a person, environment, and sociocultural context. According to Johnson a health problem or imbalance occurs from within the person's system or the environment. Her idea was that nursing's concern was to regulate maintenance of a client's balance and stability to meet the subsystem of basic human needs.

Some of Johnson's contributions to nursing thoughts are
✦ Attention to biopsychosocial responses
✦ Attention to cross-cultural values and environmental effects on behavior
✦ Focus on behavior rather than illness alone
✦ Stress reductioning

Johnson's model was intended to provide evidence of nursing as a profession, with its own sphere of responsibilities that are complementary to, but independent from, medicine (Johnson, 1968, 1980). For example, a rehabilitation nurse uses principles about roles from Johnson's model when contracting with a client or family or assisting a client in a behavioral change.

Betty Neuman

A total systems model proposed more recently by Neuman differs from Johnson's Behavioral Systems Model. Neuman combines frameworks from systems, ecology, epidemiology, and personal domains in a cybernetic open systems model with feedback loop. She brings the epidemiologic framework of levels of prevention, lines of defense, and multiple variables back into nursing. Concepts such as adaptation, stressors, whole person, and preventive intervention are woven throughout her systems model (discussed in Chapter 13) (Neuman, 1989).

The model is complex but has a capacity to be used by transdisciplinary teams across healthcare professions and throughout all levels and sites of care. For example, Neu-

man's model has been applied to long-term case management for persons with disabilities who are living in the community (Hoeman & Winters, 1990). Building on King's concepts of mutual agreement, contracting has been used to apply Neuman's Healthcare Systems Model to practice for rehabilitation nurses and to improve coping effectiveness (Chapter 13). Neuman's Healthcare Systems Model is useful in rehabilitation nursing especially for complex programs of care, lifelong care planning, and continuity from onset of injury or disease to institution or to community, which are examined further in chapters on community-based practice and case management.

Nancy Roper

The continuity of ideas is evident as theorists build on one another's work; Henderson's notions entwined with those of Orlando and Peplau are precursors of European theorist Roper's activities for daily living (Roper, Logan, & Tierney, 1980) and Gordon's functional health patterns (Gordon, 1993). Concepts from Roper and Gordon are integrated as a framework for this text.

Roper developed a model of living to conceptualize an "amalgam of activities" with activities of daily living as the criteria for the model. She views activities of daily living as all things people do in everyday life on a dependence-independence continuum. When unable to perform these activities independently, a person needs assistance. Activities of daily living are separated into those required to sustain life such as breathing, eating, or eliminating and those that allow participation in life such as communication, movement, or coping (Table 1-2).

Roper conceptualizes several dimensions and many specific activities that may be involved in each activity of living. Compounding this complexity, all of the activities are interrelated and affect total function. For example, for a particular individual, impaired mobility of the lower extremities may affect interpersonal relationships with friends and the ability to dress or gain access to the bathroom, even with a wheelchair. For another person with the same impairment, a wheelchair would result in independence in the same activities of living.

According to Roper's model, physical, psychological, and social environment; disability and disturbed physiology; degenerative or pathologic tissue changes; and accidents are examples of circumstances that may prevent a client's movement toward maximum independence. Her framework includes social and biologic aspects of living and the stages of growth and development. She uses the nursing process for nursing activities such as prevention,

Table 1-2 Roper's activities of daily living

To sustain life	To participate in life
Breathing	Personal hygiene and grooming
Controlling body temperature	Communication
Eating and swallowing	Movement
Bladder elimination	Sexuality and sexual function
Bowel elimination	Work and recreation
Sleep and rest	Accessing home and community
Maintaining skin integrity	Coping

comfort, and maximum independence in activities of daily living (Roper et al., 1980). Roper's model has been used in the United Kingdom as a framework for care in a major children's hospital (Clark, 1988).

OTHER DIMENSIONS

As with most nursing models to date, Roper's framework has not been fully developed nor have the concepts been tested. Value is added for nurses when they understand the historical development of knowledge and ongoing thoughts in nursing. Understanding the source of concepts used to assess a client, such as body image or self-care, lends credence and purpose to practice and establishes connection among thoughts, actions, and outcomes.

To this end a national group of nurse theorists developed ten dimensions or patterns of person-environment interaction:

✦ Exchanging	✦ Communicating
✦ Relating	✦ Valuing
✦ Choosing	✦ Moving
✦ Perceiving	✦ Feeling
✦ Knowing	✦ Emerging (Newman, 1986)

Other research findings on theoretic concepts indicate relationships between certain characteristics of persons who choose to become involved in taking responsibility for their own health and healthcare activities. For example, relationships between self-care and characteristics for hardiness (Pollock, 1989; Tartasky, 1993), uncertainty (Mischel, 1990; Jessup & Stein, 1985), locus of control (Rotter, 1966; Wallston & Wallston, 1982), personality types (Seigel, 1984; Kobasa, Maddi, & Zola, 1983), health beliefs (Becker, 1974), and explanatory models (Kleinman, Eisenberg, & Good, 1978), and resilience are documented in the literature. These are discussed further in Chapter 13 and in Chapter 10.

SELECTED THEORIES, MODELS, AND CONCEPTS

Nursing theorists have built on and integrated theories from other sciences. Theories from other disciplines must be used judiciously to ensure that the reality they appear to represent in non-nursing situations is the reality that exists in nursing situations. Likewise, nurses are paying attention in practice to cross-cultural issues and becoming sensitive to underlying meanings in concepts, assessments, interventions, and goal setting (Hoeman, 1989). However, in interdisciplinary and transdisciplinary practice, rehabilitation nurses often share knowledge, skills, and attitudes with other professionals using theoretical frameworks such as Piaget (Hoeman, 1993), stress/adaptation systems, Bobath, (Borgman & Passarella, 1991), or Bergstrom. These latter theorists are discussed along with methods in Chapter 14.

The following section is organized to present an integrated discussion of theories, models, and concepts from a variety of disciplines selected for a paradigm of transdisciplinary rehabilitation nursing. These are core but not exhaustive selections contributing to a dynamic scientific knowledge base. The intent of this section is to offer information that may promote understanding about how rehabilitation nurses and clients benefit from integrated conceptual frameworks. Another intent is to promote rehabilitation nurses' awareness of underlying meanings or concepts with frameworks that influence the way nurses think as they work through the nursing process in the United States and around the world.

Global Philosophy and Cultural Concepts

Rehabilitation itself is a relatively new specialty in the United States. Actually a number of factors had to coalesce over several decades until rehabilitation was recognized as a specialty. Only since 1947 was there sufficient interest in the United States to establish a board-certified rehabilitation specialty in medical practice. Nearly 30 years later, in 1974, the Association of Rehabilitation Nurses was organized, and rehabilitation nursing became a specialty within the American Nurses' Association.

Generally nurses have become familiar with rehabilitation as conceptualized and practiced in the United States, Canada, the United Kingdom, Northern and Western Europe, New Zealand, and Australia. However, a philosophy of rehabilitation has evolved unevenly throughout the world. In another large portion of the world, primary care and basic survival hold precedence. The World Health Organization (WHO) has promoted community-based rehabilitation programs. WHO also has proposed a somewhat controversial system of disability classifications that distinguishes among persons according to impairment, disabilities, or handicaps (WHO, 1985). Although used frequently in European countries, a number of advocates for persons with disabilities have questioned the WHO classification system, which is discussed further in Chapter 11 (Wood, 1986; Pfeiffer, 1992).

In fact, some countries are participating in rehabilitation initiatives or joint ventures with governmental agencies or private voluntary organizations for education and training programs. Other countries are developing their own initiatives for persons with disabilities. For example, the People's Republic of China mandated programs for governmental and private associations and foundations for persons with disabilities during a national congress held in January 1992. One program created regional demonstration projects in schools for children with special needs (Hoeman, 1992).

Globally the International Red Cross and numerous religious or private voluntary organizations work in collaboration with rehabilitation professionals and often are funded by private interest groups or U.S. government contracts. Federally funded exchange programs and international rehabilitation associations have awarded grants for international rehabilitation research, education, and practice for years.

Globally successful rehabilitation professionals are those who are prepared to assess another culture's healthcare system. This means an assessment of context, process, meaning, and explanatory models in each culture before making judgments or initiating therapeutic interventions (Hoeman, 1989). There is a temptation to base assessment on Western standards and the availability of equipment or technology. Rehabilitation may not be a societal concern or conversely may be viewed as a luxury dependent on acquiring equipment or technology.

The reference to developing countries in itself implies

some hierarchy based on technology or industrialization. Western health systems rely heavily on technology, which requires extreme resources and tests cultural ethics. This may be one reason why there are few studies evaluating how innovative nontechnical methods can be made available to people in other parts of the world. Too often efforts focus on ways to obtain technology, which may or may not be the most efficacious choice or best practice in an international setting.

With this in mind, and in an increasingly global society with diminishing resources, rehabilitation nurses may be challenged to examine theories and concepts from other cultures as well as to concentrate on sharing expertise. For example, styles of family and community caregivers or traditional methods may have application to practice in the United States. Although limited in scope, international programs represent opportunities for improving understanding and for advocating changes in social thought about the worth and place of persons with disabilities.

Social Construction of Disability

A society reflects its values in the actions of its people and through its institutions, one of which is health. The issues and directions of healthcare as a system cannot be isolated from other systems of a society or from world events. Thus the social construction of disability and availability or allocation of resources largely determines the nature of rehabilitation and beliefs about persons with chronic, disabling, or developmental disorders and also determines their subsequent treatment.

For example, at the turn of the nineteenth century, discoveries of vaccines and antibiotics eliminated many communicable diseases of children, including poliomyelitis, while medical advances and new biotechnology enabled more persons to survive formerly fatal conditions and live longer. Similarly, synthesis of medical advances, increased societal awareness about public health issues encompassing care of persons with disabilities, and veterans returned from two World Wars heightened societal attention to physical restoration as part of nineteenth-century healthcare (Gritzer & Arluke, 1985).

Slowly changing social views of persons with disabilities offered unique opportunity for them to acquire value apart from their ability to work in a society built around the "work ethic." Conversely, federally funded state social services such as special services for children, and emerging professions in physical and occupational therapies, assisted persons with disabling conditions into educational or vocational training. (See Chapter 6 for specific legislation.)

Clearly these programs reflected societal values and cultural expectations for work, but they also introduced assessment and evaluation of independent functioning into mainstream health economics. Economic strains on farming during these times pushed workers to leave an agrarian subsistence for an increasingly urban and mechanized lifestyle. A new cosmopolitan industrial population emerged at risk for increased catastrophic, traumatic, or chronic conditions. Social and economic changes in the twentieth century have resulted in persons with disabling disorders due to violence or trauma, sequela conditions such as post-polio syndrome, or immunosuppression diseases—all of which have broadened the scope of practice for rehabilitation nurses.

Disability Theories

Persons participating in rehabilitation benefit when rehabilitation nurses integrate disability theories into planning care and setting goals. Theories about disability are closely related to issues underlying a society's construction of disability.

✦ Erving Goffman

Goffman was one of the first to relate these issues when he defined the "stigma" attached to a person who visibly differed from others in a society. He learned that some persons' departures from the usual or societal norm were not visibly obvious—they might "pass" within "normal"—whereas those whose difference or disability was clearly seen became labeled as deviant. Whatever stigma accompanied a deviant state potentially became a negative trait ascribed to the person. Ultimately a person assimilated the stigma, which labeled him deviant and reinforced his "spoiled identity"; he resorted to learning strategies to manipulate or manage within limited societal acceptance (Goffman, 1963).

✦ Tamara Dembo

Closely related to Goffman's beliefs is the explanation of spread theory. According to Dembo (1969) and Dembo, Leviton, and Wright (1975), a first or strong perception is assigned as a characteristic to a person, such as someone with a disability. The characteristic is "spread" until it represents the total perception of that individual and governs responses to the person. Clients who have a limb deficiency often report others speak loudly to them during conversations, as though limb deficiency resulted in impaired hearing. Furthermore, even subtle perceptions of altered body state may be "spread" to ascribe the same, usually negative, trait to a person's personal attributes.

To continue the thought, the observer tends to attribute suffering to the person with a disability, regardless of whether the person presents suffering. In this scenario it is expected that the person with a disability must suffer, and she is devalued because of it. In turn, the person with a disability fulfills societal expectations for her public presentation of self while holding a hidden and personal experience of distress and distorted self-perception (Tait & Silver, 1989).

Social humanities of the eighteenth and nineteenth centuries demonstrated the spread of negatively ascribed mental character for persons who differed—often persons with disabilities. The Hunchback of Notre Dame, Captain Hook, and the Phantom of the Opera were labeled as socially deviant personalities, with some questions about how traits were related to their having physical disabilities. Dickens's Tiny Tim served a different purpose as a social conscience but was not allowed to survive to adulthood.

✦ Beatrice Wright

Wright, who pioneered the study of concepts within a psychology of physical disability, recognized "spread theory" but also raised social consciousness about a relationship between perception of disability and impressions about attributes of the person with a disability. She argued concepts rather than focusing on medical diagnoses. Wright's classic writings forced professionals to examine their own concerns about their own health function and status when working with persons with disabilities. Her work raised questions about underlying motives when using comparative standards based on culturally defined norms (Wright, 1964, 1983).

However, tendencies toward the social norm are persistent. Advocacy gains take time and must be reinforced in successive generations of the social consciousness. However, in the twentieth century, a great deal of rapid change in public thought is possible through media influence. Recently the U.S. media has contributed to changing the societal construction toward a positive value for persons with disabilities; ideally these changes will extend globally (Taylor, 1981).

As the United States contemplates entitlements for persons with certain disabling or developmental disorders and enacts legislation addressing access, inclusion, and normalization, the social construction of disability will continue to influence outcome. For example, in a historical study of legislation from 1900 to 1990, researchers examined issues that affected children who had chronic, disabling, or developmental disorders and traced the terms used to describe the children as an aggregate. Changes in social thought from custodial maintenance to advocacy are revealed clearly; however, they span 90 years (Hoeman & Repetto, 1992).

The classic works of Goffman, Dembo, and Wright continue to have application today (see box below). And certainly no review is complete without encouraging rehabilitation nurses to read Litman's classic critique of psychosocial theories as an approach in rehabilitation (Litman, 1979).

Rehabilitation Motivational Theories
✦ Constantina Safilios-Rothschild

Another landmark publication that influenced thinking about rehabilitation was written nearly a quarter of a century ago. Safilios-Rothschild (1970) prepared a classic sociology treatise on three levels of disability and rehabilitation: personal, social, and cultural levels.

Her thoughts integrated concepts about spread, stigma, and perceptions of disability. For instance, she established that relationships between a person's self-concept and response to a disability were dependent on values and emotions attached to the disability. That is, how and to what degree a disability affected a person's identity ultimately influenced perception of his body image. In turn, this response would be regularly reinforced by the person's relationships with others in society, particularly with those who were not disabled.

✦
SOCIAL CONSTRUCTION OF DISABILITY

- ✦ Stigma
- ✦ Social consciousness
- ✦ Spread theory
- ✦ Social system changes
- ✦ Self-actualization

Although determination of what constitutes disability differs among societies and cultures, it forms an integral part of a person's self-concept and perception of self-value, while assigning social value. Thus any assessments, plans, or implementation for rehabilitation are incomplete without addressing Safilios-Rothschild's three levels.

Safilios-Rothschild's work is currently useful when focusing on a client's reentry to the community. Her concept of social system in rehabilitation is a multidisciplinary team that itself is undergoing change to include interdisciplinary or transdisciplinary and community-based practice. While a person must experience motivation toward rehabilitation goals, the social system (i.e., team) must have a means for moving the person into the society. The culture must perceive the person's value, although persons with disabilities may present themselves as a minority with their own set of prejudices. Safilios-Rothschild's work left a legacy of understanding about relationships between self-concept and body image that upholds several nursing diagnoses (Safilios-Rothschild, 1970).

✦ Abram Maslow

Concepts of self, multiple levels, and motivation used by Safilios-Rothschild are key tenets of Maslow's attempt to explain human behavior through a hierarchy of needs. Depicted in a familiar pyramid, Maslow's basic physiologic needs form a foundation topped with successive layers of narrowing needs for safety, love and belonging, esteem and recognition, and finally peak with self-actualization.

According to Maslow a person is motivated to prioritize and direct behavior toward meeting each successive layer of individual needs. Meeting needs reduces tension only until the next level of need emerges. Similar to Erikson's notion of stage epigenesis, a person would not work purposefully toward meeting needs for any higher level unless he or she had met internal and external needs of all lower levels. This model is popular but simplistic (Maslow, 1968).

Rehabilitation nurses may find Maslow's hierarchy helpful for assessment of a client's priorities and motivation or when a client is seeking to understand what motivates his or her own behaviors or prioritize his or her energies. Predictors of self-acceptance of clients in rehabilitation have been examined using Maslow's theory (Brillhart, 1986).

Health and Wellness

One principle that has intensified and solidified nursing is concern with health, wellness, and holism beyond illness. Rehabilitation nurses recognize the importance of integrating rehabilitation nursing principles into all levels of intervention to prevent complications or further disability and to assure optimal level of independent function. Different models and concepts are essential to deal with the complexity of multiple causation, internal and external environments, psychosocial factors, and variety of settings that make up nursing practice.

✦ Halbert Dunn

Ironically many theories and models known and used by professional nurses were formally developed by members of other disciplines. As early as 1959 Dunn introduced the concept of "high-level wellness," integrating an individual's maximum potential and holistic balance into a definition of health (Dunn, 1959). This concept is basic to nursing practice.

✦ Richard Eberst

Eberst expanded on the dimensional features of the Rubik's Cube to support the dynamic, multidimensional features of health. Each person has a wellness potential ranging from low level to peak wellness and is governed by genetic, social, and environmental factors. Eberst suggested that a person who would reduce stress and achieve healthy balance must attend to synergy among all of six interactive dimensions (see box below).

Attention to balance within the whole is more productive for health than a focus on any particular dimension. Eberst's belief that wellness is a relative quality, rather than a linear or polar medical model, generated notions about the many ways to achieve health and the importance of a client's personal involvement in responsibility for health. Rehabilitation nurses regularly practice synergy consistent with Eberst's ideas and within an ecologic model encompassing environmental and biopsychosocial indicators. Within an ecologic model, an interplay of an individual's genetic and environmental status and lifestyle influences health and wellness (Eberst, 1984).

✦ The Health Belief Model

The Health Belief Model is the product of a group effort of prominent sociologic scientists in the early 1970s who shared the goal "to organize the conceptual, analytical, and research skills of the members and to direct them in a coordinated fashion toward the study of crucial problems in understanding preventive health patterns and health maintenance" (Becker, 1974). The Health Belief Model is the basis for a body of work about an individual's actions in making decisions about when, where, and how to seek health care; in choosing among health care options or alternatives; and in adhering to prescribed regimens. The original premise, derived from Lewin, was that a person would not value or take action concerning preventive health behaviors unless he or she held certain beliefs. To participate, the person must believe that:

- ✦ He or she is personally susceptible to the disease, regardless of symptoms
- ✦ Contracting the disease would have at least a moderately severe impact on his or her life
- ✦ Personal benefit through prevention or reduced severity would occur as a result of choosing or taking a certain action
- ✦ There is a low risk for barriers, such as expense, pain,

access, and psychological or sociocultural stigma (Rosenstock, 1974).

Although researchers began with preventive and acute health beliefs and behaviors in mind, the Health Belief Model has become important for understanding beliefs and behaviors associated with maintaining wellness, in tandem with chronic diseases and conditions. Characteristics of a client's decision-making, barriers that elicit resistance or influence participation in health care, and managing change over the long term are some of the challenges in rehabilitation nursing practice related to elements of the Health Belief Model. The sickness role in chronicity, adhering to and staying in treatment over time, educational interventions for self-care or prevention, client-health team interrelationships, factors influencing modification of lifestyle, and sociocultural/lay health and referral systems are only a few variables related to the Health Belief Model that are suitable for study by rehabilitation nurse researchers.

Family and Ecologic Systems Theories

Currently, rehabilitation nurses seek ways to involve individuals and families as comanagers who participate as fully as possible in planning and evaluating their care. Family systems theories are useful for rehabilitation nurses to understand family dynamics including patterns of communication, power, economics, and interaction (Bowen, 1966; Minuchin, 1980) as well as nonfunctional family relationships (Satir, 1967). The rich literature and research on family systems may assist nurses to understand the dynamics of families under stress and how to assist families to empower their members who have disabilities.

Nurses promoting a scientific basis for family nursing propose an ecologic model that covers the life span development of all family members. This notion recognizes the complexity of variables that converge when family members of different gender, generation, developmental stage, and life events interact with the environmental structures and social systems. For example, an ecologic framework exposes the fact that many family members in the United States are geographically distant from one another. Likewise adult family members tend to be fully employed, frequently relocate residences due to job or economic changes, have distinctly different socioeconomic lifestyles, may live in underserved urban or rural areas, or have variable immigrant status (Mercer, 1989).

In a seeming return to long-past patterns of care following years of acquiescence to paternalistic medicine, family members are increasingly being called on to become responsible caregivers and assist with direct care to family members who have chronic, disabling, or developmental disabilities. When traumatic or stressful life events or chronic conditions threaten, families are forced to deal with growing economic constraints manifested as controlled allocation of health services and fluctuating resources. Renewed dependence on family caregivers and full access and inclusion in a community for clients of all ages who have chronic, disabling, or developmental disabilities are examples of issues that present obvious and ethical concerns for all parties.

Our clients require care; many will not receive cure. Increasingly the nursing profession is called on by clients,

---

✦

EBERST'S SIX INTERACTIVE DIMENSIONS

✦ Mental	✦ Emotional	✦ Spiritual
✦ Physical	✦ Social	✦ Vocational

Data collected from "Defining Health: A Multidimensional Model" by R.M. Eberst, 1984, *Journal of School Health, 53*, 99-104.

other health professionals, and society to advance principles and test theoretic concepts about caring. Caregiving is one component within the broader concept of caring in nursing (Watson, 1979). Leininger expanded the literature on caring to encompass cross-cultural and universal views (Leininger, 1988), while Morse, Solberg, Neadner, Bottorff, and Johnson (1990) critiqued the literature and contributed an alternative view of caring.

Cognitive and Social Learning Theories

Social learning theorists believe individuals choose behaviors based on the ability to anticipate consequences. With that thought, community-based programs (Chapter 9) seeking educational materials about maintaining functional abilities or self-care for clients, families, and community members are markets for rehabilitation nursing services. Information about a client's abilities, motivation, and style of learning assist a nurse to plan the type of community education programs that may appeal to clients and meet the learning needs about their care.

However, these ideas reflect a basic assumption of exchange theory rationalism that clients will choose among alternatives based on anticipated outcomes, which may not always be the case. Social learning theory suggests reinforcement is the learning key to changing behavior whether directly, vicariously, or by self-management. Cognitive retraining builds on many of these principles, such as the phases of directing changes in behavior: pretraining, training, initial testing, and continued performance (Parcel & Baranowski, 1981). Patient and family education is discussed in detail in Chapter 10.

✦ Albert Bandura

The following describes anticipated steps in a social learning program. Overall, progressive learning experiences build a person's belief in his own ability to organize cognitive, social, and behavioral skills. Similarly, interactions among a person and others provide information about the person and the environment (Hergenhahn, 1982). Bandura, a pioneer of behavior modification, found four factors that influence how children learn when observing others. A child attends to the situation, retains the observation, has a certain capacity to perform the action, and identifies reward or punishments associated with performing the action. Without incentives a person may learn behaviors without performing them. However, when a person performs an action, learning and retention often are improved (Bandura, 1969).

In application, breaking behavior into small sequential steps facilitates confidence so that a person becomes comfortable with a task as well as flexible enough to transfer learning about one area to another. Resulting feelings of accomplishment or self-efficacy promote wellness and a person's ability to participate in directing care (Bandura, 1977).

✦ Jean Piaget

Social learning theories and Gestalt psychology models (Fagan and Shepherd, 1970) are classified as cognitive learning theories. Rehabilitation nurses working with pediatric populations frequently rely on another cognitivist, Piaget, whose experiments substantiated stages of cognitive development from birth through early childhood. Assessment of a child's stage of cognitive development provides information about how a child is interacting with his environment, as well as guidance for a professional about what learning materials are appropriate for that stage (Piaget, 1972; Ginsberg & Opper, 1988). Play-based learning and stimulation programs (Linder, 1990) are ways in which Piaget's research has been applied to practice, often in interdisciplinary team models beginning early with preventive intervention in special care nurseries (Hoeman, 1993). Theories and concepts pertinent for pediatric rehabilitation are discussed further in Chapter 30.

✦ Theories of aging

Cognition is an important but difficult assessment mode, especially when a client is very elderly. Among the very old, for example, accurate assessment must distinguish among dementia, depression, disorientation, alertness, communication deficits, secondary symptoms such as seen in Parkinson's disease, and normal changes of aging. An older person may become confused simply because of leaving a familiar home environment.

Complications from multiple medications or combinations of medications are common problems among elderly persons, resulting in temporarily impaired cognition. Until recently, few reliable tools were available for practice with older adults, especially the growing populations of very old persons. More guides are being developed as professionals realize a need for special assessment, intervention, and evaluation in the population.

As with assessment, theories of aging and life stage theories are not well developed for persons who are in very late aging stages. For example, Erikson's stages, concerned with ego and identity development, assign tasks for achieving life meaning through attaining wisdom and integrity in old age (Erikson, 1968), whereas Havinghurst was concerned with managing social roles and developmental stage-related tasks (Havinghurst, 1972). Both models define persons in their 50s as aged, which was in keeping with the social constructs of their time.

Nurses specializing in the growing area of gerontology are attempting to refine existing, underdeveloped theories of aging. A person's adjustment to aging and interrelationships between the aging person and her environment, social system, family system, and functional changes all have research potential. Existing tests and instruments await critical evaluation, and functional evaluations that reflect nursing practice and holistic client needs are essential.

Myths about aging and unsupported theories may be more common than nurses realize. Although unsupported by empiric research findings, the psychosocial theory of disengagement, proposing that older persons withdraw from roles, society, and personality has been advanced for 30 years (Cumming & Henry, 1961). The social context, cultural handling of aged persons, role expectations, expected life-span, and lack of other models are factors that may have promoted the notion of disengagement for so many years. However, the number of active and involved older citizens defeats the notion that "dropping out" is a normal and inevitable part of aging.

Two other psychosocial concepts regarding aging directly

contradict disengagement. The activity concept states that those who are more socially involved and active—usually by substituting new roles for those that can no longer be met—age more successfully. Continuity, the second concept, maintains that a person's acquired coping skills, which contribute to his lifestyle, personality, preferences, and ongoing roles are indicators of successful aging.

Clark and Anderson's (1967) longitudinal study of a large sample of persons who were aging successfully was perhaps more insightful as a developmental model than some theories. Analyzing data, they found persons who were able to redefine and transfer roles such as from competition to cooperation, to reassess criteria to measure themselves while accepting changes of aging, and to review life goals and ways to meet needs were happier and healthier than their age peers when in old age.

Biologic theories about aging essentially are limited to physiologic arenas. For example, notions that each person eventually depletes a given store of energy or winds down a biologic clock underlies ideas about biologic exhaustion or a time-limited life program. Stress is also viewed by some as a biologic depletion. In this view residual damage and accumulated stressors may heighten until the person does not cope effectively, and death results. With autoimmune concepts a person dies when the aging body produces antibodies against itself, resulting in cell breakdown.

Although limited, biologic concepts for aging have received a great deal of attention. More than other populations the old and very old clients may be at risk for readmission to hospitals for acute healthcare problems, in addition to their chronic or disabling conditions. This biologic view is fatalistic and defeating for elders who live longer. In spite of increased numbers of aged persons, the social construction of aging in the United States remains stagnant and restrictive. Concepts from nurse theorists such as Parse, Orem, Roy, King, Levine, and Neuman may apply to gerontologic rehabilitation nursing practice. Chapter 31 discusses how rehabilitation nurses will play key roles in working with aging populations and hopefully contribute to the scientific knowledge bases.

✦ Stress theories

Stress and coping are key concepts for rehabilitation nursing that are introduced here and discussed in context in Chapter 13. Stress is a complex, dynamic, and multidimensional phenomenon that affects all persons but touches each one differently. Research examining relationships between stress and well-being (or disease) (Friedman and Rosenman, 1974) has grown since Selye's classic work introduced stress to health sciences as a physiologic response, the general adaptation syndrome, or GAS. According to Selye the totality of changes induced by stressors is manifested in the three GAS stages: an alarm reaction, a shock phase when resistance is lowered, and a countershock phase during which defenses are activated—that is, physiologic "fight or flight."

Maximum adaptation occurs during the second stage of resistance. A proactive response is action; a person uses coping strategies during the resistance stage. If prolonged, a person may sense loss of control or communicate feelings of helplessness (Engel, 1968). When a stressor persists or

defenses are inadequate, a person becomes exhausted; adaptive mechanisms fail and disease, even death, may ensue (Selye, 1978).

Selye's model is classified as a nonspecific systemic response approach wherein stress arises within the person due to stressors. Lazarus added psychosocial categories of changes that occur as a result of response to stress to GAS responses (Lazarus, 1966). Two additional stress models are commonly accepted by researchers, although there is little agreement about how the three interrelate. In a stimulus model, stress is external to the individual, causing the person to respond to the stimulus, as with studies of stressor life events or daily hassles.

Finally, the transactional approach considers stress itself as a transaction. A person's cognitive appraisal of threat and evaluation of the challenge yield an individualized experience of stress. Stress is a product of individual appraisal of the transaction between person and environment and belongs to neither (Lazarus & Folkman, 1984). The transactional approach and appraisal are discussed in detail in Chapter 13. Longitudinal studies examining experiences and events over time are excellent designs for rehabilitation nurses conducting transactional stress research.

Change Theory

Change is a constant component of the human experience. Concepts of change theory appear in other theoretic models such as stress/adaptation or developmental theories.

✦ Kurt Lewin's change model

Lewin's classic study of change concepts was conducted in the war years of the 1940s. Lewin described change as a dynamic interplay between a person's worldview and his environment. Ideally a behavioral change would enable him to develop strategies to deal more effectively with his changing world (Lewin, 1947).

Only when a person realized a reason to change, such as discomfort with the present situation or a situation raising questions about the status quo, could he enter Lewin's "unfreezing" stage. A person is vulnerable as he "moves" toward a new level of operations and may encounter resistance or environmental restraints, which in turn may impact his motivation or problem-solving abilities. However, this is when he implements a new idea or plan designed to fit the need for change. "Refreezing" occurs when he stabilizes this process and integrates changes into his behavior, lifestyle, and relationships. A sense of closure or termination signifies the change is completed (Lewin, 1947).

✦ Ronald Lippitt's planned change approach

Planned change has become associated with improvement, choices, predictability, and problem resolution. Lippitt, Watson, and Westley (1958) prepared a classic work in which they introduced the role of a "change agent" and presented phases that occur when change is planned. Beginning with awareness of a need for change, a change relationship must be established, and criteria for change are monitored through successive phases (see Box, p. 14).

Concepts from change theories have been used in macro levels such as altering rehabilitation organizational behavior to change to a product line or managed-care culture.

IDEAL CRITERIA FOR PHASES OF PLANNED CHANGE

+ All persons and systems are involved
+ All agree about the need for change
+ Involved persons clarify the problem
+ Involved persons explore alternative solutions
+ Involved persons set goals
+ Change is instituted
+ Timing and pace of changes are monitored
+ Flexibility of the system is crucial
+ Open, ongoing communication
+ Attention to resistance
+ Stabilization period before termination (Lippitt et al., 1958)

Data collected from *The Dynamics of Planned Change*, by R. Lippitt, J. Watson, & B. Westley, 1958, New York: Harcourt, Brace, & World, Inc.

Planned change concepts may be used to improve family and client participation in rehabilitation programs and planning, or to educate colleagues working in a community nursing agency about benefits and improved outcome for clients as results of rehabilitation nursing consultations.

Even with planning, resistance to change may occur at any point in the change process, since humans tend to be reactive before they are proactive. The rehabilitation nurse may reduce resistance by identifying barriers, working with clients to overcome them, or advocating for system changes. As a change agent a rehabilitation nurse listens and learns about a client's values, lifestyle, goals, and preferences; the nurse ensures a client is informed and included in decision-making whenever possible.

Psychosocial Developmental Theories and Change

At times a person actively plans and participates in change, whereas other changes are anticipated life stage or maturational events. Growth and development theories and family development theories explain change that occurs in predictable patterns throughout the life cycle for individuals and family groups (Duvall, 1971; Hill, 1965). For this reason, most growth and development theories or models are also staging models (as discussed later), but staging models do not deal exclusively with growth and development concepts. Chapter 30 contains information about physical growth and development; however, it is important to understand psychosocial development in the context of life change.

+ Erik Erikson's stages of man

Landmark work by Erikson detailed eight stages of individual psychosocial development, each stage with a potential outcome for either successful completion or dysfunctional reworking. In his notion of epigenesis, he maintained that one must successfully complete significant psychosocial development work in one developmental stage before progressing unemcumbered to the next. Erikson began his stages with infants, who may achieve trust versus mistrust;

progress through eight stages culminating in generativity versus stagnation, then integrity versus despair. Adolescence is a key stage where identity or identity confusion occurs (Erikson, 1968).

+ Development and change

However, positive changes such as new babies or marriages, or expected changes such as death of an elderly family member, still produce stress in family coping and role relationships. When these patterns are interrupted or altered, such as when a child is born with a developmental delay or acquires a disability, families usually begin to cope by dealing with emotions and feelings of loss, which may become a "chronic sorrow" (Olshansky, 1962).

Frameworks such as Duvall's family developmental tasks are criticized as being too narrowly defined for particular socioeconomic groups and not being relevant for the diversity of many clients and families. This becomes troublesome because developmental theories tend to focus attention on identifying and monitoring delays or deviations from a set norm, and test gradients tend to be geared toward dominant cultural values and traits. Developmental models encompass cognitive, motor, biopsychosocial, moral, interpersonal, and social skills—areas in which anticipated developmental patterns or changes may vary widely according to cultural and social expectations.

For example, maternal roles are shared among several women in some cultural groups; children from an ethnic group with short stature may consistently deviate from another group norm on a standardized growth chart; or children may be weaned at later ages. Tests, evaluation techniques, and scores must be critically examined to assure they are culturally sensitive and relevant to the person or group.

Sensitivity and relevance are essential in one-to-one or small-group relationships with clients. Rehabilitation nurses work with clients to plan systematic change in response to an often unplanned disability, chronic condition, or developmental delay. Unexpected, nondirected, often nonparticipatory, unplanned change may lead to a crisis event. How a person copes with change sets directions that enable her to grow in understanding and problem-solving or conversely to create a negative stressor on her life. Although not discussed in detail here, rehabilitation nurses are encouraged to learn about conceptual frameworks for cultural diversity and group dynamics.

+ Grounded theory
Barney G. Glaser and Anslem L. Strauss

Grounded theory refers to data that are "grounded" in fact and generate theory from the fact. When no theory exists, and thus no concepts are available to be tested, grounded theory is a method used to search out factors or to relate factors to the research problem. Actually, theory is developed from data because the assumption is made that discovery is ongoing and dynamic. Data are examined and analyzed using systematic, continual comparison until hypotheses are presented for testing. This is a move from deductive to inductive modes with elements of each mode. Data, hypotheses, related factors, and theory are linked and integrated "from the bottom up." For example, Goffman's concepts about stigma were formulated inductively from grounded data.

Grounded theory is important for rehabilitation nurses who are interested in using field techniques and qualitative methods or examining daily activities within a new paradigm (Glaser & Strauss, 1973). It is especially useful for clinical-based research when there are complex uncontrolled variables such as open field research in the community, lifelong management, or synthesizing data into new paradigms.

Debates within nursing call for new or shifted paradigms, theories that will anticipate and meet the challenges and chart the direction of the profession during the changes that most certainly lie ahead. Whereas Gestalt figures illustrate the powerful tendency for one to see what one has learned to expect to see (Fagan & Shepherd, 1970), pattern recognition is thought to be one way a person transfers known data to new situations, forming a new connectedness. But first a person must discern a pattern, then recognize it. This is one basis for current attention to paradigms and paradigm shifts. Some ideas in the following sections suggest paradigm shifts for rehabilitation nurses.

✦ Rhythms and patterns as change

Chaos was a new paradigm suggesting some changes were regularly irregular. Indeed, chaos theory proposed some changes occurred over lengths of time and reproduced in patterns that were not discernible within the organizational capability of the human mind (Gleick, 1987). Changing rhythms and underlying patterns may be new paradigms of interest to nursing. Certainly rhythm theories such as circadian rhythms, culturally defined temporal cycles, sleep-rest cycles, and other recurrent patterns have gained credibility. The significance of sleep and rest patterns is discussed in Chapter 23.

Rhythms and cycles are abstractions from Rogers's model. The notion of man and his environment interacting in helicy or continuous growth and change, with reciprocity or mutual interaction, all orchestrated by nurses promoting interaction in resonancy or waves, and synchrony was a new paradigm (Rogers, 1970).

Nurses are learning to consider concepts such as Rogers's to investigate time and space and the holistic interconnectedness of mind, body, and environment as factors related to health outcome. These are challenges to unfreeze our own thinking still clinging to remnants of a traditional medical model. In a new paradigm nurses are examining their own rituals and patterns of time, space, and other boundaries—concepts about which numerous cultural groups hold differing beliefs and practices. These concepts will be tools for rehabilitation nurses to unlock secrets about the natural history of chronic conditions and the character and structure of the concept of chronicity.

✦ Chronicity as a concept

Chronicity is a concept associated more with care than with cure. That realization is becoming clearer as chronicity crosses the life path of every person. Children with chronic, disabling, or developmental disabilities such as spina bifida are surviving to adulthood, while members of an aging world population acquire chronic conditions.

Medical advances and technology enable persons to survive formerly fatal diseases or trauma while increasing the demand for services that ultimately become needs for care. Lyme disease and other immunosuppressant diseases, especially AIDS, have altered patterns of medical treatment and economics throughout the United States. Secondary or sequela disease conditions have reemerged such as poliomyelitis as post-polio syndrome.

Although changing, our society remains focused primarily on cure. Research on concepts of chronicity will assist in changing this mind-set. For example, when researchers categorized common concerns for children with chronic conditions and their families, they found more commonalities associated with chronicity than occurred among persons with the same diagnoses (Stein & Jessop, 1989).

But reliance on medical models is intensely ingrained. Persons with chronic complaints may rely so heavily on a medical diagnosis, they experience relief when given a medical label for their symptoms. A medical diagnosis legitimizes symptoms and provides a socially acceptable explanation for previous illness behaviors, even when an irrevocable condition is diagnosed. In instances such as these, only an informed public and changes in the healthcare system will create interest in concepts about chronicity. Rehabilitation nurses will have opportunity for leadership in testing concepts about chronicity and applying these findings to their practice with continuously changing populations.

✦ Staging models or theories

Staging theories offer explanations about how individuals and families adjust to loss and change. Kubler-Ross's classic study found persons grieve in stages: initial shock with anxiety and disbelief; denial and avoidance; anger accompanied by guilt and shame; realization of permanence of loss and depression; and finally resolution with relief (Kubler-Ross, 1969). This has been used extensively by rehabilitation professionals to assess and intervene with clients and their families; a person was to move sequentially and timely through the stages, then signal acceptance.

The intensity, duration, and resolution following disability may continue unresolved or recur. Individuals express and experience grief differently, may spend different amounts of time and energy in any given stage, and may enter stages in different sequences. Certain grieving practices that are culturally prescribed may aid in working through grief. When assessing response to loss with persons from cultural or ethnic groups other than one's own, differences in expression and experience of grief, distress, and emotional pain are highly probable. Similarly, children in any culture may not follow prescribed patterns of grieving. A child may engage in play or may sleep soundly to avoid painful events or may internally blame herself for losses. The experience and expression of distress and pain differ with developmental stages (Ross & Ross, 1988; Eland & Anderson, 1977).

When a person realizes loss only while envisioning few options, he may become suspended in indecision, ambivalence, anxiety, or depression. Perception is one powerful factor in coping models such as the T-Double ABC-X Model, which is discussed further in Chapter 13. A person's appraisal and perceptions of the event, values, preparation and participation in the process, resistance to change, and coping style determine his behaviors following change (McCubbin & Patterson, 1983).

Some change may occur so subtly as to be barely noticeable. Less effective change occurs when change is limited to a few exceptions to the rule or when rigid ways are totally discarded, only to be replaced with another closed system (Ferguson, 1980). Shifting a paradigm may instigate a metamorphosis, a transforming experience unfolding opportunities for growth and revival while putting aside past ways. Attention to spirituality (Chapter 28) is gaining recognition and support as an adjunct to a person's successful change and redirection.

Role Theories

Change theories may be aligned closely with role theories.

✦ Integrating Roy's concepts with role theories

Roy dealt with role changes related to loss and change when she formulated an adaptation model based on the premise that "man, as a biopsychosocial being, is interacting constantly with his changing environment" (Roy, 1980). Roy proposes illness and acceptance of a "sick role" are results of ineffective coping in four modes. The first mode involves basic physiologic needs, which must be kept in balance in response to the environment. A chronic, disabling, or developmental condition is a severe threat to maintaining basic physiological needs.

Second, a person's self-concept mode changes in response to internal and external feedback and success in performing social roles and responsibilities, which are heavily influenced by his location on the health-illness continuum. A person with a disabling condition experiences both overt and covert changes that may affect self-concept and ability to adapt. A rehabilitation nursing role is to assist a client and family to achieve positive responses to environmental stimuli, promoting adaptation. Self-concept and role mastery, the third mode, are key elements in rehabilitation.

Role mastery mode typifies the effect of illness on a person's ability to perform prescribed roles such as family roles of father, husband, or worker and community roles such as soccer coach, church elder, or politician. Family member roles will change as responses to the person's inability to perform former roles, often by accommodating tasks and duties previously performed by the person who has lost interdependence and health status.

Role mastery mode is integrated with other frameworks. Parsons described socially constructed role behaviors. One of these, a socially understood "sick role," was acceptable when one became ill, especially with acute conditions (Parsons, 1958). A role of learned helplessness may occur on three continua: universal versus personal helplessness, global versus specific helplessness, and stable versus unstable attributes that consistently influence learned helplessness deficits over time. When a person expects that outcomes are uncontrollable, he may develop deficits in motivation, cognition, or emotion. Learned helplessness is more readily applied to chronic conditions (Abramson, Seligman, and Teasdale, 1978; Quinless & Nelson, 1988). The concept was related to adaptation by role mastery as well as to ineffective response to self-care.

Rehabilitation nurses are cautioned to recall the basic theme of spread theory when using Roy's model. That is, an assessment of an individual with a disabling condition may reveal that she is bombarded with environmental stimuli that necessitate adaptations. However, the fact that a person has disabilities may not be an indicator of her overall health status. The focus must be on the person, not the disability. On the other hand, assessments frequently reveal persons who have numerous nursing diagnoses due to complex or multiple impairments, dual medical and psychiatric or developmental diagnoses, and more than one chronic condition.

The fourth mode is interdependence, wherein a change in environment may threaten interdependence related to self-concept and role mastery. A person's needs are based on her level of adaptation within the four modes. Any change in the environment may provide a threat to any one or more of the modes; when the person is unable to integrate her changed role successfully, maladaptation occurs.

One criticism of the notion of adaptation itself is that it signifies a return of the person to a certain homeostasis or former level, albeit under a new guise (Duffy, 1987). Thus adaptation in the truest sense may not be possible for a person with a disability and may limit new patterns envisioned apart from adaptation. Adaptation as a positive outcome of coping may be limited in terms of self-actualizing goal setting, must be carefully applied throughout the life-span, may have unique meanings or outcome measures for different professionals, and may be less culturally relevant than an open systems model. Adjustment may be a more appropriate and useful concept.

Several aspects of role theories important to rehabilitation nursing practice such as sick role, role mastery, and learned helplessness have been discussed in the context of other conceptual frameworks. Roles, especially transitions and changes, are also components of developmental and staging theories. Atwood addressed conflicts in roles while caring for persons with chronic or terminal conditions in their homes. She identified neglect as "the behavioral outcome of conflict between role concept and role performance" (Atwood, 1978). The conflict further involved role expectations and role performance for the client, caregiver, and family. Atwood described a selective neglect that pertained to "failure to carry out an aspect of a role because it has much lower priority than other aspects" (Atwood, 1978). Although role problems and transitions are not unique to persons with disabilities, understanding concepts from role theory is integral to professional rehabilitation nursing practice.

✦ Edwin J. Thomas's disability and role theory

Thomas identified five roles related to disability. As with other staging or sequential models, the occurrence, sequence, and pattern may vary among individuals. Beginning with the person as one who has a role as a patient with a disability, Thomas included principles from Parsons (1951) in "sick role." That is, as a patient the person attains a status that is legitimately exempt from usual social role expectations and needs care. The person is not responsible for his incapacity. However, he may employ defense mechanisms such as denial and not begin to problem-solve about his situation (Thomas, 1966).

THOMAS'S ROLES RELATED TO DISABILITY

1. Sick role
2. Functionally limited
3. Helped person
4. Disability comanager
5. Public relations expert

Data collected from "Problems of Disability from the Perspective of Role Theory," by E. Thomas, 1966, *Journal of Health & Human Behavior*, 7(2).

Second, Thomas identified the role changes resulting from functional limitations of disability (see box, above). Naming the role as "handicapped performer," a term not acceptable today, Thomas detailed the legitimate change in normal responsibilities that may be given over to others (Thomas, 1966). Accepting this role involves acknowledging that things will be this way in a client's life. There is a risk of depression and hopelessness, or learned helplessness.

Thomas's third role, "helped person," is a recipient role in conflict with societal values of self-reliance and independence. The person is expected to adjust to recipient status. Conversely and nonproductively the person may be viewed as hindering others or may be overly protected, as when the person is a child.

When the person reaches the fourth role, "disability comanager," he is an active participant in planning and deciding about his care and lifestyle. Feelings of inferiority or guilt may impede this interactive role (Thomas, 1966). As those who work with transdisciplinary teams including clients and their families as comanagers or copartners in care planning will attest, this is a challenging and pivotal stage.

Finally, Thomas described the role of "public relations expert" in which the person decides how he will present himself and explain both his role and impairment to others in society. Strategies to deal with the social world may become manipulative. Consider Thomas's role with Goffman's work on stigma where he identifies the benefits for those persons with invisible disabilities or differences who may "pass" without detection by members of society.

REHABILITATION NURSING ROLES

Trust and rapport are components so essential and basic to developing and maintaining productive relationships that they form the foundation for other life stages of Erikson's theory (Erikson, 1968). Establishing trust and rapport is prerequisite to creating helping relationships between rehabilitation nurses; persons with chronic, disabling, or developmental disorders; and their families.

Sally Thorne's Stages for Trust

Thorne describes three intense stages that are conquered before long-term helping relationships achieve trustworthiness. A person's initial encounters with a health professional simulate "blind trust" that the professional knows more information and how to solve the problem (Thorne, 1993). Over time "disenchantment" sets in, appearing perhaps when there is no cure, when there is disagreement, or if a

professional either errs or fails in some way in the client's mind. As a result many long-term helping relationships operate within the third stage: needing the health system, vacillating in opposition, but never achieving internal trust (Thorne, 1993). Families and health professionals may intend to work as comanagers of care but too often enter a "guarded alliance," but without gaining trust. Multiple family dynamics are involved, especially when clients are infants or young children or when the family holds seemingly unrealistic hope for cure.

Implications for Rehabilitation Nurses

Thus rehabilitation nurses have the opportunity and responsibility to develop instrumentation and theoretical concepts about care. Similarly, rehabilitation nurses, many of whom have case manager roles, would benefit from incorporating family systems theories and ecologic life-span developmental models into their repertoire of theory bases for practice.

However well theories or models may be orchestrated to organize knowledge into meaningful frameworks, they remain tentative explanations of phenomena that are subject to being refuted or revised. Future needs are to relate components emanating from theories with nursing metaparadigms and to reconcile nursing theories with theories from other professional disciplines and sciences.

Rehabilitation nurses know that the social construction of disability must expand to include value for persons with a wide range of chronic, disabling, and developmental conditions in an aging world population. Hardy and Conway's book is a classic comprehensive resource for understanding role theory in context of the health professions (Hardy & Conway, 1978). Rehabilitation nurses must be clear about their role and the rationale for their actions. Those nurses who scientifically test concepts from theories will make essential contributions toward advocacy, quality of life, and value clarification when allocation of resources inevitably become more pressing issues.

Rehabilitation nurses have an obligation to promote preventive rehabilitation nursing interventions not only to assure clients attain functional capacities, avoid further disability, and prevent complications but also to advocate for quality of life, socialization, and dignity. Interventions must extend continuity for older persons who receive acute care services in intensive care and acute care units, as well as in subacute and long-term care facilities, to return to the community for day care or independent living.

For example, rehabilitation nursing role functions as advocate and an "agent of change" empower a client and family to know, envision, and evaluate options, then to plan together problem-solving strategies and behaviors for achieving outcomes. A similar role function contributes to team building among professional colleagues and collaboration among various organizational departments. Not only agents of change but also professionals experiencing role changes, rehabilitation nurses practice as full members of interdisciplinary and transdisciplinary teams (Hoeman, 1993) of health professionals, community professionals, and client or family members.

Roles include educator, consultant, case manager, researcher, advocate, enabler/facilitator, leader, expert practitioner, and team member. In the next several years, rehabilitation nurses will participate in changes to transdisciplinary team roles, subspecialty roles, and advanced practice roles in multiple settings. Subspecialties include but are not limited to pediatric, pulmonary, renal, cancer and restorative, cardiac, and geriatric care and pain management. Chapter 2 discusses models for practice in more detail.

Advanced practice roles include educator, administrator, case management, practitioner, global or international expert, and expert witness or private legal consultant (McCourt, 1993). Nurses moving into advanced practice roles recognize that no health professional is uniquely prepared to manage the complex multidimensional care needs of clients with chronic, disabling, or developmental disorders. When rehabilitation nurses base practice on reputable findings from theory and outcome research, they are better prepared to articulate their roles clearly, advocate for clients, coordinate and manage care in multiple environments, and participate as collegial members of interdisciplinary teams of health professionals (Hoeman, 1993). A future advanced practice role for rehabilitation nurses will refine these and other leadership role attributes.

REFERENCES

Abramson, L., Seligman, M., & Teasdale, J. (1978). Learned helplessness in humans: Critique and reformulation. *Journal of Abnormal Psychology, 87,* 49-74.

Atwood, J. (1978). The phenomenon of selective neglect. In E. Bauwens (Ed.), *The anthropology of health.* St. Louis: Mosby–Year Book, pp. 192-200.

Backer, B.A. (1993). Lillian Wald: Connecting caring with action. *Nursing and Health Care, 14,* 122-129.

Bandura, A. (1969). *Principles of behavior modification.* New York: Holt, Rinehart, and Winston.

Bandura, A. (1977). *Social learning theory.* Englewood Cliffs, NJ: Prentice-Hall.

Becker, M.H. (Ed.). (1974). *The health belief model and personal health behavior.* Thorofare, NJ: Charles B. Slack.

Borgman, M.F., & Passarella, P. (1991). Nursing care of the stroke patient using Bobath principles: An approach to altered movement. *Nursing Clinics of North America, 26,* 1019-1035.

Bowen, M. (1966). The use of family therapy in clinical practice. *Comprehensive Psychiatry, 7,* 345-374.

Brillhart, B. (1986). Predictors of self-acceptance: Rehabilitation success for the disabled. *Rehabilitation Nursing, 11,* 8-12.

Clark, D. (1988). Framework for care: A developmental behavioral model for nursing. Part 2. *Nursing Times, 84,* 33-35.

Clark, M., & Anderson, B.G. (1967). Culture and aging: An anthropological study of older Americans. Springfield, IL: Charles C Thomas.

Cumming, E., & Henry, W.E. (1961). Growing old: The process of disengagement. New York: Basic Books.

Dembo, T. (1969). Rehabilitation psychology and its immediate future: A problem of utilization of psychological knowledge. *Rehabilitation Psychology 16,* 63-72.

Dembo, T., Leviton, G., & Wright, B. (1975). Adjustment to misfortune—A problem of social psychological rehabilitation. *Rehabilitation Psychology, 22,* 1-100. (Original work published in 1948.)

Derstine, J.B. (1992). Theory-based advanced rehabilitation nursing: Is it a reality? *Holistic Nursing Practice, 6,* 1-6.

Derstine, J., & O'Toole, M. (1987). Wellness: A theme for an elective course in rehabilitation nursing. *Rehabilitation Nursing, 12,* 33-34.

Dubin, R. (1978). *Theory building.* New York: The Free Press.

Duffy, M.E. (1987). The concept of adaptation: Examining alternatives for the study of nursing phenomena. *Scholarly Inquiry for Nursing Practice, 1,* 179-192.

Dunn, H.L. (1959). High level wellness for man and society. *American Journal of Public Health, 49,* 786-792.

Duvall, E.M. (1971). *Family development* (4th ed.). Philadelphia: J.B. Lippincott.

Eland, J., & Anderson, J. (1977). The experience of pain in children. In A. Jacox (Ed.), *Pain: A source book for nurses and other health professionals* (pp. 453-473). Boston: Little, Brown.

Engel, G.L. (1968). A life setting conducive to illness: The giving-up—given-up complex. *Annals of Internal Medicine, 69,* 293-300.

Eberst, R.M. (1984). Defining health: A multidimensional model. *Journal of School Health, 54*(3), 99-104.

Erikson, E.H. (1968). *Identity, youth, and crisis* (Chap. 3). New York: W.W. Norton.

Fagan, J., & Shepherd, I.L. (1970). *Gestalt therapy now: Theory, techniques, applications* (reprint. ed.). New York: Harper & Row.

Fawcett, J. (1989). *Analysis and evaluation of conceptual models of nursing* (2nd ed.). Philadelphia: F.A. Davis.

Ferguson, M. (1980). *The aquarian conspiracy.* Los Angeles: J.P. Tarcher.

Friedman, M., & Rosenman, R.H. (1974). *Type A behavior and your heart.* New York: Knopf.

Ginsburg, H.P., & Opper, S. (1988). *Piaget's theory of intellectual development* (3rd ed.). Englewood Cliffs, NJ: Prentice-Hall.

Glaser, B., & Strauss, A. (1973). *The discovery of grounded theory: Strategies for qualitative research.* Chicago: Aldine.

Gleick, J. (1987). *Chaos: Making a new science.* New York: Viking Penguin Group.

Goffman, E. (1963). *Stigma: Notes on the management of spoiled identity.* Englewood Cliffs, NJ: Prentice-Hall.

Gordon, M. (1993). *Manual of nursing diagnosis* (6th ed.). St. Louis: Mosby-Year Book.

Grant, J.S., Kinney, M.R., & Davis, L.L. (1993). Using conceptual frameworks or models to guide nursing research. *Journal of Neuroscience Nursing, 25,* 52-29.

Gritzer, G., & Arluke, A. (1985). *The making of rehabilitation: A political economy of medical specialization 1890-1980.* Berkely and Los Angeles: University of California Press.

Hardy, M., & Conway, M. (1978). *Role theory: Perspectives for health professionals.* New York: Appleton-Century-Crofts.

Havinghurst, R.J. (1972). *Developmental tasks and education.* New York: David McKay.

Heine, C. (1991). Development of gerontological nursing theory: Applying the man-living-health theory of nursing. *Nursing and Health Care, 12,* 184-188.

Henderson, V. (1966). *The nature of nursing.* New York: MacMillan.

Hergenhahn, B.R. (1982). *An introduction to theories of learning* (2nd ed.). Englewood Cliffs, NJ: Prentice-Hall.

Hickman, J.S. (1993). A critical assessment of critical thinking in nursing education. *Holistic Nursing Practice, 7,* 36-47.

Hill, R. (1965). Generic features of families under stress. In H.J. Parad (ed). *Crisis intervention: Selected Readings.* New York: Family Service Association of America. pp. 32-52. Families under stress.

Hinds, C. (1990). Personal and contextual factors predicting patients' reported quality of life: Exploring congruency with Betty Neuman's assumptions. *Journal of Advanced Nursing, 15,* 456-462.

Hoeman, S.P., & Winters, D. (1988). Contracting for success: case management for clients with high cervical spinal cord injury. *Guiding patients through the health care maze* (pp. 109-116) (Quality Review Bulletin, special ed.). Chicago: JCAHO.

Hoeman, S.P. (1989). Cultural assessment in rehabilitation nursing practice. In D. Gordon (Ed.), *Rehabilitation nursing. Nursing Clinics of North America, 24,* 277-289. Philadelphia: W.B. Saunders.

Hoeman, S.P., & Winters, D.M. (1990). Theory-based case management: High cervical spinal cord injury. *Home Healthcare Nurse, 8,* 25-33.

Hoeman, S.P. (Ed.). (1992). *Interdisciplinary pediatric rehabilitation delegation to the People's Republic of China.* Tacoma, WA: People-to-People Citizen Ambassador Program.

Hoeman, S.P., & Repetto, M.A. (1992). Historical research: Relevance of

USA legislation for children with special needs to nursing practice: 1903-1990. *Western Journal of Nursing Research, 14,* 102-105.

Hoeman, S.P. (1993). A research based transdisciplinary team model for infants with special needs and their families. In S.P. Hoeman, (Ed). *Interdisciplinary practice. Holistic Nursing Practice, 7*(4), 63-72.

Jessop, D.J., & Stein, R.E. (1985). Uncertainty and its relation to the psychological and social correlates of chronic disease in children. *Social Science and Medicine 20,* 993-999.

Johnson, D.E. (1968). Theory in nursing: Borrowed and unique. *Nursing Research, 17,* 206-209.

Johnson, D.E. (1980). The behavioral system model for nursing. In J.P. Riehl, & S.C. Roy, (Eds.), *Conceptual models for nursing practice* (2nd ed.). New York: Appleton-Century-Crofts.

Kim, H.S. (1987). Structuring the nursing knowledge system: A typology of four domains. *Scholarly Inquiry for Nursing, 1,* 99-110.

King, I.M. (1968). A conceptual frame of reference for nursing. *Nursing Research, 17,* 27-30.

King, I.M. (1971). *Toward a theory for nursing.* New York: John Wiley & Sons.

King, I.M. (1981). *A theory for nursing: Systems, concepts, and process.* New York: John Wiley & Sons.

Kleinman, A., Eisenberg, L., & Good, B. (1978). Culture, illness, and care: Clinical lessons from anthropological and cross-cultural research. *Annals of Internal Medicine, 88,* 251-258.

Knust, S.J., & Quarn, J.M. (1983). Integration of self-care theory with rehabilitation nursing. *Rehabilitation Nursing, 8,* 26-28.

Kobasa, S.C., Maddi, S.R., & Zola, M.A. (1983). Type A and hardiness. *Journal of Behavioral Medicine, 6,* 41-50.

Kubler-Ross, E. (1969). *On death and dying.* New York: MacMillan.

Lazarus, R.S. (1966). *Psychological stress and the coping process.* New York: McGraw-Hill.

Lazarus, R.S., & Folkman, S. (1984). *Stress, appraisal, and coping.* New York: Springer.

Leininger, M.M. (Ed.). (1988). *Care: The essence of nursing.* Detroit: Wayne State University Press.

Levine, M.E. (1967). The four conservation principles of nursing. *Nursing Forum, 6,* 45-59.

Lewin, K. (1947). Frontiers in group dynamics: Concept, methods, and reality in social science. *Human Relations, 1,* 5-41.

Linder, T.W. (1990). *Transactional play-based assessment.* Baltimore: Paul H. Brookes.

Lippitt, R., Watson, J., & Westley, B. (1958). *The dynamics of planned change.* New York: Harcourt, Brace, & World.

Litman, T.J. (1979). Physical rehabilitation: A social-psychological approach. In E.G. Jaco (Ed.), *Patients, physicians, and illness* (pp. 186-203). Glencoe, IL: The Free Press.

Maslow, A.H. (1968). *Toward a psychology of being* (2nd ed.). Princeton, NJ: D. Van Nostrand Reinhold.

McCourt, A.E. (Ed.). (1993). *The specialty practice of rehabilitation nursing: A core curriculum* (3rd ed.). Skokie, IL: Rehabilitation Nursing Foundation.

McCubbin, H.I., & Patterson, J.M. (1983). The family stress process: The double ABCX model of adjustment and adaptation. In H. McCubbin, M. Sussman, & J. Patterson (Eds.), *Social stress and the family: Advances and developments in family stress theory* (pp. 7-37). New York: Haworth Press.

Mercer, R.T. (1989). Theoretical perspectives on the family. In C.L. Gilliss, B.L. Highley, B.M. Roberts, & I.M. Martinson, (Eds.), *Toward a new science of family nursing* (pp. 9-36). Menlo Park, CA: Addison-Wesley.

Minuchin, S. (1980). *Families and family therapy.* Cambridge, MA: Harvard University Press.

Mishel, M.H. (1990). Reconceptualization of the uncertainty in illness theory. *Image: Journal of Nursing Scholarship, 22,* 256-262.

Moccia, P. (Ed.). (1986). *New approaches to theory development.* NLN Pub No. 15-1992. New York: NLN.

Morse, J.M., Solberg, S.M., Neadner, W.L., Bottorff, J.L., & Johnson, J.L. (1990). Concepts of caring and caring as a concept. *Advances in Nursing Science, 13,* 1-14.

Mumma, C. (Ed.). (1987). *Rehabilitation Nursing: Concepts and Practice A Core Curriculum for Rehabilitation Nursing* (2nd ed). edition. Evanston, IL: Association of Rehabilitation Nurses, Rehabilitation Nursing Foundation.

Nadolsky, J.M. (1987). Rehabilitation and wellness: In need of integration. *Journal of Rehabilitation, 53,* 5-7.

Neuman, B. (1989). *The Neuman systems model* (2nd ed.). East Norwalk, CT: Appleton & Lange.

Newman, M. (1986). *NANDA health as expanding consciousness.* St. Louis: Mosby.

Nightingale, F. (1860). *Notes on nursing: What it is and what it is not.* Philadelphia: J.B. Lippincott, 1946 (facsimile of first edition. London: Harrison & Sons). New York: Dover. (Original work published in 1859.)

Olshansky, S. (1962). Chronic sorrow: A response to having a mentally defective child. *Social Casework, 43,* 190-193.

Orem, D.M. (1980). *Nursing: Concepts of practice.* New York: McGraw-Hill. (Original work published in 1971.)

Orem, D.M. (1985). A concept of self-care for the rehabilitation client. *Rehabilitation Nursing, 10,* 33-36.

Orlando, I.J. (1961). *The dynamic nurse-patient relationship.* New York: G.P. Putnam's Sons.

Parcel, G.S., & Baranowski, T. (1981). Social learning theory and health education. *Health Education, 12,* 14.

Parse, R.R. (1981). *Man-living-health: A theory of nursing.* New York: John Wiley & Sons.

Parsons, T. (1951). *The social system.* New York: The Free Press.

Parsons, T. (1958). Definitions of health and illness in the light of American values and social structure. In E.G. Jaco (Ed.), *Patients, physicians, and illness* (pp. 165-187). Glencoe, IL: The Free Press.

Peplau, H.E. (1952). *Interpersonal relations in nursing.* New York: G.P. Putnam's Sons.

Perkins, J.L., Bennett, D.N., & Dorman, R.E. (1993). Why men choose nursing. *Nursing and Health Care, 14,* 34-38.

Pfeiffer, D. (1992). Disabling definitions: Is the World Health Organization normal? *New England Journal of Human Services, 11,* 4-9.

Piaget, J. (1972). *The child's conception of physical causality.* Totowa, NJ: Littlefield, Adams.

Pollock, S.E. (1989). The hardiness characteristic: A motivating factor in adaptation. *Advances in Nursing Science, 11,* 53-62.

Quinless, F.W., & Nelson, M.A. (1988). Development of a measure of learned helplessness. *Nursing Research, 37,* 11-15.

Rogers, M. (1970). *An introduction to the theoretical basis of nursing.* Philadelphia: F.A. Davis.

Roper, N., Logan, W.W., & Tierney, A. (1980). *The elements of nursing.* New York: Churchill, Livingstone.

Roper, N., Logan, W.W., & Tierney, A. (1983). *Using a model for nursing.* Edinburgh: Churchill Livingstone.

Ross, D.M., & Ross, S.A. (1988). *Childhood pain: Current issues, research, and management.* Baltimore: Urban Schwarzenberg.

Rotter, J.B. (1966). Generalized expectancies for internal versus external control of reinforcement. *Psychological Monographs, 80,* 1-609.

Roy, S.C. (1970). Adaptation: A conceptual framework for nursing. *Nursing Outlook, 18,* 42-45.

Roy, S.C. (1980). The Roy adaptation model. In J.P. Riehl & S.C. Roy (Eds.). *Conceptual Models for Nursing Practice* (2nd ed.). Appleton-Century-Crofts. NY.

Safilios-Rothschild, C. (1970). *The sociology and social psychology of disability and rehabilitation.* New York: Random House.

Satir, V. (1967). *Conjoint family therapy* (rev. ed.). Palo Alto, CA: Science & Behavior Books.

Seigel, J.M. (1984). Type A behavior: Epidemiologic foundations and public health implications. *Annual Review of Public Health, 5,* 343-367.

Selye, H. (1978). *Stress of life.* New York: McGraw-Hill.

Stein, R.E., & Jessop, D.J. (1989). What diagnosis does not tell: The case for a noncategorical approach to chronic illness in childhood. *Social Science and Medicine, 29,* 769-778.

Stryker, R.N. (1977). *Rehabilitative aspects of acute and chronic nursing care* (2nd ed.). Philadelphia: W.B. Saunders. p. 15.

Tait, R., & Silver, R.C. (1989). Coming to terms with major negative life events. In J.S. Uleman & J.A. Bargh (Eds.). *Unintended thought: The limits of awareness, intention, and control* (pp. 351-382). New York: Guilford Press.

Tartasky, D.S. (1993). Hardiness: conceptual and methodological issues. *Image: Journal of Nursing Scholarship, 25,* 225-230.

Taylor, J. (1981). Portrayal of persons with disabilities by the media. *Mental Retardation Bulletin, 9,* 38-53.

Thomas, E. (1966). Problems of disability from the perspective of role theory. *Journal of Health and Human Behavior, 7.*

Thorne, S.E. (1993). *Negotiating health care: The social context of chronic illness.* Newbury Park: CA: Sage.

Titus, S., & Porter, P. (1989). Orem's theory applied to pediatric residential treatment. *Pediatric Nursing, 15,* 465-469.

Trieschman, R. (1987). *Aging with a disability.* New York: Demos.

Wallston, K.A., & Wallston, B.S. (1982). Who is responsible for your health? The construct of locus of control. In G.S. Sanders & J. Suls (Eds.). *Social psychology of health and illness* (pp. 65-95). Hillsdale, NJ: Lawrence Erlbaum.

Watson, J. (1979). *Nursing: The philosophy and science of caring.* Boston: Little, Brown.

World Health Organization. (1985). *International classification of impairments, disabilities, and handicaps.* Geneva: World Health Organization.

Wood, P. (1986). Introduction: a second collection of papers concerning application of the international classification of impairments, disabilities, and handicaps. *International Rehabilitation Medicine, 8*(1):1-2.

Wright, B. (1960). *Physical disability—A psychological approach.* New York: Harper Brothers.

Wright, B. (1983). *Physical disability: A psychosocial approach.* New York: Harper Collins.

2

Models for Theory-Based Practice of Rehabilitation Nursing

Christina M. Mumma, PhD, RN, CRRN
Audrey Nelson, PhD, RN

INTRODUCTION

The rich variety of rehabilitation practice models provides nurses with many alternatives for developing programs and services. Diverse models of rehabilitation nursing practice have emerged to address variations in client needs, settings, providers, and collaborative efforts.

Generally rehabilitation nursing practice models are defined by the choice of setting, types and utilization of service providers, and types of services offered. At times the combination of setting, services, and providers complement each other to optimize the match between client needs and expectations. However, not all models are successful in achieving positive patient outcomes. In some cases either the settings, services, or providers are not appropriate to meet the consumer demands. In other cases the specific combination of setting, services, and providers may be incompatible. Many factors need to be considered when choosing a model for rehabilitation including cost, market, availability of providers, identified patient care demands, consumer expectations, reimbursement issues, and regulations.

A brief overview of various models for practice of rehabilitation nursing is provided, focusing on four major components: client needs, settings, providers, and collaborative efforts. An example illustrating a specific combination of setting, services, providers, and collaboration follows to illustrate one model for rehabilitation nursing.

CLIENT-CENTERED MODELS

Client-centered care is the most critical facet of rehabilitation models. These models (see Box below) often are referred to as "consumer driven" in that they emphasize the needs, thoughts, feelings, and expectations of the client. The

---

◆

CLIENT-CENTERED MODELS

Developmental level of client
Type of disability
Cultural aspects
Family as client

---

partnership between clients and healthcare providers is essential to the development of an effective rehabilitation model.

Although most rehabilitation care models attempt to address the unique needs of the persons they were designed to serve, the heterogeneity of the client mix makes this a difficult process. Specialization has emerged as one way to address these unique consumer needs. Specialization involves targeting services to particular client groups, resulting in restriction of services to a particular, more homogeneous, client population.

Specialization offers advantages and disadvantages. A recent survey of 114 facilities providing burn rehabilitation services in the United States revealed that although all facilities treated similar severity of burns, had similar lengths of hospitalization, and similar outpatient follow-up, the specialized burn facilities were more likely to report the following:

1. Organized outpatient burn rehabilitation programs
2. Available specialized burn rehabilitation personnel
3. Regular interdisciplinary inpatient staffing conferences and outpatient clinics
4. Structured educational activities (Cromes & Helm, 1992)

Rehabilitation services can be specialized based on (1) developmental level of clients, (2) type of disability, (3) cultural systems, and (4) family systems. Each of these client-centered models is described briefly.

A Focus on the Developmental Level of the Client

Rehabilitation models may provide care to client groups based on age or developmental level. The development of rehabilitation specialty programs was in part shaped by the criteria set by the Commission on Accreditation of Rehabilitation Facilities (CARF). Historically rehabilitation programs have been targeted for adults. One such program was designed in New Zealand (Roy, 1991). This adult rehabilitation program focused on unique social, psychological, and vocational needs of adults with severe disabilities.

The historical development of rehabilitation facilities for children is described by Edwards (1992). Pediatric rehabilitation nursing is a relatively new field; goals related to comprehensive and holistic care are blended with creative strategies to address the unique developmental needs of children (Selekman, 1991). Pediatric rehabilitation nurses have an appreciation for the contributions of health, social, and educational needs of their clients (Eigsti, Aretz, & Shannon, 1990). Development of a normal, age-appropriate environment with opportunities for extended parent-child interaction is critical (Richardson & Robinson, 1989). Heery (1992) described pediatric rehabilitation as a process for "restoring childhood."

Rehabilitation services for adolescents are designed to meet the critical developmental needs of teenagers including independence, socialization, and sexuality education. A model community-based adolescent rehabilitation program in Israel described three day care centers and two afternoon clubs for teenagers with cerebral palsy, mental retardation, blindness, deafness, and emotional handicaps (Hardoff & Chigier, 1991).

Geriatric rehabilitation focuses on providing rehabilitation nursing care for clients with varied gerontologic problems by evaluating and promoting restorative function (Butler, 1991). Functionally impaired elderly patients perceived to be "at risk" for nursing home placement was the targeted population for an inpatient geriatric assessment unit in a community rehabilitation hospital (Applegate, Miller, Graney, Elam, Burns, & Akins, 1990). The program focused on self-care and was aimed at improving functioning, decreasing the risk of nursing home placement, and reducing mortality. A focus on geriatric rehabilitation could result in standardization, improved treatment of the elderly, improved education of healthcare providers, and "more prestige" for this specialty practice.

A Focus on a Particular Disability

Specialized centers have emerged to care for persons with specific disabilities. For example, the model spinal cord injury systems were initiated in 1970 by the National Institute on Disability and Rehabilitation Research (NIDRR). The model systems program provides comprehensive care for persons with spinal cord injuries including services for acute care, rehabilitation, community reintegration, and long-term follow-up (Zejdlik, 1992).

The Department of Veterans Affairs (VA) advocates comprehensive, coordinated care for homogeneous groups of patients, based on disability. Regional VA centers have been developed for treatment of spinal cord injury, traumatic brain injury, and rehabilitation of blind persons.

In the 1980s numerous specialized centers were developed to provide rehabilitation, subacute care, and community reentry for persons with head injuries (Greenspan, Mackenzie, Christensen, & Robel, 1989; Finset, 1992). Rehabilitation goals for persons with cognitive impairment include provision of the least restrictive environment using the least restrictive intervention, thus promoting independence (Heacock, Walton, Beck, & Mercer, 1991).

Cancer rehabilitation (Watson, 1992; Mayer, 1992) is a relatively new specialty area for nursing practice. Cardiac rehabilitation (Gutin, Prince, & Stein, 1990; Conn, Taylor, & Casey, 1992; Pashkow, 1993; Hotta, 1991) and burn rehabilitation programs provide individuals with the training necessary to resume as much of their preexisting lifestyle as possible. Although initially prevention and control of complications is critical, reconditioning, retraining in activi-

ties of daily living, and viewing the client as a whole are critical features of these rehabilitation programs (Harden & Luster, 1991).

A Focus on Cultural Influences

A noted trend in healthcare toward increased cultural diversity has implications for rehabilitation. Patient outcomes, interactions with nurses, and responses to rehabilitation services are defined by cultural beliefs. Wenger (1992) described interpretation of cultural beliefs and behaviors as giving contextual meaning to patterns related to the lifeways of people. Transcultural nursing (Leininger, 1990) has emerged as a specialty with much to offer rehabilitation nursing practice. Hoeman (1989) urged rehabilitation nurses to examine their clients' cultural beliefs and behaviors and strategize ways to include this data in the rehabilitation process. Wenger (1992) encouraged nurses to explore migration patterns, ethnic diversity, utilization of services, and responses to healthcare interventions. Models designed to address unique cultural aspects of rehabilitation are needed.

A Focus on the Family as the Client

For treatment to be incorporated into daily life, full cooperation and commitment from the family is crucial. Although most patients have family members available to participate in the rehabilitation process, family involvement often is limited to teaching the family about patient care (Diehl, 1989). At times it is critical for the rehabilitation team to view the family as the client, rather than an individual.

Family affiliations range from the traditional nuclear or extended family units to groups established by agreement or happenstance. Regardless of the relationship each person is affected when a member becomes disabled or chronically ill (Watson, 1992). Power (1989) described a model for family involvement in the rehabilitation process. She suggested knowledge and skills that facilitate family coping ultimately benefit the client. Nurses need to pay particular attention to identifying family needs, with an emphasis on short-term intervention at specific trigger points in the rehabilitation process. Emphasizing the importance of timing, trigger points are defined as times during rehabilitation when family members are focused on specific concerns. Nursing intervention related to those specific concerns is likely to be most effective when family focus is highest.

Determining family capacity for participating in the rehabilitation process is a critical component of family rehabilitation models. Watson identified the following indicators for family involvement: willingness to help with patient care, coping patterns, knowledge of illness or disability, patient's expectations, and the family's economic status (Watson, 1989).

Several rehabilitation models focusing on the family as the client are described in the literature. Feigelman and Jaquith (1992) described a day care program for rehabilitating families with an identified youth drug abuser. Viewing drug abuse as a "family problem," the program requires behavior change in all family members.

The long-term rehabilitation of the pediatric client is necessarily a joint team-family responsibility (Eigsti et al.,

1990). Likewise, effective rehabilitation of the elderly necessitates that the healthcare team addresses the family's unique needs to assure a smooth transition to the home. Increasing concern for the well-being of caregivers demonstrates such a shift in emphasis to include the family. Addressing the physical and emotional impact of caregiving is a constant challenge for the rehabilitation nurse. Nurses play a major role in identifying caregiver problems and helping caregivers to obtain the assistance that will enable them to continue the family member's care in a home environment (Musolf, 1991).

Baum (1991) discussed strategies for addressing the needs of cognitively impaired elderly from a family policy perspective, advocating policy-level changes to promote family involvement.

SETTING-CENTERED MODELS

In addition to models that focus on client characteristics, models can be differentiated by the type of setting within which rehabilitation is practiced. Rehabilitation takes place in many settings other than the traditional inpatient rehabilitation facility. In addition to acute care facilities, rehabilitation nurses practice in long-term care settings, community-based settings, and in clients' homes (see Box at right).

A Focus on Acute Care

Before World War II minimal attention was given to rehabilitative aspects of healthcare. In 1946 physiatrist became the accepted term for physicians trained in rehabilitation medicine. It was only as recently as 1966 that CARF was founded to establish guidelines and standards for rehabilitation care (Habel, 1993).

Traditionally (obviously a very new tradition), rehabilitation care has been provided in acute rehabilitation settings. The majority of rehabilitation nurses practice in acute care facilities. A recent survey conducted by the Association of Rehabilitation Nurses revealed that 56% of respondents worked on a rehabilitation unit within a general hospital, and 23% worked in a free-standing rehabilitation facility (Habel, 1993). In 1990 there were 715 exempt rehabilitation units in acute care hospitals and 135 free-standing rehabilitation hospitals, comprising a total of approximately 18,000 rehabilitation beds (Portnow et al., 1991).

Ross (1992) mentioned the intense competition among acute rehabilitation facilities for the limited rehabilitation population. He listed some of the expectations buyers (primarily insurance companies) of rehabilitation have for acute rehabilitation settings:

- ✦ Compliance with standards of the Joint Commission on Accreditation of Health Organizations (JCAHO) and the Commission on Accreditation of Rehabilitation Facilities (CARF)
- ✦ Demonstrated patient outcomes and quality assurance
- ✦ Effective daily communication among rehabilitation team members
- ✦ Timely implementation of individualized interdisciplinary plan of care
- ✦ Minimal idle time for clients
- ✦ Case management
- ✦ Client and family involvement and satisfaction

✦

SETTING-CENTERED MODELS

Acute care
Long-term care
Community-based settings
Home care

- ✦ Coordination of resources
- ✦ Top credentials for staff
- ✦ Good price

The literature provides many descriptions of various aspects of rehabilitation nursing practice in acute rehabilitation settings. The large number of acute setting–based publications reflects the past and current predominance of this type of setting for rehabilitation care. As is discussed later in this chapter, there is a developing shift out of inpatient settings and toward delivery of rehabilitation services in the home and in other community-based settings. The mix of rehabilitation settings in the near future may look quite different than it does now.

There are reports in the literature of the development of competency-based rehabilitation nursing practice within acute rehabilitation settings. For example, Lewis, Govoni, Camp, Pierce, and Salter (1993) described the establishment of such a practice within a 172-bed rehabilitation nursing service in an acute care medical center in Cleveland, Ohio.

Other acute care settings have responded to changes within the economic and healthcare environments in a variety of innovative ways. Skipper (1993) reported the development of a utilization management system within an acute rehabilitation setting in response to such issues as increased costs of care delivery, lower reimbursement, high length of stay, and low staff morale. Their multidisciplinary approach to utilization management required careful planning and extensive communication among members of the involved disciplines. Use of the utilization management system resulted in improved quality of care and a decrease in average length of stay. Similarly, in Australia, a rehabilitation center used multidisciplinary discharge planning to assist clients to return to their communities at an optimal level of independence (Pittmann, Marton, Edwards, & Holmes, 1992).

A Focus on Long-Term Care

Only about 2.5% of rehabilitation nurses who responded to a recent job analysis survey conducted by the Association of Rehabilitation Nurses identified long-term care facilities as their practice setting (Habel, 1993). Accurate numbers of persons with chronic disability residing in long-term care facilities are difficult to determine. Certainly elderly people are overrepresented in institutional settings, with an estimated 4% to 5% of elderly individuals living in institutions (Dittmar, 1989; Friedman, 1992). There are also an unknown number of younger persons with chronic disabilities residing in long-term care facilities at any given time.

Long-term care facilities generally provide a variety of rehabilitation services to clients with disabilities. These services include but are not limited to rehabilitation nursing, rehabilitation medicine, physical therapy, occupational therapy, and speech therapy. The scheduled number of hours of therapy per week is reduced compared with acute rehabilitation facilities. The overall rehabilitation goals are congruent with those in other settings: maximum independent functioning and quality of life.

Recently the designation "subacute rehabilitation" has emerged as a model of rehabilitation care delivery. Clear, universally agreed-upon definitions of subacute rehabilitation have not yet been established. According to Mayer, Buckley, and White (1990), subacute rehabilitation facilities serve "patients whose medical treatment precludes participation in an acute rehabilitation program or who are classified as slow to progress and would not qualify for a regular rehabilitation program."

Mayer et al. (1990) described direct nursing care provided to clients in a 57-bed subacute head trauma rehabilitation center. Common medical diagnoses of clients at the center included closed head injury with quadriparesis, anoxic encephalopathy secondary to cardiac arrest, strokes, and aneurysms. Within this setting the roles of the registered nurse were primarily planner, coordinator, and evaluator of patient outcomes, as well as some direct care provision. Much of the direct nursing care was provided by nursing assistants and licensed vocational nurses (LVNs).

Inpatient settings that provide subacute and long-term rehabilitation services to clients with chronic disabilities and illnesses may be viewed in a number of different ways. For some clients these facilities may be an appropriate, cost-effective alternative to rehabilitation in a more acute setting. For other clients a subacute or long-term care setting may be one of several places of care and residence along their rehabilitation continua of care. And there may be still other clients who will be discharged home from acute rehabilitation and then later be admitted to a subacute or long-term care facility.

A Focus on Community-Based Settings

The community, rather than the hospital or inpatient setting, has become a primary treatment setting in which many persons with disabilities manage their care and daily activities. The term community-based rehabilitation has been broadly defined and applied to a wide variety of programs and settings within which clients receive rehabilitation services. Community-based rehabilitation settings include, for example, outpatient clinics, day treatment programs, independent living centers, community reentry programs, and rural outreach programs.

The purposes and goals of community-based rehabilitation have much in common with rehabilitation in other settings. Hoeman (1992) outlined the following concepts and principles basic to community-based rehabilitation:

♦ Collaboration (interdisciplinary, transdisciplinary, and interagency)
♦ Holistic and comprehensive services
♦ Self-care, maximum function, and prevention
♦ Focus on family and cultural values

♦ Client and family as a unit of service in the community

A community-based rehabilitation model involves clients and families as copartners with professionals for the accomplishment of mutually established goals. The emphasis is on short-term, long-term, and even lifelong goals that lead to improvement in quality of life as defined within that client and family's context (Hoeman, 1992).

One example of implementation of community-based rehabilitation is an outpatient program for particular client populations. Outpatient cardiac rehabilitation centers provide enhanced physiologic status, aerobic fitness, nutrition, and strengthening (Gutin et al., 1990). Outpatient pain treatment programs have been in existence for a number of years and have been described in the literature by Rosomoff (1992) and Eldar, Oren, and Goldin (1989).

Community reentry is the focus of a model program geared for the reintegration of clients with burn injuries (Goggins, Hall, Nack, & Shuart, 1990). Using "community skills training" and "community skills practice," the program demonstrated that a gradual transition between the acute care setting and active participation in family, leisure, and vocational roles enhances psychosocial and functional recovery.

Independent living centers provide short-term rehabilitation in the community. Chamberlain (1990) described such a center in England designed to rehabilitate clients with rheumatologic problems. In a thought-provoking article that challenged rehabilitation professionals to reaffirm their commitment to community, DeJong cited several highly successful independent living programs. These programs included Access Chicago, the Ann Arbor Center for Independent Living, and the Independent Living Research Utilization Program developed by The Institute for Rehabilitation and Research (TIRR) in Houston (DeJong, 1993). Fuhrer, Rossi, Gerken, Nosek, and Richards reported the results of a national survey of independent living centers and medical rehabilitation programs. The survey indicated the existence of considerable cooperation between the two types of programs. The emphasis within rehabilitation programs on functional independence is highly congruent with the independent living center focus on maintaining independent lifestyles and improving community environments (Fuhrer et al., 1990).

The rehabilitation literature includes a number of reports of rural communities that have successfully met the challenge of providing rehabilitation care in areas where resources are scarce. In the Philippines, for example, community-based rehabilitation emerged as a necessity, given that 70% of their population live in rural areas. Periquet (1989) described a community-based rehabilitation program in the Philippines in which trained volunteers were used to identify and support persons with disabilities in their own villages. A similar program might be successful in more rural areas of the United States, for example, most of the state of Alaska. A pediatric outreach service was established in England to reach high-risk children in rural and deprived areas (Spencer, 1993).

An innovative program was developed by The Rehabilitation Centre in Ottawa, Ontario, Canada, to "take rehabilitation to the people" in rural Canada (Lavallee & Crupi, 1992). The authors listed the following six problems that they maintained were central to rural rehabilitation:

+ Limited access to services for individuals with disabilities living in rural Canada and the United States
+ Individuals with disabilities living in rural areas need a variety of health services
+ Many elderly people and people with limited income living in rural areas
+ Travel to centralized rehabilitation often an overwhelming burden in terms of time and money
+ Rehabilitation requires multidisciplinary services not available in rural areas
+ Nurses make up majority of direct care providers in rural areas; often lack specialized expertise in rehabilitation

Lavallee and Crupi described the development and implementation of a mobile rehabilitation clinic to meet the rehabilitation needs of clients within rural communities in Ontario, Canada. This mobile interdisciplinary rehabilitation team was described as collaborative and dedicated to holistic practice. Lavallee and Crupi expect the mobile rehabilitation clinic to "help rural communities meet the challenges of tomorrow. It can do this because under the mobile clinic program the community as a whole becomes the client—a client for consultation, education, research, and advocacy interventions" (Lavallee & Crupi, 1992, p. 66).

A Focus on Home Care

Rehabilitation is increasingly being provided in home care settings. Home rehabilitation is generally viewed as a continuation of rehabilitation programs initiated in other settings such as acute rehabilitation facilities, outpatient programs, and long-term care settings. "Returning home" is often one of the most important desires for clients involved in inpatient rehabilitation programs. A measure of successful rehabilitation is the generalization or translation of skills to the natural setting—home. Home rehabilitation promotes client autonomy, independence, and community reintegration (Portnow et al., 1991; Preston, 1990).

In the current economic climate characterized by limited availability of financial resources for healthcare, regulatory systems such as Medicare Prospective Payment and Diagnosis-Related Groups (DRGs) have resulted in intense scrutiny of the need for and length of hospitalization. Thus hospitals have increased financial incentives to reduce costs and to discharge clients more quickly. For some clients it may be most appropriate for their entire rehabilitation program to be provided at home. Portnow et al. (1991) described a multidisciplinary home rehabilitation program designed to substitute for hospital-level care with intense comprehensive daily care. Based on their experience with this program, Portnow et al. stated that clients "are happier at home, they are more motivated, and they are able to progress to higher functional levels in a shorter time" (p. 705).

Community awareness of the availability and effectiveness of home healthcare is growing dramatically (Jaffe, 1989). There are essential differences between home care and hospital or rehabilitation facility care. Regardless of

how "client-friendly" inpatient units are designed to be, clients will quickly remind anyone listening that these settings are *not* home. Jaffe (1989, p. 173) stated very well how home care differs from hospital care:

When the patient is in the hospital, the nurse or other health care professional is in control. In the home setting the opposite is true: the patient and his family are in control. Thus, members of the interdisciplinary home care team are considered guests in the patient's home. The approach to the patient then becomes especially important. Aggressively marching into the home and demanding compliance with the treatment plan will not produce results. Careful strategic planning should occur regarding the approach to the patient and his family to ensure maximum achievement of independent functioning.

Jaffe and Walsh (1993) described the development and implementation of a specialty rehabilitation homecare program within a home health agency. The specialty rehabilitation home care team was developed to reflect the following differences between this program and traditional home healthcare:

+ Staff training in rehabilitation philosophy, team techniques, and treatment methods
+ Team conferences in the home to include client, family, treatment team, and facilitated by the rehabilitation nurse manager
+ Creative problem-solving by the team, orchestrated by the rehabilitation nurse case manager
+ Training in the transdisciplinary approach

Toward the achievement of successful rehabilitation outcomes, a key element within this program is the development of a creative mind-set on the part of each team member. As stated by Jaffe and Walsh (1993), "Creativity is generated when persons remove themselves from the 'ruts' of their training. Thus, staff are encouraged to utilize flexibility in their thinking processes in order to tap their own, along with the client's, potential" (p. 41).

PROVIDER-CENTERED MODELS

The number and type of healthcare providers is integrally linked to the model of rehabilitation practiced. Many factors are considered in determining staffing levels, particularly the supply of healthcare providers and the patient care demands for services. Staffing needs in rural settings, where healthcare providers are potentially scarce, differ from those in suburban or urban areas. Reimbursement systems and third-party payers also shape the type of providers used and thus the model of rehabilitation. Selected models whose major focus is the role of the provider of care is now discussed. Models presented here include primary care, case management, nurse-managed care, and independent practice/consultation (see Box, p. 26).

A Focus on Primary Care

Primary nursing as a care delivery system emerged more than 30 years ago as a response to the fragmentation and depersonalization of team nursing. Within a team nursing model, a team leader (usually a registered nurse) supervised a variety of team members in the total care given to an assigned group of clients (Lyon, 1993). Various members of the nursing team performed different care activities and

◆

PROVIDER-CENTERED MODELS

Primary care
Case management
Nurse-managed care
Independent practice/consultation

---

functions comprising the clients' total care. A drawback of the team nursing model was the very real possibility that each client would have multiple caregivers over the course of hospitalization, with no individual nurse clearly accountable for coordination of all care given. An essential feature of primary nursing is the professional nurse's 24-hour responsibility for care provided to clients for whom that nurse is the assigned/designated primary nurse (DelTogno-Armanasco, 1989; Lyon, 1993). A successful primary nursing system requires considerable communication and collaboration with the client and family as well as with all other health professionals involved in that client's care.

Within inpatient rehabilitation settings, primary nursing often has been implemented in a modified form in keeping with the interdisciplinary rehabilitation team approach to care. One of the authors of this chapter (Mumma) has worked in several acute rehabilitation settings that successfully used a primary nursing system. These settings all had sufficient numbers of rehabilitation registered nurses so that each primary nurse was accountable for nursing aspects of care for a maximum of three clients at any given time.

There are acute rehabilitation settings that are moving away from primary nursing models to other models of care. One such facility is Sharp Memorial Hospital in San Diego, which has implemented a case management system in place of its former primary nursing system (Loveridge, Cummings, & O'Malley, 1988). Reasons for the change mentioned by Loveridge et al. included financial constraints and decreased availability of registered nurses.

A Focus on Case Management

Case management is one of the most recent care delivery models to be embraced by nursing and the healthcare system (McBride, 1992). This model of care delivery has been defined as comprehensive, client-centered continuous care with a multidisciplinary team (Savarese & Weber, 1993). Case management is most commonly referred to in the literature as both a system and a process (Bower, 1992; Butera, 1989; Knollmueller, 1989; McBride, 1992). As a system, case management is designed for provision of services that are appropriate, timely, highly coordinated, and cost-effective. The process of case management has been described as similar to the nursing process, making use of assessment, planning, implementation, and evaluation. A unique aspect of case management is its focus on the illness or disability episode along the care continuum and often across multiple settings (Bower, 1992; McBride, 1992). An example of this would be the coordination of care for a young head-injured client by a rehabilitation nurse case

manager who receives a referral for initial assessment while the client is in an acute rehabilitation setting, and who continues to follow the client through outpatient and home settings.

Nursing case management has been implemented within a wide variety of contexts, settings, and client populations. A distinction has been made between internal case managers, or those who are hospital or facility based, and external case managers who are based in community, insurance, and independent practice settings (Patterson, 1993). Whether practicing primarily within a facility or in a community setting, the "fundamental focus of case management is to integrate, coordinate, and advocate for individuals, families, and groups requiring extensive services" (Bower, 1992, p. 1). The concept and purposes of case management are highly congruent with rehabilitation philosophies and purposes. Individual client goals related to maximizing functional ability and quality of life are integral to both rehabilitation and case management.

According to McBride (1992), "Case management in rehabilitation evolved as a means of integrating the care provided by a variety of professionals across practice settings to decrease duplication of services and omission of essential services" (p. 69). There are many descriptions in the literature of effective use of case management to meet the needs of clients with complex and/or costly healthcare problems and clients at high risk for complications. Examples include provision of case management services for homeless individuals (Savarese & Weber, 1993); for persons with Alzheimer's disease living in a rural setting (Schrader, Shelton, Dworak, & Fraser, 1993); for children undergoing craniofacial reconstruction (Schryer, 1993); for persons with high cervical spinal injury (Hoeman & Winters, 1989); and for elderly individuals at risk for institutionalization (Lyon, 1993). Chimner and Easterling (1993) described the implementation of a collaborative practice model, which included nursing case management, on a 30-bed inpatient rehabilitation unit within an acute care hospital. Benefits of this venture into collaborative practice included decreased length of stay for clients on the unit, increased client and family satisfaction with care received, and improved interdisciplinary relationships between nursing staff and therapy staff.

Lyon (1993) emphasized the need for clarification in defining and using the term case management. She identified criteria for differentiating case management from other nursing care delivery models, particularly team nursing, primary nursing, and managed care. Ginder (1990) described the process of developing case managers in a rehabilitation unit. The integration of case management, program evaluation, and marketing was described by Carey (1990).

Based on the extent of discussion of case management in both the nursing literature and the rehabilitation literature, it is a care delivery model whose popularity and usefulness will continue to grow. For many rehabilitation clients with complex healthcare needs, the most appropriate case management system may be a well-organized interdisciplinary team with a rehabilitation nurse as case manager.

In a discussion of nursing case management in rehabilitation facilities, Guinan (1993) emphasized the opportunities for nurses to make changes in the delivery of care to clients. "Through case management, nurses have been given a voice in the decision-making process that can influence future standards, the direction of the profession, and the healthcare system as it evolves" (Guinan, 1993, p. 256).

A Focus on Nurse-Managed Care

Managed care, referred to by Hampton (1993) as the basis for case management, has in common with case management the goal of promoting cost-effective, high-quality care. Also like case management, managed care emphasizes communication and coordination among members of the healthcare team. Crummer and Carter (1993) listed the following goals of managed care:

✦ Achievement of expected client outcomes
✦ Discharge within specified length of time
✦ Appropriate use of resources
✦ Collaborative practice toward attainment of client outcomes
✦ Coordination and continuity of care, involving client and family
✦ Professional development and satisfaction of clinicians

Managed care is implemented through the use of critical pathways and care maps (Crummer & Carter, 1993; Hampton, 1993; Wood, Bailey, & Tilkemeier, 1992). Critical pathways have been defined as process standards used as adjuncts to the client's plan of care. With the addition of expected outcomes to a critical pathway, client care can then be revised based on the difference between expected and actual process outcomes (Woodyard & Sheetz, 1993). Critical pathways and care maps graph a multidisciplinary care team's actions against a time line. Additionally, care maps contain key interventions and outcome index statements (Hampton, 1993). Thus critical pathways can be used to describe the course of hospitalization for clients with similar problems and treatment plans. In addition to providing a framework for communication, these tools also can be used as a framework for determination of treatment costs for particular client populations (Crummer & Carter, 1993). A rehabilitation clinical pathway was developed at the James A. Haley Veterans Hospital in Tampa, Florida, for treatment of clients with a first admission for an initial stroke (Christian et al., 1994). This clinical pathway combines features of the critical pathway and the care map to provide a time line that includes expected outcomes on a weekly basis (see Appendix 6-A, pp. 83 86).

Since the advent of a hospital-based managed care system at the New England Medical Center in the mid-1980s, managed-care systems have been described for a wide variety of settings, client populations, and nursing care delivery systems (Hampton, 1993). Wood et al. (1992) discussed a hospital-based managed-care system at Rhode Island Memorial Hospital. Within that system nurses are responsible for client outcomes during their shifts. Through the use of standardized care maps and critical pathways, they compare expected outcomes with clients' actual hospital experiences. A managed-care system on an acute orthopedic unit was described by Mosher, Cronk, Kidd, McCormick, Stockton, & Sulla (1992). The client population selected on that unit for the development and implementation of the first critical pathway was lumbar laminectomy. The critical pathway

documentation was actually used by clients, who reported that the critical pathway helped them know what their activity should be by the day of discharge. Clients described the nursing care on that unit as "very organized." Benefits of the managed-care system reported by nursing staff were improved communication between shifts, enhanced orientation of new nursing staff on the unit, and a sense of empowerment among the nurses.

Davies and O'Neill (1990) described a system of nurse-managed care on a rehabilitation ward for elderly clients in England. The main benefits noted were "partnership with patients; reduced inequalities within the team; and improved decision-making and quality of care" (p. 56).

Winters, Jackson, Sims, and Magilvy (1989) reported an improvement in quality of life for persons with multiple sclerosis cared for in a nurse-managed multiple sclerosis clinic at the Veterans Administration Medical Center in Denver, Colorado. A wide range of complementary services are provided at that clinic by a nurse practitioner, rehabilitation nurses, and home care nurses.

Within rehabilitation settings the use of managed care with primary coordination done by nurses holds promise as a means of balancing quality and cost containment. According to Wood et al. (1992), the success of managed care will continue to be measured in quality of care, length of stay, and resource utilization.

A Focus on Independent Practice/Consultation

Within the current highly complex healthcare system, and given the focus on healthcare reform, which mandates the highest possible quality of care at the lowest possible cost, opportunities abound for expansion of nursing roles and responsibilities.

Among nurse practitioners practicing from a rehabilitation nursing perspective, pediatric nurse practitioners and gerontological nurse practitioners are perhaps the most numerous. Writing from the perspective of a pediatric nurse specialist in private practice, Hays (1992) advocated for the creation of a rehabilitation environment to support optimal functioning and successful discharge of children with complex rehabilitation needs to their families.

It is also sometimes the case that an adult nurse practitioner focuses on the care of clients with chronic illness and disability (Hinton-Walker, 1993). In the future there is likely to be an increase in the number of rehabilitation adult nurse practitioners working collaboratively in practice with physiatrists, or setting up independent practices. Perhaps in the future there will be advanced nursing practice certification for "rehabilitation nurse practitioners" (RNPs).

According to Hinton-Walker (1993), advanced practice nurses, and particularly nurse practitioners, are producing a different product. What they do is not nursing according to traditional definitions, nor is it medicine. Perhaps it brings the best of each of these practice disciplines together to facilitate the accomplishment of clients' health-related goals. As stated by Hinton-Walker (1993), "Perhaps the current healthcare crisis and new political leadership will offer the profession an opportunity to fully actualize the autonomous role of the nurse practitioner in primary and community-based practice" (p. 59).

Traditionally nurse practitioners have provided primary

care in outpatient and community settings. In contrast, the advanced practice role of clinical nurse specialists has been enacted primarily in inpatient settings (Schroer, 1991). Role components within clinical nurse specialist practice include those of clinical expert, researcher, educator, and consultant (American Nurses' Association, 1986). According to Schroer the actual practices of many clinical nurse specialists and nurse practitioners are more common than different. She recommended merging the two types of advanced practice into one.

Phipps (1990) described her role as a rehabilitation nurse specialist/consultant in an acute care setting. She provides consultation throughout the hospital to assist primary care nurses to make client care decisions by providing expert opinion in collaboration with the nurse who requested the consultation.

Rehabilitation nurses also have opportunities to perform legal consultation in a variety of ways in cases involving disabling injuries. According to Faherty (1991), rehabilitation nurses having the following characteristics are particularly suited for this type of consultation:

+ Demonstrated clinical expertise in assessing and planning care for clients similar to the client in the case
+ National nursing certification
+ Supervision of nursing students as a faculty member in a school of nursing
+ Clinically current and knowledgeable regarding standards of nursing practice

A rehabilitation nurse with these characteristics would be likely to function successfully as an expert witness in depositions and trials (note that only 1% of cases go to trial), as a reviewer of client records, as someone who can offer expert opinion on the use of standards of care, as someone who can do a client assessment and develop a plan of care, and finally, as case manager for the client with a disability (Faherty, 1991).

The examples presented here are only a few of many opportunities available for rehabilitation nurses in consultation and independent practice. Such opportunities can be expected to expand considerably in the foreseeable future.

COLLABORATIVE PRACTICE MODELS

The use of treatment teams traditionally has been viewed as the optimal means for providing treatment to patients with complex rehabilitation needs. Coordinated, concurrent care by healthcare providers has been deemed critical from onset of the disability through all phases of rehabilitation.

Teams vary in their structure and function. Specifically the structure of teams addresses the composition and configuration of the team. The function of the team deals with the way teams operate, including variations in treatment intensity and delivery. Both the structure and function of teams can be critical factors in determining patient outcomes.

A team approach to rehabilitation involves a group of various disciplines united in purpose to affect rehabilitation outcomes for a client. Although the specific team mix may vary, typically specialists in nursing, medicine, physical therapy, occupational therapy, speech therapy, psychology, recreation therapy, social work, nutrition/dietetics, and orthotics provide the nucleus of the "team" in rehabilitation.

Delineation of core team members varies, depending on the unique needs of the clients they serve. For example, in pediatric rehabilitation, learning specialists are included as core team members (Eigsti et al., 1990). Regardless of the team mix and patient population served, in rehabilitation the client and family are critical team members.

Multidisciplinary, interdisciplinary, and transdisciplinary teams differ in philosophy, structure, leadership, goal-setting practices, and goal attainment strategies. These three team approaches used within rehabilitation settings are compared. A brief discussion of the future of the team approach in rehabilitation follows.

Multidisciplinary Teams

Multidisciplinary teams combine the efforts of various disciplines (Fig. 2-1). Each discipline within a multidisciplinary team submits findings and recommendations, sets their own discipline-specific goals, and works within the discipline boundaries to achieve these goals independently. Discipline-specific progress in goal attainment is communicated directly or indirectly to the rest of the team. Thus the team's outcomes are the sum of each discipline's efforts (Dean & Geiringer, 1990). Effective communication between team members is viewed as the key to success.

Many rehabilitation professionals believe that the whole is greater than the sum of its parts, emphasizing the need for integrating the efforts of team members in a holistic manner. Physical, psychological, social, and spiritual goals for each individual cannot be fully met by isolating the goals and assigning responsibility to a specific discipline. Holistic care requires the individual client be viewed as a whole, with the entire team working toward the attainment of all goals. Interdisciplinary and transdisciplinary teams strive to achieve comprehensive holistic care. These methods of team interaction have been described as synergistic in that more comprehensive outcomes are produced than any one discipline alone would be able to accomplish (Dean & Geiringer, 1990; Miller, 1991; Tice, 1993).

Interdisciplinary Teams

Collaboration replaces communication as the key to successful interdisciplinary teams (Fig. 2-2). Although membership on an interdisciplinary team is quite similar to a multidisciplinary team, the way the disciplines function is different. Rather than each discipline identifying treatment goals, the team identifies goals and strives to avoid duplication or conflict in goals. Team members are involved in problem-solving beyond the confines of their discipline (Diller, 1990). Once the "team goals" are identified, each discipline sets out to work toward goal attainment within the parameters of their discipline, collaborating when goals overlap discipline boundaries.

One obstacle to interdisciplinary efforts is that although each discipline is programmatically dedicated to the interdisciplinary team, organizationally they are aligned to their own discipline. To promote interdisciplinary team collaboration, some rehabilitation models have endorsed organizational changes to include a program director responsible for organizational leadership of several disciplines. Babicki and Miller-McIntyre (1992) describe such a rehabilitation program model.

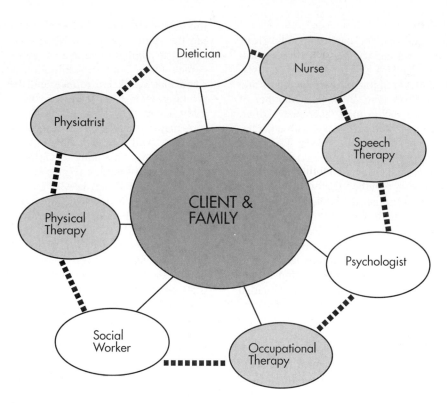

Fig. 2-1 Multidisciplinary rehabilitation team. Characterized by discipline-specific goals, clear boundaries between disciplines, and outcomes that are the sum of each discipline's efforts. Effective communication is the key to success for this type of team.

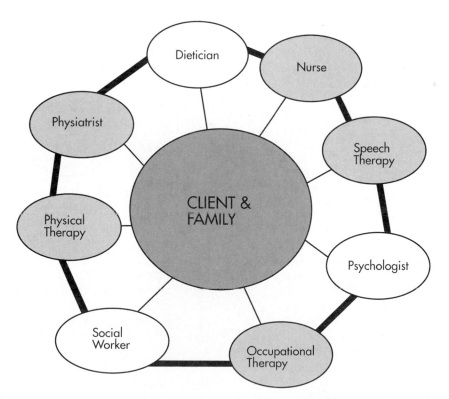

Fig. 2-2 Interdisciplinary rehabilitation team. This type of team collaborates to identify client goals and is characterized by a combination of expanded problem-solving beyond discipline boundaries and discipline-specific work toward goal attainment.

Transdisciplinary Teams

As resources shrink and patient care demands grow, healthcare providers are looking for ways to accomplish goals efficiently without jeopardizing quality. Transdisciplinary teams maximize the strengths of team members and minimize duplication in effort (Fig. 2-3). One member of the team is selected to be the primary therapist (Diller, 1990). The identified primary therapist varies with each patient, depending on the specific patient needs. The other team members contribute information and advice through this identified primary therapist. In this way the team plans implementation to reduce joint collaboration when one team member can effectively accomplish the task, regardless of discipline. Transdisciplinary teamwork involves a certain amount of boundary blurring between disciplines and implies cross training and flexibility in accomplishing tasks. Determining the range of capability of various team members is essential, and team members must be receptive and learn to cope with a wider domain of functioning. Hoeman (1993) described a transdisciplinary team model for the care of infants with special needs.

Future of Teams in Rehabilitation

The future use of teams in rehabilitation must first begin with a critical analysis of the strengths and weaknesses of this approach to care delivery. Halstead (1976), while noting the team approach is widely accepted, found little research to support that teams generate better patient outcomes. Other noted rehabilitation professionals have indicated that healthcare reform and the economic climate are working against the team approach (Diller, 1990; Melvin, 1989; Keith, 1991).

A major strength of the team method of care delivery is that it is well established, promotes good communication and collaboration among disciplines, addresses comprehensive aspects of care, energizes staff, and views the patient holistically (O'Toole, 1992).

Weaknesses of the team approach may include cost, inefficiency, and reduction in time for direct patient care. Rothberg (1981) stated that the team approach places psychological strain on staff. Problems related to role diffusion, ambiguity, status concerns, interpersonal conflicts, lack of commitment of some team members, and concerns regarding competency have been identified (Diller, 1990; Rothberg, 1981). Operationally, coordinated, cooperative, and goal-directed teamwork often is difficult to achieve.

While the comprehensive treatment team has been viewed as the foundation of rehabilitation, Diller (1990) questioned whether the team approach will erode in the face of economic constraints and healthcare reform. Accounts of

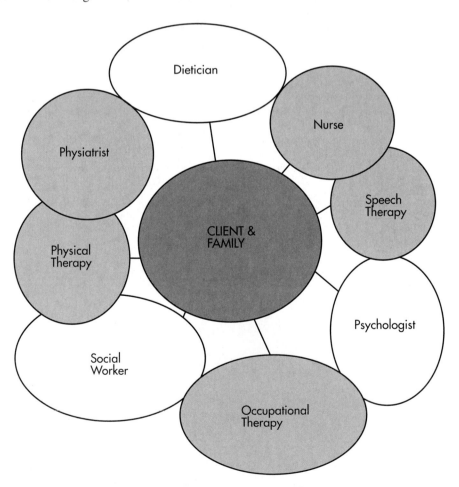

Fig. 2-3 Transdisciplinary rehabilitation team. Characterized by blurring of boundaries between disciplines, as well as implied cross-training and flexibility to minimize duplication of effort toward client goal attainment.

third-party payers opting for a limited number of specific services, rather than paying for comprehensive care, are becoming more common. As healthcare reform continues to unfold, service delivery restructuring is already under way. Keith questioned the effectiveness of comprehensive treatment teams in rehabilitation, citing cost, inefficiency, and lack of research documenting the value of teams. He advocated the development of alternate treatment models, altering the configuration of teams to make them smaller with access to consultation from other specialties, including the use of rehabilitation technicians to address the shortage of healthcare professionals (Keith, 1991). Although not everyone would agree with Keith's recommendations for the future, healthcare professionals clearly need to be creative and responsive to the changing healthcare environment.

SUMMARY

Although the rehabilitation models described provide organization for delivery of rehabilitation services, services need to be integrated, comprehensive, and appropriate. Rehabilitation nurses—diverse in expertise, roles, and work settings—play a critical role in models for rehabilitation.

◆

CASE STUDY

Joe H. is a 17-year-old high school senior who experienced a closed head injury (traumatic brain injury) about a month ago as the result of a motor vehicle accident. He was a passenger in an automobile driven by a friend of his who was giving Joe and several other friends a ride home from a party. Everyone had been drinking beer at the party. Joe's friend ran a red light, and the car was struck on the driver's side. The driver was killed on impact. The other passengers experienced minor injuries and recovered sufficiently to return to school within a few days after the accident.

Joe was transported to the hospital by paramedics, was cared for in the intensive care unit for 3 days and on a medical-surgical unit for 2 weeks. Joe's brain injury was primarily to the right frontal and parietal lobes, with diffuse cortical impairment due to concussive forces. Joe also had a fractured right femur and left radius, which were both treated with internal fixation. During his second week on the medical-surgical unit, he was assessed by a nurse case manager from the acute rehabilitation facility to determine his care needs and his readiness for transfer to rehabilitation. He has now been in the acute rehabilitation facility for 13 days. On admission he was alert and agitated with a very short attention span and behavior that seemed inappropriate to the situation and generally nonpurposeful. He is currently confused but nonagitated most of the time. He does become agitated by too much visual or auditory stimulation.

As Joe's cognition has improved, he has become depressed. He is increasingly aware of his deficits and is also grieving the death of his friend. Joe has many visitors; sometimes as many as five teenaged friends at a time want to see him. He is limited to one visitor at a time, for brief periods, to minimize agitation. His girlfriend and his mother stay with him for longer periods and assist with his rehabilitation program because they have a calming effect on him. Joe's parents are divorced, and Joe's father visits Joe only occasionally. On several of his visits, he became angry with Joe and told Joe to "shape up and start behaving." He also told Joe that the injury was his own (Joe's) fault since he had been drinking at the party and should have known better than to get in a car with a driver who also had been drinking. The psychiatric clinical nurse specialist has set up several appointments with Joe's father, but he has not kept the appointments. He also has said that he is too busy to meet with the rehabilitation team. Joe was visibly upset after his father's most recent visit and said that he did not want to see his dad for now. Joe's goal is to get home and back to school as soon as possible so he can graduate with his class.

Six weeks later, it is the decision of the rehabilitation team that Joe is ready for discharge from the acute rehabilitation facility. His case has been assessed by a nurse case manager who works with the insurance company that handles his health insurance. There has been little change in Joe's functional abilities in the past 2 weeks. He is able to walk with standby assistance and becomes unsteady after about 50 feet due to right lower extremity weakness. Joe is independent in dressing and undressing, needs standby assistance in the shower, and feeds himself. He has good urinary and bowel control. He continues to have cognitive problems, primarily distractability, impaired problem-solving and judgment. He is frustrated easily, with occasional angry outbursts. He wants to drive and to return to school. The team assessment is that he is not ready for school or driving yet, and he also is not safe alone at home all day while his mother works.

Joe is discharged from the acute rehabilitation facility to a day treatment program within a long-term head trauma rehabilitation setting. He attends the program all day, Monday through Friday, and is home with his family at night and on weekends. As anticipated, Joe makes slow, steady progress in the day treatment program and is discharged from the program after 6 months. He then lives at home and attends outpatient therapy sessions for 2 to 3 hours, 3 days/week. He returns to school the following semester and successfully completes high school. Following graduation, he passes the driving test and his parents give him a car for a graduation present. Currently he is taking community college courses and expects to move out of his parents home within a year or so. In the opinion of the rehabilitation team, including Joe and his family, Joe's rehabilitation program was a success!

Joe's overall rehabilitation program included acute rehabilitation, day treatment at a long-term head trauma facility, and outpatient rehabilitation. The mix of services used by specific clients will vary based on client needs and preferences, client insurance coverage and financial resources, and the rehabilitation resources available.

REFERENCES

Applegate, W.B., Miller, S. Granger, M.J., Elam, J.T., Burns, R. & Akin, D.E. (1990). A randomized, controlled trial of a geriatric assessment unit in a community rehabilitation hospital. *New England Journal of Medicine, 322,* 1572-1578.

Babicki, C., & Miller-McIntyre, K. (1992). A rehabilitation programmatic model: The clinical nurse specialist perspective. *Rehabilitation Nursing, 17,* 84-86.

Baum, C.M. (1991). Addressing the needs of the cognitively impaired elderly from a family policy perspective. *American Journal of Occupational Therapy, 45,* 594-606.

Bower, K.A. (1992). *Case management by nurses.* American Nurses Publishing, ANA Pub NS-32.

Butera, E. (1989). Case management and chronic illness. *ANNA Journal, 16,* 460.

Butler, M. (1991). Geriatric rehabilitation nursing. *Rehabilitation Nursing 16,* 318-321.

Carey, R. (1990). Integrating care management, program evaluation, and marketing for inpatient and outpatient rehabilitation programs. *Advances in Clinical Rehabilitation, 3,* 219-249.

Chamberlain, M.A. (1990). The disabled living centre: Its relevance to rheumatology. *Annals of the Rheumatic Diseases, 49,* 563-566.

Chimner, N.E., & Easterling, A. (1993). Collaborative practice through nursing case management. *Rehabilitation Nursing, 18,* 226-230.

Christian, J., Ochipa, C., Quigley, P., Sciabara, C., Scott, S., Smith, S., Soscia, M.J., & Williams, C. (1994). *Clinical pathway: Stroke—initial rehabilitation, first admission.* Tampa, FL: James A. Haley Veterans Hospital. Unpublished document.

Conn, V.S., Taylor, S., & Casey, B. (1992). Cardiac rehabilitation program participation and outcomes after myocardial infarction. *Rehabilitation Nursing, 17,* 58-62.

Cromes, G.F., & Helm, P.A. (1992). The status of burn rehabilitation services in the United States: Results of a national survey. *Journal of Burn Care and Rehabilitation, 13,* 656-662.

Crummer, M.B., & Carter, V. (1993). Critical pathways—the pivotal tool. *Journal of Cardiovascular Nursing, 7,* 30-37.

Davies, S., & O'Neill, M. (1990). Nurse-managed care in a rehabilitation ward. *Nursing Times, 86,* 56.

Dean, B.Z., & Geiringer, S.R. (1990). Physiatric therapeutics. The rehabilitation team: Behavioral management Part 6. *Archives of Physical Medicine and Rehabilitation, 71*(Suppl. 4), 275-277.

DeJong, G. (1993). The John Stanley Coulter lecture. Health care reform and disability: Affirming our commitment to community. *Archives of Physical Medicine and Rehabilitation, 74,* 1017-1024.

DelTogno-Armanasco, V., Olivas, G.S., & Harter, S. (1989). Developing an integrated nursing case management model. *Nursing Management, 20,* 26-29.

Diehl, L. (1989). Client and family teaming in the rehabilitation setting. *Nursing Clinics of North America, 24,* 257-264.

Diller, L. (1990). Fostering the interdisciplinary team: Fostering research in a society in transition. *Archives of Physical Medicine and Rehabilitation, 71,* 275-278.

Dittmar, S. (1989). *Rehabilitation nursing.* St. Louis: Mosby.

Edwards, P. (1992). The evolution of rehabilitation facilities for children. *Rehabilitation Nursing, 17,* 191-192.

Eigsti, H., Aretz, M., & Shannon, L. (1990). Pediatric physical therapy in a rehabilitation setting. *Pediatrician, 17,* 267-277.

Eldar, R., Oren, H., & Goldin, M. (1989). Patient assessment of care in a pain management unit. *Quality Assurance in Health Care, 1,* 229-233.

Faherty, B.L. (1991). The nurse legal consultant and disabling injuries. *Rehabilitation Nursing, 16,* 30-33.

Feigelman, B., & Jaquith, P. (1992). Adolescent drug treatment, a family affair: a community day center approach. *Social Work in Health Care, 16,* 39-52.

Finset, A. (1992). Subacute brain injury rehabilitation: A program description and a study of staff program evaluation. *Scandinavian Journal of Rehabilitation Medicine, 26*(Suppl.), 25-33.

Friedman, M.M. (1992). *Family nursing theory and practice* (3rd ed.). Norwalk, CT: Appleton & Lange.

Fuhrer, M.J., Rossi, L.D., Gerken, L., Nosek, M.A., & Richards, V. (1990). Relationships between independent living centers and medical rehabilitation programs. *Archives of Physical Medicine and Rehabilitation, 71,* 519-522.

Ginder, M.S. (1990). Developing case managers in a rehabilitation unit. *Rehabilitation Nursing, 15,* 38-39.

Goggins, M., Hall, N., Nack, K., & Shuart, B. (1990). Community reintegration program. *Journal of Burn Care and Rehabilitation, 11,* 343-346.

Greenspan, A., Mackenzie, E., Christensen, J., & Robel, C. (1989). Use of health and rehabilitation services following head injury. *Maryland Medical Journal, 38,* 239-245.

Guinan, J.K. (1993). Facility-based case management: Its role in rehabilitation nursing. *Rehabilitation Nursing, 18,* 254-256.

Gutin, B., Prince, L., & Stein, R. (1990). Survey of cardiac rehabilitation centers in New York City. *Journal of Community Health, 15,* 227-238.

Habel, M. (1993). Rehabilitation nursing practice. In A.E. McCourt (Ed.), *The specialty practice of rehabilitation nursing*: A core curriculum, 3rd ed. (pp. 1-23). Skokie, IL: Rehabilitation Nursing Foundation.

Halstead, L. (1976). Team care in chronic illness: A critical review of the literature of the past 25 years. *Archives of Physical Medicine and Rehabilitation, 65,* 74-78.

Hampton, D.C. (1993). Implementing a managed care framework through care maps. *Journal of Nursing Administration, 23,* 21-27.

Harden, N., & Luster, S. (1991). Rehabilitation considerations in the care of the acute burn patient. *Critical Care Nursing Clinics of North America, 3,* 245-253.

Hardoff, D., & Chigier, E. (1991). Developing community-based services for youth with disabilities. *Pediatrician, 18,* 157-162.

Hays, S. (1992). The need for advocating specialized care. *Rehabilitation Nursing, 17,* 172, 198.

Heacock, P., Walton, C., Beck, C., & Mercer, S. (1991). Caring for the cognitively impaired. Reconceptualizing disability and rehabilitation. *Journal of Gerontological Nursing, 17,* 22-26, 35-37.

Heery, K. (1992). Restoring childhood through rehabilitation. *Rehabilitation Nursing, 17,* 193-195.

Hinton-Walker, P. (1993). Care of the chronically ill: Paradigm shifts and directions for the future. *Holistic Nursing Practice, 8,* 56-66.

Hoeman, S. (1993). A research-based transdisciplinary team model for infants with special needs and their families. *Holistic Nursing Practice, 7,* 63-72.

Hoeman, S. (1992). Community-based rehabilitation. *Holistic Nursing Practice, 6,* 32-41.

Hoeman, S. (1989). Cultural assessment in rehabilitation nursing practice. *Nursing Clinics of North America, 24,* 277-289.

Hoeman, S.P., & Winters, D.M. (1989). Theory-based case management: High cervical spinal cord injury. *Home Healthcare Nurse, 8,* 25-33.

Hotta, S. (1991). Cardiac rehabilitation programs. *Health Technology Assessment Reports, 3,* 1-10.

Jaffe, K. (1989). Home health care and rehabilitation nursing. *Nursing Clinics of North America, 24,* (1), 171-178.

Jaffe, K.B., & Walsh, P.A. (1993). The development of the specialty rehabilitation home care team: Supporting the creative thought process. *Holistic Nursing Practice, 7,* 36-41.

Keith, R.A. (1991). The comprehensive treatment team in rehabilitation. *Archives of Physical Medicine and Rehabilitation, 72,* 269-274.

Knollmueller, R.N. (1989). Case management: What's in a name? *Nursing Management, 20,* 38-40, 42.

Lavallee, D.J., & Crupi, C.D. (1992). Rehabilitation takes to the road. *Holistic Nursing Practice, 6,* 60-66.

Leininger, M. (1990). Ethnomethods: The philosophic and epistemic bases to explicate transcultural nursing knowledge. *Journal of Transcultural Nursing, 1,* 40-51.

Lewis, M.L, Govoni A., Camp Y., Pierce H., & Salter J. (1993). Competency-based nursing in a rehabilitation setting. *Rehabilitation Nursing, 18,* 221-225, 283-284.

Loveridge, C.E., Cummings, S.H., O'Malley, J. (1988). Developing case management in a primary nursing system. *Journal of Nursing Administration, 18,* 36-39.

Lyon, J.C. (1993). Models of nursing care delivery and case management: Clarification of terms. *Nursing Economics, 11,* 163-169.

Mayer, D.K. (1992). The health care implications of cancer rehabilitation in the twenty-first century. *Oncology Nursing Forum, 19,* 23-27.

Mayer, G.G., Buckley, R.F., & White, T.L. (1990). Direct nursing care given to patients in a subacute rehabilitation center. *Rehabilitation Nursing, 15,* 86-88.

McBride, S.M. (1992). Rehabilitation case managers: Ahead of their time. *Holistic Nursing Practice, 6,* 67-75.

Melvin, J.L. (1989). Status report on interdisciplinary medical rehabilitation. *Archives of Physical Medicine and Rehabilitation, 70,* 273-277.

Mosher, C., Cronk, P., Kidd, A., McCormick, P., Stockton, S., & Sulla, C. (1992). Upgrading practice with critical pathways. *American Journal of Nursing, 92,* 41-44.

Muller, D. (1991). Multidisciplinary perspectives on disability. *International Disability Studies, 13,* 109-110.

Musolf, J. (1991). Easing the impact of the family caregiver's role. *Rehabilitation Nursing, 16,* 82-84.

O'Toole, M. (1992). The interdisciplinary team: Research and education. *Holistic Nursing Practice, 6,* 76-83.

Pashkow, F.J. (1993). Issues in contemporary cardiac rehabilitation: A historical perspective. *Journal of the American College of Cardiology, 21,* 822-834.

Periquet, A.O. (1989). Community-based rehabilitation in the Philippines. *International Disability Studies, 11,* 95-96.

Phipps, M. (1990). Rehabilitation nursing specialist practice in an acute care setting. *Nursing Administration Quarterly 14,* 12-16.

Pittman, L., Morton, W., Edwards, L., & Holmes, D. (1992). Patient discharge planning documentation in an Australian multidisciplinary rehabilitation setting. *Rehabilitation Nursing, 17,* 327-331.

Portnow, J.M., Kline, T., Daly, M.A., Peltier, S.M., Chin, C., & Miller, J.R. (1991). Multidisciplinary home rehabilitation. *Geriatric Home Care, 7,* 695-706.

Power, P.W. (1989). Working with families: An intervention model for rehabilitation nurses. *Rehabilitation Nursing, 14,* 73-76.

Preston, K.M. (1990). A team approach to rehabilitation. *Home Health Care Nurse, 8,* 17-23.

Richardson, C.J., & Robinson, S. (1989). Neonatal intensive care and pediatric rehabilitation: A joint program for care of chronically ill infants. *Journal of Perinatology, 9,* 52-55.

Rook, J. (1993). Nurse case management in rehabilitation. In A. McCourt (Ed.). *The specialty practice of rehabilitation: A core curriculum* (pp. 204-209). Skokie, IL: Rehabilitation Nursing Foundation.

Rosomoff, R. (1992). Back school programs. The pain patient. *Occupational Medicine, 7,* 93-103.

Ross, B. (1992). The impact of reimbursement issues on rehabilitation nursing practice and patient care. *Rehabilitation Nursing, 17,* 236-238.

Rothberg, J. (1981). The rehabilitation team: Future direction. *Archives of Physical Medicine and Rehabilitation, 62,* 407-410.

Roy, C.W. (1991). An integrated community and hospital service for adults with physical disability: Two years experience. *New Zealand Medical Journal, 104,* 382-384.

Savarese, M., & Weber, C.M. (1993). Case management for persons who are homeless. *Journal of Case Management, 2,* 3-8.

Schraeder, C., Shelton, P., Dworak, D., & Fraser, C. (1993). Alzheimer's disease: Case management in a rural setting. *Journal of Case Management, 2,* 26-31.

Schroer, K. (1991). Case management: Clinical nurse specialist and nurse practitioner, converging roles. *Clinical Nurse Specialist, 5,* 189-194.

Schryer, N. (1993). Nursing case management for children undergoing craniofacial reconstruction. *Plastic Surgical Nursing, 13,* 17-28.

Selekman, J. (1991). Pediatric rehabilitation: From concepts to practice. *Pediatric Nursing, 17,* 11-14, 33, 26-27.

Skipper, T. (1993). Utilization management: A rehabilitation approach to cost control. *Rehabilitation Nursing, 18,* 216-220, 230.

Spencer, N.J. (1993). Consultant paediatric outreach clinics—A practical step in integration. *Archives of Disease in Childhood, 68,* 496-500.

Tice, A.D. (1993). The team concept. *Hospital Practice, 28*(Suppl. 1), 6-10.

Watson, P.G. (1989). Indicators of family capacity for participating in the rehabilitation process: Report of a preliminary investigation. *Rehabilitation Nursing, 14,* 318-322.

Watson, P. (1992). Cancer rehabilitation: An overview. *Seminars in Oncology Nursing, 8,* 167-173.

Watson, P. (1992). Family issues in rehabilitation. *Holistic Nursing Practice, 6,* 51-59.

Wenger, A.F.Z. (1992). Transcultural nursing and health care issues in urban and rural contexts. *Journal of Transcultural Nursing, 3,* 4-10.

Winters, S., Jackson, P., Sims, K., & Magilvy, J. (1989). A nurse managed multiple sclerosis clinic: Improved quality of life for persons with MS *Rehabilitation Nursing, 14,* 13-16, 22.

Wood, R.G., Bailey, N.O., & Tilkemeier, D. (1992). Managed care, the missing link in quality improvement. *Journal of Nursing Care Quality, 6,* 55-65.

Woodyard, L.W., & Sheetz, J.E. (1993). Critical pathway patient outcomes: The missing standard. *Journal of Nursing Care Quality, 8,* 51-57.

Zejdlik, C.M. (Ed.). (1992). *Management of spinal cord injuries* (2nd ed.). Boston: Jones & Bartlett, Inc.

3

Ethical Considerations for Rehabilitation Nursing

Cheryl Graham-Eason, MS, RN, CRRN

INTRODUCTION

Professionals in all sectors of rehabilitation are facing dilemmas new to the field in greater abundance than ever, as a result of the healthcare movement in the United States and advances in biotechnical science across the globe. As integral professionals in rehabilitation, nurses are affected in their unique roles as healthcare providers in a variety of settings: hospital facilities, free-standing rehabilitation centers, home healthcare agencies, case managers, and many others. Many ethical dilemmas encountered by rehabilitation nurses arise from this healthcare milieu and must become reconciled with the principles that form the rehabilitation nurse's worldview and the rehabilitation nurse's unique advocacy role. As early as 1979 professional nurses were known to occupy a unique role in bioethical decision-making, due in part to their relationship with other persons in the process and each nurse's responsibility in this process (Lump, 1979). This chapter contains a primer of ethical theories and principles, description of rehabilitation nursing's framework in the healthcare milieu, arguments about ethical dilemmas specific to rehabilitation nursing, and models or methods of seeking resolutions for dilemmas. As answers to dilemmas become more unclear and complex, rehabilitation nurses require full understanding not only of the situation at hand but so they may reflect on and recognize the underlying processes that govern ethical decision-making.

Ethical issues are value judgments that may become laws when a society holds a certain value or belief strongly. Laws may have general relationship with an ethical issue or may be quite specific about what action members of a profession may or may not take in given circumstances (Edge & Groves, 1994). The debate about legal issues arises regularly in discussions involving ethics or values—and indeed, legal consequences are considerations in ethical decision-making. Legal issues comprise a study apart from ethics as discussed in this chapter. Chapter 5 contains information about legislation pertinent to rehabilitation nurses and reflects social action regarding issues.

ETHICS

Ethics is concerned with causing no harm or doing good. Ethics deals with what ought to be or not be in human behavior (Bandman & Bandman, 1985; Omery, 1989). Ethics is moral reasoning, or more specifically, it "is free rational assessment of courses of actions in relation to precepts, rules of conduct . . . to be ethical a person must take additional steps of exercising critical, rational judgment in his decisions" (Churchill, 1977). Ethics is reflecting on the meaning of what we do; it is clarifying and refining our decisions about what we do; it deals with engaging in difficult human problems, making decisions, and standing by them (DePender & Ikede-Chandler, 1990). Moral reasoning is a mental process that intervenes between recognition of and vocation to a moral or ethical dilemma (Omery, 1989). Moral reasoning is a process of human development that can be traced much as cognitive or social development, and it is influenced greatly by culture and values.

Ethics deals with morals or values used in decision-making when there is a dilemma; applying these values consistently requires a lifelong commitment (Quinn & Smith, 1987). Ethical values carry feeling of "good and bad," but ethical decision-making demands logical review rather than being based on feelings alone. Each professional enters a career with her own personal set of values and beliefs learned through family, education, culture, and by repeatedly facing and dealing with ethical issues common to the practice of rehabilitation nursing.

Nursing ethics is a process of reflection on nursing actions to determine professional and moral accountability (Lump, 1979). According to Carper, ethics is one of the four fundamental patterns in nursing, and within that pattern "caring as a professional and personal value is of central importance in providing a normative standard that governs the actions and attitudes of nurses toward those for whom they care" (Carper, 1978). Ethical nursing practice is based on and includes critical reflective thinking about one's duties as a nurse in relation to clients and as members of a profession fulfilling a social contract (Aroskar, 1982). Nursing ethics are based on agreement between nurse and client; that ethical decisions made within that agreement have a purpose; that the autonomy of both parties is understood and each ethical truth is true in that ethical context or situation. Further, a professional ethic, such as nursing ethics, is based on the belief that decisions made are appropriate for the profession; the specific position of one group can be judged to determine if its position is superior to another, and decisions and actions can be justified (Husted & Husted, 1991).

Rehabilitation nursing ethics is judgments about decisions to act and subsequent actions based on the rules of conduct or precepts of rehabilitation nursing practice. This practice involves the relationship of the nurse with the client, other healthcare providers, third-party payers, the nursing profession, and society at large. Professional groups publish codes and standards that facilitate understanding of current accepted practice within the profession and identify issues of concern to the profession. These codes and standards also point out ethical dilemmas that may become concerns to individuals within a profession, or in some instances may provide ethical guides when questions of professional conduct are held against minimal standards of care for professional practice.

Some codes of ethics and professional documents on clients' rights are the Consumers' Rights to Nursing Care, Code for Nurses with Interpretive Statements (Appendix 3-B), Nursing's Role in Patients' Rights and Ethics: National League for Nursing (NLN's) Principle and Issues, Volume One and Volume Two, and the International Council of Nurses Code for Nurses—which are guides for direction to the practicing nurse. A rehabilitation nurse refers to these guides in conjunction with an understanding of the specific role(s) or social contract between the professional rehabilitation nurse and society in making reasoned ethical decisions and actions within the context of the situation in which the nurse-client relationship exists. To broaden the foundation on which to make these judgments, the nurse examines theories related to ethics, principles, or the basis of questions in moral reasoning, and models of moral decision-making.

Ethical Theories

Four theoretic frameworks dealing specifically with ethics were selected for this chapter. These theories are useful because the concepts offer a view of the world that helps the nurses analyze and delimit perceptions that confound decision-making. Nurses who are informed make themselves aware of current and emerging theories before finalizing their choice of ethical theories on which their practice will be based. Regardless of theoretical framework, there is no guarantee that coming to a point of action will be easy simply because a nurse has a conceptual base and conceivably will be able to act in precisely the same manner in all dilemmas. The old phrase "on the horns of a dilemma" states the nature and difficulty of paradoxes. For instance, consider the question "What is the rehabilitation nurse's advocacy role in a situation where a client wants to refuse treatment, but the care-giver (significant other, family, professional) wants to continue treatment?" when reading the theories that follow.

✦ Deontologic

The deontologic view is that rightness or wrongness of an act does not depend on the consequence; the rightness or wrongness is inherent in the act. The concept of duty is independent of the concept of good (Beauchamp & Childress, 1989). The underlying intent of this theory is preservation of the intrinsic value or dignity of all persons including the person doing the activity. All persons have duty to do something based on a set of binding principles and rules. All persons therefore will have a clear understanding that

these rules will be followed when decisions are made, and that they have a duty to take some action based on a set of binding principles and rules.

In the case of the person wishing to refuse treatment, the nurse would be expected to act according to the moral authority of the setting. However, the moral authority of the setting might be hospital administration or physicians—or to complicate the event, both. What of the nurse's duty to the profession and practice of nursing? Using the deontologic theory can work well and agreeably where there is only one moral authority and all persons understand this. The advantage in this scenario is that it would be clear, even to the person who wanted to refuse treatment, that the decision would be to treat if that was the generally accepted practice. This theory proposes a paternalistic philosophy wherein the client is taken care of while others make the decisions. Rehabilitation nursing values do not fit well with this view. An additional dilemma occurs when a nurse practices in an environment where more than one set of duties, obligations, or authorities claim to set the moral authority or claim to be able to overrule that authority.

✦ Theologic or utilitarian theory

The utilitarian theory is based on the assumption that action taken should result in maximizing overall good (Veatch & Fry, 1987). This theory determines actions by consequences and ends, or as John Steward Mill indicated, actions are meant to promote the greatest happiness. Using this view, a nurse attempts to balance things or do things so they add up to the moral good. The nurse would ask questions about who benefits the most or the least, what are the benefits to each option, or for whom is this good. This type of reasoning necessitates asking many questions before sufficient data are available to justify the final decision; therefore answers to what is right are not as clear as when compared with deontologic-based thinking. On the positive side the rehabilitation nurse applying this theory is encouraged to explore alternatives and involve the client, leading to a closer fit with rehabilitation values for client independence.

To answer the question regarding treatment refusal, the nurse in this theoretic framework needs to determine how to act to promote the greatest good. Questions that would need to be asked are: Good for whom? Who would benefit by allowing the client to refuse treatment? What harm would result to the caregiver or perhaps the professional? Should the client refuse treatment, will the person's dependence on the caregiver, the institution, and society cause greater harm? Or would refusal of treatment mean the client would die or be moved to a low-cost institution and another person could be served?

✦ Intuitionist theory

The ethical decision-maker needs to know the rights and duties and goals of all participants under the intuitionist theoretical framework (Benjamin & Curtis, 1986). To resolve dilemmas, a nurse collects information about who benefits and asks how much and in what way do these persons or systems benefit. Concepts from this theory give equal attention to duties, goals, and rights. However, the key to intuitionist theory is that although deontologic and theologic principles are considered and all points weigh equally, practitioners are expected to rely on their own moral intuition of what is best or good. This theory is rapidly developing into what is identified as "situation ethics." Within this framework nurses understand the consequences of their own actions in terms of the universal laws that appear to exist at the time all persons involved encounter the dilemma. At first glance, this approach offers little guidance. A rehabilitation nurse may observe repeated consequences of certain actions and may build decisions on this repertoire, incorporating laws/values of the culture for this specific situation. Using this foundation in ethics may fit easier with the values of an experienced rehabilitation professional than for a beginning practitioner who may desire more definitive direction.

To answer the refusal of treatment theory, a nurse examines duties, rights, and goals of all involved in the situation to determine which offer the most good to all participants. The greatest concern is the dilemma that recurs when all rights, goals, duties, and properly gathered data weigh out equally. Whose moral intuition will be used to make the final choice? The question is whether what the nurse wants is more justified relative to what another professional, the family or caregiver, or even more so, what the client wants, in a given situation. Too often when situation ethics are used for final choices, these become questions of power, economics, productivity, and social construction of worth—which historically have not well served persons with chronic, disabling, or developmental disorders nor women, children, or the elderly.

✦ Personalized theory

The premises that exist in this theory are that all people have the capacity to grow and each has the right to choose. This capacity emerges from relationships, based on openness, responsibility, and recognition that although an individual may resist sharing, a decision to share will foster trust between the person and the nurse (DePender & Ikede-Chandler, 1990). As a result, innovative resolutions to unique problems are possible and are based on principles or the morals of the situation. This theory is called personalized because it contains no first action or universal laws that state something always must be the case. Without eliminating structure or principles, this framework allows rehabilitation nurses or other team members to choose when not to go against their own beliefs and when to compromise. One intent in this theory is to help professionals to be able to do things that go against their personal beliefs so as to support the values of the client or other professionals because of a willingness to become involved with others' views.

Relationships between a nurse and other professionals or the nurse and clients would follow a pattern of
1. Self-reflection or preparation
2. Observations such as identifying personal problems, obtaining medical data or facts, or identifying critical points
3. Gaining relational knowledge by listening to others' needs and values, as well as seeking clues that indicate the other person has potential for dealing with the problem
4. Making an ethical decision based on reflection . . . looking for unique answers to problems and basing

those on consultation with those affected by the decision (DePender & Ikede-Chandler, 1990)

Thus should a team believe that a client should participate in a recommended treatment and the client refuses, the team members would assess their own values, then assess and analyze the client's values. Before making a choice, results of the analyses would be tallied. For this framework to be helpful, a flexible approach to care and development of trust definitely is essential. One overriding concern is whether a client has sufficient participation in the process since the team members are analyzing the client's values from their own perspectives.

Choosing a Theory Model That Fits

Essentially deontology and utilitarianism are theories capable of providing direction for decision-making. Nurses might choose one as being operational for themselves based on personal philosophies of life, religious practice, secular habits, setting, political beliefs, or other factors. But when practicing rehabilitation, other precepts (discussed in the following section) may prove valuable for nurses.

The intuitionist and personalized theories offer options based on current reality; that reality as understood by all parties involved and for the situation in the specific environment or cultural context, these understood realities are reasoned to a conclusion by weighing rights and duties and goals of all parties. The state priority is to maintain the well-being of and caring for the individual. Intuitionist theoretical constructs allow for easier consideration of total good (weighing positives and negatives), whereas personalism constructs are centered more on individuals. Personalism advocates contend that its principles do not negate the rights of others, asking questions about balance as similar to intuitionist constructs and encouraging personal growth, presumptively to include ethical growth.

The personalized theory has a closer fit with rehabilitation if only because its conceptual focus is care rather than cure. As noted in the Hastings Center report, rehabilitation is "care driven" versus "cure driven" (Caplan, Callahan, & Haas, 1987); clients engaged in rehabilitation are dealing with their need to function with disabilities that are permanent. How clients learn to adjust and accomplish their goals is dependent in a great part on their values as influenced by their "subjective experience of this illness" (Caplan et al., 1987). The plan of care becomes interpersonal for the client and the care provider; it is a product of relationships that develop between a rehabilitation team member and the client. Regardless of the theoretic framework chosen for practice, each rehabilitation nurse soon realizes there are few simple, final solutions to dilemmas. Understanding ethics may offer a means to discern not necessarily right answers but moral answers where many values exist (Cunningham & Hutchinson, 1990). Each situation that gives rise to ethical concerns will be assessed and acted on separately, although previous situations will build a compendium of potential solutions coupled with the potential consequences for selecting them.

MORAL PRINCIPLES

Ethical concepts, methods of restoring, ethical standards for nursing practice, and ethical codes are founded on specific moral principles. These principles are autonomy, nonmaleficence; beneficence; justice; sanction for life (Beauchamp & Childress, 1989; Frankel, 1973; Muyskens, 1982); advocacy, loyalty, veracity, fiduciary responsibility for the client, ethic of care, nurse-client mutuality, protection of dignity, integrity, reciprocity, fidelity (Gadow, 1980; Watson, 1985; Winslow, 1984; Gilligan, 1992), and concern for community as a whole (Moccia, 1990; Gadow, 1980; Caplan, 1987; Kelly, 1981). Table 3-1 displays the generic meaning of each principle and potential dilemmas for rehabilitation nursing practice associated with each principle.

Recognizing the Dilemma

The principles (Table 3-1) are used as questions for examining ethical dilemmas; they are included in the assessment process. Some questions relate directly to a client; others relate to the nurse, nursing resources, family, or community. There will be times when all principles apply in a dilemma and times when only one or two apply. More strikingly, at times two principles will be at odds with one another, such as autonomy and nonmaleficence. For instance, a client wants to ambulate independently, but the nurse

Table 3-1 Assessment and moral principles*

Principle	Descriptor	Dilemma or concern
Autonomy	Patient has right to choose; self-determination	1. Informed consent—related to research. 2. Ventilator-dependent client feels he has no quality of life; lives in a nursing home, has no resources—financial or family. Wants to die. Questions to ask relate to whether the client has been informed of all resources.
Nonmalficience	Do no harm	Should a client be sent home with family member if it appears as though the family member is not interested or just cannot follow through?
Beneficence	Doing good	Should a head-injured client be restrained? Is this protection?
Advocacy (loyalty)	Standing for client	When dealing with adolescents or children who are comatose: Are parents always in the best position to make decisions? What is the nurse's role in the situation where the family or caregiver's decision is not consistent with philosophy of rehabilitation?
Veracity	Truth telling: client needs information before she can consent	When a client is admitted to rehabilitation, how "honest is honest" when giving prognosis while "still offering hope"?
Client fiduciary responsibility	Recognize costs to client when provided or do not provide treatments	1. Is length of stay determined by insurance? 2. Who determines level of care?
Ethic of care	Gives rise to compassion, equity, fairness, envisions problem in context—framework of relationships, dignity	Dilemma is that nurses work in situations and institutions where policies and practices may be based on paternalistic views of what is right. Nurses in rehabilitation also working with other team members who are involved with client. Nurse-client relationship here is one that takes into consideration other relationships and available resources. Does not act on what is understood common right but looks at the unique rights of the client now.
Reciprocity	Develop one's talents, integrity—be true to one's self, impartial, consistent, having respect for client's goals and values	Setting contracts with clients. They need to behave in manner consistent with plan of care. Staff members need to be fair, impartial in contract setting, and be able to keep their end of the deal. Involves having relationship. Are staff members open to compromises with clients who want to tailor a trust contract?
Fidelity	Always keep promises	Promise to keep child from ever hurting again—find out client to be returned to family that caused injury. Need to consider promises in ethical dilemma, especially in light of legal consequences or long-term outcomes.
Concern for community as a whole	Costs to the community; values of the community	1. Who will take care of indigent rehabilitation clients? 2. Client has placement problem—will end up in nursing home. Do costs that allow independence in the nursing home balance with benefits? 3. Is rehabilitation necessary when many in community do not even have access to basic healthcare needs? Is rehabilitation a basic healthcare need?
Sanction for life	Maintaining life rather than intent to end life	Persons with Parkinson's disease and others may benefit from fetal transplant neuron tissue. Is it ethically responsible to end one life to benefit another? What if fetus will be aborted anyway? Who benefits from abortion?

*Moral principles form bases for nursing practice. Dilemmas or concerns may arise for one or more principles, as with these examples from rehabilitation practice.

knows this action certainly would result in a fall. The assessment, when the nurse asks questions about whether a principle applies and how it applies, is a first phase. The answers to initial questions are integrated with information about the client's specific healthcare needs and resources and data from other team members' analyses. The questions posed here are intended to serve as guides for the ethical assessment phase but are by no means all-inclusive.

Ethical Assessment Questions Based on Moral Principles

✦ Autonomy

Was the client autonomous before the disability? Is the client old enough to function autonomously? What is the client's mental status: can the client understand what she is choosing, what the consequences will be like to live with? Does the client have enough information to make a choice among alternatives? Is the client viewed as an individual with unique needs such as religion, ethnicity, gender, and so forth (these factors contribute to a client's view of self and thus influence choice)? How much autonomy does the nurse have in this situation; how free is the nurse to act?

✦ Nonmaleficence

Will an action cause direct or indirect harm to the client? Will the client's rights be violated by an action? Will a client decision or action result in harming someone else such as another client or a family member? Is an act that seems harmful to a client, such as restraining him, appropriate for a limited time?

✦ Beneficence

Is an act of doing good in one area potentiating harm in another (e.g., to another client, to the nurse, to the family, to the institution)? Is an act of doing good in one area of concern for a particular client going to result in harm in another aspect of care to the client (e.g., providing pain medication that relieves pain but also decreases client strength and endurance)? Does an act of doing good justify not following standard procedures or rules? Are there times when exceptions to the rule are necessary?

✦ Advocacy

Who best can represent a client's desires when she is unable to so herself? Is it the nurse, and if so what resources does the nurse have to support the advocacy role, especially where there are other rehabilitation team members interested in this role? When team members cannot come to an agreement that is in accordance with the client's wishes, should the nurse encourage referral to an ethics committee (essentially another group making decisions for rather than with the client)? When a nurse is standing for a client, is she representing what she has learned the client's views are or is she imposing her own values into the situation? If the nurse's role is to advocate for the client, is this situation a time when other loyalties should come first (e.g., to the profession, to the principles of rehabilitation, to other clients, to the community, to the institution)?

✦ Veracity

How honest is honest? Can so much detail be given that the client will refuse something essential for his or her well-being? Can the truth be told and still offer hope? In research does the client clearly understand potential harms or actual benefits to self or others as a result of research? Has the client been told clearly the limits as well as benefits of treatments offered? Does the client know the alternatives?

✦ Client fiduciary responsibility

Are treatments ordered as a matter of course rather than weighing the cost/benefit ratio to client? Is equipment ordered because the insurance company will pay or because the client truly needs it? Are third-party payers controlling level of care and length of stay rather than client needs? Is the client made aware of what he will have to pay for? What resources are available to the nurse to seek support for treatment of clients who have no ability to pay (e.g., nurse lobby groups to have laws enacted to assist the handicapped or to have nursing care reimbursed so that nursing care can continue)? Should the nurse continue working in an environment where payment availability or profit is the dominating philosophy? What are the options?

✦ Ethic of care

Is the decision being made based on fairness? Would this same decision be applied in all cases or is there a prevailing bias about this client? Are all aspects of the situation known? Is the client being looked at holistically? Is the client valued as an individual? What resources are available such as nursing time; is one client getting more than his fair share and another client suffering because of it?

✦ Reciprocity

Are the rehabilitation professionals open to each other's views; is turfdom involved?

✦ Protection of dignity

Are rules of confidentiality and privacy being followed? Are clients being included in research when they might not want to be? How much information do each of the team members need to know to care for the client? Are we careful on rounds not to violate a client's privacy or dignity when sharing information with the team? When visitors are present during meals, is each client's dignity maintained or is anyone unduly embarrassed? Are persons who have incurred head trauma unduly exposed to others' view during episodes of confusion or agitation?

Identifying the Dilemma

No studies in the literature demonstrate specifically how rehabilitation nurses deal with (if at all) ethical dilemmas. Clearly this is a gap in rehabilitation nursing research. Lack of research findings does not eliminate the dilemmas. It remains imperative that rehabilitation nurses participate in ethical decision-making to ensure client-centered goals are set and to promote cohesive functions within the rehabilitation team. To accomplish this function, a nurse must recognize a dilemma when it exists (see Table 3-2). This caution is mentioned because "frequently nurses are unaware that they are involved in situations requiring consideration of ethical dilemmas" (Aroskar, 1982). One reason for nurses' lack of awareness is inadequate preparation in the basic nursing education. Findings from research on nursing education conclude that more time and emphasis on moral reasoning development in nursing education is necessary (Felton & Parsons, 1987).

Characteristics that signal a dilemma may exist have been described as

+ Problems that cause confusion—struggle over decisions (Snyder, 1992)
+ Conflicting obligations (Veatch & Fry, 1987)
+ Two moral principles apply, but each supports inconsistent actions (Jameton, 1984)
+ Ambiguity (Grier, 1983)
+ Difficulties in deciding right-to-know, determination of who has right to decide; what is quality of life, or how to distribute resources (Cresham, 1979; Bach, Campagnola, & Hoeman, 1991)
+ Cognitive dissonance or conflict between personal values with "others'" values (Gaull, 1987)
+ An uncomfortable sense of paradoxical "Catch 22"

Results from a survey indicate nurses in rehabilitation settings identified many ethical concerns regarding practice with clients (Graham-Eason, 1993).

Moral Decision-Making Models

The first scientific model that comes to mind for most nurses is the nursing process. A process developed specifically for moral decision-making contains the following four steps: (1) gather relevant information, (2) identify the dilemma, (3) decide what to do, and (4) complete the action (Purtillo & Cossell, 1981). Another model developed to prepare nurses to act on ethical decisions is the three-step ACT model: (1) *a*nticipating the objections and obstacles to action, (2) *c*larifying one's own position as part of planning action to respond to objections and obstacles, and (3) *t*esting choice by acting on it (Crisham, 1987). Snyder further states that a good way to process making a decision is to list all moral considerations on a horizontal grid—then to facilitate a final decisions list, place all practical considerations on a vertical grid. The practical consideration illuminates what options really exist (Snyder, 1985).

The final model presented here was developed by Husted and Husted (1991). This model is based on the nurse-client relationship or agreement; this agreement is founded on six bioethical standards existing within the agreement. The last step of decision-making is to be made in the ethical context of the situation. The nurse-client agreement is one of recognition of the client's uniqueness and that any nursing action must be oriented toward the client (autonomy). The client is free to choose (freedom); the client has a full understanding of the agreement (veracity); the client is not coerced (privacy); there is a final goal to the agreement (this goal is one intended to benefit the client [beneficence]); and last, the nurse will honor the terms of the agreement (fidelity). This agreement is looked at in relation to the context of the situation (what are the realities?) and the ethical context (knowing effective and justifiable ethical principles). The idea is that the nurse will be able to discern what is relevant in the dilemma or relevant to the agreement made between nurse and client.

Husted's model asks each nurse to look at the nurse-client relationship in each situation as built on an examination of the agreement between nurse and client, keeping a clear view of the standards that support the relationship and the stated purpose (solution to a dilemma) and then acting

Table 3-2 Questions posed by ARN nurses

Area	Concerns
Dignity	Who defines quality of life
	Equitable care for indigent/homeless persons
	Ability to choose to die/advanced directives
	Determination of competency
	Forcing client to participate rather than giving right to refuse
Administration	Allocation of resources: no funds—not admitted, limited funds—admitted too soon, or pushed too much or discharged too soon
	Access for funds for caregivers
	Funds for equipment
	Policies on informed consent
	Protection of nurses in abusive situations
	Team policies on control issues
	Setting up ethical review committees
Research	Should research be allowed that offers no help to clients involved?
	Should research be allowed when it causes no harm but clients are unaware of due to mental status?
	Who gives informed consent?
	Do research when funds are provided even though rationale for research is questionable?
	Privacy/confidentiality
Clinical guidelines	Professional standards—what if someone on the team is not competent or just doesn't do the job?
	Maintaining standards of excellence with little resources
	Admission criteria
	Treatment criteria (treat client as whole person, consider both psychological as well as physical wellness)
	Discharge criteria
	Determining Caregiver competence
	Team interactions
Clinical situations	Care of abusive clients
	Care of HIV clients
	Care of terminally ill clients (why do clients get transferred to die among strangers?)
	Care of abused clients
	Placement dubious

Prepared by Graham-Eason, C.

within the context of the situational and ethical context. The ethical principles used are used only in reference to the relevant factors of the situation.

The rehabilitation nurse can effectively use any of the above models or others not mentioned here. The most important fact is that some format be utilized to make decisions; that feelings must be balanced by reasoning, and this reasoning is on behalf of or support for the client's well-being.

With a model of ethical decision-making, a rehabilitation nurse may incorporate the principles of the nursing process for setting goals with clients, as well as choosing nursing interventions appropriate in a specific dilemma. Before discussing specific cases, it is necessary to understand how ethics or moral reasoning influences rehabilitation nursing practice.

REHABILITATION NURSING PRACTICE

The scope of rehabilitation nursing and standards of practice delineate what rehabilitation nurses believe and what they do. Specific statements in the scope of practice that relate to ethics are "rehabilitation nurses believe that individuals with functional disabilities have intrinsic worth that transcends their disability to make informed decisions about their futures . . . support interventions that reduce stigma of disability and help individuals re-establish and maintain control over all aspects of their lives . . . formulate nursing diagnoses based on assessment . . . promote quality of life . . . provide comfort and therapy . . . educate families and community . . . promote health conducive adjustments . . . support adoptive capabilities . . . promote achievable independence" (American Nurses' Association [ANA] & Association of Rehabilitation Nurses [ARN], 1988). This scope of practice statement also emphasizes that rehabilitation nurses participate in restoring optimal functioning and helping clients adjust or adapt to an altered lifestyle.

Standards of practice published by the ARN indicate that rehabilitation nurses maintain an awareness of their own values and belief systems. Another standard that influences a rehabilitation nurse's views regarding ethics is recognition of the nurse as an essential member of the team responsible to assure that "mechanisms exist to assume involvement of individuals, families, and significant others in appropriate team decision making."

Rehabilitation Setting

Rehabilitation nurses practice in many arenas—for example, acute care hospitals, free-standing rehabilitation centers, insurance companies, home health, subacute-level facilities, and independent living centers in addition to serving as consultants to industry, or as private practioners, and as case managers. Regardless of the arena, certain rehabilitation principles exist to some degree, and together with the societal context or rehabilitation setting, shape the worldview of the rehabilitation nurse. The anthropological concept of worldview or culture is "made up of understandings shared by persons . . . whose relationships constitute some kind of organized system . . . a cultural system can be envisioned as a set of major premises . . . from which more specific minor premises can be derived" (Peacock,

1986). It is to these patterns of thinking—a worldview of rehabilitation developed from readings and experiences in practice—that nurses refer for insight when sorting through what is known or believed to be an ethical situation. These beliefs exist in and are formed by a culture of the rehabilitation system and thus are viewed through that cultural context and from its values. Understanding the premises of what governs rehabilitation nursing practice will facilitate the decision-making process regarding what is right and what is wrong in a given situation. A rehabilitation nurse will discern the values in a situation, and the values "have intrinsic importance to moral experience or can be instrumental to attainment of what intrinsically important" (Dougherty, 1992). Again referring to the ARN standards, "Rehabilitation is based on the belief that clients should participate in the decision-making process . . . nurses face the dilemma of caring for individuals whose decision may not reflect values of independence and wellness . . . and care for individuals whose quality of life may be compromised by recent technological advances in health care" (ANA, 1988). Also, "Rehabilitation leads to patients developing to their fullest physical, social, and mental capabilities and that this should be done in the shortest possible time" (Ilis, Sedgwick, & Glanville, 1982). It is further recognized that clients in rehabilitation processes focus on their losses while losing sight of their strengths and remaining abilities; they want to be "fixed" soon and "at 110%" of their previous selves; whereas staff members in turn expect clients to regain a perspective of their self-worth in the world, however they can be (Martin, Holt, & Hicks, 1981). Rusk's traditional view proposed the role of the rehabilitation nurses "should always be one of collaboration, good judgment, empathy, and caring" (Rusk, 1977). Taken together, the sum of ethical rehabilitation is that

+ The client participates in the plan of care as fully as possible.
+ Clients will value independence and wellness.
+ Clients need to regain self-worth, as well as other physical gains.
+ Nurses collaborate with other members of the team.
+ Nurses demonstrate caring, "good" judgment, and advocacy.
+ Rehabilitation helps individuals regain lost capabilities and regain self-worth.
+ Rehabilitation happens in the shortest possible time and is cost-effective.

To function effectively in a rehabilitation practice and to determine the approach in an ethical/moral situation, a nurse internalizes the commonly held values because they will be at the center of any rehabilitation controversy.

Rehabilitation nursing culture does exist in a vacuum but alongside or overlapping other cultural contexts such as special service are various organizational cultures such as hospitals, outpatient clinics, community agencies or centers, and educational institutions. More significantly, rehabilitation nursing culture coexists within the dominant culture of general nursing and with rehabilitation medicine. Values purported by general nursing culture uphold the inherent worth of each individual with utmost regard, with access to healthcare for all as a dominant theme. Rehabilitation medicine is a relatively new field that supports restoring clients to optimal self-sufficiency and functional performance, albeit there is "no age, organ, technology, or appendage to define it" (Callahan & Haas, 1987). A distinguishing characteristic of rehabilitation professionals is that they are accustomed to dealing with clients who have irrevocable, chronic, and disabling conditions. As a specialty group, rehabilitation professionals are interested in how best to accommodate a person's quality of life, independent self-care, and ability to resume active life, and to help clients to re-evaluate functional abilities (Scofield, 1993). The underlying expectation is that society values the welfare of individuals with physical and mental disadvantages. Legislation for persons with disabilities is one means of measuring their value in a society. Chapter 5 contains information about significant legislation in the United States for persons with disabilities. Appendix 3-A is a draft of the federal government group working toward establishing ethical foundations for healthcare reform in the 1990s. This draft includes headings that refer to values of access to care, equality of care, and resource distribution. Rehabilitation nurses must recognize their own worldview, that of other members of the "team," their dominant Western culture and all of its premises, and finally, of equal importance, the worldview of each client. When the values expressed by each of these representative views coincide or agree on what the goals are and how to proceed to meet the goals, there are no di-

lemmas. When there is disregard by any one group about the values of the other, dissonance, confusion, or conflict occur and an ethical issue emerges.

Figure 3-1 is a schema of the various worldviews that may be cultural/societal influences on rehabilitation nursing practice. In this model clients bring a view of who they were before disability. This view is now influenced by disability and perceptions of the rehabilitation experiences. From these comes new identity, including the personal and professional identities that enter into the nurse-client relationships. Both nurse and clients are influenced by their personal worldviews, which encompass social subsystems: religion, education, economics, community and sociocultural values, health and disability, and individual rights. All parties are further influenced by the families or significant others. In the model dotted lines to the nurse from clients' cultures indicate the nurse will be affected indirectly, and the line to clients indicates a direct effect from these components of the relationships. The continuous line from rehabilitation team members, premises of rehabilitation, and society show direct impact on nurse-client relationships wherein clients are affected directly but are sheltered by cultural values. There are no lines between nurses and clients, because there is agreement in this model that nurses and clients are working together to achieve appropriate and acceptable ethical goals. At the end of a rehabilitation expe-

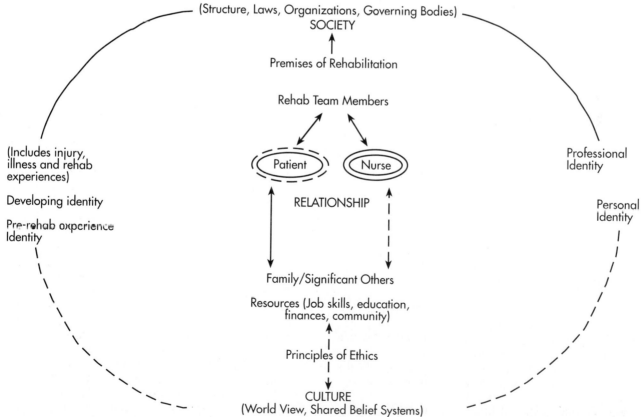

INFLUENCES ON ETHICAL DECISION MAKING

Fig. 3-1   Schema of worldviews in rehabilitation nursing practice.

rience where ethical dilemmas are resolved, or resolving, a client emerges with a new identity that supercedes the old; the person is learning to deal with the disabilities from injury or disease.

Rehabilitation Ethical Scenarios

The following are case studies of real practice situations that illustrate ethical decision-making processes. In each ethical situation the reader is encouraged to debate these case study examples in practice with colleagues. In each ethical situation the rehabilitation nurse asks the following questions:

- ✦ Is there a dilemma and is it within the rehabilitation nurse's scope of practice to participate in the decisions or actions to be made?
- ✦ What does the client want?
- ✦ Does the client know enough to choose?
- ✦ What are reasonable expectations regarding gains in self-care, independence, and wellness?
- ✦ Where do my loyalties lie?
- ✦ What resources are available and what can be made available?
- ✦ Can the nurse influence a decision so that the client may have a better quality of life; what should be risked if there is in fact a risk?

CASE STUDY 1

An unconscious female teenager, age 16 years, is dependent on mechanical ventilation support for survival. The family asks the physician to designate this daughter as DNR (do not resuscitate), and the physician agrees. The client, however, survives only to regain consciousness and discover the family's request. She becomes enraged.

With regard to Case Study 1, questions that one nurse felt need to be addressed are

- ✦ Should the client have been made a DNR?
- ✦ Should the client be upset?
- ✦ How can the nurse help the client to cope effectively with her feelings?
- ✦ Should the nurse have done more on behalf of this client when decisions for DNR were made?

From an ethical view the following information could facilitate the above answers:

- ✦ How was the client's prognosis decided? Were the appropriate data used (fairness)?
- ✦ If the prognosis was one of "no hope," should scarce resources have been utilized?
- ✦ Is the unconscious, neurologically impaired client's autonomy violated when decisions are made by others?
- ✦ Who decides quality of life?
- ✦ Was there intent on anyone's part of harming the client (maleficence)?

- ✦ Was there another client more apt to survive who was denied access to the same rehabilitation bed (fairness)?
- ✦ Does the client have enough information to comprehend the full extent of how decisions were made?

The ethical decision lies within the analysis of the answers of the questions. The nurse, however, does not examine these answers alone nor are the answers generated by the nurse. This is a team analysis involving other rehabilitation professionals with the family as designated caregivers.

CASE STUDY 2

Caring for a child with end-stage acquired immunodeficiency syndrome (AIDS) who has no planned future and no family involvement, a nurse asks, "to what benefit is a rehabilitation program for this child?"

Questions for investigation regarding Case Study 2:

- ✦ Is the program helping that child obtain some goal, being able to care more for self as one example?
- ✦ Are aspects of the program providing comfort or is it actually increasing suffering on the child's part?
- ✦ Can the child be provided with the needed care elsewhere, and if so, what role does the nurse play in seeking these resources?
- ✦ Is a good quality of life being fostered?

Ethical answers here relate to quality-of-life issues. When looking at these issues, the nurse needs to recognize that often the perception of quality of life of the individual client may be very different from the professional's perception. This was demonstrated in two studies: the first group were clients with ventilator-dependent quadriplegia (Purtillo, 1986), and the other group were clients with Duchenne's muscular dystrophy (Bach, Campagnolo, & Hoeman, 1991). In both cases the client's quality of life or satisfaction with life was significantly greater than professionals expected from or attributed to clients.

Questions posed by one nurse regarding Case Study 3:

- ✦ Should the client return to this home environment?
- ✦ Can the team actually benefit the client while in the rehabilitation setting?
- ✦ Does it make sense to continue care if the postdischarge environment does not support all of these efforts?
- ✦ What if this client wants to return to this environment?
- ✦ Does society offer this person with a disability any other alternative and at what cost to society?
- ✦ Does society value this individual with a disability as it values all other individuals—does this individual have the same rights for protection?
- ✦ Does the client have a means for reporting abuse? Would the client report abuse? Is there fear of retribution?

✦

CASE STUDY 3

A client is being discharged from a facility into a home where the family is known to be dysfunctional. There is concern and suspicion that the person with a disability is being abused.

Ethical questions to consider regarding autonomy of the client:

✦ If the client wants to go back to this situation, should attempts be made to change this?

✦ What level of independence can be attained while in rehabilitation?

✦ Does the client have enough information about alternatives?

✦ Is the nurses' role to support the client's wishes?

✦ Does the team know what to do and are they prepared to act should abuse be reported or assessed?

RESEARCH SCENARIOS

One of the most common issues in rehabilitation practice relates to informed consent. Does the client have enough information? Can the client understand the information? These questions cause greater concern when clients are asked to participate in research studies, as discussed in Chapter 4. If every human being does indeed have the right to determine what is done with their body and is entitled to a knowledgeable choice, who then safeguards that right? In rehabilitation it often may be the nurse or the nurse with other team members. With research, what ethically needs to be assured? Initially a client's competence to agree to participate is an issue for a physician to determine with contribution from nursing assessments. Second, the worth of the research is evaluated for risk versus benefits; Institutional Review Boards (IRBs) determine whether the benefits of the research will help current clients, future clients, or the profession. Third, the nurse needs to be aware of the professional role for obtaining a client's informed consent: typically, being aware of the requirement, facilitating the process, and witnessing a client's signature. Finally, a nurse advocates and protects clients' rights to privacy and confidentiality. In reality this last provision may be difficult in an environment where multiple members of the team may be interested in clients as research subjects (Bach & Barnett, 1994; Scofield, 1993). It must be said that all aspects and principles of biomedical ethics are scrutinized regarding research with clients while in a rehabilitation setting.

COMMUNITY ISSUES

The rehabilitation nurse is involved in community issues by caring for individuals and groups of individuals in the community and also as one of the "stakeholders" in healthcare reform. As nurses care for clients in the community, the nurse may find herself in the middle of issues regarding acceptance of the client with a disability. Some neighbors' willingness to help members in an independent living center may not be the same as for other neighbors; the nurse

may need to advocate for the client more than seems reasonable when the sole purpose of independent living is autonomy. The nurse will experience questions about how involved to become. Or the rehabilitation nurse may find that the client has few or no financial resources. Seeking services providing access may be difficult. The client may live outside of boundaries that would provide public transportation to a needed rehabilitation setting, or there is no appropriate setting within the client's residential boundary. How can the nurse achieve the goals set if there are no resources? Other client care questions may deal with concerns over caregiver ability to deal with equipment such as a ventilator or concerns of safety in transfer or accepting how a family chooses to care for a client. A nurse reported that one family couldn't adapt to placing a person with high quadriplegia in their tub so they "hosed" him off in the garage. Cases in the community can be decided and acted on using the same moral principles and decision-making models utilized in the institutional setting. The differences will be in degree and number, not ethical beliefs.

The second set of community concerns deals with the role of the rehabilitation nurse. The dilemma is how viable is the nurses' role; is the role necessary or can others perform our actions? If the role is necessary, what is it worth? The move toward healthcare reform is an attempt to provide quality healthcare for all; the client with disability then is entitled to needed rehabilitation services. But cost containment is also an issue. Does the rehabilitation nurse's contributions to the team equal the cost? Even though nurses don't charge fee for service, the nurse does receive a salary and does utilize supplies. Should nurses identify or classify their action and charge for these? If they do, the cost/benefit ratio could be more clearly understood by clients, family, insurance carriers, and by the Americans paying tax dollars. Some rehabilitation nurses see fee for service as an ethical issue in and of itself. These questions can be addressed by asking if the client needs an advocate to move him into an autonomous position, and is that advocate the nurse? Does the rehabilitation nursing scope give the nurse the right to provide the service? If it doesn't, then it is appropriate to withdraw. Dougherty points out that people want care at lowest cost and highest quality, and to accomplish this care providers need to become less concerned about their own interests and more concerned about national interests (Dougherty, 1992). The rehabilitation nurse needs to evaluate this issue closely and soon. If there is something that clients need from professional rehabilitation nursing, the community needs to be made as aware of it before the dollars available are distributed and none are left for nursing. The ethical dilemma is not one of nurses losing jobs but of clients being deprived of care necessary to achieve goals. It is an agreement rehabilitation nurses have made with clients: that they will be there. Is it an agreement worthy of keeping?

TEAM ISSUES

Team members offer expertise in distinct areas as well as overlapping knowledge and skill areas. The rehabilitation model does not have the traditional "captain of the ship" paternalistic relationships; it does encompass physician-client, physician-nurse, physician-therapist, nurse-therapist, nurse-client, therapist-client relationships. Due to the philosophy of rehabilitation, the team relationships also include family or significant others and dynamics with accrediting and paying institutions. For a team to deal effectively with any dilemma, the members need to develop an awareness of each other's roles—the core values of those roles. If there is a degree of clarity regarding these roles, the team members will have one less complication in dealing with ethical issues. Respect for these relationships and functions will facilitate answering questions about autonomy, advocacy, privacy, and confidentiality.

Rehabilitation team members have self-care, independence, and client well-being as ultimate goals. Clients come to the rehabilitation setting from traditional settings and home, where the degree of independence probably was different than what now will be expected. Over time teams may facilitate this dependence due to wanting to do what is best. The following six factors have been noted as causes for this dependence:

1. Number of team members is overpowering to client
2. Client fatigue
3. Client anxiety
4. Gratitude to team members
5. Fear of being considered unreasonable by team members
6. Feeling unable to change goals they are already working on (Purtillo, 1988)

To facilitate autonomy, team members can remind themselves that the client dealing with the devastating effects of the disability is doing so for the first time; recognize that it will take time for the client to develop the energy to stand alone and make choices and feel empowered to say she does not agree. While the client is gaining this strength, the team members can develop a system of checks and balances (other than those already present due to overlapping functions). The checks and balances could be as simple as deciding who is the most appropriate member to be the advocate in specific goals; who will discuss certain (if not all) aspects of the plan of care with the client to gain agreement or set contracts; or explain to the client that decisions regarding explicit goals of care will be theirs—they have real time available and changes in plans of care are acceptable.

SUMMARY

Choices in ethics are not always self-evident. The only choice in rehabilitation is what is best for the client, which may mean that in some events a particular caregiver may have to withdraw from a situation because what is best for the client is truly incompatible with their values. Choices are concomitantly influenced by society and culture: these influences may be complementary to each other or may force moral reasoning. For example, a culture that fosters the inherent worth of each human being and yet members of the culture cohabit in a society that cherishes the belief that not all have the right to the same healthcare. To provide healthcare to all is expensive; 14% of the gross national product (GNP) in the United States goes to healthcare (U.S. Department of Commerce, 1992), leading to the dilemma of how much money should be spent on an individual case when total dollars for all is limited. A greater

dilemma is who decides how much is spent on whom and for what; how much does the rehabilitation nurse participate in this decision-making process? Therefore the rehabilitation nurse learns and grows in a rehabilitation milieu that fosters precepts of caring, autonomy, and information sharing while recognizing the influences from society on the ability to provide the services connected with these precepts. What ethical role will influence healthcare at the decision-making or governmental level or institutional level? For example, who provides what care for a client, and what is the nurse/client ratio for fulfilling their social contract?

Regardless of the type of situation, the rehabilitation nurse must recognize societal and cultural pressures, the expectations of the rehabilitation environment, and what are the components of moral reasoning. The rehabilitation nurse also should recognize that the nurse-patient relationship is one that evolves—that is, as the patient deals with the identity changes as a result of the impairment, and as the client recognizes a potential for new self-worth through the views of the rehabilitation nurse. The nurse also must value the nurse-client relationship, safeguarding the client-physician trust relationship; the nurse is a conavigator on the rehabilitation ship, not a mate to the paternalistic physician "captain of the ship" theme (Payton, 1979). The nurse's repertoire of skills in dealing with each ethical dilemma will grow if the nurse remains ever alert to potential dilemmas and the consequences of decisions make for each client in each situation. Rehabilitation nurses need to be prepared for more ethical dilemmas as a result of the trends in biotechnology in healthcare and healthcare reform. For example, when to justify devices such as phrenic nerve implants; when to justify transplants; when to withhold treatment for newborns with special needs; or whether to identify the status of fetuses and for what ends.

REFERENCES

American Nurses' Association. (1985). *Code of nurses with interpretive statements*. Kansas City: Author.

American Nurses' Association, Joint Committee on Rehabilitation Nursing Practice. (1988). *Rehabilitation nursing scope of practice and outcome criteria for selected diagnoses*. Kansas City: Author.

Anonymous. (1977) Nursing's role in patients' rights. NY. NLN Publication No. 11-1671, 1-5.

Applegate, M.L., & Entrekin, N.M. (1984). *Teaching ethics in nursing: Handbook for use of the case study approach*. New York: National League for Nursing.

Aroskar, M. (1982). Are nurses' mind sets development of moral judgment among selected groups of practicing nurses? *Nursing Research, 30*, 98-103.

Aroskar, M. (1980). Ethics of nurse-patient relationships. *Nurse Educator, 5(2)*, 18-20.

Association of Rehabilitation Nurses. (1989). *By-laws Association of Rehabilitation Nurses*. Skokie, IL: Author.

Association of Rehabilitation Nurses. (1992). Unpublished minutes of Ethics Task Force and Ethics Task Force Questionnaire. Skokie, IL.

Bach, J.R. & Barnett, V. (1994). Ethical considerations in the management of individuals with severe neuromuscular disorders. *Archives of Physical Medicine and Rehabilitation, 73*, 134-140.

Bach, J., Campagnolo, D., & Hoeman, S. (1991). Life satisfaction and DMD. *Archives of Physical Medicine and Rehabilitation, 7*, 129-135.

Bandman, E.L. & Bandman, B. (1985). *Nursing ethics in the life span*. Englewood Cliffs, NJ: Appleton-Century-Crofts.

Beauchamp, T.L. & Childress, J.E. (1989). Principles of biomedical ethics. 2nd edition. New York: Oxford University Press.

Benjamin, M., & Curtis, J. (1986). *Ethics in nursing.* Oxford University Press.

Blank, R.H., & Mills, M.K. (Eds.). (1989). *Biomedical technology and public policy.* New York: Greenwood.

Caplan, A.L., Callahan, D., & Haas, J. (1987). *Ethical policy issues in rehabilitation medicine.* Briarcliff Manor, NY: A Hasting's Center Report, Special Supplement.

Carper, B.A. (1978). Fundamental patterns of knowing. Practice oriented theory part I. *Advances in Nursing Science, 1(1),* 13-23.

Churchill, L. (1977). Ethical issues of a profession in transition. *American Journal of Nursing, 77,* 873-875.

Clinton, W. (1993). Ethical foundations of health reform. Health Reform Working Draft, 9-93, pp. 11-12.

Crisham, P (1987). Moral judgment in hypothetical and nursing dilemmas. Dissertation (80-06, 592). Minneapolis, University of Minnesota.

Cunningham, N., & Hutchinson, S. (1990). Myths in health care ethics. *Image, 22,* 235-238.

Czwerwinski, B.S. (1990). An autopsy of an ethical dilemma. *Journal of Nursing Administration, 20,* 25-29.

dePender, W., & Idede-Chandler, W. (1990). *Clinical ethics: An invitation to health professionals.* New York: Praeger.

Doheny, M., Cook, C., & Stopper, C. (1982). Ethical and legal considerations. In *The discipline of nursing: An introduction.* Appleton and Lange.

Dougherty, C.J. (1992). Ethical values at stake in health care reform. *JAMA, 268,* 2409-2412.

Edge, R.S. & Groves, J.R. (1994). *The Ethics of Health Care: A guide for clinical practice.* Albany, NY: Delmar Publishers, Inc.

Ethics Task Force Questionnaire of Membership. (1992). Skokie, IL: Association of Rehabilitation Nursing. Unpublished.

Felton, G.M., & Parsons, M.A. (1987). The impact of nursing education on ethical/moral decision making. *Journal of Nursing Education, 26,* 7-11, 1987.

Frankl, V. (1973). *Ethics.* Englewood Cliffs, NJ: Prentice-Hall Publishers.

Gadow, S. (1980). "*Existential audocacy: Philosophical functioning of nursing.*" In Spicker, S. & Gadow, S. (eds). *Nursing: Images and ideals.* New York: Springer Publishing Company, pp. 79-101.

Gaull, A.L. (1987). The effect of a course in nursing ethics on the relationship between choice and ethical action in Baccalaureate nursing students. *Journal of Nursing Education, 26,* 113-117.

Gero, E., & Giordano, J. (1990). Ethical considerations in fetal tissue transplantation. *Journal of Neuroscience Nursing, 22,* 9-12.

Gilligan, C. (1982). *In a different voice.* Cambridge, MA: Harvard University Press.

Graham, C., & Royster, V. (1990). Rehabilitation of a paraplegic prisoner: Conflicts for patients and nurses. *Rehabilitation Nursing, 15,* 197-201.

Grant, A.B. (1992). Explaining an ethical dilemma: Nursing a Jehovah's Witness who believed that taking blood is expressly forbidden. *Nursing, 22,* 52-54.

Grier, (1983). Decision making process with nursing undergraduate students. Minneapolis. Presentation at University of Minnesota Research Conference.

Husted, G.L., & Husted, J.L. (1991). *Ethical decision making in nursing.* St. Louis: Mosby-Year Book.

Illis, L.S., Sedgwick, E.M., & Glonvilled, J.J. (Eds.). (1982). *Rehabilitation of the neurological patient.* Oxford: Blockwell Scientific.

Jameton, A. (1984). *Nursing practice: The ethical issue.* Englewood Cliffs, NJ: Prentice-Hall Publishers.

Kelly, L.Y. (1985). Professional ethics and accountability. In *Dimensions of professional nursing* (5th ed.). New York: MacMillan.

Ketefian, A. (1981). Critical thinking, educational preparation, and development of moral judgment among selected groups of practicing nurses. *Nursing Research, 30,* 98-103.

Lump, Sr. F. (1979). The role of the nurse in the bioethical decision-making process. *Nursing Clinics of North America, 14,* 13-21.

Martin, N., Holt, B., & Hicks, D. (1981). *Comprehensive rehabilitation nursing.* New York, McGraw-Hill.

Miya, P.A. (1984). An ethical dilemma. *Image, Journal of Nursing Scholarship, 16,* 105-108.

Moccia, P. (1990). Reclaiming our communities. *Nursing Outlook,* 73-76.

Muyskens, (1982). Moral problems in nursing: A philosophical investigation. Totowa, NJ: Roman and Littlefield.

National League for Nursing (Pub. No. 11-1671). *Nursing's role in patients' rights.* New York: Author.

Nelson, J. (1982). Authority of nursing practice. *Topics in Clinical Nursing, 4,* 22-32.

Omery, A. (1989). Values, moral reasoning and ethics. *Nursing Clinics of North America, 24,* 499-507.

Payton, R.J. (1979). Information control and autonomy. *Nursing Clinics of North America, 14,* 23-34.

Peacock, J.L. (1986). *The anthropologic lens: Harsh light, soft focus.* Cambridge, MA: Cambridge University Press.

Purtilo, R.B. (1986). Ethical issues in the treatment of chronic ventilator dependent patients. *Archives of Physical Medicine and Rehabilitation, 67,* 718-721.

Purtilo, R.B. (1988). Ethical issues in teamwork: The context of rehabilitation. *Archives of Physical Medicine and Rehabilitation, 69,* 318-322.

Purtilo, R.B. & Cassell, C.K. (1981). *Ethical dimensions in the Health Professions.* Philadelphia: W.B. Saunders.

Quinn, C., & Smith, M. (1987). *The professional commitment: Issues and ethics in nursing.* Philadelphia: W.B. Saunders.

Ridley, B. (1989). Tom's story: A quadriplegic who refused rehabilitation. *Rehabilitation Nursing, 14,* 240-256, 268.

Rosenkoetter, M.M. (1983). A code of ethics for nurse educators. *Nursing Outlook, 31,* 288.

Rusk, H.A. (1977). *Rehabilitation medicine.* St. Louis: Mosby–Year Book.

Scofield, G. (1993). Ethical considerations in rehabilitation medicine. *Archives of Physical Medicine and Rehabilitation, 74,* 341-346.

Snyder, M. (1985). *Independent nursing interventions.* Albany, NY: Delmar Publishers.

Taylor, S.G. (1985). Rights and responsibilities: Nurse-patient relationships. *Image, 17,* 9-13.

U.S. Department of Commerce. (1992). *U.S. industrial outlook.* Washington, DC: U.S. Department of Commerce, Bureau of Industrial Economics.

Veatch, R.M., & Fry, S.T. (1987). *Case studies in nursing ethics.* Philadelphia: J.B. Lippincott.

Whiteneck, G.G., et al (1985). *A collaborative study of high quadriplegia. Report to the National Institute of Handicapped Research.* Englewood, CA: Craig Hospital.

Winslow, G.R. (1984). From loyalty to advocacy: A new metaphor for nursing. Hastings Center Report, *14,* 32-40.

Wright, R.A. (1987). *The practice of ethics: Human values in health care.* New York: McGraw-Hill.

Wurzbach, M.E. (1990). The dilemma of witholding or withdrawing nutrition. *Image, 22,* 226-227.

◆

Appendix 3-A   Ethical foundations of health reform

Working group draft
Privileged and confidential

The values and principles that shape the new healthcare system reflect fundamental national beliefs about community, equality, justice, and liberty. These convictions anchor health reform in shared moral traditions.

Universal Access: Every American citizen and legal resident should have access to healthcare without financial or other barriers.

Comprehensive Benefits: Guaranteed benefits should meet the full range of health needs, including primary, preventive, and specialized care.

Choice: Each consumer should have the opportunity to exercise effective choice about providers, plans, and treatments. Each consumer should be informed about what is known and not known about the risks and benefits of available treatments and be free to choose among them according to his and her preferences.

Equality of Care: The system should avoid the creation of a tiered system providing care based only on differences of need, not individual or group characteristics.

Fair Distribution of Costs: The healthcare system should spread the costs and burdens of care across the entire community, basing the level of contribution required of consumers on ability to pay.

Personal Responsibility: Under health reform, each individual and family should assume responsibility for protecting and promoting health and contributing to the cost of care.

Intergenerational Justice: The healthcare system should respond to the unique needs of each stage of life, sharing benefits and burdens fairly across generations.

Wise Allocation of Resources: The nation should balance prudently what it spends on healthcare against other important national priorities.

Effectiveness: The new system should deliver care and innovation that works and that patients want. It should encourage the discovery of better treatments. It should make it possible for the academic community and healthcare providers to exercise effectively their responsibility to evaluate and improve healthcare by providing resources for the systematic study of healthcare outcomes.

Quality: The system should deliver high-quality care and provide individuals with the information necessary to make informed healthcare choices.

Effective Management: By encouraging simplification and continuous improvement, as well as making the system easier to use for patients and providers, the healthcare system should focus on care, rather than administration.

Professional Integrity and Responsibility: The healthcare system should treat the clinical judgments of professionals with respect and protect the integrity of the provider-patient relationship while ensuring that health providers have the resources to fulfill their responsibilities for the effective delivery of quality care.

Fair Procedures: To protect these values and principles, fair and open democratic procedures should underlie decisions concerning the operation of the healthcare system and the resolution of disputes that arise within it.

Local Responsibility: Working within the framework of national reform, the new healthcare system should allow states and local communities to design effective, high-quality systems of care that serve each of their citizens.

◆

Appendix 3-B   Code for nurses

1. The nurse provides services with respect for human dignity and the uniqueness of the client, unrestricted by considerations of social or economic status, personal attributes, or the nature of health problems.

2. The nurse safeguards the client's right to privacy by judiciously protecting information of a confidential nature.

3. The nurse acts to safeguard the client and the public when healthcare and safety are affected by the incompetent, unethical, or illegal practice of any person.

4. The nurse assumes responsibility and accountability for individual nursing judgments and actions.

5. The nurse maintains competence in nursing.

6. The nurse exercises informed judgment and uses individual competence and qualifications as criteria in seeking consultation, accepting responsibilities, and delegating nursing activities to others.

7. The nurse participates in activities that contribute to the ongoing development of the profession's body of knowledge.

8. The nurse participates in the profession's efforts to implement and improve standards of nursing.

9. The nurse participates in the profession's efforts to establish and maintain conditions of employment conducive to high-quality nursing care.

10. The nurse participates in the profession's effort to protect the public from misinformation and misrepresentation and to maintain the integrity of nursing.

11. The nurse collaborates with members of the health professions and other citizens in promoting community and national efforts to meet the health needs of the public.

4

Rehabilitation Nursing Research

Marci Catanzaro, RN, CS, PhD

INTRODUCTION

Research is an essential component of nursing practice. This chapter begins with a historical overview of rehabilitation nursing research. The relationships between practice, research, and theory are reviewed, and examples from the rehabilitation literature are used to illustrate the four levels of theory development. The challenges of conducting research in the clinical arena are addressed, and practical suggestions are offered for meeting these challenges. Finally, utilization of research findings to enhance clinical practice is discussed and trends for the future are explored.

HISTORY OF REHABILITATION NURSING RESEARCH

Assisting individuals of all ages and social and cultural groups to accomplish the tasks of daily living is a thread that can be identified in definitions of nursing beginning with Florence Nightingale (1860/1946) and continuing through the American Nurses' Association Social Policy Statement (American Nurses' Association, 1980). Nightingale also set nursing on course for research through her detailed records of the effects of nursing actions on soldiers in the Crimean War. This history notwithstanding, rehabilitation nursing research has a very short chronology. What we know as rehabilitation today had its roots following World War II. The professional organization, the Association of Rehabilitation Nurses, was founded in 1974, and the *ARN Journal* was first published the following year and later entitled *Rehabilitation Nursing*. In 1976 the first research article was published in the *ARN Journal* (Steels, 1976).

The inception of nursing research journals began in 1952 with *Nursing Research*. The first issue included an article on the adjustment of chronically ill older adults who were receiving home care (Mack, 1952). Nearly 10 years lapsed before a study more directly related to rehabilitation nursing described the development of an objective measure of decubitus ulcers (Verhoick, 1961). Forty years after the first nursing research journal began publication, a journal devoted to rehabilitation nursing research was published. In the inaugural issue of *Rehabilitation Nursing Research,* the editor noted that the emphasis on research in nursing was apparent everywhere. No longer could *Rehabilitation Nursing* address the diverse needs of all rehabilitation nurses (Puetz, 1992).

The 1990s have brought an increased interest in the research role of the rehabilitation nurse. Bachman (1990) urged nurses to work toward the goal of professional self-sufficiency by producing and using research. She noted that healthcare has become too complex for the simple authoritarian solutions that are not scientifically based. The healthcare environment is changing rapidly. The 1990s are certain to bring about unprecedented changes in the way that healthcare is defined, delivered, and reimbursed. Healthcare reform is on everyone's agenda, and cost control underlies much of the discussion about providing healthcare to all Americans. The cost/benefit ratio of rehabilitation services will become increasing important as healthcare systems evaluate what services will be provided, for whom, and under what circumstances. The contributions of rehabilitation nurse researchers will be important in demonstrating the effectiveness of public health policies aimed at preventing and reducing disability from traumatic injuries, vascular insults to vital organs, and preventable causes of cancer. Rehabilitation nurses must assume leadership roles in demonstrating the cost-effectiveness of rehabilitation nursing services during acute care rehabilitation and long-term care of those with chronic illnesses and disabilities. Clearly only those services demonstrated to be cost-effective in terms of shorter lengths of stay, decreased overall costs, and decreased utilization of expensive social and health services will be reimbursed under new healthcare systems. Research demonstrating that what rehabilitation nurses do makes a difference in patient outcomes will be essential for those services to be included in healthcare reimbursement.

Rehabilitation nurses have a long way to go in becoming recognized as professionally self-sufficient and credible voices in demonstrating the cost-effectiveness of the services they provide and rehabilitation in general. The actual involvement of rehabilitation nurses in research was explored only recently. Of the 8000 professional nurses who are members of the Association of Rehabilitation Nurses, only 186 (0.02%) responded to a survey that was included in the association newsletter about their involvement in research. Of those nurses responding, 41% reported they had no involvement in research (Hoeman, Dayhoff, & Thompson, 1993). Why did so few respond? Perhaps the vast majority of nurses who claim rehabilitation as their specialty area of practice are not involved in research. Conceivably many more rehabilitation nurses are involved in some aspect of the research process, from generating researchable questions to critically analyzing published research reports for practice implications, but did not consider themselves researchers. Those who were actively involved in the research process may have neglected to respond to the survey. Dayhoff (1993) noted that "while rehabilitation nursing practice has a rich heritage, the theoretic basis for practice is in early infancy." She encouraged nurses to seek opportunities for collaboration between clinicians and researchers that will develop theory-based practice.

Research has been praised and maligned among various groups of nurses. Some nurses believe that research is the only way in which we can improve the care of persons with disabilities, and others regard research as an ivory tower activity that has little relevance to enhancing the care that nurses provide. It is discouraging to confront the fact that, in nearly 50 years since modern rehabilitation began, so little has been learned about the scientific basis to support the assumption that rehabilitation nursing care makes a difference in patient outcomes. Conversely it is exciting to be a rehabilitation nurse today and to be in the forefront of developing a theoretic basis for our practice.

RELATIONSHIP BETWEEN PRACTICE, RESEARCH, AND THEORY

The quality and effectiveness of the care that rehabilitation nurses deliver depends on research findings. Research is the process of posing an important, answerable question derived from practice and collecting data to provide a convincing answer. Research that is based on rehabilitation nurses' experiences in clinical practice ensures that the outcome of the research will be relevant to the very essence of rehabilitation nursing: caring for individuals and groups with actual or potential disabilities. Understanding what nursing actions under what conditions produce what client outcomes will allow rehabilitation nurses to provide care that can predictably accomplish the desired patient outcomes.

Research implies a systematic approach to the study of problems. The number of research reports with implications for rehabilitation nursing has increased markedly over the years. Unfortunately many of the published studies do not build on previous knowledge in the area and remain unrelated to each other. A systematic approach to the development of a knowledge base for rehabilitation nursing practice is seriously lacking. One perspective on organizing and improving the research endeavor is to view research from the perspective of developing theory to guide nursing practice. Rehabilitation nurses can expect to build a knowledge base only through a rigorous, scholarly, and systematic scrutiny of phenomena that influence practice.

Describing Phenomena

The purpose of theory is to describe, explain, and predict phenomena. Before we can propose a theory to guide practice, we must understand the concepts involved in the theory. It is not possible to propose a theory of helping individuals cope with disability unless we understand coping, patient teaching, and outcome variables such as independence. In the first stage of theory development, therefore, we ask the question "What is this?" This question can be answered in a number of ways. Research at this level of theory development depends on literature review, open-ended questions, unstructured observations, and exploration of the phenomenon of interest in various settings.

Typically reports of research designed to answer the question "What is it?" fully identify and describe the phenomenon of interest. Descriptions may include a verbal description of a phenomenon; graphs; and reports of ranges, means, and standard deviations. The nursing and social science literature is replete with descriptions of phenomena. Many excellent studies have examined coping, adaptation, and the meaning of various disabilities and illnesses for the individual and for family members. Schneider and Conrad (1985) interviewed 80 people who experienced and managed their epilepsy outside of institutionalized settings. The people they interviewed answered the question "What is epilepsy?" from their personal perspective. They spoke of a seizure as "losing control" and as a "social event" that created trouble for others who always wanted to "call an ambulance." Those with a seizure disorder needed to engage in "preventive work" to avoid having seizures and to "attend to face" following a seizure in public. Epilepsy carries with it a social stigma in society, and those interviewed "managed information" about their condition by selectively concealing and disclosing information to others. Medication was a "ticket to normality" for many of the participants in their study, but the regulation of medication raised issues of "dependency" and "asserting control." In answering the question "What is epilepsy?" Schneider and Conrad demonstrated that epilepsy is far more than a medical diagnosis that carries a social stigma. They captured the essence of living with a seizure disorder in a way that provides insights for care providers about the experience and control of illness.

Another approach to answer the question "What is this?" is concept analysis. Forsyth (1980), in a now classic study, used the concept of empathy to illustrate the techniques of concept analysis. She utilized the case of a child hospitalized with a serious illness to portray the essential components of empathy, which included consciousness, temporality, relationship, validation, accuracy, and intensity. Each of these concepts was defined in terms of how they were or were not exemplified in an interaction between a nurse and the child's mother.

Determining Relationships

Many concepts relative to rehabilitation nursing have been described and analyzed. The next step in making these studies applicable to practice is to determine how the concepts are related to each other. The researcher asks the question "What is happening here?" Much of the rehabilitation-related nursing research has explored the relationship between concepts. For example, age is related to achieving independence in physical activity. In lower limb amputations, increased age was associated with unfavorable outcomes in physical ability (Helm, Engel, Holm, Kristiansen, & Rosendahl, 1986). Younger adults were significantly better able than older adults to achieve independence in self-care and in bowel and bladder function (Penrod, Hegde, & Ditunna, 1990). Older age was negatively associated with the level of independence at discharge following stroke in nearly 8000 individuals (Granger, Hamilton, & Fiedler, 1992). However, others have found that advancing age affected independence only in bathing, dressing, stair climbing, and transfers (Yarkony, Roth, Heinemann, & Lovell, 1988). Still other studies have demonstrated no effect of age on physical independence (Davis & Acton, 1988; Carey, Seibert, & Posavac, 1988). Acorn and Bampton (1992) related loneliness in young and middle-aged adults in a long-term rehabilitation center to age and length of institutionalization and found that loneliness was more prevalent among those who had been admitted more recently but was unrelated to the age of the person.

Gender, on the other hand, has not been demonstrated to influence independence in physical activities; however, older and uneducated women are disadvantaged in their access to rehabilitation resources (Ades, Waldmann, Polk, & Coflesky, 1992; Altman & Smith, 1990, 1992). In a phase II cardiac rehabilitation program, gender but not the demographical and diagnostic characteristics of participants was related to activity tolerance, anxiety, and efficacy in enduring exercise and activities of daily living (Schuster & Waldron, 1991).

Research designed to determine the relationship among concepts utilizes more structured observations, asks more precise questions, and uses descriptive statistics to explain the connection among the concepts. Exploring the relationship among concepts is one step further along the continuum of establishing a theoretic base for rehabilitation nursing practice. Research at this level is the first step toward explaining how we might manipulate one factor to influence another factor. Descriptive statistics including correlations, t-tests of group differences, and chi square tests of independence are useful analytic strategies.

Testing Relationships

After the phenomena are named and described and research has demonstrated that various phenomena are related, the next question that researchers ask is "What will happen if . . . ?" This stage of theory development is probably the most important because it allows us to test the theoretic relationships that were identified in the previous level of theory development. Factors believed to predict the relationship among the variables are stated and tested. Is the original theory correct? Does the theory apply to circumstances beyond those initially tested? Are there additional categories or relationships? Dille, Kirchhoff, Sullivan, and Larson (1993) used an experimental design to answer the question "What if vinyl urinary drainage bags are rinsed with dilute bleach?" Studies that ask the question "What will happen if . . . ?" are designed to impose maximum control over the concepts. The researchers randomly assigned the patients to the control and experimental groups. They measured urine colony counts weekly and evaluated the incidence of urinary tract infections between the two groups. They also assessed the aesthetic alterations and integrity of the bags and the inpatient cost of the two treatment conditions. They concluded that it was safe and cost-effective to reuse the bags for 4 weeks if they were decontaminated daily with sodium hypochlorite (household bleach).

Venn, Taft, Carpentier, and Applebaugh (1992) tested four bowel-training protocols. A major finding of their study was that the patients in the morning bowel-training groups were significantly more efficient than those in evening groups in establishing effective bowel regimens. Efficiency was highest for those assigned to a bowel-training group whose time coincided with their previous pattern. They found no significant differences between scheduled and *pro re nata* (prn) suppository use. Studies that test relationships are more challenging than studies at lower levels of theory development because they require the specification of necessary and sufficient conditions that will produce a desired outcome.

Producing Situations

The ultimate question for rehabilitation nursing practice is "How can we change the situation to bring about a desired outcome?" The last stage in theory development is goal oriented and situation producing and has been referred to as prescriptive theory. The question researchers ask is "How can I make X happen?" We must know how to change a situation to bring about the desired outcome. Studies at this level often are referred to as clinical trials in which we test the feasibility of a new treatment, determine the optimal use of a regimen or procedure, or compare the efficacy of two treatments or programs in achieving a desired outcome (Fetter et al., 1989). There are few cases in which we can confidently prescribe a rehabilitation nursing intervention and be assured that the desired outcome will occur. Testing prescriptive theory requires that the findings can be generalized beyond the specific situation. Prescriptive theory is dependent on an understanding of the mechanism of the variables studied. Rehabilitation nursing lacks the knowledge basis for understanding the underlying mechanism for nursing interventions—which precludes the conduct of situation-producing studies at this time. Studies that test theoretic relationships between concepts must be done first.

In summary, there are countless questions about the effect of rehabilitation nursing practice. Answers to these questions are laden with opinions and assumptions. Rehabilitation nursing research has concentrated on describing the concepts of interest and exploring how these factors are related. Little work has been done to establish what the rehabilitation nurse must do to bring about specific outcomes in persons requiring rehabilitation. The time is ripe for rehabilitation nurses to be proactive in developing a strong knowledge base for nursing practice and rehabilitation outcomes.

Other Approaches to Knowledge

Research directed at developing theory that will guide practice is not the only arena for rehabilitation nursing research. Important contributions to the practice of rehabilitation nursing have been made through research about attitudes of nurses and others toward persons with disabilities; nursing administration and documentation patterns that facilitate the delivery of nursing care; nurses' knowledge about rehabilitation; quality assurance; and program evaluation. The focus of this chapter, however, is on research directed toward examining the effectiveness of nursing practice on patient outcomes.

ROLES OF NURSES IN CONDUCTING RESEARCH

Research often is thought of as something that is done by other disciplines or by nurses who have doctorates and are removed from clinical practice. Every rehabilitation nurse has an obligation to improve the rehabilitative care provided to those persons with actual or potential disabilities. Involvement in research is an essential element in the improvement of rehabilitation care. Without rehabilitation nurses' involvement in research that is "productive, scientifically rigorous, and credible," this nursing specialty will "wither and die" (Wahlquist, 1982). Involvement in research can range from generating questions from clinical practice to designing and implementing complex studies that answer the question "How can I make X happen?" Reading research reports and attending research conferences and then discussing with colleagues the relevance of the findings for clinical practice are ways of participating in rehabilitation nursing research. Learning more about the research process and collaborating with other members of a research team will also enhance the development of a scientific basis for rehabilitation nursing practice.

The American Nurses' Association (1981) set forth guidelines for the investigative function of nurses. Nurses with minimum educational preparation are a valuable asset in research because they raise questions about the effectiveness of nursing interventions and participate in data collection to answer these questions. As more research education is acquired, nurses become increasingly more involved in interpreting and evaluating research for practice, conducting investigations, and disseminating research findings (Table 4-1).

Rehabilitation nurses are part of a team that has as its goal returning individuals to their level of optimum function. Collaborative relationships between nurse clinicians and researchers are essential. Nail (1990) has pointed out that clinicians in practice must be actively involved in all aspects of the research process. They identify practice problems and reformulate these problems into research questions, critique research designs, evaluate the clinical feasibility of the research protocol, assist in implementing the research protocol, raise clinical questions relevant to data analyses, and interpret the results of the study from a clinical perspective.

Hoeman, Dayhoff, and Thompson (1993) surveyed a convenience sample of 186 Association of Rehabilitation Nurses about their interest and involvement in research. Half the participants were involved in some aspects of research, "especially quality assurance activities or collecting data." They concluded by offering the following suggestions for increasing the visibility and understanding of research that are appropriate for nurses in clinical practice:

- ✦ Establish cluster groups with interest in specific methods or topics
- ✦ Conduct multisite replication of studies or research utilization projects
- ✦ Use consultants to expand knowledge and skills
- ✦ Broker networking opportunities for database and literature review systems

Conducting Research in the Clinical Arena

The clinical arena spawns many opportunities and challenges. The opportunity to explore phenomena related to rehabilitation and to examine how various phenomena are related provides a basis for understanding practice. Further exploration ultimately can lead to confidence that prescriptions for nursing interventions will influence patient outcomes in the expected direction. Unlike the laboratory, where circumstance can be rigidly controlled, the clinical area provides additional challenges related to the inability to rigidly control patient care environments. Ways of meeting these specific challenges are considered in subsequent sections of this chapter. In general, creative thinking and collaboration are useful methods for overcoming many of the demands presented by the fluidity of the clinical setting.

Many excellent research textbooks remain in print that lead researchers through the various stages of the research process (Burns & Grove, 1993; Mateo & Kirchhoff, 1991; Polit & Hungler, 1991; Wilson, 1989; Woods & Catanzaro, 1988). It is convenient to talk about the steps or stages of research, suggesting a linear sequence—whereas the actual process of engaging in research is iterative, moving back and forth between the various parts of the research process. For example, a researcher may identify a problem for study, formulate hypotheses, design the research, then reformulate the problem as more information about what is known and the realities of the clinical situation are better understood. This chapter addresses the various phases of the research process, suggests questions that need to be answered at various stages of the process, and offers suggestions for meeting some of the challenges of conducting clinical research.

Asking Research Questions

Every study begins with selecting a researchable question. Rehabilitation nurses seldom suffer from having no questions about their practice. The challenge is to decide what is of most interest. Keeping track of questions, reflecting on them, and discussing them with colleagues can make

Table 4-1 Research responsibilities of nurses

Preparation	Research responsibilities
Associate degree	Collect data
	Identify researchable problems
	Appreciate the value of research
Baccalaureate degree	Apply research findings to practice
	Share research findings
	Interpret and evaluate research for practice
Master's degree	Conduct investigations
	Facilitate access to clients
	Collaborate with other investigators
	Facilitate research
	Provide consultation
	Analyze and reformulate problems
Doctoral degree	Extend the scientific basis of practice
	Develop methods to measure nursing phenomena
	Provide leadership in research

even the most vague ideas mature into very good research opportunities.

Asking the right question is the most important part of research. The words that are used to state the question should be unambiguous, simple, and brief. The question must be understandable to those who formulate the question and to those who will ultimately be expected to utilize the research findings. The question determines how the study is designed, what data are collected, the analysis that is done, and the kind of conclusions that can be drawn. The interaction among various stages of the research process is critical when selecting a researchable question.

A research question must have an answer. It is not possible to research whether a spinal cord injury is God's punishment for a personal transgression or if the extent of neural loss in response to a traumatic head injury is less in the absence of gravity. Finding the answer to the question must be feasible.

✦ Is the question important?
✦ Will it further the knowledge base or contribute to the development of rehabilitation nursing theory?
✦ Will the answer be of interest to others, including other members of the rehabilitation team?

Framing the research question also involves consideration of the resources that will be necessary to answer the question.

✦ Is this the best time to conduct the study, and will there be enough time for completion?
✦ Will the financial resources necessary to carry out the study be available?
✦ Are others sufficiently interested in the question to cooperate either as coinvestigators or as research participants?
✦ Are there enough people available with the disease or condition being studied to ensure an adequate number of participants?
✦ Is the space and equipment available that is needed to conduct the study?
✦ Is there sufficient expertise on the research team to answer the question?
✦ What is the cost/benefit ratio of the risk of participation or nonparticipation in the study?

Even before the research question is formulated, some information about the topic is known. It is unlikely, however, that the researcher has a grasp on everything that is known about the area of interest. Again, the researcher needs to ask questions.

✦ What research has been done on the topic?
✦ Are there relevant theories or models that can guide the search for an answer to the research question?
✦ Is there other background information that would be useful?

The nursing, rehabilitation, and research bodies of literature are pivotal in asking a research question that will make a significant contribution to the care of persons with disabilities. It is crucial to know the current opinions about the topic and the implications of possible answers to the research question.

✦ Who cares about the answer?
✦ Will the answer to the research question justify the investment of time and energy needed to answer the question?

One of the major deterrents to the development of a systematic knowledge base and theory of rehabilitation nursing is the fragmentation of the research endeavor. The findings of numerous small studies with significant limitations cannot be generalized to similar situations. The rehabilitation nurse researcher would do well to step back and ask how and where the research question fits into what has already been done.

✦ Is it possible to replicate a study?
✦ How might the current research question be framed to extend previous findings?

In summary, asking the "right" research question is probably the most critical step in the research process. It must be possible to answer the question, the answer must be important, the question must build on previous knowledge, and the resources must be available to answer the question. Collaboration among members of the rehabilitation team can help to ensure that the question asked will contribute to the knowledge base of rehabilitation nursing. The way the question is asked will determine the type of data necessary to answer the question. Determining what factors predispose someone with a spinal cord injury to decubitus ulcers can be accomplished through a retrospective chart review or a prospective study of the characteristics of individuals who do and who do not develop decubitus ulcers. Asking which of several interventions will predictably prevent the development of decubitus ulcers in this population would require an experimental study with a large number of participants.

✦ Deciding what to measure

Once the research question has been asked, the next task is to decide what information is necessary to answer the research question "How will things be counted or measured, and how data will be obtained?" These decisions will depend largely on the type of question asked. Research questions that ask "What is it?" will differ considerably from those that ask "How can I make X happen?" Questions about physiologic phenomena will require different measures than psychological phenomena. Assessment of different types of mattresses will require the use of a tissue interface pressure monitor if the question is which cushion has the greatest pressure-relieving properties. However, if the question relates to patient comfort, a questionnaire about the various aspects of comfort will be more appropriate.

✦ Deciding how to measure

Reviewing the literature will provide clues about how other researchers have measured the phenomenon of interest and whether the instruments they used were reliable and valid. Compilations of research instruments is another source; for example, Strickland and Waltz have edited four volumes of instruments to measure nursing outcomes (Strickland & Waltz, 1988, 1990; Waltz & Strickland, 1988, 1990), and Frank-Stromborg (1988) have reviewed instruments appropriate for care of the person with cancer. Israel, Kozarevic, and Sartoruis (1984) have critiqued commonly used psychosocial measures for use with older adults. Instruments used to generate research data must actually (validly) and consistently (reliably) measure the phenomenon of interest. All too often researchers have not performed an adequate search for instruments or believe that their view of a situation is unique and that no existing instruments will suffice for data collection. The use of untested instruments contributes little to the knowledge base for rehabilitation nursing practice. The process of establishing the reliability and validity of new instruments is intensive and time consuming (Waltz, Strickland, & Lenz, 1991). Reliability and validity issues also are relevant for physiologic measurement. How reliable is the thermometer, the sphygmometer, the pressure transducer? How are these instruments calibrated, and when and how do they need to be recalibrated?

Deciding how data needed to answer the research question will be obtained also is important. Often the choice of study design is dependent on the quality of the clinical data available and the resources for additional data collection. Nurses in clinical practice seldom can commit their time to data collection that is not a usual part of their client care. Obtaining funding for data collection and other aspects of the research process is becoming increasingly difficult as local and national financial resources diminish.

The creative use of existing data is one solution. Often the variables of interest are routinely recorded in the client's medical record. Chart reviews may appear to be an easy source of data; however, charts often are incomplete, and the reliability of those who have assessed and recorded information cannot be ensured. Large research projects tend to collect more data than necessary to meet the specific aims of the study. These data may be available for secondary analysis. Academicians who may have students available are another source of assistance with data collection.

The researcher also needs to determine how precisely the phenomenon of interest needs to be measured. Is it sufficient to know if a urine colony count is over 100,000 organisms per milliliter, or do the specific organisms need to be identified? Is the colony count alone sufficient, or is it important to know if the client has symptoms of infection? Is it sufficient to know the presence or absence of a decubitus ulcer, or is the volume of the ulcer and its appearance necessary to answer the research question?

The outcome of a proposed intervention needs to be considered carefully. Is it reasonable to expect that the intervention will produce a large effect, in which case a measurement instrument that is sensitive to large changes will be sufficient. However, if the effect is expected to be small, more precise measurement instruments will be required. Recovery from a traumatic injury is a slow process. Progress is made in millimeters, not in kilometers. Measurement instruments must be able to measure the small gains along the way to recovery.

When deciding what to measure, the following questions need to be addressed:

+ What is the phenomenon to be counted or measured?
+ How precisely does the phenomenon need to be measured?
+ How have others measured this phenomenon?
+ Are the instruments previously used reliable and valid?
+ Are these instruments available for use at an affordable cost?
+ Is a special skill or training needed to administer or score the instrument? If so, is there someone available with those skills?
+ What is the expected effect size of the intervention?

+ Deciding when to measure

Rehabilitation is a long-term process. Determining when to measure the outcome of rehabilitation is a persistent challenge. Again, the nature of the question that was asked will define when data need to be collected. Craig (1990) was interested in the adaptations that pregnant spinal cord–injured women were required to make. She could have selected a sample of pregnant women with a spinal cord injury and followed the adaptations they made over the course of their pregnancy. Rather, she chose an *ex post facto* design in which women with a spinal cord injury who had already delivered a child were questioned about the physical and emotional aspects during pregnancy, labor, and postpartum. Dille et al. (1993) were interested in whether vinyl urinary drainage bags could be used as long as 4 weeks. Their research question required that they measure the colony count of urinary drainage bags at 1, 2, 3, and 4 weeks. Gift and Austin (1992) took 8 weeks to determine if identified differences in depression and dyspnea persisted over time following a systematic movement program for persons with chronic obstructive pulmonary disease (COPD).

Human functioning varies over time. It is well known that temperature, heart rate, and respirations vary over 24 hours. There are biologic rhythms that occur daily, weekly, monthly, and seasonally. Research that measures a rhythmic phenomenon must be planned to account for these cyclic changes. Depression is more prevalent during the winter months. A researcher who is measuring the effect of a program to decrease depression will be at a disadvantage in showing positive results if the intervention occurs during the summer and the outcome is measured during the winter.

Just as some phenomena vary in a cyclic fashion, others change over time. Developmental changes in young children are good examples of things that change permanently. Research that asks a question about how best to teach a child a psychomotor skill will be confounded by the normal development of these skills. Recovery from a traumatic injury to the nervous system evolves over time. Designing a study to measure the effect of an intervention must take into consideration the normal evolution of the phenomenon.

When research participants are available to provide data is another consideration in deciding when to collect data. Inpatients who are actively involved in therapy programs for many hours a day will not be available during those times to complete questionnaires or answer interview questions. Nurses may not be willing to come before or stay after their scheduled work period to provide data for research. Community-dwelling individuals may work, engage in leisure activities, or take vacations—making the timing of data collection a juggling act.

Research questions that require data collected at several points in time present additional challenges. Each additional data collection point represents a chance to lose research participants. Acutely ill individuals may become too sick to continue participation or they may die. Alternatively they may recover, leave the hospital, and become unavailable for further data collection. Participants may tire of answering the same questions or giving samples of bodily fluids.

Ask the following questions when deciding when to measure the phenomenon of interest:

✦ Is there a cyclic phenomenon associated with the event to be measured?

✦ Is there a normal developmental process that will confound the phenomenon of interest?

✦ What is the earliest time that the phenomenon of interest will be present?

✦ How often does the phenomenon need to be measured?

✦ At what intervals does the phenomenon need to be counted or measured?

✦ How long will it take for an intervention to make a measurable difference?

✦ How long can a change be expected to last?

✦ Is it prudent to depend on memory of past events?

✦ Are resources available to collect data at appropriate times?

✦ Will the people who need to provide the data be available at the planned times of data collection?

✦ What is the risk of people dropping out of the study before all the data are collected?

Identifying the Participants

The participants in a research project can be individuals, groups of individuals who share similar characteristics, nurses or other members of the rehabilitation team, a specific program, or an organizational entity such as a nursing unit. The research question will determine from whom the data are obtained.

The most significant limitation of the existing rehabilitation nursing research stem from the way in which the research participants were selected. The ultimate purpose of rehabilitation research is to generate knowledge that can be applied to the care of individuals with actual or potential disabilities; in other words the findings must be generalizable. Individuals who are chosen to participate in a research project because they are convenient to the investigator do not provide information that can be generalized beyond the situation from which they were chosen. It is important to think about the population of all people, events, or practice sites that represent the phenomenon of interest. Including only young white males may control for certain sociocultural factors, but the research cannot be generalized to women, to people of color, or to children or older adults.

It is rarely possible to include all possible elements of the population. It is not possible to include all adults with a urinary tract infection or all clients receiving rehabilitation. Sampling is used to select a subset of the population of interest for inclusion in the proposed study. Most often, individuals with disabilities comprise the sample in rehabilitation nursing research. Sometimes a family unit, a nurse-client dyad, a nursing care unit, shifts worked, or a geographic community make up the sample.

In general, the more representative the participants are of the larger group (population) from which they are sampled, the more generalizable will be the findings of the study. Ideally each person or other sampling element in the population of interest has an equal chance of being selected to participate. Resource limitations make obtaining a probability sample difficult. Seldom does the rehabilitation nurse researcher have access to the entire population of interest. It is not reasonable to enumerate all adults who have a specific chronic disease for the purpose of randomly selecting individuals from this population. Often the phenomenon of interest to rehabilitation nurses is rare or unpredictable, making probability sampling not feasible. For example, the occurrence of pressure ulcers in the rehabilitation setting is so low that the ability to select for study those individuals who will experience this problem is low. The use of nonprobability samples severely limits the generalizability of the study findings. We simply cannot assume that those selected nonrandomly represent the population from which they were drawn. However, nonprobability sampling is often the only feasible way of accessing research participants.

Access to research participants often presents challenges for rehabilitation nurses. Hospitalized individuals may be too sick or too busy with rehabilitation programs to participate in studies that require a significant commitment to providing information. Those who are no longer hospitalized may be difficult to access. Often community organizations can provide access to participants. For example, the people with COPD in Gift's and Austin's (1992) study were participants in a Better Breathers group of the local affiliate of the American Lung Association.

A few of the many challenges to identifying the research participants have been raised. Some strategies for meeting these challenges consist of including all individuals who meet the study criteria, not just those whom staff determine will make "good" research participants. Researchers also need to ask who has access to the potential research participants. Is permission to recruit participants needed from a physician, administrator, or agency?

Information must be obtained about the characteristics of those individuals who decline to participate. Are they of different gender, age, socioeconomic status, disability level, and so forth, than those who participated? Why did they choose not to participate? It is also important to compare the characteristics of the research sample obtained to the population they represent. Are they the same age, gender, socioeconomic group, and so forth, as the population to which the findings will be generalized.

The size of the sample is determined by balancing the confidence needed in the findings with the cost of obtaining a sample. Knowledge of the results of similar studies and the estimate of the strength of the expected relationships are necessary to determine a reasonable sample size. Rehabilitation nursing research has been plagued with problems of small sample size that do not permit meaningful conclusions to be drawn. An experienced researcher or statistician can help to determine the size of the sample and the point beyond which increasing the sample size is not cost-effective. Using a research design suited to small sample size is another strategy for conducting research in the clinical area.

Selecting the research participants presents one of the greatest challenges for researchers who are interested in generalizing their findings beyond the sample of people or events that were studied. Some questions to consider in selecting participants follow:

✦ How prevalent is the condition or event that will be studied?

✦ What is the big picture? What population is of interest?

✦ Are there representatives of this population available to the investigators?

✦ Who controls access to potential participants?

✦ What is the likelihood that those sampled will actually participate?

✦ Are sufficient resources (time, money, clients, patience) available to take the time necessary to obtain a sample?

✦ How will data be obtained about the characteristics of those who decide not to participate?

✦ How many people or events are necessary to have confidence in the findings of the study?

Protecting Participants

The foremost consideration in designing a research study is the protection of human rights. Consent to participate must be informed and voluntary. The participants must be allowed, at any time in the course of the research, to withdraw without penalty. The benefits of the research must outweigh the risks involved in participation. Finally, the investigator must be qualified to carry out the research. Except in rare circumstances, participants must sign an informed consent statement. When only medical records are used, the consent of each client is not required; however, the researcher must sign an oath of confidentiality, ensuring that identity of the individuals and their confidentiality will be protected. Research must be approved by the appropriate Institutional Review Board (IRB) before data collection can begin.

The risks and benefits of participating or not participating in the proposed study must be addressed when preparing an application for the use of human subjects in research. Invasion of privacy is almost always cited as a risk. How personal and sensitive is the information sought? Some topics such as religion, politics, sex, and human immunodeficiency virus (HIV) status are viewed by many as sensitive in nature. How essential is this information, and what are the risks to the individual that result from sharing the information? Is a proposed intervention more painful or risky than the standard of care? Is there reasonable evidence that new treatments will be better than current practice?

What are the benefits of participation? Benefits may provide participants with feedback about their performance on research instruments, a summary of the study results, an opportunity to improve some aspect of their life, and altruistic benefits such as helping others in similar circumstances. If participants are to be compensated for their participation with money or gifts, the amount of the compensation must be congruent with the demands of the research protocol and not be so great as to make people agree to participate because they need the compensation.

Withholding or withdrawing a treatment that has strong evidence for being beneficial is problematic. Ouellette and Ahn (1993) proposed a two-treatment, crossover design with participants serving as their own controls. After the study began, they faced the dilemma of removing the treatment from the first experimental group. They changed the study design so that all participants were in the control condition for the first 2 months of the study and in the experimental condition for the second 2 months.

After the human subjects application is completed, it must be submitted to the appropriate IRB. Obtaining permission to conduct a study from human subjects review boards can be difficult and time consuming. Many of the challenges stem from review boards that were constituted to review medically oriented research. Nurses who are proposing to do research in the clinical arena must be prepared to deal with these challenges. Find out who is on the IRB. Is there a nurse or someone else who is sensitive to nursing research issues and how nursing research may differ in purpose and design from medical research? Talk to key decision-makers early in the planning process to ensure that their concerns are addressed. Discuss their experience with other nurses who have gone through the review process with this IRB. Ask to review a successful application. Ally yourself with others who can exert influence on the approval of the study, either as coinvestigators, sponsors, or whatever the agency requires. Some agencies require that a physician "sponsor" nursing research. Be prepared to balance the demands of the IRB with integrity and ownership of the study.

Smoothing the human subjects review process involves asking the following questions:

✦ What is the risk/benefit ratio of participation?

✦ What forms and steps are required by this institution?

✦ Who is on the IRB?

✦ Is someone sympathetic to nursing research in a decision-making position?

✦ How often does the committee meet, and when are the deadlines for submitting applications?

✦ How long does it take to complete the entire review process and be approved to begin the study?

✦ If revisions to the application are necessary, how are these done and what review process is implemented for the changes?

✦ Where are you willing to compromise?

Selecting a Research Design

The research design is like a script for a play. Just as a play script includes the words for the actors, how they should be played, and the sequence of scenes, the research design tells what activities the researchers and participants should be performing and the order in which the activities should occur. Randomized controlled trials are considered the gold standard for clinical research. Often, however, randomized controlled trials are difficult, impractical, or unethical in the clinical setting. Other designs strengthen generalizability or address cause and effect. The level of theory development that the research question addresses will determine the kind of research design that is necessary.

Studies that aim to describe phenomena may utilize historical or document review designs, surveys, or qualitative studies that use descriptive methods for reporting data. Determining relationships requires research designs that can make connections between various conditions or events. Data collection strategies such as survey instruments, interviews, and physiologic measurements may be the same as those used in studies describing phenomena but will be designed to answer questions about relationships. Studies that attempt to test relationships and produce situations require experimental designs.

The rehabilitation nursing literature is replete with examples of study designs that allowed the investigator to describe phenomena such as attitudes toward disability, outcomes of trauma, psychosocial effects of illness or disability, perceptions of care, and so forth. Nurses considering a study to describe a phenomenon would do well to examine what a new study will contribute to the knowledge base for practice. Will the findings of a descriptive study really make an impact on practice? Is there a way to capitalize on the descriptive work that has already been done and bring about a higher level of understanding of the phenomenon? Is a review that integrates and interprets the published and unpublished data about the phenomenon appropriate (Cooper, 1989; Noblit & Hare, 1988)? What are the similarities and differences, for example, in coping with various forms of disability?

Studies that compare two or more nursing interventions are common. Many of these studies have small samples that were conveniently selected. Many failed to control for factors that might have influenced the outcome of the study, such as nonequivalent groups at the beginning of the study. Caution must be exercised when constituting two or more groups to receive different interventions. Take, for example, a study to compare the effectiveness of a group and an individual cardiac rehabilitation program. One group of men who have had a myocardial infarction come to the hospital gymnasium three times a week and participate in an individualized exercise program. Another group of men engage in their exercise program three times a week at home. If the men were not randomly assigned to the gymnasium or home exercise groups, there is a likelihood that there will be differences in these men unrelated to location that may influence the outcome of the exercise program. Think about all of the differences between the two groups of men that might make them dissimilar. For example, those men who chose to exercise at home may have physical limitations that make it difficult for them to come to the hospital—and that will confound their participation in and possible outcome of an exercise program.

When two groups are to be compared, the groups must be equivalent at the beginning of the study. Random assignment to the groups is preferred to self-selected groups. Matching participants is another way to ensure that groups are comparable; however, matching participants on characteristics important to the outcome of the study often is difficult. Some research designs, such as single-subject and case study designs, are powerful methods of conducting research when few potential research participants are available.

The challenges of conducting research in the clinical area are no more apparent than when selecting a research design to test relationships and to produce situations. Large experimental trials usually are beyond the scope of rehabilitation nursing research. There are research designs, such as multiple-case replication designs (Yin, 1994) and single-case experimental designs (Kazdin, 1982), that are appropriate for rehabilitation nursing research. One major advantage of these designs is that cases can be added together over time to produce powerful data in support of therapeutic nursing interventions.

A good exercise in the process of selecting a research design is to read reports of similar research and brainstorm with a colleague all the reasons why you should not take the study findings as the ultimate truth. How many of those reasons can you overcome in the study you are designing?

Questions that a researcher should ask when selecting a research design include the following:
+ What is the research question that is being asked?
+ Does the question require one or multiple data collection points?
+ How likely is the phenomenon of interest to change over time?
+ What are all the factors that might influence the findings in the proposed study?
+ Are there professional colleagues who will collaborate to increase the sample size?
+ Can the ideal design be implemented in your practice setting?
+ Where can you compromise on the ideal design and still maintain the scientific integrity of the study?

Writing the Research Plan

A detailed plan, or protocol, for how the study will be carried out must be articulated before the study begins. This plan will force the researchers to think through each phase of the study and anticipate problems before they arise.
+ Who is eligible to participate in the study?
+ How will eligible participants be identified?
+ How will a control group, if appropriate, be constituted?
+ What procedures will be followed to enroll the participants in the study?
+ What data will be collected?
+ Who will gather the information?
+ In what manner will the data be collected?
+ How will data be recorded and by whom?
+ Will a treatment be administered? If so, when and by whom?
+ How will the data be managed (e.g., computerized)?

Implementing the Project

It is shortsighted to expect that implementation of a research project in a clinical setting will happen exactly as it was designed. Real research participants and nurses do not follow rigid guidelines for their behavior. As part of the planning process, it is essential to bring to a conscious level the things that might change that would alter the research design and to develop contingency plans. What if staffing levels change; critical staff members no longer work on the unit; individuals with the desired characteristics disappear; new data become available about an intervention; the organizational structure of the unit changes; chart data are missing? Thinking about these questions before starting a research project will minimize surprises after the project is begun.

The adaptability of the research team is essential to meet the ever-changing healthcare environments. Each member of the team must be willing and able to recognize when a research project is not going according to the written plan and to work with other team members to evaluate the changes. Perhaps the changes are insignificant and will have no effect on the researcher's ability to answer the research question. Conceivably the alterations in data collection or applying a treatment will significantly alter the nature of the project. It is also important during implementation of research to remain alert to what is going on in the environment. For example, the outcome of an educational intervention to increase the use of bicycle helmets may be altered when the public media points out that someone was seriously injured because they were not wearing a helmet. A study of the use of prn pain medication may be influenced by the staff nurses' knowledge of the study and their increased attention to client requests for medication.

Perhaps the most important element of tracking the actual implementation of a research project is the use of a research journal. This hardbound book allows researchers to write down observations about the conduct of the research and to document decisions made during the implementation process and the rationale for changes in the research protocol. The research journal is also a good place to note insights about the research process, the study itself, or connections to other things that previously were not recognized.

Analyzing the Data

Plans for data analysis must be made as the research project is being planned. All too often researchers get to the data analysis stage and find that they do not have the appropriate data to answer the research question. If the researcher is asking whether an intervention relieves pain, a dichotomous response of "yes" or "no" will be sufficient. However, a question about degree of pain will require ordinal data that range from no pain to severe pain. Some statistic procedures require categories of data, whereas others require data points that are equally spaced along a continuum. It is relatively easy to recode ordinal data to categories; it is impossible to convert categoric data into ordinal data. The research can recode a 10-point scale of pain intensity into categories of mild, moderate, and severe. There is no way to convert mild, moderate, and severe pain into a 10-point pain intensity scale. Deciding early regarding the precision of measurement needed to answer the research question is critical. It is best to err on the side of more detail than is necessary.

The research question will determine the kind of data analysis that is required. "What will happen if . . . ?" and "How can I make "X" happen?" research questions require the use of inferential statistics that provide a precise and systematic way to generalize from the findings of an individual study to a larger population. Descriptive statistics are important when inferential statistics are used so that the reader can understand the bases for the inferential tests of significance. The clinical researcher needs to look beyond the statistical tests and the magical p-value to determine the clinical significance of the findings. A difference of 5 mm in the circumference of a stage IV pressure ulcer may be highly significant statistically but has no clinical significance.

Rarely are data collected for every variable for every research participant. Electronic equipment fails, charts are incomplete, respondents skip questions on paper and pencil instruments, data from one point in time is missing, and respondents misinterpret directions for completing instruments. Missing data can be minimized during the study by making frequent checks on the data to be sure that instruments are working properly, that data are recorded, and that people clearly understand how and when to record information. It is relatively easy to have a participant complete a missing questionnaire page or to record a physiologic

measure when the omission is noticed immediately. The researcher needs to anticipate issues of missing data and make decisions early in the research process.

+ How will missing data be handled?
+ How much data can be missing before the participant is dropped from the study?
+ Is missing data tolerable or do means need to be substituted for the missing data?
+ If means substitution is used, will the mean of the total group or the mean of the individual's other responses be used?

Analysis of research data requires resources that often are not available to practice-based rehabilitation nurse researchers. Access to computers and expertise to interpret the output from statistical programs seldom are found on nursing care units. Large institutions may have resources available to support data analysis. Collaboration with faculty from schools of nursing, biostatistics, public health, and sociology are other sources of needed assistance.

Planning for analysis of data requires that the following questions be answered:

+ Are narrative reports or descriptive or inferential statistics necessary to answer the research question?
+ Will the data necessary to answer the question be available?
+ How will missing data be handled?
+ What resources (hardware, software, consultants) are available to help with data analysis and interpretation?
+ Will there be costs involved in accessing the necessary resources?

Accessing Research Resources

Accessing the resources to conduct research in the clinical area presents a large challenge for rehabilitation nurses. Resources necessary to plan a research study may be difficult to obtain and require forethought. Designing studies that will answer questions raised by clinical practice may require consultation with seasoned researchers and statisticians. Once planned, staffing patterns are never adequate to allow time for data collection, even by the most dedicated nurses. Purchase of data collection instruments, photocopying costs, data entry, and preparation of manuscripts and posters can be costly and time consuming.

The first step in accessing resources for rehabilitation nursing research is determining exactly what is needed and the associated costs, even if the costs are going to be contributed by the agency.

+ Will access to a database be needed to identify potential research participants (e.g., medical records department or community-based agency)?
+ Who will determine whether or not someone is eligible to participate in the study, contact potential participants, and enroll them in the study?
+ Are the data collection instruments available?
+ What forms need to be purchased or duplicated?
+ Will recruitment letters, research instruments, reminder notices, or thank you notes be mailed?
+ Will the participants be compensated?
+ Is there secretarial service for typing institutional review board applications, data collection forms, and assisting in grant application and manuscript preparation?

✦ Who will prepare the IRB applications, attend committee meetings, and negotiate with the reviewers?

✦ Will data collectors be volunteers, hourly employees, or salaried employees?

✦ If data collectors work beyond the anticipated hours, how will they be compensated?

✦ Is special equipment necessary for data collection (e.g., special mattresses or cushions, ultrasound to measure residual urine volumes)?

✦ Are laboratory services or supplies needed?

✦ Where will paper, pencils, and other office supplies be obtained?

✦ Who will prepare data for qualitative or quantitative analysis (e.g., code instruments, transcribe interviews)?

✦ Who will enter the data into the computer database?

✦ Who will analyze the data and interpret the results?

✦ Are the needed computers and software available for data management and analysis?

✦ Where will the study results be shared (e.g., local, regional, or national meeting)?

✦ What resources are available to prepare slides or poster presentations of the findings?

Consultants frequently are willing to provide help in exchange for access to the data or coauthorship of a manuscript. Students in undergraduate and graduate programs customarily are searching for a research project or the opportunity to collect or analyze data that will fulfill course requirements. Faculty at colleges and universities may have large programs of research that can provide some support for smaller research studies.

Money for rehabilitation nursing research is available from organizations such as the Rehabilitation Nursing Foundation; Sigma Theta Tau, International; and the American Nurses Foundation. Local chapters of Sigma Theta Tau and other nursing organizations also may have small-grant money available. National health agencies that address the needs of a particular client population often make grants available for research. Pharmaceutical and medical equipment companies may be willing to support clinically based research that utilizes their products. Sometimes the healthcare agency has seed money for pilot studies that have promise of improving cost-effective care or obtaining future funding from another source.

Talk with colleagues. Look at funding acknowledgments in published research. Think about who might be interested enough in the findings of a study to provide resources to do the study. Obtain the funding priorities from potential granting agencies. Get whatever assistance is necessary to complete the required proposal forms. Understand any conditions for accepting the money. It is possible that the funding agency may have an agenda different from the researchers, and certain conditions for accepting the funding may bias the findings or otherwise compromise the scientific integrity of the study.

Reporting Study Results

No research is completed until the findings are shared with colleagues. Reporting results begins with those closest to the study: rehabilitation team members who have been involved in the study or who were aware of its existence. Initially findings may be shared informally, but more formal presentations are necessary if the research is expected to influence rehabilitation nursing practice. Oral presentations can be made to the staff and clients where the study was conducted; at local meetings of the Association of Rehabilitation Nurses and similar organizations; and at regional, national, or international meetings of rehabilitation groups. Poster presentations of the research findings are ideal for posting in the agency where the study was conducted and at professional meetings. Written reports of research may range from an abstract of the study and its findings to a full-length monograph or book. Most commonly research is reported in relatively brief form in a research or clinically focused professional journal.

The report of research needs to include specifics about what was done so that others can evaluate the scientific integrity of the study and determine whether the findings are appropriate for utilization. Reports of research need to acknowledge the sources of financial and other support for conducting the study. The reader of a research report should be able to answer the following questions:

✦ What was the purpose of this research?

✦ What specific objectives or aims were accomplished by this study?

✦ What was the knowledge base on which this study was based?

✦ How were the participants in the study recruited and assigned to the study groups?

✦ How many potential participants did not enter or complete the study?

✦ If two groups were used, were the groups equivalent at the start of the study?

✦ What procedures were carried out?

✦ What level of measurement was recorded for each variable measured?

✦ What safeguards were built into the study to ensure that the procedures were implemented consistently throughout the study?

✦ How were missing data handled?

✦ How were data analyzed?

✦ What do the findings mean?

✦ How do these findings relate to previous studies in the field?

✦ What is the next step in studying this phenomenon?

Utilizing Research Findings

Not everyone needs to be involved in generating research findings. Every rehabilitation nurse, however, is obligated to utilize research findings appropriately to improve the care of clients with rehabilitation needs. Perhaps the most important part of utilizing research findings is determining the applicability of the research to practice. Stetler and Marram (1976) proposed three phases in research utilization that are relevant for rehabilitation nursing: (1) validation, (2) comparative evaluation, and (3) decision-making. In the first phase, validation, the scientific merit of the study must be determined. A careful critique of the research is done that includes the problem studied, literature reviewed, setting and participants, design, instruments and measures, data analysis, and discussion and conclusions. The scientific and practice components of the research are analyzed at each phase of the critique. Killien (1988) has outlined the questions that need to be asked about each phase of the

---

EVALUATING RESEARCH FOR PRACTICE USE

A. Problem studied and literature review
   1. Scientific evaluation
      a. Is problem clearly identified?
      b. Is significance of problem discussed?
      c. Was research justified by literature?
      d. Is relationship to previous research clear?
      e. Was conceptual framework evident? Appropriate?
      f. Is specific purpose of study clear? Are variables defined? Are hypotheses stated and well founded?
   2. Practice evaluation
      a. Is this problem significant to nursing practice?
      b. Does the framework "fit" with what the nurse knows about nursing practice and the phenomenon?
B. Setting and subjects
   1. Scientific evaluation
      a. Is population described? Sample described?
      b. How were subjects recruited? Sampled?
      c. What were the sources of sampling error?
      d. Is sample size adequate?
      e. Were subjects' rights adequately protected?
      f. What was the setting for the study? Laboratory? Community? Hospital?
   2. Practice evaluation
      a. Are the clients typical? Are they similar to the clients in the nurse's setting? Could differences possibly influence results?
      b. Is the setting typical? In what ways is it similar and different from the nurse's setting?
      c. Would clients be likely to participate if this was not a study?
C. Design
   1. Scientific evaluation
      a. What type of design was used (e.g., descriptive, correlational, longitudinal, experimental, cross-sectional)?
      b. Is design appropriate to answer question asked?
      c. Are appropriate controls included?
      d. Can confounding variables be identified?
   2. Practice evaluation
      a. Would it be possible to measure the same outcomes if findings were applied in the nurse's setting?
      b. Are methods adequately described to permit replication?

D. Instruments and measures
   1. Scientific evaluation
      a. To what extent are measures valid and reliable?
      b. Were reliability and validity tested and reported in this study?
      c. Were measures adequately described to determine their relevance to study purpose and findings?
      d. Could the measures have influenced findings?
   2. Practice evaluation
      a. Is there any assurance that these measures would be meaningful and accurate in the clinical setting?
      b. Are these data collection methods feasible in the nurse's setting?
E. Data analysis
   1. Scientific evaluation
      a. How were the data distributed (e.g., frequency distribution)?
      b. Do methods answer the questions posed?
      c. Are statistical tests appropriate and applicable to questions or hypothesis?
      d. Are data presented clearly in tables?
   2. Practice evaluation
      a. Do the data fit the clinical picture?
      b. What are the probabilities that findings are due to chance? Or to some other variable?
      c. Are findings clinically as well as statistically significant?
F. Discussion and conclusions
   1. Scientific evaluation
      a. Are conclusions stated clearly?
      b. Are conclusions based on the data presented?
      c. Are limitations and alternative explanations presented?
      d. Are findings related to the original framework and purpose of the study?
      e. Are results generalized to population studied?
      f. Are conclusions appropriate, given a. to e. above?
   2. Practice evaluation
      a. Does the nurse agree with the author's conclusion?
      b. What decision does the conclusion promote?
      c. Should the literature be further examined for more information?
      d. Do the findings replicate previous findings? Suggest innovation or change?
      e. Do the findings increase the nurse's sensitivity to the problem but not lead to direct action?
      f. Does the nurse need more information from the researcher?

Adapted from Disseminating and using research findings by M.G. Killien, in *Nursing Research: Theory and Practice* (pp. 479-497) by N.F. Woods and M. Catanzaro, 1988, St. Louis: Mosby–Year Book. Copyright 1988 by Mosby–Year Book. Adapted by permission.

research process in order to validate the study (see box, p. 58).

Only if the study is found to have scientific merit is the second phase of research utilization considered. In phase 2, comparative evaluation, the study is assessed for its usefulness in a particular practice situation. Also considered is the feasibility for implementation in practice. If the study is scientifically sound and relevant to the practice situation, the final phase, decision-making, is undertaken. The nurse can decide whether or not to use the findings cognitively or directly in practice. Studies that are descriptive or that lack sufficient reliability or validity may be applied cognitively to enhance understanding of nursing practice phenomena. Decisions to apply the research to practice may confirm existing practice or require modifying or changing existing practice.

Horsley, Crane, Crabtree, and Qood (1983) developed a model for research utilization called Conduct and Utilization of Research in Nursing (CURN). The CURN project identified six phases of the research utilization process that begins with identifying the nursing practice problem that needs a solution and assessing the research base for solving the problem. The research base is evaluated in relation to the identified practice problem, the organization's practices and values, and the potential costs and benefits of adopting the knowledge. Next the scientific merit of the knowledge base is examined. Finally, a clinical trial of the innovation is conducted in the new setting and a decision is made to reject, modify, or adopt the innovation.

The complexity of implementing planned change within an organization is exemplified by the attempt by Sparkman, Quigley, and McCarthy (1991) to implement the CURN model in a general medicine unit and in a rehabilitation unit. Their attempts to address the lack of collaboration between the physicians and nurses were thwarted because one unit used primary nursing, whereas the other used a team nursing approach, and there were differences in staffing patterns. High staff turnover rates, staffing shortages, administrative changes, and the differences in activity level between the units impeded their progress in implementing the proposed changes.

Predicting the Future

What is the future of rehabilitation nursing research? The changing healthcare climate with growing concerns about the spiraling cost of healthcare, an emphasis on cost-effectiveness of care, and an outcome-oriented society is likely to change significantly the rehabilitation nursing care environment in the near future. Now is the time for rehabilitation nurses to stake a claim on the rehabilitation of individuals with long-term illnesses and disabilities. The integration of practice, research, and theory will provide a knowledge base that will ensure that rehabilitation nurses are included in whatever configuration is taken by the future healthcare system. What, exactly, do rehabilitation nurses do to help clients achieve independence in physical activities? What nursing care measures are effective in decreasing complications of disability, such as urinary tract and respiratory infections and decubitus ulcers?

Rehabilitation nursing needs to focus away from describing certain phenomena such as coping with disability or attitudes toward illness and disability. Studies need to be critically reviewed, and theories that may explain the findings across studies must be developed and tested. Studies that relate phenomena in such a way that we can begin to predict the outcome of selected client characteristics on rehabilitation is the critical next step in the development of a knowledge base for practice.

Research designs appropriate for small research samples will allow studies to build on one another. Single case studies can be conducted with small numbers of individuals and added to other cases, similarly studied, over time and at other sites. Multisite studies planned by nurses can evolve through the nurses who are employed by large healthcare corporations that operate multiple healthcare facilities. Members of the local chapters of the Rehabilitation Nurses' Association are well placed to plan multisite studies.

As the healthcare financing system changes, the charge for nursing care will no longer be included with the charge for the room. Clients will be billed for nursing service just as they are for occupational and physical therapy, laboratory tests, and consultation with the nutritionist or psychologist. What are rehabilitation nurses' services worth? What, exactly, do they contribute to the health and well-being of persons with long-term illnesses and disabilities? Answers to questions such as these will be required to ensure the future of rehabilitation nursing in a rapidly evolving national healthcare system.

REFERENCES

Acorn, S., & Bampton, E. (1992). Patients' loneliness: A challenge for rehabilitation nurses. *Rehabilitation Nursing, 17,* 22-25.

Ades, P.A., Waldmann, M.L., Polk, D.M., & Coflesky, J.T. (1992). Referral patterns and exercise response in the rehabilitation of female coronary patients aged greater than or equal to 62 years. *American Journal of Cardiology, 69,* 1422-1425.

Altman, B.M., & Smith, R.T. (1990). Rehabilitation service utilization models: Changes in the opportunity structure for disabled women. *International Journal of Rehabilitation Research, 12,* 149-156.

Altman, B.M., & Smith, R.T. (1992). Impact of rehabilitation on psychological distress: Gender differences. *International Journal of Rehabilitation Research, 15,* 75-81.

American Nurses' Association. (1980). *ANA social policy statement.* Kansas City, MO: Author.

American Nurses' Association Commission on Nursing Research. (1981). *Guidelines for the investigative function of nurses.* Kansas City, MO: Author.

Bachman, C. (1990). Producing—and using—nursing research [Editorial]. *Rehabilitation Nursing, 15,* 176.

Burns, N.G., & Grove, S.K. (1993). *The practice of nursing research: Conduct, critique and utilization* (2nd ed.). Philadelphia: W.B. Saunders.

Carey, R.G., Seibert, J.H., & Posavac, E.J. (1988). Who makes the most progress in inpatient rehabilitation? An analysis of functional gains. *Archives of Physical Medicine and Rehabilitation, 69,* 337-343.

Cooper H.M. (1984). *The integrative research review: Moving beyond metaanalysis.* Beverly Hills: Sage Publications.

Craig, D.I. (1990). The adaptation to pregnancy of spinal cord injured women. *Rehabilitation Nursing, 15,* 6-9.

Davis, C.S., & Acton, P. (1988). Treatment of the elderly brain-injured patient. Experience in a traumatic brain injury unit. *Journal of the American Geriatric Society, 36,* 225-229.

Dayhoff, N.E. (1993). Developing a vision of rehabilitation nursing practice. *Rehabilitation Nursing Research, 2,* 2.

Dille, C.A., Kirchhoff, K.T., Sullivan, J.J., & Larson, E. (1993). Increasing the wearing time of vinyl urinary drainage bags by decontamination with bleach. *Archives of Physical Medicine and Rehabilitation, 74,* 431-437.

Fetter, M.S., Feetham, S.L., D'Apolito, K., Chaze, B.A., Fink, A., Frink, B.B., Houghart, M.K., & Rushton, C.H. (1989). Randomized clinical trials: Issues for researchers. *Nursing Research, 38,* 117-120.

Forsyth, G.L. (1980). Analysis of the concept of empathy: Illustration of one approach. *Advances in Nursing Science, 2,* 33-42.

Gift, A.G., & Austin, D.J. (1992). The effects of a program of systematic movement on COPD patients. *Rehabilitation Nursing, 17,* 6-10, 25.

Granger, C.V., Hamilton, B.B., & Fiedler, R.C. (1992). Discharge outcome after stroke rehabilitation. *Stroke, 23,* 978-982.

Helm, P., Engel, T., Holm, A., Kristiansen, V.B., & Rosendahl, S. (1986). Function after lower limb amputation. *Acta Orthopaedica Scandinavica, 57,* 154-157.

Hoeman, S.P., Dayhoff, N.E., & Thompson, T.C. (1993). The initial RNF research survey: Rehabilitation nursing research interests of ARN members. *Rehabilitation Nursing, 18,* 40-42.

Horsley J.A., Crane, J., Crabtree, K., & Qood, D.J. (1983). *Using research to improve nursing practice: A guide.* New York: Grune & Stratton.

Israel, L., Kozarevic, D., & Sartoruis, N. (1984). *Source book of geriatric assessment.* Basel: S. Karger.

Kazdin A.E. (1982). *Single-case research designs. Methods for clinical and applied settings.* New York: Oxford University Press.

Killien, M.G. (1988). Disseminating and using research findings. In N.F. Woods & M. Catanzaro, *Nursing research: Theory and practice* (pp. 479-497). St. Louis: C.V. Mosby.

Mack, M.J. (1952). The personal adjustment of chronically ill old people under home care. *Nursing Research, 1,* 9-31.

Mateo, M.A., & Kirchhoff, K.T. (1991). *Conducting and using nursing research in the clinical setting.* Baltimore: Williams & Wilkins.

Nail, L.M. (1990). Involving clinicians in nursing research. *Oncology Nursing Forum, 17,* 621-623.

Nightingale, F. (1946). *Notes on nursing: What it is and what it is not.* Philadelphia: J.B. Lippincott. (Facsimile of first edition published in 1860 in London by Harrison & Sons).

Noblit, G.W., & Hare, R.D. (1988). *Meta-ethnography: Synthesizing qualitative studies.* Newbury Park: Sage.

Ouellette, F., & Ahn, D. (1993). Potential for pulmonary aspiration: Decreasing risk. *Rehabilitation Nursing Research, 2,* 61-68, 74.

Penrod, L.E., Hegde, S.K., & Ditunna, J.F., Jr. (1990). Age effect on prognosis for functional recovery in acute, traumatic central cord syndrome. *Archives of Physical Medicine and Rehabilitation, 71,* 963-968.

Polit, D.F., & Hungler, B.P. (1991). *Nursing research: Principles and methods* (4th ed). Philadelphia: J.B. Lippincott.

Puetz, B.E. (1992). Welcome to a new ARN publication [Editorial]. *Rehabilitation Nursing, 17,* 56.

Schneider, J.W., & Conrad, P. (1983). *Having epilepsy.* Philadelphia: Temple University Press.

Schuster, P.M., & Waldron, J. (1991). Gender differences in cardiac rehabilitation patients. *Rehabilitation Nursing, 16,* 248-253.

Sparkman, E.D., Quigley, P., & McCarthy, J. (1991). Putting research into practice. *Rehabilitation Nursing, 16,* 12-14.

Steels, M.M. (1976). Perceptual style and the adaptation of the aged to the hospital environment. *ARN Journal, 1,* 9-14.

Stetler, C.B., & Marram, C. (1976). Evaluating research findings for applicability in practice. *Nursing Outlook, 24,* 559-563.

Strickland O.L., & Waltz, C.F. (Eds.). (1988). *Measurement of nursing outcomes, Vol. 2. Measuring nursing performance: Practice, education, and research.* Philadelphia: Springer.

Strickland O.L., & Waltz, C.F. (Eds.). (1991). *Measurement of nursing outcomes, Vol. 4. Measuring client self-care and coping skills.* Philadelphia: Springer.

Stromborg, F.M. (1988). *Instruments for clinical nursing research.* Norwalk, CT: Appleton & Lang.

Venn, M.R., Taft, L., Carpentier, B., & Applebaugh, G. (1992). The influence of timing and suppository use on efficiency and effectiveness of bowel training after stroke. *Rehabilitation Nursing, 17,* 116-120.

Verhoick, P.J. (1961). Decubitus ulcer observations measured objectively. *Nursing Research, 10,* 211-218.

Wahlquist, G.I. (1982). Promoting research in rehabilitation nursing. *Rehabilitation Nursing, 7,* 19-20.

Waltz, C.F. & Strickland, O.L. (Eds.). (1988). *Measurement of nursing outcomes, Vol 1: Measuring client outcomes.* Philadelphia: Springer.

Waltz, C.F. & Strickland, O.L. (Eds.). (1990). *Measurement of nursing outcomes, Vol. 3. Measuring clinical skills and professional development in education and practice.* Philadelphia: Springer.

Waltz, C.F., Strickland, O., & Lenz, E.R. (1991). *Measurement in nursing research* (2nd ed.). Philadelphia: Davis.

Wilson, H.S. (1989). *Research in nursing* (2nd ed.). Redwood City, CA: Addison-Wesley.

Woods, N.F., & Catanzaro, M. (1988). *Nursing research: Theory and practice.* St. Louis: C.V. Mosby.

Yarkony, G.M., Roth, E.J., Heinemann, A.W., & Lovell, L.L. (1988). Spinal cord injury rehabilitation outcomes: The impact of age. *Journal of Clinical Epidemiology, 41,* 173-177.

Yin R.K. (1994). *Case study research. Design and methods* (2nd ed.). Beverly Hills: Sage.

5

Public Policy and Rehabilitation Nursing

Gloria T. Aubert Craven, MSN, RN, CRRN
Carol A. Gleason, RN, CRRN, CCM, LRC

INTRODUCTION

Rehabilitation, government policies, and related nursing roles are extensive subjects that fill entire books. In that light the content of this chapter is geared to motivate rehabilitation nurses to view political action as a component of their professional practice. Rehabilitation is bonded with politics, for its very origins are embedded in legislative regulations and indebted to appropriations. In order to understand how historical events have linked rehabilitation as a medical specialty with legislative actions and rehabilitation nursing practice, nurses are encouraged to read further from other sources on political action.

Although healthcare professionals and other providers have been instrumental in forming and designing legislation concerning persons with disabilities, nursing has not been involved in political action for a number of reasons: gender issues, lack of learning about implications of nursing history for current practice, reactive rather than proactive approach, low level of nursing involvement in political arenas, and poor access to governmental information.

GENDER ISSUES

Historically the majority of nurses (97%) were women. The cultural socialization of women, bolstered by a predominately female profession, did not prepare nurses to influence professional or business enterprises traditionally managed by men. Until recently women did not view themselves as powerful forces in business or politics in the United States (Mason & Talbot, 1985). Nursing pioneers, such as Lillian Wald, had personal resources and arose through a commitment to social action rather than a sense of power. Men entering nursing will alter the composition of the profession; ideally successful nurse change agents will attain stature without adopting male patterns of behavior, thus retaining an essence of nursing.

NURSING HISTORY

Nurses' appreciation of their own professional history is woefully insufficient. At the turn of the twentieth century, nurses held roles as activists in child labor legislation and hospital reform; however, nursing students do not routinely study these actions as models influencing current nursing practice. Currently, nurses are leaders in movements for programs in hospice care and for persons with immunosup-

pressant conditions or human immunodeficiency virus/acquired immunodeficiency syndrome (HIV/AIDS). In these instances nurses have responded retrospectively to social needs but only after a particular healthcare crisis illuminated a need for nursing intervention—and then little application is made to other situations. Compare this approach with the study of military strategies and movements during great battlefield encounters, examining tactics and maneuvers to be used or rejected for future encounters.

Reaction and Proaction

Nurses may become proactive in their efforts by analyzing demographic and trend data to predict health needs, identify unmet needs, and deploy nursing expertise to create as well as respond to social change. In a chain of events, statistical data project a rapidly increasing elderly population in the United States, especially for those persons older than 85 years. In turn, longevity may be accompanied by decreases in functional abilities, creating the need for increased rehabilitation services, especially for those living in the community. Clearly these indications of need are at the same time opportunities for rehabilitation nursing practice.

Political Arenas

Whether rehabilitation nurses are prepared with competencies to meet needs for services, are able to assert their practice as the appropriate professional discipline to manage or deliver those services, and have political-economic legislative support to fulfill the needs are serious concerns. It behooves rehabilitation nurses to become visible and active participants in legislation and public policy for themselves, their profession, and for the benefits of clients of all ages.

In the past nursing involvement has lagged in the legislative and regulation branches of government. This may be due in part to socialization, for political astuteness is lacking in basic nursing education content. Nurses may not become involved in political or legislative activity because the very nature of nursing practice is centered on holistic health for a client, family, and community and ignores the influence of policy on practice. Historically the considerable effects of governmental activities and legislation on the conduct of nursing practice was not analyzed uniformly in basic nursing education (Mason & Talbot, 1985), with only cursory attention given during graduate studies.

Access to Information

Timely practical information regarding legislation and regulations that affect nursing practice is difficult to monitor, time consuming, and expensive to obtain. Political action levels differ widely with nursing organizations and professional specialty groups, but individual involvement and awareness has not been fostered, even from the beginning of practice.

Until recently rehabilitation nursing held limited governmental involvement as a specialty practice, in spite of the tightly woven relationship of rehabilitation with governmental programs. However, the Association of Rehabilitation Nurses (ARN) now sends a member as a legislative representative to Washington, D.C., each year and supports a special interest group for political and legislative matters. ARN maintains liaisons with other major nursing specialty organizations and the American Nurses' Association (ANA). The newly designated National Institute for Rehabilitation Medicine within the National Institutes of Health (NIH) was accomplished with input from ARN. What remains to be seen is how actively rehabilitation nursing remains involved and whether rehabilitation nurses are awarded research funding from this resource.

HISTORICAL LANDMARKS IN LEGISLATION FOR REHABILITATION

Two main themes emerge in this review of legislative history:

1. *There have been marked changes in the social construction of disability.* A chronologic review of legislation important to rehabilitation in the United States quickly illuminates how changes in the social construction of disability has influenced healthcare delivery for persons with disabilities. Philosophic attitudes over the past centuries range widely from "caring for those who are less fortunate" to fostering independent living and mandating mainstreaming for all U.S. citizens in public places. These attitudes affect the value and utility of persons with disabilities as members of the community.

Before the twentieth century a few small groups sought reforms for those "less fortunate in society," including persons with disabilities. In 1830, for instance, a societal move toward specialized education and provisions for persons with disabilities, not legislative actions, was the impetus for founding the Perkins School for the Blind. At this time little was known about differing needs of persons with disabling conditions or about distinctions between disabilities and mental conditions. Thus this first school precisely tailored to needs of person who were blind initially was named the Massachusetts Asylum.

Advances in medicine and medical psychiatry propelled work in the mid-1900s just as social interest in welfare prompted physical and custodial care improvements in the eighteenth century. In 1854, when Dorothea Dix advocated for governmental reforms for clients who were in mental hospitals, she intended to "improve the lot of the ill and disabled." Her activism led to legislation that provided land grants to states to be used in financing mental health hospitals.

For example, since the turn of the twentieth century the evolution of legislation for children with special needs has changed slowly and only as social construction of the value of these children changed. Nearly 100 years passed, in this case, before labels of "imbecile" or "crippled children" were removed from legislative language (Hoeman & Repetto, 1992). Today client advocacy is a recognized rehabilitation nursing role.

2. *Rehabilitation as an interdisciplinary specialty profession has links with healthcare, civil rights, and social reforms aimed at access, acceptance, and inclusion of persons with disabilities in areas of education, employment, recreation, transportation, and other social systems.* Many reforms were connected to other events of the times. Lest any reader cringe at the mention of history, consider that other professions have built success on teachings from their history rather than denying its worth. Military experts still study Caesar's reports of the Gallic Wars and physicians study both history and sociology of medicine.

In fact, the federal government had close ties to healthcare services as long ago as the Revolutionary War. It was not until war veterans returned home following World War I that it became apparent to the government that war veterans surviving casualties, but injured, had rehabilitation needs. In 1914 the War Risk Act specified vocational rehabilitation training for categories of persons who incurred disability while in federal service. The National Defense Act of 1916 qualified men who served in the armed services for vocational adjustments including educational benefits. Then again in 1933, Congress passed a number of initiatives with the same philosophy of providing for veterans' needs: the Smith-Hughes Act, the Smith-Sears Soldiers Rehabilitation Act, the Veterans Administration Act, and the Civilian Rehabilitation Act. The Veterans Administration system remains a powerful force in rehabilitation.

The two latter acts established both occupational and physical therapy as treatment modalities for the rehabilitation of veterans, who were men with disabilities. This legislation set the stage for development of the therapy disciplines and their subsequent roles in rehabilitation; awareness and political activism have secured their places in rehabilitation. For example, before the 1970s, activities of daily living (ADL), wheelchair prescriptions, ambulation, and therapeutic exercises were among other modalities initiated, performed, or supervised by nurses experienced in rehabilitation.

REHABILITATION AND VOCATIONAL POTENTIAL

Perhaps you have visited a federal government building or a federally maintained historical site and noticed that the concession stand was operated by a person who was blind. The Randolph-Sheppard Act of 1936 established rights for persons who are blind to operate vending stands and perform other feasible work on federal property. The importance of being able to work in our society is evident in how case management for Workers' Compensation, ergonomics and job analysis, return to work evaluations, and Social Security payments are devised.

A year earlier the societal values of productivity and being able to work began another era of federal governmental policy. Heralded in 1935 landmark legislation for the Social Security Act united rehabilitation services with gainful employment and return to work. What began as legislation of limited provisions for "grants in aid to the states for income assistance to blind persons and services to crippled children, funds to strengthen programs for vocational rehabilitation and regulations to universalize existing state programs for worker's compensation" grew into one of the largest programs in government. In contrast to the original intent, the next 60 years of amendments to the Social Security Act have established this program as a tax revenue–based source of supplemental income assistance for most workers in the United States.

The value of a work history became evident in 1956, when amendments to the Social Security Act authorized Social Security Disability Insurance (SSDI). Persons with total and permanent disabilities were eligible to receive disability insurance when they could demonstrate a work history; without a work history eligible persons received state-administered public assistance known as Medicaid. Disability without demonstrable employment remained tied to the welfare system when the Supplemental Security Income (SSI) program began a formalized test in 1972 to determine a person's eligibility for benefits based on assured inability to become employed.

Education is the work of children. As with vocational programs, a dual track of health and education policies and regulations has persisted, at times in conflicting or paradoxical ways, to direct separate health and education programs for children of the United States. Implications from this dual legislative and funding pattern has altered the role of nursing both in school health and in rehabilitation team activities with this population (Hoeman & Repetto, 1992).

EXPANSION OF REHABILITATION SERVICES

Only since World War II have health services for the public sector become popular. In 1943 the Disabled Veterans Rehabilitation Act authorized the Veterans Administration to enact the first governmental health insurance program for both disabled and nondisabled veterans. Amendments extended rehabilitation services to persons with mental illnesses or who were "mentally retarded" and expanded the types of physical restoration services offered through state rehabilitation agencies.

However, health insurance for all persons was at best scarce. Before this act health services were paid for privately; clients often bartered goods or services for healthcare. Hospitals were considered places where persons went to die, to be isolated because of infectious disease including tuberculosis, or to become incarcerated due to mental illness.

By 1965 it was clear that special populations who required federal money and program assistance to maintain health and treat illness were composed of large numbers of persons. Legislative response to their needs was Medicare, the first federal health insurance program for persons over 65 years of age or who were disabled, and Medicaid, the state-administered health insurance program. The outcome was the beginning of the disjointed, "patchwork quilt" approach to rectifying healthcare needs for multiple and differing segments of the U.S. population. Many legislative initiatives have been proposed and enacted in attempts to provide services needed by different beneficiaries of these programs. However, without due attention and advocacy, the already severe deficiencies of Medicare and Medicaid for persons who need rehabilitation services will be more apparent in poor client outcomes (Chapter 8).

It is surprising that Medicare and Medicaid legislation passed in the political climate of the mid-1960s. Any form of national healthcare was squashed under the fearful rubric of socialized medicine, paramount to Communism itself; meanwhile civil rights activities were beginning to raise social consciousness and concerns. About this time the poliomyelitis vaccine was discovered along with medical advances that enabled persons with disabilities such as spinal cord injuries to survive and live longer than before. Future directions, especially fiscal benefits, of rehabilitation as a specialty were being debated. In some respects rehabilitation nurses who worked in hospitals or rehabilitation facilities were sheltered from the impact of Medicare and Medicaid as experienced by nurses who worked in community service agencies, such as Visiting Nurses Associations (VNAs). Unlike today, clients remained longer in hospitals, and although medical record audits and measurements of quality were being introduced, utilization review activities had not reached full force.

Legislation ran a remarkable gauntlet over the next 30 years, creating amendments with provisions that accelerated and expanded services so extensive as to mark the issues of the 1994 healthcare reform. This began in 1965 and continued through 1992, as federal monies were provided to states at an initial ratio of 75%: 25% for program development and implementation, including cooperative projects with priorities for persons with severe handicaps.

GROUNDWORK FOR ACCESS AND INDEPENDENT LIVING

By 1973 affirmative action legislation stipulated persons with disabilities could not be discriminated against in matters of employment. Persons with disabilities benefited in part from other social and civil rights movements in the United States; however, the legislation did not stipulate access or mandate accommodations in the workplace. Only when the social construction of disability changed from "caring for" to independence in living did social accommodations change. About the same time as the 1978 amendments authorized independent living centers, another significant change in social thought occurred. For the first time assistance for independent living was not tied to employment.

However, politics and policies mixed fiscal responsibilities of the federal government once again, this time decreasing federal expenditures on programs, including independent living. As a result, individual states were left with large financial burdens and commitments for federal mandates from 1980 to 1992.

Legislation concerning access has not been limited to adults. In 1987 and 1988 legislation mandated equal access to education for children with special needs through a program administered and funded largely by the states. Since provisions from this legislation are scheduled to move to entitlement status within 5 years, the programs recently have been subject to budgetary debates. The programs provide services for special needs education, with a goal of increasing independent living when a child reaches young adulthood.

Rehabilitation nurses who work with a pediatric population will recognize Title I of Part H, Early Intervention for Handicapped Infants and Toddlers, of the Individuals with Disabilities Amendments to the Education of the Handicapped Act of 1975. As Public Law 99-457 this legislation created child-centered and family-guided programs for early intervention services for infants and young children with special needs from birth to 3 years and transition to preschool programs. The goal is to fulfill each child's unique cognitive, emotional, and psychological needs to enable children to reach their educational potential. An interdisciplinary team works with families to prepare a written Individual Family Service Plan (IFSP) for achieving that potential. Related legislation, Public Law 94-142, assures that children with special needs will receive medically related services necessary to enable them to achieve the identified educational potential in the least restrictive environment when entering school (Hoeman, 1992).

However, in 1990, the ADA secured equal access for all persons with disabilities, enabling each one to become mainstreamed into daily life, regardless of employment status. Access is guaranteed to employment, recreation, transportation, and communication. Specific measures of this act, impact on the nation, and strategies for rehabilitation nursing practice are discussed in the following sections.

THE ADA

As rehabilitation professionals, have you ever given thought to the words "civil rights"? For the estimated 43 million Americans with disabilities, these words were a constant battle until the passage of the ADA of 1990 (PL 101-336). This law finally gave equality to Americans with disabilities. It enables all of us to be part of a shared vision and to partake of the "American Dream" . . . freedom and equality for all.

The purpose of the ADA was to provide a federal mandate to eliminate discrimination against persons with disabilities, enforce standards developed to protect them, enforce the Fourteenth Amendment's aspects of integration, and to keep the promise President George Bush made at the Republican National Convention: "to ensure all Americans access within our society."

The ADA is divided into the following five Titles:

I   Employment
II   Public Services
III Public Accommodations and Services Operated by Public Entities
IV   Telecommunications
V   Miscellaneous Provisions

The language in this legislation is extensive, and a review is necessary for the practicing rehabilitation nurse.

Title I: Employment

Title I prohibits discrimination of persons with disabilities in the workforce. Further, it promotes greater access to employment for persons with disabilities in concrete mandates. This division faced major debates as employers feared high costs for its implementation. The ADA is similar to the Rehabilitation Act of 1973, which was used to draft the legislation. The Rehabilitation Act of 1973 prohibited discrimination toward persons employed by programs that received federal funding. Section 503 required programs receiving $2,500 to make attempts to employ persons with disabilities. If a program received $50,000 or more and had 50 employees, a written policy to hire persons with disabilities was required. Section 504 prohibited discrimination against a qualified applicant if federal funds were received for programming.

Under the ADA discrimination by employers is prohibited; they must provide "reasonable accommodation" at company expense. This was effective July 26, 1992, in companies employing 25 or more persons. In businesses employing more than 15 and less than 25 persons, it became effective July 26, 1994.

"The term reasonable accommodation may include: (A) making existing facilities used by employees readily accessible to and usable by individuals with disabilities; and (B) job restructuring, part time or modified work schedules, reassignment to a vacant position, acquisition or modification of equipment or devices, appropriate adjustment or modification of examinations, training materials or policies, the provision of qualified readers or interpreters and other similar accommodations for individuals with disabilities" (Americans with Disabilities Act [ADA], Title I, Section 101 (9)).

These accommodations are mandated unless "undue hardship" exists. This term "means an action requiring significant difficulty or expense" (ADA, Title I, Section 101 (10)). Because this law is new, the definition of "reasonable accommodations" has not yet been tested by judicial efforts. This is a predictable event that will set a precedent over this important definition.

Section 102 prohibits discrimination "in regard to job application procedures, the hiring, advancement, or discharge of employees, employee compensation, job training and other terms, conditions, and privileges of employment" (ADA, Title I, Section 102 (a)). It is now illegal to deny jobs to qualified individuals due to a disability if—with reasonable accommodations—the duties of the job could be satisfied. In addition, physical examinations cannot be performed until after an applicant has been offered a job. Medical information cannot be included in an applicant's personnel file and must be treated as a confidential document. Managers are only to be informed of restrictions to specific work duties and not to the specific medical issues of the employee with disabilities.

Discrimination could exist if employers attempted to "screen out or otherwise deny a job . . . to an individual with a disability" unless pertinent to business and not achievable with "reasonable accommodation" (ADA, Title I, Section 103 (a)).

Section 104 prevents individuals who have successfully completed supervised drug or alcohol rehabilitation programs to be denied a job, as long as they comply with the same standards as other employees.

To understand "reasonable accommodations" the following examples are offered:

1. A clerical position includes typing, filing and answer-

ing the phone. If the applicant is wheelchair-bound, all job responsibilities could be performed if access is provided to a desk and phone. Files could be lowered to be accessible from the wheelchair, or another employee could file documents in the higher files. The "usual desk" could be rearranged to permit wheelchair access. These simple modifications enable the applicant to perform the duties listed on the job description. These accommodations are "reasonable" for the employer.

2. The above position could also include admitting clients to their room and assisting with the transfer of the client onto a bed or examining table. In this case, if no other person could complete this portion of the task, and it was an essential job function, the employer would be protected from hiring the individual.

Title II: Public Services

This section assures access to the programs and services provided by governmental agencies. This includes public transportation (via bus and rail) and alterations of existing facilities (access to bathrooms, telephones . . .). For commuter rail services, "one car must be accessible no later than five years after the enactment of this Act" (ADA, Title II, Section 242(b)(1)). New buildings now require provisions for persons with disabilities in the standards issued by the Architectural and Transportation Barriers Compliance Board.

Title III: Public Accommodations and Services Operated by Public Entities

This section of the ADA impacts three areas: (1) public accommodations in private existing businesses, (2) commercial facilities, and (3) public transportation offered in private existing businesses.

Accommodations include areas such as hotels (excluding buildings of less than five rooms, occupied by the owner with rooms for hire—for example, bed-and-breakfast establishments). It also includes schools, convention centers, bus stations, parks, banks, shopping centers, entertainment centers (theaters, stadiums . . .) to name a few. These areas were to comply with the ADA by January 26, 1992. These accommodations also must provide services incorporated into their seating (e.g., restaurants cannot segregate persons with disabilities in a particular area, as in smoking versus nonsmoking sections).

Title IV: Telecommunications

By July 26, 1993, all common carriers providing telephone voice transmission services must provide telecommunication relay services for the hearing and/or speech impaired. Individuals cannot be billed additionally for these services. The same communications services for all Americans now is ensured.

Title V: Miscellaneous Provisions

If a governmental law (local or state) exists that provides greater protection for the rights of persons with disabilities, it overrides the terms of the ADA.

The effects of this important legislation impacts everyone in healthcare. Physicians must offer the same services to all their patients, regardless of their disabilities. Their offices must be made accessible. For example, many family practices are located in converted homes. Ramps, automatic doors, elevators or chair lifts must be added to the office entry. Physicians performing employee physical examinations cannot, without further evaluation, state a former diagnosis as preventing job performance. For example, a questionable heart murmur may be offered by the client during a history. Unless there has been treatment or active follow-up, this most likely would not impair job performance and cannot be listed as a disability.

"Although professions exist because of a mandate from society to perform certain functions, and many professionals operate under legislative sanctions, there is a tendency among the rank and file members to forget this fact. There was a time when it was not considered professional to be involved in the political process. Professionals were somehow removed from the every day world in which such decisions are made. This is an innocence which can no longer be excused" (VerSteeg, 1980). Nurses and other rehabilitation professionals must be aware of these guidelines to assist their clients with the management of their disabilities. In the acute care hospital setting, the client focuses on medical stabilization, but family members may voice return to work questions. During rehabilitation, the client is made aware of her capabilities. Nurses must be able to encourage clients to reach their optimum capacity and educate them as to workplace accommodations that are legally guaranteed them by the ADA. Most clients fear isolation and rejection due to their disability. Knowing gainful employment is a goal will promote mastery of the tasks needed for increased self-reliance and respect and promote the healing process. Family support is a key factor. Maintaining communication between client and employer will assist the rehabilitation professional in establishing attainable goals.

Nurses, especially occupational health nurses and insurance rehabilitation nurses, need to be aware of the ADA. They must educate employers about the rights of persons with disabilities and coordinate job accommodations. Employers are more likely to cooperate with the rehabilitation goals of clients when nursing interventions create cost-effective outcomes. Many employers fear that there are major expenses associated with the return to work for employees with disabilities. Nurses can demonstrate the benefits of fair-employment issues, and misconceptions of this legislation can be eliminated.

Awareness of the ADA and its direct correlation to the provision of care for the rehabilitation client will assist nurses in the realization that "politics is not a spectator sport" (Craven, 1982). Political activism is essential for the optimum provision of quality nursing care.

STRATEGIES FOR AFFECTING PUBLIC POLICY

Stressing the importance of nurses' involvement in public policy does not make the process less elusive or the goal of political activism easier. The material that follows outlines strategies for effecting changes in ways that are most time efficient and effective. Nurses must develop skills in many aspects of professional practice. Expertise in clinical practice, research, education, client education, and administrative strategies are essential components of contempo-

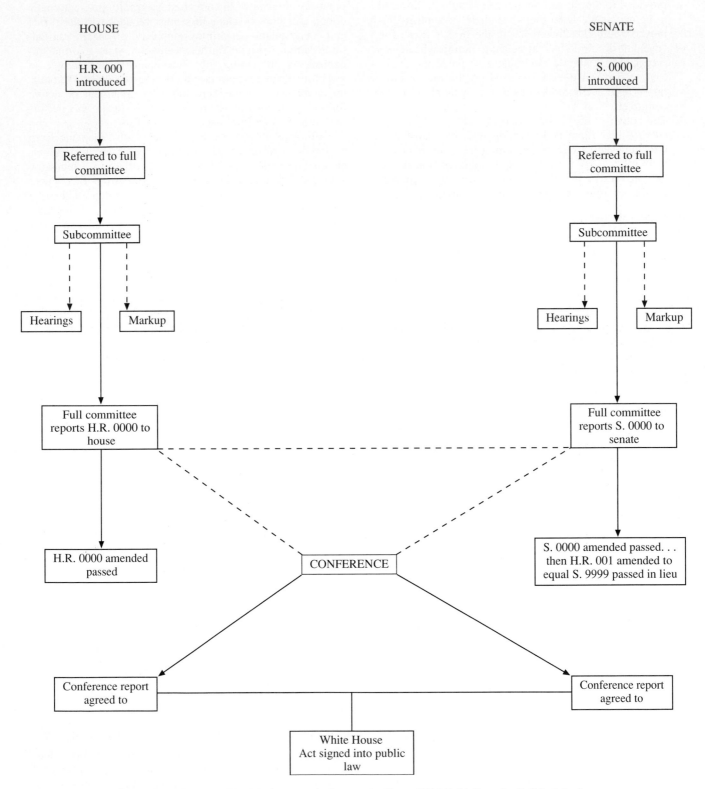

HOUSE

SENATE

H.R. 000
introduced

Referred to full
committee

Subcommittee

Hearings

Markup

Full committee
reports H.R. 0000 to
house

H.R. 0000 amended
passed

S. 0000
introduced

Referred to full
committee

Subcommittee

Hearings

Markup

Full committee
reports S. 0000 to
senate

CONFERENCE

S. 0000 amended passed. . .
then H.R. 001 amended to
equal S. 9999 passed in lieu

Conference report
agreed to

White House
Act signed into public
law

Conference report
agreed to

Fig. 5-1   The path of legislation: a typical example. From ARN Guidelines for Political Action, Compiled by 1988–1989 Legislative Committee, October 1989.

rary nursing. The connection with those areas of practice and legislation are, however, tight bonds that the practicing nurse must begin to comprehend. Expertise in rehabilitation nursing is unique within the scope of nursing practice. This knowledge must be articulated and utilized in the debates regarding legislation and regulation.

One strategy useful to the neophyte in political activism is to identify just one issue of interest per year and act on it. This allows the nurse to develop expertise in the topic, the legislation, or the regulation that it affects and learn how to create positive changes (Fig. 5-1).

Individual Involvement

Rehabilitation nurses have a unique body of knowledge. Legislators are voted into office to listen to their constituency. Nursing's voice, as a constituent, is credible and authoritative because of that knowledge base. Individual power to effect change emanates from an understanding of the impact of potential legislation based on nursing expertise. Often local city and county legislation may affect rehabilitation clients. Many cities now are struggling with implementing the mandates of the ADA. Serving on local "disability commissions" and developing a relationship with elected congressmen (federal officials) and legislators (state senators and state representatives) are roles for a rehabilitation nurse.

Most frequently nurses struggle with how to follow legislation. This, to date, has been a time-consuming and formidable task. There are some basic resources that make this task less difficult. Elected officials will inform nurse constituents of impending legislation that affects rehabilitation if they know who you are. For this reason, a relationship, either through letters, meetings, or working on campaigns is invaluable. A second source of information is that of national or local coalitions who share nursing interests. For instance, many nurses have a specialty in head injury rehabilitation. Joining the National Head Injury Foundation is one way to gain access to information about impending legislation that affects people with head injuries.

Other resources are the *Congressional Record* and the *Federal Register.* Each of these publications is composed of text of legislation introduced in Congress and impending regulatory changes. The *Federal Register* is the U.S. government's announcement of grants, legal definitions, and regulation changes for federal agencies, including the Health Care Financing Administration (HCFA). Open hearings are announced, and groups or individuals are invited to send written comments before the proposed changes become enforced. These are public documents available in any library designated a congressional depository. Some places may have an *Index to the Federal Register,* which is useful to reduce the volume of paper materials. Last, there are individual newsletters that inform nurses about legislation on a federal and state level. Subscribing makes following legislation much easier and less time consuming.

Lobbying a position is a democratic right. Lawmakers estimate any one response to a legislative issue represents concern or opinion of at least 200 other citizens; 1 in 44 voters in the United States is a nurse, which translates to more than 2 million nurse voters. The nursing profession's

political advantage is the public view of nurses as advocates for clients (and people with disabilities) and as altruistic and knowledgeable.

The issues debated always reflect three nursing concerns: quality of care, cost of care, and access for the greatest number of Americans as possible. Credibility is added to conviction if legislators know your area of practice and your professional affiliations. Expect a response to any correspondence. It is a step in building that relationship. By following the dictum of "follow one issue per year," individuals are less likely to become overwhelmed while adding a nursing perspective to the debates regarding that area of interest. Do not underestimate the power of individual activism; however, never represent an opinion as that of any organization or employer unless authorized or entitled to do so.

Organizational Involvement

Nurses are encouraged to increase their influence by joining forces with their professional organization(s). The ANA has lobbied hard to obtain the endorsement and influence of such organizations as the ARN in their political activities. There is strength in numbers. There are also the benefits of financial and human resources when coalitions are built. Whenever nursing can present a unified front in the public eye around a political issue, then the power of the profession is enhanced. There is a role to play in this strategy for each and every nurse.

Nursing organizations are increasing their involvement in the areas that unite outcomes research and public policy. One such example is the use of nurse experts on the panels of the Agency for Health Care Policy and Research (AHCPR). This agency was mandated by Congress in 1989 to develop policy guidelines for healthcare based on research from multidisciplinary panels of experts. To date, guidelines are prepared for management of acute pain and treatment of pressure ulcers. Upcoming guidelines include back pain management, treatment of acute angina, and treatment of Alzheimer's disease and related dementias.

The National Institute for Nursing is housed at the NIH. This body funds and sponsors outcome-oriented nursing research projects throughout the United States. Many findings from this body of research may contribute to public policy. Legislators are dependent on confirmable, accurate, and reproducible data when formulating their decisions for sound legislation. Nurses who use findings based on nursing research, outcomes, and standards as reliable information can effect change when they communicate with legislators around a legislative issue.

IMPLICATIONS OF SOCIETAL TRENDS AND PERSONS WITH DISABILITIES

As this chapter is being written, the politics of healthcare and healthcare delivery are riding a national wave toward healthcare reform in the United States. The country is engulfed with two overriding concerns. The public believes the administration and Congress must first control the national deficit and at the same time assure healthcare for every citizen. The cost of healthcare is greater than 14% of the gross domestic product (GDP); 14 cents of every dollar spent is toward healthcare. Estimates are for 16% of the gross national product (GNP) by the year 2000, followed by an escalating spiral of expenditures (Blendon & Hyams, 1992).

Numerous studies and polls have been used to examine healthcare problems facing the United States and the relative importance of issues to individuals. When citizens were asked to rate the country's most serious economic and social concerns, 65.1% rated the cost of medical care as the most compelling problem. In rank order AIDS (57.5%), drug abuse (55.7%), the federal deficit (52.7%), poverty (47.2%), crime (46.8%), and unemployment (46.7%) were cited (Blendon & Hyams, 1992). In fact, 82% of all personal bankruptcies in the country during 1992 were a direct result of personal healthcare expenses (Hastings, 1993).

Three separate polls by the *Los Angeles Times*/Gallup, NBC/WSJ, and "PLAN" (*p*ertinent *l*egislation *a*ffecting *n*urses) found high cost (47%, 55%, 57%) and coverage/access (27%, 37%, 39%) to be the most important healthcare problems cited in the United States. "PLAN" asked Massachusetts legislators to identify their healthcare issues of greatest concern. Their answers reflected nursing concerns: long-term care (76%), access to care (54%), AIDS/HIV (50%), health insurance reform (50%), and maternal and child healthcare (48%). Clearly both federal and state concerns pivot around the same issues. As events unfold, the tendency for a federal mandate to design the form of healthcare delivery throughout the United States is strong, but implementation strategies probably will be left to each state according to state and regional needs.

MAJOR MODELS FOR HEALTHCARE REFORM

Unlike any other time in nursing history, the economic impact of the healthcare delivery system directly influences the reimbursement and delivery of nursing care. For example, legislation in some states authorizes nurses who become licensed to practice in advanced professional nursing roles to receive direct reimbursement from third-party payers including Medicare and Medicaid.

In the debates regarding healthcare reform, two major models exist at the time of this writing: managed competition and single-payer system. Each has benefits and deficits, and the administration, Congress, and powerful healthcare lobbies are poised to argue their points. Nursing must remain the advocate for quality care and accessibility while understanding and articulating methods for effective cost controls through nursing care. Further, individual nurse's involvement will continue to be needed as the shape of services will continue to be defined on the state and local levels, where individuals have their major impact.

Managed Competition

Managed competition is the model most favored by the Clinton administration. Provisions in this model maintain healthcare reform focuses on the behavior of consumers, who become the insurers. Physicians and hospitals are not the focus of cost control. Tax incentives would encourage companies and the public to choose cost-effective health plans and allow insurers and consumers to "bid and contract" for a basic low-cost health package. The idea is that over time most providers would be compelled by competitive pressures to join organized delivery systems such as Health Maintenance Organizations (HMOs). Competition, not government regulation, would drive down the cost of healthcare.

Under this model the administration considers taxing individuals against health insurance provided by their employers; taxing the purchase of cigarettes, alcohol, and guns ("sin taxes"); and removing business tax incentives that cater to healthcare providers such as company advertising, logo gifts, or trips to conferences.

The Single-Payer Model

The single-payer model establishes the federal government as the single payer for a basic healthcare package for all citizens and residents of the United States. In this model reform for cost containment focuses on the behavior of providers and hospitals, not on consumers and patients. A single-payer model is expected to yield tremendous cost savings in administrative overhaul, since the need for multiple billing departments of insurance companies would be eliminated. In fact, this basic package would eradicate the need for a health insurance industry as we now know it. Although individuals would be able to purchase options through private insurance, these would be based on desire and ability to pay. Some estimates predict changes in this model alone could reduce healthcare costs by as much as 24%. In addition, costs would be controlled by establishing tightly regulated global budgets. Budget negotiations would occur between the government and all providers (including nurses), and spending for healthcare could not exceed those budgets. This model would be financed by the federal government, and the distribution of those funds would be designed by state and local governments. The single-payer model reflects provisions of healthcare programs in some other countries.

Unresolved Issues

Neither model is perfect, and no one has seriously studied or rectified the concerns of elders, long-term care, or rehabilitation. When nurses become informed about proposals for healthcare reform, they are prepared and educated to understand the implications of legislation. Combined with their nursing experience and clinical knowledge, they are prepared to take a stand. Legislators listen to an informed, educated, professional viewpoint. The alternative is for state and federal legislators to base decisions about legislation on information from groups whose interests are solely monetary (Hastings, 1993).

Finally, nurses are encouraged to review historical events that have led the United States to this point in healthcare for persons with chronic, disabling, or developmental conditions or disorders. Understanding how events of the past came to be, and their implications for nursing and clients, may open awareness and opportunities for political action in this changing healthcare scene and for the future. There is much to be done by nurses exercising the skills outlined in this chapter. If nurses are not involved, decisions will be made without nursing input. Use your democratic rights and activate your professional responsibility by participating.

REFERENCES

Americans with Disabilities Act (1990).

Blendon, R.J., & Hyams, T.S. (Eds.). (1992). *Reforming the system: Containing health care costs in an era of universal coverage.* New York: Faulkner & Gray. (Harvard School of Public Health, Louis Harris and Associates, Inc. Institute for the Future.)

Craven, G.T.A. (1992). An untapped resource: "PLAN" survey finds that many Massachusetts legislators want to hear more from nurses. *Boston Nurse News, 1,* 1, 6.

Hastings, K. (1993, October). *Health care reform and your role as a nurse.* Paper presented at the second annual "PLAN" seminar, Boston.

Hoeman, S.P., & Repetto, M.A. (1992). Legislation and children with special needs from 1903-1990. *Western Journal of Nursing Research, 14,* 102-105.

Mason, D.J., & Talbot, S. (Eds.). (1985). *Political action handbook for nurses changing the workplace, government, organizations and community.* Menlo Park, CA: Addison-Wesley.

Nosek, M.A. (1992). The Americans with Disabilities Act of 1990: Will it work? *American Journal of Occupational Therapy 46,* 466-467.

VerSteeg, D. (1980). The political process or the power and the glory. In B. Bullough (Ed.), *The law and the expanding nursing role.* New York: Appleton-Century-Crofts.

SUGGESTED READINGS

Anfield, R.N. (1992). Americans with disabilities act: A primer of Title I provisions for occupational health care professionals. *Journal of Occupational Medicine, 34,* 503-509.

Association of Rehabilitation Nurses. (1989). *Guidelines for political action legislative committee.* Evanston, IL: ARN.

Bowman, O.J. (1992). Americans have a shared vision: Occupational therapists can help create future reality. *American Journal of Occupational Therapists, 46,* 391-394.

Bryant, L.E., Jr. (1992). The legal impact of the Americans with disabilities act (ADA) on health information managers. *JAMA, 63,* 67-68.

Carmack, P. (1992). The ADA: New directions for the disabled and hospitals. *Health Systems Review, 25,* 12-16, 20-22.

Cavalier, W. (1986). *The history of rehabilitation.* American Association for Rehabilitation Therapy.

Chermak, G.O. (1990). A global perspective on disability: A review of efforts to increase access and advance social integration for disabled persons. *International Disability Studies, 12,* 123-127.

Coudroglou, D.S.W. (1984). Disability: The view from social policy. *Rehabilitation Literature, 45,* 358-361.

Crist, P.A.H., & Stoffel, V.C. (1992). The Americans with disabilities act of 1990 and employees with mental impairments: Personal efficacy and the environment. *American Journal of Occupational Therapy, 46,* 434-443.

Deith, B. (1988). AIDS: A rehabilitation perspective. *Occupational Health (London), 40,* 618-623.

Fagin, C.M. (1990). Cost-effectiveness: Nursing's value proves itself. *American Journal of Nursing, 91,* 16-18, 22-29.

Frieden, L. (1992). The Americans with disabilities act of 1990: Will it work? *American Journal of Occupational Therapy, 46,* 468-469.

Gostin, L. (1992). Health law. *JAMA, 268,* 364-366.

Griffith, H., Thomas, N., & Griffith, L. (1991). M.D.'s bill for these routine nursing tasks. *American Journal of Nursing, 91,* pp. 22-27.

Hablutzel, N., & McMahon, B. (1992). *The Americans with Disabilities Act: Access and accomodations, guidelines for human resources, rehabilitation, and legal professions.* Orlando: PDM Press.

Hayden, M.J. (1992). Disability awareness workship: Helping businesses comply with the Americans with disabilities act of 1990. *American Journal of Occupational Therapy, 46,* 461-465.

Harris, M. (1988). The changing scene in community health nursing. *Nursing Clinics of North America, 23,* 559-568.

Hedman, G. (1992) Assistive technology: A boon to reasonable accommodation. *National Association of Service Providers in Private Rehabilitation, 9,* 1-5.

Himmelstein, J.S., & Pransky, G.S. (1992). The ADA and you: Implication for the occupational health professional. *Journal of Occupational Medicine, 34,* 501-502.

Hyde, K.E. (1992). A new challenge for home care agencies. *Caring, 1,* 44-50.

Kalscheur, J.A. (1992). Benefits of the Americans with Disabilities Act of 1990 for children and adolescents with disabilities. *American Journal of Occupational Therapy, 46,* L419-L426.

LaVor, M.L. (1980). Section 504: Past, present, future. *Archives of Physical Medicine and Rehabilitation, 61,* 283-285.

McCarthy, J. (1992). Americans with Disabilities Act: Big impact on small business. *JAVMA, 200,* 155-156.

Pike, R. (1992). What health care institutions need to know about the ADA. *Discharge Planning Update, 12,* 9-11.

Popick, B. (1971). The social security disability program: 1. Characteristics of the program. *Journal of Occupational Medicine, 13,* 227-231.

Rybski, D. (1992). A quality implementation of Title I of the Americans with Disabilities Act of 1990. *American Journal of Occupational Therapy, 46,* 409-418.

St. Clair, S., & Shults, T. (1992). Americans with Disabilities Act, considerations for the practice of occupational medicine. *Journal of Occupational Medicine 34,* 510-517

Schaeffer, F. (1988). DRG's: A new era for health care. *Nursing Clinics of North America, 23,* 453-463.

Schelly, C., Sample, P., & Spencer, K. (1992). The Americans with Disabilities Act of 1990 expands employment opportunities for persons with developmental disabilities. *American Journal of Occupational Therapy, 46,* 457-460.

Shaller, E.H., & Rosen, D.A. (1991-1992). A guide to the EEOC's final regulations on the Americans with Disabilities Act. *Employee Relations Law Journal, 17,* 405-430.

Sharp, N. (1990). What will physician payment reform mean for nurses? *Nursing Management, 21,* 14-15.

Sherwen, L.N. (1992). Rehabilitation: The prototype for holistic health policy formation. *Holistic Nursing Practice, 6,* 84-89.

Sind, J.M., & Craft, D. (1981). Legislation affecting rehabilitation of older people: Present and future. *Journal of Rehabilitation, 47,* 85-89.

Verville, R.E. (1979). Federal legislative history of independent living programs. *Archives of Physical Medicine and Rehabilitation, 60,* 447-451.

Verville, R.E. (1988). Fifty years of federal legislation and programs affecting PM&R. *Archives of Physical Medicine and Rehabilitation, 69* (special issue), 64-68.

Watson, P.G. (1988). Rehabilitation legislation of the 1980's: Implication for nurses as healthcare providers. *Rehabilitation Nursing, 13,* 136-141.

Watson, P.G. (1979). Rehabilitation legislation of the seventies and the severely disabled. *ARN Journal, 4,* 4-6, 8-11.

Zander, K. (1988). Nursing case management: Resolving the DRG paradox. *Nursing Clinics of North America, 23,* 503-520.

Zuffoletto, J.M. (1992). New federal regulations protect disabled employees: Americans with Disabilities Act of 1990. *JAORN, 55,* 1274-1276, 1278.

6

Principles of Leadership and Management for Rehabilitation Nurses

Jean M. Benjamin, MSN, RN, CRRN
Barbara H. Warner, MS, RN

INTRODUCTION

A leader is a visionary who exudes enthusiasm. Confident because of experience and able to empower others, a leader is willing to risk for the vision. "The very essence of leadership is that you have a vision. It's got to be a vision you articulate clearly and forcefully on every occasion. You can't blow an uncertain trumpet" (Peters, 1987, p. 399). Leaders promote autonomy by creating and facilitating an environment where there is trust. Staff members believe they can accomplish anything: groundwork for empowerment, autonomy, and self-governance.

The function of a leader is to influence members of a group to move toward attaining a vision by accomplishing objectives mutually agreed upon by the group. Success with implementing the leadership role relies on purposeful interaction with other people. "The challenge is to be a light, not a judge; to be a model, not a critic" (Covey, 1992, p. 25). Although it may be possible to have a manager who is without leadership ability or an able informal leader who is not in a management position, leadership is fundamental to the effective manager. A manager uses leadership skills to transfer beliefs, values, and convictions to others and then facilitates leadership behaviors in the staff. Accessibility, visibility, and integrity are leadership characteristics of a manager who demonstrates building confidence and enthusiasm among staff.

Considering the various functions common to all managers, planning and organizing are priority functions of management as all other activities flow from them. All planning is meaningless if the manager does not operationalize the plan. On the other hand, an significant skill for a manager is the ability to realize when a plan needs to be changed and to be able to abandon the original plan—or revise it, adapt, and mobilize anew. Organizing is creative coordination: knowing how people and resources are brought together, predicting needs before the work begins. At this point managers learn to delegate effectively to get the work done and to continue to be productive when new information or unanticipated developments occur. Unfortunately the legacy of nursing leaders throughout history was to reward nurses for performing visible tasks and enumerating activi-

ties and not necessarily for low-visibility thinking, planning, and evaluating. Nurse managers, once able to sell ideas by persuading and influencing others, face additional challenges to meld nursing idealism with management realism, especially when system demands, consumer needs, and professional forces pull in opposing directions.

In the past a nurse manager was responsible for a single nursing area. With restructuring maneuvers during the early nineties, downsizing or right sizing, nurse managers may be responsible for more and varied areas including subacute levels or skilled nursing units. In the community a nurse may manage several service programs and supervise staff from multiple areas and at the same time partition resources among Medicare, Medicaid, and third-party reimbursement sources. First-line nursing managers significantly influence the work satisfaction of a large percentage of the nation's hospital employees. Efforts of these first-line managers are critical in preventing low morale and high turnover rates among staff, which are costly to the organization. Managers who have a positive understanding of the role are released from staffing and supported to develop a managerial identity, empowered to remain visible and available. The nurse manager who is visible and available for staff can affect client satisfaction. However, the manager needs to learn and demonstrate that effective time away from direct care contributes to client care.

REHABILITATION NURSE MANAGER ROLE

The nurse manager role in rehabilitation has some unique functions in addition to those traditionally expected from a frontline nursing manager. The Association of Rehabilitation Nurses (ARN) developed a role description of the rehabilitation nurse manager based on the nurse manager definition by the Association of Nurse Executives (AONE) in 1992. Functions specific to the rehabilitation setting are defined, such as promoting nursing values related to quality of life and the continuity of care into the home and community. Emphasis is on educating nurses and others to rehabilitation and supporting the interdisciplinary team model (Evans, 1994). In rehabilitation preventing further disability, maintaining current abilities, achieving maximum functional capacities, and quality of life are key considerations for clinical and managerial decisions affecting efficient and effective operations.

A substantial growth in variety of practice opportunities for rehabilitation nursing managers includes inpatient units (either within an acute care facility or a free-standing rehabilitation hospital), subacute-level units, community-based programs for special populations including university-affiliated programs (UAPs), rehabilitation clinics, community agencies or corporations that involve managed care and third-party payers. Health trends of an aging population, changing governmental roles and regulations, evolving regulatory agency expectations, increasing numbers of uninsured and underinsured persons, and growing concerns with the national healthcare delivery system offer new challenges as well as career opportunities.

Recruitment and Retention

Recruiting professional nurses to specialize in rehabilitation is a challenge, as nurses have little opportunity to learn the role functions of the specialty in basic nursing education. As a result many nurses are unfamiliar with or misinformed about the specialty of rehabilitation nursing and are not adequately educated in such concepts (Larsen, 1986). Purk's work (1993) supported this disparity, finding nurses "thus, may not seek employment in the field of rehabilitation." Nurses may associate a lack of "glamour" with rehabilitation nursing when compared with acute care nursing, especially when there are misconceptions about rehabilitation nursing practice. Nurses may not know the roles and functions of other disciplines comprising rehabilitation teams or how their roles interrelate or interface in care. The ideas of interdisciplinary teams, clients and families as active participants in care, lifelong care planning, and the focus on care rather than cure alone may not fit into a nurse's expectations about how healthcare is delivered.

When hiring any professional nurse, a recruiter asks for ideas about the nurse's interests and area of preferred practice or client population. Some nurses like a high-technology environment where clients change rapidly; others prefer to concentrate on interpersonal interactions, teaching, and counseling, which are areas where rehabilitation nurses spend considerable time and excel. Socially sensitive and culturally tolerant attitudes fit in rehabilitation nursing practice. Some unique characteristics of rehabilitation nurses are an ability to

✦ Accept others "where they are" without imposing their own expectations
✦ Work with clients and families in setting mutual goals and identifying barriers and resources, unmet needs, and strengths in the client's own environment
✦ Encourage clients and families to do whatever possible for themselves rather than the nurse to "do for the person" and remain fulfilled in a nursing role
✦ Provide care and preventive interventions as opposed to cure behaviors

As the length of stay in a facility shortens, managers and nursing staff will be challenged to know clients and their families while planning for their community reentry. Coordination and referral throughout the health system, such as with critical pathways and case management, will be nec-

essary to meet a client's increasingly complex individual care needs effectively.

In the past nurses who chose rehabilitation were often mature nurses, perhaps returning to work after several years. Experienced in nursing and in their own lives, these professionals are comfortable and secure in talking with clients and their families who are adjusting to the consequences following disability or injury and need effective coping strategies for making complex decisions. Over time some parts of rehabilitation nursing have changed. For example, technology was not a prominent feature of rehabilitation nursing, but this has changed with the nature of the client entering rehabilitation and reentering the community or long-term care residence. Mechanical ventilation, cardiac and pulmonary, and burn rehabilitation have become subspecialties. Clients with complex dual-diagnosis conditions and multiple medical needs have come into many rehabilitation nursing units. Overall, rehabilitation nurses express a high satisfaction rate for their practice and consequently a low attrition rate.

Student nurses who have received some experience in rehabilitation specialty practice during their basic education program are more likely to consider rehabilitation nursing. In some instances nurses who apply to work in rehabilitation facilities may have family or friends with a chronic or disabling condition. When interviewing nurses working in rehabilitation, Purk (1993) found only two who had selected rehabilitation nursing as their specialty—one because of the care a family member had received on a rehabilitation unit and the other because of basic education experience in a rehabilitation setting.

Including rehabilitation nursing specialty skills, knowledge, and applications within basic education curricula and expanding continuing education with rehabilitation content may improve visibility of the specialty for nursing students and create awareness among nurses practicing in other settings. Additionally rehabilitation nurses and managers have opportunities to provide continuing education about rehabilitation nursing concepts and practice throughout the continuum of healthcare services.

MARKETING REHABILITATION NURSING AS A SPECIALTY

The rehabilitation awareness campaign by the Medical Rehabilitation Education Foundation (MREF) (see Box, p. 72) places rehabilitation, an integral part of the future healthcare delivery continuum, in front of national healthcare decision-makers. Target groups are physicians, payers, employers, legislators, and the general public.

Rehabilitation nursing continues to evolve as a specialty within the nursing profession. One impact of Diagnostic-Related Groups (DRGs) during the early 1980s was shorter lengths of stay in acute care settings. More clients returned to the community with less education about their condition, poor preparation for follow-up with activities of daily living (ADL), and increased medical acuity. Some community service agencies were unprepared or inadequately staffed to meet the demands for care. Community nurses at times were unfamiliar with specific techniques or equipment required by clients returning to the community with increased acuity, technology supports, or specialized rehabilitation needs.

MARKETING AWARENESS ABOUT REHABILITATION

1989   THE ASSOCIATION OF REHABILITATION NURSES

"Rehabilitation Nurses Make the Difference!" brochure created to assist nurse managers in describing their specialty promotes education and recruitment efforts.

1992   AMERICAN CONGRESS OF REHABILITATION MEDICINE

"What is a Psychiatrist?" brochure. There is a knowledge deficit among health professionals, in general, about rehabilitation concepts, practice, goals, and cost-effective outcomes.

1992   AMERICAN HOSPITAL ASSOCIATION SPECIALTY SUBSECTION FOR REHABILITATION HOSPITALS AND PROGRAMS AND THE NATIONAL ASSOCIATION OF REHABILITATION FACILITIES (NARF) (The American Rehabilitation Association [ARA] since 1994)

"Meeting the Challenge." A national rehabilitation awareness campaign conducted by the Medical Rehabilitation Education Foundation (MREF) was established to promote better understanding of what rehabilitation is and what it does for people.

About the same time research findings documented the benefits of early intervention practices following injury from trauma or disease. Thus rehabilitation nursing principles became prominent in prevention as well as in tertiary interventions.

For the first time other nursing specialties became familiar with and began to recognize the value of rehabilitation nurses and their expertise in patient education, discharge planning, and continuity of care as well as clinical knowledge and skills, interdisciplinary teamwork, and program evaluation activities. The initial Certified Rehabilitation Registered Nurse (CRRN) credential in 1984, the steady membership growth of ARN, and the prominence of rehabilitation nurse leaders in both professional nursing and the national and global healthcare scenes demonstrate an increasing influence of rehabilitation nurses as a specialty.

WORK REDESIGN MODELS

In the seventies primary nursing essentially replaced functional nursing or assembly-line nursing and team nursing, popular in the fifties and sixties. Primary nursing may be a good fit with some rehabilitation clinical areas, as rehabilitation nurses traditionally practiced a form of primary nursing before it was labeled. Certainly the length of stay (LOS) for rehabilitation clients during the 1970s, and the extent to which nurses are involved in assessing and knowing home and community, influenced the ready acceptance of primary nursing in the rehabilitation setting.

A major debate in nursing management during the nineties concerns the ideal system for the delivery of nursing care. One positive outgrowth of the nursing shortage, which peaked during the late 1980s, was opportunity to redefine and redesign professional practice models. Fralic (1992) says that "the availability of nurses is not the singular pressing issue," but rather, "today's concern is often the high cost per nurse or the availability/affordability dilemma."

For these reasons, during the last several years there has been more experimentation and diversity in care delivery models. Care delivery models are to be client care focused, interdisciplinary or transdisciplinary, as opposed to solely addressing nursing care delivery. The ideal model will depict the way an institution organizes the delivery of care, which differs from "creating just another way that nursing operates," a critical distinction (Fralic, 1992). "Health care organizations cannot afford the same number of nurses at a dramatically higher cost per nurse" (pp. 7-8); therefore more effective systems for healthcare delivery must be designed.

The primary nursing model does bring satisfaction to nurses and patients. The patients know who their nurse is and often acknowledge and maintain contact with "their" nurse. This provides a feeling of satisfaction and a sense of accomplishment by the nursing staff.

Ter Maat (1993) found most rehabilitation hospitals used primary nursing as a model, but also noted one fifth of hospitals surveyed were using more than one form of nursing care delivery. Primary nursing facilitates the interdisciplinary model because team members identify the primary nurse who is working with the client and the family and look to that person to serve as the advocate.

Historically rehabilitation nurses have been involved in providing for continuity of care and discharge planning. By the late 1970s, and with the onset of DRGs, nurses in acute care patterned client education and discharge planning after rehabilitation nursing practice. Over the next two decades, managed care and nursing case management models catapulted to the forefront. These models seem ideal for care on rehabilitation units and in the community. The case management model, which has been used for rehabilitation clients in the community, now is being applied in the care of clients in the inpatient setting and also is being applied to tools, such clinical pathways used for tracking outcome and variance in care. Appendix 6-A provides an example of a clinical pathway, which is a clinical management tool.

Case management, discussed in Chapter 8, is an interdisciplinary process that facilitates coordination, utilization of resources, and quality outcomes in a predictable order to achieve an effective LOS. Interdisciplinary meetings in rehabilitation provide a collaborative setting for discussing any variances in a client's progress on a specific care map or clinical path to be discussed with team members.

In 1990 Medicus Systems conducted a survey of AONE members with results from 1150 returned surveys along with responses from 40 chief executive officers (CEOs) and chief operating officers (COOs) of hospitals. These executives were asked to give their opinions about care delivery models in nursing and to respond to the following statement: "The trend of case management will be the predominant approach to patient management." Sixty-nine percent of the AONE members and eighty-seven percent of the CEOs were in agreement with the statement. Regarding the statement "The patient care delivery team will expand to include more non-licensed staff," 81% of the AONE members agreed compared with 92.5% of the CEOs. The CEOs tended to favor case management and to use more unlicensed staff to deliver care than AONE executives. In results of another survey of nearly a thousand nurse executives, Wake (1990) found over half the respondents targeted case management as the model of the future.

Whatever the care delivery model used, nurses will need auxiliary helpers who are sufficiently skilled to assist with the care of clients but who will work within the criteria for unlicensed personnel set by the American Nurses' Association (ANA). Rehabilitation has used a mix of professional registered nurses (RNs), licensed practical nurses (LPNs), and some type of nursing assistants. Professional nurses who work in rehabilitation are encouraged to become certified through ARN (RN, CRRN) and to be educated with a baccalaureate nursing degree. New directions in the 1990s featured major projects around the country related to cross training, multiskilled workers, and client- and family-focused care. Caregivers trained in these models are cross trained to do everything from "direct care to changing light bulbs" in an effort to reduce the number of people and steps required to complete each task. Ideally quality of care improves, client and family satisfaction increases, and costs are reduced. The key concept in this model is "never to hand off to someone else what you can do yourself" (Brider, 1992). Thus, in a rehabilitation facility, a client in a physical therapy area would be assisted by a physical therapist for toileting, or an ancillary person from a nursing unit might transport a client to therapy or to lunch and while there assist the client with preparation for therapy or eating a meal.

In this client-focused model the organization is built around people with similar needs, a sorting that facilitates multiskilled workers in rehabilitation, where there is an existing foundation for interdisciplinary practice. This model also fits with traditional nursing goals to promote and maintain ADL skills and assure continuity of therapy interventions while the client is in nursing areas, whether day, evening, or night shifts and on weekends.

Whether client- and family-focused care models truly reduce costs is a question that remains to be answered. Certainly costs will have to be calculated using methods other than the monthly bottom line. Health executives are learning what rehabilitation nurses have known for a century: client and economic outcomes of interventions for chronic and disabling conditions require longitudinal study and analysis. The CEO at one hospital where a client- and family-focused model is being piloted estimated the hospital could reduce costs by 3% to 5% on each 40-bed unit once the system was in place throughout the hospital (Perry, 1990).

A rehabilitation hospital may be operated as an independent facility, as part of a university system, or as a rehabilitation unit within a community hospital. Each type of unit has its own set-up, mix of staff, and corresponding level of acuity for clients. The challenge is for each facility to find the best care delivery model for these variables. The same premise holds for clinics or home health agencies: the clientele, care load, staff mix, and goals of care help determine the best care delivery model.

INTRAFACILITY OR INTRAAGENCY RELATIONS

Client- and family-focused models encourage staff members to prioritize client needs, develop mutual goals, attend to problem-solving, and improve outcome because departmental barriers are reduced. Problem resolution is a process of

+ Identifying specific problems leading to breakdown in the process
+ Identifying possible combinations of solutions or alternatives
+ Selecting the most effective and efficient solutions while acknowledging effects on those involved
+ Ascertaining organizational administrative support
+ Allocating essential resources and means of distribution
+ Agreeing on evaluation and criteria for refinement before the solution is implemented
+ Assuring staff and client/family support for the resolution

Continuity of a client's care within a facility or a community agency involves coordinating activities among disciplines, observing and supporting intradisciplinary programs, and providing feedback about functions that are shared among disciplines, including observations of client functioning in all areas. Effective coordination of each client's rehabilitation program provides continuity of care among inpatient, outpatient, and home care and conserves resources.

A rehabilitation nurse manager's area of responsibility gains effectiveness and efficiency, builds trust and communication, and benefits clients when

+ Staff members establish rapport with other professionals and support services staff with whom they interact
+ Staff members maintain ongoing professional interaction that enhances reciprocal understanding of one another's knowledge, skills, and needs
+ The manager understands how support services such as central supply, laundry, food services, or maintenance are organized
+ The manager is able to recognize needs and abilities of support services
+ The manager acknowledges the contributions of support service staff to rehabilitation efforts
+ Representatives of disciplines and service areas meet to seek resolution of ineffective processes

NURSING CARE DELIVERY SUPPORT

A rehabilitation nurse manager relies on support from a variety of resources, in addition to staff members. Systems, supplies, equipment, space, and services impact care. A rehabilitation nurse manager with participation from nursing staff may identify improvements for existing or new systems as well as needs for equipment or supplies. Equipment or supply items often receive more attention as solutions to problems because they are more visible, tangible, and manageable than are systems solutions.

However, systems solutions may provide the most fertile

outcomes provided the change is for a client- or family-focused program. Basic processes in rehabilitation such as timing of bathing, bowel and bladder programs, or vital signs traditionally were scheduled according to the programs of the system rather than according to client preferences or needs. Systems problems are difficult to identify and resolve when no one discipline knows or coordinates all aspects of a client's care. This leads to discontinuity, confusion, and an ineffective, inefficient habit: "We've always done it that way." Examples of fragmented interdisciplinary systems that are opportunities to improve outcome are eating and swallowing programs (Chapter 17), or admission processes.

Equipment resources may be left unattended until budget time, when a nurse manager is called on to list and prioritize equipment needs. Ideally a manager has solicited input from the nursing staff, particularly those who use the equipment. An astute rehabilitation nurse manager

- ✦ Establishes and reviews an equipment inventory for the area, noting items owned, shared, borrowed, or leased
- ✦ Identifies equipment that may need repair or replacement due to age, frequent use, or new technology
- ✦ Schedules preventive cleaning and maintenance or repair such as for wheelchairs, shower chairs, self-propelled stretchers, or hand-held shower heads
- ✦ Replaces equipment that is obsolete or impractical
- ✦ Assures staff members understand the process for equipment repair, where it is documented, and their responsibilities
- ✦ Trains staff to habitually scan work areas for equipment or safety concerns
- ✦ Participates in environmental rounds with housekeeping or maintenance staff

Too commonly a nurse manager's first awareness of an equipment problem is a complaint from a client or family, only to discover the equipment malfunction is due to lack of report, repair, or replacement. Ideally staff and clients who use equipment are involved in evaluating new equipment before purchase and address all reports of malfunction or poor quality. Nurses and clients who problem-solve together may discover improved methods for common situations.

Another area where the rehabilitation nurse manager works with staff is in comparing usefulness and qualities of supplies of different styles or from various vendors such as for bladder care supplies, disposable pads, or antiseptic hand soap. Similarly, special qualities or varieties of supplies such as for catheterization or incontinence may not be usual stock supplies but are needed for individual clients. Another concern is matching a client's use of supplies with correct charges—for instance, ordering catheters for a client with paraplegia according to frequency of use. An increased census or change in client mix also will change supply needs.

GROWTH AND DEVELOPMENT
Self-Development

Self-learning is an important habit for the rehabilitation nursing manager to cultivate. Opportunities for self-learning are readily available; the key is to develop a strategic plan for self-learning that is balanced and planned to increase strengths as well as to improve needs. In preparing a strategic plan for self-improvement, the rehabilitation nurse manager reviews the long-range plans for the agency, department, and individual area, as these will provide valuable insights for direction. For example, if the agency is in the process of establishing a continuous quality improvement approach, the nurse manager would be well advised to seek articles, books, and programs on this process. If the department has a goal to refine its approach to program evaluation to align with other departments, the rehabilitation nurse manager could prepare by discussing approaches with the other area managers. The rehabilitation nurse manager plans for ongoing clinical and managerial development through a variety of resources such as a review of nursing, rehabilitation, and management or leadership books and journals; participation in inservices and educational opportunities; and establishing relationships with peers and supervisors.

The rehabilitation nurse manager's self-development plan schedules ongoing discussions with the direct supervisor for administrative support including time, space, materials, staff, and financial assistance. In turn, the rehabilitation nurse manager is prepared to support requests with documentation of need, features, and benefits to the staff, department, and agency or facility—and perhaps propose shared accountability.

Quality Improvement/Program Evaluation

The processes of continuous quality improvement and outcome evaluation are discussed in Chapter 7. A rehabilitation nurse manager role requires knowledge about quality improvement and outcome evaluation, skill in application, and techniques for teaching and reinforcing staff members to understand and apply these processes. Responsibilities include applications such as individualizing client goals and interventions and working collaboratively with nursing staff and other disciplines to identify specialty problems or areas for improvement. Staff members are involved in all levels of problem identification, selection of goals, measurement processes, and outcome evaluation. Concerns are identified by staff members who give direct care; staff education about quality improvement processes, demonstrations of how the processes can resolve problems, ongoing feedback and evaluation, and opportunities to initiate change assist staff members to objectively discern whether their interventions made a difference.

Nursing Staff Development

The most effective and efficient way to provide staff development opportunities for rehabilitation nursing staff remains a thorny issue for nursing managers. There is a cyclical shortage of RNs and a chronic shortage of nurses prepared to practice rehabilitation nursing. The governing priority for deciding which staff development needs are addressed in rehabilitation nursing is simply benefit to clients. Enhancement and enrichment of nursing staff competencies and abilities are justified when client care and outcome are improved.

Four fundamental objectives central to staff development are responsibilities of a rehabilitation nurse manager. The first objective is to determine educational resources that support or provide education. Educational resources may be human (e.g., yourself), other nursing personnel, other experienced rehabilitation professionals, or community speakers; material such as facility/specialty library, books/journals, equipment or supply inserts, audiovisuals; or financial, including education/travel or credentialing support.

The second objective for the rehabilitation nurse manager is to identify three types of needs by which to guide developing rehabilitation staff: client needs that drive staff development priorities, including orientation; staff needs; and facility and accreditation needs.

A third objective is to determine staff development goals and objectives. This does not mean to delineate them independently, but rather through preliminary work as a manager with supportive rationale. Meetings with staff, individually and collectively, are one means to provide a nurse manager with an opportunity to promote preliminary work and to receive feedback, additional ideas, and refinement by staff members, enhancing ownership of the goals and objectives by all. The selected goals and objectives need to concur with the agency or facility mission and with directions of the department supervisor.

The fourth objective is to create a supportive environment, beginning with the nurse manager serving as a role model. Thus manager and staff are able to demonstrate a shared initiative in increasing knowledge, skills, and the value of both.

Staff Education

A rehabilitation nurse manager may be responsible for three categories of staff education: orientation, inservices, and continuing education programs. Orientation is the process of transitioning a new staff member into a work area, the educational process, and the unit milieu. The nurse manager sets a tone with established staff about the importance of orientation and value of new employees, as well as staff, extending throughout the rehabilitation team as well. To integrate, the nurse manager intersperses classroom work with application opportunities, following principles for adult learners as discussed in Chapter 10.

Inservices comprise a second category of learning experiences provided in the work setting to assure the staff member follows the accepted practices of the facility or agency. The purposes of inservices include initial orientation or reeducation of employees, presentation of new products or procedures, and teaching skills and improved knowledge of job-related activities.

The third category of staff development is continuing education programs. Continuing education programs are planned learning experiences beyond the basic nursing curriculum. Continuing education programs may include such diverse areas as advanced assessment parameters for a specific client population, growth and development applications in rehabilitation, or exposure to ideas of rehabilitation nursing leaders. Ideally continuing education programs will offer contact hours as continuing education units (CEUs) toward maintaining certification in a nursing specialty.

Typically there are more ideas for educational activities than there is time for staff to attend or resources to provide them. Although educational activities are planned to meet staff development criteria, in reality they are offered within the context of a busy nursing unit where client needs are priorities. When educational programs are interrupted continually or not attended, the manager intervenes. Unless the manager collaborates with others to identify factors that may affect success, educational activities will remain isolated experiences for staff members without direct impact on clinical performance and client outcome.

Every educational activity is evaluated to identify how well attendees learned and the effect of learning on client outcome or clinical decision-making. Evaluation is important on several levels. In one, results of evaluation of the educational process will indicate how well the program was conducted and whether it was cost-effective. Another measure is how the participants self-reported their learning as a result of having attended the program. But over time successful education programs can be expected to change participants' behavior, or competencies, in professional practice. Otherwise educational programs cannot be defended as cost-effective or as an appropriate use of resources.

There are three reasons why nurse managers consider student experiences in a rehabilitation facility or community agency. First and foremost, student educational experiences during basic education are opportunities to expose students to the specialty of rehabilitation nursing. Second, students may become interested in rehabilitation nursing and be open to recruitment efforts. Third, when nursing students understand rehabilitation nursing principles and practices, regardless of their future area of practice, the more able they will be to incorporate rehabilitation principles and practices into other levels of nursing intervention and care. As a result clients will be prepared for rehabilitation from onset of illness or injury and throughout their health care. Ideally every eligible client will receive rehabilitation unencumbered with pressure areas, contractures, loss of potential function, and other preventable complications. The astute rehabilitation nurse manager will share a student's clinical objectives for the rehabilitation experience with nursing staff and enlist support in achieving the objectives.

Alternative models for student experiences include student rotations in clinical sites, following clients from facility to their homes, attending clinical appointments and other community-based programs, and learning to work with nurse colleagues at many points in the health system. Evaluation mechanisms include student and staff evaluations of student experiences; review of experiences, competencies, and how objectives were attained among the staff members, nurse manager, and faculty; and finally, recruitment of new graduates.

Lifelong Education for Professional Nursing

It is appropriate for nurse managers to work with staff to promote professional nursing responsibility for ongoing lifelong learning. In client and family education activities, nurses teach not only specific information but also how to apply and adapt it to the variety of situations a client and family may experience. The same is true for each rehabilitation nurse's own learning. With the rapid explosion of knowledge and technology in nursing, rehabilitation, and healthcare it has become impossible to practice as an expert professional without actively pursuing ongoing learning.

The standards for professional nursing practice include a mandate for this in the standard to acquire and maintain current knowledge in nursing practice (ANA, 1991). Within this standard are criteria that address a nurse's responsibility for participating in ongoing educational activities related to clinical knowledge and professional issues, as well as for seeking experiences to maintain clinical skills and knowledge appropriate to the practice setting.

The process that nurses use to meet this professional responsibility is very similar to the one outlined for client and family education in Chapter 10. The assessment component requires the nurse to identify learning needs, readiness to learn, and the learning style that best supports acquisition of knowledge and skills. This requires the professional nurse to evaluate critically what knowledge and skills are needed and motivators for identifying these needs. Once the assessment has been accomplished, the nurse develops a plan for how to achieve the desired learning. The plan includes identification of specific goals and objectives, available resources, learning activities that will be used, and how evaluation of the plan will take place. Finally, the plan is implemented and evaluated. For professional nurses this process of acquiring and maintaining current knowledge is ongoing with multiple components and phases of the process for different learning areas. For a rehabilitation nurse who will be involved in a new program, the learning needs may be substantial with a short time in which to meet them. That same nurse may have identified a personal learning need to become more knowledgeable about quality improvement activities in healthcare and set a time line of the next year to gain more knowledge in the area. Both of these learning needs may be being met at the same point in time but may take on very different levels of priority and implementation.

Many strategies can be used in the pursuit of lifelong professional learning and of multiple continuing education programs available in a variety of formats. Continuing education programs may be structured as seminars, workshops, and conferences attended either on site or at numerous sites across the country via satellite transmission. Increasingly continuing education also is available in independent study formats through the use of programs designed as independent study modules or through various journals. Regularly reading and critiquing journals and books, such as discussing articles in a journal discussion group, is another strategy that can be used.

Learning needs also can be met by participation in formal academic education programs. Certain career goals or positions may require completion of an academic program of study. To practice in an advanced practice role as a clinical nurse specialist or nurse practitioner requires a master's degree. Several graduate nursing programs offer specialization in rehabilitation nursing.

Education is an important component of rehabilitation nursing practice. It comprises a significant portion of what we do in providing care to individuals with disability and chronic illness. It is also a fundamental professional behavior to maintain and advance knowledge so that nurses can continue to provide quality care to our clients. The nurse manager who seeks to maintain a competent staff will encourage staff, arrange for continuing education programs, inform staff about tuition remission or similar educational supports; budget for educational activities, conferences, and professional literature; and reward and encourage staff attendance for continuing education.

Evaluation

The rehabilitation nurse manager has numerous opportunities to participate in evaluation activities. The word opportunities is used purposefully, as managers do not always view the evaluation process in a positive light. Evaluation, whether of staff, processes, or outcomes may be viewed as a task, or worse, ignored. The rehabilitation nurse manager is advised to prioritize evaluation activities, seeking ways to improve the mechanisms. Evaluation is a primary way for the rehabilitation nurse manager to measure the effectiveness and efficiency of staff members, processes, and outcomes while promoting rehabilitation expectations.

Performance Appraisal

Effective employee performance appraisal conducted by the rehabilitation nurse manager includes learning and incorporating the evaluative requirements of the specific employer. Frequently such requirements include formal written documentation, conducted minimally at the end of the probationary period and annually thereafter. Individual staff evaluations may be used by the rehabilitation nurse manager to acknowledge rehabilitation strengths of staff members: teaching skills, knowledge of specific rehabilitation diagnoses, assessment skills, or safety applications.

Staff evaluations also may identify areas for an employee's individual growth; the key in all cases is to state specific behavioral objectives. "Identify specific diet, food allergies, food or beverage preferences and dislikes, current height and weight, skin turgor, and typical mealtimes in nutritional status portion of the admission assessment" rather than "improve nutritional evaluation" gives clear and measurable expectations. Set times for completion of stated goals and follow-up evaluation with feedback to the employee allows each one to know that both responsibility and accountability are considered important. The evaluation process is clarified further by using interactive strategies such as employee input to written performance objectives; informal discussions of current employee performance status between the nurse manager and employee; and feedback from the employee to the manager being encouraged regarding progress, concerns, and needs. Intermittent informal feedback to employees, either verbal or written, is a useful managerial tool as it keeps the employee aware performance is being routinely assessed and acknowledged.

Some administrative arrangements may result in rehabilitation nurse managers providing information that will become part of evaluation for professionals who work in a nurse-managed program or area but who report to another manager. Examples include dieticians, maintenance workers, therapists, and volunteers. The manager must understand clearly the direct supervisor's expectations of these employees. When interdisciplinary teams are organized around specialty programs or product lines (e.g., a brain injury program) or team members have multiple assignments with responsibilities to several different programs (matrix), team members are evaluated for their contribution to the program(s) and for their professional competencies. As a rule professional competencies are evaluated by their own professional group standards; however, they may receive a number of program performance evaluations from supervisors within the matrix of programs in which they work. As with the manager's own employees, observations should be specific, with strengths and areas for growth clearly identified.

Process Improvement

Processes provide opportunities for the astute rehabilitation nurse manager, both for improving operations and demonstrating mechanisms of change. In rehabilitation, process evaluation opportunities include such diverse areas as the admission process, client scheduling, staff conferences, or client response to educational activities. Evaluation of processes is interdisciplinary and multidimensional, beginning with identifying the specific process outline, the needs of clinical specialties at another level, and the accomplishment of managerial expectations at a third level. Processes frequently performed by rehabilitation nurses such as client medication education and bowel or bladder management may be improved by using process evaluation techniques.

Evaluation of processes should include those individuals who participate in the processes themselves. Using medication education for clients as an example, process evaluation might include feedback from the RNs providing initial client education, LPN's comments about reinforcement activities, pharmacist's and educator's comments regarding teaching methods and educational materials, and feedback from clients. The purpose of process evaluation is to identify the most efficient ways to accomplish a process.

Outcome Assessment

Outcome evaluation analyzes the effectiveness of an activity or process. The outcome evaluation for client medication education could assess whether the activities were effective; did the client demonstrate planned outcomes such as correct route, time, and dosage of medication and an ability to describe the purpose of the medication and any side effects?

Note that process and outcome evaluations are closely interwoven, as it is difficult to identify efficient process if the desired outcome is not clear. Conversely the desired outcome may be met, but the process for achieving it might have numerous steps that could be eliminated, streamlining efficiency. It is not unusual to identify improvements in both process and outcome from the same evaluation process.

Fiscal Management

Preparation of rehabilitation nurse managers for financial management is frequently on-the-job training combined with trial and error. Often the nurse manager's first exposure to fiscal management is preparing a budget or explaining variances. There are excellent texts specifically written to assist the nurse manager in fiscal management (Finkler & Kovner, 1993); the intent of this section is to discuss key fiscal operations that a rehabilitation nurse manager can expect to perform.

Budget preparation and maintenance is the core of fiscal management. The simplistic description of budget is a fiscal plan, often for a designated period, usually annually. Budget preparation could be described as short-term fiscal strategic planning and budget maintenance as the routine evaluation of variances from the fiscal plan.

Three types of budget operations pertinent to rehabilitation nurse managers are revenue, expense, and capital. Operating budget is a term commonly used to refer to some combination of revenue and expense budgets.

✦ Operating budget
Revenue

The revenue budget provides income information for the area of responsibility, regardless of setting. Although financial report forms vary, typical contents include both current month and fiscal year-to-date information. The rehabilitation nurse manager may compare actual income versus predicted income for the current month and for the fiscal year to date to identify fiscal trends. Financial reports also often subdivide income by payer source. The nurse manager may in this circumstance review the mix of payer sources and trends over time to evaluate financial reimbursement implications. "Patient days" are the typical unit of fiscal measurement for inpatient settings and client visits; procedures and/or time increments may be used in home health or clinic settings. The rehabilitation nurse manager should be familiar with these variables.

In a facility the manager needs to be aware of decreasing total "patient days," while admissions may actually increase. The resultant impact may be an increasing workload for nursing staff, even though the average daily census is lower than previously experienced. Analyzing trends of admissions, "patient days," and LOS is important in preparing and maintaining the budget. An inexperienced nurse manager may monitor and adjust expenses compulsively based on a fixed budget, while "patient days" and reimbursements fluctuate significantly above or below expectations.

The experienced nurse manager uses the applicable unit of fiscal measurement, whether "patient days," visits, procedures, or other, to identify "break-even" points for the budget. These break-even points occur when revenues equal expenses. The nurse manager strives to increase revenues and decrease expenses while maintaining or improving effectiveness and efficiency of client outcomes. Payer sources vary in amount of reimbursement; the mix of clients by payer source affects the amount of "patient days," visits, or procedures at which the break-even point occurs. As the nurse manager gains experience, comparison of diagnostic categories and related costs is a refinement.

✦ Expense
Personnel

The expense budget reflects the rehabilitation nurse manager's prediction of annual costs for area-defined expenses. The majority of costs in the expense budget for inpatient rehabilitation nursing areas is salaries, which include fringe benefits and frequently exceed 80% to 90% of the total expense budget. This fiscal effect is due to the labor-intensive aspect of rehabilitation and the need for rehabilitation nursing staff with specialized skills and knowledge.

Shorter acute care client stays and increased survival rates of clients with selective complex diagnoses have brought increased technology and associated "know how" into the rehabilitation setting.

The goal of the function of staffing is to meet clients' needs for care with optimal quality and efficiency. Staffing is a process of determining and providing nursing staff to offer an effective number of nursing hours per "patient day;" the best mix of nursing staff personnel with the correct distribution of personnel over the 24-hour day for 7 days a week. There is no one correct staffing configuration for all rehabilitation units; differences in client populations, acuity levels, and availability of personnel make generic staffing approaches unrealistic.

✦ Acuity

Many variables affect staffing, but the primary variable is "client acuity." Acuity a measure of each client's severity of illness related to the amount of nursing care resources needed for care (Finkler & Kovner, 1993). Each facility or agency decides on a system for classifying clients into categories according to the intensity of care each one needs. In turn, the resulting acuity level indicates the mix and number of staff needed. Having reliable data from a client classification system is essential for the manager to make realistic and accountable decisions about staffing.

Ter Maat (1993) found that 67% of the rehabilitation hospitals she surveyed used a system developed within the institution and, at least from her sample, there was no indication of existence of a standard system in the rehabilitation setting. Using a nationally established client classification system does allow for comparisons of like institutions, but there are other variables to be considered when reviewing acuity data from another institution, such as client diagnosis or age. Some rehabilitation units admit clients with orthopedic or chronic pain conditions where the acuity may be lower than on a unit admitting clients using mechanical ventilators following spinal cord injury or those in coma management programs.

Administrators often are surprised to learn the acuity and recommended hours per "patient day" (HPPD) are as high as in some critical care or step-down units. Understanding that clients need more time when guided or assisted through an activity than when care is given by a caregiver is an underappreciated and unfamiliar concept. In fact, some clients may require additional resources—for instance, pediatric or geriatric clients. When an institution or agency develops or selects a client classification system, rehabilitation nurse managers ideally are key participants in decision-making. It is important for a system to represent quantifiable measures about unique functions of rehabilitation nurses, such as what they do for client education and prevention of complications. Rehabilitation nurses also perform extensive assessments concerning a client's safety, adaptability, and access to community resources, as well as participating with community agencies and services in assuring continuity of care and preventing readmission to a facility. Sometimes these functions are not weighted as highly as technologic interventions when classification systems nonspecific for rehabilitation are used to determine acuity.

Supplies/Services

The nonsalary budget includes supplies and services or direct expenses not related to employees. These items include the routine costs to the nursing areas such as medical and nonmedical supplies. It is a good idea to communicate and coordinate with other related departments when planning this part of the budget. Sometimes plans in one department affect what happens to nursing expenses, or expenses may be transferred to the nursing budget from other areas such as duplicating, maintenance expenses, meal costs, or mattress replacement costs.

The nonpersonnel budget lines (or accounts) may yield opportunities to reduce expenses and improve client care at the same time. Although some cost-effective efforts may be small in the short term, over time or in combination with others, positive results can be achieved. The rehabilitation nurse manager remains vigilant that rehabilitation needs are met in fiscal efforts. For example, client trays are being substituted for a cafeteria-style serving line in a rehabilitation facility. The intent is to reduce dietary employee full-time equivalents (FTEs) and preparation/wastage costs in a rehabilitation setting. The rehabilitation nurse manager assures the new procedure incorporates menu selection by clients and the eating area retains the atmosphere of a dining room. In another instance medications and equipment selected for bowel or bladder management protocols may have significant financial impact on the nursing department budget. These costs may be justified only if the protocols can be shown to impact client outcome positively after a client's community reentry.

The rehabilitation nurse manager also becomes familiar with charge and noncharge items for clients and their costs. Individual charges are made for those care items billed to a client as each item is used. Noncharge items affect the budget if the manager does not limit selection to those that impact client care and set ways to avoid and monitor for wastage. It is easy for an inexperienced manager to ask for a new charge item, believing the cost will be covered by the client's payment source, when in fact, the person may have a set per diem reimbursement rate, regardless of charges. Lost charges occur when chargeable items are dispensed or used but not billed to the client; this usually results in the nursing budget absorbing the cost. The astute nurse manager knows meal and snack costs, linen charges, and other facility-specific costs.

Capital Budget

Capital budget is routinely identified as equipment or building project items planned for purchase during the fiscal year that cost more than a facility-specified amount. Capital expense items are intended to be used for a designated number of years. The rehabilitation nurse manager wants to assure planned capital expenditures take into account rehabilitation needs. Examples of rehabilitation needs include considering bed height conducive to client transfer activities for new beds, effective safety lock mechanisms on wheelchair shower chairs for clients who are physically or cognitively impaired, and dining room tables that accommodate wheelchair leg rests and varying heights. Rehabilitation nurse managers often can justify a capital equipment purchase if it enhances rehabilitation activities such as installation of a tub on the unit for client bathing practice when only showers are currently available, or lifts to help prevent back injuries to staff and families. Targeting capital budget allotments for new services or planned replacement of worn equipment is within the fiscal planning requirements of the nurse manager.

Internal Fiscal Monitoring

The effective rehabilitation nurse manager uses internal monitoring to enhance fiscal control. Internal monitoring approaches vary among settings, but their purpose remains constant: to maintain current knowledge of the financial state of the area of accountability. Internal monitoring for inpatient settings could include review of storeroom or central supply utilization or routinely evaluating lost charges with staff to develop their understanding of costs and resource allocation and to encourage prudent use. Involving staff in identifying approaches to cost savings heightens their awareness of financial considerations and builds team "ownership" of responsibility. Prioritizing capital equipment purchases may also increase staff awareness of fiscal decision-making. Often nursing staff members are unfamiliar with what a wheelchair shower chair, stretcher, or lift costs. Knowledge of costs of replacement seats for wheelchair shower chairs or slings for lifts may also improve staff attention to equipment maintenance. Monthly staff meetings might include fiscal information related to monthly salary expense compared with budget, overtime usage, storeroom charges, and other expenses where there has been a significant variance between actual expenditures and the budgeted amount. Staff members may not recognize how costs in one area may reduce funds available in others when the expenses are not obviously related. A nurse manager may choose ways to monitor the budget, but there also may be internal monitoring requirements, such as a monthly budget variance report to the nurse manager's supervisor explaining variances above or below expected utilization.

Many external factors have potential to influence the budget. New regulatory expectations, such as the requirement of universal precautions in recent years, added significant monetary costs to rehabilitation units for supplies such as gloves, masks and gowns, or staff inservice training programs. Third-party payer reimbursement also affects the fiscal bottom line. First, each payer has guidelines for which services, equipment, and supplies will be paid. Second, there may be time or financial "caps" to payment, meaning a designated number of visits, days, procedures, or financial amount may not be exceeded as reimbursement above the amount is eliminated. There may also be external controls that affect costs such as federal or state requirements or limitations on services. Accreditation agencies will impact fiscal management, meeting the Commission on Accreditation of Rehabilitation Facilities (CARF) standards, for one. Fiscal management is an intricate, ever-changing set of factors that enhances or adversely affects the rehabilitation nurse manager's budget bottom line. Vigilance and creativity is necessary to effectively and efficiently maintain financial stability.

THE REHABILITATION TEAM

Composition and purposes of the rehabilitation team is discussed in other chapters of this book, such as Chapter 2. However, some information about teams is related to leadership and management issues. A team of professionals with different training, personalities, and particular expertise becomes cohesive with a common purpose and goal; the result is a smoothly functioning team that also happens to be a cost-effective team. However, individualism, independence, uniqueness of each discipline, and competition are part of a value system; too often professionals are not taught how to work together as team members. Trust and confidence in one another is preliminary to commonality; professionals meeting together weekly do not make a team.

Transdisciplinary team concepts have evolved since the emphasis in healthcare on cost savings, cross training, and client-focused care. "In this approach one member of the team acts as a primary therapist, with the other members feeding information and advice with regard to management through a single primary person" (Diller, 1990). In this current spirit of comanagement and empowerment, clients are encouraged to participate in setting goals and being involved in their plan of care. Accrediting and licensing bodies expect clients and families to participate in the rehabilitation program as active members of a rehabilitation team. Functions, interventions, and outcomes are emphasized more than discipline-specific actions in a transdisciplinary model. The cost savings and effectiveness of this model has not been demonstrated (McCourt, 1993).

However, implementing this model would take extensive education and role clarification (Hoeman, 1993). Some barriers to team activity can be related to role ambiguity and incongruent expectations, even overlapping role functions. There is a tendency for professionals either to assume too much about the knowledge, skills, and capabilities of other members of the team or to know little or erroneous information. Many problems that affect team interaction may be resolved when roles and goals are clarified. Role negotiation questions ask

- ✦ What is the target or goal of the team?
- ✦ What are the required tasks?
- ✦ What input from staff or others is required to accomplish these tasks?
- ✦ How should people work together to achieve their goals?
- ✦ Are there unique procedures and guidelines developed to carry out the task of the team?
- ✦ Where or with whom is conflict a potential?

Professionals may experience dismay or anger when others disagree with their proposed objectives or plans since many expect agreement and consider disagreement a confrontation. Conflict is inevitable, but when a team learns conflict negotiation, the outcome can be desirable, productive, and provide a sense of interdependence. Creative solutions and ideas arise varying constructive opinions, group problem-solving, and coming to consensus—which are activities that exemplify teamwork. A skilled team leader trained in conflict negotiation, group process, role relationships, and principle-centered leadership is the key to success.

Other Barriers to Teamwork

The matrix organizational structure in many rehabilitation facilities creates barriers to team functioning. In this type of complex structure, individuals report to different administrators—that is, physical therapists and occupational therapists may report to a rehabilitation administrator whereas a rehabilitation nurse reports to a nursing administrator. Although the team is central in the rehabilitation process, the matrix group has responsibilities but frequently no formal authority or budget. In settings where teams are organized around services or product lines, all team members may report to the same manager, who selects members of each service team.

Sometimes guidelines or set expectations are lacking for teams. Team members in this structure are reduced to influencing their manager for staffing, equipment, and necessary policies and procedures. Consequently it is difficult for treatment teams to make decisions that may be overruled or undersupported by their department directors. Excellent communication is imperative. Conversely teams may fail to address management concerns or needs for individual disciplines in their endeavors to address the needs of a specific client group or persons within a diagnostic category. Agencies with multiple rehabilitation teams need to establish core expectations of teams, or a multiplicity of overlapping incongruent policies, protocols, and forms may result. These, in turn, adversely affect documentation, evaluation, financial comparisons, personnel accountability, accreditation, or payer review. For example, a team may pursue a documentation approach that does not meet medical record, legal, or accreditor expectations and causes difficulty for those individuals who must work the matrix between teams. Strategies are to encourage flexibility, provide mechanisms for an individual team to investigate alternatives, and stress clear communication.

Team Building

A team-building strategy is to create a common language, a process for decision-making, and a theme, even a code name. Nurse managers can provide opportunities for staff nurses to gain skills in assertiveness, conflict management, assessment, and role definition. In this decade of proliferating knowledge and technology, specialization has made teamwork mandatory. Team building is designed to increase a group's effectiveness by improving interpersonal relationships, problem-solving abilities, communication about issues that affect efficiency, and elicit support among team members. Team building yields a more cohesive, mutually supportive, and trusting group where there are high expectations for task accomplishment with mutual respect for differences in values, personalities, and skills. Team members need time for their teamwork, to meet to discuss how their team functions. It has been said that football teams practice 40 hours a week to perform 3 hours a week; however, healthcare teams perform 40-plus hours a week without any practice. And now the client and family are to become a part of the team.

Ethical Boundaries

Client and staff interaction in the rehabilitation setting may differ from what occurs in an acute care facility. Propinquity, longer LOS, and an emphasis on wellness instead of the sick role are some of the variables that affect the therapeutic interaction. Intimate knowledge of the individual client and family over time creates a familiarity not usually available in an acute care area. Rehabilitation nurse's interactions with a client include education and counseling about daily self-care and adjustments for independent living with a chronic or irrevocable condition, which differs from technologic care or instructions about disease or postsurgical management to a client who, although ill, will recover. Many nurses were taught in basic professional education to "not get too involved" or become "too close" to a client. Setting boundaries for appropriate interaction can be difficult; in fact, nurses often deal better with issues of anger and personality conflicts between nurses and clients than with feelings of liking or fondness. Personal involvement is not the same as empathy, caring, or compassion and has the potential to be detrimental to both client and nurse (Pennington, Gafner, Schilit, & Bechtel, 1993).

Gafner and Trudeau (1990) state the most prominent contributing factors causing healthcare workers to overstep the boundaries of appropriate relationships are "unnecessary disclosure of personal information by staff; the general relaxation of a once rigid professional distance in most aspects of care; and the incapability or unwillingness of some staff to meet their personal needs off the job."

Other issues impairing the staff-client relationship as discussed by Pennington et al. (1993) are "accepting gifts and favors, doing business with patients and their families, or being coerced or manipulated by patients." These issues are sometimes more common when a person is being discharged from a facility and the client or family may want to demonstrate their appreciation. Terminating relationships in this setting is difficult, as individuals may return for care and/or follow-up for a lifetime. Staff need to be aware that even casually visiting when the person returns to the clinic may be interpreted differently than the nurse intends. Ethical considerations for professional and client relationships must be respected.

Co-dependence—that is, wanting to be liked at the expense of self-direction and doing for others what they can do for themselves—is a concept to be explored in the rehabilitation setting. Frequently this is referred to as enabling behavior. Nurses, and women especially, have been found to have co-dependent tendencies, which may be heightened in a rehabilitation setting. Since nurses teach clients to care for themselves, promote problem-solving (rather than "solution giving"), and encourage self-sufficiency, enabling situations where nurses are tempted to "help too much" may be subtle. Vulnerable staff members often are those who attempt to meet their own social and emotional needs in the work environment. Many times a staff member's own vulnerabilities interfere with the therapeutic relationship, as when both staff member and client build a personal relationship on one another's needs. In order to establish rapport with a client, staff members may disclose information about themselves, but relaying personal problems is not contributory to a professional relationship. Staff should explore their needs for affirmation with sources other than clients. In another view staff may do some caring thing to encourage a client's hopes, only to have the gesture misinterpreted by the client. A well-intentioned response to a person's loneliness too often is interpreted as a personal interest. Maintaining professional distance, however, does not mean being aloof.

Rehabilitation nurse managers can work with other team members to set guidelines for client and staff interactions. The team is an important resource, as objectivity can be offered by one's peers and colleagues. A team that has some experience in team building can be mutually supportive. When trusting and comfortable with one another, a team can provide constructive criticism while increasing awareness of all team members' behaviors. Many staff members have never had the issue of client and staff boundaries discussed in their formal education, and staff support groups can be helpful to relieve stress and discuss vulnerabilities or boundary issues. Often professionals and managers in an agency or facility are able to arrive at consensus on the philosophy or expectations for behavior, which is then supported by all departments. When all acknowledge that objectivity is essential in care, reassignment may be a consideration for a professional who can no longer be therapeutic with a client. An agreed-upon philosophy or policy then is shared with all staff members in an interdisciplinary orientation (see box below).

Examples of specific recommendations are

1. The rehabilitation agency/area/team should formulate a policy or guidelines based on their philosophy.
2. The philosophy and policy should be presented and discussed with all new employees.
3. Consistency in enforcing the policy is expected by all departments.

◆

PHILOSOPHICAL STATEMENT
EXAMPLE   *DATE:*

Competence, objectivity and concern for the best interests of the clients are primary factors considered by all health professionals and staff. This implies professional behavior in all client-staff relationships. The potential for close relationships exists in the rehabilitation setting due to the increased time the client is in the hospital and because clients usually are not "sick." Staff members need to be aware that clients may perceive a caring and concerned relationship in a different manner than staff. Personal relationships in this setting may occur, but it should be recognized that anything more than a professional relationship is not therapeutic. The staff member should not interfere with client treatments or therapies of a particular client or others on the unit. If anyone ever feels they have more than a professional relationship, or if for any reason they cannot remain objective with the client, this should be made known to the supervisor or team so that arrangements can be made for the staff member to withdraw from caring for that particular client. Staff members are encouraged to seek their supervisor for assistance in managing the situation for the benefit of the client and the employee.

---

4. Counseling/discipline needs to be consistent between departments.
5. The employee should be removed from caring for the client if a therapeutic and professional relationship is not maintained.
6. It is recommended that staff take clients out of the setting only on a planned therapeutic activity.
7. Staff will not take clients out to participate in any illegal activities (e.g., taking minors to bars).
8. Peer/team support with honest feedback is important.
9. Be sure that all clients are treated equally.

Individuals must know themselves, be aware of their own vulnerabilities and needs, and be sure that all clients are treated equally. The nurse manager has an important role in facilitating the development of guidelines for client-staff relationships, educating staff, and identifying resources for employee assistance, specifically counseling and support.

Role of the Rehabilitation Nurse Executive

The nurse executive position is the most authoritative and responsible nursing position in an organization. This individual generally is responsible for multiple areas as a top-level executive in a free-standing facility, at director level within a group of hospitals or multiple areas within a larger hospital, or as an executive director in a community agency. It is increasingly common for this nurse manager to be responsible for areas other than nursing services. The rehabilitation nurse executive is the nurse on the executive management team who is responsible for the leadership and administration of the nursing organization and for the clinical practice of rehabilitation nursing throughout the institution or agency.

The nurse executive sets the long-range vision for the departments and is able to help establish the culture of the organization. With participation of the staff, the nurse executive formulates the philosophy for the organization and subsequently the nursing department. The overall philosophy and mission of the hospital and department serve to guide strategic planning. Even individual goals and objectives flow from the overall plan.

In rehabilitation strategic planning builds on comments from interdisciplinary representation, including the medical staff. Consumer input in planning and evaluating rehabilitation programs is extremely important and beneficial and is encouraged by accrediting bodies. The effective nurse executive finds ways to assess and be knowledgeable about client, family, and community satisfaction with nursing services. Commonly used measures of satisfaction include surveys, focus groups, or even participation of former clients. The nurse executive facilitates data collection, analysis, and evaluation of the data to help provide vision for the future. External environmental criteria are part of the plan including consumers' characteristics, needs, and satisfactions. Results from client satisfaction surveys contribute data for use in strategic planning. Strategic issues have an impact on the organization and how it carries out services—for example, client, family, or community education, and developing relevant educational materials. Strategic plans of an organization may look 2 to 3 years in the future, but annual goals and objectives should be set to help achieve the long-range plan.

One role of the chief nurse executive is to develop the first-line manager, especially in this era of decentralization. An orientation plan should include not only information necessary for the new functions of the job but also assign specific time for emerging managers to develop the identity and attributes necessary to perform the role. The nurse executive is responsible for defining a nurse manager's role to the institution, the CEO, physicians, and other department heads. The nurse executive serves as a role model to the managers.

Another role of the nurse executive is to assure support for research relevant to rehabilitation nursing to improve care delivery and outcomes of care for clients. Significant findings from research are more likely to be utilized in practice with encouragement from the nurse executive. As with executives in other settings, the rehabilitation nurse executive is responsible for defining, implementing, and evaluating the care delivery system utilized in a facility; reviewing the client classification system, and justifying these with staffing and budget concerns. Continuous quality monitoring and program evaluation are crucial to the overall strategic plan for an organization. The nurse executive exercises skills in working with the leaders of other disciplines in rehabilitation to oversee the selection of program evaluation, continued assessment, and analysis of the data.

Awareness (even foreknowledge) of legislation, policies affecting people with disabilities, and reimbursement issues for services is becoming a skill required for the executive in rehabilitation. Networking and participation in professional organizations, action groups, seminars, and community projects related to nursing, rehabilitation, and individuals with disabilities builds credibility and a collegial base for an executive who is to be a leader in the organization.

REFERENCES

American Academy of Physical Medicine and Rehabilitation. (1992). *What is a physiatrist?* Chicago: Author.

American Nurses Association. (1991). *Standards of Clinical Nursing Practice.* Washington, DC: Author.

American Nurses Association. (1990). *Standards of nursing staff development.* Kansas City, MO: Author.

Association of Rehabilitation Nurses. (1994). *Rehabilitation nurse manager: Role description.* Skokie, IL: Author.

Brider, P. (1992). The move to patient focused care. *American Journal of Nursing, 9,* 26-33.

Commission on Accreditation of Rehabilitation Facilities. (1993). *Standards manual for organizations serving people with disabilities.*

Covey, S.R. (1992). *Principle-centered leadership.* New York: Simon & Schuster, p. 25.

Diller, L. (1990). Fostering the interdisciplinary team, fostering research in a society in transition. *Archives of Physical Medicine and Rehabilitation, 71,* 275-278.

Finkler, S.A., & Kovner, C.T. (1993). *Financial management for nurse managers and executives.* Philadelphia: W.B. Saunders.

Fralic, M.F. (1992). Creating new practice models and designing new roles. *Journal of Nursing Administration, 22,* 7-8.

Gafner, G., & Trudeau, V. (1990). Drawing the boundaries in staff-patient relationships. *VA Practice,* 39-45.

Hoeman, S.P. (1993). A research-based transdisciplinary team model for infants with special needs and their families. *Holistic Nursing Practice, 7,* 63-77.

Larsen, P.D. (1986). Development of educational programs in rehabilitation nursing. *Rehabilitation Nursing, 11,* 9-10.

McCourt, A.E. (ed.) (1993). The specialty practice of rehabilitation nursing care curriculum. 3rd ed. Skokie, IL: ARN Rehabilitation Nursing Foundation.

Miller, J. (1992). Patient management in the 1990's. *Interactions, 2.*

Pennington, S., Gafner, G., Schilit, R., & Bechtel, B. (1993). Addressing ethical boundaries among nurses. *Nursing Management, 24,* 36-39.

Perry, L. (1990). Hospitals seek savings by cross-training caregivers. *Modern Healthcare.*

Peters, T. (1987). Develop an inspiring vision. In *Thriving on chaos* (pp. 399-408). New York: Alfred A. Knopf.

Purk, J.K. (1993). Rehabilitation staff nurses' job satisfaction. *Rehabilitation Nursing, 18,* 249-252.

Rehabilitation Nursing Foundation. (1993). *The specialty practice of rehabilitation nursing: A core curriculum* Skokie, IL:

Ter Maat, M. (1993). An appropriate nursing skill mix: Survey of acuity systems in rehabilitation hospitals. *Rehabilitation Nursing, 18,* 244-248.

Wake, M. (1990). Nursing care delivery systems—status and vision. *Journal of Nursing Administration, 20,* 47-51.

◆

Appendix 6-A Clinical pathway: stroke—initial rehabilitation, first admission

Client needs	Week 1	Week 2	Week 3	Week 4
Medical Management (MD, RN, ARNP)	Medical problems, stroke risk factors, and appropriate treatment for these are identified; client is able to verbalize these. Client is able to participate in self-medication.	Client and family are able to verbalize medical problems and stroke risk factors. Client is able to participate in self-medication program.	Client completes self-medication program.	Client and family verbalize understanding of discharge instructions and medical follow-up.
Communication (ST, OT, RN)	Client is able to follow simple directions and simple conversation. Needs cueing 90% of the time. FIM-1	Client is able to follow simple directions and simple conversation. Needs cueing 75% of the time. FIM-2	Client is able to follow simple directions and simple conversation. Needs cueing 50% of the time. FIM-3	Client is able to follow simple directions and simple conversation. Needs cueing less than 25% of the time. FIM-4
	Client is able to respond to yes/no personal information questions. Needs cueing 75% of the time. FIM-2	Client is able to communicate basic needs. Needs cueing less than 50% of the time. FIM-3	Client is able to communicate basic needs. Needs cueing less than 25% of the time. FIM-4	Client is able to communicate basic needs. Needs cueing less than 10% of the time. FIM-5
Memory (ST, OT, RN, PT)	Client recognizes and remembers 25%-50% of time. Needs prompting more than 50% of time. Client is able to indicate awareness of memory notebook. FIM-2	Client refers to environmental cues without verbal cue 50% of time. Refers to memory notebook 25% of time without cues. FIM-3	Client refers to environmental cues. Needs prompting less than 25% of time. Refers to memory notebook 50% of time without cues. Client requires cueing to initiate memory notebook entries 50% of time. FIM-3	Client refers to environmental cues. Needs prompts less than 10% of time. Makes entries in memory notebook. Client requires cues to initiate memory notebook entries less than 25% of time. FIM-4
Problem Solving (ST, OT, RN, PT)	Client identifies that a routine problem exists, and is able to initiate sequence to correct less than 50% of the time. FIM-2	Client initiates sequence to self-correct problems 50%-75% of the time. FIM-3	Client is able to self-correct problems 75%-90% of time. FIM-4	Client is able to self-correct problems 90% of time without assistance. FIM-5
Perception Sensory/Visual (OT, PT, RN)	Client initiates correct body positioning and alignment. Client initiates environment scanning.	Client maintains correct body position and scans environment without cues, compensating for deficits 50% of time.	Client maintains correct body position and alignment and scans environment compensating for deficits 75% of time.	Client maintains correct body position and alignment and scans environment compensating for deficits 90% of time.

Continued.

Adapted from Janet Christian, MSW; Cindy Ochipa, PhD, SP; Pat Quigley, PhD, RN; Camela Sciabara, RN; Steven Scott, DO; Susan Smith, OTR-L; Mary Jo Soscia, MPH, PT; Cathy Williams, CTRS. James A. Haley Veterans Hospital, Tampa, Florida, Physical Medicine and Rehabilitation Service. Used with permission. RN, registered nurse; ARNP, advanced registered nurse practitioner; ST, speech therapist; OT, occupational therapist; PT, physical therapist; SWS, social work services; RT, registered technician; VRT, vocational rehabilitation therapist; FIM, functional independence measure; TF, tube feeding; GT, gastrostomy tube; DC, dilation catheter; PVR, postvoiding residual; ICP, intermittent catheter program; EUD, urinary device; mod, moderate; min, minimal max, maximum.

Appendix 6-A Clinical pathway: stroke—initial rehabilitation, first admission—cont'd

Client needs	Week 1	Week 2	Week 3	Week 4
Activity of Daily Living Self-Care Deficits (OT, RN, KT)	Client performs self-care activities of feeding, bathing, personal grooming, and dressing/undressing 25%-50% of time. FIM-2	Client performs self-care activities with adaptive equipment 50%-75% of time. FIM-3	Client performs self-care activities with adaptive equipment more than 75% of time. FIM-4	Client is able to perform self-care activities with set-up and supervision, using adaptive equipment. FIM-5
Dysphasia Dietary (ST, OT, RN)	Client is able to indicate awareness of swallowing difficulty. Client receives adequate nutrition via appropriate mode (TF, 6T, altered food/liquid consistency, po)	Client is able to demonstrate safe compensatory swallowing techniques with max to mod supervision.	Client is able to perform safe compensatory techniques with mod to min supervision.	Client is able to perform compensatory techniques in safe swallowing techniques.
Bowel Management Neurogenic Bowel (RN)	Client initiates verbalization of need to have bowel movement. Nursing initiates bowel management program. FIM-1	Client is continent of bowel with bowel care qod with suppository. FIM-4	Client is continent of bowel with diet supplement and/or stool softener. FIM-6	Client is continent of bowel with no accidents. FIM-7
Bladder Management Neurogenic Bladder (RN)	Client initiates verbalization of need to urinate. Nursing initiates bladder training program (DC/Foley catheter, initiate PVR, ICP) FIM-1	Client uses urinal for voiding with set-up; uses EUD at night. Accidents occur less than one time per day. FIM-2	Client is continent, using toilet during waking hours, uses urinal for night voiding only. FIM-6	Client is continent of bladder with no accidents. FIM-7
Mobility (PT, KT, OT, RN)	Client will demonstrate baseline abilities in bed and wheelchair mobility. Requires assist in bed. FIM-2 Mobility 50%-70% of time, requires assist with wc mobility 25%-50% of time. FIM-2 Client is able to perform bed, wc, chair transfers with 50%-75% assist. FIM-2 Client is able to initiate pregait activities in the parallel bars. FIM-1	Client is able to reposition self in bed 25% of time. Client is independent in wc mobility for short distances on the ward and in physical therapy clinic. FIM-5 Requires 25% assist with long-distance wc mobility. FIM-2 Client is able to perform bed, wc, chair transfers with 25% assist. FIM-2 Client is able to perform tub/toilet transfers with 50%-75% assist. FIM-2	Client performs bed positioning with less than 10% assist. Client is independent in wc mobility on the ward and to/from therapies. FIM-6 Client performs bed, wc, chair transfers with less than 10% assist. FIM-4 Client performs tub/toilet transfers with less than 25% assist. FIM-4 Client ambulates distances of 50-100 ft with assistive device and contact guard. FIM-2	Client is: ♦ Independent in bed mobility ♦ Independent in wc mobility in all terrain, inclines, curbs, and carpeting. FIM-6 ♦ Independent in bed, wc, chair transfers. FIM-7 Client performs tub/toilet transfers with less than 10% assist. FIM-4 Client ambulates independently a minimum of 150 ft with assistive device and/or orthosis. FIM-6

	Client is able to initiate gait activities with assistive device and human support outside the parallel bars. FIM-1	Client is an independent household ambulator. FIM-3	
Sexual Functioning (MD, RN, ARNP)	Client and spouse will identify sexual patterns before the stroke.	Client and spouse will understand common problems of stroke patients in sexual functioning.	Client and spouse can identify supportive resources and techniques to cope mentally and physically with sexual functioning after a stroke.	Client and spouse understand adaptive skills for sexual functioning.
Skin Integrity Potential Altered Skin Integrity Actual Impaired Skin Integrity (RN, PT, OT, ARNP)	Client and family initiate preventive skin program. Client initiates skin care program (includes preventive protocol).	Client and family are aware of risk factors for altered skin integrity. Client and family able to provide minimal assist with skin care strategies. Skin integrity: healing.	Client and family are able to inspect skin with supervision. Client and family perform at least 50% of skin care strategies with cueing and supervision.	Client and family inspect and perform skin care without supervision. Client and family perform skin care without supervision.
Discharge Planning (SWS, PT, OT, ST, RN)	Client and family identify current social service needs. Client and family identify tentative discharge needs. Client and family present model of home environment.	Client and family are aware of discharge options. Client and family follow-up on social service referrals (i.e., food stamps, public assistance).	Client and family finalize discharge plans (i.e., home, NHCU, HBHC, home healthcare agency, OP, other VA).	Client and family acknowledge discharge plans completed. Successful discharge accomplished and appropriate follow-up established.
Equipment (OT, PT, KT, RN, Prosthetics, ARNP)	Client receives initial assessment of ADL and functional status to determine basic equipment needs.	Client begins training in use of assistive devices/adaptive equipment. Client and family receive necessary equipment for use on therapeutic weekend pass; receive appropriate training in use of equipment.	Client equipment needs are adjusted according to changing status. Client and family demonstrate safe use of equipment 80% of time.	Client receives all necessary equipment for postdischarge use. Client and caregiver understand safe effective use of all equipment.
Psychosocial Needs (SWS)	Client and family participate in interview with SWS to assess psychosocial needs. Primary caregiver is identified.	Client and family receive ongoing supportive therapeutic contact.	Client and family receive ongoing supportive therapeutic contact.	Client and family demonstrate improved coping/adjustment to lifestyle change. Continue to receive ongoing supportive therapeutic contact.
Leisure (RT)	Client and/or family participate in interview to assess leisure needs. (Quality of life.)	Client and/or family indicate awareness of adapted leisure alternatives.	Client demonstrates adapted leisure involvement to be used upon discharge.	Client and/or family demonstrate knowledge of community resources for continued quality-of-life support.

Continued.

Appendix 6-A Clinical pathway: stroke—initial rehabilitation, first admission—cont'd

Client needs	Week 1	Week 2	Week 3	Week 4
Vocational (VRT)	Client and family participate in interview process to assess vocational status and potential. Client begins vocational eval. If appropriate.	Client and family participate as needed in exploring/accessing community or government agencies for services. Client continues participation in vocational eval.	Client and family participate as needed in exploring/accessing community or government agencies for services. Client and family understand results of vocational eval.	Client and family are knowledgeable in services provided by community & government agencies; understand how to access these in order to apply for appropriate vocational and/or financial assistance; participate in follow through with recommendations for vocational or financial assistance.
Education (MD, RN, PT, OT, KT, ST, RT, VRT, SWS, ARNP)	Client and family are aware of needs regarding communicating, cognition and swallowing, exercises, needs, diet, equipment, home care, disease process, and stroke risk factors. Client and family learn unit routines.	Client and family begin participation in training program on the ward and in therapies. Begin return demonstration of care.	Client and family able to perform home exercise programs and compensatory techniques safely.	Client and family able to demonstrate knowledge of needs, diet, home care, exercises, and equipment use. Client and family receive and verbalize understanding of printed discharge instructions. Client and family are aware of follow-up plans and supportive resources.

7

Total Quality Management and Outcome Evaluation

Pamela Muhm Duchene, DNSc, RN, CRRN

INTRODUCTION

The concept of quality in healthcare has been developing steadily since the late 1960s with Donabedian's seminal work outlining structure, process, and outcome components (Donabedian, 1966). Only in the late 1980s did the Joint Commission on Accreditation of Healthcare Organizations (JCAHO) specifically identify standards on quality and quality assurance as an institution-wide requirement. Assuring, defining, measuring, and evaluating quality has become a major challenge in healthcare; the quality as well as duration of life is an outcome criterion. Today cost-effective delivery of care is another feature of quality healthcare, and clinicians and administrators look to models from corporate and industrial sources for applications in healthcare.

Quality is an individual perception. As one result, in all areas of nursing, nurses are constantly being pressured to work with fewer professional staff, at a faster pace, and with sicker clients. Administrators claim that hospitals cannot afford to provide the highest level of quality care. Nurses express concern that quality will be lost. Administrators tend not to be responsive to claims that quality will suffer, since quality is an individual perception.

Some breaches in quality are apparent. A pressure sore that a client develops due to lack of turning and repositioning may be related to ineffective nursing care or inadequate client education. Aspiration pneumonia that a client experiences following failure to diagnose dysphagia may be related to a lack of substantial assessment following a stroke. Although one would not question that quality concerns exist with such examples, more often deviations from quality are subtle. Substituting a bedpan for use of the commode during the night may be viewed as conserving energy. It may also be perceived as inappropriate care, since it is more difficult for people to empty their bladders while using a bedpan. Enabling an individual to miss a therapy appointment due to fatigue may be seen as sympathetic and caring. It also may be viewed as interfering with the rehabilitation process and physical conditioning, and may result in further loss of function with slower functional gains. In rehabilitation a familiar saying is that "it takes longer for the clients to do for themselves than it takes to do for them." Perhaps the first aspect of care to slip is that of client edu-

cation and promotion of self-care. This is an area that those outside of the discipline of rehabilitation nursing may not discern.

Because quality is a subjective perception, outcomes of the care provided may be even more difficult for a layperson to discern. Outcomes of care provided are a primary focus in rehabilitation, where traditionally clinicians have sought the ability to measure and monitor small but significant gains in function and independence. In this chapter an approach to quality improvement based on general aspects of quality control including definitions of quality, standards, measurement (data collection), evaluation, and action plans and follow-up are followed by specific methods of quality improvement and a discussion of client outcomes.

DEFINITION OF QUALITY

Attempts to improve quality or even to assess it imply that we are able to identify quality and subsequently recognize variations in quality. To do so, we must be able to define basic tenets of quality. One definition of quality is "conformance to requirements" (Crosby, 1979). The problem, of course, is how to achieve agreement on a level of quality between clinicians, administrators, clients, payers, and accrediting organizations. Nurses must be cued into the perceptions of quality held by clients, physicians, therapists, and other nurses.

The characteristics identified as "quality" by clients differ from those identified by clinicians. Aspects that clients identify as quality indicators are a holistic environment with involvement of the family and client; effective communication between healthcare providers and clients; and caring, efficient, committed nurses (Taylor, 1992). These, however, are only generalizations. The most accurate method for determining the perceptions of quality held by others is simply to ask them. When clients express dissatisfaction with care, determining what quality means and attempting to correct the perceived deficiency may enable a change in satisfaction level.

For example, after her stroke, a wealthy woman showed a lack of motivation for participation in occupational therapy, particularly in participating in activities of daily living (ADL) practice. Although she had a good rapport with other members of the rehabilitation team, she overtly avoided occupational therapy. Her rehabilitation nurse met with her and explained that unless her motivational issues could be addressed, she would be discharged from the rehabilitation program. The woman explained that she had no need to work on dressing skills, since she would be hiring someone to provide her personal care. She was, however, concerned that she would no longer be able to host her tea parties for her ladies' group. The nurse reported the results of the client conference to the occupational therapist, who revised the plan of care to focus on skills necessary for serving at a tea party. Basically quality nursing care according to clients is whatever the client says it is. Some measure it by the nurse's responsiveness to questions or calls. Others measure it by the nurse's willingness to communicate with, and educate and involve, the client and family members in the plan of care. In rehabilitation nursing one significant challenge in meeting client and family expectations related to quality is to provide information and discuss expectations, which will raise the client and family's consciousness or awareness and alter their perception of quality and satisfaction.

Just as clients and family members have unique definitions of quality characteristics, members of other disciplines have views on traits indicative of quality. Identifying quality characteristics as perceived by other disciplines is essential in establishing a relationship built on peer respect. In a hospital a physical therapist, for example, may not be aware of a nurse's clinical ability but will be disturbed if the nurse's clients are consistently late for therapy appointments and will perceive the nurse as providing care lacking in quality. Clinicians in other disciplines perceive quality nursing care as effective communication, efficient follow-through, and competent carryover of therapeutic teaching. In hospital-based rehabilitation the system may make consistent communication with other rehabilitation team members difficult. For example, teams often meet early in the day or at noon, when a majority of team members are available, but when nurses are least able to leave the units. A serious conflict in peer quality definitions can occur since nurses will perceive a breach of quality by leaving clients to attend a team meeting. Likewise, team members deduce a lack of quality when nurses do not appear at the meeting.

STANDARDS OF CARE

Whatever the varying definitions of quality, nurses need to be aware of differing peer expectations and perceptions of quality. On the other hand, being cognizant of diverse perceptions is important in assuring client satisfaction as well as critical to quality standards. A standard is "a norm that expresses an agreed-upon level of practice that has been developed to characterize, measure, and provide guidance for achieving excellence"[11] (American Nurses' Association [ANA] & Association of Rehabilitation Nurses [ARN], 1994). Experts develop standards to identify acceptable norms and tolerable ranges of deviation from the norms (Rowland & Rowland, 1992). Standards mark a minimal level of practice that is acceptable. Healthcare standards are based on governmental regulations and guidelines (Medicare, Health Care Financing Administration, state public

health departments) and are set by healthcare organizations (JCAHO, 1988; Commission on Accreditation of Rehabilitation Facilities [CARF]) and consumer groups (American Association of Retired Persons, National Head Injury Alliance). Standards specific to nursing care are established by governmental agencies, healthcare organizations, and by nursing organizations such as the ANA and ARN.

Standards are used to identify quality components of general and specific aspects of nursing care with regard to structure, process, and outcome (Donabedian, 1966; Larson & Lieske, 1992). Structural standards identify the overall framework of the organization and nursing division, including the resources that will be available and the organization's rules of conduct. Requiring nurse managers of rehabilitation units to have the Certified Rehabilitation Registered Nurse (CRRN) credential is a structural standard. Process standards dictate how care is given. A policy indicating that sterile technique is needed for all intermittent catheterizations is a process standard. Outcome standards indicate what should be the client's response to treatment and nursing care. That clients with cerebral vascular accidents will demonstrate increased endurance and functional ability of two measures on a functional assessment tool is an outcome standard.

All three types of standards—structure, process, and outcome—can provide specific or precise quality indicators to be measured and monitored. However, standards may be broad statements that are not concrete but change and evolve with time, albeit slowly. There has been substantial debate in the literature, for example, on the best method for client education on intermittent catheterization (Champion, 1976; Lapides, Diokno, Gould, and Lowe, 1976; Maynard & Glass, 1987; Opitz, Thorsteinsson, Schutt, Barrett, & Olson, 1988). Research during the 1980s demonstrated that clean catheterization as completed by the client resulted in no significant differences than with sterile catheterization. However, in many client educational programs and hospitals, clean catheterization was not taught or practiced due to fear of nosocomial urinary tract infections. During the late 1980s and early 1990s, researchers have demonstrated low incidence of urinary tract infection through controlling hospital factors while teaching clean technique including the use of a private room, a private bathroom, and maintaining techniques to be used at home. The structure standard that registered nurses teach self-catheterization did not change. However, the process standard evolved from maintaining sterile technique to clean technique (with a private room and private bathroom). The outcome standard of learning self-catheterization with a low incidence of urinary tract infection did not change. Effective standards are research based and change as the knowledge of healthcare and nursing transform.

MEASUREMENT OF QUALITY (DATA COLLECTION)

If "it" can not be measured, "it" can not be controlled. Standards provide general areas of characteristics to be measured. The indicators for the standards must be measurable, or one cannot tell if a condition or situation is better, worse, or no different than expected. In the prior example, the incidence of urinary tract infections occurring in clients using clean technique for self-catheterization is an illustration of a standard-based quality measure. A urinary tract infection is a measurable event and could be identified by weekly urine cultures for individuals on self-catheterization programs.

With the prior example, the appropriate method for determining compliance with the standard is obvious, through monitoring weekly urine cultures. In many cases, however, data collection processes are less apparent. A common practice for clients with dysphagia is to place them on thickened liquids. In one rehabilitation hospital, the complaints of thirst from the clients on thick liquids sparked nurses' concern about hydration status. The existing data collection tools for the standard that clients would receive adequate nutrition and hydration included traditional intake and output (I&O) records. The accuracy of the I&O records were questioned, since many individuals including speech pathologists, occupational therapists, nurses, nursing assistants, and physicians participate in providing fluids for the rehabilitation clients. Instead of the assuming hydration could be monitored through recording I&O, urine specific gravity was identified as the indicator of hydration level to be measured.

Data collection processes typically involve client interviews, surveys, record reviews, and observations. The process must be specific and outlined in detail. Table 7-1 provides an example of the data collection process. However data are collected, the process must be realistic. For example, when nurses carrying client caseloads are also data collectors, the process must be streamlined or it will fail. In general, the lengthier and more complex the data collection tool, the more likely that noncompliance will occur. Tables 7-2 and 7-3 provide examples of practical data collection tools.

Table 7-1   Process for data collection

QUALITY ASSESSMENT AND IMPROVEMENT: PROCESS

Standard: The dysphagic client can expect adequate nutrition and hydration while on TLP.

Data collection period: _____

Process

1. Clients with dysphagia are identified by the primary nurse, speech pathologist, and physician.
2. Clients identified as dysphagic are placed on TLP.
3. Clients on TLP are assessed daily for unrelieved thirst.
4. The urine specific gravity is measured daily for all clients on TLP.
5. Results of the assessment and urine specific gravity are recorded on the data collection sheet in the client medical record.
6. At the end of the client's stay or when advanced to thin liquids, the data collection sheet is submitted to the nurse manager.
7. The nurse manager compiles the information from the individual client data collection sheets onto the summary sheet.

TLP, thick liquid protocol.

Table 7-2   Data collection tool (individual client tool)

QUALITY ASSESSMENT AND IMPROVEMENT: DATA COLLECTION CHECK SHEET

Instructions: Place one form on the record of every client with dysphagia.

Standard: The dysphagic client can expect adequate nutrition and hydration while on TLP.

Client identification number: _____

Date placed on TLP: _____

	Dates							
For all clients identified as dysphagic								
1. Assessed for thirst								
2. Indicated unrelieved thirst								
3. Urine specific gravity (indicate results)								
Initials								

Table 7-3   Data collection tool (summation tool).

QUALITY ASSESSMENT AND IMPROVEMENT: DATA COLLECTION SUMMARY SHEET

Instructions: Use the client data forms to compile these data.
Standard: The dysphagic client can expect adequate nutrition and hydration while on TLP.

Indicators	Client identification numbers							
1. Clients with dysphagia are placed on TLP								
2. Clients on TLP indicate presence of unrelieved thirst								
3. Clients on TLP tested daily for urine specific gravity								
4. No. of normal results/ no. of tests								

EVALUATING RESULTS

Since perfection is rarely achievable, the incidence of "acceptable variation" or tolerance from the optimal outcome must be identified. Although it is reasonable to expect that all clients will avoid a urinary tract infection while using self-catheterization, a standard defines what is tolerable. The point identified as acceptable variation may be set at a minimal level, 1%, 5%, or 20%. In many typical quality assessment programs, 0.1% is a number regularly used as an acceptable variation in quality. This may not be satisfactory, as illustrated in the following example of 99.9% quality (Brocka & Brocka, 1992):

+ At least 20,000 wrong prescriptions per year
+ Unsafe drinking water 1 hour/month
+ No electricity, water, or heat for 8.6 hours/year
+ No phone service for 10 minutes each week
+ Two short or long landings at each major airport per day
+ Five hundred incorrect surgical operations per week
+ Two thousand lost articles of mail per hour

In the preceding example, one gets the feeling that 99.9% good is just not good enough. This is one of the major arguments behind the movement toward a program built on the concept of continuous quality improvement, which is presented later in the chapter. However, whatever the numeric limit set to measure quality characteristics, the results must be evaluated in terms of whether the variations in quality are tolerable. For example, one area of rehabilitation nursing expertise is skin care. In many rehabilitation programs the development of even one pressure sore area is unacceptable. To meet a standard that no individual served will develop a pressure sore area, the limit may be set at zero, but that indicator would be applied to individuals developing an ulcer only while in the rehabilitation program.

When identifying the level of acceptable error, it is important to work toward improvement and set the level low enough to challenge current practice. For example, with orthopedic rehabilitation following knee joint replacement surgery, acceptable outcome standards may be identified as 70 degrees of flexion. Setting the threshold level of acceptable variance at 50% of the clients with knee joint replacement surgery achieving 70 degrees of flexion will not challenge the rehabilitation team to work toward improvement of current practice. However, setting the level at 90% of clients achieving 70 degrees of flexion will provide a goal toward which clinicians and clients will strive.

ACTION PLANS AND FOLLOW-UP

The action plan and follow-up on data collected are perhaps the most critical components of any quality assessment and improvement process (Sullivan & Decker, 1992). Once the data are analyzed, it must be determined what actions, if any, need to be taken. The action plan should include steps taken to correct the problem, individuals responsible for the actions, and target dates by which the actions should be complete. A follow-up study in which the data are collected should be planned to determine if the actions were effective in correcting the problem or in reducing the incidence of error (see Box above for an example of an action plan).

Falls are a common problem in rehabilitation settings. With many clients in rehabilitation having sensory-per-

---

ACTION PLAN AND FOLLOW-UP.
Quality assessment and improvement: action plan

Standard: The client and family can expect provision of a safe environment.

Finding: The incidence of client falls is highest during shift change.

Conclusion: During shift change, few nurses and assistants are left to answer call lights, and clients become frustrated with the delay and attempt to ambulate without assistance.

Recommendations
1. Perform round on all clients immediately before and after shift change.
2. Keep intershift report brief, and keep as many nurses and assistants on the unit as possible to answer call lights.

Action plan
1. Institute inservice with nurses and assistants on the recommended changes.
   Target date: June 1
   Person(s) responsible: Nurse manager, staff development coordinator
2. Design client education plan to reinforce need to call for assistance and to wait for assistance.
   Target date: June 1
   Person(s) responsible: Nurses and nursing assistants

---

ceptual dysfunction, mobility impairments, and short-term memory deficits, falls may occur. Falls often are associated with high-risk situations or situations that may not occur frequently, but should be monitored since any fall provides a threat of morbidity and mortality. In most rehabilitation programs, due to client risk factors, falls are monitored routinely. Although rehabilitation nurses agree that all falls should be prevented, most accept that as part of rehabilitation—as independence in self-care is increased—the risk of falls also rises. Where the process sometimes fails is in how to implement the action plan with follow-through for long-term improvement. In one rehabilitation hospital a fall prevention program was designed and implemented. Program actions included posting safety information and fall prevention strategies above each client's bed on dry erasable boards. All nurses and therapists attended inservice sessions on the program, and the fall incidence dropped to an all-time low. However, 6 months after the program had been implemented, the fall incidence was noted to climb back to preprogram levels. In analyzing why the problem did not remain resolved, the nurses noted that the information was no longer routinely posted above client beds. When the nurses and therapists were asked why they were not posting information, they stated that they could never find the special markers to use with the boards. The unit secretaries at the hospital were responsible for ordering the markers and had been told to cut down on supply expenses. As a result, due to the expense of the markers, they limited the number of markers ordered. Although the system worked, attention to maintenance was lacking, and therefore the initial outcome did not last. Unfortunately staff and administrators alike respond to short-term savings and immediate situations over long-range outcomes that may improve client quality of care, which results from a lack of vision and education to see the long-term effects. A quick cost/benefit analysis was completed to demonstrate the cost of a single fall in relation to the cost of markers for several years. Since the difference was compelling, at present there are markers in two colors mounted on every overbed board.

Keeping the ball in the air with one quality project while monitoring others is an art. It requires a careful schedule and clear delineation of responsibilities. The nurse responsible for overseeing quality monitoring must be attentive to detail and able to facilitate deadline achievement. However, one person is not capable of making a quality monitoring system work. Individuals throughout the organization must understand and invest in the quality concept (Kirk, 1992).

In rehabilitation individuals within the team must accept the quality theme. A common dilemma in hospital-based rehabilitation programs is how to provide effective, efficient transportation to and from therapy. In one hospital the nursing assistants were responsible for transportation. The therapists became concerned that clients were arriving late for therapy and causing lost therapy time. They initiated a quality monitoring project to find out how much time was lost. At the start of therapy time each day, a therapist would clock in clients and determine which nursing assistants were not completing their responsibilities in a timely fashion. The nurses reacted strongly when they were apprised of the study results during a hospital quality committee meeting. Nurses claimed therapists knew little of the nursing morning routine, which required 40 clients to be awakened, toileted, groomed, dressed, fed, retoileted, and transported to therapy in a 2-hour period. This type of monitoring creates distrust, defensiveness, and antagonism—which reduce quality of care. For resolution, nurses and therapists—knowing a problem exists—must agree the problem cannot be solved unilaterally. Such difficulties are endemic in rehabilitation organizations. Therefore, regardless of how efficient quality monitoring appears in each department, the whole organization must be considered in quality assessment. In attempting to master quality management, a variety of techniques have been used. In the following section, several of these methods are discussed, with examples as applied to rehabilitation.

METHODS OF ASSESSING QUALITY AND MAKING IMPROVEMENTS
Historical Perspectives

Before the 1940s the overriding concerns with healthcare were outcome (defined in terms of morbidity and mortality) and access (defined in terms of availability of a physician). Healthcare quality did not become a widespread public concern until the mid-1940s (Bull, 1992). With the advent of antibiotics and decline in mortality rates, people began to recognize quality-of-care issues. It seems no coincidence that this is the same period that gave impetus to medical rehabilitation.

Initially concerns with quality of care focused on process and structure. Manuals on procedures provided process guidelines, and structure standards were identified by groups such as the Joint Commission on Accreditation of Hospitals (now the JCAHO). Individuals believed that if structure and process were consistent with quality, the outcome would follow. However, little attention was paid to identifying quality outcomes (Bull, 1992). In rehabilitation quality skin care was equated with every-2-hour turn routines (process). Posting a reminder to turn every 2 hours (structure) was believed to ensure quality.

During the 1970s the efforts at providing quality care focused on process tools. The medical record audit became commonplace (Bull, 1992). It was not uncommon to retrospectively audit a sample of records of clients with a specific diagnosis and ensure that documentation reflected the correct process. For example, one might audit a 10% sample of clients hospitalized for spinal cord injury to assess use of an every-2-hour turn routine for prevention of pressure ulcers. Also included in the audit might be an assessment of whether or not a pressure ulcer developed. The information gleaned from such reviews was compiled, analyzed, and reported to organizational committees. A follow-up plan was drafted. With this example, results indicating that clients were developing pressure ulcers and that turn routines were not documented might lead to inservices and meetings with nurses to correct the problem. A second audit would be completed to determine continued status and resolution of the problem. This was based on the premise that if it was not documented (i.e., recorded), it was not done (Phaneuf, 1964).

Audits assessed one aspect of quality—primarily that of documentation. With an emphasis on what had not been done, audits were limited in utility for improvement in quality (Taylor, 1992). For example, knowing that turn schedules are not documented and that there are clients who develop pressure ulcers does not explain why the problem occurred, or what steps would be needed to correct it. The JCAHO recognized that simple audits could not impact quality or assure the delivery of quality care. During the 1980s the JCAHO published standards on development of hospital-wide quality assurance programs to focus on client care issues (see Box, p. 92 for a model of quality assurance). The adoption of the 10-step quality assurance process by JCAHO was one major step forward and took quality assurance away from a review of discipline-specific problems to a focus on the client. Table 7-4 provides the 10-step process.

THEORISTS AND CONCEPTS

As the 1990s represent a transition to the twenty-first century, a value change is occurring. More is not necessarily better, and high cost does not equate to high quality, as demonstrated by the work and writings of Deming, Juran, Crosby, and Feigenbaum. Several theories and quality improvement concepts are discussed and applied to rehabilitation nursing.

Deming

A statistician, Deming was instrumental in incorporating statistical measures into a management philosophy with the Japanese (Deming, 1986; Walton, 1986). The key aspects of Deming's philosophy are the 14 points, the seven deadly diseases, and some obstacles. Table 7-5 contains the 14 points and applications to rehabilitation.

◆

MODEL OF QUALITY ASSURANCE

◆ Identify values
◆ Identify structure, process, outcome standards, and criteria
◆ Secure measurments
◆ Make interpretations regarding strengths and weaknesses
◆ Identify options
◆ Determine action course
◆ Take action

Adapted from *Quality assurance workbook* by American Nurses' Association, 1976, Kansas City. Copyright 1976 by the American Nurses' Association. Reprinted by permission.

Unfortunately examples of the seven deadly diseases may be found in rehabilitation as well. For instance, one of the seven deadly diseases is annual review of performance (merit rating), which is done routinely for rehabilitation nurses and is required by JCAHO and CARF (Deming, 1986, Walton, 1986). It is likewise easy to apply the obstacles to rehabilitation. One of the obstacles—neglect of long-range planning—is evident in some rehabilitation programs, where a strategic plan may be absent or not followed.

One cannot apply Deming's philosophy to rehabilitation nursing unless all rehabilitation disciplines and all levels of leadership "buy in" to the philosophy. When that occurs, one would implement the 14 points throughout the rehabilitation program, assess where the seven deadly diseases existed and continuously monitor for their development, and watch out for the obstacles. Failure to "buy in" to the Deming philosophy on an organizational level results in ineffective implementation of the philosophy, since it so strongly contrasts with traditional management styles of performance appraisal and supervisory assessment.

Juran

An engineer and attorney, Juran's philosophy for quality control consists of three cornerstones (Juran, 1988). Quality improvement is the term given to the process of look-

Table 7-4   JCAHO's 10-step model of quality assurance with application to rehabilitation

Step	Rehabilitation application
1. Assign responsibility	A clinician within each rehabilitation discipline identifies an individual responsible for quality assessment.
2. Delineate scope of care	For rehabilitation nursing, scope of care would include inpatient and/or outpatient care of individuals with disabilities and chronic illnesses.
3. Identify important aspects of care	For rehabilitation nursing, important aspects of care might include skin programs, educational programs, bowel and bladder training, and carryover of therapeutic teaching.
4. Identify indicators	An indicator for an educational program might be the number of clients in a medication educational program for medications who can identify the dose of medications they are taking. Additional indicators would be identified for the times, actions, and side effects of medications.
5. Establish thresholds for evaluation	The threshold for the above indicator might be set at 90%.
6. Collect and organize data	During the data collection period rehabilitation nurses would monitor the clients' return demonstrations or quizzes. The results of these data would be submitted to the quality assessment coordinator.
7. Evaluate care	If fewer than 90% of the clients in the medication education program cannot identify the dose of medications they are taking, corrective action would be indicated.
8. Take actions to improve care	With the medication program example, actions might include revision of the program, the approach, or a review of the teaching consistency and efficacy. Nurses might evaluate the need for a self-medication program or more extensive written information.
9. Assess effectiveness of actions and maintain the gain	Improvements made in the medication education program would be reviewed through continued monitoring on a regular basis.
10. Communicate results to relevant individuals and groups	Results would be written and reported to the hospital-wide quality assessment committee, at nursing unit meetings, and at divisional meetings.

Adapted from *The Joint Commission guide to quality assurance* by Joint Commission on Accreditation of Healthcare Organizations, 1988, Chicago. Copyright 1988 by Joint Commission on Accreditation of Healthcare Organizations.

ing for errors. It is a tool and may be used on procedures, processes, and the system in general. In many rehabilitation programs the adoption of quality improvement programs is occurring. These programs are fashioned after Juran's work and also include the other two cornerstones of Juran's philosophy: quality planning and quality control. New processes are introduced through quality planning. For example, the quality improvement program for an amputee program might result in identification of a need for increased client education. Rehabilitation nurses could be identified as those responsible for education, and a revised client education program could be developed (quality planning). Assessing the clients' learning, functional skills, and satisfaction would be quality control.

Juran's trilogy of quality improvement, planning, and control is evident in many rehabilitation programs. An advantage of Juran's work is that it is in sync with JCAHO and CARF standards.

Crosby

As a podiatrist, Crosby (1979, 1988) has a medically related background, although his philosophy, like Deming's and Juran's, began with applications to industry. Also like Deming, Crosby's concepts are linked with statistical methods. A key component of Crosby's work is the idea of zero defects. In order to achieve zero defects, a quality vaccine is needed. The process of improving quality is continuous and does not rely on testing, sampling, or inspection since these methods are nonpreventive and not consistent with the "vaccine" concept. Crosby proposes 14 steps to assist organizations in arriving at zero defects. Identified is a need for management commitment to quality improvement. Also included in the 14 steps is the need for quality improvement teams, cost information, goal setting, communication, and training.

Crosby's work translates readily into rehabilitation. Many rehabilitation programs are identifying specific pro-

Table 7-5   Deming's 14 points as applied to rehabilitation

14 points	Rehabilitation application
1. Create constancy of purpose for improvement	Development of a mission statement identifying who is served, for which purposes, and by whom. Rehabilitation programs provide service to individuals with disabilities and chronic illnesses.
2. Adopt the new philosophy	The mission statement is adopted and incorporated into all aspects of care. In a rehabilitation program the mission statement should be given to clients in the program.
3. Cease dependence on mass inspection	Follow-up calls to all clients may be equated to "mass inspection." These may not be reliable and may do little to improve the rehabilitation program quality.
4. Institute training	Orientation programs to rehabilitation should include all disciplines and should be ongoing.
5. End practice of giving business based on price	Case managers sometimes shift clients to less expensive rehabilitation vendors, with price as the primary factor. This may be a disservice, although high cost is not always high quality.
6. Improve production and service constantly	As good as a rehabilitation program is, it can always be better. Any pressure ulcer is too many. The threshold for falls can always be lower.
7. Drive out fear	Fear of change must be challenged and confronted.
8. Eliminate slogans	This point relates to work targets and exhortations and is less applicable to rehabilitation.
9. Institute leadership	Leadership in rehabilitation should be team oriented for success. Just as members of the interdisciplinary team work cohesively for the client's benefit, the managers must coordinate efforts for the benefit of clinicians and clients.
10. Break down barriers	Whose responsibility is it to toilet clients during therapy treatment times? Do rehabilitation nurses have the equipment needed for gait training and promotion of self-care? These are potential points of barriers for some rehabilitation programs.
11. Remove barriers to pride of workmanship	All rehabilitation team members and the client should take pride in functional outcomes achieved.
12. Eliminate numeric quotas	The amount of nursing care received by each client should be related to the client's need more than specific nursing productivity quotas. CARF has established a 5.5-hour/patient day standard for nursing care. This is contrary to Deming's philosophy.
13. Institute a program of education and retraining	Many rehabilitation programs have "brown bag lunch inservices" in which therapists and nurses meet for interdisciplinary educational programs.
14. Take action	Too often, strategies are discussed without action plans and outcomes.

Adapted from Walton, M. (1986) *The Deming management method.* New York: Putnam Publishing Group.

gram aspects and forming quality improvement teams. As an illustration, in one hospital-based rehabilitation program, the incidence of medication errors was high. Clinicians from pharmacy, nursing, and the quality control department met and formed a quality improvement team. In measuring the problem, they found that a high frequency of sodium warfarin (Coumadin) errors existed. In fact, Coumadin errors accounted for 65% of all medication errors. The committee members completed a cause-and-effect diagram (Fig. 7-1) to identify all possible causes of Coumadin errors. In determining a plan of action, committee members identified three steps. First, the administration time for Coumadin was changed from 4 PM to 9 PM. The committee members believed that this change would effect a reduction in errors, since 4 PM was a busy time on the unit, with therapies finishing work, clients returning to their rooms and needing rest breaks, and nurses changing shifts. Second, the nurses changed the way in which they transcribed orders for Coumadin. They developed and implemented a consistent method of order transcription. Third, on the unit with the highest rate of Coumadin errors, the pharmacists implemented a unit dose program for Coumadin. On all other units the pharmacists continued to supply Coumadin as a floor stock item. Committee members communicated information on the changes and implemented the program. Results were impressive for all units. Since all units dropped to zero defects, committee members interpreted results as successful and attributed the success to the standardized time of administration (9 PM) and to the standardized method of transcription. The nurses and pharmacists abandoned the Coumadin unit dose process; results did not indicate a difference between units. Quality improvement team members communicated the results and gave formal recognition to the nurses and pharmacists involved in correcting the Coumadin error problem.

Crosby's philosophy of quality improvement includes four absolutes (Crosby, 1979, 1988). First, quality means conformance to requirements. With the Coumadin example, the nurses and pharmacists conformed to all the requirements associated with medication administration. Second, quality comes from prevention. The nurses and pharmacists had to prevent the error, since no "after the fact" correction is possible with medication errors. Third, quality performance is zero defects. The quality improvement team on the Coumadin project accepted zero errors as the target. Fourth, the price of nonconformance is quality measurement. In other words, if one cannot achieve quality, measurement must occur. Measurement of the incidence of medication errors and analysis of the errors occurred due to an indication of quality deficiency.

Feigenbaum

During work at General Electric as a quality expert, Feigenbaum (1983) introduced the term "total quality control." Feigenbaum recognized three steps as leading to total quality control: leadership, modern technology, and organizational commitment. In Feigenbaum's model quality development, maintenance, and improvement are integrated with a goal of lowest expense and highest consumer satisfaction possible. This model is directly opposed to the concept that more expense is better quality.

Extensive client, consumer, and referral source interviews are sometimes conducted when adopting total quality control programs. In one rehabilitation program, these surveys resulted in recognition that clients found the length of the walkway connecting two buildings too long. Clients who attempted to ambulate or use wheelchairs through the hall felt that the distance exceeded energy levels. Although committed to total quality control, the managers of the program recognized that the length of the hallway could not be shortened. Through involving several clinicians in the problem-solving process, they determined that benches positioned along the way could help individuals ambulating through the hallway. Since this did not assist those using wheelchairs, employees throughout the program were inserviced and given training on assisting individuals through the hallway, after determining that the individual desired assistance.

QUALITY CONTROL AND IMPROVEMENT TOOLS
Benchmarking

Basically benchmarking is a tool used to identify the national level and "best of class" level (aka best practices) as benchmarks for specific indicators. In rehabilitation the incidence of rehabilitation-acquired pressure ulcers is an indicator that sometimes is used for benchmarking. Rehabilitation nurses within the organization use the information and strive to be better than both the national level and to become the "best of class."

Audits

Although no longer the primary method used to assess quality of care, audits remain a valuable quality control and improvement tool. Additionally audits are required as a component of the quality assessment process by some regulatory and standard-setting organizations. The CARF, for example, requires a quarterly case record review and assessment of program quality for persons served. An audit may be one way of meeting CARF's standard for this review process.

Brainstorming

One technique that has been used for many years in looking at problem resolution to quality issues is brainstorming. The rules for brainstorming sessions are simple: members of the quality team suggest as many solutions and alternatives as possible without critique. During brainstorming sessions, participants gain momentum through throwing as many ideas forward as conceivable. All suggestions are written and later evaluated at a separate time.

Cause-and-Effect Diagraming

The cause-and-effect or "fishbone" diagram is a quality control tool (Fig. 7-1). It is used for identification of causes of a quality problem and often is used in combination with a brainstorming session. In using cause-and-effect diagraming, basic categories are identified that can help reduce irrelevant discussion and complaints.

Check Sheets

A fundamental tool for quality control is a check sheet used for data collection (Table 7-2). The check sheet pro-

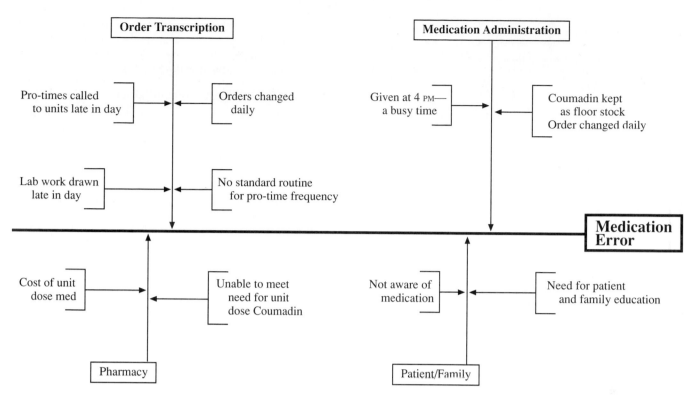

Fig. 7-1   Cause-and-effect diagram for Coumadin medication errors.

vides a standardized method of systematically collecting and recording facts. Review of completed check sheets is completed to analyze data, determine patterns, and arrive at conclusions.

Flowchart

With many quality control issues, it is difficult to determine why a problem exists. Flowcharts document all steps included in a process from start to finish (Fig. 7-2). Once the flowchart is complete, each step is reviewed for possible problems and opportunities for improvement.

Pareto Chart

Asserted in the Pareto principle is that 20% of the problems are responsible for 80% of the effects. Using a Pareto chart (Fig. 7-3) enables one to focus on the primary issues or defects rather than trying to tackle all problems. A Pareto chart is created by listing (in descending order of frequency) all problems occurring in a process.

CAUTIONS WITH QUALITY IMPROVEMENT EFFORTS
Retrospective Versus Prospective Quality Reviews

One may complete quality reviews of processes and records either after the event is completed (retrospective) or as events are occurring (prospective). Retrospective reviews typically involve closed records and collected data and are relatively easy to complete. Such reviews require time for document perusal but do not necessitate extensive tracking systems, since the individuals completing the review identify the files with appropriate information before

the data collection period. In contrast, prospective reviews require tracking of information as it occurs. This can be difficult, particularly in inpatient settings, where there are three shifts of nurses spanning 24 hours of care. However, although retrospective reviews are sometimes easier to complete, the information gleaned may be less conclusive than those data collected through prospective reviews. Clinicians find information through retrospective reviews that is easily detectable, "just waiting to be found." For example, identifying the incidence of documented complications to anticoagulation therapy through retrospective review would entail reviewing records for evidence of deep venous thrombosis, hematomas, and gastrointestinal bleeding. Such a review would not be difficult to complete. Taking a prospective look at the same issue, however, can result in a more comprehensive picture of the efficacy of anticoagulation therapy. As an example, in a prospective review of anticoagulation therapy, a data collection sheet would be developed through a team effort to identify as many components and contributing factors to complications with anticoagulation therapy as possible. The data collection sheets would be completed by members of the rehabilitation team and forwarded for analysis to the team leader or facilitator.

Costs

Although it is no longer accepted that higher quality is equated to higher cost, one must not assume that quality does not have a price. There are expenses associated with quality care. As an example, in a spinal injury program at a large free-standing rehabilitation hospital, the nurses place at-risk clients in specially designed pressure relief boots.

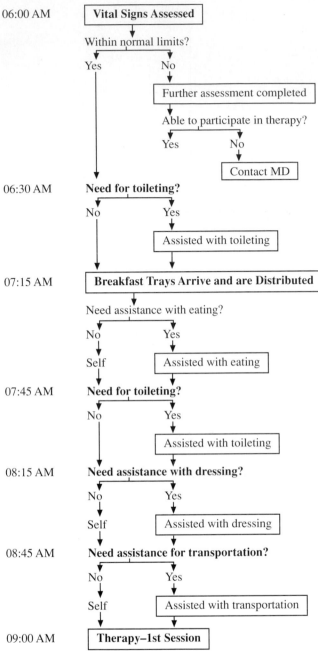

Fig. 7-2   A flowchart.

The boots cost around $150 for each boot, $300/pair. The incidence of rehabilitation hospital–acquired heel pressure ulcers is 0%. Although the cost is high, it is thousands of dollars less than the cost of time, care, and treatment associated with a pressure ulcer. It is sometimes necessary to spend a few dollars to save many.

Outcome Assessment

Most aspects of quality control and improvement apply to all healthcare programs; however, two additional methods—program evaluation and functional outcome measurement—are somewhat uncommon but key to the rehabilitation field. Program evaluation systems provide a holistic glimpse of the rehabilitation program. Functional outcome studies contribute the "so what?" data for rehabilitation, or, in other words, provide substantiation that the rehabilitation expense results in functional gains.

Program Evaluation in Rehabilitation

Program evaluation systems are required in the standards of CARF. According to CARF a program evaluation system must have measures of effectiveness, efficiency, and participant satisfaction. Program evaluation systems include programmatic objectives, with thresholds for objective attainment. On a quarterly basis individuals measure attainment of the program evaluation objectives and determine needed actions and strategies.

Many organizations develop original program evaluation systems; however, there are some commercially available systems. The Uniform Data System (UDS) is the most commonly used program evaluation system. The UDS provides effectiveness measures of functional progress through the Functional Independence Measure (FIM). The UDS provides efficiency measures by comparing charge and length of stay information for programs participating in the UDS network. Since many rehabilitation programs are members of UDS, the efficiency information is considered representative of the industry. The UDS does not provide information on participant satisfaction. This information must be gathered by the organization to complete the program evaluation system.

Functional Outcome Studies

Studies on functional outcomes provide information on the essence of rehabilitation results. Although not every individual to enter a rehabilitation program will ambulate and return home, outcome studies give data on the probability of such occurrences. Outcome studies may link the individual's length of stay in a program with the cost and efficacy of the program. Review of such information should weigh the cost of the program against the benefit of the functional gain. At one time in rehabilitation (15 to 20 years ago), the criteria for continued treatment included continued progress, even if this progress was quite slight. However, in this age of healthcare reform it is not acceptable to continue creating expense for functional gains that do not enhance the level of independence and lessen the dependence on the healthcare system.

Related to the legitimate concerns on the cost of rehabilitation and to the proliferation of rehabilitation programs and types of programs, functional outcomes from rehabilitation must be substantiated. In assessing outcomes from a rehabilitation program, one must consider the amount of experience with specific disability types and basic outcome quality indicators. Specifically the outcomes of clients with regard to quality of life, discharge disposition, and self-care independence should be appraised (Evans & Ruff, 1992).

Outcome studies are not new to healthcare or to nursing. Perhaps the first individual to consider healthcare and nursing outcomes seriously was Florence Nightingale (Bull, 1992). The outcome measure by which she looked at success was mortality. After she began work with British soldiers, she found a 30% reduction in mortality levels within 6 months (Nutting, Dock, & Dock, 1907).

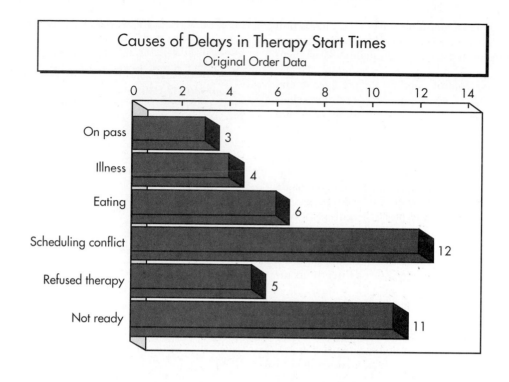

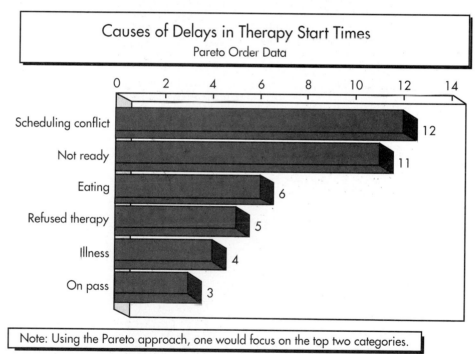

Fig. 7-3 A standard chart versus a Pareto chart.

Specific outcomes for rehabilitation nursing are still in investigation. Rehabilitation nursing care using Bobath principles has been identified as impacting or enhancing client outcomes of function and continuity of care (Borgman & Passarella, 1991). Rehabilitation nursing care incorporating client education through a self-medication program is identified as enhancing client knowledge of medication types, dosages, and routines (Thompson & Ellenberg,

1987). These studies are just two of many linking rehabilitation nursing care with a positive impact on functional outcomes and cost-effectiveness.

SUMMARY

Quality control and improvement has become an integral part of healthcare and rehabilitation nursing over the past two decades. As administrators and clinicians focus on defining quality and identifying customer satisfaction with services provided, standard-setting agencies such as JCAHO work toward redefining the quality assessment process.

Issues with quality control continue to revolve around definition, measurement, and evaluation. A primary challenge to clinicians is to transcend traditional departmental boundaries and work to refine processes. One current trend is to look at process improvement (Organizational Dynamics, Inc., 1993). In the process improvement system, process teams are formed of representatives throughout the organization including staff, leadership, and senior management. The process team is empowered to analyze and restructure a specific operation. The process team is ongoing and manages the process across traditional departmental boundaries. If carried to the extreme, an organization might have limited administrative resources and multiple process teams that report to senior management or directly to the chief executive officer.

It is imperative in the current and future climates of financial exigencies that rehabilitation nurses constantly focus on doing more, with less cost. Basic concepts of any quality control program include an organizational commitment to quality, a focus on client satisfaction, an empowerment of clinicians and staff members, a loss of department "territoriality" or specific links between quality threats or improvements and client outcome, and rewards for quality improvement (Schroeder, 1992). Rehabilitation nursing has made some steps toward identifying positive outcomes of rehabilitation nursing on clients. But there is extensive work needed in identifying and monitoring the outcome of rehabilitation nursing care.

REFERENCES

American Nurses' Association. (1976). *Quality assurance workbook.* Kansas City: Author.

Borgman, M.F., & Passarella, P.M. (1991). Nursing care of the stroke patient using Bobath principles: An approach to altered movement. *Nursing Clinics of North America, 26,* 1019-1035.

Brocka, B., & Brocka, M.S. (1992). *Quality management: Implementing the best ideas of the masters.* Homewood, IL: Business One Irwin.

Bull, M. (1992). Quality assurance: Professional accountability via continuous quality improvement. In C. Meisenheimer (Ed.), *Improving quality: A guide to effective programs* (pp. 3-20). Gaithersburg, MD: Aspen.

Champion, V. (1976). Clean technique for intermittent self-catheterization. *Nursing Research, 25,* 13.

Crosby, P. (1988). *The eternally successful organization.* New York: McGraw-Hill.

Crosby, P. (1979). *Quality is free: The art of making quality certain.* New York: McGraw-Hill.

Deming, W. (1986). *Out of the crisis.* Cambridge, MA: MIT Press.

Donabedian, A. (1966). Evaluating the quality of medical care. *Milbank Memorial Fund Quarterly, 44,* 194-196.

Evans, R.W., & Ruff, R.M. (1992). Outcome and value: A perspective on rehabilitation outcomes achieved in acquired brain injury. *Journal of Head Trauma Rehabilitation, 7,* 24-36.

Feigenbaum, A. (1983). *Total quality control* (3rd ed.). New York: McGraw-Hill.

Joint Commission on Accreditation of Healthcare Organizations. (1988). *The Joint Commission guide to quality assurance.* Chicago: Author.

Juran, J. (1988). *Juran on planning for quality.* New York: Free Press.

Kirk, R. (1992). The big picture: Total quality management and continuous quality improvement. *Journal of Nursing Administration, 22,* 24-31.

Lapides, J., Diokno, A.C., Gould, F.R., & Lowe, B.S. (1976). Further observations on self-catheterization. *Journal of Urology, 116,* 169-171.

Maynard, F., & Glass, J. (1987). Management of the neuropathic bladder by clean intermittent catheterization: 5-year outcomes. *Paraplegia, 25,* 106-110.

Nutting, M., Dock, A., & Dock, L. (1907). *A history of nursing.* New York: G.P. Putnam's Sons.

Opitz, J., Thorsteinsson, G., Schutt, A., Barrett, D., & Olson, P. (1988). Neurogenic bladder and bowel. In J. DeLissa (Ed.), *Rehabilitation medicine* (pp. 492-518). Philadelphia: J.B. Lippincott.

Organizational Dynamics, Inc. (1993)(personal communication).

Phaneuf, M. (1964). A nursing audit method. *Nursing Outlook, 12,* 67.

Rowland, H., & Rowland, B. (1992). *Nursing administration handbook.* Gaithersburg, MD: Aspen.

Schroeder, P. (1992). Future perspectives on quality. In C. Meisenheimer (Ed.), *Improving quality: A guide to effective programs* (pp. 334-340). Gaithersburg, MD: Aspen.

Sullivan, E., & Decker, P. (1992). *Effective management in nursing* (3rd ed.). Redding, MA: Addison-Wesley.

Taylor, C. (1992). Overcoming skepticism about quality improvement. In J. Dienemann (Ed.), *Continuous quality improvement in nursing* (pp. 125-129). Washington, DC: American Nurses Association.

Thompson, T., & Ellenberg, M. (1987). A self-medication program in a rehabilitation setting. *Rehabilitation Nursing, 12,* 316-319.

Walton, M. (1986). *The Deming management method.* New York: Putnam.

II

FOUNDATIONS OF REHABILITATION NURSING

8

Case Management

Patricia L. McCollom, RN, MS, CRRN, CIRS, CCM
Dorothy Sager, RN, CRRN, CIRS, CCM

INTRODUCTION

As a changing healthcare delivery system has been called on for accountability for economic as well as outcome improvements, the concept of case management emerged as a key strategy for effectively controlling costs in healthcare, primarily through expert coordination of care. Case management is not a profession in itself, but rather a functional area of practice within one's profession, which more often than not has interdisciplinary relationships. Case management processes benefit clients, families, and community by assisting those who become chronically ill, injured, or disabled to reach their potential for independence and satisfaction with quality of life. The process of case management enables clients to achieve autonomy through advocacy, communication, education, identification of resources, and facilitation of services. Clients are interested in access to care that will enable them to remain functionally independent and to manage lifelong health problems (Preston, 1994).

ORIGINS OF CASE MANAGEMENT

Case management began in the early 1900s with people interested in coordinating community services, followed by legislation impacting the public sector, and propelled by insurance industries into the private sector. Although this chapter focuses on external case management, many healthcare institutions are adopting principles of the model for use in internal case management programs and methods, such as care maps. (Chapter 2 and Chapter 6 contain samples of a critical pathway and a care map.) Some case managers work with multilevel systems of care and cross from institution to community, following a client for community referrals or readmission to the institution.

INNOVATIVE COMMUNITY SERVICE PEOPLE

Coordination, continuity, and quality of care have been hallmarks of quality practice since the early history of the health professions. In 1907 Mary Wadley established the first medical social work department at Bellevue Hospital in New York. In that context, social workers functioned as case managers. Around 1910, before occupational therapy became a discipline, pioneering nurses such as Susan Tracy educated clients and families about activities of daily living, eventually opening another avenue of case management. By 1942 Sister Kenny, a nurse who became famous for her work with poliomyelitis, pioneered techniques that promoted physical therapy as a unique discipline. Case management gained credibility and professionals began to practice the concept.

ENABLING LEGISLATION FOR THE PUBLIC SECTOR

The Vocational Rehabilitation Act of 1943, which funded professional training and research for persons with disabilities, helped to establish the vocational counselor case manager. This area was strengthened by the Workers' Compensation Rehabilitation Law of 1960, which detailed provisions governing vocational rehabilitation services to the injured employee. (Mumma, 1987) (Chapter 5 details other significant legislation including Medicare and Medicaid.)

INSURANCE INVOLVEMENT AND THE PRIVATE SECTOR

In 1945 Liberty Mutual Insurance Company hired the first nurse case managers in the insurance industry, with the goal of assisting injured workers to return to work. Then in 1970 Insurance Company of North America (INA) opened the first private sector rehabilitation company, International Rehabilitation Associates, and hired case managers to coordinate the care of injured persons and those with disabilities. Crawford and Company, the largest adjusting company, followed into this field soon after. Thousands of smaller companies have been spawned from these pioneers since 1970.

INTERNAL AND EXTERNAL CASE MANAGEMENT

Since the events described above, medical, vocational, and social welfare legislation have resulted in a need for both internal and external case management in a wide variety of practice settings. External case managers from numerous disciplines work in private practice, corporations, insurance companies (Arneson, 1993), managed care organizations, hospitals, and rehabilitation and vocational entities in additional to public or community settings such as mental health clinics, maternal child health services, or nursing centers, among others. External case management is discussed in more detail later in this chapter.

Similarly, case management practice within facilities has evolved rapidly over the past 5 years. Internal case managers may recommend services, treatments, or procedures and may refer to therapies and other disciplines for interventions (Mann, Hazel, Geer, Hurley, and Podrapovic, 1993). Internal case management is considered advanced practice because the practitioner is expected to predict critical pathways for care, analyze care maps for variance, lead other health professionals through the process, use all available resources for the client's best interest, and demonstrate improved outcome for clients, as well as cost-effectiveness. Care maps are tools that are designed so they can be used by multiple disciplines as often found in rehabilitation team program models or matrices (e.g., traumatic brain injury or stroke programs). When case management tools are used to document care according to national standards, managers are able to provide research opportunities, improve client outcomes, and reduce costs through reduced variances and length of stay, and manage resources from preadmission to community re-entry (McCollom, 1991; Kreutzer and Wehman, 1990).

Case managers serve diverse groups of individuals who are in need of medical, vocational, psychosocial, and other coordinated care. They plan with clients and families to broker services and resources to achieve mutually agreed-upon goals throughout the healthcare delivery system (Marr and Reid, 1992).

CASE MANAGEMENT

The evolution of case management has dramatically advanced efforts to provide quality, cost-efficient healthcare. Examples are cost and quality issues for technology, chronicity, an aging population, changes in reimbursement, new survivors and newly emerging conditions, community-based trends, and demands from informed consumers. Case management was defined as "the movement of an individual client through the rehabilitation process, and includes management and coordination of all services needed to successfully achieve the rehabilitation goals" (Parker & Hansen, 1981).

Beginning with this definition and bolstered by positive outcomes, the case management concept was endorsed and clarified by the American Hospital Association (AHA) in a White Paper published in 1987: "Case management is the process of planning, organizing, coordinating and monitoring the services and resources needed to respond to an individual's health care needs." AHA differentiated case management from "managed care" by defining managed care as a cost containment strategy (AHA, 1987).

As the leaders in the healthcare system continued to seek solutions to control soaring costs, case management was identified as an alternative means of care delivery. However, no common definition for case management existed; there were no common criteria for professionals who conducted case management. "Case manager" was a title claimed by persons working in the insurance industry, by nurses working both within and outside of facilities, by physicians working as primary providers in Health Maintenance Organizations (HMOs) and Preferred Provider Organizations, (PPOs) and by social workers dealing with community-based psychiatric care programs or elder care in the community. As legislation for healthcare developed, the term "case management" continued to appear as a mandated service but without a clear definition.

In February 1991 representatives from 36 professional associations came together to discuss the status of case management and the potential for consensus regarding issues surrounding the definition and practice of case management. Following a year's research a steering committee of the National Task Force on Case Management presented the following definition:

"Case Management is a collaborative *process* which assesses, plans implements, coordinates, monitors and evaluates options for services to meet an individual's health needs through communication and available resources to promote quality, cost-effective outcomes."

The group clearly established that the process of case management focuses on appropriate use of available resources and on client outcomes.

In addition to the definition of case management, the National Task Force on Case Management designed a model of case management that has become widely accepted. As shown, the traditional team has expanded to include the payer. Case management (Fig. 8-1) aims to achieve quality and cost-effective healthcare through a process, employing specific strategies, all resulting in a balance among concerned parties.

Rehabilitation and Case Management

Case management has been established in a number of community health service programs; the concept is adapted readily to rehabilitation nursing. A coordinated effort among all care providers and across disciplines correlates with the model for the long-accepted "rehabilitation team." The payer, as a participant on the team, has the opportunity to contribute to positive outcomes, since decisions about expenditures are based on specific individualized case knowledge (Whitman, 1991).

It has been said that "no one wants to be a case, and no one wants to be managed." The role of the family as a support framework is critical to the success of rehabilitation. The process of case management contributes to client and family involvement, since long-term needs of both the client and family must be identified to attain the objective of appropriate use of available resources. With the increased communication inherent in case management, the client and family have greater knowledge about care options (Campbell, 1988; Elliot and Smite, 1985). Clients and families also have opportunities to direct energy toward rehabilitation because case management processes promote education, vocation, and advocacy.

◆

SOURCES OF ASSESSMENT DATA

- ◆ Client interview
- ◆ Medical records
- ◆ Family interview
- ◆ Home visit
- ◆ Physician meeting
- ◆ Communication with the treatment team
- ◆ Employer

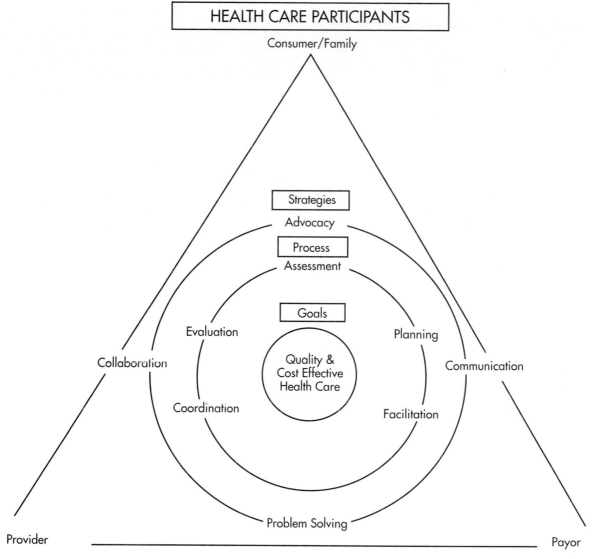

HEALTH CARE PARTICIPANTS

Consumer/Family

Strategies
Advocacy
Process
Assessment
Goals
Evaluation   Planning
Collaboration   Quality &   Communication
                    Cost Effective
                    Health Care
Coordination   Facilitation
Problem Solving
Provider   Payor

Fig. 8-1 Case management: a process directed at coordinating resources and creating flexible, cost-effective healthcare options in collaboration with the treatment team for individuals and their families to facilitate optimum healthcare outcomes.

Case Management Process and Roles

The specific activities of the case manager blend with the stages of the nursing process or clinical reasoning process to form a framework for nursing case management (Nursing Assessment and Management of the Frail Elderly Project, 1987). Referring to the case management model developed by the National Task Force on Case Management, the process involves assessment, planning, facilitation, coordination, and evaluation.

Assessment requires a systematic, comprehensive appraisal of the individual's health status including abilities, limitations, psychosocial status, coping skills, medical treatment received to date and anticipated care, current therapeutic prescriptions including medications, and health and work histories (see Box, p. 102). Additionally an assessment must consider the family status, number of persons within the household and the role of each, financial resources, sup-

port networks available or able to be developed, coping levels of those within the support network, and environmental issues such as accessibility or home safety (Pickerell, 1993; Hegeman, 1988). Assessment provides the basis for development of a case management plan. Education and vocation opportunities are explored with the client toward meeting long-term goals, identifying transferable skills, conducting job analysis or work reengineering, or for building on interests and aptitudes.

Planning involves addressing action necessary to meet the individual's needs across the entire episode of illness, bridging all healthcare settings and extending into the community (see Box, p. 104). The plan itself must identify actions required of the various participants: client, family, care providers, payers. Further, the plan indicates treatment alternatives and associated cost/benefit analysis.

OUTCOMES OF CASE MANAGEMENT PLAN

✦ Communication among all concerned parties
✦ Definition of short- and long-term goals
✦ Recommendations for additional/alternative services
✦ Identification of potential barriers

Facilitating and Coordinating

The case manager, having initiated the process of case management through assessment and planning, becomes the activist to facilitate and coordinate the services necessary to met the identified healthcare needs. These activities may be described as linking the client and family with providers or services through collaboration, negotiation, and communication—ideally on a regularly scheduled basis.

Evaluation

Finally, all phases of the process of case management must be monitored, updated, revised, and modified through ongoing evaluation. This component of the process is dynamic as the client's condition changes or as resources are consumed. Evaluation provides the basis for quality assurance and comparison with planned outcomes.

The process of case management, as described, may occur in a facility, within the insurance industry, or in community health programs. The variety of practice settings have raised barriers inhibiting a common definition and transdisciplinary standards of performance for case management. Transdisciplinary threads identified through research are those activities defined as components of the case management process. Clearly case management practiced according to national standards results in efficient coordination of services and improved communication about needs and outcomes.

The National Task Force for Case Management developed a strategic plan for a model for case management (Fig.

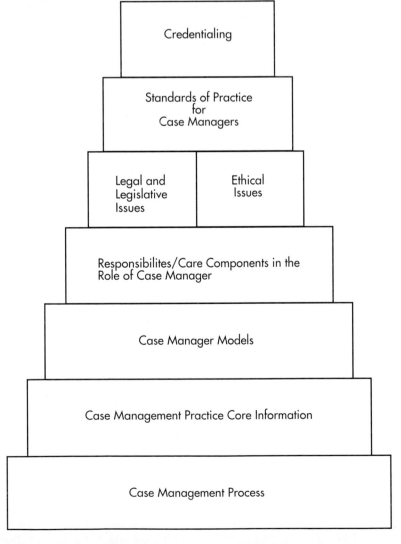

Fig. 8-2   Case management: industry-wide, multidisciplinary, integrated effort.

8-2), beginning with process and building to credentialing.

Certification is a process to validate a professional's expertise and adherence to a set of recognized industry standards. Certification is a means to designate that an individual case manager possesses the education, skills, and experience required to render appropriate services based on sound principles of practice. The first national examination for the Certified Case Manager (CCM) credential was offered to eligible case managers in May 1993. Approximately 5,000 eligible professionals completed the first certification examination; in November 1993 12,000 case managers sat for the certification examination (National Task Force on Case Management, 1992).

Other certifications important to rehabilitation nurses are the Certified Rehabilitation Registered Nurse (RN, CRRN) credential, the Certified Rehabilitation Counselor (CRC) credential, and the Certified Insurance Rehabilitation Specialist (CIRS) credential.

Unlike state licensure, certification is voluntary and is awarded by nongovernmental agencies, such as the Certified Insurance Rehabilitation Commission, the Certified Rehabilitation Counselor Commission, the Association of Rehabilitation Nurses, and the American Nurses' Association. Generally, certification requires a minimum period of practice and/or education in the specialty, as well as letters of reference, position descriptions, continuing education units (CEUs), and a written examination. Certification is valid for a number of years established by the certifying organization, with renewal based on earning set numbers of CEUs, contributions to the specialty, and practice in the field, or retaking the examination.

Future demands for case management will be unlimited. Case management can be expected to be expanded beyond insurance companies, hospitals, long-term care facilities, and industry—and it will extend to national health services as they are developed to satisfy the requirements of current healthcare reform efforts.

Increased awareness of the advantages of case management, together with a recognized need for cost-effective, quality medical care, and the importance of proper coordination of services will prompt tremendous growth in the case management specialty. As the healthcare system evolves, case management becomes critical to meeting the needs of the population throughout their life-span. These needs develop from an aging population, the underserved, an increase in diseases such as acquired immunodeficiency syndrome (AIDS) and tuberculosis, and the segment of the population covered by the Americans with Disabilities Act (ADA; Falik, et al., 1993).

As stated in the White Paper addressed to the National Health Care Task Force of the Clinton administration by the National Coalition of Associations for the Advancement of Case Management:

Clearly, these federal health objectives require coordination of all health services, knowledge of the full continuum of services available, the ability to assist people in moving efficiently through the health system, and the ability to facilitate full community integration regardless of health status. Case management is a logical process for addressing these needs.

Health care reform and the changing population of health system users will create new challenges. Proactive use of case management can anticipate needs, design solutions and facilitate changes that will benefit the efficacy and cost-effectiveness of the health system. The need for case management service will grow in the future.

To be effective, case management must also be used in order to properly meet the individual's needs, to optimize the quality of care, and to provide cost containment. Although less frequently utilized to date, three additional components of case management are injury and illness prevention, early intervention, and computerized outcome studies.

An effective information reporting program is essential for all participants in the prevention and early intervention program. Case managers who step up to this higher level of service will see increased satisfaction at the referral source, earlier referral of cases after injury or illness—and they will achieve better documented and more cost-effective outcomes. Table 8-1 provides a sample case management plan (McCollom, 1991).

Goals are met when optimum treatment or service is rendered by the most appropriate providers within a predetermined period at reasonable cost. In the future case managers, management information systems, and data about client outcome will be partnering to optimize America's healthcare delivery system.

Note: Mary Pickerell, RN, CRRN, is acknowledged for her comments and contribution regarding this chapter.

CASE STUDY (see Table 8-1)

Through review of the prototype case management plan (Table 8-1), the process can be further viewed as a method for organization of needed care, a tool for evaluation of services, and a framework for resource allocation.

INITIAL ASSESSMENT:

A.B. (client) was observed and his family interviewed for assessment purposes on August 3, 1991.
Date of injury: January 10, 1991
Medical diagnosis: Status post–severe head injury; emergency and intensive care treatment completed at Comprehensive Medical Center, Chicago, Illinois. Coma is noted in medical records as 31 days. Acute rehabilitation was declined due to continuing coma. A.B. currently is receiving post–acute brain injury treatment.

CURRENT STATUS:

Age: 17
Sex: Male
Marital status: Single
Living relatives: Father, mother, brother, paternal grandparents
Role in family: Oldest child
Occupation: Student
Recreational interest: School sports: participated in football, music
Housing: A.B. requires total care for his health, wellness, and safety. He is maintained at QC Care Center, participating in post–acute neurobehavioral brain injury treatment.

A.B. responds inconsistently to verbal, visual, and environmental stimuli. He participates in a full rehabilitation program daily. A.B. is wheelchair dependent for mobility with full assistance required for transfer; the right side is nonfunctional with hypertonicity of the right upper extremity; physical therapy promotes sitting balance, range of motion, and walking with adaptive devices (with two-person assistance). Daily psychological therapy focuses on verbal and visual stimulation; visual perception cannot be assessed at this time. Speech therapy focuses on consistent use of a voice output communication aid.

A.B. experiences generalized seizures one to two times daily; continuous drooling was noted, right side of mouth. Skin breakdown at the coccyx and right hip has required hospitalization on one occasion (July 1991). A.B. is dependent in mobility, dressing, and personal hygiene. He is independent in oral intake with prompting and adaptive equipment. A gastrostomy for feeding was closed surgically March 1991.

HEALTH HISTORY

A.B. had the usual childhood diseases; fractured his left wrist June 1987; is allergic to house dust, molds; and completed desensitization October 1983.

CURRENT MEDICATIONS:

(as noted on chart)

EDUCATION:

One semester tenth grade; A.B. to attend special education, Community High School, fall 1991

WORK HISTORY: Not applicable

FAMILY STATUS

A.B.'s parents have been actively involved in all facets of their son's care. His mother has resigned from work as a legal secretary to participate in care. Both parents have participated in brain injury education programs provided by the facility; they are attending the Head Injury Association support group weekly. A.B.'s father is employed as a regional supervisor for sales of farm equipment (annual salary is $40,000); health and accident coverage is Blue Cross/Blue Shield of Illinois. A.B. has $2000 in a savings account. Owing to personal savings, A.B. has been declared ineligible for Supplemental Security Income (SSI) Medicaid funding.

MEDICAL RECORDS REVIEWED

Comprehensive Medical Center
  1. Records of emergency care
  2. Consultation reports
  3. Operative reports
  4. Discharge report to QC Care Center
QC Care Center
  1. Monthly conference reports
  2. Neuropsychological evaluation completed July 1990

ADDITIONAL INFORMATION

A meeting was held August 5, 1991, with the following in attendance: J. Jerry, MD; K. Olson, speech therapist; T. Davis, PhD, psychologist; M. Goode, MSW social worker; T. Strong, PT. The following needs were discussed: (1) further evaluation of uncontrolled seizures, (2) assistance to family for home modification; and (3) clarification of insurance benefits.

CONCLUSIONS

  1. Due to cognitive and functional deficits resulting from severe head injury, this client is dependent on others for health, well-being, and safety and will require total direct care for the remainder of life.
  2. Due to severe head injury, this client will require various medication for life.
  3. Due to this client's medical diagnosis of status post–severe head injury, certain periodic professional monitoring will be required for life.
  4. Due to the client's at-risk health status, episodic medical care is predicted for life.

Table 8-1   Case management plan (see case study on p. 106)

Conclusion 1:   Due to cognitive and functional deficits resulting from severe head injury, this client is dependent on others for health, well-being, and safety and will require total direct care for the remainder of life

Care provider	Purpose	Expected time frame	Current cost	Comments
QC Care Center, Anywhere, USA	Provide direct care and prescribed treatment	2/26/91-10/18/96 (to age 21).	$590 per diem (plus medications)	Costs vary per 6 months, based on prior 6 month's expenses No overnight passes allowed unless full per diem rate is guaranteed; current payer does not guarantee, which prevents this therapeutic effort
Long-Term Quality Living Center, Concern, USA	Provide direct care and prescribed treatment	10/18/96-potential, lifetime	Projected at $600/day (per facility president)	
ALTERNATIVE				
Home care attendant	Provide direct care and prescribed treatment	10/18/98-potential, lifetime 14-16 hours/day, 365 days/year	Nurse aide through agency $17/hour	Agency services recommended to avoid family responsibility for payment for Social Security, vacation time, other benefits for paid attendant

Conclusion 2:   Owing to severe head injury, this client will require various medication for life.

Current prescription	Dosage	Purpose	Current cost	Comments
Sodium warfarin (Coumadin)	5 mg daily except Sunday; 2.5 mg Sunday	Prevent deep venous thrombosis (anticoagulant)	$44.33/100 tablets $43.79/100 tablets	Costs obtained from Town Clinic Pharmacy, a multistate chain
Carbamazepine (Tegretol)	100 mg 3 times daily (chewable)	Seizure control (anticonvulsant)	$16.89/100 tablets	
Phenytoin (Dilantin infantabs)	50 mg, 3 tabs at bedtime	Seizure control (anticonvulsant)	$6.22/100 tablets	
Bisacodyl	10-mg suppository every 3rd day	Prevent constipation (stimulant laxative)	$10.99/box of 100	
Diazepam (injectable)	5 mg as needed (IM)	For seizure lasting over 5 minutes	$7.88/10-mg syringe, prepackaged	Diazepam unavailable in 5 mg dosage; therefore 5 mg will be wasted when medication is used and charge will be for 10 mg
Citrucel	1 tsp twice daily	Prevent constipation (side effect of anticonvulsant)	$15.78/30-oz bottle	
Milk of magnesia	30 ml twice daily as needed.	Prevent constipation (side effect of anticonvulsant)	$6.39/26-oz bottle	

Conclusion 3:   Due to this client's medical diagnosis of status post–severe head injury, certain periodic professional monitoring will be required for life.

Professional care	Frequency	Purpose	Current cost	Comments
Physical medicine evaluation	Annually/life	Prevent complications Promote/maintain function Adjust therapeutic prescriptions	$100/examination	

Continued.

Table 8-1 Case management plan—cont'd

Professional care	Frequency	Purpose	Current cost	Comments
Neurologic examination	Annually/every 5 years as prescribed/life	Monitor status Adjust medications Prevent complications	$75/examination	
Neuropsychological evaluation	Every 5 years or as prescribed/life	Monitor status Specify neurobehavioral interventions Prevent complications	$850/examination	
Blood sample evaluation	Every 6 months throughout time anticonvulsants are prescribed/life	Monitor blood chemistry levels altered by use of anticonvulsives Prevent complications of long-term use of anticonvulsants Monitor blood levels of medication	$42 (CBC) $88 (SMA-12) $18 (blood level of carbamazepine)	
Dental treatment	Every 3-6 months for life	Monitor side effects of anticonvulsants Prevent complications	Hygienist: $45/examination Dentist: $55/examination	Additional treatment for revision of problems associated with side effects will increase cost
Speech evaluation/therapy	Annual evaluation, pending outcome of long-term 5-sessions-weekly program (current treatment) for life	Increase communication skills Improve consistency in response to environment Maintain achieved function	$500/full evaluation $85/session	Home program will be followed on a daily basis to promote quality of life, increase function, and maintain functional level achieved
Occupational therapy evaluation/treatment	Annual evaluation, pending outcome of long-term 5-sessions-weekly program (current treatment) for life	Increase upper extremity motion/function Attempt to promote functional independent behaviors Attempt to promote appropriate responses to environment Long term: maintain achieved function	$500/full evaluation $75/session	
Physical therapy evaluation/treatment	Annual evaluation, pending outcome of long-term 5-sessions-weekly program (current treatment) for life	Increase balance mobility, lower extremity functioning Attempt to promote functional, independent behaviors Prevent complications of of mobility Long term: maintain achieved functioning	$500/full evaluation $85/session	

Conclusion 4: Due to this client's at-risk health status, episodic medical care is predicted for life.

Professional care	Time frame	Purpose	Current cost	Comments
Orthopedic evaluation/treatment	As needed/life	Due to immobility of right arm/shoulder, hand may become painful or contracted and require treatment	$75/examination; treatment for contractures requires extensive physical therapy or surgery 1 week's hospitalization with surgery: $7,000	

Table 8-1 Case management plan—cont'd

Professional care	Time frame	Purpose	Current cost	Comments
Orthopedic evaluation/treatment *cont'd.*		Seizure disorder and spastic hemiparesis (balance is impaired), falls may result in fractures	Blue Cross/Blue Shield reports usual and customary charges for treatment of a fractured fibula without manipulation as $150-$175, physician charges only	
		Medical records reveal current heel cord tightening and resulting brace prescription	Brace: ankle-footorthosis $354/leg	Costs quoted from American Orthotics
Emergency care	As needed/life	Due to seizure disorder, potential exists for status epilepticus (continuous seizures)	$500/emergency examination and treatment	Status epilepticus represents a medical emergency

Conclusion 5:   As a result of severe head injury, certain durable medical equipment will be required for ongoing care of this client.

Equipment	Purpose	Repair/replace	Current cost	Comments
Wheelchair: padded armrest, leg rests, footrests, vertical projection on wheels	Mobility throughout home, community	Replace every 5 years	$2,100	"Quickie" standard light wheelchair
Tires		2 front tires: usual life, 1 year	$66/pair	
		2 rear tires: usual life, 1 year	$109/pair	
Maintenance	Prolong functioning	Annual	$50	
		Replacement every 2 years		
		Seat	$35	
		Back	$35	
		Armrest	$25 each	
Electric wheelchair	Mobility for use during greater distances or with diminished energy with aging; potential exists for this client to be self-mobile	Replace every 5-10 years	$10,000	
Parts		Drive belt; 2 sets/year	$25 each	
		4 tires; usual life, 1 year		
		2 front tires	$25 each	
		2 rear tires	$40 each	
		Wheelchair bearings: 2 sets last 2 years	$60 each	
		Wheelchair batteries: 2 last 2 years	$175 each	
		Battery charger: replace once during life of chair	$115 each	
Maintenance	Prolong functioning	Routine maintenance check of wheelchair	$75 annually	
		Upholstery repair/replacement every 2 years		
		Seat	$35/2 years	
		Back	$35/2 years	
		Armrest	$25/2 years	

Continued

Table 8-1   Case management plan—cont'd

Equipment	Purpose	Repair/replace	Current cost	Comments
Seat cushion (Jay cushion)	Prevent skin breakdown	Replace every 2-4 years	$295 for jell-type cushion (can range up to $400 depending on type of cushion)	
Cushion covers	Protect equipment, skin	2-3/year	$25 each	
Voice output communication aid	Interaction with environment	None/lifetime expectancy	$825/Intro-Talker	Lifetime expectancy; batteries, charger included
Right forearm support walker	Mobility; maintain function	Replace every 3-5 years	$78.95 (walker) $25/forearm attachment	ABC Supply Catalog
Wheelchair tray	Balance support; placement of communication aid	Replace every 5-10 years	$100	Custom made to accommodate needs
Assistive feeding devices	Independence in eating	Replace every year		
Plate guard			$5	Costs obtained from ABC Supply Catalog, Fall 1991
Adaptive utensil			$10.50 (universal cuff)	
Cup			$19.95	
Shower chair	Personal hygiene	Replace every 5-10 years; requires antitip bars and brakes	$677.75	Superior Medical Supply

Conclusion 6:   As a result of severe head injury, certain medical supplies will be required for this client's ongoing care.

Supply item	Number used	Purpose	Cost	Comments
Disposable Briefs, medium (Attends)	6/day	Collection of body waste	$44.95/package of 72	May not be needed if current toilet training efforts are successful

Conclusion 7:   Due to this client's cognitive and functional status, he will never be a candidate for participation in gainful competitive employment.

School grades A-B; anticipated enrollment at the University of Illinois; Intended major, International Business.

College Placement Council, Salary Survey, September 1989, indicated the following beginning salary offers to bachelor degree graduates:

Business/Accounting	$2,102/month	$25,233/year
Political Science	$1,940/month	$23,280/year

Conclusion 8:   Housing adaptation and modification will be necessary for this client's home, should he remain in a private home.

Accessibility needs	Comments
ANSI standard specified entrance/exits, two areas of dwelling	Costs for home modification vary according to geographic location and the status and style of the home to be modified.
Doorway widths: 36 inches	
Hallway widths: 48 inches	
Pocket doors Bathroom: 5-foot central radius, minimum	
Security system	Cost: $2,000 (per market)
Central heating/air (to maintain body temperature control)	
Wheelchair-accessible shower	Modification costs: $1,500-$5,000
Should a garage be available to this client, an automatic door opener would allow exit/entry without exposure to inclement weather	Information regarding accessibility standards and accessible housing design have been forwarded to client's parents; cost estimation for an accessible addition is $36,000

Table 8-1 Case management plan—cont'd

Conclusion 9: Family counseling is recommended to promote adjustment and adaption to their child's/siblings' catastrophic injury.

Professional care	Purpose	Cost	Comments
Psychological counseling	Stress management Communication Family stability Promote healthy environment for siblings Maintain healthy environment for continuing care for this client	$65-$95/hour	Counseling services should be available to each family member, individually, as well as group sessions; counseling may be necessary intermittently throughout this family's existence

Conclusion 10: This client *may* become a candidate for additional post–acute brain injury rehabilitation services in the future.

Treatment	Time frame	Current status	Therapeutic interventions	Current cost
Post–acute neurobehavioral injury treatment	6-18 months (or as prescribed by physician; determined by progress)	Limitations Cognitive Behavioral Physical Social	Individual therapy to promote verbal, cognitive, behavioral responses.	ABC Facility, 2 locations; $12,000/month
			Individual therapy to promote physical, psychological, social functioning	Neurobehavioral Treatment Program, Anywhere, USA $25,000/month
				Note: Treatment may include a 30-day evaluation only, to determine this client's ability to participate due to severity of injury

Conclusion 11: Due to limitations, this client requires transportation assistance for mobility throughout the community.

Equipment	Purpose	Cost	Comments
Vehicle: van	Safe and efficient transportation	$18,000 minimum $3,000 installation of customized interior	Does not include insurance, taxes, maintenance; replacement schedule related to mileage driven
Wheelchair lift	Allows ease of entry to vehicle for individual requiring wheelchair	$3,275 (cost includes installation)	Price obtained from Minneapolis firm
Power door opener		$600-$800	
Power lock down	Secures wheelchair in position for transportation; safety mechanism	$1,050 installed	
Remote system opener		$500	
Drop floor *or*		$1,220-$2,450	Cost varies per manufacturer of van purchased, depth of needed drop, and whether drop is for driver only or driver and passenger
Raised roof		$2,000	Cost revisions quoted by Pete Smith, Smith Medical Services, specialist in van modification *Note:* Due to rural residence public transportation is unavailable

Continued

Table 8-1 Case management plan—cont'd

Conclusion 12: Due to this client's health status and complex needs, ongoing case management services are recommended to assure continuity, consistency, and coordination of required care.

Service	Purpose	Cost	Comments
Case management	Plan, organize, coordinate and monitor services and resources on an ongoing basis to respond to healthcare needs Promote optimum conditions for care service provisions Assist family to think of care of client after their death or disability; advanced medical directives should be formulated for client	$55-$108/hour	Expect 2-10 hours/month for case management services, until other services are established and stabilized; quarterly monitoring should then cover needs, with 5 hours/quarter expected

Conclusion 13: Due to wheelchair dependency, clothing modification is required to prevent skin complications; multiple clothing changes are necessary due to instability in self-feeding.

Modified clothing

Modified clothing is essential for this client to maintain health. Standard clothing does not protect the individual who is wheelchair dependent.

Shoes must be sturdy: hard toes are preferred to prevent unknown damage to feet.

Slacks and shirts must be altered to allow room to prevent skin pressure (seams that bind may produce skin breakdown, which may lead to infection and generalized illness).

Modification costs vary: The seamstress used by this firm states alteration costs as, slacks, minimum of $20; shirts, $10.

Due to this client's limited and uncontrolled ability to self-feed or toilet independently, clothes must be washed repeatedly and therefore do not last as long as with normal wear.

CBC, complete blood cell count; SMA-12, sequential multiple analysis—12 different tests; AFO, ankle-foot orthosis; ANSI, American National Standards Institute.

REFERENCES

Arneson, B. (1993). Case management services and long-term care insurance benefits. *Journal of Case Management, 2,* 66-69.

Ballew, J.R., & Mink, G. (1986). *Case management in the human services.* Springfield, IL: Charles C Thomas.

Bower, K.A. (1992). *Case management by nurses.* Kansas City, MO: American Nurses Publishing.

Campbell, C.H. (1988). Needs of relatives and helpfulness of support groups in severe head injury. *Rehabilitation Nursing, 13,* 320-325.

Diller, L., & Ben-Yishay, Y. (1987). Outcomes and evidence in neuropsychological rehabilitation in closed head injury. In H.S. Levin, J. Grafman, and H.M. Eisenberg (Eds.), *Neurobehavioral recovery from head injury* (pp. 146-165). New York: Oxford University Press.

Dixon, T.P., Goll, S., & Stanton, K.M. (1988). Case management issues and practices in head injury rehabilitation. *Rehabilitation Counseling Bulletin, 31,* 332.

Do, H.K. (1988). Head trauma rehabilitation: Program evaluation. *Rehabilitation Nursing, 13,* 71-75.

Elliot, J., & Smith, D. (1985). Meeting family needs following severe head injury: A multidisciplinary approach. *Journal of Neurosurgical Nursing, 17,* 111-113.

Falik, M., Lipson, D., Lewis-Idema, D., Ulmer, C., Kaplan, K., Robinson, G., Hickey, E., & Veiga, R. (1993). Case management for special populations: Moving beyond categorical distinctions. *Journal of Case Management, 2,* 39-45, 74.

Gwyther, L.P. (1988). Assessment: Content, purpose, outcomes. *Generations: Case Management, 12,* 11-15.

Habermann, B. (1982). Cognitive dysfunction and social rehabilitation in the severely head-injured patient. *Journal of Neurosurgical Nursing, 14,* 220-224.

Hegeman, K.M. (1988). A care plan for the family of a brain trauma client. *Rehabilitation Nursing, 13,* 254-258.

Hembree, W.E. (1985). Getting involved: Employees as case managers. *Business and Health, 11.*

Kreutzer, J.S., & Wehman, P. (Eds.). (1990). *Community integration following traumatic brain injury.* Baltimore, MD: Paul H. Brookes.

Levin, H.S. (1987). Neurobehavioral sequelae of head injury. In P.R. Cooper (Ed.), *Head injury* (2nd ed., pp. 442-446). Baltimore: Williams & Wilkins.

Lezak, M.D. (1978). Living with the characterologically altered brain injured patient. *Journal of Clinical Psychiatry, 39,* 592-598.

Marr, J.A., & Reid, B. (1992). Implementing managed care and case management: The neuroscience experience. *Journal of Neuroscience Nursing, 24,* 281-285.

Mann, A.H., Hazel, C., Geer, C., Hurley, C.M., & Podrapovic, T. (1993). Development of an orthopaedic case manager role. *Orthopedic Nursing, 12,* 23-27.

Mauss-Clum, N., & Ryan, M. (1981). Brain injury and the family. *Journal of Neurosurgical Nursing, 13,* 165-169.

McCollom, P.L. (1991). *Case management guide, the individual with brain injury.* Little Rock: ICMA/Systemedic.

Mullahy, C.M. (1990). Empowering the case manager. *Continuing Care, 9,* 14, 16, 18-20, 30.

Mumma, C. (Ed.). (1987). *Rehabilitation nursing: Concepts and practice.* Evanston, IL: Rehabilitation Nursing Foundation.

National Task Force on Case Management (1992). Unpublished data.

Nursing Assessment and Management of the Frail Elderly Project, 1987. Curriculum of eight models on Case Management NAMFE Project, Kansas City, KS.

O'Hara, C.C., & Harrell, M. (1991). *Rehabilitation with brain injury survivors: An empowerment approach.* Gaithersburg, MD: Aspen.

Parker, R.M., and Hanson, C. (1981). *Rehabilitation counseling.* Boston: Allyn & Bacon.

Pickerell, M. (1993, November 6). *External medical case management.* Paper presented at the Association of Rehabilitation Nurses Annual Educational Conference. Denver, CO.

Preston, K. (1994, April). ARN president's message. Our role as case managers: The collective results of individual practice. *ARN Newsletter,* pp. 1, 7.

Rosenthall, M. et al. (1983). *Rehabilitation of the head injured adult.* Philadelphia: F.A. Davis.

Smith, S.S. (1985). Traumatic head injuries. In D.A. Umphred (Ed.). *Neurological rehabilitation* (pp. 249-288). St. Louis: Mosby–Year Book.

Whitman, M. (1991). Case management in head injury rehabilitation. *Rehabilitation Nursing, 16,* 19-22.

Williams, M.H. (1990). The self-help movement in head injury. *Rehabilitation Nursing, 15,* 311-315.

Zander, K. (1988). Nursing case management resolving the DRG paradox. *Nursing Clinics of North America, 23,* 503-520.

9

Community-Based Rehabilitation Nursing

Lisa Cyr Buchanan, MS, RNC, CRRN

INTRODUCTION

Scientific advances, an aging population, and improved technology have created a milieu where increasing numbers of individuals of all ages are living with chronic disabilities. When these individuals attempt to re-enter the community, they continue to experience numerous barriers and gaps in services. Traditionally healthcare providers have focused on illness and the physical needs of clients. Ensuring successful community re-entry for clients involves attending to diverse variables that impact on this process including geographic location, family support systems, access to community resources, financial resources, attitudinal barriers, and access to healthcare services.

A goal for community re-entry is to foster independence. Careful assessment of the changing needs of persons with chronic disability or developmental disorders across their life-span and as they re-enter the community purposefully directs funding and support services to ensure proper and efficient use of funds. When society views persons with disabilities as dependent persons, public policy will continue to allow wasteful funding, discrimination, and impediments to community and environmental access (Rubin & Millard, 1991).

The role of the rehabilitation nurse is paramount to the success of community reintegration. Successful community re-entry can be implemented when clients are involved in the discharge plan, when they are encouraged to maintain control over their environment, and when they are encouraged to take responsibility for their health maintenance plan and behaviors. In addition, collaboration with home healthcare providers will promote client involvement and successful community re-entry.

AN OVERVIEW OF COMMUNITY-BASED PRACTICE

In the United States the complex healthcare needs of clients living in various community sites or at home, restrictive reimbursement systems, competition between providers, economic trends, legislative mandates, and skyrocketing healthcare costs have been responsible for the creation of models designed to ensure the provision of comprehensive, efficient, cost-effective healthcare services. Three of these models are case management, community-based rehabilitation (CBR), and managed care (Chapter 2 and Chapter 8 provide more information about these models.) Basic principles common to these models are coordination of services; promotion of self-care and independence; enhancement of quality of life; collaboration between providers, families, and clients; attention to quality of care; and a focus on client outcomes (Hoeman, 1992; McBride, 1992). CBR nursing practice broadens this scope to include a focus on the family and social support networks, considers the impact of the community environment, incorporates cultural values, has a theory base, promotes lifelong planning for living and coping with a disability, and emphasizes the need to mesh the practice base with home healthcare (Hoeman, 1992).

Participation as a healthcare provider in CBR nursing practice demands that the practitioners adeptly define a scope of practice. Integral to defining a scope of practice is the development of a knowledge base that includes the following:

1. Rehabilitation philosophy
2. Anatomy and physiology
3. Group dynamics
4. Importance of family in the rehabilitation process
5. Interdisciplinary approach
6. How to access community services and resources
7. Educator role
8. Discharge planning
9. Legislated entitlements and rights
10. Early intervention
11. Transition and normalization
12. Research and utilization or application to practice
13. Case management

Hence CBR nursing practice is a challenging arena for delivering complex rehabilitation services to clients and their families.

THE NEUMAN MODEL AND COMMUNITY-BASED PRACTICE

A major goal of CBR practice is to promote prevention and health maintenance. This goal can be demonstrated through the use of Neuman's conceptual model for developing care plans for patients re-entering the community.

Neuman's Healthcare Systems Model emphasizes the interplay between the total person, the environment, health, and nursing as a systems approach and demonstrates a strong reciprocal relationship between a person and the environment. Integral to the model are the nursing role func-

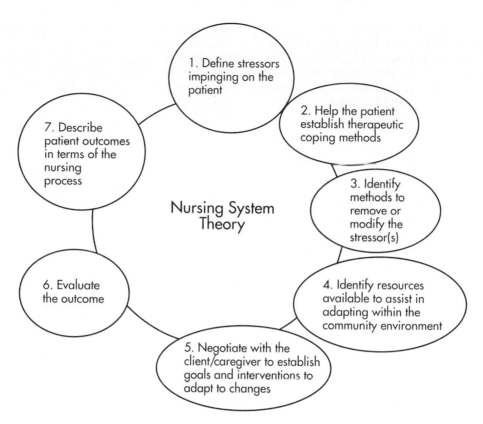

Fig. 9-1   Nursing system theory.

tions to identify internal and external stressors, define the level of prevention and degree of tolerance or resistance, define nursing interventions appropriate for each level and determine when intervention is appropriate (Fawcett, 1984). Neuman (1989) emphasizes that all persons seek and require stability within this system and will react differently to stressors.

Clients with disabilities are bombarded with a multiplicity of stressors during the transition to the home environment. An understanding of systems theory (Fig. 9-1) can help the nurse in CBR nursing practice.

The Person with Chronic Disability or Developmental Disorders

There are over 23 million persons in the United States who have disabilities, and almost 11.5 million have severe disabilities (Gottlieb, Vandergoot, & Lutsky, 1991). Stroke, musculoskeletal/orthopedic, traumatic brain injury, and spinal cord injury (SCI) represent the majority of the disabling conditions in the United States, with musculoskeletal diseases being the primary cause of disability (Rehabilitation Nursing Foundation [RNF], 1993). These numbers will increase as the global population ages. By the year 2000 over 19 million persons in the United States will be over the age of 65 years and coincidentally 1 out of every 14 persons will be female (Preski & Burnside, 1992). RNF reports that more than 118,000 persons will be over the age of 100 years by the year 2000. Groch (1991) reports that 32.5 millions persons in the United States have physical limitations due to chronic health problems.

✦ **Community-based rehabilitation services.** Over 5 million of the elderly persons in the United States are hospitalized annually, with 59% requiring rehabilitation services. The length of stay in hospitals and on rehabilitation units has decreased from 52.2 days in 1978 to 29.1 in 1990. However, there are still deficits in CBR services for 28 million persons in the United States who are not receiving needed rehabilitation services (RNF, 1993). These trends will have economic, medical, and social consequences. In fact, there are rapidly increasing numbers of persons living in the community who will require some type of rehabilitation services for the rest of their lives. In a milieu of decreasing resources and increasing numbers of those requiring community resources, rehabilitation nurses and other allied health professionals must become skilled at ensuring successful re-entry and become politically active to assure services to persons with disabilities are continued.

✦ **Mental health and community-based rehabilitation**

There is also a trend toward community re-entry for those with psychiatric disabilities. In the United States there were 560,000 persons in mental health institutions during 1955, compared with 120,000 persons currently (Dibner & Murphy, 1991). Statistics demonstrate over 2 million persons suffer from chronic mental illness, and over 20% of the U.S. population will experience mental illness during their lifetime (Jones, Gallagher, Kelley, & Massari, 1991).

Persons with psychiatric disabilities often have limited access to rehabilitation services in the community. This population usually has reduced earnings; their rehabilitation rate is lower than for those with physical disabilities; and fewer are accepted for vocational rehabilitation programs (Andrews et al., 1992; Cushion, 1992; Hirsch, 1989; MacGilp, 1991). Due to the financial constraints, those with mental disabilities often lack sufficient funds to purchase basic items and have limited social contacts (MacGilp, 1991). According to MacGilp there is a dearth of community follow-up. Many persons with mental disabilities are unable to demonstrate knowledge about their medication regimen and as a result take their medications incorrectly.

✦ Dual diagnoses

Persons with combined cognitive and physical disabilities have needs that challenge attempts at community reintegration. Psychiatric problems often prevent access to programs designed to address physical disabilities and vice versa. It is imperative that a total assessment of cognitive and physical abilities be completed. Healthcare providers may focus on the obvious disabilities when planning for community re-entry and neglect more subtle impairments. This selective neglect may set the client up for failure in the community environment. Rehabilitation nurses may need to consult with other interdisciplinary team colleagues when planning community re-entry for persons with multiple disabilities. Managing the complex nature of these conditions requires expertise in more than one professional discipline, and conditions may be rare or unique. As a result a rehabilitation nurse or other team member may have limited knowledge or a lack of experience with unusual or dual disabilities.

✦ Pediatric clients

Age discrimination occurs throughout the life-span of persons with disabilities including when they attempt to access rehabilitation services. Only in the past decade have there been federally legislated programs and services, home- and community-based services, or funding for assistive devices for persons with disabilities of all ages. Parette and VanBiervliet (1991) report that recent laws have finally recognized the need for assistive technology, medically related services, and adapted devices for infants and children. However, a number of unmet needs for infants and children with disabilities include transportation, lack of funding to purchase assistive equipment, and lack of information provided to families relative to training and practice sessions with new equipment. Parette and VanBiervliet report a lack of training opportunities for professionals to provide necessary technology services to the pediatric population.

✦ The elderly

Persons who are elderly and have disabilities face many gaps in services while residing in the community. This is frequently coupled with attitudinal barriers (Middleton & McDaniel, 1990). This group is primarily female and has the highest number of disabilities (Mayer, 1991; Preski & Burnside, 1992). Strategies for providing rehabilitation services to this population in the community should first determine the preillness activity level; identify factors impeding participation in the rehabilitation program such as impaired sensory perception/stimulation, mobility restric-

tions, and the environment; and promote wellness. The success of community reintegration for the elderly will be dependent on meeting social, emotional, physical, and cognitive needs; mutual goal setting; and promoting social independence (Mayer, 1991; Middleton & McDaniel, 1990).

✦ Culture

There are cultural barriers to accessing healthcare services. The cultures of the clients, family, institution, and the medical system impact every clinical interaction. These cultural differences may prevent the delivery of adequate healthcare services. The beliefs, attitudes, behaviors, and values of every individual will impact on the interplay between each of these individuals within the healthcare system (Fitzgerald, 1992). It is imperative that rehabilitation healthcare professionals understand the influence of cultural beliefs on the rehabilitation process; identify individual beliefs, attitudes, and values that may impact on client outcomes; and develop strategies to incorporate these beliefs in the rehabilitation process in order to promote the provision of adequate healthcare services.

✦ The environment

CBR nursing practice should begin with assessing the needs of clients in the community. Care plans and services must be individualized. The services and resources required for each person will vary greatly and be impacted by a multitude of factors (Paulson, Dahl, and Wasch, 1993).

✦ Geographic location

Rural communities frequently have difficulties assisting clients in accessing services and resources because the areas are underserved by healthcare professionals and have inadequate resources. There is frequently a lack of public or private transportation, limited accessible housing, architectural barriers in the community, limited employment opportunities, few social groups, limited home care services, limited access to attendant care, no participatory recreational or sports events, and attitudinal barriers. Services may be available in the urban setting, but demand may exceed availability. (Chapter 5 details provisions from the Americans with Disabilities Act.)

Rehabilitation nurses have a responsibility to ensure that clients receive necessary services regardless of the setting. Concurrently it is paramount that the available services are not abused by clients who do not truly require them.

Identifying Barriers to Community Re-entry

An absence of accessible transportation, poor access to trained attendants, and restricted availability of affordable and accessible housing have been identified as the three major areas that create barriers for persons with disabilities returning to the community (Bergland & Clark, 1991; Fanning, Judge, Weihe, & Emener, 1991). The CBR nurse is in a position to identify and assist in modifying these barriers.

✦ Transportation

A dearth of accessible and affordable transportation has a major impact on the ability of persons with disabilities to live independently. Barriers to transportation impact the ability to work, use of public facilities, access to healthcare services, participation in recreational and social activities, and the pursuit of public or private education. Access to these activities and services is imperative if persons with disabilities are to participate in life activities necessary for successful community re-entry. Barriers to transportation can make the difference between community re-entry or institutionalization.

Communities have been mandated to provide accessibility on buses, airlines, and trains (Dittmar, 1989). Practitioners in CBR nursing practice can play a vital advocacy role in promoting access to transportation. In part, this role demands that practitioners educate the community regarding the needs of persons with disabilities.

✦ Attendant care

The cost and availability of attendant care remains a major problem for a number of persons with disabilities (Fanning et al., 1991). Many persons with disabilities are unable to live independently in the community without assistance with personal care and household activities.

Funding for some attendant care may be linked with eligibility for income assistance by Medicaid in certain programs. The waiting lists for these programs may be long. Lack of training programs for attendants is another major issue. Few states regulate these attendant services appropriately. Individuals hiring attendants must provide on-the-job training. Either the client or family members have to be able to manage hiring and firing, training, scheduling, and payroll for the attendants. In some instances this may be required when the care is funded by federal or state monies. Similarly, attendant care services for infants and children are underfunded by federal and state monies in some states. These conditions differ throughout the United States. Rehabilitation nurses who work in CBR familiarize themselves with the administrative codes, mandates, entitlements, and regulations for the state in which they practice.

The current availability of accessible housing in most communities is inadequate to meet the need. One study cited the reasons as insufficient supply, inaccessibility, architectural barriers in the home, long waiting lists, not affordable, and poor location. State and federal mandates have attempted to meet the housing requirements of persons with disabilities through legislation (Fanning et al., 1991). Housing needs and options need to be meshed with consumer need, accessibility, and adequate funding. Persons with disabilities generally prefer home or integrated independent living situations to institutions and segregated housing (De-Jong, 1993; Fanning et al., 1991; Spencer, 1990). Independent living has been associated with promoting the general well-being and self-esteem of persons with disabilities; however, discrimination continues even when housing is erected to accommodate them under federal mandates.

✦ Employment

Employment is equated with life satisfaction, provides people with an identity, and allows for financial independence (Kiernan & McGaughey, 1992). There have been fewer numbers of persons with disabilities accepted into the vocational rehabilitation process during the past 15 years due to budget constraints and mandates that these services be provided to persons with severe disabilities. There has

been an increase in the number of persons with severe physical disabilities and a concurrent decrease in the number of persons with severe psychiatric disabilities who have returned to the competitive employment marketplace (Andrews et al., 1992). The unemployment rate for persons with psychiatric disabilities may be as high as 85% (Hirsch, 1989). A minority of companies have policies in place for hiring those with psychiatric disabilities (Jones et al., 1991). Companies frequently favor hiring those with physical disabilities over persons with psychiatric disabilities (Greenwood, Schriner, & Johnson, 1991; Jones et al., 1991). Even when companies do hire persons with disabilities, there is a shortage of well-trained job coaches to provide the necessary training and supervision (Grossi, Test, & Keul, 1991).

The return to work after a disability is impacted in part by the type and severity of the disability, educational level, age, gender, and preinjury wages (Tate, 1992). Hirsch (1989) cites studies that define variables affecting return to work for those with psychiatric disabilities: living arrangement; dependability; ability to work with others, to complete work tasks, and to accept supervision.

Increasing numbers of persons in the United States have physical and mental disabilities. Companies need to consider which variables impact return to work outcomes and develop programs that promote successful re-entry into the competitive labor market.

✦ Financial constraints

Sufficient financial resources are essential to meet household expenses; purchase equipment, attendant care, homemaker services, and medical care; arrange for respite care; complete home modifications; purchase/rent an emergency response system; and pursue educational opportunities. Frequently the spouse may have to relinquish employment in order to assume the caregiver role at the same time that the person with disability may have lost gainful employment. This scenario creates a heavy financial burden on the family. Ultimately the cost of caring for a family member with a disability at home may exceed financial resources. These circumstances increase the stress placed on the caregiver role.

✦ Caregiver concerns

The burdens on the caregiver and the family often are ignored or minimized. When a person with a chronic, disabling, or developmental disorder returns to a home environment, there is a major impact on the caregiver and family system (Power & Dell Orto, 1980; Schmidt et al., 1986; Stroker, 1983; Watson, 1992). Lack of adequate preparation and training, information, skills, respite care, support services, support networks outside the home, and finances create unconscionable stress and strain on the caregiver. (Chapter 13 discusses caregiver burden and family systems.) Many of these needs can be identified during the discharge planning phase when institution staff and community providers collaborate and include the client and family in planning (Rhoads, Dean, Cason, & Blaylock, 1992). Lack of knowledge regarding care and community resources predictably and unnecessarily impedes successful community re-entry. When identified before a client receives discharge to the community, most issues and concerns can be addressed and often resolved.

Defining Interventions

Skillful rehabilitation professionals will be able to identify variables impinging on the plan for community re-entry; conduct a thorough assessment; participate in mutual goal setting; and intervene on a level that promotes patient success, self-reliance, and independence (see Box below).

✦ Discharge planning

Successful community re-entry involves skillful discharge planning. Outcomes for clients and their families improve with interdisciplinary collaboration including professionals from institution and home healthcare agencies, the primary physician, the client and family or caregiver(s), and a social worker. The home care team may be expanded to include those who are not classically part of an inpatient team such as the clergy, school nurse, psychologist, audiologist, nutritionist, Department of Human Services staff, neighbors or similar network persons, and extended family members. The goal of the team is the same whether in the institution or community: to work collaboratively in meeting the physical, emotional, social, vocational, cultural, spiritual, and economic needs of clients, caregivers, and/or family members in the community environment.

According to Rhoads et al. (1992), many families feel unprepared to care for family members at home. Concern over medication management, difficulty deciphering or following written instructions, reluctance or inability to perform direct care skills, and poor awareness of community resources were identified as problematic areas for clients and caregivers. Rhoads et al. propose a model that will address these issues for clients and caregivers regarding the acquisition of skills and knowledge for providing direct care and assessing community resources (Table 9-1). Institutional-based providers and home healthcare providers should elect to implement this model to promote successful community re-entry. This model also will assist the team

Table 9-1 Functions of care providers

Hospital based	Home healthcare based
Initiate community resource referrals	Follow-up on all services requested
Teach home care skills	Follow-up on demonstration of skills
	Adapt equipment as needed to facilitate caregiver's ability to give care with ease
Provide medication education	Follow-up with all medications
Follow-up with admitting and discharge medications	Follow-up on cost of medication and client's ability to obtain them
Obtain home assessment data	Assess home environment to determine if client is able to adapt environment to meet needs at home
Assess adequacy of financial resources	Identify financial resources that client is using and assess their adequacy
Assess knowledge base of client/caregiver	Evaluate caregiver's knowledge base regarding information taught in the hospital
Involve caregiver in discharge process; involve home healthcare nurse early in discharge plan	Provide necessary skilled care procedures according to caregiver's ability to provide skilled care services; reassess as care becomes more the client's/caregiver's responsibility
Initiate list of available emergency services and transportation resources	Follow-up on need and use of emergency services and transportation alternative resources
Coordinate clinic visits	Follow-up on clinic visits
	Identify respite care alternatives
	Assess safety measures in home

From "Comprehensive discharge planning: A hospital-home healthcare partnership" by C. Rhoads, J. Dean, C. Cason, and A. Blaylock, 1992. *Home Healthcare Nurse, 10,* p. 17. Copyright 1992 by J.B. Lippincott. Reprinted by permission.

✦

DISCHARGE PLANNING ASSESSMENT

Community resources available and/or needed
✦ Respite care
✦ Home healthcare services
✦ Support services/groups
✦ Support from family/friends/clergy
✦ Disability-related information
✦ Transportation
✦ Early intervention services
✦ School services
✦ Outpatient rehabilitation services
✦ Contingency plan if caregiver is ill or unavailable
✦ Attendant care

Client/caregiver knowledge base
✦ Caregiver training for direct care needs
✦ Emergency services
✦ Financial resources
✦ Equipment care and repair
✦ Infection control procedures

Home evaluation

Access to community environment

Home pass assessment before discharge

HOME AND COMMUNITY ASSESSMENT
Access considerations

Outdoors

Parking and distance from entrance

Location of mailbox

Storage of vehicle and access to home from the storage area

Access to home: width of doors; ability to turn key, open and close doors; need for ramps, handrails

Lighting in entrances

Community buildings used regularly; access to these buildings

Access to private or public transportation: distance from home, cost, assistance required, ability to operate own vehicle safely

Parking areas marked for handicapped; adequate space to maneuver

Width, height of incline of ramps, sidewalks

Indoors: General

Thresholds, floor obstructions, steps inside home

Arrangement of furniture and ability to use

Location of telephone

Ability to raise/lower windows

Floor coverings: slippery, scatter rugs; can a wheelchair be maneuvered

Location of all rooms; ability to maneuver a wheelchair or assistive device

Location of fuse box

Ability to control heat

Width of walkways, doorways, halls: space to maneuver

Access to outlets; ability to change light bulbs

Type of furniture and ability to use safely

Elevator: threshold, timing of door, adapted for hearing and visual impairments

Indoors: Kitchen

Access to stove, sink, cupboards, storage, work space, refrigerator, contents, other appliances

Countertop and sink height; opening under sink for wheelchair access

Ability to operate faucets, use microwave, reach knobs on stove

Convenient arrangement of appliances

Indoors: Bathroom

Height of sink and toilet, shower/tub, and location of faucets

Space for maneuvering wheelchair or assistive device

Threshold for shower

Ability to use facilities safely

Presence, location of grab bars, securely anchored

Indoors: Bedroom

Height of bed

Access to closet, ability to reach rods, storage area

Firmness of mattress

Ability to transfer in and out of bed safely; adequate space around bed

Arrangement of furniture: space to maneuver

SAFETY CONSIDERATIONS
General

House number clearly visible and readable for quick identification during an emergency

Locks secure; deadbolts; ability to use

Ability to see and talk to visitor at the door without being seen

Steps, porch, front door lighted and protected from the weather

Nonslip doormat

Ability to use telephone, emergency response system

Ability to control water temperature

Wiring, outlet covers for children

Smoke detectors: type, location, access

Lighting in rooms, hallways; access to control lights inside and outside the home

Ability to respond to a fire emergency: fire exits/access, use of stairs instead of elevator, use of fire extinguisher, fire drills

Use of oxygen: precautions and appropriate signs in the home

Access to telephone, radio, television while in bed

Use of space heaters: type, location

Location of knobs on stove, safety around stove, cleanliness of stove; ability to use good judgment when cooking

Ability to dispose of infectious materials safely

Safe play area

Ability to transport food from kitchen to table

Ventilation in all rooms

Pest-free method of trash storage

in identifying and understanding the diverse and complementary functions of each player. It is vital for rehabilitation professionals to understand the differences in their roles in order to complement each other throughout the discharge planning phase. This will promote collaboration, communication, unity, and coordination between providers, in addition to successful community re-entry.

Thorough discharge planning must include consideration of the home and community environment (see Box, p. 119). This will facilitate rehabilitation professionals in obtaining a complete database for planning community re-entry. The discharge planning team may elect to postpone discharge until modifications in the home are completed.

The client, family, and/or caregivers should be given the opportunity to have a home pass before discharge (Henderson & Pentland, 1991). This will assist in pinpointing variables that must be addressed before discharge to promote a successful transition to the community. Implementing a model for discharge planning that utilizes the home pass may

1. Enable the client and caregiver to practice their skills in the home setting
2. Allow documentation of the client/caregiver's perception of the client's ability to function in the home environment
3. Boost the morale of the client/caregiver
4. Identify actual and possible problems that would need to be addressed before discharge
5. Assist the rehabilitation practitioner to evaluate the client/caregiver's actual abilities
6. Provide information to the rehabilitation team about the client's mood and motivation during community re-entry (Henderson & Pentland, 1991)

Comprehensive discharge planning can have an impact on preventing readmissions to hospitals. Implementing client and caregiver involvement in the planning process for community re-entry; using home passes, intensive home assessment, extensive client/caregiver teaching; and coordinating and securing community resources and services before discharge from an institution will contribute to successful community reintegration. The rehabilitation professional has a vital role in identifying individual needs, developing a knowledge base about the availability of community resources and services, developing methods for accessing services, and planning for ongoing evaluations in the community to ensure that the services are adequately meeting changes in individual needs. These strategies will help to prevent hospital readmissions and subsequent institutionalization.

✦ Attendant care options

Funding sources for attendant care may be obtained through a variety of programs. The client usually will be required to meet eligibility requirements specific to each program. Some of these programs include Medicare; Medicaid; Workers' Compensation; private healthcare insurance such as Blue Cross/Blue Shield, Health Maintenance Organizations, Preferred Provider Organizations; Medicare Supplemental Benefit Plan; auto liability policies; and Veterans Administration benefits. A number of persons with disabilities are ineligible for these programs or require extended hours of care that are not covered by these programs.

Hence the burden of caregiving again lies with family members. It is imperative that rehabilitation professionals assist clients and caregivers to identify individual needs relative to attendant care requirements—specific tasks requiring assistance, number of hours per day—and to obtain the resources required to promote independent community living.

Caregiver stress and strain can increase dramatically if an infant or child is returning to the home and has developmental needs and/or a disability (Ahmann & Lipsi, 1992). These families will have special needs. They will require support services to provide respite care for the caregiver to have time alone and to allow time for caregiver/parents to spend time with siblings. Siblings in the home may feel neglected. Thus attendant care services may be vital for meeting the needs of the client and the entire family unit.

Home healthcare agencies can provide extensive attendant care services to persons with disabilities. The client must meet the eligibility requirements for individual programs through Medicare, Medicaid, Blue Cross/Blue Shield, and other third-party payers. Medicare, Medicaid, and other third-party payers require that home healthcare services be provided on a part-time or intermittent basis. The plan of treatment must be established and approved by a physician.

Medicare

Persons under age 65 years of age wait 2 years after the onset of a disability to be eligible for medical benefits under the federal Medicare program. To qualify under Medicare for home healthcare, the client must have a skilled need defined by requiring skilled assessments of a medical condition; teaching needs; injections; Foley catheter care; case management on a short-term basis; wound care; physical therapy; speech therapy; or an ongoing need for occupational therapy once nursing, physical therapy, or speech therapy staff have established a plan of care. The person must be homebound—that is, confined to the home due to a normal inability to leave the home, there is a considerable and taxing effort to leave; and absences from home are infrequent or of short duration or for the purpose of receiving medical care (Health Care Financing Administration [HCFA], 1989). Thus a client with a psychiatric problem, who has no physical limitations, would be considered homebound when the illness is manifested by a refusal to leave the home or if it would be unsafe for the person to leave the home unsupervised. Additional conditions must be met by the client and the home health agency providing the services for coverage for home health services. A client is allowed to have frequent absences from the home when the purpose is to receive medical care.

Medicaid

Individual state Medicaid programs have home health services eligibility requirements. Generally the three primary conditions include the following: (1) the medical condition of the client must be able to be treated safely at home; (2) the condition must require the skilled services of a registered nurse, physical therapist (PT), occupational therapist (OT), speech therapist (ST), medical social worker (MSW), or, when unskilled services are medically necessary, a home health aide; and (3) the services obtained cannot be reasonably obtained outside the client's place of residence.

The 1978 Amendments to the Rehabilitation Act of 1973 and the Rehabilitation Comprehensive Services and Developmental Disabilities Amendments of 1978 mandated independent living services for persons with disabilities (Bergland & Clark, 1991). These programs provide long-term supportive services to promote each client's re-entry into the community and participation as community members. Attendant care has been one of the support services funded through federal and state monies, according to a state's rules and regulations. The attendants are hired by the person with a disability to assist the person to live independently. An attendant may be the key to unlocking community living for many persons with chronic disability or development disorders who otherwise would reside in an institution or nursing home.

In most instances attendants provide any care that is directed and approved by the person who has hired them. Many persons with disabilities have complex care requirements even living at home. Since attendants are not employees of certified home healthcare agencies, there are no regulations defining scope of practice. On the other hand, persons with disabilities need access to this type of care. Rehabilitation nurses advocate for clients' independence in living while ensuring that attendants have adequate training and are qualified to provide the required level of care for each client. Rehabilitation nurses are in a position to lobby for formal training, supervision, and certification of attendants.

✦ Health contracts

Home healthcare providers have defined the need to develop health contracts with clients before their discharge into the community. The purpose of a contract is to delineate the responsibilities of all participants, establish expected outcomes and methods for achieving mutually agreed-upon goals, and is expressly client centered (Hoeman & Winters, 1988). The health contract is not a legal document. The terms of a contract set a time line and contain a method to measure the results. Hoeman and Winters recommend a written contract over a verbal contract to prevent miscommunication and ambiguity.

Hoeman and Winters (1988) outline the five steps for developing a health contract:

1. Assess needs
2. Establish mutually agreeable goals
3. Explore resources and strengths
4. Implement the plan
5. Evaluate the contract

Consideration is given for differences in values and beliefs, and the client must be intellectually and emotionally able to enter into a contractual agreement.

There is a trend toward sending clients home with higher acuity and complex healthcare needs. Many are frail elderly persons or those with chronic, disabling conditions who may have few support systems. Home healthcare agencies have increased demands on them to provide complex, comprehensive services using high technology. Frequently community-based agencies provide care to persons who have difficulty managing their own care, and in fact many persons continue to participate in behaviors, which if eliminated, might prevent multiple medical and nonmedical problems. A client's reluctance, inability, or resistance to participating in self-care and preventive health behaviors may form the basis for establishing a contract with that person.

Clients have an obligation to be responsible for their behaviors, be able to establish goals, and achieve a desired outcome for their healthcare. The health contract is one method to promote self-directed community-based care.

Health contracts can be effective for clients who are admitted into services but who wish to limit the care they receive. Establishing a contract enables all parties to address the issue of refusal of care before the care is initiated and to appropriately define the responsibilities of each care provider. This promotes communication, defines the roles of each party before discharge to the community, clearly outlines expected outcomes, defines the limitations of care, and establishes agency liability. The contract will assist in eliminating gray areas for agencies when the ethical, moral, and legal issues are addressed before care is provided. Each provider then has the option of deciding against admitting the client into care. This then allows the client and family time

Table 9-2 Housing options for the disabled.

Type	Description
Congregate	Segregated community living developed for individuals with mobility impairments
Residential	Support services shared by a group of persons with disabilities living in proximity; services managed by others
Independent living center	Persons with disabilities assisted with housing referral, attendant referral, attendant training, advocacy, equipment repair, and other services; services not managed in a single setting
Institution	Person receives individualized care according to nursing care plan 24 hours/day
Boarding home	Private or state run; person usually required to perform own personal care and must demonstrate ability to be mobile in environment with or without assistive device
Supervised environmental living facility	Supervised apartment program for chronically mentally ill persons; provides comprehensive, supportive, and rehabilitative services to promote community re-entry
Integrated housing: private residence or rental	Independent living; may receive support services from the community such as home healthcare, attendant care
Group home	Supervised living environment; persons with similar disabilities live together

to seek services elsewhere if necessary. As advanced directives and specific orders such as DNR (do not resuscitate) become common, rehabilitation nurses will find their roles as advocates become more complex with moral issues and with fully informed consent about allocation of services and resources for persons with chronic, disabling, and developmental disorders. (Chapter 3, discusses foundations for these role functions in more detail.)

Funding for nursing home placement in some parts of the United States is the easiest to obtain but is the most expensive, although this may differ throughout the country. Persons with disabilities consider nursing homes the least desirable housing option (Spencer, 1990). An array of independent living arrangements are made available to persons with disabilities along with the necessary community-based support services (Table 9-2). Spencer states that our society supports excessive resources for institutional care versus community-based care. Clearly rehabilitation nursing may be advocate for public policy changes and healthcare reforms that propose revisions in the reimbursement structure for providing housing to persons with disabilities.

✦ Independent living programs

The advantages of independent living programs (ILPs) were to promote community reintegration and participation in community activities and to provide long-term community-based support services (see Box below). The services provided by individual programs have varied across the country. Some types of services offered include the following:

1. Attendant referral and training
2. Housing referral
3. Consumer advocacy
4. Equipment loans and repair
5. Disability awareness and social acceptance programs
6. Reduction of barriers
7. Employment/vocational services
8. Peer counseling
9. Information and referral services
10. Driver training
11. Temporary housing
12. Transitional or permanent residential housing (Means & Bolton, 1992; Nosek, Roth, & Zhu, 1990; Tate, Maynard, & Forchheimer, 1992)

✦

FACTORS IMPACTING INDIVIDUAL DECISIONS LEADING TO CHOICES OF INDEPENDENT LIVING ALTERNATIVES

- ✦ Financial resources
- ✦ Type of disability
- ✦ Geographic location
- ✦ Availability and need for social support systems
- ✦ Availability of attendant care in the community
- ✦ Need for skill acquisition and training
- ✦ Availability and affordability of transportation services
- ✦ Ability to manage own finances
- ✦ Ability to hire, train, and supervise attendants

Despite these noble intentions, many programs fall short of their goals to provide these services to persons with disabilities.

Research findings demonstrate that collaboration between a medical rehabilitation program and an ILP positively prepares patients for community re-entry (Tate et al., 1992). Participation in a "hospital to community" program assisted clients who had a new disability to gain control in their lives, enabled them to acquire "significantly more knowledge about disability and independent living issues," and decreased the degree of psychological distress postinjury. CBR nurses or case managers develop similar collaborative programs for persons with disabilities who are returning to the community.

It is imperative that the newly emerging ILP models strive to embody the philosophy of the early models: to provide client advocacy, promote community reintegration and participation, be consumer based, provide a range of services above and beyond housing, and serve persons with a variety of disabilities (Nosek et al., 1990).

Effective ILPs are proactive, rather than reactive, when identifying and eliminating social, environmental, and economic barriers in the community. Those that remain static may become self-serving, which is a gross injustice to persons with disabilities. Staff who are trained, available, and knowledgeable are needed for supervision and consultation about meeting the complex needs of persons with disabilities as they re-enter their homes and communities.

Not surprisingly, integrated, residential housing opportunities are preferred by persons with disabilities (Fanning et al., 1991; Spencer, 1990). Legislation to make housing available and accessible—the Housing Act of 1959—provided mortgage loans for construction of housing projects for the elderly and those with disabilities. Fourteen years later the Rehabilitation Act of 1973 (Section 504) prohibited discrimination against those with disabilities in the sale or rental of federally subsidized housing. Then the Housing and Community Development Act of 1974 provided mortgage assistance to lower income families (RNF, 1987).

Barriers to desirable housing such as transportation, affordability, accessibility, attendant care, and financial assistance programs (Fanning et al., 1991) create limited and/or desirable housing options (Table 9-2), which may be rectified through policy changes, legislation, and advocacy.

✦ Employment and education options

Whether a client returns to work following a disabling event is dependent in part on the type and severity of the disability, as well as the person's educational level, age, sex, and preinjury wages (Tate, 1992). Increasing numbers of persons in the United States are surviving with chronic, irrevocable disabilities. Businesses and companies are beginning to consider which variables have an impact on a person's return to work and to develop programs that enable employees to return to the labor market. CBR nurses are active in case management to ensure programs are in place and are meeting the needs of persons with disabilities who desire to return to the workforce.

Employee assistance programs

Employee assistance programs (EAPs) have been used during the past decade in an effort to return injured workers to their work environment bolstered with selected training and supports. Methods used in EAPs include supervisory training, peer training, employee education, and counseling supports. Early EAPs targeted employees who were substance dependent; programs then were expanded for employees who were experiencing stress due to family, work, or fiscal problems; and most recently for workers with disabilities (Kiernan & McGaughey, 1992).

The passage of the Americans with Disabilities Act (ADA) of 1990 has had an impact on these EAPs. This legislation expanded the Rehabilitation Act of 1973. The original act prevented businesses receiving federal funds from discriminating against qualified persons with disabilities in employment practices only. The ADA of 1990 is designed to prevent discrimination against persons with disabilities in the private sector. The areas defined now include employment, telecommunications, transportation, and public services and accommodations (Satcher and Hendren, 1992). (Chapter 5 provides details about the ADA.)

Supported employment

The 1986 Amendment to the Rehabilitation Act of 1973 provided grants to states for the development of supported employment programs for persons with physical and psychiatric disabilities. Supported employment is defined as "providing competitive work in integrated settings (a) for individuals with severe handicaps for whom competitive employment has not traditionally occurred, or (b) for individuals for whom competitive employment has been interrupted or intermittent as a result of a severe disability and who, because of their handicap, need ongoing support services to perform such work" (Hirsch, 1989). The components of supported employment include the following:

1. Integrated work settings
2. Job-site training and advocacy
3. Paid employment
4. Ongoing monitoring and support
5. Job retention
6. Services provided for those with severe disabilities (Hirsch, 1989; Rogan & Murphy, 1991)

Supported employment programs are preferred over sheltered workshops because of the philosophy of providing persons with disabilities with real work environments (Rogan & Hagner, 1990; Rogan & Murphy, 1991), whereas sheltered workshops may be a form of segregation (Rogan & Hagner, 1990).

There are several models for providing supported employment in the workplace. Some of these are job coaches, individual placement, and competitive employment. In these models workers are paired with a staff person (some are called job coaches). This staff person is available for skills training, advocacy, support, and for ensuring that the quality of the work meets the outcomes desired by the company. As the worker's independence increases, the role of the job coach diminishes (Grossi et al., 1991; Hirsch, 1989). Unfortunately there is a paucity of qualified job coaches (Grossi et al., 1991; LeRoy & Hartley-Malivuk, 1991).

Supported employment programs match the individual to an integrated employment setting rather than promoting placement alone (Rogan & Hagner, 1990; Rogan & Murphy, 1991). Concurrently as staff become trained, this will lead to positive outcomes for individuals who work in sup-

ported employment situations (LeRoy & Hartley-Malivuk, 1991; Szymanski & Danek, 1992).

Disability management programs

The emphasis in disability management programs is to return workers to the jobs they had before any injury, illness, or accident (Gottlieb et al., 1991). It would behoove corporations to implement disability management programs as a cost-containment measure. Reduced absenteeism, lower Workers' Compensation costs, reduced healthcare and rehabilitation costs represent savings to employers (Roessler & Schriner, 1991). The components of a disability management program should include financial support; prevention activities; postdisability services such as an assessment of medical, psychological, social, and return-to-work needs, case management, job analysis, and job modification; and a follow-up evaluation of the program outcomes and subsequent modifications (Gottlieb et al., 1991; Roessler & Schriner, 1991).

Although a vital component in the success of rehabilitation programs, few return-to-work alternatives have been offered by companies (Gottlieb et al., 1991), perhaps related to inaccurate information or company policy. The employment provisions of the ADA of 1990 became fully effective July 1994. Companies are mandated to ensure that their hiring practices and policies are nondiscriminatory against persons with disabilities. Many companies do not agree with the employment components of this act (Satcher & Hendren, 1992), which has major implications for workers with disabilities and corporations who are out of compliance with this legislation.

Rehabilitation professionals may play key roles in facilitating successful implementation of ADA legislation. Developing educational programs for employers, training company personnel, and providing on-site consultation will assist personnel to implement policies and practices in the best interest of both company and workers.

Vocational rehabilitation

Over the years a number of legislative mandates have addressed the vocational rehabilitation (VR) services for persons with disabilities. Initially the Smith-Fess Act of 1920 mandated vocational training opportunities for those with disabilities. Later the Vocational Rehabilitation Act Amendments of 1954 and 1965 expanded services for those with mental disabilities, as well as awarding federal grants for the development of statewide service delivery systems. The Social Security Act Amendments (1954 and 1972) established permanent VR programs. The Rehabilitation Act of 1973 (amended 1974 and 1976) mandated that vocational services be made more available to individuals with severe disabilities. The Rehabilitation, Comprehensive Services and Developmental Disabilities Amendments of 1978 provided federal funding for vocational services that included counseling, case management, physical rehabilitation services, therapeutic treatment, equipment, and employment programs (Rubin & Roessler, 1983).

The purpose of VR is to provide support and training services to individuals with disabilities that will enable them to return to a competitive work environment. Such services may include vehicle and home modifications, work hardening programs, meeting transportation requirements, assessing the job market, defining vocational limitations, job training and/or modification, job placement, and educating employers (RNF, 1993). Ironically, federal mandates requiring that VR programs increase services to those with severe disabilities have resulted in fewer VR applications processed for those with nonsevere disabilities. The concurrent budget cuts in VR programs have caused a serious gap in services for a significant segment of the population with disabilities (Andrews et al., 1992).

Rehabilitation professionals have a professional obligation to assist persons with disabilities to obtain vocational services when appropriate, advocate to eliminate the disparities that continue to exist, and educate employers about the merits of employing persons with disabilities.

Early intervention is a concept for infant and child programs for those with special needs. As a concept early intervention also may be in order for adults following catastrophic injuries or when preventing further disability or complications. In this CBR section the focus is on pediatric programs.

Early intervention programs

Increasing numbers of infants and children are dependent on medical technologies, are medically frail, and have physical and mental disabilities. Many of these infants and children have developmental complications, frequently due to premature birth. Any of these problems can be superimposed and create a challenge for providing early intervention services. A thorough assessment of these infants and children must include all areas of development; identify family issues, resources, and abilities; and provide for a multidisciplinary approach to care (Ahmann & Lipsi, 1992).

A thorough assessment will promote comprehensive planning and intervention that will meet the complex needs of these infants and children. This will in turn enhance developmental potential, which should be the long-term goal for early intervention programs (EIPs). Other benefits of EIPs include financial savings: children usually complete their education through high school, and children with special needs usually can be integrated into regular classes (Roberts, 1991).

Children from birth to 3 months make up an age group typically underserved by community EIPs (Roberts, 1991). It is important to evaluate the availability of services in the school environment—for example, adaptive equipment, electronic equipment needed for learning, augmentative communication aids, special seating arrangements, and telecommunication devices—in addition to personnel in interdisciplinary teams composed of nurses, PTs, OTs, and speech-language therapists, plus special educators and social workers.

Godfrey (1991) outlines priorities for EIPs: "(1) protecting physical health; (2) promoting optimal psychosocial development; and (3) facilitating motor, cognitive, and communicative development and self-care skills." EIPs need to be community based, family and child centered, and provide for cultural differences if these priorities are to be met (Fullmer & Majumder, 1991; Godfrey, 1991; Roberts, 1991). The literature is replete with discussions regarding the importance of family-centered rehabilitation (Power & Dell Orto, 1980; Watson, 1992; Wright, 1983). This concept

historically has been missing in EIPs, in part due to the medical model approach.

Few EIPs have recognized the need to integrate healthcare services into early intervention and education programs (Godfrey, 1991). There are increasing numbers of infants and children who require technology-related services, which in turn can interfere with a child's developmental stages (Ahmann & Lipsi, 1992).

In general, early intervention services have been fragmented, have failed to incorporate family-centered care, had little emphasis on a multidisciplinary approach, neglected to provide services to the most needy age groups, and segregated children with special needs in educational settings (Davern & Schnorr, 1991; Godfrey, 1991; Roberts, 1991). There has been varying emphasis on the importance of providing these services in a home environment (Godfrey, 1991), although some programs have a home-based model. Early intervention services must be meshed with healthcare needs in order to adequately meet the needs of this population. Comprehensive planning for services can take place once a thorough assessment is completed through an interdisciplinary approach (Ahmann & Lipsi, 1992; Godfrey, 1991). Parents and families are becoming participants in planning and implementing programs for their children and in writing goals that agree with their lifestyle, preference, and cultural values. The Individual Family Service Plan (IFSP) is one means of activating the process of parental comanagement and empowerment (Hoeman, 1993).

Public and private schools and day care centers have a major role to play in coordinating early intervention services. The services provided by nurses and therapists include developmental testing, health screening and assessment, community referrals, language and communication development, cognitive development, training for adaptive skill development, development of fine and gross motor skills, psychosocial skill development, assisting children to build friendships, family assessments, development of self-care skills, and conducting ongoing assessments of the age level at which each child is functioning (Ahmann & Lipsi, 1992; Davern & Schnorr, 1991; Godfrey, 1991; Roberts, 1991).

Rehabilitation professionals are in a position to assist in meeting the goals of EIPs: providing infants and children with preventive healthcare services and developing instructional guidelines with parents and caregivers to implement these preventive healthcare services. These goals can be met in the planning and intervention phases as long as no boundaries exist between healthcare and the developmental and educational needs of the recipients of EIP services and their families (Godfrey, 1991). (Chapter 30 provides additional discussion of this topic.)

THE REHABILITATION NURSE AS CLIENT ADVOCATE

The National League for Nursing stated that Nursings' Agenda for Health Care Reform lists strategies for universal access to health care, cost effective services, and consumer responsibilities. Healthcare reform is necessary for funding many support services that enable persons with disabilities to live in the community. Under the present reimbursement structure, CBR may not be reimbursed. Ideally the delivery of services is based on need rather than criteria for reimbursement alone.

Rehabilitation nurses have the opportunity to activate innovative approaches toward supporting healthcare reform. First, they can work to change the concept of long-term care to include infants and children, the mentally ill, the chronically ill, persons with disabilities, and the frail elderly. A long-term care concept is a holistic approach to care, ensuring a wide range of services are provided according to individual needs for prevention, health maintenance, and care during acute or chronic illnesses and disability (ANA, 1993).

Second, nurses can promulgate the concept that healthcare reform means universal access, cost-effectiveness, and consumer responsibility (ANA, 1993). Nurses provide cost-effective services to individuals across their life-span and in a variety of settings (Brown & Grimes, 1993; Safriet, 1992). The shift of government spending from crisis intervention to health promotion and maintenance eventually will keep healthcare costs from rising at the current, out of control rates.

Third, nurses who are creative about CBR programs may incorporate existing community services such as Visiting nurse associations, (Hekelman, Stricklin, Brown, & Aemagno, 1992) informal networks of volunteer community groups, and other programs in addition to assistance from neighbors, friends, family, clergy, and service groups. Alternative funding for financial support (Jamieson, 1991) may be a challenge since community-based nursing practice traditionally has been limited, with funds allocated to hospital-based care and under reimbursement constraints. Innovative approaches to providing community services may open opportunities in community re-entry for persons with disabilities.

Last, nurses will expand their roles into a variety of settings depending on individual client needs (Buchanan, 1992; Cyr, 1990; Lister & Thayer, 1992 (Meister, Feetham, Girouard, & Durand, 1991)) for a smooth transition to the community. Thus a facility-based rehabilitation nurse conceivably could practice across community agencies and in a client's home (Pitts-Wilhelm, Nicolai, & Koerner, 1991).

It is vital that rehabilitation nurses broaden their scope of practice in order to be empowered over their practice (Naylor & Brooten, 1993), increase autonomy, receive direct third-party reimbursement, and continue to develop independent practice (Schoen, 1992) in line with Nursing's Agenda for Healthcare reform (ANA, 1992).

CBR nurses participate in community planning activities, assisting persons with disabilities to have access to information about support networks, equipment, vendors, community resources, advocacy services, legal services, and medical care. Information about how to access services and resources, along with referrals to community resources, empowers clients in community re-entry.

Many localities have failed during the planning phase to eliminate or even to reduce architectural barriers. They have not provided public housing, public transportation, employment opportunities, or information services to persons with disabilities of all ages (Couch, 1992; Dattalo, 1992; Fullmer & Majumder, 1991; Groch, 1991; Parette & VanBiervliet, 1991) and have few identifiable city and town offices overseeing programs (Groch, 1991). When assessment and planning phases are neglected, CBR services also are neglected.

A RESEARCH AGENDA FOR COMMUNITY-BASED REHABILITATION NURSING

Progress in nursing research has been slow in the area of CBR practice. Dramatic changes will be occurring during this century and into the next as the country develops and implements strategies for financing national healthcare.

Multiple issues are charges for research in CBR nursing practice where findings will demonstrate nursing expertise to consumers, professional colleagues, and to the nation. The uncertainty of how our nation will finance healthcare reform will create a competitive environment among an array of healthcare providers. Conducting research and using findings will assist nurses in meeting the goals of the profession. Research findings (see Box below) will establish a much needed credibility with consumers, provide clients with further rehabilitation services that have a scientific basis, improve client outcomes, and mesh high-quality rehabilitation care with cost-effectiveness.

CONCLUSION

After a century of progress, there remains a propensity to promote dependency of persons with disabilities. Persons with disabilities become handicapped by limitations, such as persistent architectural barriers in our communities. Communities across the nation have much work still to be done to remove these barriers. Legislative mandates alone will not create the change. The social construction—our attitudes about persons with disabilities—are the first change. As a nation we continue to communicate our devaluation of disabilities through barriers that exist despite federal mandates.

When value is placed on enabling persons with chronic, disabling, or developmental disorders to be independent, they have the opportunity to live in the community as active and productive members who are seen for their abilities and not for their disabilities. This can be accomplished

---

RESEARCH IS NEEDED TO

✦ Measure the cost effectiveness of rehabilitation nursing practice in multiple-practice areas including case management
✦ Establish norms to evaluate rehabilitation services according to a client's functional outcomes
✦ Determine the optimal time frame for offering rehabilitative services after the onset of disability
✦ Develop and evaluate methods for measuring client outcomes in a variety of settings
✦ Define the variables having the greatest impact on health-seeking behaviors
✦ Evaluate nursing models and their impact on client outcomes
✦ Determine the efficacy of the team approach on client outcomes

through CBR programs that promote independence, remove environmental and attitudinal barriers, and increase consumer involvement and control over policies that directly affect their lives.

Innovative approaches rehabilitation nurses may use with clients and families to promote successful community re-entry include the following:

1. Involvement in mutual goal setting
2. Activism for public policy changes
3. Expansion of scope of practice
4. Involvement in all levels of discharge planning
5. Development of methods for evaluating practice outcomes

6. Adoption of a unified stand on practice issues
7. Support of healthcare reform
8. Promotion of third-party reimbursement for nurses in advanced practice
9. Development of a comprehensive clinical knowledge base

Rehabilitation nurses possess the ability to access information, facilitate community resources and services, and ease transition for persons with disabilities who are returning to their communities. They may return as active and productive members of society, or they may return simply because they belong to their community.

◆

CASE STUDY*

S.T. is a 30-year-old white male who sustained a C3-C4 spinal cord injury (SCI) as a result of a motor vehicle accident. During his hospitalization S.T. experienced numerous episodes of pneumonia, which led to the placement of a permanent tracheostomy button. S.T. also battled depression and had a temporary gastrostomy tube placed when he refused to eat. He developed a severe pressure sore that required surgical intervention. S.T. has limited social and family support systems. S.T. eventually did complete the acute rehabilitation phase of recovery. Due to medical problems, depression, lack of funding, and lack of available accessible housing, S.T. remained institutionalized at the medical center for 4 years. S.T. required total assistance in activities of daily living.

Discharge planning consisted of obtaining subsidized housing, hiring attendants who received some training before S.T. was discharged, obtaining Medicaid funding for attendant care up to 54 hours/week, and providing a referral to a home health agency 3 days before discharge.

S.T. experienced several problems during the initial transition to the community.

IMPAIRED PHYSICAL MOBILITY:

S.T. was at risk for complications including skin breakdown, joint contractures, decreased sensory stimulation, respiratory infections, and decreased muscle tone and mass. S.T. had the occurrence of open areas on his bilateral metacarpophalangeal joints due to contractures and reddened bilateral areas on his hands due to ill-fitting resting splints. S.T. had tried a number of mattress devices that were ineffective in preventing skin breakdown while at the medical center. Medicaid denied coverage for the alternating-pressure mattress that was effective. S.T. utilized a water mattress over his hospital bed mattress at home. S.T. developed a stage III ulcer over his ischial tuberosity 2 months after discharge. This required myocutaneous muscle flap surgery and a 6-week hospitalization. A second hospitalization was required 3 months after discharge for another stage II ulcer at the site of the previous skin flap. This required an additional 4-week hospitalization for treatment.

GOALS:

1. Maintain skin integrity.
2. Client/attendants will participate in risk assessments and prevention of pressure ulcers.
3. Client/attendants will describe etiology and prevention measures.

INTERVENTIONS:

1. Provide referral to occupational therapist to repair splints.
2. Advocate for the alternating-pressure mattress needed by contacting Medicaid office and state representative's office.
3. Discuss and evaluate client's seating system with rehabilitation team.
4. Provide detailed instructions to client and caregivers regarding etiology, prevention measures, and rationale for interventions; skin inspection every 2 hours or with each position change; prevention of shearing, promotion of optimal circulation; range-of-motion exercises to increase blood flow to all areas; nutritional requirements; and instructions to not rub reddened areas.

ALTERED PATTERNS OF URINARY ELIMINATION/REFLEX INCONTINENCE:

S.T. uses an external catheter attached to a leg bag or overnight drainage bag. S.T. experienced an occasional urinary tract infection (UTI). A Foley catheter was placed temporarily when S.T. developed two stage II areas on his penis. The external catheter was changed daily. S.T. developed a UTI after the Foley catheter was placed. This was treated with carbenicillin.

GOALS:

1. Client will have residual urine volume of less that 50 ml.
2. Attendants will use triggering methods to initiate reflex voiding.
3. Client/attendants will identify and report signs and symptoms of a UTI.
4. Attendants will demonstrate correct technique for application of external catheter and skin care measure.
5. Client/caregiver will demonstrate knowledge about side effects of medications.

INTERVENTIONS:

1. Plan a teaching and demonstration/redemonstration session with attendants regarding skin care and application of external catheter and triggering methods.
2. Provide a teaching session regarding medications and signs and symptoms of a UTI.
3. Establish a schedule for checking postvoid residuals.
4. Promote optimal hydration.
5. Provide instructions to avoid fluids that act as irritants and diuretics such as coffee, alcohol, tea, hot chocolate, and cola drinks.

---

*The nursing diagnoses used in the case study are NANDA-approved from *Nursing diagnosis: Application to clinical practice* (4th ed.) by L. Carpenito, 1992, Philadelphia: J.B. Lippincott.

CASE STUDY—cont'd

IMPAIRED HOME MAINTENANCE MANAGEMENT

S.T. transfers to electric wheelchair via a Hoyer lift. He is unable to participate in meal preparation, housekeeping activities, take medications independently, use the telephone, access emergency services, leave his apartment independently, use the television or radio without assistance, control heat, access the fire alarm, lock or unlock doors, and so on. No environmental control unit is available. No arrangements were made for home modifications before hospital discharge. S.T. has insufficient funds to pay for modifications or equipment.

GOALS:

1. Attendants will demonstrate ability to perform skills required to maintain client in his home environment.
2. Client will demonstrate ability to reside safely in his own apartment.
3. Client will demonstrate ability to contact appropriate community resources to obtain necessary adaptive equipment and home modifications.

INTERVENTIONS:

1. Provide referrals to appropriate community agencies to expedite process for obtaining a sip and puff telephone, electronic door opener, and emergency response system.
2. Provide referral to advocacy group for persons with disabilities.
3. Instruct client/attendants regarding community resources; obtain application for environmental access loan/grant for technology assistive devices if funding is available from other resources.
4. Provide referral to community agency for homemaker services.
5. Plan for 24 hour/day care until technology assistive equipment is in place.
6. Contact housing authority for approval for application of electronic door opener.
7. Ensure barrier-free access to door inside and outside the home (e.g., snow removal).
8. Evaluate access to community environment and lobby local government for necessary changes.

INEFFECTIVE INDIVIDUAL COPING

S.T. is withdrawn and nonverbal. He reportedly has never developed friendships easily and has not initiated participation in social activities since his discharge. S.T. initially had refused to participate in the rehabilitation process during hospitalization, experienced depression, and had difficulty with participation even after agreeing to the process.

GOALS:

1. Client will verbalize feelings about his emotional state.
2. Client will demonstrate ability to make decisions and take appropriate actions regarding his care in the home environment.
3. Client will accept support from the home health nurse and appropriate community resources.

INTERVENTIONS:

1. Provide ongoing assessment of coping status.
2. Assess for causative factors.
3. Teach problem-solving techniques.
4. Provide referral for MSW services for counseling through the home healthcare agency if agreed to by the client.

5. Facilitate emotional support from others.
6. Provide referral for peer counseling.
7. Assist with attainment of control over environment.
8. Provide support for demonstration of functional coping behaviors.
9. Identify activities that the client previously enjoyed and develop a plan with the client to gradually increase participation in these activities.

POTENTIAL ALTERED RESPIRATORY FUNCTION:

Portable suction equipment, which was sent home at the time of discharge, was malfunctioning. Attendants had received no training on suctioning techniques. S.T. experienced frequent upper respiratory infections (URIs). Nebulizer treatments were ordered qid. S.T. developed pneumonia after discharge and required hospitalization. He has an allergy to dust and lives in a dry environment with forced hot air heat and rugs on the floor. S.T. lives in subsidized housing and is dependent on personal care attendants to do household chores.

GOALS:

1. Client will maintain airway clearance.
2. Attendants will demonstrate ability to perform assisted cough maneuver.
3. Client/attendants will verbalize knowledge of methods for maintaining airway clearance, signs and symptoms of infection to report, ability to use suction equipment, and actions and side effects of medications.
4. Client will receive nebulizer treatment as ordered.

INTERVENTIONS:

1. Contact vendor to maintain suction equipment.
2. Plan for teaching and demonstration/redemonstration session on suction technique and equipment care, procedure for nebulizer treatments and equipment care, signs and symptoms of infection to report, proper body alignment, assisted cough maneuver, nutrition and hydration principles, tracheostomy button care, and action and side effects of medications.
3. Obtain a vaporizer per physician order.
4. Provide referral for homemaker services as stated under the Home Maintenance diagnosis.
5. Remove allergens from the environment.
6. Instruct attendants to vacuum and dust two to three times a week until homemaker services are in place.
7. Consult with respiratory therapist as needed.
8. Provide instructions regarding use of incentive spirometer.
9. Conduct thorough skilled respiratory assessment one to two times per week.

Evaluation of goal attainment in the established plan between the client and home healthcare nurse is paramount. The care may require modifications in order to promote successful community re-entry. Recommendations for the evaluation of outcomes in this case study may include the following:

1. Frequency, number, and duration of hospitalizations
2. Client/attendants demonstrate mastery of skills taught
3. Frequency, type, location, and stage of skin breakdown
4. Participation in social, recreational activities
5. Ability to exert control over own care and environment
6. Occurrence of UTIs
7. Occurrence of URIs and/or pneumonia
8. Evidence of coping skills

REFERENCES

Ahmann, E., & Lipsi, K. (1992). Developmental assessment of the technology-dependent infant and young child. *Pediatric Nursing, 18,* 299-305.

American Nurses' Association. (1993). *Report on long-term care and the developmentally disabled to ANA institute of constituent members on nursing practice.* Washington, DC: Author.

Andrews, H., Barker, J., Pittman, J., Mars, L., Struening, E., & LaRocca, N. (1992). National trends in vocational rehabilitation: A comparison of individuals with physical disabilities and individuals with psychiatric disabilities. *Journal of Rehabilitation, 58,* 7-16.

Bergland, M.M., & Clark, D.W. (1991). The community independent living program: An educational model. *Journal of Rehabilitation, 57,* 43-46.

Brown, S.A., & Grimes, D.E. (1993). *A meta-analysis of process of care, clinical outcomes, and cost-effectiveness of nurses in primary care roles: Nurse practitioners and nurse midwives.* Washington, DC: American Nurses' Association.

Buchanan, L.L.B. (1992). A rehabilitation clinical nurse specialist: Evaluation of the role in a home health care setting. *Holistic Nursing Practice, 6,* 42-50.

Carpenito, L.J. (1992). *Nursing diagnosis: Application to clinical practice* (4th ed.). Philadelphia: J.B. Lippincott.

Couch, R.H. (1992). Ramps not steps: A study of accessibility preferences. *Journal of Rehabilitation, 58,* 65-69.

Cushion, B. (1992). Mental health: Long-term needs. *Nursing Times, 88,* 34-35.

Cyr, L.B. (1990). The clinical nurse specialist in a home healthcare setting. *Home Healthcare Nurse, 8,* 34-39.

Dattalo, P. (1992). An evaluation of an area-wide message relay program: National implications for telephone system access. *Journal of Rehabilitation, 58,* 50-54.

Davern, L., & Schnorr, R. (1991). Public schools welcome students with disabilities as full members. *Children Today, 20,* 21-25.

DeJong, G. (1993). Health care reform and disability: Affirming our commitment to community. *Archives of Physical Medicine and Rehabilitation, 74,* 1017-1024.

Dibner, L.A., & Murphy, J.S. (1991). Nurse entrepreneurs, *Journal of Psychosocial Nursing, 29,* 30-34.

Dittmar, S.S. (1989). *Rehabilitation nursing: Process and application.* St. Louis: Mosby–Year Book.

Fanning, R.A., Judge, J., Weihe, F., & Emener, W.G. (1991). Housing needs of individuals with severe mobility impairments: A case study. *Journal of Rehabilitation, 57,* 7-13.

Fawcett, J. (1984). *Analysis and evaluation of conceptual models of nursing.* Philadelphia: F.A. Davis.

Fitzgerald, M.H. (1992). Multicultural clinical interactions. *Journal of Rehabilitation, 58,* 38-42.

Fullmer, S., & Majumder, R.K. (1991). Increased access and use of disability related information for consumers. *Journal of Rehabilitation, 57,* 17-22.

Godfrey, A.B. (1991). Providing health services to facilitate benefit from early intervention: A model. *Infants and Young Children, 4,* 47-55.

Gottlieb, A., Vandergoot, D., & Lutsky, L. (1991). The role of the rehabilitation professional in corporate disability management. *Journal of Rehabilitation, 57,* 23-28.

Greenwood, R., Schriner, K.F., & Johnson, V. (1991). Employer concerns regarding workers with disabilities and the business-rehabilitation partnership: The PWI practitioners' perspective. *Journal of Rehabilitation, 57,* 21-25.

Groch, S.A. (1991). Public services available to persons with disabilities in major U.S. cities. *Journal of Rehabilitation, 57,* 23-26.

Grossi, T.A., Test, D.W., & Keul, P.K. (1991). Strategies for hiring, training and supervising job coaches. *Journal of Rehabilitation, 57,* 37-42.

Health Care Finance Administration. (1989). *Medicare Home Health Agency Manual* (HCFA P11R222). Washington, DC: U.S. Government Printing Office.

Hekelman, F.P., Stricklin, M.L., Brown, K., & Alemagno, S. (1992). Clinical research in home care: A report of the Visiting Nurses Associations of America, *Journal of Nursing Administration, 22,* 29-32.

Henderson, E.J., & Pentland, B. (1991). Home pass assessment in neuro-rehabilitation practice. *Journal of Advanced Nursing, 16,* 1439-1443.

Hirsch, S.W. (1989). Meeting the vocational needs of individuals with psychiatric disabilities through supported employment. *Journal of Rehabilitation, 55,* 26-31.

Hoeman, S.P. (1993). A research-based transdisciplinary team model for infant with special needs and their families. *Holistic Nursing Practice, 7,* 63-72.

Hoeman, S.P. (1992). Community-based rehabilitation. *Holistic Nursing Practice, 6,* 32-41.

Hoeman, S.P., & Winters, D.M. (1988). Case management for clients with high cervical spinal cord injuries. In Fisher, K., & Weisman, E.E., (eds). *Case Management: Guiding patients through the health care maze* (pp. 109-115). Chicago, IL: Joint Commission on Accreditation of Healthcare Organizations.

Jamieson, M.K. (1991). Block nursing: Practicing autonomous professional nursing in the community. In Goentzen, I. (ed) *Differentiating nursing practice into the twenty-first century* (#G-182). MO: American Academy of Nursing.

Jones, B.J., Gallagher, B.J., Kelley, J.M., & Massari, L.O. (1991). A survey of Fortune 500 corporate policies concerning the psychiatrically handicapped. *Journal of Rehabilitation, 57,* 31-35.

Kiernan, W.E., & McGaughey, M. (1992). A support mechanism for the worker with a disability. *Journal of Rehabilitation, 58,* 56-62.

LeRoy, B.W., & Hartley-Malivuk, T. (1991). Supported employment staff training model. *Journal of Rehabilitation, 57,* 51-54.

Lister, E.M., & Thayer, M.B. (1992). Private practice: The time is now. *Pediatric Nursing, 18,* 295-298.

McBride, S.M. (1992). Rehabilitation case managers: Ahead of their time. *Holistic Nursing Practice, 6,* 67-75.

MacGilp, D. (1991). A quality of life study of discharged long-term psychiatric patients. *Journal of Advanced Nursing, 16,* 1206-1215.

Mayer, A. (1991). Rehabilitation round the clock. *Nursing Times, 87,* 65-66, 68.

Means, B.L., & Bolton, B. (1992). A national survey of employment services provided by independent living programs. *Journal of Rehabilitation, 58,* 22-26.

Meister, S.B., Feetham, S.L., Girouard, S., & Durand, B.A. (1991). Creating and extending successful innovations: Reach Project Practice and policy implications. In *Differentiating nursing practice into the twenty-first century* (#G-182). MO: American Academy of Nursing.

Middleton, R.A., & McDaniel, R.S. (1990). The (re)habilitation needs of the older non-disabled handicapped person: Expanding the role of the rehabilitation professional. *Journal of Rehabilitation, 56,* 23-27.

National League for Nursing (1991). Nursing's Agenda for Health Care Reform. New York: Author.

Naylor, M.D., & Brooten, D. (1993). Theories and functions of clinical nurse specialists. *Image, 25,* 73-77.

Neuman, B. (1989). *The Neuman systems model* (2nd ed.). East Norwalk, CT: Appleton & Lange.

Nosek, M.A., Roth, P.L., & Zhu, Y. (1990). Independent living programs: The impact of program age, consumer control, and budget on program operation. *Journal of Rehabilitation, 56,* 28-35.

Parette, H.P., & VanBiervliet, A. (1991). Rehabilitation assistive technology issues for infants and young children with disabilities: A preliminary examination. *Journal of Rehabilitation, 57,* 27-36.

Paulson, C., Dahl, R., & Wasch, W.K. (1993). Eliminating architectural barriers: A multidisciplinary approach. *Topics in Geriatric Rehabilitation, 9* (2), 59-73.

Pitts-Wilhelm, P., Nicolai, C.S., & Koerner, J. (1991). Differentiating nursing practice to improve service outcomes. *Nursing Management, 22,* 22-25.

Power, P.W., & Dell Orto, A.E. (1980). *Role of the family in the rehabilitation of the physically disabled.* Baltimore, MD: University Park Press.

Preski, S., & Burnside, I. (1991). Clinical research with community-based older women. *Journal of Gerontological Nursing, 18,* 13-18.

Rehabilitation Nursing Foundation. (1987). *Rehabilitation nursing: Concepts and practice* (2nd ed.). Skokie, IL: Author.

Rehabilitation Nursing Foundation. (1993). *The specialty practice of rehabilitation nursing: A core curriculum* (3rd ed.). Skokie, IL: Author.

Rhoads, C., Dean, J., Cason, C., & Blaylock, A. (1992). Comprehensive discharge planning. *Home Healthcare Nurse, 10,* 13-18.

Roberts, R.N. (1991). Early intervention in the home: The interface of policy, programs, and research. *Infants and Young Children, 4,* 33-40.

Roessler, R.T., & Schriner, K.F. (1991). Partnerships: The bridge from disability to ability management. *Journal of Rehabilitation, 57,* 53-58.

Rogan, P., & Hagner, D. (1990). Vocational evaluation in supported employment. *Journal of Rehabilitation, 56,* 45-51.

Rogan, P., & Murphy, S. (1991). Supported employment and vocational rehabilitation: Merger or misadventure? *Journal of Rehabilitation, 57,* 39-45.

Rubin, S.E., & Millard, R.P. (1991). Ethical principles and American public policy on disability. *Journal of Rehabilitation, 57,* 13-16.

Rubin, S.E., & Roessler, R.T. (1983). *Foundations of the vocational rehabilitation process* (2nd ed.). Austin, TX: PRO-ED.

Safriet, B.F. (1992). Health care dollars and regulatory sense: The role of advanced practice nursing. *Yale Journal on Regulation, 9,* 149-220.

Satcher, J., & Hendren, G.R. (1992). Employer agreement with the Americans with disabilities act of 1990: Implications for rehabilitation counseling. *Journal of Rehabilitation, 58,* 13-17.

Schmidt, S.M., Herman, L.M., Koenig, P., Leuze, M., Monahan, M.K., & Stubbers, R.W. (1986). Status of stroke patients: A community assessment. *Archives of Physical Medicine and Rehabilitation, 67,* 99-102.

Schoen, D.C. (1992). Nurses' attitudes toward control over nursing practice. *Nursing Forum, 27,* 27-34.

Spencer, J.C. (1990). An ethnographic study of independent living alternatives. *The American Journal of Occupational Therapy, 45,* 243-251.

Stroker, R. (1983). Impact of disability on families of stroke clients. *Journal of Neurosurgical Nursing, 15,* 360-365.

Szymanski, E.M., & Danek, M.M. (1992). The relationship of rehabilitation counselor education to rehabilitation client outcome: A replication and extension. *Journal of Rehabilitation, 58,* 49-56.

Tate, D.G. (1992). Workers' disability and return to work. *American Journal of Physical Medicine and Rehabilitation, 71,* 92-96.

Tate, D.G., Maynard, F., & Forchheimer, M. (1992). Evaluation of a medical rehabilitation and independent living program for persons with spinal cord injury. *Journal of Rehabilitation, 58,* 25-28.

Watson, P.G. (1992). Family issues in rehabilitation. *Holistic Nursing Practice, 6,* 51-59.

Wright, B.A. (1983). *Physical disability: A psychosocial approach* (2nd ed.). New York: Harper & Collins.

10

Outcome-Directed Teaching and Learning

Susan L. Dean-Baar, PhD, RN, CRRN, FAAN

INTRODUCTION

Teaching and learning are inseparable from quality healthcare. In the rehabilitation setting the process focuses on the individual's need to incorporate adaptive behavior into his or her lifestyle. The ultimate goal of the process is to assist the individual with a chronic, disabling, or developmental disorder to reach a maximum level of functioning and self-care. In rehabilitation the educational process fosters self-care by helping the client or family acquire new information, develop new skills, competently apply knowledge and skill to functional activities, develop adaptive behaviors to manage the illness or disability, and to prevent further disability (Diehl, 1989). It is the responsibility of each member of the rehabilitation team to be knowledgeable in both rehabilitation techniques and the teaching-learning process in order to provide individualized, client-centered learning experiences.

Changes in technology have made many learners in rehabilitation more sophisticated consumers of the teaching-learning process. The fast-paced changes in society have had an impact on every individual's life regardless of age. Individuals come already familiar with the use of many mechanisms that can be used to assist in gaining new information about a topic of interest. Children now learn by computer-assisted instruction (CAI) in preschool, and adults can tap into a variety of educational resources via video-cassette, computer programs and networks, and television programs. Distance learning, augmentative communication, and the information highway are learning pedagogy of the next decade.

These changes in society, and the underlying philosophy in rehabilitation of enabling clients to learn how to be as independent as possible, may influence the teaching-learning process in rehabilitation. They also influence the responsibility of the professional nurse for maintaining current knowledge to provide effective care to clients. This chapter focuses on the components of the teaching-learning process in rehabilitation and its application to nursing practice.

PRINCIPLES OF TEACHING-LEARNING

Client education in rehabilitation is based on principles of teaching-learning from fields such as psychology and physiology. This section focuses on the principles related to the developmental level of the client and the role of memory in learning. Client and family education information and interventions are found in most chapters throughout this book.

Developmental Level

In providing the educational component of the rehabilitation process, one must consider the developmental level of the client and tailor the teaching-learning experience to the appropriate level. In addition, rehabilitation requires the nurse to consider problems or stressors that may be expected to occur as a part of the normal developmental process at various stages of the life cycle and to incorporate this in the educational planning. Knowledge of development and its application to learning is important to the development of individualized client teaching-learning plans (Falvo, 1985). The Box on p. 131 outlines approaches that might be used by rehabilitation professionals during various life stages.

Knowles (1984) has outlined a model for adult learning that has gained wide acceptance. His model is based on five key assumptions. First is the concept of the learner as self-directed rather than a dependent, passive learner. Second, an adult learner brings both a greater quantity as well as quality of previous experiences that serve as a vast resource for the adult learner in new learning situations. This results in a need to develop highly individualized learning plans. Third, adults become ready to learn when they experience a need to know something in order to perform more effectively in some aspect of their lives. Fourth, adult learners have a life-centered, task-centered, or problem-centered orientation to learning. They learn so that they can perform a task or solve a problem, not simply for the sake of learning. Fifth, adult learners are more strongly motivated by internal motivators such as self-esteem, recognition, better quality of life, and greater self-confidence. External motivators such as a better job or salary do influence adult learners but not as strongly as internal motivators.

Using principles of adult learning places the teacher in the role of facilitator of learning and designer and manager of the learning processes and procedures. Seven elements have been identified in designing the learning experience. The first element involves setting the climate for learning. This includes both the physical environment as well as the psychological atmosphere. The physical environment includes arranging furniture so that it is conducive to discus-

◆

CLIENT APPROACHES FOR TEACHING-LEARNING DURING VARIOUS PHASES OF THE LIFE CYCLE

LIFE STAGE	CLIENT/CAREGIVERS	APPROACH OF REHABILITATION PROFESSIONALS
Prenatal	Client	Open-minded approach with no preconceptions; nonjudgmental; give emotional support to both parents; work within parents' framework
Infancy	Parents	Foster security by giving positive feedback regarding parents' ability to care for child; no nagging or lecturing; take seriously what may appear to be small problems
Toddler	Client	Encourage child in warm, matter-of-fact manner; use no analogies when giving explanations in accurate, simple terms
	Parents	Nonjudgmental approach; continue support and positive reinforcement
Preschool	Client	Encourage child to express fear; give no false promises; explain procedures before doing them
	Parents	Provide guidance and encouragement
Later Childhood	Client	Give explanations in simple, logical way; approach child in confident, optimistic manner
	Parents	Provide continued guidance and support
Young Adult	Client	Offer empathetic, nonjudgmental attitude
Middle Adult	Client	Offer empathetic, nonjudgmental attitude
Later Years	Client	Approach client as unique, not stereotyping because of age; keep awareness that aging is a multidimensional process in which multiple factors affect functioning; capitalize on client's strengths; refrain from using first names unless invited to do so; speak clearly and concisely; avoid being patronizing

Reprinted from *Effective Patient Education: A guide to increased compliance,* 2nd edition (p. 128) by D.R. Falvo, 1994, Rockville, MD: Aspen Publishers. Copyright 1994 by Aspen Publishers. Reprinted by permission.

sion and interaction and minimizes the message that the learner is to be a passive recipient of knowledge. The psychological atmosphere includes a climate of mutual respect and trust, collaboration, supportiveness, openness and authenticity, pleasure, and humanness.

The other elements include involving the learners in mutual planning of the learning experience, diagnosing their own learning needs, formulating their learning objectives, and designing the learning plan. The last two elements involve helping the learner carry out the learning and involving the learner in evaluating the learning.

There are strong applications of this model to the teaching-learning process of clients and their families in rehabilitation. The assumptions and elements of this model can be used as a framework to develop individualized meaningful learning experiences in rehabilitation. Full use of the model requires learners who are willing and comfortable in taking responsibility for directing their own learning. At times this may not be true either because of the clients' previous experiences in educational settings; because of their response to the disability or illness they are presently experiencing; or because of cognitive or related impairment. Pratt (1988) has provided a framework for looking at teaching-learning situations based on the degree of direction and support needed by the learner. The framework identifies four general categories of educational situations based on the amount of direction and support needed by the learner (see Box, p. 132). In one category learners need both direction and support because they lack both competence in the content (previous experience/knowledge that is related and can be built on) and commitment or confidence in their ability to learn the content. In a second category the learner needs direction because of a lack of competence in the content but needs less support because of confidence or a commitment that the new information can be mastered. In both situations the teaching-learning process requires a more teacher-directed approach because of the need for a high degree of direction. In a third category the learner needs support but can be fairly self-directed in determining content needs and requires less direction. In the fourth category the learner is at least moderately capable of providing her own direction and support. In these last two categories the teaching-learning process requires a more learner-directed approach because of the lower need for direction.

This approach supports the principles of adult learning but allows for the reality that in some situations learners may be unable or unwilling to assume responsibility for their own learning. It allows the rehabilitation nurse to assess with the client the specific teaching-learning needs and

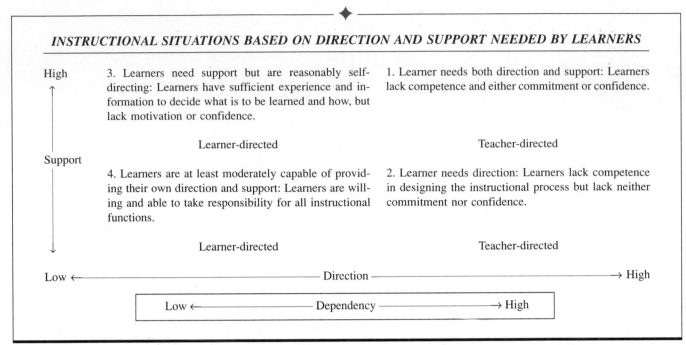

INSTRUCTIONAL SITUATIONS BASED ON DIRECTION AND SUPPORT NEEDED BY LEARNERS

High

3. Learners need support but are reasonably self-directing: Learners have sufficient experience and information to decide what is to be learned and how, but lack motivation or confidence.

1. Learner needs both direction and support: Learners lack competence and either commitment or confidence.

Learner-directed

Teacher-directed

Support

4. Learners are at least moderately capable of providing their own direction and support: Learners are willing and able to take responsibility for all instructional functions.

2. Learner needs direction: Learners lack competence in designing the instructional process but lack neither commitment nor confidence.

Learner-directed

Teacher-directed

Low ←———————————— Direction ————————————→ High

Low ←————————— Dependency —————————→ High

Used with permission of author. Adapted from "Andragogy as a relational construct," by D.D. Pratt, 1988, *Adult Education Quarterly, 38,* p. 167.

develop a plan that draws on the expertise of the rehabilitation nurse in content areas that the client may be totally unfamiliar with such as bowel and bladder programs. The plan also can be individualized to provide the appropriate level of support depending on the level of commitment and confidence expressed by the client or family. Theoretic bases for learning and related concepts are discussed in Chapter 1.

Role of Memory in Learning

Learning is a critical element of the rehabilitation process. Memory is the physiologic basis of learning. Two major memory systems have been identified: the declarative and procedural memory systems (Boss, 1986). The declarative system is also known as informational memory. It includes memory related to information, facts, and knowledge about things. Learning can occur in this system with just one exposure to the information. The hippocampus, amygdala, and cortical–sensory association areas of the cerebral cortex are thought to be important structures for declarative memory. (Chapter 26 discusses memory in detail.)

The declarative memory system can be subdivided into short-term, recent and long-term memory. Short-term memory is also referred to as immediate or working memory. The ability to focus attention is critical to effective short-term memory. The declarative memory system requires a conscious activation by the individual. The recticular activating system (RAS) allows for the ability to focus attention. There is limited storage capacity in this system, and it is vulnerable to distraction. A decrease or loss of immediate or short-term memory can be caused by dysfunction in the recticular formation or its tracts ascending to the cortical–sensory association areas. (The RAS is discussed in Chapters 23, 24, and 26.)

The recent memory system is important for getting short-term or immediate memory to long-term memory. Recent memory is distraction stable, and the individual can attend to other things and not lose what is in recent memory. It is a function of the hippocampus, amygdala, and the limbic system. The hippocampus is believed to play a role in consolidating memories by sorting stimuli for relevant information, coding and classifying information with already stored information that appears related, and orchestrating rehearsal with other stored memories—which is needed to complete the transfer to long-term memory. The amygdala contributes emotion to memory and cooperates with association areas to help integrate and appreciate new information. The limbic system is involved with visual recognition, symbol recognition, and spatial perception.

The long-term memory system provides the storage of information or memories in cortical association areas from days to years. Cortical association areas in the left hemisphere store memories related to language, mathematic calculations, and abstractions. The right hemisphere stores memories in a holistic fashion including visual, auditory, and spatial components. An example of this is memories of music.

Reduction in or loss of long-term memory can be due to problems in several areas. There may be a failure in the transfer of information or in the consolidation process. Difficulties also may occur with retrieval and recall or because of the physical loss of memory stores.

The procedural memory system includes memory of responses, not of information. It is the memory of "how" to do something. Included in this are such things as skills and habits. It is thought that the procedural memory system involves an interaction between the motor cortex and the subcortical areas of the basal ganglia, especially the tail of the caudate and the caudal putamen. Memories are established only by actually performing or engaging in the skills or operations. Although no neural pathways connecting the declarative and procedural systems have been found, the procedural system can be used to compensate for losses in the declarative system. Learning can be facilitated by conditioning responses or developing patterns to form habits that do not rely on declarative information.

TEACHING-LEARNING PROCESS IN REHABILITATION
Assessment

Assessment involves identifying learner needs, determining the client and family's readiness to learn, and learning style. The client and family's readiness to learn includes assessment of motivation, cognitive ability, and developmental level. Other learner characteristics that need to be assessed include cultural background, accessibility to caregivers, and potential to teach others.

✦ Identifying learning needs

Learning needs are identified in many ways. Evidence of the need might be brought to the attention of the nurse teacher by the client, a family member, friend, member of the health team, or a number of other individuals associated with the client. The need might be made obvious through a direct request or through observation of the individual's physical and emotional states or identified during assessment. This assessment of learning needs should begin as a part of the initial admission or intake assessment.

Four categories of potential problems may affect a client's learning needs. The first category is the client's physical functioning with regard to the present illness or disability and any limitations from a previous illness or disability. The rehabilitation nurse assesses basic activities for present and past physical functioning: mobility, transfer activities, dressing, eating, elimination, and personal hygiene. Questions such as "Which hand do you eat with?" or "Do you use any kind of assistance when you walk?" or "Where is the bathroom in your house?" will elicit clues to learning needs.

The client and family's understanding of any past and present illness and disability includes how they discern relationships that may exist between illnesses and lifestyle. For example, does the client who has had an amputation understand the relationship between peripheral vascular disease and smoking? Does a client understand the relationship between cardiac disease and decreased endurance following stroke? An individual's knowledge level may not relate to the length of time he has had an illness or disability. Increasingly diagnosis and treatment of many illnesses and conditions occurs in an office, outpatient, or ambulatory care setting where teaching is inconsistent and learning is left untested. In addition, the rapid expansion of knowledge and technology related to many conditions may render an individual's previous knowledge about a disease incomplete or obsolete.

The second category deals with social needs. How much the learner and the family have been compromised by the disability must be determined. For example, if the learner provided total financial support of the family before the dis-

ability, major adjustment problems for the client and family member correspondingly change plans for finances and for the future. The type of living arrangements (whether the client rents or owns) and the structural arrangement of the home are significant. Does the client have to climb stairs to enter the home or to get to the bedroom or bathroom? Who will be at home with her? Is she married? Does she have children? Answers to these and similar questions target social learning needs.

The third category encompasses psychological needs, which are assessed for a number of reasons. The stress imposed by illness and disability can be of such magnitude that psychological counseling is needed before learning can take place. The need for counseling might be manifested in the client's self-esteem and perceived ability to control learning outcomes. The psychological status of an individual may influence the ability of the client to participate in the learning process. For instance, with depression or high anxiety a client may believe that participation in the learning process will have little or no influence over the outcomes, diminishing learning potential. In addition, intellectual functioning may be impaired because of brain trauma or deterioration from disease.

The fourth category focuses on vocational problems. The disability might have produced unemployment or loss of job-related skills. Vocational counseling and training may be determined as a need of the client or family member. When learning needs of the client and family are assessed, goals are determined jointly by the client, family member, and nurse teacher. Obviously some needs identified cannot and are not intended to be met by the nurse teacher. However, the nurse's role is to advocate for clients to ensure learning needs that enable clients to reach their educational potential are addressed and to know what has and is being taught by other team members.

✦ Assessing a client's readiness to learn

Readiness for learning is defined here as the capability to expend energy and focus attention for a given purpose. The definition contains three elements necessary for learning. First, clients must be physiologically capable of participating in a learning experience. Second, the purpose of the learning experience must be such that intellectually clients can see its relevance to their needs. Third, the purpose also must have emotional appeal so clients are willing to participate actively. Assessing these areas is important to understanding factors influencing the motivation of clients and family members.

The physiologic capacity to learn depends not only on neuromuscular functioning but also on limitations from previous illness or injury. Any limitations that impair a client's capacity to learn are significant. Examples of such limitations include joint stiffness from arthritis, diminished visual or auditory acuity, or decreased cardiac reserve. Immediate basic needs such as relief from pain, anxiety, or the need to void always take priority over learning needs.

Emotional readiness to participate actively in the learning process is enhanced greatly by positive life experiences, beliefs, and values. This readiness can be impaired by helplessness, hopelessness, negative beliefs about the disease process or injury, or unpleasant past experiences with the same or similar disease state. Lack of readiness to learn also might be due to the client's stage of adaptation to any perceived loss he has experienced. Denial and anxiety are two common responses that may influence a client's readiness to learn (Vance, 1992). Clients who are anxious or in denial may state they have never been provided with information that the rehabilitation team or other healthcare providers are known to have given to the client. When these common reactions are identified, the nurse considers them in developing the teaching-learning plan. Intellectually the learner must have the cognitive ability to understand the relationship between learning and future well-being. Assessment of the learner's cognitive and intellectual ability includes information about orientation, attention span, concentration, perception, and memory (Redman, 1993).

Data collected from the learner, the learner's significant others, the nurse's own observations, and the observations of other members of the interdisciplinary team are used to assess the three elements of readiness to learn for each client, as well as to identify information needed in developing the teaching-learning plan. During the same process, the nurse provides information to the client and significant others to clear up misunderstandings related to chronicity, disability, or rehabilitation. Include data about

+ Life experiences that have an impact on learning
+ Responses of the client and family (both physiologic and emotional) to previous illnesses
+ Psychosocial adaptation
+ Normal daily activities before the disabling event
+ Willingness to achieve rehabilitation
+ Perception of rehabilitation potential
+ Belief about health and healthcare

+ Assessing a family's readiness to learn

Readiness of the family to participate actively in the learning process enhances the client's potential for rehabilitation. Information gleaned from family members related to family relationships and attitudes before the onset of disability provides information about the client's support systems. Families with close relationships are more likely to have supportive attitudes and behavior toward disabled family members, enhancing clients' prospects for rehabilitation and returning home. Conversely, in families where hostility, alienation, or other negative attitudes prevail, the support system is likely to be less effective. Another important factor in the selection process is how the learner feels toward the family member designated as the "backup" learner. Compatibility between or among the individuals will facilitate successful carryover of learning.

In assessing a family's readiness to learn, learners should be chosen with the realization that they may be the primary learner or may serve as backup to the primary learner. From the beginning it is essential that backup learners understand that they are to provide assistance only with activities the learner is unable to perform. The family member's potential to understand and follow through with learning also needs to be considered. In addition, the degree of reliability of the family member must be considered. This may begin to demonstrate itself early in the rehabilitation process in areas such as follow-through with appointments with team members and in keeping promises made to clients.

Family members who frequently miss appointments, are late for scheduled appointments, or who promise to do things for the client without following through may be demonstrating behaviors that indicate they are not ready to learn or may be unreliable in providing care to the client.

Knowledge and understanding of the illness or disability by the family tends to increase their supportive behavior. The nurse who provides information relating to both the illness or disability, as well as the recovery and learning process, enhances the participative efforts of family members. Through continuous and open communication, much of the family's anxiety can be anticipated and allayed. As a result more energies on the part of family members are available to support the individual with the disability and the learning endeavor.

+ Assessing learner style

The success of the teaching-learning process be influenced by the learning preferences of the client and family members. A nurse tailors the learning experiences to support the learning preference of the client, using a variety of methods (Craft, 1987). Individuals have a range of preferences influenced by previous learning experiences. Some individuals prefer to learn by doing; others need to read or hear about the content before actually doing. Another dimension to consider is whether clients need an overview of the total content to be learned so that they can see the whole picture and how the pieces fit together, or whether the whole picture overwhelms them and they prefer to deal only with the individual pieces and let the whole picture emerge as each piece is mastered.

Assessing the learner's preference allows the nurse to choose which learning materials and strategies best support the preferences of the client. For some clients this may mean providing demonstrations before written materials; for others the best approach may be to supply written materials for the client to go over before the actual demonstration. Some clients will prefer visual formats, and others may prefer a stronger use of auditory formats. It may be helpful for frequently used patient education materials to be available in several formats to support the client in learning in a way that is most comfortable and familiar. This may mean that written materials could be audiotaped similar to the use of the talking books format. Recognizing the differences in learning preferences and developing materials that can be matched to preferences can positively influence the learning outcomes, especially in an environment of competing demands for the client's energy and decreasing lengths of stay.

+ Other learner characteristics

Assessment of a client and family's cultural background can be an important consideration in developing a mutually satisfying learning experience. Cultural and ethnic factors may influence many aspects of learning in rehabilitation. For instance, cultural factors may impact on the dietary considerations of the client, the decision about acceptable family caregivers, or the beliefs about the cause and course of the illness or disability. Clients whose primary language is other than English may benefit from materials prepared in their native language. When available, tutors or translators who are acceptable to the client or other language assistance aid programs are provided.

As early as possible in the rehabilitation process, caregivers who will work with a client are identified and their learning needs assessed for many of the same areas just discussed. An early and preliminary assessment by the rehabilitation nurse and team of the care needs a client is likely to have at discharge includes the client's accessibility to caregivers. This assessment will help identify the type and amount of care that caregivers, family, or other members of the client's support system will be taught. At times there may be no family or support system members to provide necessary care, and the nurse needs to be prepared to teach other individuals who may be hired as attendants to the client. The client's potential to teach others about their care is particularly important to clients who, because of their functional ability, are dependent on others to implement the actual care required. Being as independent as possible is enhanced when the client is able to direct others in providing necessary care. Examples include skills in giving sequential, step-by-step directions, the ability to be assertive in communicating needs, and knowledge about the disease or condition.

✦ Age-related characteristics

A great deal of rehabilitation nursing education for clients and their families is directed toward adult learners in an effort to meet practical application and utility in everyday life as opposed to academic, diadactic teaching. Although family members generally fall within the category of adult learners, clients who are younger or older benefit from education that is directed to their learning styles and needs. (Chapters 30 and 31 discuss specific characteristics of pediatric and elderly clients in more detail.) It is worthwhile to incorporate a sensitivity to age-related learner characteristics into any teaching program. Learning by elderly persons, for instance, may be affected by sensory impairments, altered cognitive processes, fatigue, comfort such as with seating or position, need for more frequent toileting, room temperature, type or amount of medication, or nutritional requirements. Intergenerational language, acronyms, jargon, or even speaking too rapidly may become barriers to learning. On the other hand, the notion that educators may attribute slowness and lowered competence to persons simply because of age is a myth. Simply enunciating clearly and speaking slowly may enable many older persons to learn adeptly.

As a rule more data are available, either from school assessments or developmental evaluations, about the learning potential and special needs of pediatric clients than for elderly persons. Learning through developmental age-appropriate play is the ideal means for teaching children. Excellent play therapy and teaching programs are available; most involve the family and a transdisciplinary team approach. Teaching and learning are evaluated using each child's achievement of developmental tasks, as well as chronologic age, neurologic function, and specific skills needed for learning. For example, motor development skills or hand-eye coordination may be psychomotor requirements for a task, whereas cognitive ability is required for problem-solving or self-directing a procedure. For teaching self-care

to a school-aged child consider the following guidelines:

- ✦ Involve family and assure cultural sensitivity and relevance
- ✦ Teach with the intent that the child will perform his/her own care or self-direct the care
- ✦ Provide developmentally correct information
- ✦ Use audiovisuals, dolls or stuffed animals, games, computer-assisted programs
- ✦ Schedule within the child's attention span
- ✦ Avoid naptime, mealtimes, or times that compete with visitors or peers
- ✦ Assure privacy and minimize distractions
- ✦ Assure a comfortable, well-lit, ventilated environment
- ✦ Position, seat, and otherwise prepare the child
- ✦ Use adaptive or assistive devices as adjuncts to learning
- ✦ Consider the meaning of the content to the child
- ✦ Anticipate questions, concerns, fears, or common errors
- ✦ Monitor the child's psychosocial response as well as performance
- ✦ Develop learning aids to use apart from formal sessions
- ✦ Use behavior modification or other techniques with team approach
- ✦ Use principles of sequential learning
- ✦ Incorporate self-care and hygiene into learning content
- ✦ Ask the child how he or she feels about the content and process
- ✦ Seek opportunities to enhance the child's self-esteem and build confidence
- ✦ Communicate with community-based colleagues about the process (Hoeman, 1991)

Planning

Planning the learning experience involves developing goals and objectives, identifying resources, developing content, identifying learning activities, and planning for evaluation. The format for writing the plan is part of the actual teaching-learning plan. Any number of different formats may be used; whatever format is chosen, clearly display the interdependency of the parts. The goals and objectives depend on learner needs; the content depends on the goals and objectives; the resources needed; and the learning activities used depend on the content; and evaluation of the plan depends on all of these.

✦ Developing goals and objectives

Since the learning experience is designed to assist the client to develop adaptive behavior and to function at maximum potential, the learner must participate actively in determining both the goals and the objectives to be achieved. Learners who do not understand clearly that the objectives lead to the achievement of the goals will have difficulty complying with instruction (Grief & Mataruzzo, 1982). For example, "applies (unassisted) a straight leg brace" is a behavioral objective that can help achieve the goal of "ambulates independently."

The family also should play a major role in identifying the goals and objectives. Family theory indicates that stress or change affecting one family member affects other family members as well (Friedman, 1992). Trieschmann (1974) maintains that failure of persons with disabilities to rehabilitate "may often be traced to lack of family involvement in the rehabilitation process." Consequently family involvement in planning the learning experience enhances the client's potential for rehabilitation and helps assure that the goal—that is, the overall purpose of the learning experience—is realistic.

Before specific goals and objectives can be established, the nurse teacher determines the behavioral domain in which learning needs to occur and whether impairment exists in the domain. Learning that is reflected in human behavior occurs in three domains. The cognitive domain activates thought processes, enabling the client to recognize the need for retraining, as well as to grasp the concepts (mental constructs) relative to the disability and lifestyle (Bloom, 1956). The ability to conceptualize is basic to problem-solving, and the learning process leading to rehabilitation is a problem-solving process.

The psychomotor domain concerns the client's ability to perform physical skills within the parameters set by the state of their neuromuscular systems. In addition, learning to perform a skill depends on the ability to envision mentally how the skill is performed. Taxonomies to describe the psychomotor domain has been developed—one example uses a perceptual approach to describe the differences in the psychomotor domain. The perceptual domain involves the ability to extract information from the multiple stimuli presented to the sense organs. It can involve the simultaneous interpretation of stimuli from multiple senses (Moore, 1970). The affective domain involves attitudes, feelings, values, and emotions (Krathwohl, Bloom, & Masia, 1969). Expressions of this domain permeate all client behaviors and must be incorporated into the learning process. Activity in this domain has a heavy impact on readiness to learn.

Upon determining the domain or domains in which learning is to occur, the nurse teacher and client are ready to establish the goals that should be achieved by the learning. These goals are broken down into behavioral objectives, using action verbs that enable the observer to measure whether the objective has been reached. Refer to the Box below for examples of verbs suggested by Mager (1975). By using Mager's principles for preparing instructional objectives, the objectives will be stated in behavioral terms and can be understood clearly by the learner, family members, and each member of the instructional team.

◆ Identifying resources

When selecting resources for the teaching-learning process, the following factors must be considered:
- ◆ Objectives to be achieved by the process
- ◆ Client's functional ability
- ◆ Client's intellectual capability, including reading ability

The objectives to be achieved by the process dictate to a large measure the resources appropriate for the experience. The learning required for each objective should be broken down into small units. Based on the small units, resources for learning can be selected. For example, an objective that involves knowledge acquisition (cognitive domain) would be met primarily through the use of media, whereas a skill might be taught more effectively through demonstrations. In making the selections, the nurse teacher must consider not only the domain in which the learning is to occur but other factors as well. If reading is required in the learning process, then reading level must be assessed to ensure that the teaching aid is appropriate. Media requiring the sense of sight are ineffective for the visually impaired individual unless alterations, such as enlarging print, can be made. Likewise, audiovisuals require adequate sight and hearing. All senses of the client capable of actively participating in the learning process should be stimulated to do so.

Not all clients need or are able to learn in all three domains. The cooperation and active participation of a learner in the learning process are contingent on the ability to comprehend, remember, and organize information and behavior. Interference with one or more of these processes affects the resources to be used and dictates levels of learning achieved.

If the learning process is to result in follow-thorough with a prescribed regimen, clients must have access to resources outside the healthcare setting specific to their living environment and be acquainted with appropriate resources as a part of the learning process. It may be necessary to use resources that closely resemble the living environment, such as bathrooms and beds, on discharge from an institution to facilitate the learning of bowel and bladder management. In some situations, vendors deliver durable medical equipment or supplies to a client's home to be used for teaching-learning.

Members of the interdisciplinary team are excellent resources for determining what is appropriate and available for learners. The social worker is usually the most knowledgeable about community resources. The psychologist and

---

EXAMPLES OF BEHAVIORAL VERBS FOR SPECIFIC DOMAINS

COGNITIVE VERBS	AFFECTIVE VERBS	PSYCHOMOTOR VERBS
Recognize	Select	Use
State	React to	Write
Identify	Solve	Operate
Organize	Choose	Perform

speech and language pathologist may be very helpful in determining specific approaches to be used to maximize client cognitive abilities and minimize client cognitive impairments. Librarians in medical libraries can provide information about resources and materials available from governmental agencies and organizations for persons with disabilities. Many community hospitals have a consumer health education section open to use by the public or community practitioners. Special interest organizations, such as the Multiple Sclerosis Society, will send materials or loan media, and audiovisual equipment is available on loan from similar resources. Some facilities have speakers' bureaus available to conduct group learning sessions on specific topics. Informal networking with other professionals and clients also provides an extremely effective means for learning about resources.

✦ Developing content

Based on the goals and behavioral objectives, the knowledge and tasks required to achieve each objective are analyzed—that is, each area of knowledge or task to be learned is broken down into logical steps. The steps proceed from the simplest part of the information or task to the most complex.

To analyze the task, the nurse asks questions related to each objective. What does the learner have to do or know to accomplish the objective? In this manner specific information or tasks can be identified. From the assessment of the client, the nurse can determine if the specific behaviors required to perform the task have been previously learned by the client. Breaking tasks down into content is extremely important because it determines the appropriate learning activities. Omission of this step can result in failure of the client to learn.

✦ Identifying learning activities and strategies

After the content needed to achieve the goals and objectives is identified clearly, the next step is to identify the teaching activities to be used to facilitate mastery of the content. For example, learning the names of specific objects is a cognitive learning skill. An appropriate activity for this type of learning would be to have the client repeat the names of the objects while looking at the objects. To learn such a skill as catheterization, on the other hand, an appropriate activity might be to practice each subtask until the client can perform it without difficulty. From the content the nurse teacher determines the domain from which learning will occur. Finally, learning activities are based on the content and the domain with a target date for achieving each objective.

The plan should sequence all activities according to priority of learning needs. The following types of learning needs can be considered when sequencing activities:

- ✦ Acute learning needs: knowledge, skill, or attitudes needed to avoid danger (e.g., a client requiring insulin)
- ✦ Preventive learning needs: knowledge, skill, or attitudes needed to alleviate or diminish the potential for disease and injury (e.g., foot care for the diabetic client)
- ✦ Maintenance learning needs: knowledge, skill, or atti-

tudes needed to adapt to changes in usual functioning (e.g., a client with compensated congestive heart failure)

Many strategies are available for use in the teaching-learning process. Matching the objectives, resources available, content to be covered, and learning characteristics of the client leads to a correct choice. Teaching strategies should be evaluated so that they support the achievement of the learning objectives. Demonstrations, either in person or by video, may be one of the most effective strategies for teaching psychomotor skills. Knowledge or cognitive content is taught using a variety of strategies such as written materials, oral discussion, videos, CAI, role playing, games or simulations, and less frequently by presentation.

Video education offers advantages such as consistency of content and the ability of the learner to review the content as often as necessary (Alexiewich, 1990; Curtis, 1990). Clients and families always benefit with opportunities to discuss the content with a nurse to clarify specific content, answer any questions, and identify early any misunderstandings or misconceptions about the material. Computerized learning, such as CAI and interactive computer videodiscs, is another strategy that has blossomed in rehabilitation (Lynch, 1991). Computers are increasingly being used with individuals with brain injury to assist in rehabilitation of cognitive skills such as memory, problem-solving, visual-spatial skills, and language-related functions (Kurlychek & Levin, 1987; Robertson, Gray, Pentland, & Waite, 1990). Similarly clients who are unable to speak verbally or who have functional impairments may be able to communicate using computer adaptations that translate vocal sounds into words or construct vocal words from other means of computer input. Clients with progressive neuromuscular conditions or spinal cord injury may be candidates for these computer program adaptations.

Written materials are developed or evaluated so that clients comprehend the material. Formulas such as the SMOG and FRY readability formulas (Doak, Doak, & Root, 1985) will help evaluate the degree of difficulty and the readability, of written materials. Readability level is, however, only one aspect of written materials that needs to be evaluated. Interest and experience with the content also will influence comprehension and language. These same considerations are used to evaluate material prepared in an audio format, such as audiotapes.

✦ Plan for evaluation

The method for evaluating how successfully each objective has been achieved also is stipulated. Since the behavioral objectives are stated using action verbs, they can be used in the evaluation. Simply ask the learner to do whatever the behavioral objective states she is able to know as a result of participating in the learning strategy.

Methods of evaluation are coordinated with the type of learning. For example, motor skills are evaluated readily through observation. The subtasks identified in the task analysis can be used to develop a checklist or scale for rating the behavior. Each component of the rating tool identifies a specific behavior that culminates in the achievement of the desired objective. Cognitive skill, on the other hand, cannot always be observed and might require evaluation through verbal or written questions. Behavior in the affective domain is probably the most difficult to measure simply because learners can choose not to express their true feelings. Learning in this domain is best observed when learners are unaware of the evaluation being made. Expression of feelings may differ across cultural, generational, social, and other groups. Assessments based on expression or affect require multiple observations and are validated with the client and family to prevent erroneous assumptions or personal interpretation.

✦ Interdisciplinary implications

Teaching-learning plans in rehabilitation need to focus on the client and family learning needs. Many of the learning needs will have teaching implications for multiple disciplines. Whenever possible, consideration should be given to developing teaching-learning plans that coordinate and integrate all of the involved disciplines. For example, when developing a plan for bowel and bladder management, the identified learning needs that rehabilitation nursing is primarily responsible for may include normal functioning, bowel and bladder management programs including such areas as medication, timing, skills such as suppository insertion or catheterization, and adaptation to routines and lifestyle preferences at home. The rehabilitation nursing component of the plan should be coordinated with the occupational therapist's plan for learning related to management of clothing during toileting and the physical therapist's plan for learning related to toilet transfers. In the community the nurse or rehabilitation nurse consultant will accomplish teaching all areas in collaboration with therapists, if they are available.

Implementing the Plan

When implementing the written plan, the nurse makes decisions about a climate conducive to learning and the benefits of group versus individual instruction. The teaching-learning process can take place in any setting; however, the setting should be such that distractions are kept to a minimum. Distractions impair the learner's ability to concentrate on the learning task; those with attention disorders will be unable to work at learning. To prevent distractions, learning should take place in a self-contained area in which other clients, visitors, or personnel are limited. A client's personal modesty is another concern; content and demonstration are private unless the client gives permission for others to be present or within hearing or viewing distance.

The learning climate should be comfortable, with seats that allow for appropriate positioning and flexibility in movement. Provide indirect lighting to avoid glare, and adjust room temperature to activity. Color and texture of the walls and other surfaces should be "coordinated" to assist in differentiation between surfaces and fixtures (Brever, 1982). Temperature may affect persons with impaired sensation or those sensitive to hot or cold weather. Clients are offered opportunity for toileting, fluids, or other personal comforts during learning sessions.

Time is another important element to consider in implementing learning experiences. The length of time the learner can concentrate attention on a given activity is a major factor in determining the time of day, length, and frequency of the learning sessions. Clients who have diminished physical strength and energies might learn more efficiently early in the day or following a rest period. It is also important to recognize that time between sessions is needed to assimilate what has been learned. Without time for assimilation, the learner's endeavors are more likely to lead to failures than successes. Such an error in implementation can result in loss of desire to continue the learning process.

The environment itself can be used to assist in focusing the client's attention on what is to be learned (Redman, 1993). Different types of learning media in the environment such as posters, booklets, and practice equipment tend to gain the attention of the learner and lead to the exploration of the meaning and significance of the aids. Assistive devices such as a bathtub seat, utensil holder, or hygiene and grooming aids can be placed in view to stimulate not only learning but encouragement as well. The environment can be arranged to provide appropriate facilities for learners to practice relearned skills, such as dressing and shaving, at a time of their own choosing. The nurse teacher is available if needed. Such an arrangement encourages independence and reestablishes routine for the learner. In the community, volunteer groups, capable family or friends, or professionals are able to construct and redesign home facilities to meet the client's needs. Teaching for home is based on a home assessment to assure continuity.

The learning environment includes attention to comfort, setting, media, climate, time, distractions, rewards, and ambiance. The learning environment should provide positive reinforcement (reward) for new behaviors to encourage learners to repeat the behaviors. Initially the reinforcement should follow each time the behavior is performed until the behavior is learned well, then reinforcement is intermittent (Grief & Mataruzzo, 1982). Rewards can take many forms. Perhaps the most common is praising the learner. Other incentives, such as special outings or food treats, unless medically contraindicated, can provide variety. Each learner responds differently to different rewards. The nurse teacher should identify which rewards provide the most incentive to the learner.

An atmosphere that conveys warmth and acceptance promotes a positive attitude and a desire to learn. An equally important quality of the atmosphere is an attitude that encourages learners to begin at their level of need and progress at a comfortable rate to learn what they want to learn. Such an attitude promotes success. As learners are guided to new achievements, they gain greater self-confidence and become more self-motivating. Because it requires change in beliefs and behaviors, learning normally produces a mild level of anxiety, which can be useful in motivating the client; however, severe anxiety is incapacitating (Redman, 1993). For this reason, goals are set mutually, reasonably, and realistically. Anxieties decrease as the fear of failure is diminished. Through interactions with the nurse teacher and the environment and through increased self-motivation, learners develop positive feelings about their self-worth.

✦ Group versus individual learning

Group learning provides an opportunity for clients to interact with other learners. This learning environment helps to avoid feelings of isolation and also encourages learners to maintain contact with reality. Opportunity for sharing information with others on common mutual problems provides a supportive atmosphere. The stimulation derived from group concern can bring hope and encouragement to strive toward skillful performance of the adaptive behaviors. The experience of finding others willing to relate to the individual with a disability often helps to improve social skills and assertiveness needed after the learning period.

The group learning environment is arranged to enable the nurse teacher to provide guidance, demonstrations, and reinforcements to individual learners without interfering with the activities of the other learners. Such an arrangement provides the ideal teaching-learning experience. The success of group learning is dependent on effective planning and implementation (Pasquarello, 1990).

Group learning is also a cost-effective and more efficient use of staff time for teaching-learning; however, not all clients and families are candidates for group learning. Those who are distracted easily or who have difficulty managing multiple sources of stimulation may do better in individual learning situations. Learning preferences also need to be considered, since some individuals prefer not to participate in group learning activities. The specific learning needs of the client and family also will influence the decision to use individual or group learning activities. Group learning usually is designed to include content that is needed by the "average" client or family. It is used frequently to provide the foundation or basic knowledge necessary for further individualization to a specific client or family. The identification of the specific learning needs would indicate whether a client is referred to a group educational session or whether the learning needs would be best met in an individual approach. Even in situations where it is appropriate to include clients in group activities, it is always important to provide an opportunity for clarification of content and application of the content to the individual.

Evaluation

The purpose of evaluation is to determine the effectiveness of the teaching-learning process. Evaluating the process is accomplished by determining if the goal has been achieved by comparing and measuring behavioral outcomes that have been stated as objectives. If the client can perform the activities stated as objectives, then the goal was achieved. If he or she cannot, then the nurse teacher should ask and answer each of the following questions:

✦ Was the goal realistic?
✦ If not, how should the goal be altered to become realistic?
✦ Were the learning activities appropriate for the client's learning abilities?
✦ Should the content be retaught?

Anytime that evidence suggests the teaching plan is not working, the plan should be reviewed for deficiencies and appropriate corrections made. Evaluation of the plan is continued informally throughout all phases of the teaching-learning process. For the teaching-learning process in rehabilitation to be completely successful, the client and appropriate others need to be able to transfer the learning that occurs to the home or community setting. The client who

is able to successfully learn how to perform intermittent catheterization independently in the rehabilitation setting but who cannot perform the catheterization in the home setting ultimately has failed. The nurse teacher must assist the client with learning how to adapt specifics learned to situations likely to be encountered. A useful strategy in evaluating whether this level of learning has occurred is to use role playing and other simulation activities to present the client with "what if" situations that allow the nurse teacher to estimate the degree to which the learning will transfer to other situations.

The evaluation process is threefold. It should include both teacher and client evaluations of client progress and teacher and client evaluation of the teaching plan. Results of the evaluation should be used in future learning processes designed for the same learners, as well as for different learners. In addition, professional nurses have the responsibility to evaluate their own teaching critically to look for areas of strength in addition to areas that need improvement. This may be accomplished by self-evaluation, asking clients for their evaluation of the teaching, and as a part of a peer review process.

✦ Documentation

Documentation of the teaching-learning process consists of two parts: (1) the teaching plan and (2) objective and measurable data describing movement of the client toward goal achievement. When the plan to be implemented is determined, it should become a part of the client's permanent record and conveyed to all members of the treatment-instructional team. Knowledge and availability of the plan encourages all team members to support the development of behaviors leading to the predetermined goal. Progress notes describing the client's behavior in measurable terms enable team members to track progress and continuously evaluate the effectiveness of the teaching plan. Notes should include descriptions of behavior demonstrating change in all domains: cognitive, psychomotor, and affective.

Standardized teaching-learning forms may provide a mechanism to include documentation of the plan, as well as evaluation of the plan in the same place in the patient record. This approach is most useful when it allows for specific individualization of learning objectives and inclusion of specific strategies to be used with a client. These forms also can be used to ensure that teaching focusing on reinforcement and follow-through with interdisciplinary teaching is included in the nursing plan of care. Another important purpose that standardized forms can serve is the documentation of time spent in teaching-learning activities that can then be used for patient classification systems and/or reimbursement. The uniqueness of each individual must be preserved, even with standardized plans.

KNOWLEDGE DEFICIT VERSUS NONCOMPLIANCE

A common discussion within nursing is the appropriate label for several diagnoses that occur when focusing on the learning needs of clients. This is particularly true when the original teaching-learning plan has been implemented and evaluation reveals that it has not been as successful as anticipated. Evaluation of the teaching-learning process may reveal that the objectives are not being achieved as planned or that there is difficulty with the transfer of learning to other situations. When this occurs, only careful analysis will reveal what the problem may be. Specifically the question is whether the problem continues as a lack of knowledge or whether appropriate knowledge is present but is not being used fully.

Knowledge deficit is defined as "the state in which an individual or group experiences a deficiency in cognitive knowledge or psychomotor skills regarding the condition or treatment plan (Carpenito, 1993). It has been argued that knowledge deficit itself is not a nursing diagnosis but is rather an etiologic or contributing factor for other diagnoses or problems (Jenny, 1987). Assessment or evaluation findings that may lead the nurse to determine that a knowledge deficit is present include the client verbalizing a deficiency in knowledge or skill, requesting information, expressing inaccurate perceptions of his health status, incorrectly performing a desired or prescribed health behavior, demonstrating the inability to integrate the treatment plan into daily activities, or exhibiting or expressing a psychological alteration such as anxiety resulting from misinformation or lack of information (Carpenito, 1993).

At times evaluation reveals that appropriate knowledge is present but is not being used. When this occurs, further evaluation needs to take place to determine the contributing factors. There has been much discussion about the negative connotations of the terms compliance and noncompliance when used to describe client behavior and responses to the teaching-learning process, and in managing and following through with recommendations and teaching provided by healthcare providers. A common criticism is that these terms imply that the client is passive and lacks autonomy and that the healthcare professional is coercive and paternalistic (Blevins & Lubkin, 1990). Other terms such as adherence, concurrence, and cooperation have been suggested because they imply choice, mutuality of goals, and a patient-provider relationship based on respect and trust (Rankins & Stallings, 1990). In a client-centered empowering mode, the alternative terms are available and acceptable, so that compliance and noncompliance are replaced in most instances.

The definition of noncompliance as a nursing diagnosis is "the state in which an individual or group desires to comply but is prevented from doing so by factors that deter adherence to health-related advice given by health professionals (Carpenito, 1993). This diagnosis as defined would not be appropriate for a client who has made an informed autonomous decision not to comply. Thus this diagnosis would be appropriate only when further assessment indicated that the client wanted to comply but was unable to. Many factors could contribute to a client's inability to adhere to recommendations and follow through with learning. These might include side effects from medications or other treatments, a complex or not well-understood regimen, the financial cost of the recommendations, poor self-esteem or body image, nonsupportive significant others, lack of access to resources or supplies in the community, or the inability to perform a task or skill because of the effects of the disability (poor memory, motor or sensory deficits). In

situations where the client would like to follow through but is unable to do so, the nurse needs to consider additional interventions aimed at alleviating the identified reason. For instance, the interventions might be focused on increasing the self-esteem of the client, managing the side effects caused by medications or other parts of the treatment plan, referrals to appropriate community agencies, identifying less costly alternatives, providing additional teaching or simplifying the regimen, or modifying the way a skill or task is performed to accommodate effects of the disability.

In those situations where the client makes a deliberative and informed decision not to follow the plans or regimen, the nurse assesses whether the client's perception of his health needs and his own situation is understood clearly by the nurse and other healthcare providers. These may provide insight as to the reason for the client's decision. Perhaps it is important for the client to be control, or the client may rely on others for following a regimen. Understanding this might result in modifying the approach used to one that reinforces independence and decision-making by the client in all aspects of life and supports the client's ultimate right to make decisions. Over the course of time, this could lead to a more trusting relationship and an increased openness by the client to consider recommendations made by the nurse.

Another reason a client may choose not to follow through may be because they believe the benefits of following the recommendations are not sufficient to warrant the time, energy, cost, or discomfort associated with the recommendations. We may not agree with the client, but it is important to respect the choices made. We can continue to provide information and our rationale in a supportive, nonjudgmental way with hopes that the client may change her mind (Chapter 9 provides a discussion of contracting.)

COMMON CHALLENGES IN REHABILITATION

Much of the teaching that occurs in rehabilitation is focused specifically on accommodating the cognitive, sensory-perceptual, and motor impairments resulting from a disability or chronic illness. Members of the rehabilitation team need to work together to identify the specific strategies that will work for best for each client. A few of the commonly occurring problems and teaching strategies to accommodate impairments in these areas are discussed. Detailed information on interventions and approaches to treating cognitive, sensory-perceptual, and motor impairments are found in other chapters in this book. Safety is a key consideration in all teaching-learning activities, whether in a facility or in the community.

Cognitive Impairments

Individuals with brain injuries due to trauma or stroke may present with a variety of cognitive impairments. In teaching clients with cognitive impairments, consider adapting content and strategies to facilitate learning and using additional assessment information from neuropsychological testing, if available, to assist in making appropriate adaptation. One of the important areas to discuss with other members of the rehabilitation team is the short- and long-term prognosis for the individual client. This information may be critical in deciding whether the primary learner will be the client, a family member, or another individual who will assume primary caretaking responsibilities.

The major emphasis in adapting the teaching-learning process for individuals with cognitive impairments is to focus on the use of areas of cognitive functioning that are intact or less severely impaired to compensate for impaired areas of functioning. Ideally members of the rehabilitation team pool assessment data to determine the strategies most likely to facilitate learning. For instance, an individual who has difficulty independently accessing information from memory may be able to recall necessary information with memory cues such as visual pictures or words. This individual may be able to use lists as prompts to remember all the things required to complete an activity, such as cooking a meal. A visual aid, such as a chart listing all the medications taken in a day, may assist an individual to be independent in medication administration. For some individuals the chart may contain simple symbols to indicate the reason for the medication and have a pill attached to the chart so the individual can visually match the pill with the time of day to be given. The individual or caregiver is instructed to take the chart to the pharmacist each time the prescription is filled. The example pill is changed when the medication changes, as when a generic equivalent that appears different from the pill previously used is substituted.

In cases where the cognitive impairment is related to attention and concentration, the nurse may need to structure the environment to minimize stimuli that could interfere with a client attending to the task at hand. An individual who is easily distracted may not be a good candidate for group teaching sessions and may even require a very structured one-on-one approach with minimal extraneous stimuli in the environment. Teaching-learning sessions may need to occur in a room with no other activity taking place and a "do not disturb" sign placed on the door. (Chapter 12 provides additional ideas.)

In cases where the cognitive impairments are severe, and the degree of recovery is not expected to be rapid or significant, a family member or significant other may become the primary focus of the teaching-learning process. When the learner understands the cognitive abilities of a client and knows methods to compensate for impairments, the ingredients to facilitate the highest level of self-care for the client are in place.

Sensory-Perceptual Impairments

Sensory-perceptual impairments may be present in many rehabilitation clients. Modifications in the teaching-learning process may need to occur to accommodate these deficits. The visual sensory-perceptual problems that frequently occur in the rehabilitation population present as visual field cuts, blurred vision, and double vision. An individual with a visual field cut will need to have teaching-learning materials presented in the intact visual field. Individuals with blurred or double vision that cannot be corrected through interventions such as patching one eye may need teaching-learning materials presented in formats other than visual presentations. Materials may need to be presented in an auditory format through verbal presentation and discussion or by use of audiotapes. Depending on the extent of blurred vision, this can sometimes be accommodated by use of large and bold print in teaching-learning materials.

Individuals with impaired touch may need to learn how to perform an activity such as self-catheterization by using intact visual cues and more rigid plastic catheters instead of more flexible rubber catheters. The rehabilitation client may need to use mirrors or positioning to visualize the urethral orifice. The more rigid catheter provides greater sensory input so the client can better feel the catheter. Use of visual cues to compensate for sensory impairments is an important strategy for other impairments. For instance, learning safe independent transfers for an individual with impaired proprioception may require that the client learn to compensate visually to be sure that his feet are flat on the floor and positioned correctly. An individual with impaired temperature may need to learn to use a thermometer to test the temperature of water before bathing to prevent injury (Chapter 16 provides additional information.)

Motor Impairments

Motor impairments in a rehabilitation client may affect the way in which psychomotor skills need to be taught. Two major areas need to be considered. First, creativity and adaptive equipment may need to be used to enable an individual with a motor impairment to learn and successfully perform a skill. An individual with spasticity may need to learn which positions are best for self-catheterization. These may best be accomplished through a series of planned trials, noting which positions are most comfortable and tend not to trigger the spasticity. Adaptive equipment may be helpful in learning how to be independent in many areas of activities of daily living. Occupational therapists are a key resource in suggesting equipment that encourages greater independence in areas such as dressing, eating, and hygiene. Independence in medication administration may be possible by replacing safety caps on bottles with specialty caps designed for individuals with weakness or those with pain, as sometimes experienced by individuals with arthritis.

The second area that needs to be considered in teaching a client with motor impairments is the individual's ability to direct others in performing any necessary skill. This may involve teaching and practicing with the client to give specific and sequential directions to another person about how to assist or actually perform a necessary skill. Clients who need to be able to direct others should be given the opportunity to demonstrate this ability to appropriate members of the rehabilitation team before discharge from the rehabilitation program. The rehabilitation nurse can role play with the client as a strategy to master giving directions to others. In a role play strategy, the nurse would do only those things directed to be done by the client. The nurse and client could then evaluate how successful the client had been and decide if the directions were adequate or if they needed to be clearer either in the degree of specificity or the sequencing of the steps.

◆

CASE STUDY

Mr. Scottie Blaylock fell on the ice and suffered a left intertrochanter fracture, which required a left open reduction with internal fixation (ORIF). He is 67 and has a history of osteoarthritis but no other significant medical problems. The symptoms associated with the osteoarthritis have been well controlled with indomethacin. He works full-time selling appliances in a large department store. He lives alone in a two-story home with two stairs into the house. The bedrooms and full bathroom are on the second floor of the house. His wife died 3 years ago, and his children all live more than 200 miles away. Because of his living arrangements, he is admitted to the inpatient rehabilitation unit for an intense 10-day rehabilitation program with the plan to discharge him to his home and eventually return to work.

The nursing assessment indicates that Mr. Blaylock is very interested in learning how to care for himself and be as independent as possible. He has only a cursory knowledge of osteoarthritis and his medication regimen, stating that "after a couple of years of telling my doctor that my knees and hips hurt and were stiff, he told me to take this medicine and it's been a lot better since . . . when I remember to take it." He also is still experiencing some mild to moderate postoperative pain and mentions how tired he is since surgery. His surgical record indicates that he did lose significant blood during surgery, and on admission to the rehabilitation unit his hemoglobin level is 8.5 g/dl and hematocrit is 34%. He completed high school and tells the nurse that he enjoys reading mystery novels. He also discusses a woman that he and his wife used to play cards with who broke her hip and had to go to a nursing home for 6 weeks; he wonders why he is doing so much better already. Further discussion reveals that the woman had needed a total hip arthroplasty. The nurse explains the differences in the procedure he had and the one his friend had and assures him that his mobility restrictions won't be as great. He also tells the nurse that he learns best by talking and reading about things that interest him and rarely watches television.

The nurse discusses with him the following areas that the assessment indicates should be included in the teaching-learning plan: postoperative pain control, osteoarthritis management, medications, activity tolerance, mobility skills, self-care skills, and discharge planning. He agrees that these are areas he would like to learn more about. Together they develop specific objectives to be accomplished for each of these. The learning objectives for activity tolerance include that Mr. Blaylock will be able to

1. Describe reasons for lowered activity tolerance at this time
2. Describe the need to balance rest and activity
3. Identify a plan for balancing rest and activity when he gets home

4. Recognize signs of overactivity
5. Demonstrate measures to conserve energy with daily activities at home

Each objective is placed on the teaching sheet, which also includes areas to document learner characteristics (e.g., preferred learning style, reading ability), teaching method, learner response, and achievement of objectives.

Based on the assessment data that indicated that Mr. Blaylock prefers to learn by talking and reading about things, the nurse decides to rely on these two strategies. Written materials from the unit's learning resources are used, and the nurse recommends that Mr. Blaylock consider purchasing *The Arthritis Helpbook* (Lorig & Fries, 1986) as a reference that might be helpful for him to have now and in the future. For each topic the nurse verbally provides an overview of the content, provides Mr. Blaylock with the appropriate written materials, answers any immediate questions, and then gives him time to look over the materials. At the next teaching interaction, she provides more information, answers any questions he has, and uses questions to evaluate Mr. Blaylock's learning. After each teaching interaction the teaching sheet is updated.

All teaching is planned to be completed 2 days before discharge so that no new materials are presented at the very end of the rehabilitation program. This allows for time to reinforce any areas that Mr. Blaylock is still having trouble with. The nurse's evaluation shows that he has grasped the basics well but is still having some difficulty integrating the parts. He understands the principles of energy conservation and balancing rest and activity, but when he describes his plan for home he is doing everything he needs to do before noon each day. The nurse has him write down all of the activities that need to be accomplished and then works with him to develop an actual schedule. He says that it is important to him to get dressed early in the day even if he isn't going anywhere, but he is very tired if he tries to take his shower, get dressed, and then eat breakfast. The nurse encourages him to problem-solve other ways of getting all this done without becoming fatigued. He decides to take his shower in the evening before retiring.

Because of the limited support that Mr. Blaylock has in the area, a home health referral is made for nursing follow-up and home therapy for 3 weeks before beginning outpatient therapy. The nurse includes a copy of the teaching sheet from Mr. Blaylock's record, a list of resources given to him, and summarizes the areas that will need reinforcement. In addition, Mr. Blaylock will be seen in the follow-up clinic approximately 1 month after discharge, and the effectiveness of the teaching-learning plan will be evaluated further at that time.

REFERENCES

Alexiewich, D. (1990). Evaluation of a videotape: Orientation of patients to rehabilitation. *SCI Nursing, 7,* 31-33.

Blevins, D., Lubkin, I.M. (1990). Compliance. In I.M. Lubkin (Ed.). *Chronic illness: Impact and interventions* (2nd ed.). Boston: Jones and Bartlett, pp. 155-178.

Bloom, B.S. (Ed.). (1956). *Taxonomy of educational objectives: the classification of educational goals. Handbook I: Cognitive domain.* New York: David McKay.

Boss, B.J. (1986). The neuroanatomical and neurophysiological basis of learning. *Journal of Neuroscience Nursing, 18,* 256-264.

Brever, J.M. (1982). *A handbook of assistive devices for the handicapped elderly: New help for independent living.* New York: Haworth Press.

Carpenito, L.J. (1993). *Nursing diagnosis: Application to clinical practice* (5th ed.). Philadelphia: J.B. Lippincott.

Craft, M. (1987). Selecting and using teaching strategies, resources, and materials for client education. In H.L. Van Hoozer (Ed.), *The Teaching Process.* Norwalk, CT: Appleton-Century-Crofts.

Curtis, M. (1990). Videotapes: Are they helpful in the practice setting. *Journal of the American Academy of Nurse Practitioners, 2,* 172-173.

Diehl, L.N. (1989). Client and family learning in the rehabilitation setting. *Nursing Clinics of North America, 24,* 257-264.

Doak, C.C., Doak, L.G., Root, J.H. (1985). *Teaching patients with low literacy skills.* Philadelphia: J.B. Lippincott.

Falvo, D.R. (1985). *Effective patient education.* Rockville, MD: Aspen.

Friedman, M.M. (1992). *Family nursing: Theory and assessment* (3rd ed.). Norwalk, CT: Appleton-Century-Crofts.

Grief, E., & Mataruzzo, R.G. (1982). *Behavioral approaches to rehabilitation: Coping with change.* New York: Springer.

Hoeman, S.P. (1992). Pediatric nursing. In G. Molnar (Ed.). *Pediatric rehabilitation* (2nd ed.). Baltimore: Williams & Wilkins, pp. 202-219.

Jenny, J. (1987). Knowledge deficit: Not a nursing diagnosis. *Image, 19,* 184-185.

Knowles, M.S. (1984). *Andragogy in action.* San Francisco: Jossey-Bass.

Krathwohl D.R., Bloom, B.S., & Masia, B.B. (1969). *Taxonomy of educational objectives: the classification of educational goals. Handbook II: Affective domain.* New York: David McKay.

Kurlychek, R.T., & Levin, W. (1987). Computers in the cognitive rehabilitation of brain-injured persons. *Critical Review in Medical Informatics, 1,* 241-257.

Lorig, K., & Fries, J.F. (1986). *The arthritis helpbook* (2nd ed.). Reading, MA: Addison-Wesley.

Lynch, W.J. (1991). The Macintosh as a tool in rehabilitation. *Journal of Head Trauma Rehabilitation, 6,* 64-66.

Mager, R.F. (1975). *Preparing instructional objectives* (2nd ed.). Belmont, CA: Fearon.

Moore M.R. (1970). The perceptual-motor domain and a proposed taxonomy of perception. *Audio Communication Review, 18,* 379-413.

Pasquarello, M.A. (1990). Developing, implementing, and evaluating a stroke recovery group. *Rehabilitation Nursing, 15,* 26-29.

Pratt, D.D. (1988). Andragogy as a relational construct. *Adult Education Quarterly, 38,* 160-181.

Rankins, S.H., & Stallings, K.D. (1990). *Patient education: Issues, principles, practices* (2nd ed.). Philadelphia: J.B. Lippincott.

Redman, B.K. (1993). *The process of patient education* (7th ed.). St. Louis: Mosby–Year Book.

Robertson, I.H., Gray, J.M., PentLand, B. and Waite, L.J. (1990). Microcomputer-based rehabilitation for unilateral left visual neglect: A randomized controlled trial. *Archives of Physical Medicine and Rehabilitation, 7,* 663-668.

Trieschmann, R.B. (1974). Coping with disability: sliding scale of goals. *Archives of Physical Medicine and Rehabilitation, 55,* 556-560.

Vance, J.L. (1992). Learning readiness in rehabilitation patients. *Rehabilitation Nursing, 17,* 148-149.

11

Functional Evaluation

Margaret Kelly-Hayes, EdD, RN, CRRN

INTRODUCTION

The general goals of rehabilitation are to improve function, promote independence and life satisfaction, and preserve self-esteem (Brummel-Smith, 1990). For rehabilitation nursing these goals are extended to include achieving and maintaining an acceptable quality of life, ensuring that the client's specific needs are addressed, and promoting adaption by clients and families to life changes while optimizing wellness (McCourt, 1993). The process by which these goals are met consists of comprehensive evaluation and planned interventions designed to meet the needs of the individual. Recent advances in rehabilitation enhance the scientific basis on which comprehensive evaluation and related goals now are based. They include conceptualization and definition of disablement, reliable assessment of human performance, refinement of functional measures, and objective measurement of rehabilitation outcomes. In rehabilitation nursing these gains in theory-based evaluation have influenced the nursing process and on several levels form one of the major cornerstones of practice.

The conceptualization and determination of functional performance are central to the nature and direction of planning, performing, and evaluating restorative care. For nursing a traditional approach to the assessment of a client's functional abilities often has been qualitative and subjective. With professional encouragement for certification and standards in rehabilitation evaluation, formal assessment is incorporated into the nursing process using refined instruments that produce reliable and valid data. Subsequent monitoring and evaluation of function is contingent on reliable baseline assessment information. Functional evaluation can be viewed as an extension of the traditional components of nursing assessment and thus provides a framework for an orderly review of essential components deemed important to independent life. It is a more useful overall indicator of ability to perform independently and maintain a meaningful life than disease categories alone. Recent reports that formal assessment may be more reliable than clinical impressions helps establish the role of evaluation as an essential component in providing rehabilitative care.

The concept of functional evaluation has been an integral part of the rehabilitation nursing process. Nurses have assessed capacities of clients to meet their personal needs. They have traditionally assimilated this type of information in developing nursing plans. Today we know that a nursing assessment of function, based in part on validated and objective measures, is an asset to the client, the nursing staff, and contributes in a meaningful way to the interdisciplinary process. It has a direct influence on nursing diagnosis, nursing intervention, and every nursing-specific outcome criterion.

Expansion of functional evaluation parameters have been guided by changes in the concept of rehabilitation, the populations being served, and the functions of the rehabilitation team. The incorporation of functional evaluation in the interdisciplinary process of rehabilitation provides a common denominator for the team effort, an essential component in rehabilitation. The rehabilitation team provides the collaborative effort, with each member accountable for his or her own professional specialty-regulated interventions. Regardless of the client population being served, the rehabilitation team provides an interdisciplinary patient evaluation, a discipline-specific assessment, a determination of commonly agreed-upon goals, and an evaluation of the plan initiated. Functional evaluation is an integral component of each of these elements and falls within the responsibility of nursing as well as for the rehabilitation team in general.

This chapter addresses functional evaluation primarily from a nursing perspective. It defines the conceptual basis for disability evaluation, the terminology, and the purpose and essential components of functional evaluation. In addition, this chapter presents and describes several specific assessment measures commonly used by rehabilitation professionals including nurses, which have proven to be valid, reliable, and sensitive to changes expected from rehabilitative interventions. The types of instruments described in this chapter include measures of global disability, instrumental activities of daily living (I-ADL), and quality-of-life measures. Presently, functional evaluation practices vary widely, and no single measurements have become universally accepted. Because the goals of assessment change over time, the type, frequency, and goals for utilization of information change. All of the measures cited here are appropriate for inclusion in a client-centered assessment system, and their utilization fosters the utilization of acceptable measures as a central component in nursing.

DISABILITY FRAMEWORK FOR EVALUATION

The focus of rehabilitation is to provide interventions to improve function and to limit the impact of disability. The spheres of measurement to evaluate these interventions in rehabilitation have evolved from the conceptual framework of disablement. The term disability has been defined as the "expression of a physical or mental limitation in a social context—the gap between a person's capacity and the demands of the environment" (Pope & Tarlov, 1991). Although by definition the term disability assumes interaction between the individual and the environment, the word is frequently equated with separate and specific impairments. The relationship between severity of disability and independent living is apparent; however, many times the terms impairment, disability, and handicap are used interchangeably without consideration of their specific differences. These inconsistencies can pose obstacles to the design and evaluation of interventions.

The conceptual process from which we define disability has developed over the past 25 years. The two main architects of the disability model were Nagi (1965, 1969, 1976) and Wood (1980). These two theorists, although in many ways similar in the elements of the construct, differ in identifying the locus of responsibility. Nagi describes three major potential consequences of active pathology or disease: (1) impairment or physiologic abnormalities; (2) functional limitations, which he describes as sensorimotor abilities such as walking or dressing; and (3) disability, which he defines as an inability or limitation in performing expected social roles and activities such as in relation to work, family, or independent living. Disability occurs when there are conditions that interfere with the performance of an individual in personal, social, or culturally expected roles. The World Health Organization (WHO, 1980) International Classification of Impairments, Disabilities, and Handicaps (ICIDH) developed by Wood extends Nagi's construct to also include the concept of "handicap" (Table 11-1). Wood (1980) defined handicap as "a disadvantage for a given individual, resulting from an impairment or disability, that limits or prevents the fulfillment of a role that is normal (depending on age, sex, and social and cultural factors) for that individual." Although handicap in the WHO model is similar to disability in the Nagi model, the Nagi model has

the advantage of removing the negative connotation associated with the word "handicap." The disability model described by Nagi is more in accordance with rehabilitation viewpoint in that it emphasizes the difference between impairment, limitations, and disability and the importance of quality of life. For this reason, the Nagi model is more frequently referenced in the rehabilitation community (Pope & Tarlov, 1991).

MEASUREMENT OF DISABILITY IN REHABILITATION

Applying disability theory and definitions in rehabilitation has been a difficult task due to the complexities related to physical limitations. Surveying disability trends in the United States, Colvez and Blanchet (1981) defined disability in terms of physical mobility, physical independence in basic activities, and ability to carry out one's normal activity. Charlton, Patrick, and Peach (1983) expanded the measurement of disability to also include psychological status, ability to communicate, and ability to work. The approach devised by Kane and Kane (1981) conceptualized health and disability as a hierarchical structure: the first level is general health or the absence of illness, the second level is basic performance of self-care and mobility activities that are critical for independence, and the third level is the ability to perform and maintain those complex activities and roles associated with a meaningful life. Kane and Kane's conceptualization of disability addresses the wide range of functional performances from basic self-care to community reintegration. Utilizing their hierarchical approach to disability, rehabilitation interventions can be targeted to treatments and outcome measures at the levels of impairment, limitations, and disability. Assessment then becomes the keystone for planned interventions and should include all parameters that affect "active life" functioning. Following the guidelines set forth within the concept of the disablement model, functional evaluation by definition should include the wide range of disability measures that addresses maximizing function within a physical loss.

With the expanded scope of rehabilitation, there has been

Table 11-1   Comparison of the conceptual models of disability

WHO INTERNATIONAL CLASSIFICATION OF IMPAIRMENTS, DISABILITIES, AND HANDICAPS

"Disease"	Impairment	Disability	Handicap
The intrinsic pathology or disorder	Loss or abnormality of psychological, physiologic, or anatomic structure or function at organ level	Restriction or lack of ability to perform an activity in a normal manner	Disadvantage due to impairment or disability that limits or prevents fulfillment of a normal role

NAGI SCHEME

Active pathology	Impairment	Functional limitation	Disability
Interruption or interference with normal processes, and efforts of the organism to regain normal state	Anatomic, physiologic, mental or emotional abnormalities or loss	Limitation in performance at the level of the whole organism or person	Limitation in performance of socially defined roles and tasks within a sociocultural and physical environment

Summarized from *International classification of impairments, disabilities, and handicaps (A manual of classification relating to consequences of disease)* (p. 23-43) by the World Health Organization, 1980, Geneva: Copyright 1980 by the World Health Organization. For Nagi's scheme, see Nagi (1965).

an increase in the number of domains routinely assessed as part of the rehabilitation process. Today it is common practice in rehabilitation services to utilize a large number of assessment instruments to document impairments, basic activities of daily living (ADL), performance of complex ADL, and quality of life. The combination of these instruments provides the evaluation of critical components that make up independent active life. For rehabilitation nursing the scope of assessment includes physical, cognitive, affective, social, and quality-of-life measures.

ASSESSMENT MEASURES: GENERAL CONSIDERATIONS

Information from assessment instruments can be utilized for several purposes, the most common being descriptive, evaluative, and/or predictive. Descriptive measures document the type and severity of impairments, functional limitations, or disabilities at a given point in time. Evaluative components measure clinical changes over time, and predictive components are utilized to establish goals and plan treatments. The overall goal is that an assessment instrument be practical, simple to administer, and yield meaningful results that can direct the rehabilitation process.

The guiding principles in choosing a functional assessment instrument include that the instrument be a valid measure of the function being tested, that previous studies document adequate reliability, and that the measurement should be sensitive enough to document clinically important change (Kane & Kane, 1981). These characteristics are defined as follows:

+ *Reliability.* Interobserver reliability is the technique where two individuals administer the same test to the same client and obtain similar results. Test-retest reliability refers to whether repeated use of a measure yields consistent results in the absence of a change in the client.
+ *Validity.* Validity is the ability of an instrument to measure what it is intended to measure. An instrument's criterion validity is determined by comparing its results with a standard accepted within the field.
+ *Sensitivity.* The sensitivity of an instrument is its ability to detect clinical change.
+ *Sensibility.* Sensibility refers to the instrument's overall importance, relatedness to what is being measured, and ease of use.

The nature of the observed disability influences choices in measurement instruments. The assessment instrument employed should be able to measure disability, monitor progress, enhance communications, measure effectiveness of treatment, and document benefits of rehabilitation interventions. Since assessment instruments are used repeatedly during the course of rehabilitation, the results should be reliable and a valid measure for the disability being treated.

It is important to remember that the method of test administration influences the data obtained, and those who administer the test distinguish between the concepts of capacity and performance. Methodologic differences in obtaining the assessment measures and the type of populations being assessed are two sources for the discrepancies. Often measures do not clearly differentiate between the presence of a functional impairment that makes an activity im-

possible to carry out and the actual performance of an activity. In a Framingham study of noninstitutionalized cohort members, performance of ADL was shown to have an integral cognitive component (Kelly-Hayes, Jette, Wolf, D'Agostino, & Odell, 1992). In addition, Nagi (1965) has documented that disability, unlike functional limitations, has a major social component. Since disability reflects performance within a sociocultural context, one could expect that daily performance would be strongly influenced by social factors as well physical factors.

The distinction between functional limitations and disability is of importance (Kelly-Hayes et al., 1992). Should assessment determine capacity or daily performance? Behavior that is executed in an ideal setting under controlled circumstances may not be an accurate measure of the extent of disability experienced. In the real world situation, lack of motivation and environmental factors can impede the carrying out of certain activities conducted independently in the rehabilitation setting. This needs to be evaluated in considering independence and final placement after rehabilitation.

Domains and Definition of Functional Assessment

The expanded scope of rehabilitation has led to the increased domains of assessment. In providing rehabilitation services today, a large number of assessment instruments are utilized to document impairments, basic ADL, performance of complex ADL, and quality of life. These measures can be generic to rehabilitation in general or disease specific, depending on the intended use of the data. In general, most documentation of disability is determined utilizing generic tools.

The general purposes of functional assessment are to determine physical functional status, document the need for interventions and services, devise a treatment plan, and assess and monitor progress. A measure of physical functioning can be derived from many different combinations of items. One of the earliest definitions of functional assessment, defined by Lawton (1971), describes objective measurement in a variety of areas such as physical health, emotional status, and quality of self-maintenance. More recently Granger (1987) stated that "functional assessment is a method for describing abilities and limitations to measure an individual's use of a variety of skills included in performing tasks necessary to daily living, leisure activities, vocational pursuits, social interactions, and other required behaviors." Quantitative measurements across multidimensional function areas are apparent in both definitions, demonstrating that assessment is not unidimensional but rather evolves along with the underlying philosophy of rehabilitation today.

Within the domain of measurement of function, there is considerable agreement that self-care and mobility are central to rehabilitation. This narrow focus of self-care and mobility, however, does not adequately describe the actual range of interventions in rehabilitation. Although these functional skills are important parameters in reducing dependence on others, the repertoire of behaviors required to lead a meaningful life is obviously much broader. Most rehabilitation programs also incorporate measures of cognitive, emotional, perceptual, social, and vocational function-

UNIFORM DATA SYSTEM FOR MEDICAL REHABILITATION
INPATIENT CODING SHEET

1. Facility Code

2. Patient Code

Admission Assessment

22. Admit Form
1-Home 2-Board and Care 3-Transitional Living
4-Intermediate Care 5-Skilled Nursing Facility
6-Acute unit of own facility 7-Acute unit another facility
8-Chronic Hospital 9-Rehabilitation Facility 10-Other
12-Alternate Level of Care Unit

23. Prehospital Living Setting
Use codes listed for item 22.

24. Prehospital Living With
(Complete only if item 23 is coded 1-Home.)
1-Alone 2-Family/Relatives 3-Friends
4-Attendant 5-Other

25. Prehospital Vocational Category
1-Employed 2-Sheltered 3-Student 4-Homemaker
5-Not Working 6-Retired-age 7-Retired-disability

26. Prehospital Vocational Effort
(Complete only if item 25 is coded 1,2,3 or 4.)
1-Full-time 2-Part-time 3-Adjusted workload

Discharge Assessment

27. Discharge to
1-Home 2-Board and Care 3-Transitional Living
4-Intermediate Care 5-Skilled Nursing Facility
6-Acute unit of own facility 7-Acute unit in another facility
8-Chronic Hospital 9-Rehabilitation Facility 10-Other
11-Died 12-Alternate Level of Care Unit

28. Discharge Living With
(Complete only if item 27 is coded 1-Home.)
1-Alone 2-Family/Relatives 3-Friends
4-Attendant 5-Other

(For Items 29-38 See Follow-Up Coding Sheet)

39. Functional Independence Measure (FIM)

ADMISSION   DISCHARGE

Self-Care
A. Eating
B. Grooming
C. Bathing
D. Dressing-upper body
E. Dressing-lower body
F. Toileting

Sphincter Control
G. Bladder management
H. Bowel management

Transfers
I. Bed, chair, wheelchair
J. Toilet
K. Tub, shower

Locomotion
L. Walk/wheelchair — Walk Wheelchair Both
M. Stairs

Motor Subtotal Score

Communication
N. Comprehension — Auditory Visual Both
O. Expression — Vocal Nonvocal Both

Social Cognition
P. Social interaction
Q. Problem solving
R. Memory

Cognitive Subtotal Score

Total Motor and Cognitive Score

FIM Levels

NO HELPER

| 7 | Complete independence (timely, safely) |
| 6 | Modified independence (device) |

HELPER

Modified Dependence

5	Supervision
4	Minimal assistance (Subject = 75% +)
3	Moderate assistance (Subject = 50% +)

Complete Dependence

| 2 | Maximal assistance (Subject = 25% +) |
| 1 | Total assistance (Subject = 0% +) |

(NOTE: Leave no blanks; enter 1 if not testable due to risk)

Complete Both Pages

Source: Uniform Data System for Medical Rehabilitation (1993), UB Foundation Activities

Fig. 11-1 Uniform Data System for medical rehabilitation: inpatient coding sheet.

ing. Clearly rehabilitation nursing is involved with all of these areas with function and quality-of-life issues important in goal setting.

Functional Assessment Instruments for Adult Disability

Comprehensive functional assessment is an essential clinical management component. It expands across disease categories and physical impairments to address the resultant disability targeted by rehabilitation efforts. The rationale or goal of treatment interventions guides in the choice of instrument employed.

Most disability or ADL scales measure a combination of activities including feeding, dressing, bathing, mobility, and continence. ADL scales are usually hierarchical in their arrangement, from basic functions such as feeding to higher level functions of stair climbing. Some of the more recently developed scales include measures of functional communication and social cognition. Information is obtained by observing actual performance, rather than a capacity demonstrated in an artificial setting such as in therapy.

SELECTED DISABILITY SCALES

The following section of this chapter identifies and describes several validated scales within the domains related within the field of rehabilitation that are appropriate to be integrated within rehabilitation nursing practice.

The instruments recommended in this chapter are in general use in the rehabilitation community and have had substantial testing for reliability, validity, and sensibility. They are practical and valid for incorporation into rehabilitation nursing assessment. The yield from using standardized instruments results in evolving toward objective methodology for nursing assessment.

Although there have been over 50 functional assessment instruments developed in rehabilitation, the most widely utilized scales are the Functional Independence Measure (FIM) (Fig. 11-1) and the Barthel Index (Mahoney & Barthel, 1965) (Table 11-2).

The FIM, developed by the Uniform Data System, provides uniform language, definitions, and measurements that describe the components of disability (Fig. 11-2). The conceptual basis is that the level of disability should indicate the burden of care or the cost to the individual or society for that person not to be functionally independent. The measure is used to establish criteria for admission, discharge, and maintenance of rehabilitation gains. The instrument can be administered by those who practice rehabilitation and who have been certified in its administration. Ideally it should be administered by one specialty discipline, thus far with nursing taking a leadership position.

The FIM measures disability in the following performance categories: feeding, grooming, bathing, dressing the upper body, dressing the lower body, toileting, bladder management, bowel management, bed/chair/wheelchair transfers, toilet transfer, tub/shower transfer, locomotion, communication, and social cognition. Utilizing a seven-level scale, a FIM score ranges from a maximum of 126 points, representing complete independence in all performance areas, to the minimal score of 18, representing dependence in all areas evaluated. The WeeFIM is an adaptation of the FIM designed to meet the specific needs of children. For example, assessment includes developmental categories (Fig. 11-3).

The Barthel Index measures performance ability in mobility, self-care, and continence. It is a weighted scoring system, ranging from 0 to 100. A score of 100 indicates complete independence in all 10 domains measured, and 0 indicates complete dependence in all 10 domains. To be considered independent, the client will not require assistance at any time.

There are a number of valid and reliable scales that document basic ADL. Most are administered by trained clinicians, although there are some that are subjective judgment based. The utility of these instruments is that they provide a description of minimum physical functioning and can be appropriately utilized to follow broad measures of a clinical course.

Table 11-2   Barthel index

	With help	Independent
1. Feeding*	5	10
2. Moving from wheelchair to bed and return (includes sitting up in bed)	5-10	15
3. Personal toilet (wash face, comb hair, shave, clean teeth)	0	5
4. Getting on and off toilet (handling clothes, wipe, flush)	5	10
5. Bathing self	0	5
6. Walking on level surface	10	15
If unable to walk, propelling wheelchair (score only if unable to walk)	0	5
7. Ascending and descending stairs	5	10
8. Dressing (includes tying shoes, fastening fasteners)	5	10
9. Controlling bowels	5	10
10. Controlling bladder	5	10

From "Functional Evaluation: The Barthel Index" by F.I. Mahoney and D. Barthel, 1965, *Maryland State Medical Journal, 50,* p. 62.
*If food needs to be in cup, score as "with help."

UNIFORM DATA SYSTEM FOR MEDICAL REHABILITATION
WeeFIM ASSESSMENT CODING SHEET

Rehabilitation Patient

1a. Facility Code

1b. Facility Care Class (Pediatric Care Only)
2-Inpatient 6-Clinic 7-Home 8-School

2. Patient Code

2. Admission Date
MONTH   DAY   YEAR

Assessment

21. Assessment Type   1-Admit 2-Interim 3-Discharge 4-Follow-up

22. Assessment Date
MONTH   DAY   YEAR

23. Admit From Setting
(Same as item 24)

24. Living Setting
1-Home 2-Acute Unit of own facility 3-Acute Unit of other facility
4-Chronic Hospital 5-Rehabilitation Facility 6-School Based Program
7-Home Care 8-Alternate Level of Care 9-Board and Care
10-Transitional Living 11-Intermediate Care 12-Skilled Nursing 13-Other 14-Died

25. Living With   (Only if item 24 is coded 1-Home)
1-Two Parents 2-One Parent 3-Relatives
4-Foster Care 5-Shelter 6-Other

26. Educational Category
1-Not a student 2-Early Intervention Program
3-Pre-School 4-Regular School 5-Other

27. Educational Setting   (Only if item 26 is coded 2, 3 or 4)
1-Regular Class 2-Special Class 3-Home Based
4-Day Care/Nursery School   (Only if item 26 is 2 or 3)

28. Information Source   (Only for followup or outpatient)
1-Patient 2-Family 3-Other 4-Clinician

29. Assessment Method   (Only for followup or outpatient)
1-In person 2-Telephone 3-Mailed Questionnaire

30. Health Maintenance   (Only for followup or outpatient)
1-Own Care
2-Unpaid person or family   Primary
3-Paid attendant or aide
4-Paid, skilled professional   Secondary

31. Therapy (Only for discharge, followup or outpatient)
1-None 2-Outpatient therapy 3 Home based paid professional therapy
4-Both 2&3 5-Inpatient Hospital 6-Long-term care facility
7-Other combinations 8-School based

32. Therapy Services (Only for discharge, followup or outpatient)
1-None 2-Physical Therapy 3-Occupational Therapy
4-Speech Therapy 5-Physical & Occupational
6-Physical, Occupational & Speech 7-Other Combinations of 2, 3 or 4

33. Other Diagnoses
(ICD-9 codes)

a. ___ . ___   d. ___ . ___
b. ___ . ___   e. ___ . ___
c. ___ . ___   f. ___ . ___
               g. ___ . ___

34. Functional Independence Measure (FIM)

MOTOR

Self-Care
A.   Eating
B.   Grooming
C.   Bathing
D.   Dressing-Upper Body
E.   Dressing-Lower Body
F.   Toileting

Sphincter Control
G.   Bladder Management
H.   Bowel Management

Transfers
I.   Chair, Wheelchair
J.   Toilet
K.   Tub, Shower

Locomotion
L.   Walk/Wheelchair/Crawl
     ○ Walk
     ○ Wheelchair
     ○ Crawl
     ○ Combination
M.   Stairs

COGNITIVE

Communication
N.   Comprehension
     ○ Auditory
     ○ Visual
     ○ Both
O.   Expression
     ○ Vocal
     ○ Nonvocal
     ○ Both

Social Cognition
P.   Social Interaction
Q.   Problem Solving
R.   Memory

(NOTE: Leave no blanks; enter 1 if not testable due to risk)

FIM LEVELS	
NO HELPER	
7	Complete Independence (Timely, Safely)
6	Modified Independence (Device)
HELPER	
Modified Dependence	
5	Supervision
4	Minimal Assistance (Subject = 75% +)
3	Moderate Assistance (Subject = 50% +)
Complete Dependence	
2	Maximal Assistance (Subject = 25% +)
1	Total Assistance (Subject = 0% +)

Source: Uniform Data System for Medical Rehabilitation (1993), UB Foundation Activities

Fig. 11-2   Uniform Data System for medical rehabilitation: FIM assessment coding sheet.

TABLE
FUNCTIONAL INDEPENDENCE MEASURE (FIM)

L E V E L S			NO HELPER
	7 Complete Independence (Timely, Safely)		
	6 Modified Independence (Device)		
	Modified Dependence		HELPER
	5 Supervision	4 Minimal Assist (Subject=75%+)	
	3 Moderate Assist (Subject=50%+)		
	Complete Dependence		
	2 Maximal Assist (Subject=25%+)	1 Total Assist (Subject=0%+)	

	ADMIT	DISCHG	FOL-UP
Self Care			
A. Feeding	—	—	—
B. Grooming	—	—	—
C. Bathing	—	—	—
D. Dressing - Upper Body	—	—	—
E. Dressing - Lower Body	—	—	—
F. Toileting	—	—	—
Sphincter Control			
G. Bladder Management	—	—	—
H. Bowel Management	—	—	—
Mobility Transfer:			
I. Bed, Chair, W/Chair	—	—	—
J. Toilet	—	—	—
K. Tub, Shower	—	—	—
Locomotion			
L. Walk / wheel Chair	W C —	W C —	W C —
M. Stairs	—	—	—
Communication			
N. Comprehension	a V n —	a V n —	a V n —
O. Expression	a V n —	a V n —	a V n —
Social Cognition			
P. Social Interaction	—	—	—
Q. Problem Solving	—	—	—
R. Memory	—	—	—
TOTAL			

Fig. 11-3   Functional Independence Measure.

The selected disability scales that meet the criteria for validity and reliability standards are contained here in Table 11-3. This table is a listing and description of selected ADL scales that are currently in use in rehabilitation.

Measures of Disabilities in Complex Activities of Independent Living

Beyond the basic performance of ADL, the ability to accomplish certain activities that make independent living possible are categories under the title of I-ADL or extended ADL (E-ADL). Such activities include a variety of tasks not limited to but including using a telephone, shopping, preparing meals, and managing money. These skills are often part of rehabilitation retraining but are difficult to evaluate until the individual returns home. I-ADL scales may be rated by either an interviewer or by the individual, depending on the disability and circumstances. These scales can often be invalid or insensitive to change unless directly rated. They also do not take into account safety as a feature of performance. Table 11-4 lists and describes three I-ADL scales utilized in rehabilitation services.

Cognitive Assessment

Cognitive status evaluation should be an integral part of the rehabilitation assessment. The ability to acquire and retain new information, the underpinning of the rehabilitation process, can be obtained by observation of the client's interactions, responses to questions, and general knowledge. In addition, incorporation of a mental status test as part of

the assessment process can serve as a guide in planning outcome goals and identifying those at risk for difficulty in adapting to disability. Measurement tools for cognitive function can be self-administered, observer rated, or structured interview. The Mini–Mental State Examination (Folstein & McHugh, 1975) has been widely used in a variety of populations, is well validated, reliable, and brief (Table 11-5).

Affective Functioning

Affect and mood are among the most powerful determinants of successful rehabilitation. Depressive symptoms can often be exacerbated by loss of physical well-being and independence. In some conditions such as stroke, depression actually may be a feature of the disease. Berkman et al. (1986) studied the association between depression and functional disability in elders. She found that depression varied by health characteristics, with individuals having major functional disabilities demonstrating higher levels of depression. Although depression is known to affect outcome, there is little consensus on how to screen and measure for it. If not recognized and treated, depression can have a profound negative impact on all rehabilitation efforts (Table 11-5).

Assessment of Family Functioning

Family structure and functioning play an important role throughout the rehabilitation process. They become very important in discharge planning and for the client to return

Table 11-3 Measures of disability

Scale	Description and type of scale	Reliability, validity, and sensitivity	Time and administration	Comments
Barthel Index (Mahoney & Barthel, 1965)	Ordinal scale with scores from 0 (totally dependent) to 100 (independent); 10 weighted items: feeding, bathing, grooming, dressing, controlling bladder, controlling bowels, toileting, chair/bed transfer, mobility, and stair climbing	Well-documented reliability and validity; not sensitive to minor changes at higher levels of ADL functioning	Clinician observation <40 minutes Appropriate for screening, formal assessment, monitoring, and maintenance	Widely established measure for disability; excellent reliability and validity
Kenny Self-Care Scale (Schoening & Iverson, 1968)	Ordinal scale with 17 specific activities under six major categories: bed, activities, transfers, locomotion, personal hygiene, dressing, and feeding; measured on 5-point scale: 0 = dependence to 4 = independence; range of scores from 0 to 24	Documented reliability and validity; reasonable sensitivity	Clinician observation or judgment >30 minutes Appropriate for formal assessment, monitoring, and maintenance	Range of inclusive categories, geared to rehabilitation assessment; ratings can be subjective
FIM (Granger, Hamilton, & Sherwin, 1986)	Ordinal scale with 18 items, seven-level scale with scores from 18 to 126; areas of evaluation include feeding, self-care, controlling sphincter, mobility, locomotion, communication, and social cognition	Well-documented reliability and validity; able to detect minor changes with seven levels; physical and cognitive components able to detect increments of change	Clinician observation <40 minutes Appropriate for screening, formal assessment, monitoring, maintenance, and program evaluation	Widely accepted in rehabilitation; broad measure of ADL and social cognition; standardized interobserver reliability by certification of clinicians
PECS (Harvey & Jilinet, 1981)	Ordinal scale with 115 items in a six-step scale ranging from total dependence to total independence; major headings include medicine, nursing, physical mobility, ADL, communication, medications, device utilization, pay, neuropsychology, social issues, therapeutic recreation, procedures nutrition, pain, pulmonary	Documented reliability and validity; broad range of categories relating to rehabilitation services	Discipline-specific evaluations <60 minutes most disciplines Appropriate for formal assessment, monitoring, maintenance, and program evaluation	Extensive number of items evaluated; focus on long-term needs and program evaluation
LORS/LAD (Carey & Posavac, 1978)	Five-interval subscales assessing ADL, mobility, communications, cognitive ability, memory, measured on 5-point scale from 0 = unable to perform activity to 4 = able to perform activity	Documented reliability and validity; specific to physical and cognitive measures in rehabilitation setting	Clinician observation 10 minutes/subscale; >60 minutes total Appropriate for screening, monitoring, maintenance, and program evaluation	Measures broad functional outcome categories; provides separate score for subscales; does not measure bladder or bowel incontinence

PECS, Patient Evaluation and Conference Systems; LORS/LADS, Level of Rehabilitation Scales/LORS American Data System.

Table 11-4 Measures of instrumental activities of daily living

Scale	Description and type of scale	Reliability, validity, and sensitivity	Time and administration	Comments
Functional Health Status (Rosow & Breslau, 1966)	Guttman Scale; 25 questions determining ascending dependency; questions include out-of-home activities such as going to the movies, walking half a mile, and doing heavy work	Documented reliability and validity	Interviewer <30 minutes Appropriate for maintenance in community setting	Simple measure design with general functioning questions; limited utility for persons with disabilities; difficult to validate in institutional setting
OARS I-ADL (Duke University, 1978)	Multidimensional assessment tool containing 105 questions in five domains: social resources, economic resources, mental health, physical health, and ADL	Documented reliability and validity	Interviewer >10 minutes Appropriate for maintenance in the community	Measures broad base of information necessary for independent living; complex domains assessed
PGC I-ADL (Lawton, 1972)	Guttman Scale; questions on using telephone, walking, shopping, preparing food, housekeeping, laundry, public transportation, medication	Validity (Rubenstein, 1984); reliability (Lawton, 1972, 1988)	Interviewer <30 minutes	Strength: measures broad base of information necessary for independent living

OARS, Older Americans Resources and Services; PGC, Philadelphia Geriatric Center Morals Scale.

Table 11-5 Cognitive, affective, and family measures

COGNITIVE STATUS

Scale	Description and type of scale	Reliability, validity, and sensitivity	Time and administration	Comments
Mini–Mental State Examination (Folstein & McHugh, 1975)	Measures seven domains including orientation, registration, calculation, recall, language, and visual construction	Valid, reliable, and sensitive	Interviewer 10 minutes Screening instrument	Several functions with summed scores; education considerations
ASSESSMENT OF AFFECTIVE DISORDERS				
CES-D (Radloff, 1977)	Measures severity of depressive symptoms; 20 items	Valid, reliable, and sensitive	Self-rating or interviewer 15 minutes Screening instrument	Brief, easily administered; effective for screening possible depression
FAMILY FUNCTION				
FAD (Epstein, Baldwin, and Bishop, 1985)	Measures of family roles, problem-solving, communication, behavior control, and general functioning	Valid and reliable	Interviewer 30 minutes Appropriate for discharge and maintenance in the community	Assessment subjective

CES-D, Center for Epidemiologic Studies of Depression; FAD, Family Assessment Device.

Table 11-6   Measures of quality of life

Scale	Description and type of scale	Reliability, validity, and sensitivity	Time and administration	Comments
MOS 36-Item Short Form Survey (Ware & Sherbourne, 1992)	Assesses eight health domains including physical and social activities, mental health, general health perceptions, vitality, and discomfort	Tested validity and reliability	Interviewer: in person or phone <30 minutes Appropriate for maintenance in community setting	All items are well standardized; widely used in the community
SIP (Carter, Bobbitt, Bergner, and Gilson, 1976)	Subscales evaluate the following areas: ambulation, self-care, emotions, communications, alertness, habits, home and recreation, vocation, and social interactions	Tested validity, reliability, and sensitivity	Interviewer: in person or phone <30 minutes Appropriate for maintenance in community setting	Comprehensive evaluation; behavior rather than subjective health items; focus on community life

MOS, Medical Outcome Study; SIP, Sickness Impact Profile.

to the community. Critical factors to be assessed include family and caregiver involvement, living environment and community access, and family roles and problem-solving skills. For assessing family function, one standardized tool is the Family Assessment Device (FAD) (Table 11-5).

Quality-of-Life Measures

Quality-of-life measures denote a wide range of capabilities, symptoms, and psychosocial characteristics that describe function and satisfaction with life. Components of quality of life include social roles and interactions, functional performance, intellectual functioning, perceptions, and subjective health. Indicators can include standards of living and general satisfaction with life. Although there is controversy over the measurement of quality of life, it is a powerful indicator of successful rehabilitation.

There have been several measures developed, but only a few of these have been well validated. Two measures that assess a broad range of health dimensions and are widely used are included here in Table 11-6.

Timing of Assessment for Rehabilitation Clients

Systematic assessment of impairments and disability is the major means of describing, monitoring, and evaluating specific interventions essential at each stage of the recovery process (Fig. 11-4). The primary objective of identifying at what point in time and at what phase of the disability assessment should occur includes identifying who would most likely benefit from rehabilitation therapies, prescribing specific therapies, monitoring the recovery process, and determining the long-term benefits of interventions.

Assessment begins with the initial clinical contact with the client, usually at the time of admission either to an inpatient facility, an outpatient facility, or to a rehabilitation program in the community. Often the first examination is a screening for impairments and disability related to the condition for treatment. A detailed evaluation is performed at the time of the formal assessment into a specific program. This assessment can be used to validate the appropriateness of the referral, formulate treatment goals, confirm the management plan, and to provide a baseline for monitoring change. The client's progress should then be assessed at periodic intervals during rehabilitation. Assessment should include a baseline and then a subset of the baseline, which are particular targets of intervention. Well-established reliable measures are essential to achieving valid comparisons among clients with similar problems. After discharge from rehabilitation, assessment is performed to monitor adaptation to the community and for maintenance of functional gains made during rehabilitation.

DIRECTION FOR REHABILITATION NURSING

The movement in nursing toward developing methodologies for assessment, evaluation of interventions, administrative planning, and documentation of effectiveness parallel the general efforts of all disciplines involved in rehabilitation. Ditmar (1984) identifies these purposes of functional evaluation in rehabilitation nursing as

1. Systematic identification of functional limitations requiring preventive, maintenance, and restorative actions
2. Recognition of client's learning needs
3. Documentation of feedback about progression toward goal achievement
4. Allocation of nursing time, dollars, staff
5. Coordination of care
6. Systematic nursing research and objective evaluation of care
7. Facilitation of placement decisions
8. Provision of objective data on which to analyze costs, benefits, and quality of care
9. Assistance for accreditation bodies, program evaluation, and third-party payers

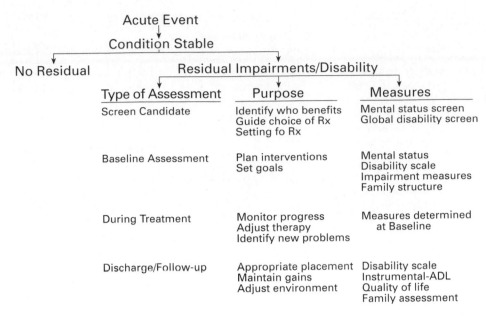

Fig. 11-4   Stages of assessment.

Rehabilitation nursing is based on the belief that rehabilitation is a process of restoring and maintaining a client at optimal physiologic, psychological, vocational, and social health. Functional evaluation is a critical component of this process. Measurement of function, therefore, is an essential element of rehabilitation nursing practice. The nursing process is linked to functional assessment and nursing diagnosis. The nurse arrives at a disability-related nursing diagnosis after a comprehensive assessment is performed. Assessment, planning, implementation, and evaluation of nursing practice are major components of evaluation of all interventions. The assessment of the client's functional abilities has a direct influence on nursing diagnosis, interventions, and outcome evaluation.

Formalized functional evaluation should be an integral part of rehabilitation nursing practice. The contributions of nursing can then be standardized and judged by colleagues, documenting the contribution made by the profession to overall rehabilitation goals. Rehabilitation nurses should view assessment instruments as they would other essential clinical information. They should be familiar with the strengths, weaknesses, and precision of the instrument they incorporate into their assessment. Changes in rehabilitation practice demand that nursing utilize the appropriate documentation to reflect current standards.

REFERENCES

Berkman, L.F., Berkman, C.S., Kasl, S., Freeman, D.H., Jr., Leo, L., Ostfeld, A.M., Coroni-Huntley, J., & Brody, J.A. (1986). Depressive symptoms in relation to physical health and functioning in the elderly. *American Journal of Epidemiology, 124,* 372-388.

Brummel-Smith, K. (1990). In B. Keep, K. Brummel-Smith, and J.W. Ramsdell (Eds.). *Geriatric rehabilitation.* Austin, TX: PRO-ED.

Carey, R.G., & Posavac, E.J. (1978). Program evaluation of a physical medicine and rehabilitation unit: A new approach. *Archives of Physical Medicine and Rehabilitation, 59,* 330-337.

Carter, W.B., Bobbitt, R.A., Bergner, M., & Gilson, B.S. (1976). Validation of an interval scaling: The sickness impact profile. *Health Services Research, 11,* 516-528.

Charlton, J.R.H., Patrick, D.L., & Peach, H. (1983). Use of multivariate measures of disability in health surveys. *Journal of Epidemiology and Community Health, 37,* 296-304.

Colvez, A., & Blanchet, M. (1981). Disability trends in the United States population 1966-76: Analysis of reported causes. *American Journal of Public Health, 71,* 464-470.

Ditmar, S. (1984). Functional assessment in nursing. In C. Granger & G. Gresham (Eds.). *Functional assessment in rehabilitation medicine* (pp. 194-209). Baltimore: Williams & Wilkins.

Duke University Center for the Study of Aging and Human Development. (1978). *Multidimensional functional assessment: the OARS methodology.* Durham, NC: Duke University.

Epstein, N., Baldwin, L., & Bishop, D. (1985). The McMasters family assessment device. *Journal of Martial and Family Therapy, 9.*

Folstein, M.F. & McHugh, P. (1975). Mini-Mental State: A practical method for grading the cognitive state of patients for the clinician. *Journal of Psychiatric Report, 12,* 189-198.

Granger, C.V. (1990). Health accounting—Functional assessment of the long-term patient. In Kottke, F.J. & Lehmann, J.F. (eds.) *Krusen's handbook of physical medicine and rehabilitation* (4th ed). Philadelphia: W.B. Saunders.

Granger, C.V., Hamilton, B.B., & Sherwin, F.S. (1986). *Guide for the use of the uniform data set for medical rehabilitation.* Buffalo, NY: Uniform Data System for Medical Rehabilitation Project Office.

Harvey, R.F., & Jilinek, H.M. (1981). Functional performance assessment: A program approach. *Archives of Physical Medicine and Rehabilitation, 62,* 456-460.

Kane, R.A., & Kane, R.L. (1981). *Assessing the elderly: A practical guide to measuring.* Lexington: Lexington Books.

Katz, S., Lord, A.B., Moskowitz, R.W., Jackson, B.A., & Jaffe, M.W. (1963). Studies of illness in the aged. The index of ADL a standardized measure of biological and psychological function. *JAMA, 185,* 914-919.

Kelly-Hayes, M., Jette, A., Wolf, P.A., D'Agostino, R., & Odell, P. (1992). Functional limitations and disability among elders in the Framingham study. *American Journal of Physical Rehabilitation, 82,* 841-845.

Lawton, M.P. (1971). Assessing the competence of older people. In E. Kent, K. Kastenbaum, R., and S. Sherwood (Eds.). *Research planning and action for the elderly.* New York: Behavioral Publications.

Lawton, M.P. (1972). Assessment, integration, and environment for older people. *The Gerontologist, 10,* 38-46.

Mahoney, F.I., & Barthel, D. (1965). Functional evaluation: The Barthel index. *Maryland State Medical Journal, 14,* 56-61.

McCourt, A. (Ed.). (1993). *Rehabilitation nursing: Concepts and practice—a core curriculum* (3rd ed.). Skokie, IL: Rehabilitation Nursing Foundation.

Nagi, S.Z. (1965). Disability concepts revisited. In M.B. Sussman (Ed.), *Sociology and rehabilitation* (pp. 100-113). Washington, DC: American Sociological Association.

Nagi, S.Z. (1969). *Disability and rehabilitation: Legal, clinical and measurement.* Columbus: Ohio State University Press.

Nagi, S.Z. (1976). An epidemiology of disability among adults in the United States. *Milbank Memorial Fund Quarterly, 54,* 439-467.

Pope, A.M., & Tarlov, A.R., (Eds.). (1991). *Disability in America: Toward a national agenda for prevention.* Washington, DC: National Academy Press.

Patient Evaluation and Conference System, Inc. (PECS). Wheaton, IL: Marionjoy Rehabilitation Hospital and Clinics.

Radloff, S.L. (1977). The CES-D scale: A self-report depression scale for research in the general population. *Applied Psychological Measurements, 1,* 385-401.

Rosow, I., & Breslau, N. (1966). A Guttman health scale for the aged. *Journal of Gerontology, 21,* 556-559.

Shah, S., Vanclay, F., & Cooper, B. (1989). Improving the sensitivity of the Barthel index for stroke rehabilitation. *Journal of Clinical Epidemiology, 42,* 703-709.

Schoening, H.A., & Iversen, I.A. (1968). Numerical scoring of self-care status: A study of the Kenny self-care evaluation. *Archives of Physical Medicine and Rehabilitation, 46,* 221-229.

Stewart, A.L., Greenfield, S., Hays, R.D., Wells, K., Rogers, W.H., Berry, S.D., McGlynn, E.A., & Ware, J.E. (1989). Functional status and well-being of patients with chronic conditions: results from the medical outcome study. *JAMA, 262,* 907-913.

Ware, J.E. Jr., & Sherbourne, C.D. (1992). The MOS 36-item short form survey (SF-36) I. Conceptual framework and item selection. *Medical Care, 30,* 473-483.

Wood, P.H.N. (1975). *Classification of impairments and handicaps.* Geneva: World Health Organization.

Wood, P.H.N. (1980). The language of disablement: A glossary relating to disease and its consequence. *International Rehabilitation Medicine, 2,* 86-92.

World Health Organization. (1980). *International classification of impairments, disabilities, and handicaps (A manual of classification relating to consequences of disease).* Geneva: Author.

12

Self-Care and Activities of Daily Living

Anaise (Sis) Theuerkauf, MEd, RN, CRRN, CCM

The concept of self-care has a broad definition in rehabilitation nursing practice, encompassing bathing, mouth care, dressing, menstrual management, grooming, toileting, and other personal care or hygiene areas. Applying cosmetics, shaving, or giving oneself a manicure or pedicure are self-care activities of daily living (ADL), which become noteworthy when they cannot be performed independently at will.

Traditionally rehabilitation nurses were knowledgeable about teaching dressing or grooming skills as well as bowel, bladder, or skin/wound management. Over time a variety of health professionals incorporated ADL functions into their roles, and nurses ceased to learn all but minimal ADLs in basic education and performed fewer in practice. With trends toward transdisciplinary practice, client participation in self-care, and community-based programs, nurses are re-activating their traditional roles in ADL (Connelly, 1993). Not only are nurses case managers or coordinators of care, but in underserved rural or urban areas, a nurse may be the professional with ADL competencies who is consistently represented on the health team. Community-based programs, such as community nursing agencies, request rehabilitation nursing consultation and technical assistance with ADL for the increased numbers of clients returning to live in the community with increased acuity.

In the past a client who entered a rehabilitation institution found personal preparation for the day was structured and dictated by the schedules and routines of the institution. Today self-care activities are directed by a client's strengths, abilities, preferences, lifestyle, and participation. For example, a person who has impaired cognition learns using a functional approach in an environment where each activity is performed with consistent structure and order. Physically dependent, a client with a spinal cord injury learns preplanning as a strategy to facilitate independence in everyday life. When learning to dress while in bed, this client learns to arrange clothing items in a drawer where they are accessible from the bed. In their own homes clients with arthritis may arrange bedroom and bath for easy access and schedule activities to avoid fatigue or painful episodes.

Just as in earlier years, ideal rehabilitation nursing units allocate space for a home environment or demonstration unit where clients and families, and perhaps community nurses, are able to work in living areas to demonstrate competence or solve problems with functional approaches to daily living (Jacus, 1981). Rehabilitation institution–based nurses make referrals to community nurses who conduct home evaluations; rehabilitation nurses serve as consultants to community nursing agencies. Shortened stays for clients in rehabilitation institutions challenge professional team members to find ways to assure clients and families are prepared to follow through with ADL skills when they re-enter the community.

Self-care activities discussed throughout this chapter may be taught in a rehabilitation, subacute, or long-term care unit; in community settings such as adult day care programs, group homes, or senior centers; or increasingly in a client's home or independent living arrangement. As detailed in Chapter 9, a complete institutional residence or home evaluation is essential to quality in planning for optimal self-care and independence in ADL. Minor rearrangements may free major access in a home, such as simply removing throw rugs, placing beds with no locking systems against a wall to prevent rolling during transfers, installing bathroom grab bars, adapting everyday household items, or adding a ramp to the entrance door.

Definitions of Self-Care

Self-care activities necessary for participation in everyday life in Roper's schemata (Chapter 1) include personal hygiene, grooming, and dressing. Self-care is more than a learned group of skills. It is a process that allows the client and family their first opportunity to acquire the ability to function effectively after injury or disease and assume responsibility for personal healthcare. When the focus is client centered, sensitive to lifestyle and preferences, it is their opportunity to accept or reject techniques and practices offered to them. Facilitated learning and an openness to questions challenge a client to accept responsibility for his or her actions. Teaching self-care activities in a nonjudgmental atmosphere assists clients to take a step toward knowledgeable consumerism (Theuerkauf & Carpenter, 1992).

Orem defines self-care as "the practice of activities that individuals initiate and perform on their own behalf in maintaining life, health and well-being" (Orem, 1980). She identifies five methods that nurses use to assist clients: doing for, guiding and directing, providing physical and psychological support, providing a developmental environment, and teaching. As described in Chapter 1, Orem's nursing intervention has three nursing systems—wholly compensatory, partly compensatory, and supportive-educative—

which rehabilitation nurses use to assess and assist clients for independence in self-care.

Teaching Self-Care in Activities of Daily Living

As discussed in Chapter 10, client and family education may be provided in a variety of ways. At its least effective level, a paternalistic professional gives information to a client with expectation of blind acceptance and compliance. Little problem-solving, learning, adaptation, or independence occur, and home living is thwarted. "The management of one's personal self-care is critical to one's sense of self-worth and independence" (DeJong & Wenker, 1979). Performing self-care is a very personal matter beginning with rituals, habits, timing, and methods of carrying out these activities learned from families at a very young age. Additionally physical conditions in a home, such as the available toilets, plumbing, water, and the number of family members using facilities, all influence ways in which a client approaches self-care in ADL.

Other factors affecting self-care activities are internal or external rewards for either independence or dependence. For instance, in Western society an individual may be judged according to kindness, interpreted as doing things for others. Unfortunately the more independent a client becomes, the less attention she may receive, resulting in a negative response, perhaps regression. When teaching a client about ways to independence, be alert for perceived withdrawal of attention. The practice of "partnering" clients' "old injuries" with newly admitted clients may enable a nurse to remain supportive, akin to a cheerleading role, with the more independent client, while working with one who has more dependency needs. At times the mere physical presence of another individual can be a strong reinforcer. Judicious use of peer role models from a facility or the community may hold built-in rewards and reinforcements for both the role model who has reached a high level of independence and for the person with a newly acquired injury or impairment.

Education for Self-Sufficiency

Another practice that can have a negative effect on an individual who seeks greater independence and self-sufficiency is placing too much emphasis on the performance of skills and techniques, rather than on the control and direction of the care. With a severe functional loss, such as a spinal injury at the C-4 level, an individual may be construed to be totally dependent. Findings from research increasingly support independence as a state of mind, as well as a measure of physical functioning. For the individual who has impaired self-care abilities, directing self-care, interviewing, and selecting caregivers or personal assistants creates self-sufficiency and offers control over daily life events.

Sessions for training clients in effective skills for managing caregivers and personal assistants include content about interview processes, advertising for assistance and checking references or qualifications, managing finances, Workmens' Compensation or related legal matters, and assertiveness training—in addition to content regarding information about correct procedures or techniques and how to work with technology or maintain adaptive equipment.

Goal Development

Rehabilitation goals are directed toward helping the client achieve and maintain maximum independence and safe performance of self-care activities. Achievement of some independence in the performance of these skills is one measure of successful rehabilitation. The real measure of success should be focused on the client's ability to live an independent, successful life as he perceives it (Rogers, 1982).

Both long- and short-term goals are part of self-care. A goal is simply an expectation that may be constructive and attainable or unrealistic and extreme. Goals may center on the immediate such as "Will I live?" or "Will I be able to get out of this bed?" Short-term goals are related to long-term success. When short-term goals are too ambitious and stymie early success, a person may become discouraged and stop trying. On the other hand, short-term goals set too simply may lead to easy achievement—which may cloud realistic expectations for future challenges and mask the work necessary to achieve successful quality of life (Zejdlik, 1992).

Health professionals may rely too heavily on rehabilitation system goals rather than focusing on the client's goals. Although this attitude is changing, a rehabilitation nurse may unwittingly limit goals for a client's recovery by setting goals based on past experiences with other clients. For example, it may be realistic to set goals expecting a 10-year-old child with a spinal cord injury at the C-7 level to become functionally independent, while losing sight of other factors that affect the accomplishment of that goal. A client's working mother with two other children to care for may choose to dress the child herself; choosing time efficiency over self-care goals.

Goals that focus on the person, not the disability, promote higher satisfaction with quality of life. A client's long-term goals may be the same as if there were no disability or chronic condition (Zejdlik, 1992). Independence and autonomy in functional abilities (Morgan & McClain, 1993; Pedretti & Zoltan, 1990) and future aspirations are optimal criteria for short-term, long-term, or lifelong goals.

CONDITIONS ALTERING ABILITY TO PERFORM PERSONAL HYGIENE AND GROOMING ACTIVITIES
Condition-Specific Variations

Alterations in a client's ability to perform self-care in personal hygiene and grooming activities are related to a variety of conditions or impairments listed in Table 12-1. In some instances a single disease process may hamper ability, whereas in other instances multiple processes contribute to the client's limited self-care ability. Functional limitations also may be associated with cognitive impairment in ability to reason, solve problems, or communicate. It is difficult to teach a client who has impaired reasoning or problem-solving the importance of everyday hygiene such as not sharing toothbrushes, combs, or other items.

◆ Sensory variations

Safety is an ongoing concern for all clients. Alterations in sensory function may restrict vision, hearing, or touch and may cause a client to be vulnerable to accidents and injuries while performing self-care activities. Water temperatures or slippery floor surfaces may not be apparent to

Table 12-1

Conditions affecting self-care	Disorder
Paralysis or paresis of a hand	CVA, SCI, cerebral palsy, MD, TBI, arthritis
Decreased sensation of a hand or arm	SCI, TBI, CVA
Incoordination of upper extremities	Cerebral palsy, TBI
Perceptual deficits such as body image disturbances, spatial disorientation, and apraxia	Amputations, CVA, TBI
Hemianopsia	CVA
Limited range of motion; surgical procedure causing musculoskeletal limitation	Arthritis, SCI, CVA
Poor or weak hand grasp	SCI, MD, MS, arthritis
Amputation of an upper extremity	Amputation of an upper extremity
Limited endurance	Arthritis, MS, MD, SCI
Spasticity, ataxia, tremors	Parkinson's disease

CVA, cerebrovascular accident; SCI, spinal cord injury; TBI, traumatic brain injury; MD, muscular dystrophy; MS, multiple sclerosis.

a client. Poor balance may mean that a client performs personal hygiene and grooming activities while in a lying or sitting position to prevent injury from falls. Optokinetic nystagmus, an ocular movement reflex, was found to reduce a person's ability to perform personal hygiene and grooming activities independently (Duckworth, 1986). Using upper extremity dressing independence to indicate functional skill level, persons with right hemisphere brain damage following stroke accompanied by defective optokinetic nystagmus did not improve as well during rehabilitation as did those without optokinetic nystagmus. They also required a caregiver and were less likely to return to live at home (Dudgeon, DeLisa, & Miller, 1985).

✦ Limited mobility variations

Complete or partial assistance may be needed temporarily to limit client frustration and conserve energy. Persons with limited range of motion (ROM) and strength may have restricted movement of the head with limited ability to look up, down, or from side to side. Likewise limited ROM may alter a person's ability to raise or bend the arms and legs, and altered coordination may restrict ability to direct movement of the extremities. When fine motor movements of the hand are impaired, self-care items, personal appliances, and clothing may need to be adapted.

Location and Extent of Impairment as Variations

Before beginning an assessment, a rehabilitation nurse uses knowledge of the disease process or outcome expectations for the condition to understand the unique functional potential for each client and to probe areas of concern that may be overlooked. The assessment guidelines in Table 12-2 provide a sample of functional potential for a person according to level of spinal cord injury, as well as simple

Table 12-2 Functional assessment for activities of daily living (complete spinal cord injuries)

C-1–C-3
- Ventilator support needed
- Absence of movement in upper and lower extremities, absence of neck control
- Cardiac pacer or stimulator necessary

C-4
- Ventilator support may be needed (phrenic nerve is located at the C4 level)
- Shoulder shrug and neck control are present

C-5
- Involvement of both hands; hands are nonfunctional without assistive devices; client can learn to use his mouth for fine motor activities such as opening wrapper; contracted closed fists sometimes are more functional
- Absent or extremely weak triceps; without triceps use client will need to rely on pulling-type movements instead of pushing movement in performing dressing and other self-care activities; loops can be sewn onto pants or clothing to allow an individual with a C5 injury to hook her hand to her wrist in the loop to attempt a pulling movement, which is initiated by her biceps
- Severe weakness in trunk and lower extremities

C-6
- Involvement of upper extremities and hands
- Normal or good triceps (4 or 5 on testing scale)
- Generalized weakness of the trunk and lower extremities, interfering significantly with trunk balance and ambulation

C-7
- Involvement of upper extremities present
- Normal or good finger flexion and extension
- Grasp and release normal except for absence of intrinsic hand function responsible for the ability to spread fingers apart, which is not generally viewed as a functional activity
- Generalized weakness of trunk and lower extremities
- Poor balance

T-1–T-5
- Total abdominal paralysis or poor abdominal muscle strength (0-2 on testing scale); absence of abdominals greatly impairs client's ability to dress, undress, and perform other self-care activities because abdominals are the "balance muscles"
- No useful trunk sitting
- Normal upper extremity function

T-6–T-10
- Normal upper extremity function present
- Upper abdominal and spinal extension musculature sufficient to provide some element of trunk sitting

T-11–L-2
- Upper body function and extremities normal
- No quadriceps or very weak (quadriceps up to 2 on testing scale)

T-2–S-5
- Quadriceps in grades 3-5
- Ambulation with some support possible, requires strong upper body and a high level of conditioning (Zejdlik, 1992; Theuerkauf & Stewart, 1993)

Table 12-3 Parts of the brain

FRONTAL LOBE	PARIETAL
Expressive language	Body senses
Motor planning	Orientation
Emotion	Sensation
Creativity	Academic skill
Drive-motivation	Spatial relations
Impulse	
Abstract thought	**OCCIPITAL**
Sequencing	Vision
Reasoning	Visual perception
Judgment	
Initiation	**BRAINSTEM**
	Involuntary activities
TEMPORAL LOBE	Vegetative functions
Hearing	Digestion
Music	Sleep/wake
Understanding	Temperature
Receptive language	Respiratory center
Memory	Circulatory center

CEREBELLUM

Muscle coordination
Balance coordination

*An understanding of the various control centers of the brain will assist in developing appropriate self-care activities for individuals with traumatic brain injury as well as those with lateralized disabilities (CVA, etc.), which are summarized in this table.
CVA, cerebrovascular accident.
Information compiled from Ann Stewart. Kimberly Quality Care Rehabilitation Manual, 1993.

techniques to assess specific functions used when learning self-care activities.

Similarly knowing where a lesion lies relative to the various control centers in the brain and its extent may help a nurse to predict potential problem areas for a client. Table 12-3 compares functional abilities with their corresponding locations in the brain. Careful assessment determines whether a self-care deficit may be due to structural damage to an area of the brain or whether there is a perceptual, cognitive, or behavioral problem or a combination of deficits (Mossman, 1976). The underlying cause and extent of a person's impairment warrants a specific treatment plan to manage problems related to the limitation. For instance, a client who is able to physically perform the activities necessary for dressing does not dress independently when unable to initiate the activity. Consequently the treatment plan for this client would include developing appropriate cues so the client becomes aware of the problem. At that point a client may develop a personal external cueing system.

✦ Energy conservation variables

The level of energy available to a client is another factor that will fluctuate with movement along the illness trajectory and according to symptoms for the disease. Clients who have impaired respiratory or circulatory function may experience fatigue while performing self-care activities due to reduced stamina. With rheumatoid arthritis, for instance, joints characteristically become inflamed, but the eyes, heart, lungs, spleen, liver, blood vessels, kidneys, and digestive system also may be affected singly or in combination (Jackson & Neighbors, 1990). Rheumatoid arthritis presents multiple clinical problems that vary according to the stage of the disease, affecting functional abilities. The following three stages of rheumatoid arthritis occur:

1. Acute stage: joints are inflamed with typical symptoms of local swelling, redness, restricted ROM, and perhaps fluid accumulations in the joints. Activity is restricted.
2. Subacute stage: acute symptoms begin to subside and a client may resume self-care activities.
3. Chronic stage: signs of inflammation and instability are absent. Self-care activities are limited by pain, joint disorders, and muscle weakness (Lin, 1981).

Many progressive neuromuscular diseases and chronic conditions require clients to use energy conservation and work simplification techniques. Multiple sclerosis, Parkinson's disease, lupus erythematosus, muscular dystrophies, amyotrophic lateral sclerosis (ALS), cardiac and respiratory conditions, and arthritic diseases are a partial listing. A nurse assesses an individual's preinjury strength and endurance, current capabilities, and potential for regaining function (Sarver & Howard, 1982). When working with persons who have disorders requiring energy conservation, both client and team goals are prioritized.

NURSING ASSESSMENT

The client's presenting appearance gives a nurse information about his or her ability to perform self-care in hygiene and grooming and the client's own estimate of ability to perform these activities. Cues from the health history obtained before the physical and functional assessment provide information about current health practices and past and present health problems.

Subjective Assessment

During the history, information is gathered about the client's past self-care activities with attention focused on hygiene, grooming, and dressing. This interview is an excellent opportunity to gather more than historical information. When an interview is structured appropriately, it can be a chance to evaluate the client's perception of the disability, coping mechanisms, and other underlying information. A client who is comfortable will feel free to add information as the nurse allows the client the majority of the speaking. The nurse pays close attention to what the client says, what is not said, and how information is transmitted through body language, eye contact, and expressions (Kimberly Quality Care, 1991). Sessions may be shortened and resumed later for clients who cannot physically tolerate a complete assessment or who become irritable or agitated. When a client is easily distractible or holds a short attention span, structure the environment to minimize stimulations. In these ways behavior becomes another indicator to be used in developing the "how to" of teaching self-care activities. Behaviors are excellent indicators of a client's potential for achieving goals in a rehabilitation milieu. Suggested behavioral patterns to evaluate are

1. Problem-solving. When a client demonstrates a strength in openness to suggestions about ways of overcoming obstacles to self-care, ask: "If someone failed to place your wheelchair close to the bed, how would you reach it?"

2. Communication. Since communication is a reciprocal process, a client or family's ability to communicate effectively is essential data that may be gathered partly before a client's communication can be evaluated during an interview process.

3. Energy and enthusiasm. Ask a client, "Tell me how you feel about regaining independence in dressing?" or "What does it mean to you to be independent in toileting?"

4. Decisiveness. Decisiveness is a strong indicator of a client's ability to overcome the difficulties in relearning a skill such as dressing. Indecisiveness may indicate brain damage such as may follow stroke, which must be distinguished from inability to initiate an activity such as with traumatic brain injury or other stroke responses. The client with Parkinson's disease exhibits characteristic behaviors when unable to initiate a movement activity. Ask a client to complete this sentence: "I will be able to . . ."

5. Rationalization and projection. A client may present these defense mechanisms as an inability to accept responsibility for future outcomes or for the present. Lead with an open-ended statement: "You stated that your accident was caused by . . ."

6. Organizational planning—sequencing. Greet the client and ask, "How do you start your day?"

7. Maturity and interpersonal skills. Maturity is difficult to evaluate. Age and stage-related developmental tasks are partial criteria; or simply evaluate a client's demonstrated willingness to accept change and consider others. Lead with, "You will be sharing dressing areas with others; can you suggest ways that may avoid conflicts?"

Open-ended questions empower a client, as well as provide an opportunity for the nurse to gather information about a client's perception of how to participate in the rehabilitation process. A client is asked what a self-care behavior or action means to her, as well as when or under what circumstances it is important to perform, or not to perform, the activity. All areas of self-care from eating to dressing and personal care may be assessed in order to identify a client's preferences and lifestyle as well as to encourage participation. Questions are provided later in this chapter for eliciting information for self-care assessment; these questions follow corresponding information about the anatomy and physiology of hygiene and grooming for self-care.

✦ Pediatric history for self-care

When obtaining the history of a pediatric client, information is gathered from a parent or primary caregiver and the child. Assessment guides, tests, or instruments used for an infant, child, or young adolescent are age, culturally, and developmentally adjusted. Sole reliance on a parent for information may mask essential information about the child and family life, as well as void a valuable opportunity to evaluate self-care learning potential (Molnar, 1992).

Objective Assessment

After obtaining a history, the nurse physically examines the client for the following:

Hair: cleanliness, odor, texture, color, and distribution of hair; note infestations and scalp dryness or lesions.

Nails: cleanliness, color, and texture. Inspect nail contour for Beau's line (Fig. 12-1), condition of cuticles, and clubbing of fingertips.

Mouth: odor, color, and moisture of lips. Inspect inside the mouth for xerostomia or dry mouth, leukoplakia or other lesions, spots, or patches. Clients with impairments may have malocclusion, altered biting patterns, or nervous behaviors that injure the oral mucosa.

Teeth: cleanliness, plaque, occlusion, missing teeth, dental caries, restorations, sharp edges, chips, cracks, or loose teeth. Tooth color may indicate poor personal hygiene, food stains, or health risks such as cigarette smoking. Inspect dentures and prostheses for chips, fit, sharp edges, or loose parts.

Dress: fit and utility of apparel for cleanliness, condition, and appropriateness of clothes for climate as well as the client's age and lifestyle, finances, and culture.

Movement: unusual or out of place movement such as spasticity and tremors; test range of joint motion, strength, and dexterity; posture and balance are important for self-care. Assess hand-eye coordination and dominance.

Sensation: alterations in sensation may be barriers to a client's performing self-care activities. Paresis and reduced or absent sensation indicate safety precautions, including use of transfer belts, during self-care activities. Here, as with mobility exercises, the risks and benefits of restraints for safety must be weighted against maintaining independence for each client, including institutional or agency restraint policy.

Following the objective assessment, a nurse assesses a client's unique abilities for self-care through direct observation of the client performing personal hygiene and grooming activities. Additionally a nurse assesses a client's cognitive level and alertness and notes any impaired or altered posture, pattern, balance, or strength in mobility.

Assessing Conditions Common to Rehabilitation for Activities of Daily Living

The next section of this chapter contains specific assessment information pertinent to designing ADL programs for persons with a variety of conditions commonly encountered in rehabilitation nursing practice.

✦ Neuromuscular and spinal cord assessment

Understanding neuromusculoskeletal function enables a rehabilitation nurse to teach self-care activities more com-

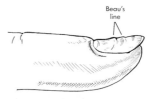

Fig. 12-1   Beau's lines.

OTHER NEUROMUSCULAR ASSESSMENTS

✦ Muscle strength: quality of controlled movement, not the quantity
✦ ROM: active versus passive
✦ Presence of pain according to client
✦ Fine motor and gross motor abilities
✦ Muscle tone: flaccidity, spasticity
✦ Kinesthetic perception: the body's place in space
✦ Balance: test for postural control during specific activity such as toileting; managing in bed, tub, or shower; ambulating; driving; sitting at a computer; or sitting in a wheelchair for sports or travel
✦ Body build and posture
✦ Alertness and cognition (Sine, Holcomb, Rausch, Liss, & Wilson, 1981)

Information compiled from Ann Stewart. Kimberly Quality Care Rehabilitation Manual, 1993.

pletely. Although not always responsible for a conducting a neuromuscular assessment, a rehabilitation nurse may use simple tests to assess the amount and type of information a client will need to maximize self-care (Denton, 1984). The boxes, above and at right, list tests for neuromuscular and spinal cord injury assessment of self-care functional abilities with illustrations about techniques.

✦ Hemiplegia

Functions of the brain such as communication, spatial awareness, or mathematic performance are "lateralized." This means the control centers for a particular function are located in one hemisphere of the brain. For example, the control center for speech is located in the left hemisphere of the brain. When assessing hemiplegia, a nurse looks beyond merely identifying and observing deficits. For example, when assessing a client with hemiplegia following stroke, a nurse would use the strength and coordination of the person's unaffected side as baseline data for learning how to modify self-care skills the person formerly performed with the affected side or with both hands. Since the person has sustained injuries to one hemisphere of the brain, the tendency is for the person to process more information using the intact hemisphere. If the client has sustained damage to the left hemisphere, where speech and communication are controlled, the nurse will rely on communication such as pictures, symbols, gestures, or visual cues other than verbal means to help a client to relearn self-care skills. The nurse seeks a client's "learning strengths" based on the intact hemisphere to evaluate self-care skills. (Chapter 16 and Chapter 25 provide additional information.)

✦ Traumatic brain injury

Specific motor/physical skills, impaired balance, poor coordination, generalized weakness, and level of endurance are assessed for a client with traumatic brain injury (Rosenthal, Griffen, Bond, & Miller, 1990). Particular attention to assess cognitive and perceptual status is beneficial because these may affect the outcome for clients learn-

---

SIMPLE ASSESSMENTS AND TECHNIQUES OF SELF-CARE POTENTIAL FOR PERSONS WITH NEUROMUSCULAR OR SPINAL CORD INJURY CONDITIONS

GRIP TEST

Shake hands with client. Grip right to right and left to left. Evaluate both thumb and finger function for normal grip. Spasticity, contractions, and decreased strength will all impact on self-care activities. If pincher grasp is present (movement of first finger to thumb), client should be able to perform many self-care activities with modification.

TRICEPS TEST

Have client straighten arm over head then bend arm at the elbow, moving hand behind head. The examiner places hand against forearm. Client lifts forearm against resistance. This test will evaluate an over-the-head movement as well as general range of motion, triceps strength, and deltoid strength. Some individuals will be able to push against resistance, but due to severe spasticity or decreased range of motion the movement is not functional, preventing client from having functional movement over the head. Absence or extreme weakness of the triceps will make pushing movements such as pushing clothing down impossible without adjustment of the hand position to involve the biceps.

BALANCE TEST

While "spotting" client from behind, ask her to move to the front of the seat of the wheelchair or straight-back chair and fold arms across chest with the elbows pointing forward, away from the body. Watch the abdominal area to evaluate abdominal control and strength. If these appear stable, gently push client from side to side or front to back and observe for compensatory movements. Weak or absent abdominal control will make sitting balance—is necessary in dressing—difficult to maintain. This will require compensatory positioning when teaching dressing, as well as other activities that require leaning over a sink.

SPINAL COLUMN MOBILITY TEST

With hips stationary, ask client to look behind himself or herself by rotating as far as he can. Evaluate both neck and trunk rotation. Inadequate trunk rotation will make upper extremity dressing difficult and probably will necessitate teaching over-the-head pull-on technique even with button-up shirts, coats, and dresses (Theuerkauf, 1992).

---

ing self-care activities and hygiene following traumatic brain injury. Similar perceptual problems may occur following cerebrovascular accidents (CVAs) and brain injury as described in the following list:

1. Agnosia is an inability to recognize a common object such as a comb, toothbrush, mirror, or item of clothing. A common self-care or grooming item is placed before a client; the person is requested to select and

pick up the named item and then to tell or demonstrate its use. Agnosia variations include tactile agnosia when a client is unable to recognize an object through touch or handling (Zoltan, Siev, & Freishtat, 1986).

2. Apraxia is an inability to perform a learned activity even when the person has motor ability to do so. When assessing self-care abilities, the rehabilitation nurse examines individual activities to identify particular difficulties due to apraxia. For example, a client with constructional apraxia has limited ability to perform purposeful actions using self-care items such as brushing teeth, combing hair, or shaving. This person may be unable to understand verbal commands or to carry them out and can be expected to have difficulty with sequencing of steps in an activity. A simple assessment is to ask a client to take a brush and brush the hair. Second, ask a client to copy a picture of a house on another paper. Incomplete lines or incorrect proportions indicate possible constructional apraxia (Zoltan et al., 1986).

3. Disturbed body schemata occur when a client becomes unaware of body structure and may not be clear where the body begins or ends. Ask a client: "Show me your left knee" and then "Place the left foot on the floor" (Zoltan et al., 1986).

4. Disturbances of body image may be manifestations of unilateral neglect. Ask a client to draw a picture; drawing half a picture indicates neglect is probable.

5. Figure-ground and depth perception problems occur when a person has difficulty differentiating foreground from background. Although some decrease in depth perception occurs with aging, the disturbance is more severe with a client who has cognitive impairment. Easily and often distracted, a client may have a short attention span for learning or carrying out self-care activities. Ask a client to pick up a white washcloth spread flat on a white sheet; observe for distractibility.

The following cognitive abilities are evaluated:
+ Attention to task (as a skill essential for a client to learn dressing skills)
+ Orientation to environment (lack of orientation usually precludes self-care)
+ Sequencing (does the client use the proper order of steps when applying makeup or when dressing?)
+ Ability to generalize to other learning situations
+ Initiation (beginning a task without verbal prompting)

+ **Pediatric assessment**

When assessing a client who is a child, the general areas previously discussed are included along with disability-specific assessments. With a child, the following three points govern assessment:
+ Movement is assessed according to expectations for the child's chronologic age; cultural differences and developmental age are considered.
+ Functional mobility is assessed specific to the level and the type of disability.
+ Neurologically influenced movement is assessed, including both fine and gross motor function (Molnar, 1992).

Childhood developmental activities that have an impact on a child's potential for independent self-care are listed in Table 12-4 for categories of age, self-help, gross motor, fine motor, and play.

NURSING DIAGNOSES

Nursing diagnoses reflect a client's strengths and limitations for self-care activities based on assessment. Interventions are governed by client preferences, scientific nursing knowledge, and nursing experience. Table 12-5 lists nursing diagnoses and interventions commonly used with self-care and ADL. NANDA nursing diagnoses (Gordon, 1993) related to personal hygiene and grooming activities include:

+ **Self-care deficit.** A client who is unable to perform personal self-care activities due to limitation resulting from impaired motor, sensory, or cognitive function or in combination may be diagnosed with impaired self-care. Is the client unable or unwilling to perform these ADL? Can the client manipulate devices such as a toothbrush, comb, hairbrush, or razor as needed to perform hygiene activities? Are assistive devices available that enable these activities? Is the client able to manipulate objects such as toothpaste dispenser, deodorant, cosmetics, shampoo, tampon, or sanitary pad? Is the client able to don, fasten, wash, obtain, and replace articles of clothing? What about incontinence pants or pads, sheath or Texas catheters, or similar aids? Planning should include strategies to enable the individual to perform these tasks with optimum responsibility and minimum assistance (Hudson, 1983).

+ **Impaired bathing/hygiene and self-care.** The bases for this diagnosis may be perceptual, sensory, or motor impairment resulting in an individual becoming unable to wash, regulate water, or gather items for hygiene such as preparing to bathe. Planning includes safety precautions against injuries, as well as a consistent routine in a private environment.

+ **Altered self-dressing/grooming.** An individual who lacks motor ability, activity tolerance, cognitive/perceptual capabilities or lacks adequate strength may not be able to perform all or part of a grooming or dressing activity. Planning to select manageable clothing, allowing time to dress, coaching sequences in donning clothing, and encouraging independence in dressing may improve outcome.

+ **Activity intolerance due to fatigue.** When a client experiences fatigue with a chronic or disabling condition, activity intolerance alone may restrict participation in or completion of personal hygiene and grooming activities. Grooming hair requires strength and endurance for holding the arms above the head for a time. Persons with conditions such as arthritis may not be able to perform this activity without planned rest. Planning for rest periods may pace a client until the component steps of these activities can be relearned and endured. Assistive devices may enable a client to maintain independence.

+ **Impaired knowledge.** A client may have poor personal hygiene or grooming as a result of a chronic, disabling, or developmental disorder; perceptual, sensory, or motor impairments may interfere with ability to perform tasks. Although strategies to increase knowledge about personal care and to develop skills are therapeutic interventions, knowledge alone does not predict improved personal care activity frequency or outcome.

Table 12-4 Normal childhood development having impact on self-care activities

Age (years)	Self-help (Sanford, 1973)	Gross motor (Denton, 1984)	Fine motor (Denton, 1984)	Play (DeJong & Wenker, 1979)
0-1	Picks up object Feeds self cracker Fusses to be changed after bowel movement	Plays in standing Sits independently Has no differentiation of head and neck	Holds bottle without help Uses grasp reflex Uses radial digital grasp with extended wrist	Places hands and toys in mouth
1-2	Can unzip zipper Pulls up socks Unwraps object	Has good walking and running skills Demonstrates equilibrium reactions in standing Reaches well with arms while standing	Drinks from small glass Needs help releasing cup Demonstrates accurate placement of forms Finger-feeds self	
2-3	Removes coat or dress Dries own hands Gets drink unassisted	Stands on one foot (5 seconds)	Washes and dries hands	Plays interactive games
3-4	Unbuttons buttons Dresses with supervision Undresses	Stands one foot (10 seconds) Walks up and down stairs Marches	Imitates	Shares toys Talks while playing Concept of 2
4-5	Laces shoes Can cut with knife Washes face and hands unassisted	Jumps over objects Climbs stairs with alternating steps		Concept of 3 Role plays Likes to play with others
5-6	Dresses without assistance Begins brushing teeth supervised	Has gross motor control and body awareness	Demonstrates hand preference Draws well Prints simple words	Likes dramatic play Likes group play Plays purposefully
6-7	Continues improving dress Bathes independently Brushes teeth independently Combs hair supervised	Shows better gross motor coordination Rides a bike		Enjoys active games Is competitive Identifies with sex peers in group
8-9	Knows differences and similarities Dressing like others is important	Arms lengthening and growing	Has better manipulative skills	Is loyal to "gang"
9-10	Plans future actions Solves problems		Eyes are almost mature	Enjoys sports and hobbies Appreciates reality over fantasy (may begin as early as 7 years)
7-12			Enjoys game characteristics of play School is important Has some awareness of rules and boundaries Demonstrates beginnings of group orientation	
12-16	Acquires basic habits such as regular bathing, tooth care, hair care		Play takes on mature function Teamwork and cooperation are emphasized Is very concerned about following rules	

Based on information from Sanford, 1973; Denton, 1984; DeJong & Wenker, 1979.

Table 12-5 Examples of nursing diagnoses and nursing interventions for the client with deficits in personal hygiene and grooming activities

Nursing diagnosis	Nursing intervention
SELF-CARE DEFICIT	
Bathing/hygiene	Collaborate with occupational therapist and other disciplines to accomplish goals
Hair grooming	Teach use of adapted devices: long-handled comb, brush
	Teach use of external modifiers: handles, universal strap
	Teach use of assistive devices: around the neck mirror, shampoo tray, shower hose
	Teach use of appliances: hair blower, electric comb, electric razor, battery razor, razor with universal strap
Mouth	Lubricate mouth, use mouthwash
	Teach proper brushing and flossing
	Refer to physician and dentist when lesions found
Teeth	Teach dental hygiene and use of adapted devices: one-handed dental floss holder, handles on toothbrush, modified electric toothbrush, water-Pik, toothpaste squeeze key, toothpaste pump dispenser
	Collaborate with occupational therapist and other disciplines to accomplish goals
	Refer to dentist
Menstrual management	Teach different positions to facilitate insertion of tampon or placement of pad
	Teach ways to adapt underwear
	Teach use of assistive or adapted devices
DRESSING/GROOMING	
Nails	Teach use of adapted devices: external modifiers, handles on clippers
	Refer to podiatrist when necessary
Shaving	Teach to organize equipment in safe area
	Teach use of assistive and adapted equipment when needed
Application of deodorant	Teach different positions to use for ease of application
Application of makeup	Teach one-handed techniques for opening containers, tubes
	Teach use of neck mirrors, stand-up mirrors
	Give appropriate feedback
KNOWLEDGE DEFICIT	
Personal hygiene	Plan varies according to area of deficit
	Consider client's abilities, values, developmental level, interest, past experience, readiness to learn
	Involve family
	Plan time to teach
	Use appropriate methods to teach according to client's preference and learning ability
	Collaborate with other team members to plan and implement client and family education
Grooming	Teach use of specially designed equipment, clothing
	Teach use of clothing closure devices: snaps, zippers, Velcro, hooks
	Teach use of assistive devices: spray shoe polish dispenser, electric shoe polisher, buttons, elastic, shoehorn, reacher
	Teach modified dressing techniques
	Refer to occupational therapy
	Collaborate with occupational therapist and other disciplines to accomplish goals
ACTIVITY INTOLERANCE	Plan specific activity schedule with client, nursing staff, and other team members according to client's physical, physiological, psychosocial abilities
POTENTIAL FOR INJURY	Teach about safety hazards as result of perceptual or physical deficits
	Involve family as necessary in use of safety measures for personal hygiene, dressing activities
	Collaborate with other team members to plan, teach, and implement safe use of assistive and adapted devices and special techniques

✦ **Potential for injury.** This diagnosis is becoming increasingly important to rehabilitation nurses whose clients may have impairments due to perceptual, sensory, or motor deficits; lack of awareness of safe self-care practices; or lack of attention to environmental hazards. Premorbid personality, family or social system, lifestyle, risk-taking behavior, or substance abuse may heighten the potential for a client to have this nursing diagnosis. Planning incorporates assistive devices, adaptive equipment, and information about prevention and safety.

GOAL DEVELOPMENT AND PLANNING

Rehabilitation goals are directed toward helping a client achieve and maintain maximum independence and safety in self-care activities. Realistic goals are those mutually determined with the client and family. Success of a client's rehabilitation is influenced by support received from the family when included from the beginning of the rehabilitation process. Support and instructions from rehabilitation team members will help the family assist the client in achieving maximum independence throughout life.

Goals for self-care activities in personal hygiene and grooming flow from nursing diagnoses to define clearly what the client, family, and nurse intend to accomplish. Setting priorities for goal accomplishment may motivate a client to continue and attempt the next goal (McCourt, 1993). (Chapter 10 provides additional discussion of the influence of readiness and teachable moments.) Broad outcome statements for maximum independence in personal hygiene and grooming activities are for a client to be able to

- ✦ Perform personal hygiene and grooming activities at the highest level of function possible
- ✦ Understand when and how to use assistive devices or adaptive equipment
- ✦ Plan for rest periods before fatigue occurs
- ✦ Understand the role of personal hygiene and grooming in promoting good health and maintaining and restoring positive self-esteem in body image
- ✦ Practice personal hygiene and grooming activities safely within one's own environment

SPECIFIC GOALS FOR CHRONIC OR DISABLING DISORDERS

The following goals are important for specific disability groups.

Goals with Spinal Cord Injury

✦ **C1–C4.** At this level of functional disability, self-directed care is paramount. A person who relies on others for physical care, gains when taught how to function assertively in a personal attendant relationship. Independence is the ability to control the environment, direct care, and plan for the future. (Chapter 13 and Chapter 27 provide additional information.)

✦ **C5–C7.** The goals for these levels will vary depending on intact functional ability and individual determination. For a person injured at C-6 or C-7, the goal of physical independence is a possibility with a substantial commitment to work and challenge.

✦ **T-1–T1-2.** Functional independence at wheelchair level is within reach with education and commitment, barring any presence of outside forces. Some persons with paraplegia may ambulate aided by braces, stimulators, or computers. However, practicality and true functional outcome remain questions.

✦ **L-1–S-4.** Individuals with lower spinal cord injuries may ambulate with crutches and braces. But as with other paraplegic conditions, many choose to use wheelchairs when energy conservation is an issue.

Function and Appearance

Research findings about the behavior of adolescents and young adults with disabilities indicate they are concerned with feeling "normal." They attempt to normalize in three areas: physical appearance and function, physical and emotional independence, and social skills and interpersonal relationships (Rogers, 1982). Attempts at "normalcy" in appearance may account in part for certain clients with quadriplegia who resist using assistive devices.

Goals with Hemiplegia

In reverse, the primary goal for a person with hemiplegia, as well as anyone working with hemiplegia, is to communicate openly along perceptual channels. The perceptual difficulties experienced following hemiplegia are so subtle as to be overlooked (Chen Sea, Henderson, & Cermark, 1993). Healthcare professionals themselves err by giving oral instructions to a person who has severe aphasia but who appears to have independent functional abilities (Rosenthal, et al., 1990).

Programs of self-care for a person with hemiplegia build on full physical and cognitive development of the intact side. By activating strengths of the intact cerebral hemisphere, an individual uses that side, as well as assistive devices, to overcome functional impairments from the hemiplegia. For instance, a person with difficulty understanding verbal communication through language may benefit by strengthening learning through visual or computer programs, including augmentative communication. Any return to motor function is an additional asset (The Arthritis Foundation, 1969).

Goals Following Traumatic Brain Injury

Goals for the individual with traumatic brain injury relate to the level that the individual is able to achieve. Table 12-6 displays goal setting according to a recognized scale for levels of cognition. Just as in spinal cord injuries, these goals vary considerably and rely on several factors. Individuals who have sustained a brain injury often have significant motor and cognitive difficulties but may recover with little or no physical impairment. A client may have motor capabilities to perform all self-care skills but continue to need verbal cueing; this in itself can cause difficulty. Although an individual may appear unimpaired, a client may have significant cognitive and behavioral difficulties that require one-on-one assistance (Hagen, 1984). "Skilled care" needs as interpreted by insurance companies may not be apparent. Finding support may be difficult and place added burden on the family. Subsequently, in brain injury rehabilitation programs, as well as programs that deal with other disabilities, goal development and setting must be client and family focused.

Table 12-6 Basic goals based on Rancho levels of cognition

Level	Goal
I, II, III, IV	Activate a response Decrease agitation Increase awareness
V, VI	Activate purposeful and appropriate response
VII, VIII	Increase ability to perform ADL with little or no direct supervision

Information compiled from Ann Stewart. Kimberly Quality Care Rehabilitation Manual 1993.

Goals with Altered Strength and Endurance

In dealing with persons who have altered strength and endurance, the primary goal is to control the environment. This might be done by arranging both activity schedules and the physical environment to allow for rest within the daily schedule. Monitored programs can be designed to increase endurance and stamina gradually, according to individual tolerance and goals.

Disease processes such as arthritis have different stages that require different goals throughout the program. However, a consistent and properly paced exercise program can make the difference between recovery with good function of the joints and recovery with "burned-out . . . joints" (Phipps, 1995).

Goals for the individual with Parkinson's disease, both in learning self-care activities and later in life, encourage a client in gaining effective coping skills (see Chapter 13). Frustration occurs when family or friends do not allow a client to do as much as possible, often because completing activities takes a long time and may become tedious. Caregiver goals are to encourage the client, to allow the client to perform as many activities or parts of activities as possible (Morgan & McClain, 1993). Caregivers may remind the client about performance aids such as completing activities in one continuous movement or "nose over toes" when arising from a seated position.

Goals with Limb Deficiencies

Goals for individuals who have limb deficiencies, often due to surgical amputation, vary according to the site, degree, and status of the amputation and the overall health of the individual (Yetzer, Kauffman, Sopp, & Talley, 1994). Generally three primary goals are (1) a client's acceptance of the amputation, (2) integration of the prosthesis into the client's body image, and (3) utilization of the prosthesis to achieve the highest functional level of independence. Dressing skills for persons with lower limb deficiencies may be hampered by imbalance due to shifts in center of gravity. When these affect balance, a person may not be able to lean forward or backward safely without assistance. Persons with upper limb deficiencies may benefit from modified clothing, assistive devices, environmental control units, and adaptive equipment. Adapted switch toys and computer programs are widely available for children who have limited or absent upper limb function. Both fixed and motorized

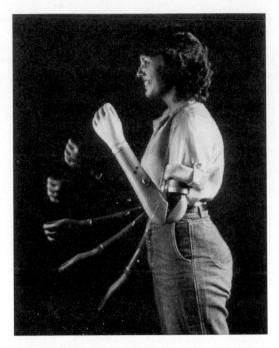

Fig. 12-2 The Utah arm is a myoelectric elbow and hand system developed to enable clients with above and below elbow amputations to function independently and with high levels of skill in their daily activities and work. The Utah myoelectric arm features proportional control. (From Rehabilitative/Restorative Care by S.P. Hoeman, 1990, St. Louis, Mosby–Year Book. Copyright 1990 by permission; Photos courtesy of Motion Control, division of 10 MED. Inc., Salt Lake City, Utah.)

prostheses are available for individual client's needs and lifestyles (Fig. 12-2). The art and science of prosthetics has entered a new era of cosmetic appearance, utility, function, comfort, and fit.

Goals with Pediatric Clients

The long-term goal for the pediatric client is self-care management and includes family-centered goals. However, the ultimate goal is effective transition into community-based programs and return to the appropriate educational environment that will allow continuation of mastery of self-care activities. Ultimately that very mastery of self-care skills will place the child in the least restrictive environment (Hoeman, 1992).

REHABILITATION NURSING INTERVENTIONS

After the initial client assessment, the nurse is able to develop an individualized plan with the client's strengths and limitations in mind. Interventions are chosen with client and family input to promote maximum health, independence, and safety and are based on nursing knowledge and accepted standards of practice.

Therapeutic intervention to self-care may involve teaching a client and family the problem-solving process, supplementing self-care abilities by providing assistive or adapted devices when necessary, and educating the client and family regarding safe and effective performance of self-care skills (see Box, p. 167).

PRINCIPLES USED WHEN TEACHING ANY ACTIVITY OF DAILY LIVING

1. Know procedure thoroughly before starting to teach client.

2. Know client's abilities and limitations, and do not expect achievement beyond ability. Expect to provide extended supervision, since client may forget part of the procedure from one day to the next.

3. Provide encouragement, but do not pressure client to perform. When difficulty is experienced, provide help to try another activity that can be performed, then return to the first procedure later.

4. Use assistive or adapted devices if client does not have the use of muscles needed to perform task. Provide proper equipment for activity and allow sufficient time and space so client does not feel rushed or restricted.

5. Be flexible. Adapt procedures with help and suggestions of client and family. If one method does not work, try another.

6. Ensure that everyone who works with client is aware of what is being taught. Each person involved in teaching should teach the same way, follow the same steps, and use the same terms.

7. Give instructions as simply as possible, using short sentences and repeating them often. If client has difficulty understanding a sentence, it should be reworded. Gestures should be used to clarify directions, especially with clients who have language problems.

8. Repeat procedure each time client would normally perform activity (Mossman, 1976).

Teaching Children

Teaching self-care activities to pediatric clients requires a unique approach. A child is not merely a small adult but a person with growing functional development (Rosenthal et al., 1990; Hoeman, 1992). The following hints should be helpful in teaching self-care activities to pediatric patients:

1. Use age-appropriate teaching techniques, such as toys and games for younger children
2. Begin teaching self-care activities at the preschool level (Molnar, 1992), when dolls or puppets in play situations are effective
3. Use rhythm and rhymes to instill patterns for self-care activities
4. Pay attention to patterns of growth and development, particularly with a child following a traumatic brain injury (Pedretti & Zoltan, 1989)
5. Similarly, attend to patterns of cognitive development
6. Keep fun in learning

Another technique for teaching ADL at any age is sequential steps that break tasks into small units. A person completes as many units of a sequence as possible, even though the nurse may assist with some units. Clients should be reminded of safety precautions with each activity they are

learning. Frequent repetition of instructions, demonstration of the activity by the nurse or therapist, practice with each step of the activity, and the evaluation of performance assists in learning. Limiting distractions in the environment makes it easier for the client to concentrate on the instructions and to practice the component steps of the activity.

Specific Techniques for Personal Care
✦ Personal hygiene

Hand-washing—especially before eating meals and after toileting—and individual towels, washcloths, and personal articles have become essential to personal hygiene. Avoid soap and products that interfere with the natural pH of the skin; apply lotion after washing to prevent chafing or irritation and to promote skin integrity (Chapter 15). Clients who have an active lifestyle may use alternate methods for hand-washing, such as individually wrapped towelettes that can be dropped into backpacks or purses and used when sinks or bathrooms are unavailable. The large-sized boxes of towelettes at bedside are convenient for hand-washing before and after toileting.

Ask clients or families about special rules, customs, or rituals they may use in self-care activities. There are various ethnic or cultural beliefs and practices about washing and bathing activities that may vary further with individuals or families. As a rule never remove amulets, pins, necklaces, or bracelets without permission of the client or family. Never cut hair or nails without permission; never dispose of hair, nail trimmings, or other body remnants except as directed by a client or family member (Hoeman, 1990).

✦ Hair

Hair consists of threads of hard keratin that project through the epidermis from epithelial bulbs located in the dermis; only the hair shaft is visible. Beneath the dermis, the root is encased in a hair follicle. Muscles in the dermis attached to the hair follicles contract to conserve heat when the body temperature is lowered, resulting in "gooseflesh" skin (Phipps, Cassmeyer, Sands, & Lehman, 1995). Two types of body hair are the pigmented vellus hair over large body areas and the longer, coarser, and pigmented terminal hair. The entire body—except for palms of the hands, soles of the feet, and parts of the genitalia—is covered with hair. Hair grows at varying rates and sheds 20 to 100 strands a day.

Characteristics of hair differ among ethnic groups. For instance, hair appears coarse when the shaft is flat and may twist on itself to form whorls or loops. A dull sheen may be caused by a concentration of microscopic air bubbles that diffuse and reflect light, giving a matte appearance. Hair pulled back tightly in elaborate styles for long periods may become fragile, resulting in alopecia, or may become damaged by styling in corn rows or by pick combing or using hot combs (Owens, 1984).

Hair changes commonly occur with aging; changes in melanin production cause hair to thin and gray. Testosterone controls hair distribution in both sexes, resulting in diminished pubic and axillary hair and loss of scalp hair in men with aging. As estrogen decreases, older women may discover hair on the chin and upper lip (Hudson, 1983). Men have increased hair on the ears and in the nostrils. Hair growth patterns and distribution reflect health; abnor-

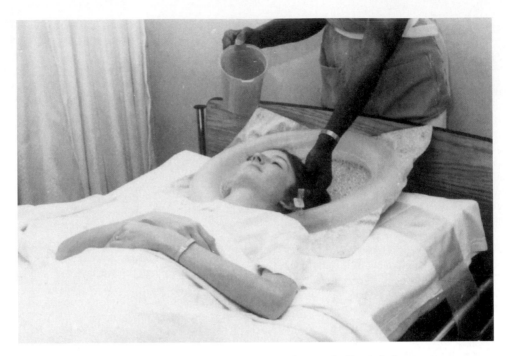

Fig. 12-3   Shampoo tray being used to wash client's hair.

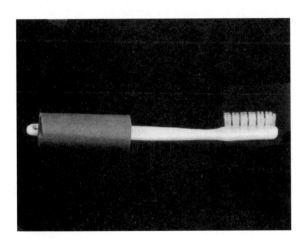

Fig. 12-4   Toothbrush with adapted handle.

mal hair loss, excessive hair growth, or changes in hair texture may be caused by hormonal imbalance, general ill health, infection, chronic liver disease, or drugs.

Combing and brushing the hair daily prevents tangling and matting, and biweekly shampoos maintain clean hair unless the hair is oily and needs to be shampooed more frequently. Persons of some ethnic groups lubricate, stretch, loop, braid, or straighten their hair. Careful brushing minimizes breaking hair strands; combing hair while wet using a wide-toothed comb will reduce tangling; rolling or braiding rather than pulling while styling is less apt to result in alopecia (Sims, 1976). When unable to sit or balance at a sink or in a shower, a client may need assistance to shampoo. A shower tray or a clean pan, even a bedpan, placed behind the head can collect rinse water while the person lies on a stretcher or in bed for a shampoo (Fig. 12-3).

The person who has left-sided paresis or is hemiplegic may have difficulty combing the back section of the hair and may tend to neglect the left side. Suggesting through verbal cues may be an effective strategy. For example, a rhyme about "brush the back" may cue the behavior. However, a person with right-sided hemiplegia who develops agnosia may construe the comb to be a toothbrush and put the comb into the mouth. When use of the comb is demonstrated, this client will learn proper use of the comb quickly. Built-up handles on self-care or assistive devices enable a client to grip items securely so they are easier to handle (Fig. 12-4). When a client has difficulty with grip, the universal cuff will hold combs or brushes as well as other self-care items. Looped straps attached to brushes create a space where a person, including a person with C5 or C6 spinal cord injury, could slide a hand through and then brush the hair (Fig. 12-5).

Should a client's hair be infested with lice or nits, treat with gamma benzene hexachloride (Kwell) shampoo or other specific medication. Regular shampoos can be used within 24 hours after treatment. A fine-toothed comb used for several days will remove remaining nits. All personal hair care items as well as towels, washcloths, and linens are washed and reserved for individual use.

✦ The mouth and teeth

The mucous membrane of the mouth is a continuation of the skin in the body orifices. Mucous membranes secrete mucus, salt, and enzymes to protect the mouth from harmful organisms. Additionally these membranes absorb nutrients into the body and provide support for the teeth as they masticate food in the initial stage of digestion (Normal & Snyder, 1982). Each tooth is composed of a crown, a root, and a pulp cavity. The dentin is the internal part of the crown covered with hard enamel. Covered with bony ce-

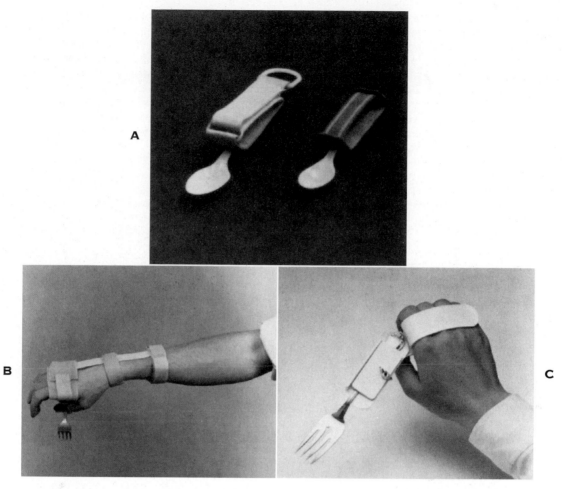

Fig. 12-5 **A,** A universal cuff can grip many self-care items. **B,** Universal cuffs may be combined with wrist splints for support and stability. **C,** This universal cuff uses a C-clip and a different style pocket.

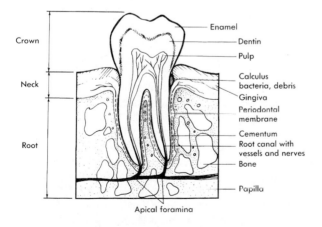

Fig. 12-6 Cross-section of normal tooth.

mentum, the root is embedded in the jaw, and the center pulp cavity contains blood vessels and nerves (Fig. 12-6).

Two major consequences of poor oral hygiene are dental caries and periodontal disease. Dental plaque, a thick putty-like material composed of salivary deposits, food particles, and bacteria forms around the neck of the tooth. If dental plaque is not removed regularly, anaerobic bacteria react with sucrose in the plaque to form an acid that attacks the surface enamel of the tooth, causing dental caries. Untreated caries may reach nerves in the pulp of the tooth, causing pain, infection, or abscess. Plaque irritates soft tissue as gingivitis, which in turn can destroy soft tissue and supporting bone with loosening and subsequent loss of the teeth.

The oral mucosa of elderly patients is thin and less resistant to disease. Because the elderly often experience tooth loss from neglect or disease, some form of denture may be needed. Dentures are supported by the bones of the jaw, or alveoli dentales. These bones are absorbed slowly throughout life, often causing difficulty with the fit of dentures and consequent problems with speech and mastication. Absence of teeth and loose-fitting dentures contribute to poor nutrition. Chronic illness, lowered resistance, and medication regimens may make dental treatment for the elderly a hazardous procedure.

Good oral hygiene contributes to physical and mental well-being. Daily flossing and brushing with a soft toothbrush with end-rounded bristles removes food particles and

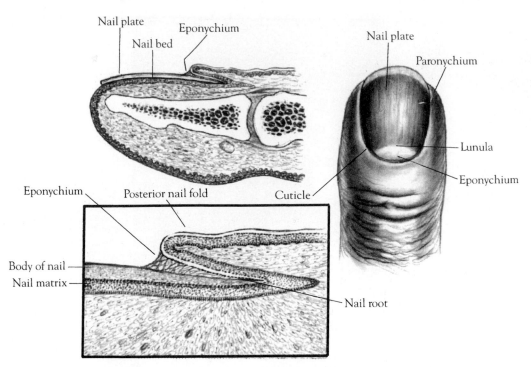

Fig. 12-7 Structures of nail. (From Mosby's Clinical Nursing, 3rd ed, by Thompson, 1993, St. Louis, Mosby–Year Book. Copyright 1993 by permission.)

plaque, strengthens the gums, and prevents plaque formation and tooth decay. When a client is unable to perform mouth care, stand behind the client who is seated, with instructions to tilt the head backward as if to look at the ceiling. The caregiver then supports the client's head in a position to perform mouth care.

Dentures are cleaned with a soft brush and dentifrice after a client finishes eating. When the dentures are removed at night, allowing the oral mucosa to recover from any irritation, a client rinses the mouth to remove food particles. Dentures are examined every 6 months for proper fit or replacement needs.

A client who has limited or absent function in one hand grasps a toothpaste tube close to the top and uses the thumb and index finger of the unaffected hand to turn the cap. With minimal grasp, a client stabilizes the tube between the knees and uses the sides of both hands to twist; pump tubes of toothpaste now are available. As with other self-care items, an electric toothbrush and water-Pik can be adapted for independent handling.

Good oral hygiene and regularly scheduled dental examinations are practiced and taught as part of the rehabilitation process. When toothaches, dental caries, or other mouth problems are present, the client should be referred to a dentist. With alteration in a client's ability to perform oral hygiene, the nurse collaborates with a dentist, dental hygienist, and occupational therapist to modify procedures or design adaptive devices.

♦ Nails

Nails are hard flattened keratin cells that grow as a nail plate at a rate of about 1 ml/week. Nails help protect the fingers from injury. If the matrix is injured, the nail may grow in a split or distorted manner; if the matrix is de-

stroyed, the nail is permanently lost and replaced by stratum corneum of the epidermis (Phipps et al, 1995) (Fig. 12-7). Some common problems affecting the nails are paronychia, ingrown toenails, and onychauxis. Paronychia, or inflammation of the tissue around the nail, often is the result of an infected "hangnail." Ingrown toenails may result from a familial trait, improper cutting, or wearing tight ill-fitting shoes. Onychauxis, or hypertrophy or thickening of the nails, is associated with aging, nutritional disturbances, repeated trauma, or degenerative diseases. With the degenerative disease, the nail plate may become thickened, discolored, and difficult to trim.

Appearance of the nails may change with age and ill health. As aging occurs, nails have a tendency to become thick and brittle. Brittleness, roughness, or a change in shape of a nail may indicate metabolic disease, nutritional imbalance, or digestive disturbance; Beau's lines (temporary horizontal grooves in the nails) suggest an internal disorder. The nail bed may reveal cyanosis or be used to assess circulation when a cast or elastic bandage is in place.

Fingernails are trimmed in a curve, using an emery board to file rough edges. Soaking dirty nails before using a nailbrush will ease removal of soil underneath the nails, but only mild soap is used because harsh soap may dry the nails and cause them to become brittle. Suction cups attached to a table or countertop stabilize a nailbrush, adapted file, and nail clipper when gross motor skills or only one hand is available to hold an item (Fig. 12-8). Soak toenails, then cut straight across. An orange stick is used gently to remove dirt without injuring underlying skin. Those clients who have thickened nails, calluses, or ingrown toenails or who have diabetes or peripheral neuropathy may be referred to a podiatrist.

When a client has limited ROM or pain in the hands or

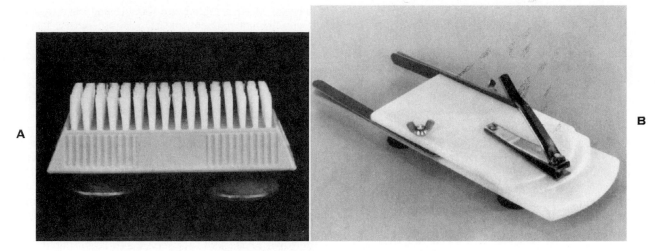

Fig. 12-8 **A,** Nailbrush stabilized with suction cups. (From Rehabilitation Nursing: Process & Application by Dittmar, 1989, St. Louis, Mosby–Year Book. Copyright 1989 by permission.) **B,** Many assistive devices are available to enable clients to participate in self care activities. A client who is able to use one hand can cut his own nails with this assistive nail clipper. (From Rehabilitative/Restorative Care by S.P. Hoeman, 1990, St. Louis, Mosby–Year Book. Copyright 1990 by permission; Reprinted by permission of © Bissell Healthcare Corporation/Fred Sammons, Inc.)

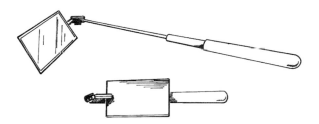

Fig. 12-9 Long-handled skin inspection mirror.

when a client's hands are fixed in a closed position or grasp, use care to open, wash, and dry the skin; with the feet, gently dry skin between the toes to prevent moist maceration of the skin (Graham & Morley, 1984). This client may have difficulty with balance or with reaching the toes, requiring adapted devices or total assistance. Loss of sensation in the extremities may result in a client not being aware of early signs of infection, ingrown toenails, or dry and cracked tissue surrounding the nails or the nails themselves. Clients who have impaired vision may use a stabilized magnifying glass or require assistance with nail care.

✦ Menstrual management

One of the most difficult self-care tasks for women with lack of sensation, spasticity, loss of strength and dexterity, or loss of movement is menstrual management. To insert a tampon or place a sanitary pad, a woman must be able to pull her pants down or her skirt up, her underwear down, position herself, remove and dispose of the soiled pad or tampon, wipe and wash the perineal area, unwrap a new pad or tampon, place the pad or insert the tampon, get up from the toilet, and pull up underwear and pants or pull skirt down (Duckworth, 1986).

Recommendations to assist the woman with a disability to manage self-care with menstruation include adapted positions, underwear, tampon or pad, mirrors, and knee spreaders. Duckworth (1986) recommends the following adapted positions. A woman using a wheelchair who can slide her pants down and who has good hand dexterity may manage tampons by sitting on the front edge of the wheelchair seat but is unable to maneuver sanitary pads far enough under and back. To assist with placing sanitary pads, she may lean against the back of the chair while bridging the hips upward, then slide the pad posteriorly. The woman who cannot lean over may manage using a raised toilet seat with a front opening in order to place the tampon or pad. She may use a long-handled mirror (Fig. 12-9) if she lacks sensation or a knee spreader if she cannot abduct her legs. Safety is an issue if inserting a tampon increases spasticity; if balance is poor, she may lean to one side holding onto a bar or wheelchair side. Both positions allow a tampon to be inserted, but the person must be able to transfer from wheelchair to toilet. When pulling pants down and up remains a problem, some women find it easier to transfer to a bed to change pads or tampons.

Those who have problems with coordination, such as women with cerebral palsy, may have to kneel to stabilize themselves. This position can be quite distasteful if used in public facilities that are littered or unclean, or embarrassing if there are wide gaps under the cubicles. Women with no spasticity or loss of balance may be able to stand to manage pads or tampons, especially if a grab bar is installed within reach.

Underwear may be adapted by replacing the crotch flap with one that has a Velcro fastening and loops, or by placing an unsewn flap extending from the back of the crotch or the back waistband to the front waistband. Another version is to sew loops to the side of underwear, enabling a woman with lack of hand dexterity to pull underwear up and down by using the loops. Most women and those who lack dexterity prefer pads with stick-on backs to belts, which are uncomfortable and difficult to fasten (Duckworth, 1986).

✦ Shaving

Shaving the face is an important aspect of cleanliness and grooming for men. In most instances a daily shave is required, but the frequency also depends on the rate of hair growth and personal habit. Electric razors help clients taking anticoagulant medications and clients with restricted movement or unilateral paresis to avoid nicks or cuts. Some clients may retain or grow a beard or moustache to convey a masculine appearance even though facial hair may require daily washing and frequent trimming to be neat and clean. Both men and women use depilatory creams and lotions to remove excessive hair unless these irritate the skin; electrolysis may be used as a permanent method of hair removal. Women who shaved their legs and axillary hair before disability will continue these as part of personal hygiene and grooming and a positive body image.

✦ Applying deodorant

Deodorant, either spray or roll-on and unscented, can be applied when a client is in the supine position. When one extremity is flaccid or spastic, use the other extremity to raise the first extremity to a position above the head, then use the unaffected hand to apply deodorant to the axillary area. Alternatively a client seated at a table moves the flaccid arm forward and reaches underneath to apply deodorant.

✦ Applying cosmetics

Application of cosmetics also is important grooming that contributes to body image and well-being. Women who regularly wear cosmetics are encouraged to do so to enhance appearance and protect the skin. Cosmetic jars can be opened with one hand when the base of the container is stabilized to a countertop with suction cups. A client is taught to grasp a tube near the screw top using an unaffected hand, then use the thumb and index finger to twist loose the cap; or flip the top of snap caps. The degree, location, and type of motor, sensory, or perceptual deficits influence success. Nurses and therapists should give support and honest feedback. Although correctly applied cosmetics may enhance a client's appearance, incorrectly applied cosmetics may result in odd, even grotesque, facies.

✦ Dressing

Wearing personal clothing signifies an active lifestyle, rather than sick role, during rehabilitation. Assessment of a client's ROM, coordination, finger dexterity, sitting balance, strength, and stamina preceeds dressing interventions. Restricted ROM limits the client's independence in dressing but usually can be surmounted with modified clothing, dressing techniques, and assistive or adapted devices. Some clients are able to master a one-handed shoe tie (Fig. 12-10). Others choose slip-on shoe styles. Shoe styles may be dictated when they serve protective, corrective, or adaptive purposes for individual clients.

Clothing that is attractive, comfortable, easy to manage, and reasonably priced has become readily available for persons with disabilities. Personally selected clothing styles reflect a person's positive body image and independence. Persons who rely on a wheelchair for mobility are encouraged to evaluate clothing for practicality when sitting as well as for style. For instance, clothing should hang free from wheels. Modern fabrics are durable and easy to care for; styles include gussets, pleats, reinforcements, fastenings, and openings for comfort and ease. Slacks, shorts, or other pant styles are comfortable, modest, and nonrestricting during physical therapy sessions. Other adaptations are loose-fitting stretch fashions; full shirts to fit over the hips; trousers or slacks with a front zipper and elastic waistbands, and brassiers with front closures and elastic straps.

Bras are a particular problem for women. Often a regular back-fastening bra is easier to manage than a front-closing bra. The bra is put on backward, being fastened in the front, and then turned around (Fig. 12-11). If the hooks are a problem, Velcro tape can be placed over the hooks. However, Velcro is difficult to manage with only one hand and the hook edges may irritate the skin. Some clients have success with a clothespin snapped to hold the bra to the underpants or slacks. This serves as a stable holding hand while the unaffected hand is used to close the hooks.

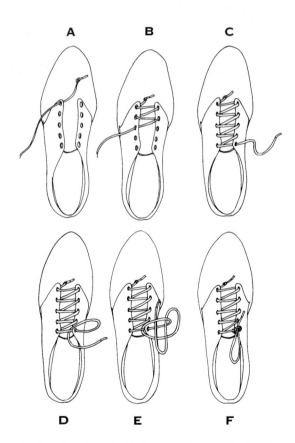

Fig. 12-10 Technique for lacing and tying a left shoe for a person with right hemiplegia. **A,** Tie a knot on one end of the shoestring. Begin to lace the open end of the shoestring through the eye at the left side. **B,** Lace the shoestring across the tongue of the shoe, alternating sides. Be sure to lace in under each eye and over to the opposite side of the shoe. **C,** The laced shoe should look like this. **D,** Loop the end of the shoestring under the top row of lacing. Leave the loop open. **E,** Insert the folded end of the shoestring through the open loop. Pull the folded end toward the ankle and the inside of the leg. **F,** Tighten the loop. Be sure the shoestring is not too long so client will not trip over the loose end. (From Rehabilitation/Restorative Care by S.P. Hoeman, 1990, St. Louis, Mosby–Year Book. Copyright 1990 by permission.)

A bra that is very stretchable lycra can be stitched closed. It is put on by stretching it over the head and pulling it down into place. This is an easy method for persons with upper extremity disabilities such as hemiplegia, amputations, spinal cord injuries, and multiple sclerosis. A person with arthritis may not be able to move her shoulders enough to put a bra on over her head. She may, however, be able to step into the bra and pull it up from her feet.

Clothing worn by the client before the disability can be altered so openings and fastenings are easy to reach and simple to manipulate. Velcro, larger hooks, large buttons, large snaps and zipper pulls, loops, or extensions adapt clothing to maximize an individual's independence in dressing. Assistive devices such as long-handled shoehorns and stand-up mirrors are among the many items that aid in dressing activities (Fig. 12-12).

The nurse and occupational therapist collaborate to modify dressing techniques according to individual needs. Modified dressing techniques include dressing while in bed or using a wall or doorjamb for support when balance or stamina are altered. As a rule when dressing, the affected extremity is inserted first into clothing. An average dress-

Text continued on page 178.

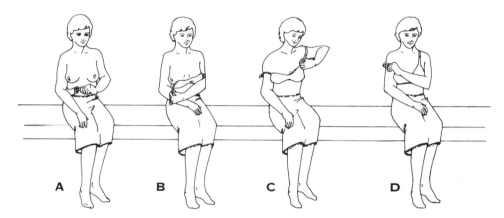

Fig. 12-11 Dressing in a bra. **A,** Client must be able to sit and balance safely. She puts the bra on backwards around her waist. Be sure cups are positioned correctly. If she cannot fasten the hooks, Velcro may work instead of hooks. Use a safety strap if needed. **B,** She turns the bra to the front. She uses her unaffected hand to insert the affected arm into the strap. **C,** She inserts her unaffected arm into the other strap and position bra. **D,** She uses her unaffected hand to position the strap on the affected side and to adjust the bra. (From Rehabilitation/Restorative Care by S.P. Hoeman, 1990, St. Louis, Mosby–Year Book. Copyright 1990 by permission.)

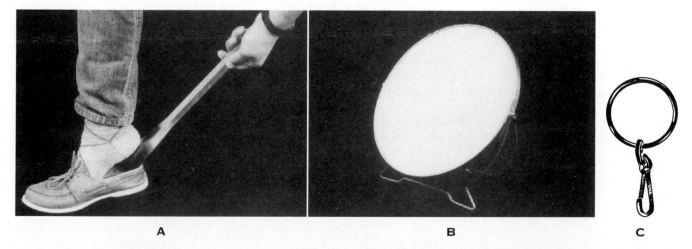

Fig. 12-12 Assistive/adapted dressing devices. **A,** Long-handled shoehorn. **B,** Stand-up mirror. **C,** Zipper pull.

◆

DRESSING AIDS AND TECHNIQUES FOR SPECIFIC CONDITIONS

A. Persons with limited ROM such as with arthritic conditions
   1. Use large buttons or zippers with a loop on the pull tab
   2. Replace buttons, snaps, and hooks with Velcro or zippers
   3. Use garments made from stretchable fabrics
   4. Eliminate bending to tie shoelaces; use elastic shoelaces or other adapted shoe fasteners
   5. Use stocking aids
   6. Pick up items from the floor before donning them and after removal, and remove clothes from hangers using reaches
   7. Push stockings off heel of foot using dressing sticks
B. Persons who have neurologic disorders (when dressing while seated in a wheelchair, put on clothing in the following order: stockings, undergarments, braces [if worn], pants, shoes, shirt or dress)
   1. To put on stockings while in bed, pull one leg into flexion, or to a cross-legged position in a chair (Fig. 12-13), slip sock over foot and pull on; avoid elastic tops or garters (Pedretti & Zoltan, 1989)
   2. To put on pants and underwear in bed, pull or roll to a sitting position
      a. If balance, health status, and mobility permit lean forward to work pant legs over feet, then pull pants up to hips
      b. While retaining the grip at the pant waist, client lays back onto bed and rolls from hip to hip while pulling the garment up over the buttocks (Fig. 12-14)
   3. To put on pants and underwear in a wheelchair, client slides to the front of the seat, then leans against the seat back
      a. Pull one leg into a flexed position and put foot into pant leg; put foot through pant leg and pull rest of pants up past knee on that side; repeat with other leg
      b. Work pants up as high as possible in this forward seated position and gather excess pant material in front
      c. Perform a "push-up" and raise the buttocks, thighs, and pant tops from the seat while repositioning self to back portion of wheelchair seat
      d. Hold pant waist and slide or "butt-walk" down into pant tops; repeat lift/slide until pants are positioned properly
      e. To remove pants, undoing from fasteners while sitting in the forward part of the wheelchair seat, hook the waistband with the thumbs and perform another "push-up" while backing out of the pant top, repeat as necessary

4. Shirts, sweaters, and dresses that open down the front should be donned while in the wheelchair; some clients may need to modify traditional methods because of balance deficits
   a. Open garment on lap with collar facing toward chest and opening up
   b. Put arms into sleeves and pull up over elbows
   c. Put garment on over head, pull the back down, adjust and button
5. If putting on shoes while in bed, bend at the waist from a sitting position and put shoes on immediately after donning pants, if dressing in a wheelchair
   a. Cross legs above knee, lean over at the waist and rest torso on lap, then pull shoe on with both hands; return to upright sitting, repeat with other leg

or

   b. Slide to front of wheelchair seat and lean back onto seat back; pull one leg into a flexed position with one hand, put shoe on foot with free hand (Pedretti & Zoltan, 1989)
C. Persons who have hemiplegia or hemiparesis (when client has balance problems, encourage dressing while seated in a sturdy armchair or a locked wheelchair, organize clothing and arrange within easy reach or use reaching devices)
   1. Put on shirts using either techniques mentioned for persons with neurologic impairment or by inserting the affected arm first (Fig. 12-15)
   2. Put on pants by crossing the affected leg over the other leg; work affected foot through pant leg, but do not pull pants past knee or it may become difficult to insert the other leg; to pull pants up several methods are possible
      a. If able to do so safely, client may stand to pull pants over the hips; to prevent pants from sliding down before they are fastened, place affected hand into a pocket or hook a finger/thumb into belt loop
      b. Position pants as high as possible while in seated position, elevate the hips by pushing down on floor with other leg and lean back against chair; pull pants up, then lower the hips back into chair to fasten pants (Fig. 12-16 illustrates dressing in pants while seated)
   3. Remove pants using method mentioned for persons with neurologic conditions; instruct client to sit to the front of the seat, unfasten pants, hook thumbs in waistband, and then back out of pants
   4. Another way to put on shoes is to cross the legs while in a seated posture

Continued.

DRESSING AIDS AND TECHNIQUES FOR SPECIFIC CONDITIONS—cont'd

As a general rule when working with individuals who have hemiplegia, insert the affected extremity into clothing first. Modified dressing techniques also may include dressing while in bed or using a wall or doorjamb for support when balance or stamina are altered.

D. Persons with perceptual problems
  1. When teaching client with visual agnosia, encourage client to feel parts of clothing that will assist in recognizing the object—for example, client may trace the line of buttons on the front of the shirt or practice drills to name different pieces of clothing (Zoltan et al., 1986)
  2. Clients with dressing apraxia may benefit from using the following techniques
     a. Instruct client who has difficulty positioning a garment, to place the garment facedown on the bed or lap with buttons facing down or zipper facing down
     b. Use labels to distinguish front from back, and right from wrong side
     c. When buttoning a shirt, begin at the bottom matching the lowest buttonhole
     d. Use touch to determine whether the button is pushed through the buttonhole (Zoltan et al., 1986)
  3. When teaching clients who have disturbances of body scheme, always touch the body part when instructing client to place clothing on that part; it may be necessary to continue this touching through the dressing activity (Fig. 12-16)
  4. Clients who have unilateral neglect need to have the neglected side stimulated
     a. Place clothes on client's neglected side, then teach scanning techniques to enable client to "find" clothes
     b. While dressing, client is instructed to pay attention to the neglected side
     c. Initially frequent cueing to continue dressing that side will be necessary
     d. Use the same sequence of dressing, because this will become a "built-in cueing" system, triggering client to the neglected side at a certain point in the dressing routine
     e. Finally, always speak and teach client while at the affected side
  5. Clients with figure-ground visual difficulty benefit from organizing drawers and separating types of clothing items
     a. Client must be taught to slow down and carefully look for items of clothing that may be "lost"

  b. Lay clothes out on a background that is unlike the color or pattern of the clothing
  c. Keep clutter from the self-care area (Zoltan, Sieva & Freishtat, 1986).
  6. Clients with cognitive deficits such as memory problems, inattention, poor judgment, lack of insight, limited problem-solving ability, difficulty with abstraction, and poor mental flexibility can benefit from using an approach to dressing skills focusing on
     a. Being consistent
     b. Using verbal cueing
     c. Using self-cueing: vocalizing step-by-step sequence for dressing
     d. Scanning the environment
     e. Controlling the amount and duration of stimuli
     f. Using memory aids such as cue cards with the steps of dressing listed (Stewart, 1993); tape cue cards to a bathroom mirror or top of a wheelchair lapboard
     g. Acknowledging family and client preferences and lifestyle
E. Persons who have amputations of limbs (person with upper extremity amputations may use some of the same one-handed methods employed by clients with neurologic conditions; persons with lower extremity amputations, however, may have dynamic standing balance impairments that interfere with pulling up pants [Pedretti & Zoltan, 1989]; most other dressing procedures can be performed while seated)
  1. Pants may need to be pulled up in bed using the "hip roll" from side to side
  2. If client has sufficient body strength, "bridging" techniques may allow enough room to pull up the pants while in bed or in a chair (Fig. 12-17)
  3. Remove pants by unfastening while seated and merely using supported standing to let them fall
  4. Older persons or those with diabetes who have incurred amputations may have problems donning or doffing shoes and socks and managing shoelaces; clients may need to use techniques or assistive devices such as shoehorn or sock aid (Pedretti & Zoltan, 1990)
  5. An extended shoehorn may also be used to push shoe and sock from the foot
F. Persons who have cognitive problems
  Table 12-7 details interventions for persons who have cognitive problems listed according to nursing diagnosis

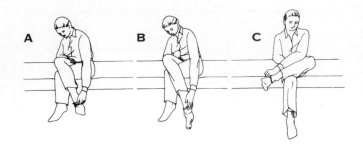

Fig. 12-13 Applying socks. (Check client's ability to balance safely before beginning.) **A,** The client sits to cross his affected leg over his unaffected knee. He must be able to reach his affected foot without leaning over and losing his balance. **B,** Using his unaffected hand, the client pulls the top of the sock completely over his toes. He works the sock over his foot until his toes are into the toe of the sock. He pulls the top of the sock at the front, then at the back to pull the sock on over his heel and ankle. **C,** The other sock is applied by using the same technique. The client uses his unaffected hand to pull the sock onto the unaffected foot. Reverse the procedure to remove socks. To remove: Grasp the top of the sock. Pull it down the leg, over the heel, and off the foot. (From Rehabilitation/Restorative Care by S.P. Hoeman, 1990, St. Louis, Mosby–Year Book. Copyright 1990 by permission.)

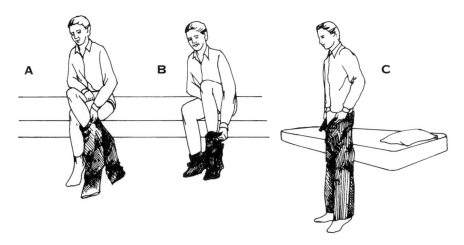

Fig. 12-14 Dressing in pants while standing to balance. **A,** Check client's ability to sit or stand and balance safely. Sitting on the bed, he uses his unaffected hand to lift his affected leg across his unaffected knee. He pulls his pants leg completely over his affected foot and ankle. If he cannot lift or cross his leg, assist him or elevate his affected leg on a box or stool so that he does not lean over. **B,** He inserts his unaffected leg fully through the other pants leg. He uses his unaffected hand to pull the pants up on both legs as high as he is able. **C,** If he can safely stand, he holds onto the pants and the waist with his unaffected hand. He pulls the pants on and adjusts the waist and zipper. He never bends over to pull his pants. (From Rehabilitation/Restorative Care by S.P. Hoeman, 1990, St. Louis, Mosby–Year Book. Copyright 1990 by permission.)

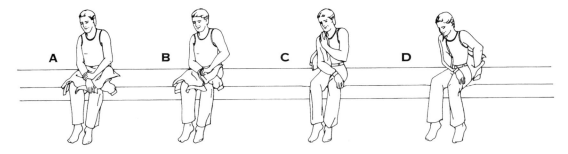

Fig. 12-15 Dressing in a shirt (or button-style dress). **A,** Check your client's ability to balance before beginning. The client who has one side of the body affected should sit down to put on a shirt or shirt button–styled clothing. Lay the shirt inside-up with the collar at his knees. **B** and **C,** He uses his unaffected hand to lift the affected hand into the armhole and to pull up the sleeve over his affected shoulder. **D,** He uses a tossing movement to place the shirt and other sleeve behind him. He can reach behind him with his unaffected hand and insert it into the shirt sleeve to finish dressing. (From Rehabilitation/Restorative Care by S.P. Hoeman, 1990, St. Louis, Mosby–Year Book. Copyright 1990.)

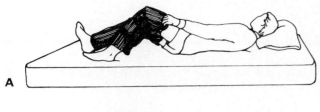

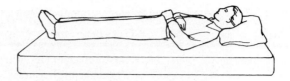

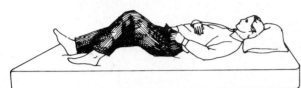

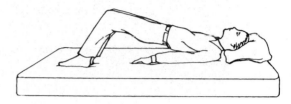

Fig. 12-16 Bridging for dressing. **A,** If he cannot stand, he lies down on the bed. He flexes his unaffected knee, keeping the foot flat on the bed. **B,** As he pushes down on the bed, his hips will elevate. He can uses his unaffected hand and arm to pull up his pants and fasten them. (From Rehabilitation/Restorative Care by S.P. Hoeman, 1990, St. Louis, Mosby–Year Book. Copyright 1990.)

Fig. 12-17 Bridging is a useful technique for clients who can lift their hips and bear weight on their shoulders. This technique may be used by some persons following amputation. (From Rehabilitation/Restorative Care by S.P. Hoeman, 1990, St. Louis, Mosby–Year Book. Copyright 1990.)

Table 12-7 Cognitive management strategies (Stewart, 1993)

Nursing diagnosis	Nursing intervention
Impaired alertness and mental fatigue	✦ Plan daily schedule to take advantage of client's peak periods of alertness ✦ Divide tasks for the day into short 5- to 15-minute segments with frequent scheduled rest breaks ✦ Do not overstimulate client ✦ Emphasize the sensory stimulation (vision, hearing, smell, touch or taste) to which client best responds ✦ Allow extra response time ✦ Plan activities that include client's preinjury interests as much as possible ✦ Expect variability in alertness from day to day ✦ Repeat commands and stimuli frequently ✦ Enlist family support in strategies ✦ If alertness level becomes deeper or prolonged, report to physician
Attention problems	✦ Stimulate attention with what interests client ✦ Be sure to have client's attention before giving commands, providing information ✦ Use demonstration as well as verbal and written instructions Keep distractions to a strict minimum: *structure* environment ✦ Start with tasks client can easily achieve ✦ Use verbal praise and other positive reinforcers ✦ Hemiinattention or unilateral neglect: continually cue client to attend to the neglected side ✦ Perseveration: constantly cue client to the flow of activities ✦ Reinforce the completion of each step in task sequence ✦ Encourage telephone conversation to promote communication skill and attention
Confusion and disorientation	✦ Establish consistent schedule of caregivers for client ✦ Maintain maximum structure and stability in client's environment ✦ Limit stimulation: promote quiet, nonstimulating environment ✦ Explain fully what you are about to do with the client: no surprises ✦ Redirect client by suggestion or demonstration: don't confront confusion ✦ Use frequent reorientation to time, date, place, identity of others in the environment ✦ Use clocks, posters of daily schedule, calendar, etc. ✦ Remain calm, quiet, and confident to reduce client fear

Continued.

Table 12-7 Cognitive management strategies (Stewart, 1993)—cont'd

Nursing diagnosis	Nursing intervention
Memory problems	✦ Assist client to use the memory notebook to promote short-term memory ✦ Try to pair new learning with old—e.g., if you want client to remember where she went for dinner last night, remind client that the kind of food (pizza, burgers) is one of client's favorites ✦ Frequent cueing and rehearsal of new information is helpful ✦ Present material in different ways: written, pictures, verbally, and by demonstration ✦ Be *consistent* with memory training Proceed from simple to complex, promoting success ✦ If client is bilingual, present material to be remembered in both languages
Communication problems	✦ Establish a means of communication with the client if at all possible: speech, communication device, eye blinks, head nods, finger or eye movements, yes/no indicators ✦ Caregivers and family should encourage client to speak; they tend to become frustrated or embarrassed with the effort and withdraw *Approach to the aphasic client* ✦ Make direct eye contact ✦ Be relaxed and unhurried ✦ Speak slowly and distinctly and in a normal tone of voice ✦ Give client one brief thought to process at a time ✦ Allow client plenty of time to "process" communication, to understand what is said and to formulate and produce a response ✦ Use appropriate gestures to convey meaning Cardinal rule: *never* pretend to understand what client has said; it's better to be honest and ask questions for clarity Don't interrupt client or try to finish the sentence for client; exception: if client becomes frustrated looking for a word or phrase, you may need to supply it ✦ Try to find meaning in jargon or nonsense language spoken by the client with receptive problems ✦ Client will not communicate as well when upset or fatigued ✦ Discourage telephone conversation—client will not comprehend or perform as well
Impaired ability to carry out a plan of action	✦ Always explain activities to be done by client clearly and simply ✦ Provide continual cueing to the steps of the task ✦ Encourage client to participate in organizing and planning a new task ✦ Try to increase the complexity of instruction toward a single direction or command
Impaired abstraction and judgment	✦ Early recovery: approach must be at simple, concrete tasks within client's grasp ✦ Try to explain things to client in as concrete terms as possible; use familiar situations and recognizable objects ✦ Always explain the reasons for activities client is to do ✦ Computer games are helpful in developing abstracting ability
Impaired ability to integrate new tasks and skills into behavior	✦ Try to build new learning on old, overlearned tasks when possible ✦ Encourage new skills and tasks that apply in many areas of activity ✦ Remind client to do the new things daily ✦ Try to balance the difficulty level of the task with client's ability: too simple is insulting and produces boredom; too difficult is depressing and results in failure ✦ Client will require visual cues, demonstration, and verbal cues until new learning has been achieved ✦ Be a cheerleader: use praise and rewards as incentive to learning

Information compiled from Ann Stewart. Kimberly Quality Care Rehabilitation Manual, 1993.

ing time that exceeds 30 to 40 minutes with a procedure that consistently frustrates a client is a signal for the nurse, therapist, or family member to offer assistance.

Clients who spend time in spica casts may buy or make extra large shirts that pull over the head, skirts or pants with wide tops (hip size plus 10 or 12 inches) and drawstring or elastic waists. Antiembolic stockings worn on the unaffected leg, are countered with a boot for the other leg (Mather, 1987).

Both clients and families are advised about the danger of hypothermia and hyperthermia with a client's altered sen-

sation. During inclement weather a client may take fewer baths to avoid lowering body temperature through evaporation and wear sweaters and footware indoors. When outside, the client dresses for inclement weather by layering clothing, wearing a hat and gloves. Exertion in cold weather should be avoided. When finances are an issue in maintaining home heating, a social worker assists clients to contact local or government agencies that offer assistance with heating bills or to clarify arrangements for emergency heat or electrical services in advance to forestall any discontinued services.

Hyperthermia, or increased body temperature, is just as damaging as hypothermia because it leads to dehydration. Clients with sensory deficits and their families may not be aware of the physical problems caused by extremes of environmental temperature. Education includes recognizing factors that may influence a client's perception of the environment; monitoring body temperature; dressing in cool, lightweight cotton clothing in summer; remaining indoors on extremely hot days; wearing protective headgear; and drinking liquids to prevent dehydration.

A wide variety of footgear is available to meet specific needs for clients. For example, the stocking a client wears may be prescribed by his physician. Special stockings are often prescribed to support a client's circulation or to reduce edema in his legs. These stockings usually are made of lightweight, pliable lycra and are used by a client who needs mild support. Heavier, brown-colored stockings, made from a stiffer elastic, are used to provide firmer support. These stockings, which are measured and sized to fit each wearer, most often are worn by clients who have spinal cord injuries. Socks and knee-high nylons should not have elastic tops because they may be too tight around the leg. Similarly tube socks with long areas of elastic will irritate the skin and cause circulation problems as they become too tight at the top after being worn for long periods.

Support stockings are expensive. They must be hand-washed in warm, not hot, soapy water. They are then thoroughly rinsed and hung to dry. The stockings must be washed and hung at least every other day in order to retain their shape and elasticity. (Do not place stockings in the dryer or they will lose their elasticity.) Your client will need several pairs of stockings to rotate and a spare pair (Hoeman, 1990).

Care of prosthetic socks is an important daily hygiene task. Prosthetic socks must be changed daily or as often as necessary to prevent perspiration buildup. Perspiration collects on the socks and causes skin breakdown to begin. The person with a relatively new prosthesis tends to require more changes of prosthetic socks due to swelling of the residual limb. The socks come in different sizes and thicknesses. A supply of prosthetic socks (several sizes and thicknesses) must be available for your client as he may change the socks two to four times in a day (Hoeman, 1990).

Wool socks can be washed, but they are dried slowly away from direct heat. Nylon socks are machine washed and dried. Good quality socks will not have seams. If your client uses socks with seams, the seams should run from side to side. They should not run front to back across the suture line. Your client may even wear several prosthetic socks at the same time. He may use extra socks to create various levels of thickness inside the socket of the prosthesis. This may be necessary because of some shrinking of the amputated leg over time. Persons with upper limb amputations traditionally use a thick sock. Some clients elect not to use socks. The nurse, client, and prosthetist will decide if this is workable (Hoeman, 1990).

The following section details methods or techniques for dressing with a variety of special conditions. Clothing that has front openings are easiest to use for all of the disability categories mentioned here. Pants may need to be one size larger because of seated postures, muscular weakness or incoordination, and/or urinary collection systems. Because many techniques require moving the skin over fabric, furniture, or materials, skin integrity is an important concern for clients who are learning dressing modifications or techniques. Jeans are the choice of most young people and may be worn if they are the wide-leg, full-cut styles. The back center seam may cut into the person's skin as it is very stiff and heavy. This often is a problem for the person who has a spinal cord injury, if moved or positioned by someone holding onto the jeans. This can cause skin breakdown from rubbing and pressure. Jeans must be kept wrinkle free.

✦ Donning and doffing a prosthesis

Donning and doffing are the terms used to describe the process of putting on and taking off a prosthesis. To don, or put on, a prosthesis is one of the first tasks learned during rehabilitation following amputation of a limb. The person usually wears a special sock over the dressing of the amputated area. The seam of the sock is arranged so that it does not touch the suture line at the amputation site, nor should wrinkles touch the suture line at the amputation site, as these could cause skin irritation and blister. As the size of the residual amputated limb decreases over time, additional socks will be needed for correct fit (Hoeman, 1990).

Some prostheses have Velcro straps or other fasteners to keep them in place once they are donned. Your client may have to stand to adjust the prosthetic leg. Other maneuvers may be necessary to get the leg set into the prosthesis.

Prostheses and covers will vary, and clients will require different amounts of assistance. Figure 12-18 shows a series of photographs with a client who can independently don an above-the-knee prosthesis and its cosmetic cover.

Doffing is usually taught at the rehabilitation center or hospital. Each client is taught techniques to suit her special needs. Always make sure your client is in a position with good balance and in a safe environment for donning or doffing the prosthesis. Your client may feel more secure and in control if the prothesis is stored near her bed or chair within reach. The client should follow instructions from the center or the therapist about handling and storing the prothesis when it is not in use (Hoeman, 1990).

Some clients have more than one prosthesis, such as an upper body prosthesis that ends with either a hook or a solid hand. Check for specific instructions for use and care. Avoid using any products that contain grease or solvents. Do not immerse the prosthesis in water or remove the covering (Hoeman, 1990).

✦ Bathing and toileting

Independence in toileting is a major goal for clients, so that in spite of the potential difficulties, any who are able to use the bathroom are encouraged and assisted to do so. Because persons who are wet, soapy, and loosely dressed are moving on or off the toilet or in and out of the tub or shower, it is no surprise the home bathroom is a place where most accidents occur. Many accidents may be prevented by attention to safety during personal hygiene, grooming, and toileting.

Many safety measures are structural: countertops with space for grooming items; no electrical razors or hair dryers near water; electrical outlets near the mirror positioned away from the sink; insulated or covered hot water pipes

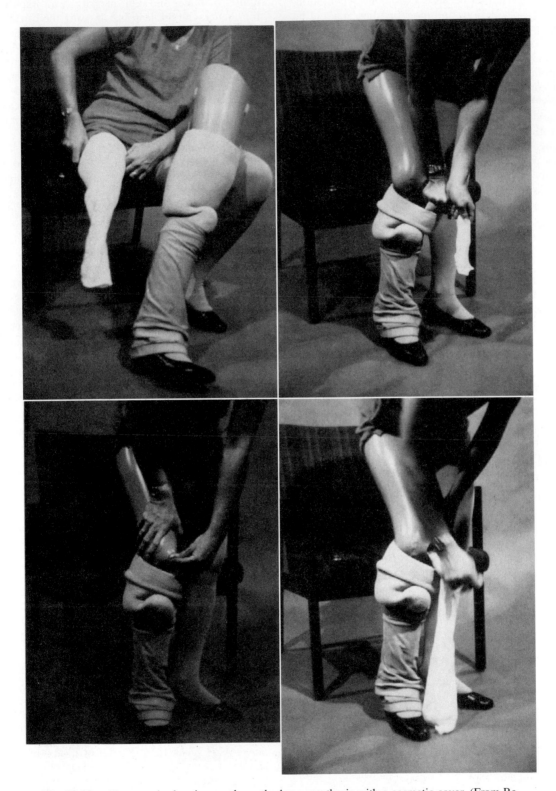

Fig. 12-18 The steps in donning an above-the-knee prosthesis with a cosmetic cover. (From Rehabilitation/Restorative Care by S.P. Hoeman, 1990, St. Louis, Mosby–Year Book. Copyright 1990; photo courtesy of Otto Bock Orthopedic Industry Inc., U.S.A.)

Continued.

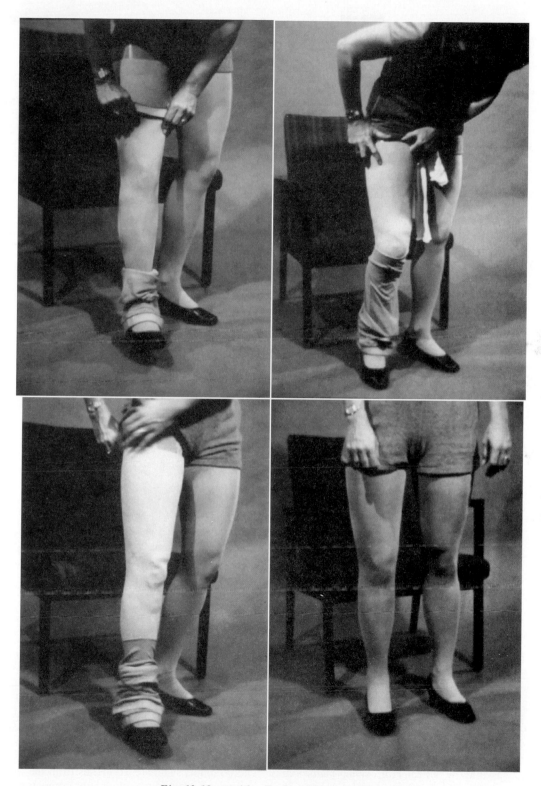

Fig. 12-18, cont'd For legend see p. 180.

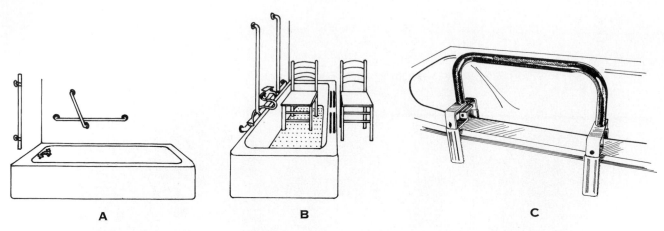

A   **B**   **C**

Fig. 12-19   **A,** Grab bars are placed within reach for a seated or standing transfer into a tub. Grab bars must be firmly attached into the studwalls. **B,** A homemade shower seat, nonslip bath mat, and grab bars promote bathroom safety. The tub chair legs are cut to reduce the height of the chair so the seat is level with the chair placed outside the tub. **C,** Bathtub bars. (**A** and **B** from Rehabilitation/Restorative Care by S.P. Hoeman, 1990, St. Louis, Mosby–Year Book; copyright 1990.)

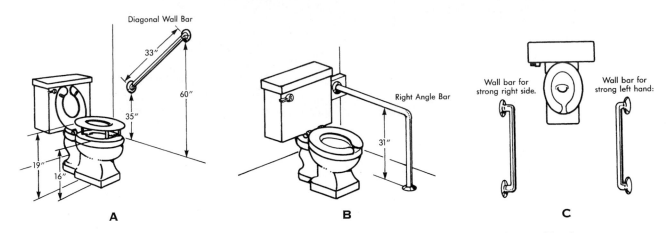

A   **B**   **C**

Fig. 12-20   Safety wall grab bars. **A,** Diagonal wall bar. If commode seat is too low, making it difficult to get up, it may have to be raised by using a raised toilet seat. Be sure it is secure. **B,** Right angle bar. **C,** The wall bars should be securely fastened to avoid a fall and should be at a 45-degree angle. They should be 2 to 4 inches away from the wall on the patient's strong side when he is sitting. (From Rehabilitation/Restorative Care by S.P. Hoeman, 1990, St. Louis, Mosby–Year Book. Copyright 1990.)

such as under the sink; nonslip surfaces; controlled shower or tub water temperature; installed safety bars; and removal of loose articles such as rugs, towels, and clothing. Small baskets or bags for wheelchair storage may be the safest way to carry miscellaneous items to the bathroom when space is limited or shared (Fig. 12-19).

Access is another concern in most home bathrooms where space to turn around or complete a transfer is cramped or inaccessible by wheelchair. When bathroom doors are too narrow for wheelchairs to pass, they may be removed, enlarged, or converted to sliding doors for access. Sink countertops, mirrors and electrical outlets, bathtub rims, and tub enclosures frequently are not sized, styled, or placed at proper height for use from a wheelchair or trans-

fers. Lowering a sink with countertop and mirror and opening space under the counter allow a client to sit in a wheelchair while grooming.

Safety rails or "grab bars" are essential equipment for bathing and toileting areas. Figure 12-20 shows proper placement for bars installed into wooden wall studs near a commode. A client may use bars to lower into sitting or pull up on bars to rise from a tub or toilet seat. Since most home toilets seats are 16 inches from the floor, an elevated toilet seat with adjustable height armrests securely attached to the commode or toilet may enable some clients to rise and sit independently from the toilet.

When transferring from the wheelchair to the toilet, a client may use a pivot transfer or in some instances use a trans-

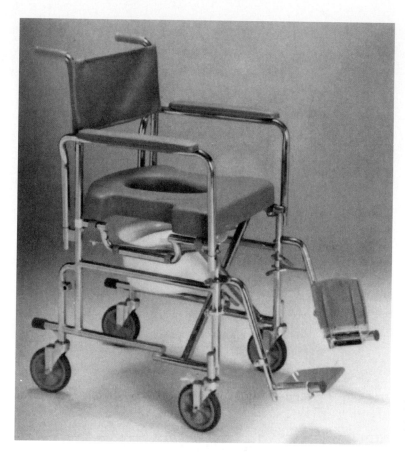

Fig. 12-21 Commode chair with wheels and underseat bucket. (From Rehabilitation/Restorative Care by S.P. Hoeman, 1990, St. Louis, Mosby–Year Book. Copyright 1990; Courtesy of Everest & Jennings, Inc.)

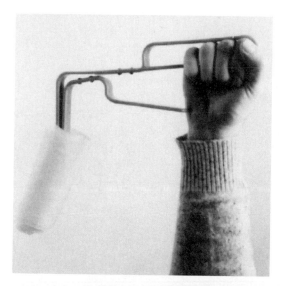

Fig. 12-22 A toilet paper holder assists client to cleanse himself after toileting. (From Rehabilitation/Restorative Care by S.P. Hoeman, 1990, St. Louis, Mosby–Year Book. Copyright 1990; reprinted by permission of © Bissell Healthcare Corporation/Fred Sammons, Inc.)

fer board to move from one seat to the other. If the toilet seat is more than 2 to 4 inches away from the lip of the tub, place a sturdy chair outside the tub to serve as a "landing place" during transfers. Safety precautions include locking chair wheels; universal precautions and client hygiene;

maintaining skin integrity; and a client's balance, alertness, and motivation. A transfer belt is recommended when assisting clients to move about the bathroom. An elevated seat will assist with a pivot transfer, but when using a transfer board, the toilet seat is at the same height as the wheelchair seat (Fig. 12-21). The same is true for transfer to a bedside commode. Many styles of bedside commodes are available with locking casters or wheels, elevated seats, armrests, underseat buckets, and seat cushions.

Many assistive devices and aids are available for bathing assistance. Personal assistive devices include premoistened wipes, extended toilet paper holders (Fig. 12-22);long-handled mirrors, brushes, and sponges; shampoo dispensers; and universal cuffs or Velcro wrist tabs for holding toilet paper, soap, razor, brush, or bath mitt (Fig. 12-23). Benches and tub seats are available in a wide variety of sizes, heights, styles and colors, and adjustable features. A larger seat is preferred when assisting a client to move and bathe. Bath mats, rubberized or nonslip tub and floor materials, hand-held shower hoses, automatic water temperature control settings, bath mitts and soap bags filled with nonallergenic products, and items held to the wall by suction cup are available. Should bathing in a tub become too unmanageable for a client, a walk-in shower stall, with or without a shower seat or chair, is a good choice. A client who is functionally dependent may use a shower table, such as this burn unit shower table (Fig. 12-24) as a safe means of hygiene. A client's modesty, privacy, and dignity are important considerations with any toileting or bathing approach.

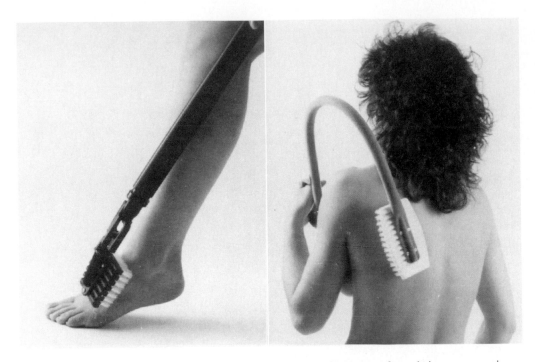

Fig. 12-23 Long handles on combs and brushes enable clients to perform their own grooming activities. (From Rehabilitation/Restorative Care by S.P. Hoeman, 1990, St. Louis, Mosby–Year Book. Copyright 1990; courtesy of Lumex, Division of Lumex, Inc.)

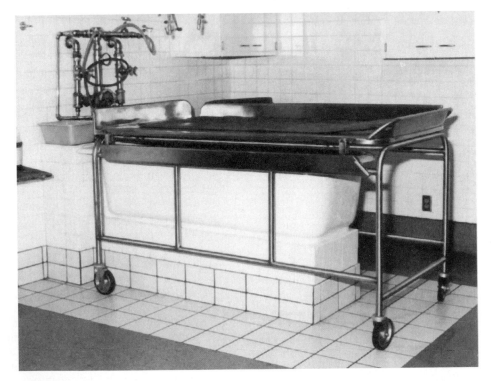

Fig. 12-24 Shower table used for daily hydrotherapy, debridement, and hygiene. (From AACN Clinical Reference for Critical Care Nursing, 3rd ed, by Kinney, 1993, St. Louis, Mosby–Year Book. Copyright 1993.)

Supplemental Assessment for Self-Care and Activities of Daily Living

A. Personal Hygiene and Grooming
   1. Tell me about any health concerns related to your hair, nails, teeth, mouth, or menstrual management (if applicable)?
   2. How would you compare your ability to care for your hair, nails, teeth, mouth, and menstrual management (if applicable) now, with the way you did before your injury? (One subject may be covered at a time.)
   3. When was your last dental examination?
   4. Do you shave? How often do you shave? Tell me about the process; what is different now?
   5. Do you use deodorant? Do you have difficulty applying it?
   6. Do you wear cosmetics? Do you require assistance to apply cosmetics?
B. Hair
   7. Tell me about your hair care practices. Are there any differences now?
   8. Have you noticed any unusual hair loss or hair growth?
   9. How would you describe the condition of your hair?
C. Mouth and Teeth
   10. Tell me about your dental history (probe for gum soreness, lesions, taste, or mouth odor).
   11. How would you describe your procedure for mouth care? Has your disability affected it?
   12. Do you have difficulty chewing? Wear dentures? If you do wear dentures, when do you remove them; how are they cleaned; where and how are they stored when not worn?
D. Nails
   13. Have you noticed any change in your nails (appearance or texture)?
   14. How do you take care of your nails?
   15. Do you have any difficulty cutting your nails?
E. Menstrual Management (if applicable)
   16. What position do you use to insert tampons or place pads?
   17. Do you use any adaptations to your underwear?
   18. Do you use any additional equipment, such as a mirror to insert tampons or place pads?
   19. Do you have any difficulty inserting tampons or placing pads?
F. Dressing
   20. Do you have any difficulty dressing?
   21. Do you require any assistance dressing (help of another person, assistive devices)? What do you do about laundry?
   22. What type of clothing do you prefer?
   23. Do you have any difficulty obtaining or caring for your clothing?
   24. Do you have any concerns about your clothes or about dressing now?
   25. Do you feel your disability will change your dressing style? How?
      Assess fit of shoes and adaptive or assistive devices.
G. Safety
   26. Have you had any accidents or received any injuries while performing personal hygiene and grooming activities?
   27. What safety measures do you take while performing these activities?
   28. Tell me about your main safety concern(s) now. *Coordinate with home or living arrangement assessment data.*
H. Psychosocial Functioning
   29. Tell me about your family patterns of personal hygiene. Are there any special requirements or ways of performing personal care?
   30. Has your disability affected your family? How?
   31. Tell me about your decision to learn self-care using rehabilitation techniques.
   32. What are your feelings about your family being involved in your care?

REHABILITATION TEAM INTERVENTION

The nurse collaborates with the client, family, and other rehabilitation team members to plan, implement, and evaluate interventions and accomplish the goals that have been mutually established in relation to personal hygiene and grooming. Other team members who work closely with the client and family in these areas of function are the physiatrist, dentist, occupational therapist, physical therapist, social worker, and prosthetist or orthotist. In the traditional multidisciplinary approach to rehabilitation, each team member had a very specific role working with specifically designated tasks. In the interdisciplinary approach to rehabilitation, activities are broken down into skills needed to provide the client with the highest level of functional independence. The team then works together to facilitate the whole picture. The treatment plan focuses on the activity and not on isolated roles of the therapist or nurse. Each member of the team brings certain strengths to the process of understanding the whole picture. Physiatrists diagnose the client's condition and prescribe treatment. They must have knowledge of the biophysical, physiologic, and psychological responses to various treatments used by the treatment team. Treatment prescriptions should be individualized and specific for each client. They should contain enough detail to inform the team about the goal to be accomplished and include instructions for treatment to be continued by the client, who hopefully has been a contributing member of the treatment team.

Approach to Therapy

In the traditional multidisciplinary team approach, the occupational therapist carries out training in many of the ADL and designs special assistive and adaptive devices to assist the client in these activities. The prescription received from the physiatrist may specify personal self-care areas that need particular attention. In the interdisciplinary approach the occupational therapist would work closely with all team members before developing assistive devices to ascertain their effectiveness. An example would be that a certain type of splinting might prevent independence in dressing if the client were using loops as a means of pulling up pants.

A physical therapist supervises a program of therapeutic exercise. Before carrying out a prescription for therapeutic exercise, the therapist will perform a complete evaluation of the client's function including a manual muscle test, evaluation of ROM, assessment of bones and joints, and evaluation of coordination. Depending on the client's diagnosis, family assistance, the physician's prescription, the results of the evaluation, and the treatment team's goals, the therapist establishes a program to improve strength, balance, ROM, coordination, and stamina.

Traditionally social workers assist the client in exploring sources for financial aid for equipment and supplies, home modifications, and heating. Their roles have expanded and may cover other case management responsibilities. Social workers, together with other team members, help resolve problems that may interfere with the client's and family's function and ADL.

The prosthetist fits clients who have upper and lower extremity amputations with artificial limbs when loss of limb interferes with independence and threatens body image. Upper extremity myoelectric prostheses can now be operated with batteries connected to electric motors, allowing these limbs to be functional in performing ADL. A team consisting of the client, prosthetist, physiatrist, rehabilitation nurse, physical therapist, occupational therapist, orthotist, and vocational counselor can best determine the prosthesis that is suitable for the client's needs. The orthotist designs braces according to individual client needs. The braces are used to apply force to an extremity and assist, resist, align, or stimulate function of the extremity. A lengthy inpatient stay may not be necessary following a person's single limb amputation. The client can access necessary services on an outpatient basis.

The rehabilitation plan for achieving maximum functional independence in personal hygiene requires assessment and evaluation by all team members. They meet together regularly and reevaluate the plan with the client and family to determine progress in meeting the established goals. Other professionals may join or assist a team as client needs dictate.

OUTCOME CRITERIA

Outcome criteria for the client diagnosed with functional deficits in personal hygiene and grooming activities include the following:

1. The client and family will perform the client's personal hygiene and grooming activities at an optimum level of function.
2. The client and family know when and how to use assistive and adaptive devices when these are prescribed.
3. The client and family will anticipate fatigue and plan rest periods before fatigue occurs.
4. The client will possess positive self-esteem and body image.
5. The client and family will perform personal hygiene and grooming activities safely within their own environment.

FUTURE DIRECTIONS

Shorter hospital stays, limited policy coverage for acute rehabilitation, or absence of coverage together have moved acutely ill clients through the system much faster than in the past. This trend has placed a new burden on the system to prioritize rehabilitation goals. Unfortunately these problems have also placed individuals in an environment that focuses on teaching when they are scarcely ready to learn. At times self-care skills acquisition can suffer because

"there isn't time." One way of diminishing this problem is to bring therapy to the clients on the units. This technique is being used in many rehabilitation facilities throughout the country. This can be a true multidisciplinary approach if all members of the team are involved. This approach further places heavy responsibility on rehabilitation nursing to move from the traditional role of nursing to the more modern role of a rehabilitation team member.

Some institutions have met the shortened stay crisis by offering "therapy" 7 days a week. Again this relies heavily on nursing for initiation, carry-through, and delivery of teaching of the self-care activities.

The Role of Home Care

Transition programs from facility to home have been initiated by a small group of home health companies. The face of home health is changing. It is no longer synonymous with a sitter service or a hospital without walls but can be an equal partner in returning the client to his highest level of functional independence. The home health caregiver must become educated in facilitation and teaching of self-care skills, just as the nurse in the facility must expand her skills in those areas.

The client who is returning home generally experiences a great deal of anxiety and may regress regarding independence. That client needs a knowledgeable cheerleader who can help build his confidence and empower him to problem-solve appropriately in his "new" environment.

As home care agencies develop the ability to work with specialized programs such as rehabilitation, facilities can begin to discharge clients home earlier, thereby providing a tremendous cost savings to the consumer. This early discharge with appropriate caregivers also allows for the utilization of specialized outpatient clinics at the rehabilitation facilities.

Providing Care at Home

A great deal of emphasis is placed on the family delivering self-care activities. Unfortunately when the client returns home, the family caregiver finds that it is too time consuming for the client to perform these activities, and it is easier to do these activities for the client. This becomes another strong argument for the use of trained caregivers in the home environment.

These caregivers are generally paraprofessionals working under the direction of a nurse. This arrangement can further assist the client and/or her family to further develop management skills as well as other skills necessary in acquiring private caregivers if that is appropriate.

Clients and their families should be encouraged to interview anyone who will be delivering services to them. They should evaluate home care companies for (1) knowledge in rehabilitation philosophy, (2) ability to facilitate client performance of self-care skills (either physical performance or in verbal direction of self-care), and (3) ability to give a time frame when the client will be independent in performance of the self-care skills or in direction of the activity (Marelli, 1994).

The client or family member should be able to indicate to the agency that they see the agency involvement as only a part of the continuum and not an end in itself. Generally by the time the client is ready for discharge to the home, the agency should be offering LPN or home health agency level support. Too heavy of a reliance on therapies or RNs may be an indicator that the agency does not have a "caregiver delivered, client-driven" program. The program would be managed by the RN at the agency. Multidisciplinary teams can exist in the home as they do in the facility. The client is a significant member of this team and needs to have an "equal voice." Activities traditionally practiced at home can be moved to a more functional environment such as a department store dressing room.

To provide a true continuum of care as well as a smooth transition to the home, the home care agency nurse should be involved in the hospital staffings. This allows her to be knowledgeable as to the client's status at discharge. Early participation in hospital conferencing can also assist with the acquisition of supplies and equipment so as to eliminate lag time before the client actually begins the home program.

SUMMARY

The rehabilitation nurse is in a unique position to assist the client in achieving an optimum level of independence in personal hygiene, grooming activities, and self-care. Through nursing assessment of the client's ability to perform these activities, the nursing diagnoses are formulated and interventions are planned and implemented. The nurse collaborates with other rehabilitation team members to assist the client and family in use of assistive and adapted devices and specialized techniques to function safely at an optimum level in these activities. When the client can be independent in performing some or all of these activities, body image or self-esteem are enhanced, therefore helping the client regain control of his life.

REFERENCES

Berliner, H. (1986). Aging skin Part 1. *American Journal of Nursing, 86,* 1138-1141.

Chen Sea, M-J., Henderson, A., & Cermak, S.A. (1993). Patterns of visual spatial inattention and their functional significance in stroke patients. Archives of Physical Medicine & Rehabilitation, 74, 355-360.

Connelly, C.E. (1993). An empirical study of a model of self-care in chronic illness. *Clinical Nurse Specialist, 7,* 247-253.

DeJong, G. (1979). Attendant care as a prototype independent living service. *Archives of Physical Medicine and Rehabilitation, 60, 482.*

Dewis, M.E. (1989). Spinal cord injured adolescents and young adults: The meaning of body changes. *Journal of Advanced Nursing, 14,* 389-396.

Denton, B. (1984). *Child Development.* School of Allied Health Professions. Master's thesis, unpublished. Department of Occupational Therapy.

Denton, B. (1984), Fall, Louisiana State University Medical Center, Shreveport.

Duckworth, B. (1986). Overview of menstrual management for disabled women. *Canadian Journal of Occupational Therapy, 53,* 25-29.

Dudgeon, B.J., DeLisa, J.A., & Miller, R.M. (1985). Optokinetic nystagmus and upper extremity dressing: Independence after stroke. *Archives of Physical Medicine and Rehabilitation, 66,* 164.

Gordon, M. (1993). *Nursing diagnosis: Process and application* (2nd ed.). New York: McGraw-Hill.

Graham, S., & Morley, M. (1984). What foot care. *American Journal of Nursing, 84,* 889-891.

Hagan, C. (1984). Language disorders in head trauma. In A. Holland (Ed.), *Language disorders in adults.* Austin, TX: College Hill Press.

Hoeman, S.P. (1992). Pediatric rehabilitation nursing. In G. Molnar (Ed.)., *Pediatric rehabilitation* (2nd ed., pp. 202-219). Baltimore: Williams and Wilkins.

Hoeman, S.P. (1990). *Rehabilitation/restoration in the community.* St. Louis: Mosby–Year Book.

Hudson, M.F. (1983). Safeguard your elderly patient's health through accurate physical assessment. *Nursing, 13,* 58-64.

Jacus, C.M. (1981). Working with families in a rehabilitation setting, *Rehabilitation Nursing,* 6(3)10-14.

Jackson, J.E., & Neighbors, M. (1990). *Home care client assessment handbook.* Rockville, MD: Aspen.

Kimberly Quality Care. (1991). *The art of interview.* Kansas City: Author.

Marrelli, T.M. (1994). *Handbook of home health standards and documentation guidelines for reimbursement* (2nd ed.). St. Louis: Mosby–Year Book.

Mather, M.L.S. (1987). The secret to life in a spica. *American Journal of Nursing, 85,* 56-58.

McCourt, A.E. (Ed.). (1993). *The speciality practice of rehabilitation nursing: A core curriculum* (3rd ed.). Rehabilitation: Nursing Foundation. Skokie, IL.

Molnar, G.E. (1992). *Pediatric rehabilitation* (2nd ed.). Baltimore: Williams and Wilkins.

Morgan, K.J., & McClain, S.L. (1993). *Core curriculum for home health care nursing.* Gaithersburg, MD: Aspen.

Mossman, P. (1976). *A problem oriented approach to stroke rehabilitation.* Springfield, IL: Charles C Thomas.

Normal, V., & Snyder, M. (1982). Assessment of self-care readiness. *Rehabilitation Nursing,* 7(3), 17-21.

Orem, D. (1980). *Nursing concepts of practice.* New York: McGraw-Hill.

Owen, R. (1984). *Language development.* Columbus: Charles E. Merril.

Pedretti, L.W., & Zoltan, B. (1990). *Occupational therapy practice skills for physical dysfunction.* St. Louis: Mosby–Year Book.

Phipps, W.J., Cassmeyer, V.L., Sands, J.K., & Lehman, M.K. (1995) *Medical-Surgical Nursing: Concepts and Clinical Practice,* 5th ed. Mosby–Year Book, St. Louis.

Rogers, S. (1992). The spirit of independence: The evolution of a philosophy. *American Journal of Occupational Therapy, 36,* 709-715.

Rosenthal, M., Griffen, E., Bond, M.R., & Miller, D.J. (1990). *Rehabilitation of the adult and child with traumatic brain injury* (2nd ed.). Philadelphia: F.A. Davis.

Sanford, A.R. (1973). *Learning accomplishment profile.* Chapel Hill, NC: Training Out Reach Project.

Sarver, S.C., & Howard, M. (1982). Planning a self-care unit in an inpatient setting. *American Journal of Nursing, 32,* 1112-1114.

Sims, N. (1976). *All about health and beauty for the black woman.* New York: Doubleday.

Sine, R., Holcomb, D.J., Rausch, R.E., Liss, S.E. & Wilson, G.B. (1981). *Rehabilitation techniques: A self-instruction guide* (2nd ed.). Rockville, MD: Aspen.

Stewart, A. (1993). *Care of traumatic brain injury. Rehabilitation manual, CEU program.* Boston: Kimberly Quality Care.

The Arthritis Foundation. (1969). *Home care program in arthritis.* New York: Author.

Theuerkauf, S., & Carpenter, P. (1992). *GUMBO Training Manual,* Bulletin 1830 (Rev). Baton Rouge: Louisiana State Department of Education.

Theuerkauf, S., & Carpenter, P. (1992). Return to the real world. A spinal cord injury. *Journal of Home Health Care Practice,* 4(4), 14-23.

Theuerkauf, S., & Stewart, A. (1993). *Kimberly Quality Care rehabilitation manual.* Kansas City: Kimberly Quality Care.

Wells, R., & Trostle, K. (1984). Creative hairwashing techniques for immobilized patients. *Nursing, 14,* (1), 47-51.

Yetzer, E.A., Kauffman, G. Sopp, F., & Talley, L. (1994). Development of a patient education program for new amputees. *Rehabilitation Nursing,* 19, 355-358.

Zejdlik, C.P. (1992). *Spinal cord injury management* (2nd ed.). Boston: Jones and Bartlett.

Zoltan, B., Siev, E., & Freishtat, B. (1986). *The adult stroke patient: A manual for evaluation and treatment of perceptual and cognitive dysfunction.* (2nd ed.). Thorofare, NJ: Slack.

13

Coping with Chronic, Disabling, or Developmental Disorders

Shirley P. Hoeman, PhD, RN, CRRN, CNAA, CCM

INTRODUCTION

"Stress" and "coping" are reflected in expressions of the 1990s: "stressed out" and "I can't cope with this!" In rehabilitation nursing the complex concepts of stress and coping are important to client outcomes. Many assessment and outcome evaluations include measures based on connotative definitions of stress and coping. The large amount of empiric literature about these concepts contains gaps and controversies since studies use a variety of methods dealing with a broad array of health and illness topics, rendering findings that cannot be compared or generalized.

The content for this chapter was chosen to enhance the scope, depth, and variety of strategies available to rehabilitation nurses as they facilitate adjustment and improve outcomes that reflect the unique needs and lifestyle for each client and family. Understanding relationships of stress with a person's quality of life, wellness, and capacity for independent function and knowing how to intervene to promote effective coping are major interests for rehabilitation nurses. Coping effectively with stressors following disability or living with chronic conditions tests personal reserves and stretches social and economic resources. Thus clients and families are challenged in multiple ways to manage chronic, unpredictable, irreversible, progressive, comorbid, or recurrent conditions. This means learning more about stressful circumstances and conditions under which health breaks down, since stress itself is not synonymous with illness or disability. This chapter begins with theoretic discussions and proceeds to assessment and practical interventions.

PARAMETERS OF STRESS AND COPING

Psychological stress is "a particular relationship between the person and the environment that is appraised by the person as taxing or exceeding his or her resources and endangering his or her well-being" (Lazarus & Folkman, 1984). A conceptual framework includes stress initiators—namely specific stressors—mediators, buffers or catalysts, and stress concepts, particularly coping. To date the following three theoretic views of stress are generally recognized.

Early behaviorists wrote about uniform responses to an external stimulus; touch a hot stove and draw back from pain. Other researchers experienced marginal success and methodologic problems when they explored relationships

between life events and health outcome (Dixon, Dixon, & Spinner, 1989) or questioned how life events might serve as precursors of stress (Dohrenwend & Dohrenwend, 1980). To some extent stress may be a part of the human condition—an essential, constructive ingredient in human activities. However, a stressor does not evoke the same response in every person, nor does a certain stimulus always become appraised as a stressor.

Second, stress is viewed as an internal condition generated as a result of a noxious stimulus. The abbreviated discussion that follows demonstrates how findings about the physiology of stress influence nursing assessment and interventions regarding coping with stressors. Identifying stress as the nonspecific physiologic response, Cannon (1914, 1935) described a "fight-or-flight" response and Selye (1956) detailed a universal general adaptation syndrome (GAS), which concentrated on the effects of biophysical stress on the body. Although individual responses are the same, unique factors or characteristics influence progress and outcome of the GAS and the specific nature and extent of changes in response to stress.

The GAS has three stages: an alarm reaction, a stage of resistance, and a stage of exhaustion. The alarm stage is further divided into an initial shock resulting from the noxious agent's effect on body tissues—lowered blood pressure, for one. Next the countershock phase of the alarm reaction is characterized by physiologic defense activities—blood pressure and body temperature rise and the adrenal cortex becomes activated.

During the stage of resistance, physiologic efforts are dedicated to resisting or adapting to the noxious agent, perhaps ignoring other potentially threatening agents. Tissue resistance triggers the nervous system and the endocrine glands. The adrenal and pituitary glands produce antiinflammatory, proinflammatory, and catatoxic hormones that attempt to resist or adapt to the noxious agent (Trieschmann, 1987). Symptoms of illness reflect the body's attempts to adapt to stressors. All of these responses may be modified by other factors such as heredity, individual coping experiences and reactions, health status, and diet. Should this stage persevere, stressors may accumulate and superimpose on the system, further reducing capacity for adaptation and signaling exhaustion.

When resistance fails, exhaustion sets in and finally death. Perhaps the body becomes exhausted from defensive reactions or from giving in to agents, physiologically producing excessive or insufficient adaptive hormones. Either way an impact of chronic or repeated stressors is for the "worn down" person to develop one of the "diseases of adaptation." Selye categorizes arthritis, hypertension, allergic and hypersensitivity conditions, circulatory and heart diseases, digestive problems, and other diseases as diseases of adaptation (Selye, 1956; Trieschmann, 1987). Research about the relationship of sequence of stressors, chronic stressors, and exhaustion with long-term disability is a priority for nurses.

In a third view stress is brought about from a person-environment transaction. An individual and the environment integrate in a dynamic and reciprocal exchange wherein both physiologic and psychological stressors are neither process nor outcome. An individual's appraisal, a cognitive evaluation of a person-environment transaction, and coping are key mediators of stress in transactional models (Lazarus & Folkman, 1984). The person manages stress arising from a person-environment transaction using a process of complex, multiple component coping strategies that are influenced by mediating factors and resources. This process is discussed more thoroughly in this chapter.

Nursing Conceptual Frameworks and Stress

The transactional view is consistent with constructs from nursing frameworks, fitting with Orem's or Rogers's theories and Leininger's cultural model (Chapter 1). Neuman (1989) defines stressors as "tension producing stimuli or forces occurring within both internal and external environmental boundaries of the client system." Because Neuman's model is holistic and considers proximal and distal environmental stressors, it is useful as a comprehensive assessment guide for rehabilitation nursing practice (Wein, 1985).

Neuman envisions the client structure set within concentric lines of resistance and defense. Nursing interventions occur at primary, secondary, and tertiary levels to correspond with the level of penetration by the stressor. When a stressor is identified before onset, primary interventions may retain the person's stability. When a stressor occurs and the person reacts, secondary interventions strengthen internal and external resources, manage any symptoms, and set mutual priorities. At the tertiary level, interventions prevent further stressor damage and reconstitute the person's system.

However, when an individual, family, or community experiences too many changes in succession, when stressful events accumulate or recur, or when the meaning of loss is overwhelmingly painful, the system may experience overload. In effect the system's perception of tolerable stress exceeds the available resources; meanwhile expectation of reality is contradicted by events. The system may break down or collapse (Neuman, 1989).

A transactional view of stress blends with concepts of theorists from other disciplines in useful ways. For example, Smelser (1963) defined social stressors as system disruptors; Rosenstock (1974) outlined a health belief model; and Knowles (1973) identified motivational factors associated with adult learning. In management, proactive personal and corporate management skills are guided by transactional principles for decision-making and effective coping in a changing world (Covey, 1989).

♦ Stressors

Accurate assessment of effective coping for a client and family is more likely when a rehabilitation nurse understands the components of stress. In the following section findings from research are used as a basis for discussion of selected stressors and person-environment factors influencing appraisal of stress. Stressors are life transitions and events, temporal stressors, loss and change, health status, daily hassles, environment, and the rehabilitation system itself. Person-environment factors are knowledge and self-efficacy, uncertainty, and individual and family characteristics. These are followed by variables associated with stressors such as self-esteem, locus of control (Rotter, 1966), and hardiness.

Life transitions and happenings. Life transitions are anticipated developmental changes experienced by most persons and their families (Figley & McCubbin, 1983) as they adjust, adapt, and cope with life transitions. Normative life events, such as menopause, are accompanied by health/illness stressors—which vary among individuals (Werner, 1993). Cultural rites of passage signal life transitions, such as recognizing physical and psychosocial changes during puberty as a child's passage into adolescence. Roles, responsibilities, and opportunities are expected to change with life transitions. However, when events do not occur when or as expected, they may become stressful.

Conversely, unpredictable, sudden, and life-threatening stressors resulting in serious or multiple consequences become catastrophies. Associated with traumatic events or with unusual stressors, such as after a natural disaster, catastrophies disrupt and damage family patterns and imprint involuntary and voluntary memories of the event, such as with posttraumatic stress disorder. Lifelong adjustment or adaptation may be necessary for clients in rehabilitation and their families who encounter impairments, alterations, disruptions, or other catastrophic stressors (Figley & McCubbin, 1983).

♦ Temporal stressors

The timing of events and relationship with other current or past events in the person's life influence stress tolerance. Some life events become stressful because they occur "off time," when unexpected in life; others are stressful because they did not occur "on time." As a result the person is bereft of support and camaraderie of peers, misses satisfaction of achieving an anticipated milestone, and musters few anticipatory coping resources (Neugarten, 1979).

Chronic sorrow was conceptualized from data about family experiences and reemergent feelings of loss when developmental and social milestones were not achieved as expected in a child with cognitive delays (Olshansky, 1962). The concept has been expanded to include families with a child who has chronic or disabling conditions (Fraley, 1990; Thomas, 1987; Wikler, Wasow, & Hatfield, 1981) and to recognize chronic sorrow as a normative factor associated with the concept of chronicity.

A great deal remains to be learned about how stressors

persist and vary over time, and the specific conditions that influence outcomes. Although stressors may be persistent, what is perceived as stressful can be expected to change during the course of a chronic condition. Survivors of myocardial infarction (MI) (n = 52) were found to experience stress 1 month postinfarction. Clients reported some stressors existed before the MI and persisted afterward. However, stress related to the MI itself was manifested as distress based on a client's cognitive appraisals of harm, loss, or threat (Miller, Garrett, Stoltenberg, McMahon, & Ringel, 1990).

In other research clients (n = 40) who had received renal transplants within 4 years completed a 35-item Likert-type scale that listed potential stressors and stress management strategies. Clients selected fear of rejection of the transplant, uncertainty of outcome, and concern about costs as most stressful. Although fears of familial or social rejection were low, concern about others' expectations for a client to resume former roles was highly stressful.

Perceptions of stress changed over time, although participants used problem-solving approaches with stressors. Notably clients within 2 years posttransplant perceived more control over factors affecting outcome and reported overall lower stress than those 2 to 4 years posttransplant. Clients between 2 and 4 years posttransplant indicated increased use of affective methods of prayer, viewing all sides objectively, and maintaining control to cope (Sutton & Murphy, 1988).

Adjustment to chronic and disabling conditions is a lifelong process for clients and families, which requires interventions far beyond brief crisis intervention. Over a third of families with a member who had a stroke reported unsatisfactory adjustment 5 years following the incident (Holbrook, 1982). Clients with spinal cord injury acknowledged adjustment issues persist years after they re-enter the community. Persons with ineffective social, psychological, and vocational adjustment were among those who did not survive. On the other hand, 4 years following an initial 11-year study of changes and factors in adjustment (Crewe & Kraus, 1990), clients with spinal cord injury (n = 135) repeated the Life Situation Questionnaire (LSQ). As these clients aged, their sitting tolerance and thus vocational opportunities improved and hospitalization decreased. These findings raise questions about relationships of health-activity variables, vocational success, and adjustment (Krause, 1992).

Family members who care for a relative who has psychosocial changes following a traumatic brain injury (TBI) may develop maladaptive behaviors. Family caregivers (n = 51) surveyed at intervals over 2 years were found to have increased medication use and substance abuse and decreased employment and financial status. Spouses of clients with TBI needed mental health and respite services and socialization (Hall et al., 1994).

In a critique of theory and "clinical lore," Wortman and Silver (1989) found a number of long-held beliefs about coping with loss and related responses were not based on results from empiric research. They question the veracity of widely held assumptions about distress, grieving, and depression inevitably following loss, including disability. How often are nursing interventions based on untested assumptions, while significant findings from research languish in the literature and are not utilized? Rehabilitation nurses are encouraged to examine health beliefs critically and test them clinically.

✦ Loss and change

Loss and change with recurrent or unresolved grieving are corollaries to chronicity. Grieving may be a prerequisite to adjustment for some, but judging a chronic or disabling condition to be the source of a client's grieving may impede holistic assessment. Experiencing chronic or disabling disorders does not guarantee a client immunity to other stressful life events such as loss or injury of family, friends, or pets. However, acquired cognitive impairment or altered cognition may influence a person's perception of loss (Sachs, 1984).

With real or perceived loss, there is an element of psychosocial pain that may alter perceptions of basic needs, independent functioning, or cognition. Rehabilitation nurses encounter clients who are coping with change, loss, and physical and psychosocial pain in scenarios wherein a person's, family's, or community's perception of what is real, or what is tolerable, differs from what is occurring. As a result symptoms of family disintegration may appear: disequilibrium, confusion and dissonance, anxiety, fear, isolation, and embarrassment. When reality of loss and change exceed the resources or capabilities for effective coping behaviors, overload may collapse the entire family system (Neuman, 1989). Ultimately communications, relationships, commitment, resources, and goals may disintegrate. The daily reality of chronicity prevents closure on loss and initiates stressors.

✦ Health status

There is little debate that actual or potential loss of health status is stressful. Conversely stressors may lead to loss of well-being and reduced immunity. In one study clients believed stress about threats to health had greater impact on health outcome than stress from potential life happenings or anticipated maturational changes (Ferketich & Mercer, 1990). A review of nursing research found the impact of acquiring disease to be more stressful than actual experiences associated with procedures or hospitalization (Barnfather & Lyon, 1993).

Actual or potential threats to health, roles, self-efficacy, or empowerment follow catastrophic events. Clients' (n = 50) descriptions of powerlessness while hospitalized for acute spinal cord injury revealed feelings of powerlessness occurred at various times during hospitalization but were significantly more intense and frequent with increased acuity. Clients over age 60 and those whose injury resulted in quadriplegia reported the most powerlessness (Richmond, Metcalf, Daly, & Kish, 1992).

✦ Daily hassles

Researchers do not agree about how stressful events are experienced and perceived by individuals and families. For instance, what are the amounts and kinds of stress generated by daily hassles, especially when hassles recur over long periods? Are daily hassles relevant indicators of overall stress or tolerance levels (Weinberger, Hiner, & Tierney,

1987), or will chronic stressors produce responses and yield health outcomes that differ from those associated with acute, time-limited stressors? How do stressors associated with daily hassles relate to stressors initiated by disability or dependency for lifelong care?

Rehabilitation nurses can be instrumental in researching questions about stressors, while in practice promoting strategies that enable clients to embrace hope, holistic self-concepts, and empowerment as part of adjustment to loss (Pereira, 1984).

✦ Environment

Environmental stressors may be excruciatingly obvious to one person and seemingly invisible to another. Nurses are sensitive to potential stressors and anticipate ways to improve a client's comfort: reducing noise, controlling temperature, eliminating chemical and other irritants, removing offending media, or replacing uncomfortable furniture. Barriers in access, time, or space are stressors. Simply placing a prosthesis within reach, arranging items in a client's preferred style on the table, or installing a wheelchair ramp at home extends personal control over the environment.

Other clients may rely on computer or mechanical technology, assistive devices, and adapted equipment to support independent functioning for activities of daily living (ADL) or to promote learning in the least restrictive environment. Even technologic assistance necessary to sustain life is a potential stressor. Malfunction or breakdown, repair or refurbishing, maintenance, reassessment to fit a client's changing needs, or costly replacement may become daily hassles.

Barriers to services and geographic access are significant stressors for those who live in underserved urban areas, or for the one-third of older Americans who live in rural areas. Older rural residents report greater physical impairment, chronic conditions, and less access to services than urban counterparts (Preston & Mansfield, 1984). The rural elderly experience high levels of stress that contribute to reduced health status and impede optimal independent functional abilities.

For example, visual impairment, altered upper extremity function, or progressive neuromuscular changes may mean lost driving privileges for a rural resident—contributing to potential loneliness and isolation and reduced access to food, medications, or health maintenance services (Johnson, Waldo, & Johnson, 1993). Community nurses who work with children at home on Medicaid Model Waivers or with elderly persons with functional limitations are aware of the impact of environmental barriers. Parents cite transportation as a major stressor in obtaining access to service needs (Hoeman, 1992b).

✦ Rehabilitation system

The rehabilitation system itself may introduce stressors. Client and family attitudes and beliefs about the intent of the rehabilitation process and about their place in the system may be incongruent or incompatible with those of rehabilitation professionals. Team members may obtain satisfaction from helping rather than enabling, the system may be designed to ease its own stressors, or steps in the process may be habitual rather than planned (Hoeman, 1990b).

Goals to have clients and families participate in the rehabilitation process mean different things to clients and families than to team members when the time comes for implementation, regardless of whether the goals deal with individual preferences in daily care or larger issues about community living or resource allocation (Nyhlin, 1990).

Implementing a plan driven by meeting clients' needs means to foster coping strategies that enable clients to self-manage their lifestyle—rather than teaching them how to negotiate the rehabilitation system—and will improve outcome.

As advocates for improved outcomes, rehabilitation nurses are encouraged to examine their own practice and the rehabilitation system for cultural barriers. Persons who are not fluent in English may misinterpret information and receive inaccurate assessment, especially when a client has speech or language deficits. Rehabilitation system processes may be stressful for clients and families when their cultural perception of the meaning underlying a process differs from the intent. More difficult to discern are cultural stressors that may arise from a number of traditionally held assumptions on the part of rehabilitation team, specifically assumptions that professionals, clients, and families share coping strategies toward achieving the same rehabilitation outcomes. Professionals may assume that persons who enter rehabilitation are seeking independence in ADL, when in fact some families may uphold cultural values and roles that conflict with self-care (Hoeman, 1989).

Ways of expressing stress may differ. In an ethnography of young males on a spinal cord unit, researchers argued swearing behavior by clients who had incurred traumatic spinal cord injury was a temporary coping strategy for despair, altered body image, and impaired functional abilities resulting from disability. Swearing replaced crying as a more culturally acceptable mode of emotional release for young males. The swearing behavior may represent a strategy for coping with an altered life plan and a renegotiation of hope (Laskiwski & Morse, 1993).

✦ Person-environment factors

Nurse researchers are working to learn more about the characteristics of appraisals and perceptual phenomena, relationships among perception, concepts of stress and coping, and definitions for the appraisal process. For example, "a critical evaluation of immediate experience" has been a suggested reference for the concept of appraisal. Although underdeveloped, two perceptual themes are sensory experiences and a cognitive position from which to evaluate experiences and responses (England, 1993). The content of debates on stress and coping paradigms is lengthy and complex. Several factors in appraisal of person-environment transactions are discussed in the following material.

✦ Knowledge and self-efficacy factors

Knowledge about a disability or health condition is crucial to self-efficacy for caregivers and family members as well as for clients. Being informed about procedures and routines, and becoming knowledgeable about what will occur and why, promotes self-direction in care. Thus a client must be able to perceive the elements of what is being learned and perform the changed action while cognitively participating in the transaction (psychosocial and cognitive actions). A person's cognitive, social, and behavioral skills integrate with the environment at complex levels, such as judgment and transaction, to create usable knowledge. Finally, the person must be able to accomplish the action. When the goal is to learn changes promoting self-efficacy, a client makes the changes while the nurse supplies the concepts to be learned and practiced (Bandura, 1982). Ideally effective coping and empowerment are enhanced through learning, whereas powerlessness may impede a client's learning essential knowledge.

Swedish researchers investigated how adults with insulin-dependent diabetes mellitus (n = 55) managed their disease. Addressing biologic, psychological, and social areas, investigators used the components needed for a sense of coherence in Antonovsky's (1972) model, with comprehensibility, manageability, and meaningfulness as variables. When nurses directed client education toward a person's own abilities from a personal point of view—incorporated individual preferences, and accommodated lifestyle and habits—a client was found to use effective coping strategies to manage diabetes, maintain health, and follow educational guidelines (Wikblad & Montin, 1992).

✦ Uncertainty factors

Uncertainty about progress and outcome in chronic, disabling, or developmental disorders is a troublesome but familiar concept in rehabilitation. A study of women with rheumatoid arthritis (n = 23) explored the experience of living with continual uncertainty such as learning about relationships among length of illness, degree of uncertainty, and appraisal of uncertainty. Findings suggest women who perceive high levels of uncertainty concerning immobility, pain, or impaired functional abilities following rheumatoid arthritis may appraise uncertainty as danger. If correct, an appraisal of danger would increase anxiety, fear, physiologic responses, and ineffective coping behaviors (Bailey & Nielsen, 1993).

Certainty and predictability are valued in Western cultures where persons are uncomfortable with not knowing what to expect and with not knowing how to influence what is expected. Preferred thinking is linear, organized, controlled, and precise. Valued traits are self-efficacy, control, goal direction, and time management, whereas not knowing when or how is less acceptable. Thus when clients face chronic, disabling, or developmental disorders that have uncertain outcomes, they initially want to know how to cure the problem to counteract system breakdown. When chaotic rhythms (Mishel, 1990) are used to illustrate the nature of uncertainty, clients may be able to shift their paradigms to think in terms of possibilities, diversity, randomness, or nonlinear relationships.

Uncertainty as a concept has gained international interest. A Swedish researcher used a qualitative approach to learn how persons who had diabetes mellitus accompanied by severe complications dealt with uncertainty of outcome. Basic coping strategies used by clients were normalizing their lives, explaining events in their lives to make sense of the situation, coming to terms with their changing status, accepting increased dependence on the healthcare system, and adjusting while "keeping going" in spite of the uncertainty and related barriers. Overall these persons managed well within their limitations.

An unexpected but important finding was that some uncertainty was introduced needlessly into clients' lives by policies or routines embedded in the health system. Attention to the uniqueness of each client's entire system, rather than illness alone, was suggested for improving coping effectiveness (Nyhlin, 1990).

Mishel documented four situations that hinder a client who lives with uncertainty (see Box below); each situation reinforces the societal belief that stressors associated with uncertainty and a person's responses are in some way unacceptable, disruptive, and abnormal.

For example, a client with a chronic condition who is the parent of a teenager may delay the teenager's psychological adjustment to the uncertain outcomes from the client/parent's chronic condition. Thus family members in this situation are unprepared to support one another effectively or think toward possibilities.

Even when clients are prepared, support needs may change over the disease trajectory. Researchers tested relationships between uncertainty and coping style of adults recovering from nonemergency coronary artery bypass surgery (n = 129). Clients expressed concern about treatment, possible complications, future self-care ability, and return to former life roles consistent with uncertainty stressors. Clients were found to be preoccupied with uncertainty, manifested as ambiguity, about their health status 1 week after surgery. Six weeks after surgery, their concern transferred to uncertainty about the treatment and the health system of care, manifested as complexity. Clients also used emotion-based coping, such as wishful thinking and avoidance (Redeker, 1992).

However, causal relationships are not simple; complex dimensions of physical, environmental, and personality influence adjustment. For example, a person with multiple sclerosis (MS) must deal with loss and uncertainty as well as with disease progression; however, having MS has not

---

✦

FOUR SITUATIONS ASSOCIATED WITH UNCERTAINTY

1. Members of a person's support system do not promote options or think about possibilities.
2. Health professionals may insist only curative measures are acceptable outcomes and deny opportunities to assist a client with adjusting to uncertainty.
3. Isolation may curtail interaction with social supports, further restricting the person's worldview.
4. A person with a chronic condition who is a primary caretaker may delay others from developing skills they eventually will need to cope effectively with the caretaker's condition (Mishel, 1990).

Adapted from "Mishel Reconceptualization of the Uncertainty in Illness Theory", *Image, 22,* 256-262. Adapted by permission.

been demonstrated in itself as a strong predictor of difficulty with adjustment (Marks & Millard, 1990).

✦ Individual and family characteristics

Client education, age, intelligence, culture, emotional status, philosophic or spiritual beliefs, previous coping experience (Holaday, 1984), gender, roles, personality traits, and status as client are related to cognitive knowledge and coping strategies. Psychosocial behavior assessment is founded on the unique way in which each individual looks at or finds meaning in a situation. As a process, perception varies with

- ✦ Context, meaning, and value attached to the particular stressors
- ✦ Lifestyle changes such as altered role performance or financial changes
- ✦ Sociocultural variables
- ✦ Sensory inputs
- ✦ The mix of stressors with coping capabilities

The relationship of physiologic pain with the experience of psychological pain is evident in persons who develop conditioned responses to a stressor triggering back pain, then subsequently alter their personal appraisals of what is occurring. When the body and mind reach agreement that a person is unable to perform independently, society releases or absolves certain responsibilities and temporarily sanctions a "sick role." However, a client who "learns helplessness" makes dependence a choice, which may be a consequence of coping. Nurses attuned to complex, multidimensional relationships among various stressors and health outcome continue to heighten their awareness and integrate systems information into their assessment skills.

✦ Variables

Variables associated with stressors themselves are discussed in the following section and are listed in the following Box.

✦

VARIABLES ASSOCIATED WITH STRESSORS

- ✦ Intensity
- ✦ Duration
- ✦ Timing
- ✦ Predictability
- ✦ Uncertainty of process or outcome
- ✦ Knowledge about stressor

Individual or family characteristics influencing appraisal

- ✦ Self-esteem
- ✦ Hardiness
- ✦ Locus of control
- ✦ Sociocultural beliefs and practices
- ✦ Developmental stage, age, or gender
- ✦ Behavior patterns
- ✦ Vulnerability and resilience
- ✦ Quality-of-life experiences

✦ Self-esteem

Self-esteem is a variable influencing how a person appraises stressors, as well as an individual attribute for effective coping, learning self-care, developing relationships, and maintaining hope. Four antecedents of self-esteem are

- ✦ Power to control one's behavior and influence others
- ✦ A sense of being loved, respected, and belonging
- ✦ A sense of personal moral values
- ✦ A belief in one's competency in expected roles for self and by others (Coopersmith, 1981)

On the other hand, three disturbances of self-esteem negatively affect coping behaviors. In one, a person lowers previously healthy self-esteem due to a situation or event that has challenged the self-identity. Situational loss of a family member, altered body image, changed roles in family or workplace, overwhelming life responsibilities, or acquiring a disability may lower self-esteem (Antonucci & Jackson, 1983). Changes in body image following disease or injury require a client to adjust to threats to self-esteem as well as to loss and change (Drench, 1994). Restoring self-esteem may be prerequisite to effective coping for an individual and family.

Every person has developed and refined certain mechanisms that are used to keep things the way they are or to manipulate how the person wants them to be. However, persons who use defensive coping hide behind behavioral mechanisms to cover their true self-appraisal. Defense mechanisms tend to be patterns for avoiding the truth about what is happening as well as for shielding self from discomfort, blame, shame, loss of self-esteem, and protecting from other unpleasant fears.

Commonly used defense mechanisms are

- ✦ Rationalization to substitute for the real reason behind actions
- ✦ Projection with blame
- ✦ Displacement of anger or frustration
- ✦ Fantasizing to avoid reality or delay action
- ✦ Withdrawal for isolation
- ✦ Denial permeating physical and psychosocial-emotional health
- ✦ Overcompensating for deficits or losses
- ✦ Avoidance roles that become insulating masks, such as for defensive low self-esteem, addictive behaviors, or negative self-images

Defense mechanisms are learned and reinforced through family and social relationships and carried out in lifestyle choices. However, a person who has low self-esteem predisposing disability or chronicity, such as from devaluing experiences, may engage in chronic negative self-appraisal, which in turn may lead to negative appraisal of stressors and ineffective coping. The person who has chronic low self-esteem may experience powerlessness and hopelessness, feeling unworthy or devalued.

Often a person with chronic low self-esteem has developed maladaptive or self-destructive behaviors, which only serve to reinforce a poor self-image. Verbally self-deprecating, this person may ignore self-care and health maintenance, participate in nonsupportive interpersonal relationships, engage in addictive patterns such as overeating, smoking, or alcohol and substance abuse; and be at risk for personal safety. Viewing life options has been difficult, so the person uses distorted thinking; thus a self-appraisal of a situation following a disabling or chronic condition only becomes more negative.

✦ Types of behavior patterns

A person's stress behavior has been portrayed as an impetus that spurs an athlete to victory, sustains a student through an examination, and encourages one toward a challenging goal. Certain personality types are associated with behavior and stressors. Thus a person who manifests psychological factors consistent with a Type A behavior pattern is said to respond to her environment with driving, intense, and impatient behavior. Internalizing both overt and covert stressors, clients ultimately drive themselves to stress-provoked cardiac disease and recurring or fatal cardiac incidents (Jenkins, Zyzanski, & Rosenman, 1976).

For example, angina pectoris is known to be a stress-aggravated condition that is related significantly with Type A behavior pattern characteristics in individuals (Haynes & Feinleib, 1982). In part, perception of stressors, including environmental stressors, govern individual coping responses (Rosenman, 1982).

One explanatory model proposes stress mediators or buffers. Perception is processed as information and mediates stressors between psychosocial or environmental stimuli and physiologic reactions (Dembroski, 1978). This may account for the person with Type B behavior who experiences stressors differently from the person with Type A behavior—namely, by not perceiving an environmental stimulus as stressful or challenging. Situations involving moderate competition, reduced control of events, or slow meticulous detail work elicit typical impatient behaviors from a person with a Type A pattern (Matthews, 1982); however, some life situations may elicit Type A behaviors from almost anyone.

Despite numerous studies, no unique physiologic mechanisms have been found to explain why Type A behavior emerges when certain persons are challenged with their environment. Little is known about cultural differences, socioeconomic factors, amount or type of challenge, what discrete values are criteria for sorting persons into types, and the consequences of stifling behavior patterns in certain individuals (Siegel, 1984). Anger and hostility potentially are precursors of undesirable outcomes. Thus preventive interventions aim to reduce intensity of psychosocial and emotional responses, partly through changing appraisal of events.

✦ Hardiness and vulnerability

Early research on hardiness began with workplace stressors and created interest in the burnout syndrome. In fact, hospital staff nurses were found to be particularly at risk due to their negative perceptions of job conditions coupled with ineffective, counterproductive coping strategies (Chiriboga & Bailey, 1986).

A series of research studies have investigated individuals who remained healthy after being challenged by high levels of stress, while other persons became ill or injured. The question is whether certain personality characteristics—hardiness for one—enable a person to resist multiple stressors without succumbing to physical or psychological impairment. Referring to Antonovsky's (1972) concept,

appropriate resources may resist, buffer, or balance the potentially destructive effects of stressors; in Neuman's Systems Model (Neuman, 1989), persons may have or develop a type of stress resistance to reduce their vulnerability.

Hardiness, a constellation of stress-resistant tendencies, has been debated in the recent literature. One question is whether hardiness is a mediator between stress and adjustments. A longstanding view held hardiness to have three key dimensions: commitment, control, and challenge. Researchers found persons who exhibited commitment were actively involved in their own lives and expressed a sense of purpose or direction. Those who believed they could influence, perhaps not prevent, the way events in their life progressed were seen as having control, rather than feeling powerless. They viewed challenge as stimulating, necessary, and as opportunity for personal growth or skills development (Kobasa, 1979; Kobasa, Maddi, & Kahn, 1982; Kobasa, Maddi, & Zola, 1983). These dimensions are similar to those found in individuals who identify an internal locus of control.

What is termed hardiness may influence how events are cognitively appraised and coping occurs, thus enabling a person to effectively resist health threats arising from stressors. It would follow that persons with hardiness predictably resist illness, whereas persons who are vulnerable, with low hardiness, may have lowered resistance to stressors and increased health problems (Pollock, 1986, 1989). Hardiness may or may not be a factor determining whether a person incurs a chronic, disabling, or developmental condition.

Hardiness is a motivating mediator for persons who exhibit strong psychosocial adjustment and problem-solving skills. Families whose child had a developmental disability were able to maintain effective family coping, social networks, self-appraised satisfaction, and family integration when they had strong hardiness attributes (Failla & Jones, 1991).

At this writing, the concept of hardiness is receiving critical review. Is hardiness an integrated construct or three separate dimensions; must all dimensions be present to be effective? Can hardiness be present, absent, or occur in increments; can hardiness be nurtured? Findings from research into these questions will be important to therapeutic interventions in rehabilitation nursing (Wagnild & Young, 1991).

Resilience, an ability to defuse a potential stressor into a nonstressor event, may be due in part to an ability to "bounce back," which is integrated into personality. Those who view change as opportunity while valuing commitment and enjoying challenge, along with a sense of humor, tend to recover rapidly or "bounce back" from loss or failure (Kobasa, 1979; Kobasa et al., 1983).

Locus of control. The concept of locus of control is related closely to the control dimension of hardiness and intertwines with other factors influencing coping. The major constructs are two opposing views of how one's life events and corresponding behavior are controlled. One view is an inner or intrinsic locus of control identified by persons who believe they have some degree of influence over life events and how they choose to respond. They may expect to achieve greater life satisfaction by actively engaging in effective coping strategies.

On the other hand, those who perceive an external locus of control frequently are ineffective in coping because of beliefs that external forces, persons, or events control what happens in their lives. Since these persons do not believe it is within one's ability to change the course of events, depression may result.

Sensitivity to values and context are essential when examining this construct. Many persons hold highly valued cultural or spiritual beliefs that influence locus of control and worldview. Some researchers have attempted to substantiate relationships between a person's perceived locus of control and effectiveness of coping with chronic illness. However, locus of control was never intended to be the only measure of a person's response to illness. Furthermore, many scales and definitions differ from the original work (Rotter, 1966) on the construct and have been used collectively, without distinguishing among or separating the findings, or findings were reported as outcomes based on locus of control data when other instruments were used in measurement. Discussion of the topic is found in a critique of the research (Strickland, 1978).

Schussler (1992) examined locus of control as a part of a larger study involving 205 persons with chronic conditions. He used and confirmed eight different illness concepts as identified in clinical patients: "illness as challenge, enemy, punishment, weakness, relief, strategy, irreparable loss or damage, and value" (Lipowski, 1979).

When classifying clients' individual meanings about and attitudes toward illness, persons who had a sense of control and acceptance regarding their illness used more problem-solving approaches. Emotional-based coping strategies typified persons who did not accept their illness or viewed it as out of their control (Schussler, 1992). Western medicine's emphasis on cure has led our society to expect curative results. When cure is not forthcoming, a person senses reduced control and loss of equilibrium. Others, including professional care providers, may become disenchanted with the person's inability to become cured and impatient with needs for care, then angrily blame the person for the circumstances (Hoeman, 1990).

✦ Sociocultural influences

In a global matrix study, nurses from diverse cultural backgrounds (n = 50) were selected randomly and assigned to care for clients also from multiple cultures. Each nurse made varied assessments of clients' expressed pain. Not only were assessments of a client's pain found to differ among nurses from various cultures, but each nurse assessed pain differently in clients of several other cultures. Major discrepancies occurred among nurses assessing whether a client was experiencing pain or was distressed. All nurses made incorrect assessments of psychological distress, rather than actual pain, as expressed by clients who were from cultures other than the nurse's own (Davitz, Sameshima, & Davitz, 1976).

Incomplete or inaccurate assessment of cultural perceptions, expressions of pain, anxiety, or distress may impede a client from reaching optimal rehabilitation goals. Demographic upswings in the United States toward diversity and immigrant groups necessitate culturally relevant and sensitive assessment guidelines for nurses. Immigrants to a new country have more difficulty with psychological coping as a group than the general population (Hitch & Rack, 1980; Meleis and Lipson, 1992). In rehabilitation discerning signs of pain, distress, or psychosocial problems is compounded when a client with aphasia or impaired cognition speaks a native language. At times folk beliefs and practices are misunderstood, leading to confusion, eroded trust, and unanticipated consequences.

When clients and families do not speak English or are not familiar with Western medical procedures, unintentional cultural assumptions may lead to errors and create stress. For example, culture-bound conditions, such as susto, have no equivalent meaning in Western medicine; or Western diagnoses cannot be translated into the person's native language because there is no comparable term. As a result confusion, avoidance, distress, or even conflict may emerge. Similarly health professionals are cautioned to use discretion when translating health data or obtaining an interpreter to remedy a language difficulty. Many topics or issues simply are not discussed or are restricted to family, gender, or social class discussions.

However, all stressors or coping behaviors cannot be attributed out of hand to cross-cultural differences. Within the United States, intraethnic diversity, cultural norms, and social or gender structures also influence stressors for clients. Findings from a study of members of a Black community in the rural South revealed differences in coping styles, stressors, and stress symptoms among men and women within the same cultural group (Dressler, 1985). When a person has a chronic, disabling, or developmental disorder resulting in diminished cognitive, physical, or affective function, cultural criteria are compounded.

✦ Perceptions of quality of life

Researchers found a relationship between effective coping and quality of life for clients whose spinal cord injury occurred more than 2 years ago. On the other hand, a client's effective coping has not been shown to improve quality of life in of itself, nor is it known whether teaching coping skills to clients improves their quality of life (Nieves, Charter, & Aspinall, 1991).

A nurse's perception of the impact of stressors on clients may differ from a client's view. When nurses evaluate their own perceptions about how clients experience and express stress, they gain insights that enable them to better accommodate each client's unique appraisal of stressors. In an Australian study young adults with cerebral palsy rated their perceptions about severity of problems associated with their disability. When results were compared with ratings by their close relatives and by persons in the public, the young adults rated their quality of life higher and their problems as less severe than did the others (Gething, 1985).

Adults (n = 40) living in the community, who required mechanical ventilation and were dependent for ADL, were surveyed about their perceptions of their quality of life. Using the same attitudinal scale, 40 community health nurses rated their own quality of life. The nurses repeated the scale, this time rating how they believed clients in the sample would rate their (the client's) quality of life.

Nurses and clients had similar views of their own lives. Nurses imputed clients would rate the quality of their (clients') lives negatively; instead the nurses predicted poorly because clients thought quite positively about their own lives. A larger study surveying interdisciplinary health professionals supported these findings (Bach, Campagnolo, & Hoeman, 1991). These clients were coping more effectively, participating in activities, and describing a higher quality of life than health professionals believed possible.

This is a timely finding because nurses and other health professionals are instrumental in decision-making about allocation of resources or a client's potential ability for community living. A client's appraisal of her own quality of life must be clear to avoid professionals imposing or projecting their own perceptions on assessments of clients, often without mutual appraisals. As cost controls gain greater influence in decision-making about who receives various levels of health care, finances and resource allocations will become powerful stressors. The question of quality of life may incorrectly diminish questions about sanctity of life.

✦ Developmental influences

Understanding the unique influences of developmental stages on appraisal and coping is important for rehabilitation nurses, who often provide care to clients of more than one age group and their families. Learning to approach each client and family's unique appraisal of stressors from their developmental standpoint enhances and sharpens a nursing assessment. The following section contains sample content across stages of the life-span for infants and young children, adolescents, middlescents, and aged persons. Very young infants and adolescents frequently are overlooked as age cohorts in life-span assessments of psychosocial concepts.

Infants and young children. Consider a young child who does not comprehend the idea of psychological pain until he has achieved sufficient cognitive and psychosocial development. This child cannot appraise a stressor beyond an understanding of physical pain and may express and experience pain differently from an older child or adult. Over two decades nursing research findings have exposed misperceptions about children coping with pain (McCafferty & Beebe, 1989) and the plight of children who experienced pain because they were undiagnosed and undermedicated (Eland & Anderson, 1977). As a result nurses have expanded their scientific knowledge about multiple facets of childhood pain and improved outcomes in pain management for infants and children.

Very young infants, including those who are very low birthweight, prematurely newborn, or medically fragile, are at risk for ineffective coping patterns from birth. These special care infants use behavioral cues to communicate with their environment. However, their parents have multiple stressors that are compounded when their infant does not respond in ways they have come to expect. For example, stimulation from light, sound, changing clothing, or being held may stress a premature or very-low-birthweight infant—stimulations that would benefit an uncompromised infant (Hoeman, 1992a).

For these families loss may be perceived or become reality. Theoretically they may experience chronic sorrow and uncertainty about outcome throughout their infant's developmental stages; some infants do not survive. Family members who have gained competency have more reassurance

about their relationships with their infant whether or not the baby survives. Ideally a competent family includes parents, siblings, and those extended family members who are actively involved (Hoeman, 1992a).

Adolescence. The flurry of physical and psychosocial changes during adolescent years is well documented. As with younger children, assessment based on an individual adolescent's developmental stage is more valid than chronologic age. To add complexity, symptoms or complications of chronic conditions may progress, diminish, or reappear as a child develops. Because wide variations of changes during adolescence occur differently for each emerging person, it is not surprising that preadolescents and adolescents cope differently with chronic or disabling conditions. Adolescents' coping strategies do differ from those used by their parents; adolescents tend to use more emotion-based coping methods (Keller & Nicolls, 1990).

A study compared adolescents who had cystic fibrosis with their parents concerning how far into the future each was willing to project about the adolescent's life plans. Regardless of uncertainty about progression of the cystic fibrosis, adolescents projected plans ahead significantly longer, possibly due to an emerging developmental stage of self-identity. Adolescents and families were working through the illness at differing paces, but each group's responses were consistent with trajectory patterns for chronic illness (Strauss & Glaser, 1975; Yarcheski, 1988).

It follows there would be differences in how young persons in adolescent substages use coping skills to participate in care, manage their care, and learn about their condition. However, in practice, these discriminations may not be clear without careful assessment. In a study examining how preadolescents and adolescents cope with insulin-dependent diabetes mellitus, researchers found younger persons displayed more overt verbal behaviors such as yelling and arguing. Older adolescents, who had a wider range of freedom, began avoidance behaviors associated with poor internal control such as smoking, drinking alcohol, or staying away from home. Some adolescents may acquire traumatic injuries as a result of previous ineffective coping with stressors, and now face stressors from the disability (Grey, Cameron, & Thurber, 1991).

Adolescents in the 1990s are challenged by sets of stressors that differ from past generations. Technology, availability of substances, freedom of expression, multiple career choices, public violence, and confrontation of moral values are among the trademark stressors of the decade. The psychosocial development of adolescents enables them to expand their worldview to take in global issues and plan for their future, while leaving them vulnerable to stressors over which they have no sense of control.

A major life event, buildup of multiple stressors, or world events stretch the coping resources of adolescents. Concerns for the preservation of the environment, high-technology wars, and natural disasters are greater stressors to adolescents than commonly realized. Adolescents may be reluctant to share their concerns or hopes with persons other than their peers.

Personalized stressors such as loss of a family member, friend, or pet; moving to a new location; real or imagined rejection by peers; failure at school or sports; group or community threats to safety; and family conflicts or violence may have undesirable consequences. Use of illicit substances; eating disorders; poor school performance; and high-risk behaviors such as sexual activity, driving without a seatbelt or motorcycle helmet, or daredevil stunts are maladaptive attempts at coping and are behaviors that add stressors.

Suicide, the ultimate expression of hopelessness, is a leading cause of death among adolescents around the world. Suicide and attempted suicide among adolescents have been correlated with stressors from chronic conditions and life events (Greene, Werner, & Walker, 1992). Not all ineffective coping behaviors are due to illness or disability; some may be typical conflicts of adolescent development behaviors, apart from chronicity. Holistic assessment focuses on the changing developing individual, not on the disease or disability.

Middlescence and transition. Transitions between various levels of services—whether early intervention into preschool or adolescence into university or vocational training programs—signal adjustment to a new stage. As people with disabilities develop throughout the life-span, they may have difficulty locating health professionals who will manage their care. For example, a child with a developmental delay may visit a developmental pediatrician and work with an interdisciplinary team until reaching adolescence or young adulthood. These clients then are "too old" for the pediatric team, only to find adult or family team practitioners are neither trained nor comfortable with their care. The very system available to assist this person becomes another source of stressors.

Likewise persons who encounter newly identified chronic conditions such as fibromyalagia or complications from untreated Lyme disease, or persons seeking restorative care following cancer surgery or requiring specialized care skills for renal or burn care must develop coping strategies for consequences of conditions with little-known trajectories. And coping strategies are needed on multiple levels in middlescence, when clients may themselves be caring for aging parents, supporting their young adult children and perhaps grandchildren, as well as negotiating their own health status. As they near midpoint in their lives, they may acquire additional chronic or disabling conditions from among those that emerge during middle life.

Aging and comorbidity. "Thus the essential problem of aging is not only how to treat declining biological-organic function but also how to adapt the environment to allow the person to be as functional as possible—to work around or compensate for the altered biological function" (Trieschmann, 1987).

The numbers of persons who become aged with a disability and those who have age-related disabilities and chronic conditions are relatively new but burgeoning population groups. Members of these groups often experience comorbidity by having more than one chronic or disabling disorder. Some are challenged with reemerging syndromes or sequela diseases and experience unique stressors. Consider those who survived poliomyelitis in childhood only to develop post-polio syndrome as adults. Whatever coping strategies they have employed during and following the initial manifestation of the disease now are being threatened.

Stress arises from potential loss of functional ability and independence, role changes, relationship strains, economic hardship, or worsening of symptoms. The person not only ages but with sequela to a disabling condition that was thought to be arrested.

When a client's lifestyle is modified to accommodate aging processes consider access to services; socialization in a mentally healthy environment; adequate income for nutrition, medications, and recreation; social and spiritual support; education about health promotion and management of any health conditions or medications; and opportunities for continuing life pursuits within limitations and abilities (Fig. 13-1).

Whether in facilities or community, rehabilitation nurses are encountering clients who are aging and have greater acuity, cormorbid conditions, altered or impaired sensory function, altered cognition, and limited functional abilities. Rehabilitation and restorative care promotes effective coping by attending to

◆ Preventing further physical or psychosocial disability or complications

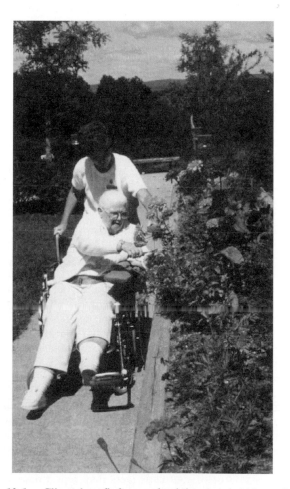

Fig. 13-1 Clients benefit from maintaining their hobbies and interests. Assist your client to be as independent as possible while enjoying their environment and activities. (From *Rehabilitation/ Restorative Care,* by S.P. Hoeman, 1990, St. Louis: Mosby–Year Book. Copyright 1990 by Mosby–Year Book. Reprinted by permission.)

+ Encouraging client and family participation and direction
+ Providing safe, stimulating, and unrestrictive environments
+ Assuring attention to primary care and health maintenance
+ Employing assistive devices or adaptive equipment and other means to maximize functional abilities
+ Utilizing therapeutic interventions and exercises for the highest level of independence in ADL
+ Advocating for quality of life and dignity for each individual

Far too little is known about effects of health maintenance, access to services, resources, independent function, and/or effective coping strategies on outcomes for persons who are aging or whether there are relationships with chronic conditions or disability. The Agency for Health Care Policy and Research (AHCPR) is in the process of developing and disseminating clinical practice guidelines prepared by panels consisting of consumer representatives and professionals from multiple disciplines. The guidelines provide a synthesis of research and knowledge in a particular area, such as pressure ulcers or cancer pain. Recommendations for standardized protocols for management of chronic diseases and mental conditions, preventive care, and age-related information are featured in each guideline. (Chapter 31 contains additional discussion of rehabilitation and restorative care of the older person.)

ASSESSMENT

Assessment of an individual or family's effectiveness in coping is a complex, multidimensional process that encompasses cognitive, affective, and psychomotor domains. A sophisticated subjective assessment is crucial, especially as more rehabilitation nurses are working independently, such as with case management or as community-based consultants.

Assessment of Coping Effectiveness
+ **History and subjective data**

A history is used to assess a client's effectiveness in coping including insight into their appraisal of stressors, underlying meanings, and ways of coping. The following section contains suggestions and sample queries for eliciting subjective data about coping effectiveness during the course of therapeutic conversation between nurse and client or family.

+ **Suggestions**
+ An interview may include questions to elicit a client's descriptions of beliefs about health and illness, potential causes of the condition, remedies that have been tried, what will help, who can or should help improve things, and how long before relief is expected.
+ Parents or significant caregivers may report data for infants or persons with impaired communication or cognition. However, ascertain reliability of the person's report and validate with other assessment data from the individual, family, or social system.
+ Select a model for assessment or combine several. Begin by asking the person about her perception of what

are personal stressors and what strategies she uses in coping.
+ What is the developmental stage, both individual and family? Draw a health and social genogram to depict family patterns, identify resources, or pinpoint difficulties with adjustments during life transitions, events, or happenings.

+ **Sample queries**
+ What was the nature and extent of the loss? What does this situation or event mean to you? Have you or your family or friends experienced similar events before? If so, what did you do? Are these resolved, recurrent, or unresolved? How does your family handle stressful events or situations?
+ Who was/is involved or affected? What is your role in this event? What do you think you are able to do about it?
+ What has changed specifically due to this loss or event? For example, ask about changes in lifestyle, role relationships, health, self-perception including body image, occupation, functional independence, social system, quality of life, behavioral patterns, financial status, attitude or worldview, and vocation or education.
+ If you could change three things now, what would they be or why were these selected? What do they mean to you?
+ Describe what is stressful to you. How would you describe your feelings; are you anxious or fearful? Do you feel helpless or hopeless? How would you describe the way you typically handle stressful situations or deal with loss? (After the client responds ask about the use of alcohol or controlled substances; other addictive responses such as food or sexual activity; diversional activities; exercise; emotive behaviors such as crying, anger, acting-out, leaving/withdrawal.) Do you engage in these behaviors now?
+ What do you think will happen as a result of this stress or this event? What are your major concerns other than this stressor?
+ Do you have a lot of daily hassles? How do you respond to annoyances? What is most important to you at this time?
+ How will this event affect your worth as an individual; who else will be affected by this?
+ Why do you think this event happened? Are you or someone else able to control what is happening or is there anything that can be done to change things? What kind of control do you believe you have over what happens?
+ Do you believe you know enough about what has occurred? Are you uncertain about any aspect of the situation or your condition? Where do you go for help and for information? Has this event affected your ability to make decisions or the way in which you make decisions? Have others questioned your decisions more than usual; what do they propose for you to do?
+ How have you and/or the family managed? What have you tried? Who or what is helpful to you? What do you think will be helpful to you now? Are there things you believe you should not do or things you must do?
+ What will be the greatest difficulty for you since this stress or event has occurred? How would you have de-

scribed another person with your (condition or injury) before your now being in this situation? Are you concerned about how others will view or respond to you; about who may reject you; or what others may say about you? What would you "call" someone like yourself?

✦ Will you be able to follow the medical and healthcare plan? Can you perform or direct your own care? Do you have a caregiver or attendant? Do you have questions about your condition or care plan? What do you envision for your future (next day, week, or year, as appropriate)?

✦ Do you have pain? Since the event have you experienced difficulty or changes in patterns of sleeping, eating, grooming, sexuality, working, concentrating, communicating, self-care skills, emotions, thoughts, physical functions or sensations, or other feelings?

✦ What are environmental stressors or barriers for you?

✦ What are your specific strengths and resources? For example, family, pets, sense of humor, sense of control and self-determination, religious faith, education, income or employment, living arrangement, assistive devices or equipment, interests or hobbies, service agency supports, acceptable caregiver, other social supports, and personal goals with hope.

✦ Objective data

Objective data obtained by examination, observation, inspection, and direct report are correlated with subjective, psychosocial data.

✦ Verify medications, health products, or therapeutic items.

✦ Elicit the person's description and definition, or denial, of the stressor event. Note whether the person is able to describe concerns in present sense, use proactive approaches, or verbalize need for assistance. Assess whether the person is able to depict the situation and roles of self and others accurately.

✦ Observe affect, alertness and mood, or nonverbal signs such as crying, lack of eye contact (unless culturally inappropriate), withdrawal responses, irritability or anger, inappropriate behavior, nervous manifestations (e.g., picking, twitching, or tapping), or signs of socioemotional deprivation. A child may sleep, suck the hands or toys, avoid response, or engage self in play; attempt several observations apart from clinical examination, such as in the playroom or with other children while in the waiting area. For older clients assure they are not tired or hungry from travel, waiting, or needing medications before assessment.

✦ Inspect physical appearance for poor grooming or hygiene, bruises, cuts, hair pulling, or other nervous self-inflicted injuries; assess for abuse or neglect by others. Observe gums and mucosa for biting lesions.

✦ Assess self-destructive manifestations such as weight gain or loss, eating disorders, substance abuse, changes in health maintenance, or self-reported actions.

✦ Measure weight, vital signs, and blood pressure.

✦ Conduct review of systems referring to the following list of signs or symptoms that have been associated with ineffective coping responses; this list is not ex-

haustive. All signs or symptoms are evaluated in context of the whole person and family.

✦ Physical data regarding effective coping

Possible physical manifestations of stressors are racing pulse, palpitations, dizziness or fainting, shortness of breath, hyperventilation, nausea, indigestion, "burping," refluxlike symptoms, burning sensations, changes in tongue or mucosa, difficulty swallowing, constipation, diarrhea, irritable bowel signs, urinary frequency, localized itching, headache, pain or geographic pain, "nervous twitches," fatigue, neckache, posture, grinding or clenching teeth, or skin eruptions.

Acute episodes such as strep throat have been found to follow stressful events; chronic conditions such as arthritis or lupus may be exacerbated with stress.

✦ Evaluate sensory manifestations such as ability to concentrate, memory loss, confusion, changes in speech patterns, changes in communication style or amount, depressive reactions, pain or discomfort, altered hearing, or visual disturbances. Compare assessment with data about location, severity, duration, and type of injury or impairment.

✦ Inspect injured area, altered or impaired body part, or functional disability. Concurrently assess client's perception of body image and whether client looks at his body or withdraws; verbal comments; and destructive or inappropriate mood swings.

Family Systems

An early assessment of the family is essential to effective coping, growth, and future goal setting. Family genograms with psychosocial entries, assessment of open versus closed boundaries, identified problems or concerns, and recent loss or change provide important family data. Although rehabilitation nurses frequently work one-on-one with a client, nursing process and outcome must be based on each person as a part of a family, a social network, and

---

ASSESSMENT OF FAMILY SYSTEM MALADJUSTMENT

✦ Regular neglect of family duties or carrying out of responsibilities

✦ Tense communication among family members, which is expressed by irritability, resentment, criticism, or frequent arguments

✦ Regular neglect of the client's care or treatments by family members as if the condition were denied as not existing

✦ Family members other than the client may exhibit physical symptoms, become anxious or overburdened by caregiver responsibilities, and develop emotional responses (Power, 1985)

community system. All family members experience some degree of risk when the system is threatened by illness or disability (especially critical when the client is a child).

Most families experience multiple stressors from various sectors of their lives. Stressors may occur simultaneously; family members develop at different stages, hold unique appraisals, and have personal response times and coping styles. Few families analyze their management style, patterns of communication or action, or coping strategies in preparation for a crisis event. In fact it may be difficult for a family under great stress to identify and mobilize their resources and strengths. Families may be dysfunctional before the stressor event at hand or overwhelmed by the situation. A family system has maladjusted coping behaviors when the criteria listed in the Box on p. 199 are evident.

Many older adults return to the community following a stay in a hospital or rehabilitation facility with functional or cognitive impairments that require them to live with family members. Family systems may become dysfunctional when family members become caretakers for an older family member who has a disability or chronic condition. The Box below lists indicators of potential dysfunction in a family.

Ideally rehabilitation nurses will forge collegial relationships with community health nurses or serve as consultants in the community. In these roles, nurses can use results of home assessments and family system evaluations as a basis for working with clients to develop preventive interventions and plans to improve outcome for clients and families.

Other signals may alert a nurse that an individual family member (or system) may collapse or is breaking down. Several or many of the indicators listed in the Box below, right may appear.

ASSESSMENT MODELS FOR STRESS AND COPING

The following section presents selected theoretic models for assessment of stress and coping. While state of the art, these are neither exhaustive nor conclusive models.

Patterns of Psychosocial Reactions

A number of patterns of psychosocial reactions to stressors have been proposed. It is useful to learn the composition of these patterns because they reappear in the literature as researchers use them for developing instruments or constructing research questions about stress or coping. Additionally the patterns aid nurses in assessment and care planning. The following patterns describe reactions to onset of disability, challenges of coping, and maintaining hope with loss.

Eight patterns of psychosocial reaction to onset of disability are suggested in one model: shock, anxiety, denial, depression, internalized anger, externalized hostility, acknowledgment, and adjustment (Livneh & Antonak, 1990). However, researchers were unable to rank the reactions in a predictive hierarchy (Antonak & Livneh, 1991). These expand on the familiar stages of grieving (Kubler Ross, 1969), which is discussed in Chapter 1.

Strauss et al. (1984), followed by Miller (1983), proposed 13 tasks that challenge coping skills of the chronically ill. These are normality, lifestyle, knowledge, self-concept, social relationships, grieving, role changes, physical discomfort, compliance, death, social stigma, control, and hope.

Moos proposed a sequence of seven coping behaviors used by individuals, families, and professionals when significant loss has occurred, each based on maintaining hope consistent with coping level. Intervention begins with telling the truth and continues by offering support based on a client's behavior during reality negotiation. According to Moos's schemata, clients isolate or dissociate feelings about a stressor; seek knowledge as a means of relieving tension or anxiety when due to uncertainty or misconception; remain personally competent supported by emotional support from family, friends, or professionals; learn self-care skills to confirm personal capability and effectiveness; set concrete but limited goals; interact with friends, family, and professionals to rehearse alternative processes or outcomes; and ultimately find a purpose, pattern, or meaning in the events of the stressor event and its outcome (Moos, 1981).

INDICATORS OF POTENTIAL DYSFUNCTION IN A FAMILY

+ Knowledge is deficient about condition, care, or resources.
+ Caregivers are overly burdened with responsibility.
+ Another family member avoids or denies his own health-care needs until the client is able to function well.
+ Conflict overshadows care decisions.
+ Unresolved conflicts reemerge and become active.
+ Warmth or caring is lacking.
+ The older person is not a part of decision making (Kemp, 1986).

INDICATORS OF POTENTIAL INDIVIDUAL BREAKDOWN

+ Chronic fatigue
+ Anger leading to cynical, sarcastic, or irritable behaviors
+ Impatience and exhaustion
+ Anxiety and fears bordering on paranoia
+ Disturbed sleep and rest patterns
+ Distress in role relationships
+ Illness and accidents or injuries
+ Maladaptive behaviors such as depression, substance abuse, avoidance or isolation, inattention to personal care, or eating disorders
+ Potential for suicide
+ Depleted or inaccessible resources
+ Perceived low options

These pattern models do not take into account individual or family differences in coping skills, resources, capabilities for dealing with stressors, meanings of stressors, developmental stage, or cognitive appraisal. Since chronicity invariably becomes a family matter, family models are useful in assessment.

✦ The T-double ABC-X model of family adaptation

One frequently referenced model that attempts to deal with the full dimensions of stress, coping, and perception is the Double ABC-X Model of Family Adaptation, which has been reconfigured and revised as the T-Double ABC-X (McCubbin and McCubbin, 1987). The T-Double ABC-X Model distributes assessment over time beginning with a family's precrisis situation. When a stressor impinges on a family, both the existing resources (a) and family perception (c) of stressor (a) plus resources (b), produce the family's unique definition of the crisis (x).

Following the crisis event, when the stressor (a) becomes compiled with other stressors (a + A), coping occurs. How a family chooses to cope is influenced by a combination of all elements: precrisis and postcrisis stressors (a + A), the existing and new resources (b + B), family perception of the crisis (c), and all available resources at a given time. Outcome is stated as a level of adaptation (x), making it possible for a family to achieve either homeostatic adaptation or a higher level called bonadaptation. A third alternative is maladaptation, which in itself represents a compounded crisis situation (McCubbin & McCubbin, 1987).

This model has proven to be a useful tool that allows for a combination of precrisis factors. When using this model, it is important to preserve meaning of an event in social or cultural context, attention to beliefs and values, and a mechanism for feedback. Adaptation has been used as an outcome in rehabilitation; however, adaptation relates more to homeostasis than to metamorphic changes. The client, family, and rehabilitation team must agree adaptation describes their mutual goals as an optimal level of outcome. The following model provides an additional view.

✦ Salutogenic model

Rehabilitation professionals may choose an adjustment model rather than a classic adaptation model. Antonovsky (1972) conceptualized the "salutogenic" model wherein an individual or family, unable to cope with stressors over a prolonged period, "breaks down" and encounters a chronic condition. Characteristics of chronicity such as uncertainty, permanency, or impaired function fuel ways of coping. When stressful demands on the individual are compounded, unresolved issues accumulate and a person's ability to maintain balance breaks down, adding health risks.

Recommendations for alleviating "breakdown" are to promote an individual's sense of self, foster socialization and social support, support effective coping behaviors, and attend to affirming client-professional relationship (Antonovsky, 1972). Emphasizing coping behaviors that promote adjustment enables clients to build on strengths and resources. For example, health professionals promoted adjustment for nonhospitalized clients who had inflammatory bowel disease (IBD) by reinforcing their effective coping patterns and reaffirming their sense of control. These cli-

ents used problem-solving to identify behaviors for achieving lifestyle satisfaction (Kinash, Fischer, Lukie, & Carr, 1993).

Not all reinforcement for adjustment originates with health professionals. Persons who assumed roles as constructive "support agents" among groups of Jewish-Israeli adults with chronic illnesses were found to have assisted themselves as well as others with adjustment to chronicity (Ben-Sira, 1984).

Indicators of strong adjustment include positive mood, quality-of-life satisfaction, effective problem-solving coping strategies, internal locus of control, and functional family systems. Adjustment signals competency with interpersonal, social, psychosocial, emotional, and vocational roles suitable for community re-entry. However, acknowledgment of reality may precede adjustment.

Acknowledgment means a client cognitively recognizes the trajectory of a condition and realizes it will have permanent impact (Dunn, 1975). It follows that adults who survived extensive burn injuries were found to be better adjusted when they confronted their difficulties rather than avoiding them and used problem-solving to define coping strategies (Roberts et al., 1987).

✦ An adapted trajectory model

This model is an adaptation of Hill's Family Systems Intervention Model combined with Strauss and Glaser's (1975) chronic illness trajectory. Hill's model arose from the family systems research and served as a foundation for the T-Double ABC-X Model. Hill viewed an individual's or family's initial response to a stressor as disruption or disorganization that resulted from an attempt to recover or resolve the stressor event. As the person or family attempts to resolve disorganization, they will chose a pattern and level where they regroup (Hill, 1965).

Hill compared the process to a rollercoaster ride, beginning with precrisis onset, dipping to the lowest level, and then rising to a level of reorganization as the person experiences each situation. Time, depth, and width of the dip are process measures and the level the person attains is an outcome. Each family member travels a personal ride through crisis but intertwined with the shared family system trip. The nursing process in this model is applied to the complex system that results when Hill's adapted model is superimposed on the illness trajectory for a chronic condition regarding effective coping (Hill, 1965), which suggested uncertainty as a concept.

The conceptual model of the chronic illness trajectory was developed from a grounded theory approach over 30 years ago. The underlying principle is that "chronic conditions have a course that varies and changes over time. This course can be shaped and managed" (Corbin & Strauss, 1991). The phases of the chronic illness trajectory are

1. Pretrajectory
2. Trajectory onset
3. Crisis
4. Acute
5. Stable
6. Unstable
7. Downward
8. Dying

A line drawing of the chronic illness trajectory would show the process of a particular disease over time. Barely visible at onset, the line would change to become distinct and curved toward crisis and acute levels until reaching temporary stability. From that point the line would progress and end, according to the natural history of the condition. Outcomes vary for individuals and for various chronic conditions, but a particular condition tends to adhere to a typical pattern when plotted over time.

Thus a person's health status might plummet, steadily edge downward, zig-zag down with intermittent plateaus, maintain status quo, or improve. At each change of position on the trajectory, a person would have the opportunity to reassess and prepare coping strategies, although it may be uncertain when symptoms would appear or ebb (Strauss & Glaser, 1975).

This combined model may be useful when a client has knowledge deficits to assist with preventive interventions or with reality negotiation, or to promote effective coping behaviors, even when there is uncertainty. In practice, clients and families have responded to the visual guide presented by this model, and some choose to set goals, plan community re-entry, and complete selected life tasks as they plot their course on the trajectory (Hoeman, 1992b).

Although a client in rehabilitation may experience a chronic, irreversible, progressive, or recurrent loss, tracing a natural history of the condition with a client may be helpful for establishing a sense of control, hope, and reality. Combining models reinforces assessment of the whole person. Resources vary and developmental or adaptive skills are acquired differently; therefore disability alone does not determine whether a child, adolescent, adult, or aged person engages in effective coping. This model incorporates cognitive appraisal and meaning of the stressor as with transactional approaches.

The Process of Coping

The process of coping is linked to the framework of stress and the concept of stress tolerance. Coping responses are assessed in relation to their effects. Research indicates that effective coping for individuals and their families is a key indicator of how they will adjust to changes that occur following disability, especially reintegration or community re-entry (Ben-Sira, 1982).

Coping has been defined as "constantly changing cognitive and behavioral efforts to manage external and/or internal demands that are appraised as taxing or exceeding the resources of the person" (Lazarus & Folkman, 1984). An individual may be coping simultaneously with numerous combinations of stressors. Coping behaviors are manifested through cognitive function, motor actions, affective responses, and psychological defense mechanisms.

Coping is a process, not a judgment about whether or how an individual personally responded, or did not respond, to stressors. It is not as if one could choose not to cope or did not cope. It has been said that no action is a very powerful form of action. Coping responses are assessed according to their relationships with health outcomes; it is the effect of the coping response, not the response itself, that is assessed. Thus the consequences of ineffective coping are maladaptive outcomes. Understanding coping as a concept with dynamic, multifaceted, and unique characteristics is an essential competency for rehabilitation nursing.

Nursing Diagnoses

NANDA has approved nursing diagnoses for
+ Coping, Defensive
+ Coping, Ineffective Individual
+ Coping, Family: Potential for Growth
+ Coping, Ineffective Family: Compromised
+ Coping, Ineffective Family: Disabling (NANDA, 1994)
+ Caregiver Role Strain (Burns, Archbold, Stewart, & Shelton, 1993)

Nurse researchers have agreed that coping is both a nursing diagnosis and a key concept for nursing inquiry. And they agree with other scientific disciplines that relationships among stress or stressors, coping, adaptation, and biopsychosocial factors somehow influence health outcomes. However, there are gaps in the research literature about how, why, when, to whom, and under what circumstances effective coping is elicited. Researchers question whether a short-term crisis, managed within several months time, may differ from an event requiring long-term coping and stress tolerance behaviors—and if so, how daily hassles may become more hazardous to health than maturational crises or major life events.

Researchers also are interested in learning what coping behaviors are associated with certain preventive and prescriptive interventions for specific populations. For example, when initially diagnosed with MS, clients manage their stress with responses that range from relief to fear to denial. Outcomes are improved by assessing a client's coping behaviors and then matching interventions to fit the person's responses, including practical suggestions for dealing with issues that commonly occur for clients with MS (White, Catanzaro, & Kraft, 1993).

The crucial test is the relationship between the coping response and the health outcome. For example, rehabilitation nurse researchers found a positive relationship between effective coping with selected social, physical, and psychological factors and perceived quality of life for persons who were functionally disabled following spinal cord injury. Factors were selected from the stress-transactional system developed by Lazarus and Launier: physical and social environment, demographic characteristics, major life changes, chronic illness, perceived support, attitude toward illness, and self-esteem (Lazarus & Launier, 1978; Nieves et al., 1991).

Ways of Coping

Coping skills develop into patterns or strategies a person uses to manage environmental, economic, and cultural demands and to meet physical and psychosocial-emotional needs. A client's coping behaviors enable a nurse to understand patterns of behavior by offering insight into what a person might do based on individual ways of coping. This lends insight into motivation when setting mutually agreed-upon goals. Clients and their families may use different or alternative pathways to achieve their goals. Within the context of a client's values, capabilities, preferences, and cultural norms, coping patterns may or may not be effective, promote growth, or be productive. The response cannot be evaluated apart from the outcome. Apart from pathologic responses such as suicide, the effectiveness of a response is determined by its relationship with health outcome.

Productive coping patterns lead to resolution and new behavioral responses, such as constructive ways of adapting to changes or completing a developmental task or improved future problem-solving. Findings reported in nursing research literature indicate that most persons with health-related stressors use a combination of emotion-based and problem-solving coping styles. Lazarus and Folkman (1984) identified the following coping styles and related characteristics for an individual or a family:

1. An *emotion-based coping style* generally characterizes an individual displaying affective signs of distress, emitting an emotional signal, and presenting resigned acceptance of the situation. Both the response to and anticipation of the stressor are part of the person's biopsychosocial self as well as of the emotional expressions. Emotional coping behaviors may be culturally prescribed expressions. When a client from an ethnic or cultural group other than one's own displays emotional reactions to a stressor, assess the behavior within cultural context but do not automatically ascribe a client's emotions to cultural behavior. Emotion-based coping strategies, especially in combination with problem-solving strategies, have been included in findings from nursing studies.

2. *Problem-solving coping style* characterizes a person seeking information as well as support. The person evaluates the reasons why a transaction is stressful and the degree or extent of stress it represents. This person attempts to act in a problem-solving manner and identifies alternative rewards. Prior experience with problem-solving may indicate how well a person manages subsequent stressors. Personality, cultural norms, family lifestyle, and resources are factors that influence how effectively a person uses problem-solving to cope. In addition, problem-solving coping strategies are used in many instances to work through a specific event or situation or in combination with emotion-based styles.

3. Effective coping often is accomplished through an *appraisal-based coping style,* which integrates concepts using logical analysis and mental preparation, cognitive redefinition, and at times cognitive avoidance with denial. Uncertainty about definition or outcome of a stressor creates its own imbalance and prevents resolution or closure, which may impede effective coping.

Understanding a client's appraisal of stressors may be essential to synthesizing meaning underlying his actions. Clients and families may make choices that at times cannot be fathomed by health professionals. They may use alternative pathways to meet needs or achieve goals, attach meaning to seemingly unimportant events or rituals, or view situations differently from team members.

Consider that under some conditions, a client may appraise any change as preferable to the present stressful situation. When a person has achieved developmental tasks, recognizes options, identifies resources, has positive self-image or self-esteem, and has those qualities described as hardiness and resiliency, an individual is more apt to engage in reality appraisal and effective coping. In rehabilitation nursing practice the impact of self-image influenced by others and by social construction of a condition cannot be ignored or forgotten. Self-image in turn influences appraisal. (Chapter 1 details theories related to these concepts.)

At times the variable stressors associated with irreversible chronic conditions that have remission and exacerbations may confound coping. Smith and Wallston used domains of Lazarus and Folkman's theory to study coping, appraisal, and adaptation for 239 persons with rheumatoid arthritis over a 4-year period. They suggest variability found in a client's positive or poor adjustment may be interwoven with the cyclic nature of the disease process. When clients appraised themselves as experiencing helplessness, depression was predictable. Similarly a passive style of coping with pain was associated with impaired psychosocial status; however, clients who perceived adequate socioemotional support used support as a buffer for psychosocial impairment (Smith & Wallston, 1992).

Clients who are capable of problem-solving when in remission were found to experience ineffective coping episodes when perceiving increased stress. Rehabilitation nurses who are able to predict ineffective coping episodes may be able to institute therapeutic interventions in time to avert maladaptive behaviors. These findings support additional research about empowering clients toward consistency in problem-solving coping behaviors. However, inadequate resources, multiple or competing stressors that overwhelm resistance, and environmental or perceptual barriers limit a person's problem-solving abilities and thus reduce the capacity for change.

In summary, analyzing a decade of nursing literature on coping, clients used many approaches to cope with illness. Jalowiec identified the following five main types of coping that were mentioned in the nursing research:

✦ "Trying to remain optimistic"
✦ "Using social support"
✦ "Making use of spiritual resources"
✦ "Trying to maintain some control"
✦ "Trying to accept the situation" (Jalowiec, 1993)

Ineffective Coping Behaviors

At times ineffective coping behaviors may appear to alleviate an immediate stressor for persons who hold themselves in low esteem, display poor decision-making abilities, have altered or negative perceptions of body image, or identify an external locus of control. Ultimately these choices may limit opportunity to develop patterns of effective coping. Often this person adopts internal labels that devalue such as poor self-esteem, powerlessness, or helplessness. In the following section, giving-up–given-up complex, defensive coping, personality disorders, and substance abuse are discussed.

✦ Giving-up–given-up complex

Results of ineffective coping have been observed clinically. Engel described a syndrome entitled "giving-up—given up" complex. He documented an observable sequence of behaviors that, although not causal, may contribute to illness. In other words the person psychologically concedes inability to cope with stressors as a precursor to illness; failure to cope produces physiologic changes that alter immunity.

The five characteristics of the giving-up–given-up complex are as follows:

1. Affect of giving up to helplessness or hopelessness
2. Depreciated image of oneself
3. Loss of gratification from relationships or roles in life
4. Disruption of the sense of continuity between past, present, and future
5. Reactivation of memories of earlier periods of giving up (Engel, 1968)

Engel's classic is relevant for predicting client needs in current rehabilitation nursing practice and examines these characteristics in detail. For example, he suggests reactivated feelings of past hopelessness due to unresolved grieving may account for an excessive response to some reminder of the lost person, even years later. Similarly Engel ties concepts, such as perceived control and self-image, into a usable construct.

Some ineffective coping behaviors may be due to alterations or impairments following a disabling disease or injury, as depression following disability may initiate helplessness, in effect triggering Engel's syndrome (Friedland & McColl, 1992). Depression following stroke is particularly difficult to assess. Clinical depression must be differentiated from lowered mood states that may occur with loss, or distress over altered functional abilities or self-care, or from labile emotions secondary to impairments such as may follow stroke.

Ongoing rehabilitation nursing assessment may be necessary to distinguish among a client's severe clinical depression, major or minor stroke-related depression, or mood disorders. The location of brain injury and the type and degree of loss influence the type of depression; the resulting classification of depression affects intervention and outcome in persons with poststroke depression (Bruckbauer, 1991).

Defensive Coping

Defensive, or false, coping is an ineffective coping style. Individuals may seek continual approval and caring from others rather than working on coping tasks. This person releases his own pain to hurt others, while relying on defense mechanisms to falsify his ineffective coping (i.e., "fake it or make it"). Manipulative strategies may become habitual when defense mechanisms are used repeatedly to respond to anxiety. When this combination of behaviors forms a nonproductive pattern, the person may obliterate effective coping options.

Personality Disorders

In many instances a personality disorder may have preexisted or contributed to the disabling condition. Personality disorders comprise an important behavior pattern because as a rule persons who have personality disorders have not been excluded out of hand from rehabilitation units or community settings when they have rehabilitation care needs. Recent presentations for audiences composed of rehabilitation professionals have addressed topics of violence among clients, staff, and others. Complete psychosocial and personality assessment is important for understanding the nature of a client's condition and planning the appropriate level and type of care.

When adults who had incurred traumatic head injury (n = 102) were examined during the first year postinjury, researchers found greater improvements in physical functioning than in psychosocial functioning. Although problems varied with severity of injury and time of examination, preexisting personality characteristics remained evident. Using four psychosocial measures, researchers suggest not all psychosocial manifestations such as headaches, fatigue, anxiety, or irritability necessarily are products of the head injury (McLean, Dikmen, & Temkin, 1993).

The basis for behavior of a client with a personality disorder differs from that of a person who develops agitated behavior patterns following altered or impaired cognition, but one does not exclude the other. An individual whose personality is inflexible or immature, lacking empathy and personal or social awareness, prone to anxiety or depression, and unsure of self-identity can be expected to have experienced multiple stressors and furthermore to have met stressors with ineffective coping strategies. This individual may be disruptive to others, antagonistic to self-care or learning about the condition, and ultimately require mental health intervention.

Teaching or transferring effective coping skills to clients may represent important learning for persons who are dependent on others, such as home health aides or personal attendants, for part or all of their care. Challenges of physical dependency, sensory impairment, psychological adjustment, and pressures for clients to re-enter their lives on all levels may be met with psychosocial pain that evokes therapeutic or maladaptive coping strategies.

Substance Abuse

Clients with disabling conditions may be at risk for maladaptive coping behaviors, especially alcohol abuse, and reduced rehabilitation outcomes. While testing validity of a screening tool (CAGE—*c*ut down, *a*nnoyed by criticism, *g*uilty about drinking, *e*ye-opener drinks) to determine tendency toward alcohol abuse for persons who had spinal cord injury, a researcher learned clients who had previously abused alcohol and/or drug substances had a higher risk for medical complications, notably spasticity, than their peers (Tate, 1993).

Increasingly rehabilitation nurses will need to understand substance abuse behaviors in clients who seek rehabilitation services, including clients whose substance abuse and related risky or thrill-seeking behaviors preceded their disability (Pires, 1989). Lifestyle behaviors are a factor influencing outcome once these persons return to the community. Substance abuse may increase a client's vulnerability and chance of re-entering an abusive relationship, as well as influence physical and psychosocial health status.

Seemingly opposite to thrill seeking, another type of behavior pattern is one that leaves a person repeatedly vulnerable to stress-induced illness or injury. Characterized by a focus on maintaining homeostasis in an unchanging, predictable, and orderly environment, this person does not seek thrills. Challenges are viewed as problems and become personalized, so that a number of stressors spill over indiscriminately flooding stress into many areas of the person's life. When in overload, this client may engage in substance abuse or other addictive behaviors coupled with learned helplessness or resort to giving up.

Potential for ineffective coping patterns crosses all boundaries of lifestyle and life-span for individuals and families. Loss due to impairment or disability may place an individual (and family) at risk for ineffective coping. Coping abilities may be impaired following cognitive impairment following disease or traumatic injury, such as with TBI. Premature or "substance-exposed" infants, older persons with progressive conditions such as Parkinson's disease (PD), or caregivers who have stressor overload may experience altered coping behaviors.

Family Coping

Stressors faced by families who have a member with a chronic, disabling, or developmental disorder may appear formidable. When the client is an infant or child, the family system is increasingly at risk for ineffective coping and potential breakdown. These families are accosted with multiple stressors and demands from internal and external sources. Stressors and demands that do not appear in any logical or orderly fashion may accumulate and intensify. The literature holds conflicting reports concerning increased incidence of divorce or separation for these families, but there is little disagreement about the multiple stressors that impact all parts of the family system.

Siblings of a child with a chronic, disabling, or developmental disorder often are ignored but are at risk for not having their basic and primary care needs met and for developing ineffective coping behaviors. Siblings manifest behavioral problems or compensation when they compete for attention and their own needs in a stressed and overly taxed family system (Breslau & Prabuki, 1987; Gibbons, 1992).

Surprisingly McCubbin (1989) found little difference in "pile up" of stressors for white middle-class single and two-parent families who had a child with cerebral palsy. Although single-parent families had fewer financial resources, they were more adaptable with flexible role functions. This finding requires further study using families of other ethnic and economic compositions and children with other diagnoses and examining uncontrolled variables related to social supports and family dynamics. However, results highlight caution about planning care or interventions based on popular but untested assumptions.

Research findings reinforce important differences, and individuality of family caregiver responses are based on characteristics resulting from the person's injury. Age, gender, serverity, deficit type and manifestation, social presentation, accompanying impairments, and the person's own adjustment to traumatic head injury influence family coping responses (Graffi & Minnes, 1989).

Families who have a member with a traumatic head injury may be able to accommodate physical impairments and altered functional abilities more readily than they can adjust to the person's cognitive deficits and resulting personality and behavioral changes. As the client's altered cognition manifests its features over extended periods, stressors mount to create new family crises. With adjustments to altered roles, for instance, spouses need assistance adjusting to altered role patterns. Likewise children align and realign their own growing and developing roles to accommodate a parent who has changed personality and behaviors within an already stress-laden family system. Adolescents and young adults may be thrust into roles of parenting their parents, and so it continues.

Too often the unrelenting, continual nature of family caregiving may be minimized when planning community-based care. Many families who care for a member with a chronic, disabling, or developmental disorder view their options for alternative caregiving arrangements as negative choices. When cognitive, psychological, and behavioral problems occur, such as with Alzheimer's disease, a family is more likely to consider institutional placement. These problems also increase potential for abuse, often as a result of breakdown of an exhausted, frustrated, and unrelieved caregiver (Wilson, 1989).

Families in the rural South who cared for relatives with disabilities in their homes identified financial assistance, medical care, and vocational services as priorities. Although the families expressed concerns about interactive relationships and displayed various levels of effective coping strategies, their attention was directed primarily toward basic survival needs, consistent with Maslow's theory (Arnold & Case, 1993).

Certainly with trends toward improved access, changing health economics and allocations of services, and independent community living it is essential to assess and build on each family's strengths and resources to maximize effective coping. This may mean providing basic needs as well as attending to psychosocial functioning. Although additional research is needed, support from social systems, peers, and extended family is a prevailing element in caregiver resistance to stressors.

Selected Assessment Instruments

Many coping and stress measurement instruments are available. Rehabilitation nurses must be careful to choose assessment instruments that are valid, reliable, and appropriate and be cautious to interpret results in context. Data that are measured, gathered, analyzed, or reported must be drawn from instruments known to be valid, reliable, and relevant regarding members of cultural or ethnic groups; those who comprise special populations; or persons with chronic, disabling, or developmental conditions. Rehabilitation nurses serve as client advocates when data, or results of data analysis, are used to to define resources, interventions, and expected outcome. Qualitative interviews are not listed but are an important and useful means of eliciting information about coping beliefs and practices. Content in this chapter could be used in part for underlying concepts when constructing a qualitative assessment. Table 13-1 contains a sample of assessment tools available for measuring concepts of stress and coping.

Goals

Goals are for families or individuals to be able to
✦ Activate strengths and resources
✦ Remove barriers to effective coping

Table 13-1 Selected assessment instruments

Title	Design	Intent	Concepts	Validity
Schedule of Recent Experiences (and similar cumulative stress scales)	Client selects own events that have occurred recently from a list of potentially stressful life events, each with a weighted numeric value for social adjustment; then a total stress score is calculated.	Stressors from life events may accumulate until health is compromised. The higher the total score, the greater the probability for illness or accident.	Stressors include marriage, divorce, loss such as death or employment, holidays, and a large mortgage.	Neither validity/reliability have been established. Nonetheless, the schedules are familiar and popular. (Holmes & Rahe, 1967)
Jalowiec Coping Scale (JCS)	Select a place on a 4-point ordinal scale to describe response to each of 60 coping strategies.	Developed by nurses to assess clients' coping "styles."	Concepts are broad categories: palliative, optimistic, emotive, self-reliant, supportive, fatalistic, evasive, and confrontive.	JCS has content validity, construct validity, and tested as reliable. (Jalowiec, Murphy, & Powers, 1984)
Revised Ways of Coping Checklist (WCCL) (Vitaliano, 1987)	Answer questions about ways of coping using a Likert-type scale to record responses.	The revised checklist measures "how" coping occurs.	Five subscales are avoidance, blamed self, wishful thinking, problem focused, and seeks social support.	Has been evaluated in a variety of populations to reduce demographic bias. Construct- and criterion-related validity and reasonable internal consistency reliability have been demonstrated. (Vitaliano, Russo, Carr, Maiuro, & Becker, 1985)
Mishel Uncertainty in Illness Scale (MUIS) (Mishel, 1987)	Self-selections from multiple cues about uncertainty arranged on a Likert-type scale.	Used in nursing research on relationship of uncertainty with chronic or disabling conditions.	Constructs include multiple cues for ambiguity about whether the illness is vague or clear and complexity as self-perception of treatment and the system of care. (Mishel & Braden, 1988)	Has demonstrated reliability and validity; Mishel reconceptualized the concept. (Mishel, 1990)
Ways of Coping Checklist (Revised) (Lazarus & Folkman, 1984)	Describe a situation, then circle the extent to which you used each of the listed items in coping in that situation; a Likert-type scale.	This is the most commonly used tool in psychosocial studies and elicits responses for a given situation. Measures individual coping processes.	Eight strategies for coping with 67 items. Strategies are confrontive coping, planned problem-solving, social support, distancing, self-control, escape-avoidance, accepting responsibility, and positive reappraisal.	Has satisfactory ratings for internal consistency and reliability.
Coping Health Inventory for Parents (CHIP) (McCubbin et al., 1983)	Identify how parents cope and whether specific interventions or resources are helpful in managing family life during a child's illness or chronic condition.	Health inventory form that deals with family system issues when a child is ill or has a chronic condition.		Related instrument is Coping Health Inventory for Children (CHIC) (Austin, Patterson, & Huberty, 1991)

Instrument	Description			Comments
FACES-III (Olson, Portner, & Lavee, 1985)	Self report and evaluation scales for family assessment.	FES (Moos, 1984), a related scale, is a similar instrument.	Screen a family for health resources and function.	Recognized scale in common use.
Rosenberg Self-Esteem Scale (RSE) (Rosenberg, 1965)	Self-rating of self-esteem using a Guttman scale.	Used to test self-esteem in high school students, adults, and a variety of ethnic groups.	Scale of 10 items concern person's own rating of self-esteem.	Frequently used; reliable and holds construct validity across various groups.
Coping Strategies Questionnaire (CSQ) (Rosenstiel & Keefe, 1983)	Respond to questions about coping with pain; a self-report on 6 cognitive and 2 behavioral coping strategies.	Individuals also rate perceived control over pain and ability to decrease pain.	List of coping strategies: divert attention, reinterpret pain, coping self-statements, ignore pain sensation, pray/hope, catastrophize, increase activity level, and increase pain behaviors.	Factor analysis sorts answers into response patterns, but no reliability or validity has been established.
Beck Anxiety Inventory (Beck, Epstein, Brown, & Steen, 1987)	Respond by rating degree to which or "how much" each common symptom of anxiety bothers person on that day and over the preceding week. Select from "not at all" to "severely" per a Likert-type scale.	Quick and easy. Used frequently in clinical settings to screen anxiety levels.	Responses to 21 items yield numeric scores. Total scores correspond with several levels of mood depression, mood disturbance, or normal mood.	No reliability or validity test results are available.
African-American Women's Stress Scale (AWSS) (Watts-Jones, 1990)	Measures gender and cultural differences in stress and coping.	A beginning preliminary scale for a specific group.	Examines relationships between stressors and unique physical and psychological impairments that may be characteristic for African-American women.	Included to document and represent the need for research in stress and coping with diverse and multicultural groups. No validity or reliability is known.

+ Establish health maintenance and safety programs
+ Identify and resolve issues
+ Gain access or referral to resources, services, and activities that promote independence
+ Prevent further disability or complications
+ Rectify knowledge deficits and enhance capabilities
+ Be involved and empowered in planning and decision-making processes
+ Use culturally, developmentally, and personally appropriate intervention methods
+ Develop coping responses/behaviors that lead to improved health outcomes

INTERVENTIONS TO PROMOTE EFFECTIVE COPING BEHAVIORS

Interventions with persons and families are those processes that promote and improve effective coping strategies and stress management outcome for achieving both short- and long-term goals, perhaps lifelong. Interventions are instituted as preventive or therapeutic actions when nursing assessment and diagnosis indicate potential or actual stress intolerance or ineffective coping for an individual or family. The initial intervention is to reconfirm and clarify each person's appraisal and meaning for the stressor situation and affirm, then enable, potential for growth. Throughout a rehabilitation nurse works with the person or family to improve trust and rapport and guide open, honest communication.

Two categories of interventions are discussed: intervention concepts, such as humor and social supports, and specific techniques for interventions, such as relaxation. Rehabilitation nurses may select any or several interventions to promote effective coping strategies with their clients and families. However, interventions do not stand alone without a conceptual basis for practice.

Intervention Concepts
+ Enhancing empowerment and hope

Empowerment and hope are related concepts. Empowerment for clients and their families is a process that enables them to recognize and mobilize their strengths and resources, gain knowledge and develop skills and attitudes to improve their capabilities and confidence, formulate effective coping strategies, gain mastery over their environment, and effect change consistent with their goals and values. Empowerment encourages self-direction and determination; it is essential to hope.

With chronic conditions empowerment is necessarily a long-term process. Individual or family motivation to sustain as well as invest in a plan of care is dependent in part on their energy, social support, coping strategies, and resources. Similar to steps in change theory, a client is motivated to seek and maintain health when able to appraise readiness, change, and then integrate change (Fleury, 1991).

With empowerment a client or family experiences hope and feels capable; the antethesis is powerlessness. Those who are powerless are at risk to become helpless and eventually hopeless—the final stage before breakdown or death. Empowerment must flow from interpersonal or spiritual sources as well as from individuals, health professionals, or caregivers. In reality health systems are not organized to empower clients and their families, even when included as participants of interdisciplinary teams. The idea of clients and families as team members is well intentioned but often inoperative when professionals muddle or devalue client participation. Until systems are truly client driven, not systems driven, empowerment will be an issue for clients and families. Community-based services, where families are active participants, may position health professionals to experience conflict about relinquishing power in decisions and relationships (Hoeman, 1993).

Hope is a significant factor in effective coping, especially spiritual hope. Allport theorized that a person needed to have some type of unifying religious belief or a philosophy in order to cope effectively with potential and actual stressors that occur in a person's life (Allport, 1951). This dimension of coping is only beginning to be studied by nurse researchers. A number of studies have findings supporting prayer, faith, and religious belief as significantly related to hope (Herth, 1989).

Since hope is a construct of empowerment, it follows that those persons with spiritual hope have been found to be better able to set goals, have stronger family relationships, and develop religious and social supports. Either unrealistic hopefulness or unjustified hopelessness may become ineffective coping strategies and impede therapeutic interventions—such as when a client alters, rejects, or ignores a treatment plan (McGee, 1984).

Caring remains an essence of rehabilitation nursing. However, there are variations among individual, cultural, and lifestyle appraisals of what constitutes appropriate or meaningful caring. Nurses who validate the effect of their interventions and caring with their clients may find their clients have reduced stress and are better able to follow through with self-care (Keane, Chastain, & Rudisill, 1987). Over several decades health professionals gradually have come to regard principles from holistic health, recognize client utilization of traditional or alternative patterns of healing, and acknowledge the mind-body-spirit connection in health. (Chapter 28 discusses these principles in more detail.)

Promoting Healthy Humor

Humor is a noninvasive approach with combined physiologic and psychosocial components. Humor may be an intervention to break a person's concentration on stressors, aid in expression of internalized emotions, enhance learning capabilities, and contribute to effective coping simply by altering a person's appraisal of resources against stressors.

Physiologically laughter results in increased production of catecholamine in the brain, which releases endorphins. Blood pressure and vital signs increase until muscles contractually respond, then when muscles relax, both readings measure lower than initial rates (Robinson, 1983). Laughter potentially alters hormone levels, may benefit the body's immune system (Seigel, 1986), stimulates circulation, promotes spiritual hope, and assists in temporary pain relief (Cousins, 1979).

In group psychology humor-provoking laughter is recognized as a tension release technique because laughter has cultural potential to diffuse conflict or anger, salvage embarrassment, promote camaraderie, or relieve stress. However, when attempts at humor or laughter are not shared or viewed positively by all persons, the effects may be detrimental rather than beneficial.

Negative humor may be used as a substitute for effective confrontation or complaint. It may emerge as sarcastic humor to mask anger or hostility or perpetuate stereotypes and label victims. Negative humor demeans a targeted person or group (Balzer, 1993) just as humor directed negatively toward a disabling condition ultimately devalues the person with the disability. A philosophy that persons who are disabled direct negative humor at themselves as an ingroup coping mechanism without detrimental effects holds an underlying message. All negative humor subliminally carries degrading effects that reinforce devalued status, cynicism toward future outcome, and stigma for a person who has a disability (Cassell, 1985).

Similarly humor that is not culturally, ethnically, generationally, and spiritually sensitive is counterproductive and destructive to relationships and effective coping. Noted comedians state that "timing is everything." However, when a nurse assesses a client or family member to have distress, high anxiety, or depressive states a humorously intended message may be transmitted as convoluted and counterproductive.

The detrimental types of humor just described differ from therapeutic interactive laughter that is shared among clients and professional staff. A study of clients and nurses in a rehabilitation hospital found that joined laughing may establish trust and rapport. When clients and staff laugh together, there is opportunity to create an environment conducive to trying new activities, permitting failures, encouraging participation in recreational or lighthearted events, and assisting families and clients to do things together (Schmitt, 1990).

Laughter has been rediscovered and legitimized as an adjunct therapeutic intervention to promote effective coping. Stress reduction and coping methods used by hospitalized persons (n = 20) who had MS were studied. In addition to findings related to the increased stress experienced by persons with MS, "keeping a sense of humor" and "learning something new" were frequently mentioned individual coping strategies which correlated with individual resiliency (Buelow, 1991).

Multiple stressors and limits of coping of family caregivers who provide support, resources, and care at home for family members who have chronic, disabling, or developmental disorders have become a concern for health professionals. Community-based nurses working with such families have identified humor as one component in on-site respite to prevent caregiver burnout. One program for family caregivers experimented with content designed to enable caregivers to look at the humor, even absurdities, in their situation. Since multiple role changes and role overload exemplify caregiver stressors, each one is encouraged to find an activity that suits personal humor style and can be enjoyed several times a week (Pasquali, 1991). Overall evidence encourages research about humor and laughter as vehicles to improve outcome for clients and their families.

However, rehabilitation nurses who work with persons who have cognitive, functional, or organic impairment assess a client's emotional status for potential adverse responses before initiating humor as an intervention. For example, persons with diagnoses of epilepsy, presenile dementia, and amyotrophic lateral sclerosis purposefully were excluded from a case study using auditory laughter stimulation to reduce stress with persons who have aphasia. However, clients who had aphasia following a cerebrovascular accident (CVA) demonstrated some improvement in information processing and problem-solving. The researchers speculated about the influence of right versus left hemisphere deficits on client responses to laughter therapy (Potter & Goodman, 1983).

Social Support

Research findings document social support as an important predictor of coping effectiveness and stress tolerance. Social support is a stress mediator that may intervene to "buffer" the stressors that may attend health-threatening situations. Persons who have strong and resourceful social supports may ward off or reduce the impact of stressors, preventing illness or injury or assisting effective coping behavior (Broadhead et al., 1983).

How relationships between social support and stressors work, and what other variables, such as distress or premorbid personality, are significant, is unclear. Effective family functioning may be a key mediator. Family functioning before a child's TBI, interrelated with severity of the injury, was found to be predictive of a child's adjustment postinjury (Rivara et al., 1993).

Thus individualized interventions regarding social support are based on careful, multiple assessments that take place in cultural context, over time, and in a variety of situations. Premorbid personality, lifestyle, and associations will be key factors in adjustment, not only because a person may return to them as social support but because there may be rejection or abandonment. Some persons may compensate by selecting or even rejecting social relationships and situations that differ from former affiliations, whether out of convenience, because of lowered self-esteem, or alternatively for a sense of superiority rather than devaluation. In contrast, strong social support may impede a person when barriers are embedded in the support system.

Social support may be emotional, spiritual, physical, educational, vocational, or recreational. Elements of the construct of social support include the following:

✦ Family
✦ Support groups
✦ Extended family
✦ Peer groups
✦ Church members
✦ Interest-sharing networks
✦ Social recreational groups or clubs
✦ Friends, neighborhoods
✦ Professional organizations
✦ Service groups

Clearly there are differences in the amount, kind, and level of supportive contact among elements on this list. Social support networks can be categorized as (1) relational social support provided by persons one can "count on," care about, or love and (2) social facilitative support, such as obtained through a service organization or agency.

The caring relational support network begins when a person asks a friend or relative what he has done about a similar problem or for recommendation of a health practitioner before deciding to obtain healthcare services. A classic study of the "lay referral structure" describes the route a person travels, moving for advice from family opinions through other friends and acquaintances until a professional is reached (Friedson, 1960). Firm rules, cultural or ethnic values, traditions, beliefs, and expectations govern both context and process of health help-seeking behavior and the use of social support.

When sudden events or traumatic injury occur, the caring social help-seeking process may be short circuited because of reduced opportunity for choices. At those times social facilitative social support may be available depending on eligibility and access. Persons who need social support but are without suitable networks may seek help for stress and distress through healthcare delivery systems.

Social facilitative support services tend to document the person's need for support but may be lacking when called on to design interventions. This is true especially when the person has consistently inadequate or unproductive social support. Too often persons seek emergency care, when in reality their needs are related to ineffective means of coping .with stressors rather than having emergency medical conditions. Conversely persons with disabilities or developmental delays frequently encounter healthcare staff who are unprepared to deal with their illnesses in light of their disabilities. Merely needing support does not generate it; having support does not guarantee it is effective or constructive; and lacking support does not mean that appropriate support is always the obvious, available, or capable source when the intended outcome is to improve a person's health.

Counteracting Loneliness and Isolation

Loneliness is a condition of our times. Within the supportive confines of rehabilitation centers, living in independent living centers, living at home with family—with or without disability—people in the United States are lonely. As aggregates, adolescents and young adults report some of the highest rates of loneliness across the life-span (Acorn & Brampton, 1992). When lonely, a person feels loss, isolation, depression, and other stressors. Being with other people does not assure a person will not be lonely. Thus simply placing a person in a specialty support group or assembling community services may be inadequate or counterproductive.

Social support may generate, buffer, mediate, or directly effect coping; findings in the literature are both inconsistent and contradictory. In one instance a person whose social support is caring and available may have a stronger buffer than one who relies on a list of resources and persons (Cohen & Hoverman, 1983). Social support associated with personal or family characteristics such as hardiness has been found to contribute significantly toward well-being in women who had rheumatoid arthritis (n = 122) (Lambert, Lambert, Klipple, & Mewshaw, 1989). Social support may protect against depression or deteriorating psychosocial or emotional functioning for persons who have crises in their lives or have lost functional abilities such as with arthritis or chronic pulmonary or heart disease.

On the other hand, chronically ill persons who have effective coping strategies may not require intervention with social support (Patrick, Morgan, & Charlton, 1986). Social support did not have a direct effect on coping effectiveness in one study of cognitively unimpaired clients in wheelchairs who lived in the community (McNett, 1987).

Coping and Social Support

Constructive social support promotes effective coping outcomes throughout the life-span. In a study of mothers (n = 153) and their children with chronic, disabling, or developmental disorders such as cerebral palsy, chronic obesity, juvenile rheumatoid arthritis, diabetes mellitus, or spina bifida researchers examined each child's adjustment. These children consistently have more behavioral problems, not necessarily clinical maladjustments, than others of their age group. Children who received caring social support from both family and peers benefited because they were more likely to resist behavioral problems. However, those who received either peer or family support, but not both, did not adjust as well (Wallander & Varni, 1989).

Peer groups have been used with adolescents and young adults for educational and psychological purposes in a variety of settings. Some individuals work or learn well in groups, whereas others become angry, confused, or intimidated.

The stringent test of coping will occur in the community as more clients return to live at home, in an independent living arrangement, or in other community settings. Persons with physical disabilities may enhance their self-esteem, perception of quality of their lives, and other adjuncts to effective coping when they have social support in the community, especially when interactive and communicating with an extensive network.

SUPPORTING FAMILIES AND CAREGIVERS

In another view social support for caregivers has become an issue. Continual requirements and long-term commitment with limited resources are a reality for many caregivers. The very nature of caregiving may create social isolation with few support contacts for a primary caregiver. Even family members may distance themselves from the caregiver out of denial, avoidance, or guilt—further impacting family systems. As follows from earlier discussion, when there is a high degree of uncertainty about a client's condition, social support tends to dwindle and caregiver-client isolation increases.

For example, support groups for relatives of persons with severe deficit head injuries were evaluated by Campbell. Family support groups were found to contribute toward educational and psychological needs of participants, including meeting some of their unique needs, and as a forum for discussing future problems and health concerns. However, in spite of the information exchanges, there was less satisfaction for meeting a family member's social needs (Campbell, 1988). Rehabilitation nurses working in the community are well aware of interplay between well-being and endurance of caregivers and a client's ability to manage living at home.

In spite of these stressors, family caregiving is assumed to offer qualities unavailable in other settings, such as affection. Available family support may dwindle as the person ages while still requiring assistance. Rehabilitation nursing assessments and interventions have become focused on the family as a unit, including the person who has a disability, in response to the complex nature of chronic conditions and in realization of importance of the family system in determining outcome. Assessments that anticipate, and interventions that prevent, breakdown in coping effectiveness or buffer stressors may be key contributions from rehabilitation nursing (Riffle, 1988). Rehabilitation nurses assess and quantify strengths and needs of family support according to economic, emotional, social, and physical care support patterns (Brillhart, 1988).

Not all families provide good care; not all can withstand the stressors of caregiving. Although a majority of persons who survive a stroke live at home with their families, it is apparent that family caregivers are themselves at risk for ineffective coping. At the same time a person becomes depressed following a stroke, the caregiving family may experience individual or family anxiety, coalesce about the identified client, or become dysfunctional due to disrupted patterns of roles, communications, or operations (Evans, Griffith, Haselkorn, et al., 1992).

Family caregivers most often are wives or mothers who initially perceive family caregiving as their responsibility or are nominated because they are available. In these circumstances a woman already may be fulfilling multiple roles such as parent, employee, or community volunteer. A caregiver may receive minimal or no assistance from organized social support (Wood, 1991).

What begins as tasks may become burdens imposed on caregivers, without respite. Conflicts may arise about regimens, procedures, equipment, or routines between family members and health professionals, creating a guarded alliance (see Chapter 1). Generational and cultural differences concerning expectations of family and social supports may be assets or concerns. Family caregiving beliefs are not homogeneous practices across any ethnic group and may falter under economic pressures.

Ultimately each caregiver is faced with sorting personal, ethical, and moral belief systems about responsibility and the nature of caregiving and relationship with the person requiring care. A caregiver's combined experience of benefits and stresses may reflect personal moral development and the level of burden (Klein, 1989). The issues surrounding families as caregivers have raised ethical questions about limits of morality from some health ethicists (Callahan, 1988).

The expectation that a family caregiver role will be valued in a society that has attributed little moral support, or contributed few resources or mechanisms to meet demands of family care, may be idealistic. Family caregiving, apart from economic necessity, may become achievable only when resources and interventions can be applied meaningfully to real life situations.

DesRosier, Catanzaro, and Piller (1992) describe coping strategies used by women living in their homes as caretakers of husbands who are homebound due to disease progression from MS. Some gender differences between adjustment of husband and wives as primary caregivers occur, such as use of informal and formal support systems—

but both experience similar multiple stressors and role strains.

Similarly parents who have a child with cystic fibrosis face the responsibilities of family functioning, parenting, and special demands of a child with a chronic condition. Even when families are able to cope effectively, they experience high levels of multiple stressors and need multiple financial, social, and structural supports (Stullenbarger, Norris, Edgil, & Prosser, 1987).

Even when social supports and community resources may be available and acceptable, they may be inaccessible to the caregiver who is unable to leave a spouse at home without supervision. As time passes, social contacts and activities essentially disappear for this caregiver. Eventually the couple communicate only with each other and no longer engage in activities or maintain contact with friends (DesRosier et al., 1992).

Family caregiving may produce stressors on role relationships, producing multiple conflicts and threats to self-esteem, well-being, safety, and health. In one study caregivers responded to stressors by socially distancing themselves from the client, angrily restricting their outside activities, and holding back from what they wanted to do themselves (Sayles-Cross, 1993). Caregiver issues ranged from needs for control to perceived loss of autonomy extending from simple daily activities to major life events.

For many family caregivers, as responsibilities grow, time for outside communication is restricted and resources dwindle. Caregivers report social isolation, loneliness, fatigue, and reduced satisfaction with quality of life. Many caregivers have chronic or disabling conditions themselves; community health nurses recognize caregivers are at risk for breakdown. However, clients benefit from family caregiving; simply having a spouse enabled persons who survived stroke to score significantly higher on the Barthel Index following rehabilitation (Baker, 1993).

SPECIFIC TECHNIQUES FOR INTERVENTION
Health Contracting

Health contracting is an agreement—in this instance between a health professional or team and a client or family—to set goals and conditions and assign responsibilities toward meeting an expected outcome. When client and professional are able to set realistic goals and gain satisfaction from achievement, each becomes empowered. Although a contract may address an entire plan of care, more often it is used to identify responsibilities and to focus on goals for a particular action.

Not all situations are appropriate for contracting, since a client must be cognitively and emotionally capable of informed consent. Contracts may be verbal or written, but do not replace the need for other documentation. The Box on p. 212 displays the steps in developing a health contract and basic assumptions.

Basic assumptions underlying a health contract include the following:

♦ Client accepts primary responsibility for care and outcomes.

♦ Client intends to achieve maximum self-direction in care, although self-esteem and assertiveness may be low.

◆

STEPS IN DEVELOPING A HEALTH CONTRACT

---

1. Assess needs
   · Clarify values
   · Identify unmet needs
   · Complete the assessment
2. Establish mutually agreeable goals
   · Use behavioral verbs
   · Define priorities
   · Set achievable goals
3. Explore strengths and resources
   · Seek access and remove barriers
   · Name strengths and support systems
   · Resolve ineffective coping strategies
4. Implement the plan to be
   · Client and family centered
   · Professionally accountable
   · Culturally sensitive and relevant
   · Appropriate for objectives
   · Cost-effective
5. Evaluate the contract with client to decide
   · How well goals were met
   · Why goals were met or not met
   · Future items or modifications
   · Closure or termination of contract

+ Intervention will be preventive as well as secondary or tertiary.
+ Differences in cultural or religious beliefs, values, and ways will exist.
+ Health professionals agree to arrange necessary basic resources and support (Hoeman & Winters, 1988).

ALTERNATIVE HEALING

At times a nursing assessment and plan for care will differ from a client's or family's view of what is or what should be done. Families may have lifestyle preferences, religious beliefs, or family system patterns that do not match a nursing or team care plan. Increasingly, traditional or alternative practices are being introduced into mainstream healthcare, whereas formerly these practices were conducted privately and apart from Western medicine. Openness is essential, but health professionals are not required to participate in practices or to refute their own moral or religious beliefs.

When client and health system practices differ, assess whether the client's alternate plan
   + Is legal and safe
   + Can be documented
   + Can be incorporated into the rehabilitation plan
   + Is reasonable
   + Has detrimental effects
   + Is discussed with the full rehabilitation team
   + Is feasible

   + Is ethical
   + Promotes rehabilitation goals
and whether a client
   + Is informed and knowledgeable about the consequences

SELF-REGULATING TECHNIQUES OR MODALITIES

Medical procedures and treatments are highly visible and often costly but do not constitute the bulk of techniques used by persons for their healthcare. Nursing has long promoted wellness and prevention and the body-mind-spirit connection, and emphasized the essential nature of caring for health. Similarly cultural or ethnic groups may have preferences for traditional methods, persons may employ or refuse a technique for religious purposes, or lifestyle may dictate whether risks are negotiable. Sales of over-the-counter drugs, adaptive devices, or self-treatment books and materials confirm that clients refer to lay network sources apart from the health system. Periodically certain self-regulating techniques or alternate strategies for healing gain popular use, but more research is needed to test the merit of these interventions. The newly designated Center for Alternative Medicine at the National Institutes of Health (NIH) is one avenue to support research into the viability and benefits of numerous alternative health practices.

Sutterley conceptualized approaches used in self-regulation of stressors into five categories: meditative approaches, visualization approaches, kinesiology and somatic approaches, group approaches, and personal approaches encompassing diet with nutrition and physical exercise or activity. She associates these approaches with Nightingale's concept of the potential for the person to heal and nurses as facilitators in the process (Sutterley, 1979). These categories are used in the following material as a framework for nursing interventions using self-regulators. However, without self-efficacy and motivation, unsupervised self-regulatory modalities are not feasible; execution of intervention is related to effective coping strategies.

Meditative Types of Approaches

Meditative approaches encompass mystical mantras, formalized programs, religious ceremonies, and personal relaxation methods. During meditative approaches a person positions comfortably in a quiet, stimulus-free environment. Once settled, the goal is to focus meditation intending to passively "let go" of distracting thoughts. Following meditation, the body enters a state of hypometabolism and reduced stress. Examples of meditative approaches are self-suggestion exercises, concentration exercises such as yoga, spiritual meditations, certain imagery activities such as concentrating on being heavy or warm, or group meditation approaches that guide feelings toward growth.

Visualization or Imagery

Visualization approaches include self-hypnosis techniques, guided or creative imagery such as visualizing and imagining a healthy body, behavior modification modalities, or various therapies such as music or art. For example, imagery coping strategies have been used in treatment of migraine (Brown, 1984) and relaxation with guided imagery with surgical stress and wound healing (Holden-Lund, 1988).

Kinesiology and Somatics

Rehabilitation nurses are familiar with kinesiology and somatic approaches to reducing stress in their own practice such as biofeedback, therapeutic touch, therapeutic massage, progressive relaxation, or acupressure and shiatsu.

Biofeedback is a method of autonomic nervous system control via self-regulation. The client is given ongoing data, such as would be presented by auditory or visual signals emitted from electromyelograms or electroencephalograms, about her biologic functioning, such as heart rate or body temperature. Clients attempt to perceive the workings of their internal biologic systems and then to control them by incorporating themselves in the system as a "feedback loop." Although somewhat controversial, biofeedback has gained acceptance as a treatment used in combination with or as an adjunct to other modalities. Clients seek relief of migraines and other painful conditions and increased control over hypertension, cardiac arrhythmias, asthma, and similar conditions (Lubkin, 1986).

Nurses have expressed an interest in therapeutic touch as an adjunct to treatment, but a great deal of research is needed before clear efficacy is determined. Regardless, both clients and nurses find the concept of healing through the transfer or exchange of energy appealing and important for reducing anxiety. Specific instances and documentation for therapeutic touch are adjuncts to rehabilitation nursing practice when both client and nurse are prepared to participate as interacting energy fields to promote physical, emotional, and spiritual well-being for the client (Payne, 1989).

A basic program of relaxation techniques was found to be beneficial in stress reduction for persons with spinal cord injury in a rehabilitation facility (Bertino, 1989). Slow-stroke back massage added comfort and produced physiologic signs of relaxation when used as a nursing intervention with clients in a hospice program (Meek, 1993). Examples of steps in performing four exercises for relaxation are detailed in the Box on pp. 214-215. The exercises are intended to induce relaxation through slow rhythmic breathing; simple touch, massage, or warmth; peaceful past experiences; and active listening to recorded music (McCafferty & Beebe, 1989).

Other techniques such as functional integration and therapies using devices (e.g., transcutaneous electrical nerve stimulation [TENS]) are practiced by physical or occupational therapists, exercise physiologists, and other practitioners. Forms of Chinese traditional medicine and techniques from a number of other cultures should not be mistaken as folk medicine, although the traditional approaches often include spiritual and dietary components and herbal medicines. Individuals may subscribe to dietary programs for stress reduction including herbal medicine, culturally prescribed treatments, vitamins, and other remedies, in addition to special nutrition plans prescribed by health professionals. Creative nutrition plans that incorporate individual and cultural or religious preferences may add pleasure and reduce stressors for persons with impaired swallowing or restricted food choices.

These are too lengthy to discuss in this chapter, but nurses are encouraged to investigate the client's use of traditional approaches. Other techniques, such as reflexology or yoga, receive mixed reception from health professionals. Each person must have a clear perspective about expected results and how these are related to the entire rehabilitation program.

Group Sessions

Nurses often lead group sessions for stress management, such as assertiveness training used to prepare persons with disabilities for empowered re-entry to the community. Peer groups for feedback and problem-solving and self-help groups for addictive or self-destructive behaviors or codependency are available in both professional and lay community groups. Findings from a study of elderly couples (n = 73) at 6 to 12 months following stroke revealed that groups with a psychoeducational component promoted social support from family, community groups, or peers and effective coping strategies for both spouse and client (Robinson-Smith, 1993).

Organized group training programs with content about assertiveness, time management, conflict resolution, advocacy and patients' rights; those promoting self-esteem through attentive listening, respect, and dignity; and those exploring community living options with clients and their families help to empower and foster a sense of order. In addition to pet therapy, individual and group reminiscing techniques have been used to reduce depression, improve memory, identify life events, and target interventions with elderly clients (Burnside, 1990; Tourangeau, 1988).

Exercise and Recreational Activities

Stress reduction and prevention are dual goals from holistic approaches that incorporate nutrition and physical exercise. Regular exercise over time reduces heart rate and blood pressure, combats the "hazards of immobility" by stimulating metabolism and circulation, promotes flexibility and range of motion, and contributes to improved self-image.

Organized sports and exercise programs range from wheelchair basketball to aqua therapy, equine therapy, aerobic exercises, various yoga forms, T'ai Chi; and art, music, or dance therapy (Fig. 13-2). Sets of therapeutic exercises, some age specific, are used commonly by rehabilitation nurses practicing in the community for preventive and therapeutic interventions with clients. Persons with arthritis may experience relaxation after performing an exercise program tailored to their range of motion but mindful of their fatigue.

Pet Therapy as Social Support

The importance of social support in alleviating stressors was discussed earlier in terms of family, friends, and community groups. Rehabilitation nurses are able to assist clients with their interaction skills, coping behaviors, and self-image—all of which contribute to gaining social support. However, nurses cannot choose or locate friends or manage family functions. A nurse can, however, intervene by introducing clients to another type of friend—namely, animal friends. Whether pets, companion animals, guide dogs for the blind, or simian helpers (Fig. 13-3), pet therapy has become established as a therapeutic intervention. Clients

---

◆

RELAXATION EXERCISES

Exercise 1: Slow rhythmic breathing for relaxation

1. Breathe in slowly and deeply.
2. As you breathe out slowly, feel yourself beginning to relax; feel the tension leaving your body.
3. Now breathe in and out slowly and regularly, at whatever rate is comfortable for you. You may wish to try abdominal breathing.
4. To help you focus on your breathing and breathe slowly and rhythmically (a) breathe in as you say silently to yourself, "in, two, three"; (b) breathe out as you say silently to yourself, "out, two, three."

or

Each time you breathe out, say silently to yourself a word such as "peace" or "relax."
5. Do steps 1 through 4 only once or repeat steps 3 and 4 for up to 20 minutes.
6. End with a slow deep breath. As you breathe out say to yourself, "I feel alert and relaxed."

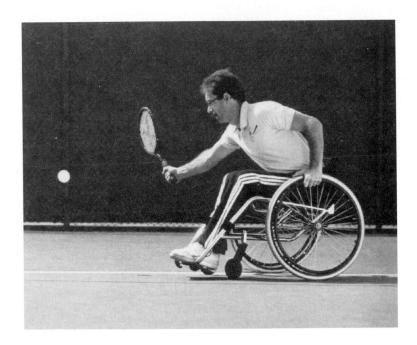

Fig. 13-2 Wheelchair sports activities are gaining popularity throughout the world. (Courtesy of Everest & Jennings, Inc. From *Rehabilitation/Restorative Care,* by S.P. Hoeman, 1990, St. Louis: Mosby–Year Book. Copyright 1990 by Mosby–Year Book. Reprinted by permission.)

Fig. 13-3 Simian monkeys have proved to be ideal helpers for persons with disabilities. (Courtesy of *New Jersey Rehabilitation Magazine.* From *Rehabilitation/Restorative Care,* 1990, St. Louis: Mosby–Year Book. Copyright 1990 by Mosby–Year Book. Reprinted by permission.)

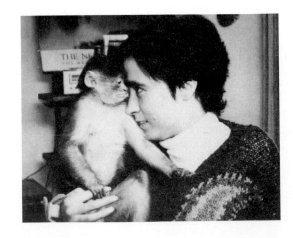

◆

RELAXATION EXERCISES—cont'd

Exercise 2. Simple touch, massage, or warmth for relaxation

Touch and massage are age-old methods of helping others relax. Some examples follow:

1. Brief touch or massage (e.g., handholding or briefly touching or rubbing a person's shoulder).
2. Warm foot soak in a basin of warm water, or wrap the feet in a warm, wet towel.
3. Massage (3-10 minutes) may consist of whole body or be restricted to back, feet, or hands. If the client is modest or cannot move or turn easily in bed, consider massage of the hands and feet.

   · Use a warm lubricant (e.g., a small bowl of hand lotion may be warmed in the microwave oven, or a bottle of lotion may be warmed by placing it in a sink of hot water for about 10 minutes).
   · Massage for relaxation is usually done with smooth, long, slow strokes. (Rapid strokes, circular movements, and squeezing of tissues tend to stimulate circulation and increase arousal.) However, try several degrees of pressure along with different types of massage (e.g., kneading, stroking, and circling). Determine which is preferred.

Especially for the elderly person, a back rub that effectively produces relaxation may consist of no more than 3 minutes of slow, rhythmic stroking (about 60 strokes per minute) on both sides of the spinous process from the crown of the head to the lower back. Continuous hand contact is maintained by starting one hand down the back as the other hand stops at the lower back and is raised. Set aside a regular time for the massage. This gives the client something to look forward to and depend on.

Exercise 3. Peaceful past experiences

Something may have happened to you a while ago that brought you peace and comfort. You may be able to draw on that past experience to bring you peace or comfort now. Think about these questions:

1. Can you remember any situation, even when you were a child, when you felt calm, peaceful, secure, hopeful, or comfortable?
2. Have you ever daydreamed about something peaceful? What were you thinking of?
3. Do you get a dreamy feeling when you listen to music? Do you have any favorite music?
4. Do you have any favorite poetry that you find uplifting or reassuring?
5. Have you ever been religiously active? Do you have favorite readings, hymns, or prayers? Even if you haven't heard or thought of them for many years, childhood religious experiences may still be very soothing.

Additional points: Very likely some of the things you think of in answer to these questions can be recorded for you, such as your favorite music or a prayer. Then you can listen to the tape whenever you wish. Or, if your memory is strong, you may simply close your eyes and recall the events or words.

Exercise 4. Active listening to recorded music

1. Obtain the following:

   · A cassette player or tape recorder. (Small, battery-operated ones are more convenient.)
   · Earphone or headset. (This is a more demanding stimulus than a speaker a few feet away, and it avoids disturbing others.)
   · Cassette of music you like. (Most people prefer fast, lively music, but some select relaxing music. Other options are comedy routines, sporting events, old radio shows, or stories.)
2. Mark time to the music (e.g., tap out the rhythm with your finger or nod your head). This helps you concentrate on the music rather than your discomfort.
3. Keep your eyes open and focus steadily on one stationary spot or object. If you wish to close your eyes, picture something about the music.
4. Listen to the music at a comfortable volume. If the discomfort increases, try increasing the volume; decrease the volume when the discomfort decreases.
5. If this is not effective enough, try adding or changing one or more of the following: massage your body in rhythm to the music; try other music; mark time to the music in more than one manner (e.g., tap your foot and finger at the same time).

Additional points: Many clients have found this technique to be helpful. It tends to be very popular, probably because the equipment is usually readily available and is a part of daily life. Other advantages are that it is easy to learn and is not physically or mentally demanding. If you are very tired, you may simply listen to the music and omit marking time or focusing on a spot.

with allergies or families with infants may not be candidates (Hoeman, 1990).

Some institutions have on-site pets or regularly arranged visits by pets. Cognitive retraining programs use pet care as a means of imparting responsibility, including sequenced learning of care activities, for clients before community re-entry. Pets are nonjudgmental about body image or impaired language skills; pets contribute to trust relationships and provide both social and sensory stimulation, even opportunities for persons to exercise when walking a pet (Wille, 1984). However, when a pet becomes ill, injured, lost, or dies this signifies a major stressor event for a client and family.

Each reader is aware of a family where the family pet is considered a family member. Convincing findings from research about the animal-human bond and pets as significant others have documented what many professionals already suspected—that pets may be significant in reducing stress, dealing with loss, and promoting coping for certain clients but not for everyone. Individual preferences and rights must be respected (Carmack, 1991).

Reframing or Cognitive Redirecting

Reframing is a useful intervention because it has potential to influence a person's appraisal of a stressor and redirects coping strategies. An overview is presented here, but use of reframing techniques requires planning and skill. Reframing is complicated because personal paradigms are set for certain expected worldviews. A person's worldview is shaped over a lifetime by many factors, assumptions, and beliefs that filter how information is received and perceived. When a person reframes, the concepts and emotions associated with a stressor must change. In other words the person takes a "snapshot" of the stressor event and fits it into another frame of context or meaning while retaining the facts of the situation; in effect a paradigm shift.

For example, Canadian researchers studied mothers whose adult children had developmental delays (n = 147) as they learned to reframe issues related to their adult children. Researchers found the mothers were able to improve their own coping effectiveness and broaden their base of support. Thus as a consequence of reframing their value orientation about their children, they reframed their own larger worldview (Cameron, Armstrong-Stassen, Orr, & Loukas, 1991).

Reframing is a powerful tool when used successfully to make changes in personalities and behaviors because it involves changing value orientation. For example, in a classic study of how persons encountered aging, those who were able to reframe their values and change the direction of their goals had more life satisfaction as they aged. Those who exchanged values of competition for cooperation and socialization as they aged had greater life satisfaction (Clark & Anderson, 1967).

Techniques for reframing in four phases are to
1. Challenge the client's worldview
2. Agree change is needed
3. Place change in context
4. Follow-up with feedback

Initially the nurse challenges the client's worldview by offering a reverse but nonconfrontational scenario. The intent is to get the client to recognize there are other plausible or improbable views. This phase must occur before a client becomes open to the next stages. When the client and nurse are able to acknowledge the same problem, they both can agree that change is needed. In the next phase client and nurse seek to come to agreement that mutual goals are contingent on a change in worldview and/or behavior. Before they are able to set goals, they identify components of the problem that either do not align with or contradict the proposed change. What is appropriate in the current situation is the focus. Reinforcement and encouragement from the nurse promotes effective coping strategies and the client's self-esteem.

For instance, "I know it has been difficult having a child with developmental delay at home along with three other small children. You have done a good job. Now that she is older, it would be appropriate in the current situation to send her to day care for several mornings each week."

In the third phase the nurse uses embedded directives that synchronize with the shift in context about the event. At this point the nurse must offer realistic strategies and tangible activities that will enable the person to experience and apply the change. Computer-assisted programs for education or play therapy for a child bring the context into the reality. The nurse who uses reframing interventions anticipates time for follow-up and feedback phases. Changes in worldview are difficult to accomplish and to maintain. Reframing one situation may or may not influence others.

Developmentally Targeted Interventions

Developmental stage as well as chronologic age may dictate choice of interventions for both families and individuals. The predominant thought in the literature is that coping behaviors will change for a person across her life-span and with other changes in her life. However, on occasion an intervention may target a life event. The following section contains sample interventions across the life-span.

✦ Special care infant interventions

Special care infants are surviving and living at home with families in unprecedented numbers. Families and many health professionals have not been prepared to deal with the unique characteristics of these infants. A special care infant communicates an overly stimulated state when the respiratory pattern changes, skin becomes either pale or flushed, or he engages in tremorous or startle movements; the infant may turn away becoming limp or floppy or stiffen, extending the arms, legs, and fingers. Some infants hiccup or spit up apart from feedings and actually adopt a worried or grimacing countenance. An infant may have uncoordinated eye movement when trying to avoid direct contact with others, often refusing nourishment (Hoeman, 1992a).

An infant may attempt to calm himself by reducing the intensity of a stimulus such as avoiding eye contact, yawning or sneezing, or retreating into a drowsy light sleep. Since most infants experience imbalance while lying supine, he may extend his limbs in an attempt to gain a side-lying position or push his lower limbs or back against a firm support to stabilize them. Parents who recognize and interpret these behaviors are prepared to assist their infant to cope.

The initial hurdle is to assist caregivers in realizing a premature, medically fragile, or special care infant's reactions are to stimulation, not a measure of the infant's dislike for a family member. Caregivers can assist infants to cope with overstimulation by giving them a respite from stimulation. Provide "time out" by simply holding him quietly, placing your hand on the soles of his feet when he tenses and extends his legs, or swaddling—which comforts many infants. If holding is too stimulating, slowly move him to a fetal tuck position on his abdomen with a blanket roll at the feet, or position him side-lying with a small blanket roll at both his back and feet to maintain him in a relaxed position. Holding him and letting him hold one of your fingers may be enough, or use a soft, calm voice.

Should an infant continue to cry, gently stroking his body or giving a pacifier to encourage sucking may quiet him. Do not interject more than one sensory input at a time; either quiet voice, touch, or relaxed face with or without eye contact is sufficient until he relaxes. He tires quickly, so allow him to sleep when he is restful; as he arouses, slowly alert him to his environment or your face.

Parents need assistance to remain patient, to understand their infant's subtle cues, and to gain confidence in their own abilities to care for this infant. Because gains occur in such minute increments with these infants, videotaping allows families to view progress they are not able to perceive while visiting their baby. The entire family, siblings, and extended family will become comfortable and invested in helping the infant and their family unit to develop long-term effective coping skills and strategies. Manual documentation systems, logs, records, and memory aids may help a family to realize the small gains, the increments that are not apparent at the time but which become evident through documentation or the videotaping.

✦ Adolescent interventions

A first step in intervention with adolescents is to recognize the potential for the multiplicity of stressors associated with this developmental stage. Then arrange time needed to build trust and rapport with the person. Adolescents may be hesitant to share their concerns, tend to minimize or deny them, or be unable to clearly verbalize them. Other interventions specified in the following material also contribute to a young person's attaining developmental tasks for adolescence. Rehabilitation nurses may promote effective coping skills with an adolescent client by assisting her in

- ✦ Learning that past mistakes are part of growth, by reviewing past successes and reaffirming personal worth, while gaining understanding that she is not responsible for some events that are not controllable or not within her control
- ✦ Prioritizing and assigning a relative worth to stressors
- ✦ Defining lifetime relaxation techniques or hobbies, such as physical or cognitive games for effective time out or energy expenditure
- ✦ Promoting assertiveness, reducing knowledge deficit by her participating in self-care including knowledge about the condition, adaptive devices or equipment, and educational or vocational options
- ✦ Providing access to peer and support groups or networks for services and socialization

- ✦ Facilitating family counseling and identifying buffers when stressors become threatening
- ✦ Facilitating a spiritual life
- ✦ Helping her to identify a trusted adult confidant she respects (This person must be able to foster effective coping behaviors and offer her a sense of balance. Too often health professionals or family members are reluctant to release an adolescent to another relationship, but when chosen carefully this intervention may be one of the most beneficial for lifelong coping effectiveness.)

✦ Geriatric interventions

As rehabilitation nursing expands and develops subspecialty and advanced practices, new information will be needed for specific assessment and intervention. One group growing rapidly in size and in use of rehabilitation nursing services is the geriatric population. As noted with caregiving, when older persons in a family develop chronic or disabling conditions, the entire family system experiences stressors. When a family system is dysfunctional, ineffective coping may result in abuse or neglect of the older person.

Maintaining functional abilities is a concern for older persons and their families. In many instances older persons are becoming caretakers for their family members who are very old. Impaired cognition is another issue when working with older persons. Nurses may enhance an older person's self-efficacy and effective coping strategies by helping with memory-related skills (McDougall, 1993). Forgetfulness and other memory complaints may originate from environmental conditions, medications, or sources other than impaired cognition. Nonetheless, attitudes about changes in cognitive behaviors may lead older persons needlessly to doubt their abilities, relinquish control over personal affairs, become socially isolated, and lead to neuroses or depression—in short, to negatively affect their quality of life. (Chapter 31 provides additional content.)

Documentation Techniques as Interventions

Written logs of activities and responsibilities, daily records of activities, exercises, or dietary programs are ways of discussing a client's progress or targeting difficulty with maintaining a schedule. Time structuring, a list of specific tasks or activities to be completed within a certain period, such as a daily rehabilitation schedule, may be practical intervention techniques to assist persons who have aphasia to deal with chronic depression. Pleasurable activities, personal time, and social visits are part of the schedule. Researchers found consistent use of visual cues and positive reinforcement by family and friends improved a client's self-concept (Tanner, Gerstenberger, & Keller, 1989).

Preventive Intervention as a Philosophy

Preventive intervention may be an often overlooked and underrated rehabilitation nursing opportunity for improving client outcomes. Specific indications for preventive intervention arise from nursing assessment and diagnoses. As findings from nursing and health sciences research reveal more about stress and coping, more occasions for preventive intervention will become evident. Rehabilitation nurses are encouraged to adopt an attitude of advocacy by predicting or recognizing indicators for how a client or family may cope. Outcome of interventions for clients who have a chronic or disabling disorder and their families may be influenced by the timing as well as the nature and source of support (Woods, Yates, & Primomo, 1989).

Early identification of situations that are becoming increasingly stressful may prevent system breakdown or role relationship conflicts. Siblings of a child with a chronic, disabling, or developmental disability; spouses of persons who have had a stroke; and special needs children who enter schools under mainstreaming policies all benefit from preventive interventions (Damrosch & Perry, 1989; Power, 1989). Modeling parenting activities and developmentally appropriate play therapy, participating in family picnics or community outings, and parental support groups are interventions to prepare and empower parents (Hoeman, 1992a; Ziolko, 1991).

Preventive intervention is cost-effective. Family functioning after a member's disability was found to be significantly correlated with the long-term adjustment of the caregiver (Evans, Bishop, & Ousley, 1992). Having a caregiver is an essential resource for maintaining independent function and community living, for many persons with disabilities are at risk. Preventive intervention strategies such as assuring respite care, use of day care and similar support services, screening assessment for caregiver depression or burnout, and referrals for maintaining a caregiver's health are all preventive interventions. Trickle-down effects from altered role relationships are key concerns.

CASE STUDY

NURSING DIAGNOSIS: STRESS AND COPING WITH A PROGRESSIVE NEUROMUSCULAR CONDITION

Mr. J is a 75-year-old man diagnosed with PD 23 years ago. No longer able to operate his watch repair shop because of his hand tremors, he and his wife sold the business and lived on business profits, payments from a preexisting disability insurance policy, and their investments. Within 2 years he developed increased tremors of the hands and tongue, "pill rolling" with his fingers, and a shuffling gait. He refused medication, embarking instead on his own regimen of nutrition, vitamins, herbal remedies; a tonic of honey, water, and cider vinegar. Always self-disciplined, he performed daily exercise. His wife prepared his diet and joined him in activities to "keep mentally alert." Although he had difficulty walking and slurred speech, little changed for 6 more years. The Js traveled and met with friends, and Mr. J continued to drive their car.

At age 62 things changed dramatically. He began L-dopa concurrent with his own regimen. Mr. J used a cane; a wheelchair or Amigo cart in public. The Js moved to a one-level ranch-style house accessible for Mr. J's wheelchair; he walked "on good days." After his urinary frequency, difficulty turning in bed, and nightmares interrupted sleep for both Mr. and Mrs. J, he slept in a separate bedroom. Larger and more frequent doses of L-dopa did not control periods of bradykinesia, cogwheeling, and rigidity. "Freezing," which impaired self-care with ADL and drooling, caused him embarrassment and anxiety. He contacted a physician who would prescribe anti-Parkinson's drugs in combinations and newly released medications.

At age 70 Mr. J took a "drug holiday" at home; a decision not supported by his wife or physician, both of whom described Mr. J as "demanding and stubborn" concerning his health regimen. He was rushed to the hospital after experiencing dyskinesia, hypotension, pain, confusion, nausea, and incontinence. Mrs. J was depressed and anxious about how she would continue to care for him. He returned home unable to perform bathing or dressing but able to walk "on good days." Although he could feed himself, everything was slowed including his speech. His overall health status was excellent, except for dental care needs since he had not visited a dentist for 15 years. He played games for stimulation, but fewer friends came to visit and Mrs. J became his main contact. Ironically Mr. J drove the car to his biweekly physical therapy sessions.

Mrs. J continued care for her husband until he fell during the night several times. Unable to assist him off the floor, she called 911 for help. The Js refused visiting nurse services as "charity care," so Mrs. J hired the first in a succession of three "helpers" who were to assist Mr. J with his personal care, meals, and exercises three times a week. When the third helper left, Mrs. J, who had experienced a mild stroke earlier the same year, decided that Mr. J should move to a nursing home. The Js' long-term care policy covered most costs. Mrs. J would visit regularly and Mr. J would receive therapy, medical supervision, and assistance with ADL. Reluctantly Mr. J agreed to a trial stay in the nursing home, provided he came home on Saturdays.

After a month at the nursing home, Mr. J was functioning at a higher level: walking more, sleeping through the night, and experiencing fewer speech problems. Mrs. J began to attend local social activities and rejoined her bridge and garden clubs. Mr. J came home on Saturdays but increasingly objected to returning to the nursing home on Saturday nights. He began to complain about the nursing home food and being lonely for his own home. When Mrs. J stated she could not take care of him at home, he accused her of "putting him away." However, both Mr. and Mrs. J are reluctant to have help in the home, especially live-in help. They state they want privacy and are fearful and distrustful of outsiders.

This week Mr. J informed his wife that he is coming home. He arranged a driving assessment and plans to resume driving. Although he has difficulty with ambulation, he insists the reflexes required for driving are intact. Mrs. J sought advice from a cousin whose husband lived at home following a stroke and as a result has hired an independent rehabilitation nurse as case manager. Eventually the Js worked with the nurse to write a health contract identifying their goals and responsibilities based on the following nursing diagnoses and process (Table 13-2).

Table 13-2   Nursing diagnosis and process

Nursing diagnosis	Assessment	Interventions	Outcomes
Ineffective coping due to denial and anger	Inability to adjust to changes; unrealistic expectations from self and others; lack of control over disease process; lack of problem-solving; fear of abandonment by spouse.	Write health contract, elicit Mr. J's perception and appraisal, then institute reframing and decision-making techniques, discuss methods for coping with loss and change, remove barriers to self-care. Evaluate marriage relationship.	Adherence to written contract, empowerment for decision-making, and improved interpersonal relationships.
Knowledge deficit	Stress from rejection or denial of disease process and drug therapy; lack of acknowledgment of wife's health condition.	Empower client by educating about disease trajectory; inform of local PD support groups; educate regarding wife's health condition; educate about medications and drug holidays, assistive devices, speech therapy, and relaxation techniques.	Revise regimen; recognize wife's role and responsibilities; employ assistive devices and techniques to reduce stressors; verbally describe treatment program. (Refer to Chapter 10 for discussion of education and teaching.)
Caregiver role strain; potential for breakdown of trust in the marriage relationship	Caregiver has history of stroke, restricted socialization, primary responsibility for client's care and safety.	Arrange respite care when Mr. J returns home; educate about services and support groups; teach relaxation techniques and interpersonal skills; assure safety in home; inform community emergency services; evaluate relationship.	Reduced stress from daily responsibilities; resumption of club activities; use of personal relaxation techniques; monitoring of health status
Altered health status (dental)	Regular checkups and overall excellent health status apart from signs and symptoms of PD, except for dental caries, reddened gums with bleeding, chipped teeth, and malocclusion resulting in damage to lips and oral mucosa.	Provide information about dentist skilled in working with clients who have conditions such as PD.	Dental appointments for preventive and restorative care.
Alterations in urinary pattern; frequency, incontinence	(Refer to Chapter 21 for discussion of bladder elimination.)		
Impaired mobility; potential for altered skin integrity	Reduced ability to initiate movements voluntarily or to move from bed to chair or commode; rigidity, tremor, bradykinesia, cogwheeling, "pill rolling," and shuffling gait. Potential for injury, falls, damage to skin.	Teach ROM exercises, teach exercises specific for coping with immobility due to PD (e.g., position "nose over toes" to rise from chair, stepping over imaginary mark to initiate walking, or rocking side to side to move legs); evaluate need for special mattress and trapeze bar in bed; observe for edema; consider OT and/or PT	Prevent complications or further immobility, maximize comfort and sense of control; adherence to regimen.

Continued

Table 13-2 Nursing diagnosis and process—cont'd

Nursing diagnosis	Assessment	Interventions	Outcomes
		consultations for ambulation, fine motor movements. (Refer to Chapter 14 for discussion of mobility.)	
Disturbed sleep pattern; safety issues	Inability to sleep through the night; nightmares, falls.	Negotiate use of siderails or other devices, bedside urinal; relaxation and ROM before bedtime; medications as ordered.	Establish rest and sleep patterns with minimal interruptions. (Refer to Chapter 23 for discussion of sleep and rest.)
Social isolation; potential for reduced satisfaction with quality of life	Physical, social, and spiritual isolation, reduced stimulation and access to information or contact with others; caregiver has responsibility for all interactions.	Institute community programs such as day care centers, senior center, van transportation, attendant services, church programs, meals on wheels, partners for "thinking games," support groups, exercise or therapy programs; respite for wife. Obtain realistic evaluation of ability to drive.	Encourage maximum stimulation and independence in social interaction; reduced stressors in marriage relationship; improved quality of life.

Other problems for nursing diagnosis and process: (1) Impaired communication, slurred speech; (2) self-care deficit, ADL; (3) threats to community re-entry, driving, refusing attendant services; (4) potential for altered nutritional status, family dysfunction, financial problems, and chronic condition for caregiver

OT, occupational therapist; PT, physical therapist; ROM, range of motion.

Preventive intervention may include those interventions to improve outcome for clients who have chronic lowered self-esteem. In this instance premorbid or preinjury personality and lifestyle are important factors. Ensuring a client's safety; eradicating substance abuse; preventing self-injury or suicide; identifying barriers and strategies to be overcome or dealt with; eliminating self-defeating behaviors and language; and training in assertiveness, vocational skills, and interpersonal relationships are appropriate interventions that require long-term monitoring and follow-up. Referral to community-based services and access to resources are essential (Norris, 1992).

Access enhances self-esteem and allows clients another dimension of control over their own life. Rehabilitation nurses have advocacy roles in identifying then working to eliminate all types of barriers that inhibit successful community reintegration for clients (Avillion, 1986). Organized medicine must acknowledge the cultural bias toward cure at the expense of care. The trend for clients to be discharged from institutions with shortened lengths of stay and greater acuity creates both stressors and opportunities for clients and rehabilitation nurses. The opportunity for nurse-to-nurse referral and collaborative efforts has never been more needed and possible.

REFERENCES

Acorn, S., & Brampton, E. (1992). Patients' loneliness: A challenge for rehabilitation nurses. *Rehabilitation Nursing, 17,* 22-25.

Allport, G.W. (1951). *The individual and his religion.* New York: Macmillan.

Antonak, R.F., & Livneh, H. (1991). A hierarchy of reactions to disability. *International Journal of Rehabilitation Research, 14,* 13-24.

Antonovsky, A. (1972). Breakdown: A needed fourth step in the armamentarium of modern medicine. *Social Science and Medicine, 6,* 537-544.

Antonucci, T.C., & Jackson, J.S. (1983). Physical health and self-esteem. *Family and Community Health, 6,* 1-9.

Arnold, M., & Case, T. (1993). Supporting providers of in-home care: The needs of families with relatives who are disabled. *Journal of Rehabilitation, 3,* 55-59.

Austin, J.K., Patterson, J.M., & Huberty, T.J. (1991). Development of the coping health inventory for children. *Journal of Pediatric Nursing, 6,* 166-174.

Avillion, A.E. (1986). Barrier perception and its influence on self-esteem. *Rehabilitation Nursing, 11,* 11-14.

Bach, J.R., Campagnolo, D.I., and Hoeman, S.P. (1991). Psychosocial aspects of long term mechanical ventilatory support for patient with Duchenne muscular dystrophy. *American Journal of Physical Medicine and Rehabilitation, 70,* 129-135.

Bailey, J.M., & Nielsen, B.I. (1993). Uncertainty and appraisal of uncertainty in women with rheumatoid arthritis. *Orthopedic Nursing, 12,* 63-67.

Baker, C.A. (1993). The spouse's positive effect on the stroke patient's recovery. *Rehabilitation Nursing, 18,* 30-32.

Balzer, J.W. (1993). Humor—a missing ingredient in collaborative practice. *Holistic Nursing Practice, 7,* 1-90.

Bandura, A. (1982). Self-efficacy mechanism in human agency. *American Psychologist, 32,* 122-147.

Barnfather, J.S., & Lyon, B.L. (Eds.) (1993). *Stress and coping: State of the science and implications for nursing theory, research, and practice.* Indianapolis: Center Nursing Press of Sigma Theta Tau International, Inc.

Beck, A.T., Epstein, N., Brown, G., & Steen, R.A. (1988). The Beck Anxiety Inventory. An inventory for measuring clinical anxiety: Psychometric properties. *Journal of Consulting and Clinical Psychology, 56,* 893-897.

Ben-Sira, Z. (1982). Life change and health: An additional perspective on the structure of coping. *Stress, 3,* 18-28.

Ben-Sira, Z. (1984). Chronic illness, stress, and coping. *Social Science and Medicine, 18,* 725-736.

Bertino, L.S. (1989). Stress management with SCI patients. *Rehabilitation Nursing, 14,* 127-129.

Breslau, N., & Prabuki, K. (1987). Siblings of disabled children: Effects of chronic stress in the family. *Archives of General Psychiatry, 44,* 1040-1046.

Brillhart, B. (1988). Family support for the disabled. *Rehabilitation Nursing, 13,* 316-319.

Broadhead, B., James, S., Wagner, E., Schoenback, V., Grimson, R., Heyden, S., Tibblin, G., & Gehlbach, S. (1983). The epidemiologic evidence for a relationship between social support and health. *American Journal of Epidemiology, 117,* 521-537.

Brown, J.M. (1984). Imagery coping strategies in the treatment of migraine. *Pain, 18,* 157-167.

Bruckbauer, E.A. (1991) Recognizing poststroke depression. *Rehabilitation Nursing, 16,* 34-36.

Buelow, J.M. (1991). A correlational study of disabilities, stressors, and coping methods in victims of multiple sclerosis. *Journal of Neuroscience Nursing, 23,* 247-252.

Burns, C., Archbold, P., Stewart, B., & Shelton, K. (1993). New diagnosis: Caregiver role strain. *Nursing Diagnosis, 4,* 70-76.

Burnside, I. (1990). Reminiscence: An independent nursing intervention for the elderly. *Issues Mental Health Nursing, 11,* 33-48.

Callahan, D. (1988). Families as caregivers: The limits of morality. *Archives of Physical Medicine and Rehabilitation, 69,* 323-328.

Cameron, S.J., Armstrong-Stassen, M., Orr, R.R., & Loukas, A. (1991). Stress, coping, and resources in mothers of adults with developmental disabilities. *Counseling Psychology Quarterly, 4,* 301-310.

Campbell, C.H. (1988). Needs of relatives and helpfulness of support groups in severe head injury. *Rehabilitation Nursing, 13,* 320-325.

Cannon, W. (1914). The interrelations of emotions as suggested by recent physiological researchers. *American Journal of Psychology, 25,* 256-282.

Cannon, W. (1935). Stresses and strains of homeostasis. *American Journal of the Medical Sciences, 189,* 1-14.

Carmack, B.J. (1991). The human-animal bond: Implications for professional nursing. *Holistic Nursing Practice, 5,* 1-87.

Cassell, J.L. (1985). Disabled humor: origin and impact. *Journal of Rehabilitation, 51,* 59-62.

Chiriboga, D.A., & Bailey, J. (1986). Stress and burnout among critical care and medical surgical nurses: A comparative study. *Critical Care Quarterly, 9,* 84-92.

Clark, M., & Anderson, B.G. (1967). *Culture and aging: An anthropological study of older Americans.* Springfield, IL: Charles C Thomas.

Cohen, S.C., & Hoverman, H. (1983). Positive events and social supports as buffers of life change stress. *Journal of Applied Social Psychology, 13,* 99-125.

Coopersmith, S. (1981). *The antecedents of self-esteem.* Palo Alto, CA: Consulting Psychologists Press.

Corbin, J.M., & Strauss, A. (1991). A nursing model for chronic illness management based upon the trajectory framework. *Scholarly Inquiry in Nursing Practice: An International Journal, 5,* 155-174.

Cousins, N. (1979). *Anatomy of an illness as perceived by the patient.* New York: W.W. Norton.

Covey, S.R. (1989). *Seven habits of highly effective people.* New York: Simon & Schuster.

Crewe, N.M., & Krause, J.S. (1990). An eleven-year follow-up of adjustment to spinal cord injury. *Rehabilitation Psychology, 35,* 205-210.

Davitz, L., Sameshima, Y., & Davitz, J. (1976). Suffering as viewed in six cultures. *American Journal of Nursing, 76,* 1296-1297.

Damrosch, S.P., & Perry, L.A. (1989). Self-reported adjustment, chronic sorrow, and coping of parents of children with Down syndrome. *Nursing Research, 38,* 25-30.

Dembroski, T.M. (1978). Reliability and validity of methods used to assess coronary prone behavior. In T.M. Dembroski, S.M. Weiss, J.L. Shields, S.G. Haynes, & M. Feinleif (Eds.), *Coronary-prone behavior* (pp. 95-106). New York: Springer-Verlag.

DesRosier, M.B., Catanzaro, M., & Piller, J. (1992). Living with chronic illness: social support and the well spouse perspective. *Rehabilitation Nursing, 17,* 87-90.

Dixon, J.P., Dixon, J.K., & Spinner, J. (1989). Perceptions of life-pattern disintegrity as a link in the relationship between stress and illness. *Advances in Nursing Science, 11,* 1-11.

Dohrenwend, B.S., & Dohrenwend, B.P. (1980). What is a stressful life? In H. Selye (Ed.), *Selye's guide to stress research. Vol. 1.* New York: van Nostrand.

Drench, M.E. (1994). Changes in body image secondary to disease and injury. *Rehabilitation Nursing, 19,* 31-36.

Dressler, W.W. (1985). The social and cultural context of coping: Action, gender, and symptoms in a Southern Black community. *Social Science and Medicine, 21,* 499-506.

Dunn, M.E. (1975). Psychological intervention in a spinal cord injury center. *Rehabilitation Psychology, 22,* 165-178.

Eland, J.M., & Anderson, J.E. (1977). The experience of pain in children. In A. Jacox (Ed.), *Pain: A sourcebook for nurses and other health professionals* (pp. 453-473). Boston: Little, Brown.

Elliot, G.R., & Eisendonfer, C. (1982). *Stress and human health.* New York: Springer.

Engel, G.L. (1968). A life setting conducive to illness. *Annals of Internal Medicine, 69,* 293-300.

England, M. (1993). Implications of knowledge claims for continued study of perception. In J.S. Barnfather & B.L. Lyon (Eds.), *Stress and coping: State of the science and implications for nursing theory, research, and practice.* (pp. 151-170). Indianapolis: Center Nursing Press of Sigma Theta Tau, International.

Evans, R.L., Griffith, J., Haselkorn, J.K., Hendricks, R.D., Baldwin, D., & Bishop, D.S. (1992). Poststroke family function: An evaluation of the family's role in rehabilitation. *Rehabilitation Nursing, 17,* 127-131.

Evans, R.L., Bishop, D.S., & Ousley, R.T. (1992). Providing care to persons with physical disability. *American Journal of Physical Medicine and Rehabilitation, 71,* 140-144

Failla, S., & Jones, C.J. (1991). Families of children with developmental disabilities: An examination of family hardiness. *Research in Nursing and Health, 14,* 41-50.

Ferketich, S.L., & Mercer, R.T. (1990). Effect of stress on health status during early motherhood. *Scholarly Inquiry for Nursing Practice, 4,* 127-149.

Figley, C.R., & McCubbin, H.I. (1983) *Stress and the family: Vol. II. Coping with catastrophe.* New York: Brunner/Mazel.

Fleury, J.D. (1991). Empowering potential: A theory of wellness motivation. *Nursing Research, 40,* 286-291.

Folkman, S., & Lazarus, R.S. (1980). An analysis of coping in a middle-aged community sample. *Journal Health and Social Behavior, 21,* 219-239.

Fraley, A.M. (1990). Chronic sorrow: A parental response. *Journal of Pediatric Nursing, 5,* 268-273.

Friedland, J., & McColl, M.A. (1992). Disability and depression: Some etiological considerations. *Social Science and Medicine, 34,* 395-403.

Friedson, E. (1960). Client control and medical practice. *American Journal of Sociology, 65,* 374-382.

Gaynor, S.E. (1991). The long haul: The effects of home care on caregivers. *Image, 22,* 208-212.

Gething, L. (1985). Perceptions of disability of persons with cerebral palsy, their close relatives and able bodied persons. *Social Science and Medicine, 20,* 561-565.

Gibbons, M.B. (1992). A child dies, a child survives: The impact of sibling loss. *Journal of Pediatric Health Care, 6,* 65-72.

Graffi, S., & Minnes, P. (1989). Stress and coping in caregivers of persons with traumatic head injuries. *Journal of Applied Social Science, 13,* 293-316.

Greene, J.W., Werner, M.J., & Walker, L.S. (1992). Stress and the modern adolescent. *Adolescent Medicine: State of the Art Reviews, 3,* 13-28.

Grey, M., Cameron, M.E., & Thurber, F.W. (1991). Coping and adaptation in children with diabetes. *Nursing Research, 40,* 144-149.

Hall, K.M., Karzmark, P., Stevens, M., Englander, J., O'Hare, P., & Wright, J. (1994). Family stressors in traumatic brain injury: A two-year follow-up. *Archives of Physical Medicine and Rehabilitation, 75,* 876-884.

Haynes, W.G. & Feinleib, M. (1982). Type A behavior and the incidence of coronary heart disease in the Framingham Heart Study. *Advances in Cardiology, 29,* 85-95.

Herth, K. (1989). The relationship between level of hope and level of coping response and other variables in patients with cancer. *Oncology Nursing Forum, 16,* 67-72.

Hill, C.E. (1978). Differential perceptions of the rehabilitation process: A comparison of client and personnel incongruity in two categories of chronic illness. *Social Science and Medicine, 12,* 57-63.

Hill, R. (1965). Generic features of families under stress. In H.J. Parad (Ed.), *Crisis intervention.* New York: Family Service Association of America.

Hitch, P.J., & Rack, P.H. (1980). Mental illness among Polish and Russian refugees in Bradford. *British Journal of Psychiatry, 137,* 206-211.

Hoeman, S.P. (1988). A system designed for paradox: hospital based home health care nursing in the United States. *Recent Advances in Nursing, 20,* 92-104.

Hoeman, S.P., & Winters, D.M. (1988). Case management for clients with high cervical spinal cord injuries. In K. Fisher & E. Weisman (Eds.), *Case management: Guiding patients through the health care maze* (special ed., pp. 109-115). Chicago: Joint Commission on Accreditation of Health Organizations.

Hoeman, S.P. (1989). Cultural assessment in rehabilitation nursing practice. *Nursing Clinic of North America, 24,* 277-289.

Hoeman, S.P. (1990). *Rehabilitation/restorative care in the community.* St. Louis: Mosby–Year Book.

Hoeman, S.P. (1988) Nursing roles and the multidisciplinary rehabilitation team. Presentation at Society for Applied Anthropology Conference, Tampa, Florida.

Hoeman, S.P. (Ed.). (1992a). *The Parent Infant Project manual for professionals and parents.* Morristown, NJ: U.S. Department of Energy.

Hoeman, S.P. (1992b). Community based rehabilitation. *Holistic Nursing Practice, 6,* 32-41.

Hoeman, S.P. (1993). A research based transdisciplinary team model for infants with special needs and their families. *Holistic Nursing Practice, 7,* 63-72.

Holaday, B. (1984). Challenges of rearing a chronically ill child. *Nursing Clinics of North America, 19,* 361-368.

Holbrook, S.E. (1982). Stroke: Social and emotional outcome. *Journal of the College Physicians London, 16,* 100-104.

Holden-Lund, C. (1988). Effects of relaxation with guided imagery on surgical stress and wound healing. *Research in Nursing and Health, 11,* 235-244.

Holmes, T.H., & Rahe, R.H. (1967). The social readjustment rating scale. *Journal of Psychosomatic Research, 11, 213-218.*

Jalowiec, A., Murphy, S.P., & Powers, M.J. (1984). Psychometric assessment of the Jalowiec Coping Scale. *Nursing Research, 33,* 157-161.

Jalowiec, A. (1993). Coping and illness: Synthesis and critique of the nursing coping literature from 1980-1990. In J.S. Barnfather, & B.L. Lyon (Eds.), *Stress and Coping: State of the Science and Implications for Nursing Theory, Research and Practice* (pp. 65-83). Indianapolis: Center Nursing Press of Sigma Theta Tau, International.

Jenkins, C.D., Zyzanski, S.J., & Rosenman, R.H. (1976). Risk of new myocardial infarction in middle-aged men with manifest coronary heart disease. *Circulation, 53,* 342-347.

Johnson, J.E., Waldo, M., and Johnson, R.G. (1993) Research considerations: Stress and perceived health status in the rural elderly. *Journal of Gerontological Nursing, 19,* 24-29.

Kammer, A.D., Coyne, J.C., Schaefer, C., Elazarus, R.S. (1981). Comparison of two modes of stress measurement: Daily hassles and uplifts versus major life events. *Journal of Behavioral Medicine, 4,* 1-19.

Keane, S.M., Chastain, B., & Rudisill, K. (1987). Caring: Nurse-patient perceptions. *Rehabilitation Nursing, 12,* 182-184.

Keefe, F.J., & Williams, D.A. (1990). A comparison of coping strategies in chronic pain patients in different age groups. *Journal of Gerontology, 45,* 161-165.

Keller, C., & Nicolls, R. (1990). Coping strategies of chronically ill adolescents and their parents. *Issues in Comprehensive Pediatric Nursing, 13,* 73-80.

Kemp, B. (1986). Psychosocial and mental health issues in rehabilitation of older persons. In S.J. Brody & G.E. Ruff (Eds.), *Aging and rehabilitation: Advances in the state of the art.* New York: Springer, 122-158.

Kinash, R.G., Fischer, D.G., Lukie, B.E., & Carr, T.L. (1993). Coping patterns and related characteristics in patients with IBD. *Rehabilitation Nursing, 18,* 12-19.

Klein, S., Sr. (1989). Caregiver burden and moral development. *Image, 21,* 94-97.

Knowles, M. (1973). *The adult learner: A neglected species* (2nd ed.). Houston: Gulf.

Kobasa, S.C. (1979). Stressful life events, personality, and health: An inquiry into hardiness. *Journal of Personality and Social Psychology, 37,* 1-11.

Kobasa, S.C., & Maddi, S.R. (1979). Existential personality theory. In R. Corsini (Ed.), *Current personality theory* (pp. 243-246). Itasca, IL: Peacock.

Kobasa, S.C., Maddi, S.R., & Courington, S. (1981). Personality and constitution as mediators in the stress illness relationship. *Journal of Health and Social Behavior, 22,* 368-378.

Kobasa, S.C., Maddi, S.R., & Kahn, S. (1982). Hardiness and health: A prospective inquiry. *Journal of Personality and Social Psychology, 42,* 168-172.

Kobasa, S.C., Maddi, S.R., & Zola, M.A. (1983). Type A and hardiness. *Journal of Behavioral Medicine, 6,* 41-51.

Kraus, J.S. (1992). Longitudinal changes in adjustment after spinal cord injury: A 15-Year study. *Archives of Physical Medicine and Rehabilitation, 73,* 564-568.

Kubler-Ross, E. (1969). *On death and dying.* New York: Macmillan.

Lambert, V.A., Lambert, C.E., Jr., Klipple, G.L., & Mewshaw, E.A. (1989). Social support, hardiness and psychological well-being in women with arthritis. *Image, 21,* 128-131.

Larsen, P.D. (1986). Development of educational programs in rehabilitation nursing. *Rehabilitation Nursing, 11,* 9-10.

Laskiwski, S., & Morse, J.M. (1993). The patient with spinal cord injury: The modification of hope and expressions of despair. *Canadian Journal of Rehabilitation, 6,* 143-153.

Lazarus, R.S., & Folkman, S. (1984). Stress, appraisal, and coping. New York: Springer-Verlag.

Lazarus, R.S., & Launier, R. (1978). Stress related transactions between person and environment. In L.A. Pervin & M. Lewis (Eds.), *Perspectives in interactional psychology* (pp. 287-322). New York: Plenum.

Lipowski, Z. (1970). Physical illness, the individual, and the coping process. *Psychiatric Medicine, 1,* 91-102.

Livneh, H., & Antonak, R.F. (1990). Reactions to disability: An empirical investigation of their nature and structure. *Journal of Applied Rehabilitation Counseling, 21,* 13-21.

Lubkin, I.M. (1986). *Chronic illness: Impact and interventions.* Boston/Monterey: Jones and Bartlett.

Marks, S.F., & Millard, R.W. (1990). Nursing assessment of positive adjustment for individuals with multiple sclerosis. *Rehabilitation Nursing, 15,* 147-151.

Matthews, K.A. (1982). Psychological perspectives on the Type A behavior pattern. *Psychological Bulletin, 91,* 293-323.

McCafferty, M., & Beebe, A. (1989). *Pain: A clinical manual for nursing practice.* St. Louis: Mosby–Year Book.

McCubbin, M.A. (1989). Family stress and family strengths: A comparison of single two-parent families with handicapped children. *Research in Nursing & Health, 12,* 101-110.

McCubbin, M., & McCubbin, H. (1987). Family stress theory and assessment: The T-Double ABCX Model of Family Adjustment and Adaptation. In H. McCubbin & A. Thompson (Eds.), *Family assessment inventories for research and practice* (pp. 3-32). Madison: University of Wisconsin Press.

McCubbin, H.I., McCubbin, M.A., Nevin, R.S., Cauble, A.E., Wilson, L.R., Warwick, W. (1983). CHIP-coping health inventory for parents: An assessment of parental coping patterns in the care of the chronically ill child. *Journal of Marriage and Family, 45,* 359-370.

McDougall, G.J. (1993). Older adults' metamemory: Coping, depression, and self-efficacy. *Applied Nursing Research, 6,* 28-30.

McGee, R. (1984). Hope: A factor influencing crisis resolution. *Advances in Nursing Science, 6,* 34-44.

McLean, A., Dikmen, S.S., & Temkin, N.R. (1993). Psychosocial recovery after head injury. *Archives of Physical Medicine and Rehabilitation, 74,* 1041-1046.

McNett, S.C. (1987). Social support, threat, and coping responses and effectiveness in the functionally disabled. *Nursing Research, 36,* 98-103.

Meek, S.S. (1993). Effects of slow stroke back massage on relaxation in hospice clients. *Image, 25,* 17-21.

Meleis, A.L., Lipson, J.G., & Paul, S.M. (1992). Ethnicity and health among five Middle-Eastern immigrant groups. *Nursing Research, 41,* 98-103.

Miller, J.F. (1983). *Coping with chronic illness: Overcoming powerlessness.* Philadelphia: F.A. Davis.

Miller, P., Sr., Garrett, M.J., Stoltenberg, M., McMahon, M., & Ringel, K. (1990). Stressors and stress management 1 month after myocardial infarction. *Rehabilitation Nursing, 15,* 306-310.

Mishel, M.H. (1987). Mishel Uncertainty in Illness Scale. Unpublished manuscript.

Mishel, M.H., & Braden, C.J. (1989). Finding meaning: Antecedents of uncertainty in illness. *Nursing Research, 37,* 98-103, 127.

Mishel, M.H. (1990). Reconceptualization of the uncertainty in illness theory. *Image, 22,* 256-262.

Mischel, M.H. (1990). Reconceptualization of the uncertainty in illness theory. *Image, 22,* 256-262.

Moos, R. (1981). *Family environment scale.* (form RO. Palo Alto, CA: Consulting Psychologists Press.

Neugarten, B.L. (1979). Time, age, and the life cycle. *American Journal of Psychiatry, 136,* 887-894.

Neuman, B. (1989). *The Neuman systems model* (2nd ed.). Norwalk, CT: Appleton & Lange.

Nieves, C.C., Charter, R.A., & Aspinall, M.J. (1991). Relationship between effective coping and perceived quality of life in spinal cord injured patients. *Rehabilitation Nursing, 16,* 129-132.

Norris, J. (1992). Nursing intervention for self-esteem disturbances. *Nursing Diagnosis, 3,* 48-53.

Nyhlin, K.T. (1990). Diabetic patients facing long-term complications: Coping with uncertainty. *Journal of Advanced Nursing, 15,* 1021-1029.

Olshansky, S. (1962). Chronic sorrow: A response to having a mentally defective child. *Social Casework, 43,* 190-193.

Olson, D., Portner, J., & Lavee, Y. (1985). *FACES-III.* Minneapolis: Family Social Science, University of Minnesota.

Pasquali, E.A. (1991). Humor: Preventive therapy for family caregivers. *Home Healthcare Nurse, 9,* 13-17.

Patrick, D.L., Morgan, M., & Charlton, J.R.H. (1986). Psychological support and change in the health status of physically disabled people. *Social Science and Medicine, 22,* 1347-1354.

Payne, M.B. (1989). The use of therapeutic touch with rehabilitation clients. *Rehabilitation Nursing, 14,* 69-72.

Pereira, B.A., Sr. (1984). Loss and grief in chronic illness. *Rehabilitation Nursing, 9,* 20-22.

Pires, M. (1989). Substance abuse: The silent saboteur in rehabilitation. *Nursing Clinics of North America, 24,* 291-296.

Pollock, S. (1986). Human responses to chronic illness: Physiologic and psychosocial adaptation. *Nursing Research, 35,* 90-95.

Pollock, S.E. (1989). The hardiness characteristic: A motivating factor in adaptation. *Advances in Nursing Science, 11,* 53-62.

Potter, R.E., & Goodman, N.J. (1983). The implementation of laughter as a therapy facilitator with adult aphasics. *Journal of Communication Disorders, 16,* 41-48.

Power, P.W. (1985). Family coping behaviors in chronic illness: A rehabilitation perspective. *Rehabilitation Literature, 46,* 78-83.

Power, P.W. (1989). Working with families: An intervention model for rehabilitation nurses. *Rehabilitation Nursing, 14,* 73-76.

Preston, D.B., & Mansfield, P.K. (1984). An exploration of stressful life events, illness, and coping among the rural elderly. *Gerontologist, 24,* 490-494.

Redeker, N.S. (1992). The relationship between uncertainty and coping after coronary bypass surgery. *Western Journal of Nursing Research, 14,* 48-68.

Richmond, T.S., Metcalf, J., Daly, M., & Kish, J. (1992). Powerlessness in acute spinal cord injury patients: A descriptive study. *Journal of Neuroscience Nursing, 24,* 146-152.

Riffle, K.L. (1988). The relationship between perception of supportive behaviors of others and wives' ability to cope with initial myocardial infarctions in their husbands. *Rehabilitation Nursing, 13,* 310-314.

Rivara, J.B., Jaffee, K.M., Fay, G.C., Polissar, N.L., Martin, K.M., Shurtleff, H.A., & Liao, S. (1993). Family functioning and injury severity as predictors of child functioning one year following traumatic brain injury. *Archives of Physical Medicine and Rehabilitation, 74,* 1047-1055.

Roberts, J.G., Browne, G., Streiner, D., Byrne, C., Brown, B., & Love, B. (1987) Analysis of coping response and adjustment, stability of conclusions; burn injury. *Nursing Research, 36,* 94-97.

Robinson, V. (1983). Humor and health. In P.E. McGhee and J.H. Goldstein (Eds.), *Handbook of humor research. Vol. 2.* (pp. 109-124). New York: Springer-Verlag.

Robinson-Smith, G. (1993). Coping and life satisfaction after stroke. *Journal of Stroke and Cerebrovascular Disease, 3,* 209-215.

Rosenman, R.H. (1982). Role of Type A behavior pattern in the pathogenesis and prognosis of ischemic heart disease. *Advances in Cardiology, 29,* 77-84.

Rosenberg, M. (1965). *Society and the adolescent self image.* Princeton, NJ: Princeton University Press.

Rosenberg, M. (1979). *Man conceiving the self.* New York: Basic Books.

Rosenstiel, A.K., & Keefe, F.J. (1983). The use of coping strategies in low back pain patients: Relationship to patient characteristics and current adjustment. *Pain, 17,* 33-44.

Rosenstock, I.M. (1974). *The health belief model and personal health behavior.* Thorofare, NJ: Charles B. Slack.

Rotter, J.B. (1966). Generalized expectancies for internal versus external control of reinforcement [entire issue]. *Psychosocial Monographs, 80*(1).

Sachs, P.R. (1984). Grief and the traumatically head-injured adult. *Rehabilitation Nursing, 9,* 23-27.

Sayles-Cross, S. (1993). Perceptions of familial caregivers of elder adults. *Image, 25,* 88-92.

Schmitt, N. (1990). Patients' perception of laughter in a rehabilitation hospital. *Rehabilitation Nursing, 15,* 143-146.

Schussler, G. (1992). Coping strategies and individual meanings of illness. *Social Science and Medicine, 34,* 427-432.

Selye, H. (1956). *The stress of life.* New York: McGraw-Hill (revised edition 1975).

Seigel, B. (1986). *Love, medicine, & miracles.* New York: Harper & Row.

Siegel, J.M. (1984). Type A behavior: epidemiologic foundations and public health implications. *Annual Review of Public Health, 5,* 343-367.

Smelser, N. (1963). *Theory of collection behavior.* Boston: Butterworth.

Smith, C.A., & Wallston, K.A. (1992). Adaptation in patients with chronic rheumatoid arthritis: Application of a general model. *Health Psychology, 11,* 151-162.

Strauss, A.L., Corbin, J., Fagerhaugh, S., Glaser, B., Maines, D., Suczek, B., & Wiener, C.L. (1984). *Chronic illness and the quality of life.* St. Louis: Mosby–Year Book.

Strauss, A.L., & Glaser, B.G. (1975). *Chronic illness and the quality of life.* St. Louis: Mosby–Year Book.

Stullenbarger, B., Norris, J., Edgil, A.E., & Prosser, M.J. (1987). Family adaptation to cystic fibrosis. *Pediatric Nursing, 13,* 29-31.

Strickland, B.R. (1978). Internal-external expectancies and health-related behaviors *Journal of Consulting and Clinical Psychology, 46,* 1192-1209.

Sutterley, D.C. (1979). Stress and health: A survey of self-regulation modalitics. Stress management issue. *Topics in Clinical Nursing, 1,* 1-29.

Sutton, T.D., & Murphy, S.P. (1988). Stressors and patterns of coping in renal transplant patients. *Nursing Research, 38,* 46-49.

Tanner, D.C., Gerstenberger, D.L., & Keller, C.S. (1989). Guidelines for the treatment of chronic depression in the aphasic patient. *Rehabilitation Nursing, 14,* 77-80.

Tate, D.G. (1993). Alcohol use among spinal cord-injured patients. *American Journal of Physical Medicine and Rehabilitation, 72,* 192-195.

Thomas, R.B. (1987). Family adaptation to a child with a chronic condition. In M.H. Rose & I R.B. Thomas (Eds.), *Children with chronic conditions: Nursing in a family and community context* (pp. 29-54). Orlando: Grune & Stratton.

Tilden, V.P., & Galyen, R.D. (1987). Cost and conflict, the dark side of social support. *Western Journal of Nursing Research, 9,* 9-18.

Tourangeau, A. (1988). Group reminiscence therapy as a nursing intervention: An experimental study. part 1. *AARN Newsletter, 44,* 17-18.

Trieschmann, R. (1987). *Aging with a disability.* New York: Demos Publications.

Vitaliano, P.P., Russo, J., Carr, J.E., Maiuro, R.D., & Becker, J. (1985). The ways of coping checklist: Revision and psychometric properties. *Multivariate Behavior Research, 20,* 3-26.

Vitaliano, P.P. (1987). Manual for revised ways of coping checklist (WCCL). Seattle, WA: Stress and Coping Project.

Wagnild, G., & Young, H.M. (1991). Another look at hardiness. *Image, 23,* 257-259.

Wallander, J.L., & Varni, J.W. (1989). Social support and adjustment in chronically ill and handicapped children. *American Journal of Community Psychology, 17,* 185-201.

Watts-Jones, D. (1990). Toward a stress scale for African-American women. *Psychology Women Quarterly, 14,* 271-275.

Wein, A.G. (1985). Rehabilitation assessment—A nursing perspective. *Rehabilitation Nursing, 10,* 25-27.

Weinberger, M., Hiner, S.L., & Tierney, W.M. (1987). In support of hassles as a measure of stress in predicting health outcomes. *Journal of Behavioral Medicine, 10,* 19-31.

Werner, J.S. (1993). Stressors and health outcomes: Synthesis of nursing research, 1980-1990. In J.S. Barnfather & B.L. Lyon (Eds.), *Stress and coping: State of the science and implications for nursing theory, research and practice.* (pp 11-38). Indianapolis: Center Nursing Press of Sigma Theta Tau, International.

White, D.M., Catanzaro, M.L., & Kraft, G.H. (1993). An approach to the psychological aspects of multiple sclerosis: A coping guide for healthcare providers and families. *Journal of Neurologic Rehabilitation, 7,* 43-52.

Wikblad, K.F., & Montin, K.R. (1992). Coping with a chronic disease. *The Diabetes Educator, 18,* 316-320.

Wikler, L., Wasow, M., & Hatfield, E. (1981). Chronic sorrow revisited: Parent vs. professional depiction of the adjustment of parents of mentally retarded children. *American Journal of Orthopsychiatry, 51,* 63-70.

Wille, R. (1984). Therapeutic use of companion pets for neurologically impaired patients. *Journal of Neuroscience Nursing, 16,* 323-325.

Wilson, H.S. (1989) Family caregiving for a relative with Alzheimer's dementia: Coping with negative choices. *Nursing Research, 38,* 94-98.

Wood, F.G. (1991). The meaning of caregiving. *Rehabilitation Nursing, 16,* 195-198.

Woods, N.F., Yates, B.C., & Primomo, J. (1989). Supporting families during chronic illness. *Image, 21,* 46-50.

Wortman, C.B., & Silver, R.C. (1989). The myths of coping with loss. *Journal of Consulting and Clinical Psychology, 57,* 349-357.

Yarcheski, A. (1988). Uncertainty in illness and the future. *Western Journal of Nursing Research, 10,* 410-413.

Ziolko, M.E. (1991). Counseling parents of children with disabilities: A review of the literature and implications for practice. *Journal of Rehabilitation, 57,* 29-34.

14

Independent Function: Movement and Mobility

Mary Frances Borgman-Gainer, EdD, RN

INTRODUCTION

Movement science is a multidisciplinary field of study of normal movement. The parent disciplines include biology, computer science, physics, physiology, psychology and nursing. Theories formulated in movement science help to provide the "why" certain practices of movement are effective rather than the "how" a health provider, such as a nurse, performs the practice. A professional rehabilitation nurse keeps abreast of scientific advances in movement science because the development of new knowledge affects practice and characterizes the orientation of scholars and researchers within the discipline. In the future movement science will be one of the foundations of rehabilitation nursing as nurses understand principles of movement before pathokinesiology, the study of movement dysfunction (Moskowitz, 1991).

Traditionally rehabilitation nursing was influenced by classic motor development theorists such as Stockmeyer, the Bobaths, Knott, and Voss. These theorists identified specific development sequences and incorporated certain behaviors of early motor development into various treatment programs, primarily those used by physical therapists and occupational therapists. According to classic theorists motor development occurs as a process of maturation of the central nervous system. The corollary to this theory is that when neural maturation is completed, the motor developmental process terminates. Thus mature behaviors of young adulthood comprise the standard by which older and younger individuals are evaluated.

LIFE-SPAN MOTOR DEVELOPMENT THEORY

An emerging concept of motor development theory is the life-span concept built on the assumption that age-related changes in motor behaviors are lifelong phenomena. With this in mind the concept of neurologic maturity as the marker of completed developmental processes must be re-examined. Using a life-span concept, maturity is just a passing point in time that has no added value over infancy, the middle years, adolescence, or any other age.

With contemporary motor development theories, behavioral change is a result of interactions among intrinsic factors, such as physical growth or neural maturation, and extrinsic factors, such as supportive and risk environments. In the life-span theory not only are interactions among intrinsic and extrinsic factors examined but also processes of change for all ages. The life-span perspective provides the opportunity to examine a broad range of change processes such as maturation, learning, and aging.

In order to illustrate the different viewpoints of these concepts, one can review the phenomenon of physical growth. This phenomenon is almost synonymous with the traditional concept of development by which one grows taller and heavier from infancy into childhood. Growth as well as development is portrayed as a progressive process, characterized by increases in size or through advancement in some area. However, throughout adolescence, middle age, and adulthood, a person's height and weight change. Declines, losses, or regressions are natural trends of developmental change too often ignored. Some motor behaviors are lost and new motor actions are acquired, whereas other behaviors remain stable from infancy to old age despite change.

The literature provides examples of research findings to support the life-span concept of motor development (Public Health Service, 1990). For example, "righting tasks" are a major component of functional physical independence. To be able to move from a supine to a sitting position, to roll over and to get to a standing position are all expressions of physical independence. Traditionally, early appearing righting movements were considered to be under control of the subcortical nuclei. With central nervous system maturation, the cerebral cortex is believed to exert control over the primary forms of righting, and the mature integrated behaviors of righting are evidenced. If central nervous system damage occurs, righting abilities often are lost or more primitive patterns of righting are utilized. VanSant's (1990) research found healthy adults did not conversely demonstrate what had been characterized as "mature" forms of behaviors. In fact, an inordinate amount of variability in movement was observed for a variety of tasks related to righting (VanSant, 1990).

Incorporating a life-span perspective into principles of movement and into rehabilitation nursing concepts affects the daily practice of nursing. First, the assessment of movement patterns clients use to perform tasks should be compared with expected patterns for their age-specific groups. Age, gender, body size and body shape, as well as activity level are considered when teaching information relative to movement. Second, the variability in human performance may be the characteristic that describes normalcy. Varying the situational demand introduces variability into client performance; thus a client's ability to cope effectively with varying demands may describe movement pattern categories for differing client populations.

In summary, the life-span approach to movement science provides a framework within which continued development of a person's motor abilities may be examined. The broadened life-span perspectives support research about factors that have not been considered traditionally as part of age-related changes in behavior. This conceptual framework reveals natural variability in movement patterns among and between individuals across their developmental life-span.

Models of Central Nervous System Control

Two models of central nervous system control are reported in the literature: the reflex-hierarchical model and the system model. In the reflex-hierarchical model the central nervous system is thought to be organized as a strictly vertical hierarchy; primitive reflexes, such as stretch reflexes, are controlled at the spinal cord level. The asymmetric and symmetric tonic neck and knee labyrthine reflexes are controlled by the brainstem, and righting reflexes are controlled by the midbrain. Last, the equilibrium reactions are controlled hypothetically by the highest level of central nervous system, the cerebral cortex. Therefore, in the reflex-hierarchical model, motor development moves from reflexive to voluntary control as a child matures. Thus the emergence of independent balance and locomotion depends on the maturation of sequentially higher levels of the central nervous system hierarchy, which yield higher levels of behaviors—equilibrium reactions, for instance.

Many rehabilitation techniques are based on this assumption about normal reflex maturation and development. For example, proponents of neurodevelopmental treatment (NDT) suggest that posture and movement designed to inhibit primitive reflexes, such as bilateral midline activities, inhibit the asymmetric tonic neck reflexes. Pediatric assessment techniques, based on a reflex-hierarchical model, are attempts to determine a child's developmental level through reflex tests and tests of voluntary control. For instance, developmental protocols (e.g., Chandler, Andrew, & Swanson, 1980; Milani-Comparetti & Gidoni, 1967; Fiorentine & Brazelton, 1973) were created to provide a systematic approach to evaluating essential parameters of function in children including muscle tone, primitive reflexes, automatic reaction and voluntary movements (Winstein & Knecht, 1990). If there were a lack of balance control, it was thought to be due to the presence of primitive reflexes constraining the emergence of higher level righting and equilibrium reactions. The treatment of a child with developmental delays would center on sensorimotor techniques that would stimulate the child through progressively higher levels of reflexes and reactions.

Another model of motor control is Bernstein's (1967) system or the distributed control model. The body is modeled as a mechanical system with mass that is subject to gravity and inertial force. Because these forces change as one moves, the same motor program gives different movement depending on the position one occupies. In this model the concept of a human is as an active agent in a continuously changing environment to be examined as a physiology of activity, not only as reactions. According to the systems model the nervous system is a part of a flexible complex of systems and subsystems each sharing in the control process. Movement is an emergent outcome from complex interactions of multiple systems.

The research question is whether the vertical hierarchy hypothesis (that as children mature, higher nervous system centers take over function from more primitive reflex systems, and that as adults age, higher centers deteriorate while lower level systems emerge) is valid. Recent research findings show that although there is some reemergence of spinal reflexes in the older adult, all other similarities in function between the different musculoskeletal and nervous subsystems can be explained by developmental changes in the functional status of each independent system.

The systems model provides great flexibility and gives potential for understanding balance changes across the life-span and therapeutic interventions for individuals with balance dysfunction. However, since research data using the model are limited, effective approaches to assessment and treatment of some postural problems likewise are limited.

Research Bases for Practice

Technology research has provided a tremendous amount of information about the generation, control, and acquisition of movement. Neurophysiologists, neuropsychologists, and human movement scientists have contributed to the effort. In order to use the information, models of movement have been developed as working hypotheses from which rehabilitation nurses and other team members extrapolate ideas and apply them in their own therapy practice. Originally, neurorehabilitation treatment focused on peripheral control of movement by which therapists attempted to control movement output by controlling sensory input. Newer data indicate a greater emphasis on treatment involving the central control processes. In addition, research data show tremendous variability in the way persons of all ages use their nerves, muscles, and bodies to accomplish the same task. Nursing care of the client with a movement and/or mobility disability is extremely complex. Even for clients with the same diagnosis, there may be no definite protocols. The question can be asked, "How can a nurse remain competent to care for clients?" The answer lies in continuous study of critical thinking and with reasoning about clinical entities and therapeutic nursing skills based on research and advanced practice of nursing. Assessment includes knowledge about normal movement and observation of components of movement that are altered or impaired for each person. This competency skill requires rehabilitation nurses to develop observational and reasoning skills through education, practice, and research.

NORMAL MOTOR MOVEMENT

Normal movement is a person's ability to interact with the environment in a flexible and adaptable way. Mobility involves initiating a movement pattern for each limb, coordinating these patterns among limbs, adapting the strength and speed of the movement pattern to counteract the resistance and/or sensory conditions encountered in the tasks, and maintaining body balance despite changes in the center of gravity as the limbs move in relation to the trunk. Additionally the ability to move presumes the following capabilities: (1) sensing the environment, (2) processing the information perceived in the sensed environment, (3) remembering prior movement sequences and selecting appropriated responses, and (4) implementing the appropriate motor response.

A Conceptual Model of Movement

◆ **Environmental demand is sensed.** Purposeful movement does not occur in the absence of a perceived need to move, usually generated from within the person or by an external stimuli. For instance, vision is a powerful stimulus influencing both movement and the limbic system as the seat of emotion and motivation, which may trigger movement patterns. A purposeful movement is organized and planned before its initiation (Squires, 1983).

◆ **Long-term memory is searched.** All voluntary movement is based on previously acquired movement patterns. The memories of how the effort to move felt and the result achieved by the effort guide the present movement. The idea to move initiates a search of the long-term memory centers for the memory trace of the planned activity, and then it notifies the programming center to start strategy development.

The movement plan is the concept of an action that concludes a number of simple motor programs and nonprogrammed parts. Motor programs are abstract representations of a movement pattern coded on a form that defines relative timing, amplitude, and force but not specific muscles. The most practiced motions are those most embedded in memory and available for use or for modification (Squires, 1983).

◆ **A program is developed.** Some movements—walking or writing, for example—are more highly programmed than others. The plan of the action is stored in several different motor programs, each specifying a part of the act. The chief characteristic of a programmed movement involving muscle coordination is the temporal relationship between the muscles and a specific skill.

Motor programs command the automatic parts of a motor skill and brainstem, the cerebellum, the cerebral cortex, and the basal ganglia all contribute to control of the automatic postural aspects of the program. The motor programs are modified to fit certain circumstances by strategies that specify certain parameters of a movement. A strategy can be compared with a set of instructions that facilitates or inhibits particular alpha and gamma motor neurons and interneurons to fire at specific frequencies at certain times. Various types of movement and environmental factors require unique control strategies, and these differ among people (Squires, 1983).

◆ **Movement is executed, monitored, and adapted.** The body has two motor systems. One system controls gross body and limb movements, and the other system controls skilled movement. Both systems execute movement via the anterior horn cells—the final motor pathway to the effector muscles. The anterior horn cell, or alpha motor neuron, connects via its axon to several muscle fibers within a muscle. This unit is called a motor unit and is the basic unit of muscular control. When the alpha motor neuron is depolarized and fires, all the muscle fibers of that unit contract. The number of motor units activated in a contraction are recruited according to size: the smallest are recruited first and

---

> ◆
> ### *A CONCEPTUAL MODEL OF MOVEMENT*
>
> 1. Environmental demand is sensed or a wish to move is generated.
> 2. Long-term memory is searched for prior motor patterns to fit situation.
> 3. A pattern is developed and forwarded for execution.
> 4. The movement is executed as programmed, monitored, or adapted.
> 5. Knowledge of results of the success of program is received and correlated with other sensory information.
> 6. The program is stored in memory for future use (Squires, 1983).

---

the largest last. The smaller centers are low-threshold, slow-twitch motor units, and the large units are high-threshold, fast-twitch motor units.

The proximal limb musculature is usually an open-loop system, and the distal musculature is a closed-loop system. Open-loop movements are programmed movements and ballistic and energetic in nature. Closed-loop movements are not programmed but are consciously or unconsciously controlled from moment to moment and are characteristically slow in nature. Unlearned movements and skilled movements are examples of closed-loop movements (Squires, 1983).

◆ **Knowledge of results is received and correlated.** A movement can be executed exactly as programmed and yet be inaccurate as far as accomplishing the goal. Knowledge of the results means the person has an awareness of the outcome of movement in relation to the goal. This knowledge of results is crucial to motor learning (Squires, 1983).

◆ **The program is stored in memory.** Movements are generated from past experiences if successes have been recognized and are stored in long-term memory. If the information is lost from short-term memory, it does not become a part of long-term memory and learning does not take place. The learned motor skill must be practiced to be retained at a level of expertise (Squires, 1983).

MOTOR DYSFUNCTION DUE TO CENTRAL NERVOUS SYSTEM DEFICIT
Cortical Lesions

Cerebral cortical areas have the following specific functions:

1. Primary motor cortex assumes execution of movement. It translates program instruction from other parts of the brain into signals that specify which muscles should control the programming.
2. Supplementary motor area controls the programming of complex sequences of rapid discrete movements.
3. Premotor area is active in assembling new motor programs.
4. Posterior parietal areas direct attention to objects of interest in visual space, form strategies for eye and arm movements, and guide arm movements in space.

5. Prefrontal cortex performs cognitive functions related to movement.

The motor dysfunction resulting from acquired cortical lesions depends on the site and extent of the lesion. Diffuse lesions (closed head injury) may result in damage to the surface and deeper structures of the brain. The motor dysfunction may result in swallowing and breathing deficits (brainstem injury), righting and equilibrium responses (midbrain and basal ganglia), coordinated deficits (cerebellar injury), motor planning (cerebral palsy). Circumscribed cortical lesions (cerebrovascular accident [CVA], gunshot, penetrating wounds) result in dysfunctional planning limited to the function controlled by the damaged tissue. Negative symptoms of cortical damage are the decreased abilities for sufficient motor units to perform movement. Positive symptoms include exaggerated reflexes such as spasticity. Motor control is abnormal not only because of motor deficits but also because of deficits in sensory, cognitive, and perceptual processing.

Cerebellar Lesions

The cerebellum specifies the movement parameters and initiates preprogrammed movements including dysmetria, rebound phenomenon, and dysdiadochokinesia. A positive symptom is intention tremor.

Table 14-1   A review of the skeletal structure and function

PURPOSE

+ Protects vital organs such as the brain, heart and lungs

FUNCTION

+ Acts as the hemoregulatory system by producing red blood cells in the marrow of the long bones
+ Facilitates movement by muscles contracting the bones
+ Is a storage area for salts and minerals

GROSS DESCRIPTION: TOTAL OF 206 BONES

+ Axial skeleton: skull, spinal vertebrae, ribs, sternum and hyoid bones
+ Appendicular skeleton: other structures of the upper and lower extremities

MACROSCOPIC DESCRIPTION: POROUS SUBSTANCE CONTAINING LIVING CELLS AND BLOOD

+ Spongy bone (cancellous bone): contains large spaces (trabeculae) filled with red marrow, which is responsible for producing new blood cells (hematopoiesis)
+ Compact bone (dense bone) contains few spaces and consists of a series of concentric rings

MICROSCOPIC DESCRIPTION: BLOOD VESSELS AND NERVES FROM THE PERIOSTEUM (DENSE, WHITE BONE COVER) PENETRATE THE COMPACT BONE THROUGH VOLKMANN'S CANAL

+ Blood vessels from Volkmann's canals connect with blood vessels and nerves of the medullary, or marrow cavity, and those of the haversian canals
+ Haversian canals run lengthwise throughout bone and are surrounded by lamellae
+ Lamellae are rings of hard calcified material and osteocytes are found in spaces (lacunae) located between the lamellae
+ Each haversian canal with surrounding lamellae, lacunae, and osteocytes is called a haversian system or osteon
+ With osteons, bone tissue is constantly created and reabsorbed (ossification)

Table 14-2   A review of bone classification and types of diarthroses

BONE CLASSIFICATION

+ Long: consists of a shaft (diaphysis) and two ends (epiphyses) (e.g., femur, radius)
+ Short: consists of spongy tissue covered with a thin layer spongy bone (e.g., carpals, tarsals)
+ Flat: consists of spongy bone encased in compact bone (e.g., scapula)
+ Irregular (e.g., vertebra)
+ Sesamoid (e.g., patella)
+ Gross bone joints: junction between bones
+ Synarthroses: fixed joints (e.g., skull)
+ Amphiarthroses: slight movement (e.g., symphysis pubis)
+ Diarthroses: freely movable

TYPES OF DIARTHROSES (ARTICULAR CAVITY ENCLOSED BY A CAPSULE OF FIBROUS ARTICULAR CARTILAGE)

+ Pivot: round, pointed, or concave surfaces fitting into a shallow depression causing a rotation movement
+ Hinge: spool-like surface fitting into a concave surface permitting flexion and extension (e.g., elbow, knee, ankle, and interphalangeal joints)
+ Saddle: opposing concave and convex surfaces permitting flexion, extension, abduction, and adduction (e.g., carpometacarpal joint)
+ Condyloid: composed of oval-shaped condyle fitting into an elliptical cavity capable of flexion, extension, abduction, and adduction (e.g., radiocarpal joint)
+ Gliding: consists of flat articulating surfaces producing flexion, extension, abduction, and adduction (e.g., intercarpal and intertarsal joints)
+ Ball and socket: consists of a ball-like head fitting into a cuplike depression (e.g., shoulder and hip)

OSSIFICATION BONE FORMATION AND REABSORPTION

+ Kept in balance via the regulation of local stress, vitamin D, parathyroid hormone, and calcitonin
+ Local stress (weight-bearing) stimulates local bone reabsorption and formation
+ Loss of weight-bearing or local stress results in loss of calcium from the bone
+ Vitamin D increases the amount of calcium by mobilizing calcium from the bone
+ Parathyroid hormone regulates the concentration of serum calcium by producing movement of calcium from the bone
+ Calcitonin increases the production of bone

Lesions of the Basal Ganglia

The major diagnosis seen is Parkinson's disease, where there is a delay and slowness in initiating and carrying out movement. Positive symptoms include rigidity and tremors at rest caused by other structures released from the inhibitory control of the basal ganglia.

NORMAL ANATOMY AND PHYSIOLOGY OF MOVEMENT

Movement consists of the action of muscles on bones and joints. It may involve an involuntary, reflex process or a process of conscious, deliberate choice. The review of anatomy and physiology in this chapter focuses on bones, muscles, joints, and nerve pathways for producing voluntary and involuntary motions. Readers should have a sound background in anatomy and physiology; therefore this review is presented in table format. Table 14-1 presents a review of skeletal function. Table 14-2 presents a review of bone classification and types of diarthoses. Table 14-3 presents major joints and movements commonly employed in rehabilitation nursing.

Muscle Structure and Function

Muscle tissue constitutes 40% to 50% of total body weight. Muscle tissue is characterized by irritability, contractility, extensibility, and elasticity. In other words, muscle tissue is capable of responding to stimuli, shortening and thickening, and stretching and returning to its original shape after being stimulated. Muscles produce motion, maintain posture, and produce heat through contraction. The three types of muscle tissue are skeletal, visceral, and cardiac. The focus of this chapter is skeletal, or striated, muscle.

Skeletal muscles are attached to bones, connective tissue, other muscles, soft tissue, or skin by tendons or aponeuroses. Tendons are cords of fibrous connective tissue; aponeuroses are broad, flat sheets of connective tissue.

The muscles are composed of parallel groups of muscle cells referred to as fasciculi and are encased in fascia, which is a fibrous tissue. Muscles may consist of both red and white muscle fibers. Red muscle fibers contain a large amount of myoglobin, a hemoglobinlike protein pigment that transports oxygen from the blood capillaries to the muscle cells for metabolism. White muscle fiber contains little myoglobin and is characterized by quick extended periods of contraction.

A sarcomere is the contractile unit of a muscle. When a nerve impulse reaches the motor end-plate located in a sarcomere, the neuron releases acetylcholine, causing an electrical charge in the sarcolemma of the muscle fiber. This charge travels over the sarcolemma and is eventually conveyed to the sarcoplasmic reticulum. When the impulse reaches the sarcoplasmic reticulum, calcium ions are released from storage into the surrounding sarcoplasm. The calcium ions move to myosin cross bridges and activate the myosin. Myosin catalyzes the breakdown of adenosine triphosphate (ATP) into adenosine diphosphate and phosphate (ADP and P). The calcium ions also permit the tropomyosin-troponin complex to split from the thin myofilament so that the free receptor site of action is permitted to attach to the myosin cross bridge. The energy released from the breakdown of ATP is used for the attachment and movement of the myosin cross bridges and thus the sliding of myofilaments. As the thin myofilaments slide past the thick myofilaments, they are drawn toward each other, causing the sarcomere to shorten and the muscle to contract. When the calcium concentration in the sarcomere falls at the end of the nerve impulse, the myosin and actin filaments no longer interact, and the sarcomere returns to its original resting state.

ATP is synthesized by skeletal muscle from oxidation of glucose to water and carbon dioxide during low levels of activity. During high levels of activity, sufficient oxygen may not be available, and the glucose is metabolized primarily to lactic acid, as well as some ATP. Therefore, dur-

Table 14-3 Classification of joints and movements

Name	Type	Movements
Atlantoaxial	Pivot	Pivoting or partial rotation of head
Shoulder	Ball and socket	Flexion, extension, abduction, adduction, rotation, circumduction
Elbow	Hinge	Flexion, extension
Radioulnar	Pivot	Supination, pronation
Wrist	Condyloid	Flexion, extension, abduction (ulnar deviation), adduction (radial deviation)
Carpal	Gliding	Gliding
Hand		
Metacarpals	Hinge	Flexion, extension, abduction, adduction
Thumb	Saddle	Flexion, extension, abduction, adduction, rotation, circumduction, opposition
Hip	Ball and socket	Flexion, extension, abduction, adduction, rotation, circumduction
Knee	Hinge	Flexion, extension
Ankle	Hinge	Dorsiflexion, plantar flexion
Foot		
Between tarsals	Gliding	Inversion, eversion
Between metatarsals, phalanges	Hinge	Flexion, extension, adduction, abduction

ing high levels of activity, increasingly large amounts of glucose are required and must be supplied by glycogen stored in the muscle. Muscle fatigue may occur from the rapid rate of work of the muscle, resulting in depletion of glycogen and energy and in the accumulation of lactic acid. Creatinine phosphate stored in the muscle cell also may be converted to ATP when necessary.

At any one time some cells in a muscle are contracted while others are relaxed, resulting in muscle tone. Tone is a requirement for maintaining normal posture. If there is less than normal muscle tone, the muscles are characterized as flaccid or flabby and floppy. If the flaccid tone continues over a long period, muscle atrophy may occur with consequent loss of muscle mass. Such conditions may result from neurologic or muscular disorders or from prolonged inactivity, including bed rest. Spasticity occurs when the muscle tone is greater than normal and causes dysfunctional posture and positioning. Again, neurologic disorders or muscle diseases may be responsible. Contracture formation is a serious consequence of spasticity.

Muscle fibers can produce either isotonic or isometric movement of the muscle. In isotonic contraction the muscle shortens, with no increase in tension within the muscle. In isometric contraction the length of the muscle remains constant, but the tension or force generated by the muscles is increased. Isometric contractions do not result in body movement, whereas isotonic contractions do produce movement.

In every movement there is a prime mover, or agonist, causing a particular movement. Muscles assisting the prime mover are known as synergists. Muscles opposing a prime mover are known as antagonists. The antagonist relaxes while the prime mover contracts.

In flexion of the forearm the biceps is the prime mover, or agonist, and contracts. The antagonist in this case, the triceps, relaxes while the synergists, the deltoid and the greater pectoral, hold the arm and shoulder in a position suitable for flexing the forearm by also contracting. Synergists assume a special importance in the paralyzed individual who may be able to retrain synergists to perform the function of a weakened primary mover.

Skeletal muscles derive their names in several ways. These muscles may be named according to the action produced (flexor), location (femoral), or point of insertion or attachment (sternocleidomastoid). The name of the muscle also may indicate the shape of the muscle body (trapezius), the number of muscle divisions (biceps and triceps), and the direction of the muscle fibers (rectus or transversus).

Nervous System Structure and Function

Voluntary motor activity involves the cerebral cortex, the descending pathways of the spinal cord, and the anterior horn of the spinal cord. Voluntary motor impulses originate in the motor strip just before the central sulcus of the brain. The impulses travel through the hemispheres to merge in the internal capsule and then continue downward through the brainstem. When the pyramidal or upper motor neuron fibers (alpha motor neurons) reach the medulla oblongata, the majority decussate, or cross to the opposite side, to descend through the spinal cord in the lateral white column known as the lateral corticospinal tract. In this way the mo-

tor cortex of the right side of the brain controls muscles on the left side of the body and vice versa. On reaching the spinal cord, the impulses synapse with association neurons, which then synapse with alpha motor neurons in the anterior gray horn. The lower motor neurons exit at all levels of the cord to terminate in skeletal muscle (Fig. 14-1).

About 15% of the upper motor neurons do not cross at the medulla but descend on the same side to the anterior white column, becoming part of the direct, or uncrossed, corticospinal tract. These corticospinal fibers of upper motor neurons cross at the spinal cord level to the opposite side of the origin of their pathway before synapsing with lower motor neurons. The anterior corticospinal tract provides skeletal muscle impulses primarily for muscles that control the neck and part of the trunk.

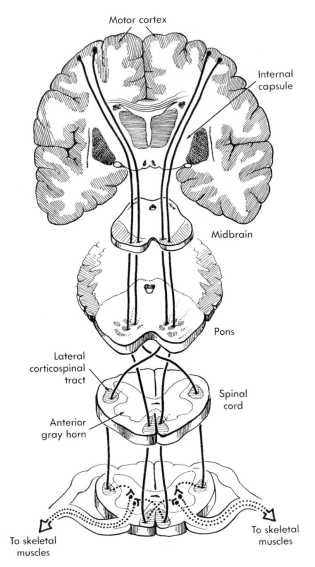

Fig. 14-1 Voluntary motor impulses from the cortex to skeletal muscles. Impulses arising in the cortex descend directly through the anterior corticospinal tract or cross at level of the medulla and descend through the lateral corticospinal tract to anterior horn cells.

Motor Dysfunction Due to Central Nervous System Deficit

The upper motor neuron therefore is the only path between the cerebral cortex and cranial nerve nuclei and the spinal cord. The lower motor neuron is the neuron that actually terminates in a skeletal muscle. Since it is the final common pathway, loss of function of the lower motor neuron through disease or trauma results in flaccid paralysis or loss of both reflex and voluntary movement. If injury or disease occurs in the upper motor neuron pathway, the result is continued muscle contraction evidenced by spastic tone and exaggerated reflexes.

Clients who experience a CVA may become hemiplegic as a result of upper motor neuron damage. Hemiplegia is loss of function of the arm and leg on one side of the body. Those who have experienced poliomyelitis develop a lower motor neuron flaccid paralysis because the anterior spinal cord is affected. Both upper and lower motor paralyses may occur in spinal cord injury in which both the descending pathways and anterior horn cells are disrupted. When both legs are paralyzed, the resulting condition is referred to as paraplegia; when both arms and both legs are paralyzed, the resulting condition is referred to as quadriplegia.

The extrapyramidal system provides input from the cerebellum and basal ganglia to the muscles, resulting in smooth, accurate, and coordinated muscular activity. Impulses that arise in the cerebellum and basal ganglia are transmitted downward through the white matter of the spinal cord. The principal extrapyramidal tracts include the rubrospinal, tectospinal, and vestibulospinal tracts. Dysfunction in the cerebellum or in the extrapyramidal tracts may result in loss of coordinated, controlled voluntary movements. Activities may become disjointed and choppy. Coarse tremor may appear; gait may be ataxic, staggering, and with a wide-based step.

Dysfunction in the basal ganglia or extrapyramidal pathways associated with the basal ganglia results in disturbances of posture and movement and marked muscular rigidity. Coarse tremor may occur; other involuntary movements, such as athetosis or chorea also may develop. Athetosis is characterized by slow, writhing, twisting motions, and chorea is manifested by spasmodic, grotesque motions of the trunk and extremities with facial grimacing. Table 14-4 delineates clinical signs of disrupted motor functioning at three levels of the nervous system.

RECOVERY OF MOVEMENT

Recovery of movement is defined as an attainment of a goal the organism was capable of accomplishing before neural injury. Recovery can occur due to the following reasons: (1) takeover of function by spared tissue, (2) morphologic reorganization, and (3) adaptive and learned changes in strategies for information processing.

Recovery from cortical lesions due to physical mechanisms usually follows a developmental sequence from reflex to voluntary control, from mass to discrete movement, and from proximal to distal control. Recovery can stop at any level along the continuum and is not wholly predictable. The speed of spontaneous recovery provides a clue to the ultimate level of functions. Any cells in the brain that have been destroyed will not regenerate, and the functions for which they were responsible will be diminished.

Diseases of the cerebellum or basal ganglia are degenerative and recovery due to neural changes is not expected.

Table 14-4 Clinical signs of disrupted motor function at three levels of the nervous system

Level	Clinical signs	Examples of causative disorders
Suprasegmental	Weakness or paralysis of voluntary movement Increased muscle stretch reflexes; reflex arc intact (after "spinal shock") Some muscle atrophy secondary to disuse EMG normal	Spinal cord lesions such as trauma, infarct, tumor, and hemorrhage
Segmental	Weakness or paralysis of voluntary movement Decreased or absent muscle stretch reflexes (reflex arc disrupted) Marked muscle atrophy secondary to denervation ($\downarrow$ trophic factors) EMG changes: fibrillation, giant polyphasic action potentials (denervation supersensitivity)	Brainstem lesions affecting cranial nuclei: tumors, infarct, hemorrhage Cerebellopontine angle tumors compressing cranial nerves Polyneuropathies such as Guillain-Barré syndrome, alcoholic polyneuropathy, diphtheritic polyneuropathy, and toxic chemical polyneuropathy
Myoneural junction	Weakness or paralysis of voluntary movement Muscle stretch reflexes intact No muscle atrophy EMG diminished: muscle able to contract when directly stimulated; pattern of $\downarrow$ contraction varies with disorder	Chronic: myasthenia gravis (may have acute episodes of life-threatening myasthenic or cholinergic crisis); Eaton-Lambert syndrome (myasthenic symptoms associated with carcinoma); acute: botulism, curare, succinylcholine, "nerve gas," organophosphate insecticides

From *Neurological Disorders* by Chipps, 1992, St. Louis: Mosby–Year Book. Copyright 1992 by Mosby–Year Book.

Improvements are usually due to functional compensation through rehabilitation. The central nervous system seems to have tremendous recuperative potential. Since neural connections differ for clients with brain lesions, potential associated with neural plasticity in the rehabilitation of persons with central nervous system lesions is a frontier for discovery.

ACQUISITION OF MOVEMENT

Normal movement is thought to have its origin in genetically wired configurations of neurons. Most motor systems are modifiable, providing the base for the development of acquired skills. As the fetus and infant mature, the genetically based movement patterns become more elaborate as the nervous system develops.

The spinal reflexes are the lowest level of control, and they lose dominance as the brainstem reflexes emerge. The latter reflexes are supplemented by the higher level righting and equilibrium responses. Reflex maturation proceeds caudocephally; thus spinal reflexes develop before the brainstem, and the brainstem develops before the midbrain and so forth. Both reflex and voluntary control proceed cephalocaudally and proximally to distally. To illustrate this, the upper extremity exhibits a withdrawal reflex before the lower extremity, voluntary head movement is learned before voluntary trunk movement, and shoulder control is learned before hand control.

Movement and posture are intertwined developmentally. Early mobility patterns such as kicking, waving, banging, and rocking are largely without purpose—although they are temporally organized but are not random movements. Mobility is developed into a synchronous coactivation of flexor and extensor muscles, which provides the stability of posture. Visually directed reaching and hand function develop from a visual regard of the hand to release of a grasp and finally to individual finger control. These maturationally developed sequences provide the basis for learning motor skills or purposeful goal-directed activity.

There is greater variability from person to person in learned motor skills than in maturationally acquired motor patterns. As a person practices a skill, the variability of his own performance decreases. Learned motor skills are characterized by automatic movement, a large part of which does not need conscious attention for correct execution. Automaticity is due not only to physical capability but also to efficient cognitive control processes. The rehabilitation nurse keeps the variability of each person in mind.

NEUROPHYSIOLOGIC AND DEVELOPMENTAL TREATMENT APPROACHES

There are five recognized programs of treatment for clients with motor control problems due to brain damage. These programs are as follows: (1) Root Approach, (2) Bobath Neurodevelopmental Approach, (3) Brunnstrom Approach, (4) proprioceptive neuromuscular facilitation (PNF), and (5) Carr and Shepherd Approach of Motor Relearning. Table 14-5 outlines the major focus and emphasis of each approach, and the Bobath Neurodevelopmental Approach is discussed in more detail in the following section.

Bobath Neurodevelopmental Approach

Whatever neurophysiologic and developmental treatment approach is used, it is vital that the entire rehabilitation team use the basic premises related to a specific approach. Since many nurses are using the Bobath Neurodevelopmental Approach in the care of stroke patients, the following review of these premises is in order:

1. Sensation of movements are learned and not the movement per se.
2. Basic postural hand movement patterns are learned that are later elaborated on in order to become function skills.
3. Every skilled activity takes place against a background of basic pattern of postural control, righting, equilibrium and other protective reactions.
4. When the brain is damaged, abnormal patterns of posture and movement develop that are incompatible with the performance of normal everyday activities.
5. The abnormal patterns develop because sensation is shunted into these abnormal patterns.
6. The abnormal patterns must be stopped not so much

Table 14-5 Focus and emphasis of contemporary neurophysiologic and developmental treatment approaches

Areas of focus/emphasis	Neurophysiologic and developmental treatment approaches				
	Root	Bobath	Brunnstrom	PNF	Carr
Focus: patient attention in movement			X	X	X
Focus: importance of eliciting goal desired movement	X	X			
Uses primitive reflexes to elicit movement			X		
Activity inhibits primitive reflexes	X				
Redevelops movement and posture in developmental sequence	X	X	X	X	
Emphasizes development of basic movement and facilitates underlying skills	X	X	X	X	X

by modifying the sensory input but by giving back to the client the lost or underdeveloped control over her motor output in developmental sequence.

7. The basic patterns of posture and movement, the righting and equilibrium responses, are elicited providing the appropriate stimuli while abnormal patterns are inhibited.

8. In this way the client experiences normal motor patterns.

9. The sensory information from these correct motor patterns is absolutely necessary for the development of improved motor control.

NURSING ASSESSMENT OF MOVEMENT

The nurse's physical assessment includes general impression, range of joint motion, muscle tone and strength, deep tendon reflexes, proprioception and position sense, balance and coordination, and gait assessment. In the assessment outlined in the Box on pp. 233-236, a nursing assessment builds on basic physical assessment and presents assessment criteria specific to movement assessment.

♦

NURSING ASSESSMENT OF MOVEMENT

I. General impression
   A. During interview assess client's external appearance
   B. Observe client for posture, especially for stooped shoulders; asymmetry; unevenness of length of extremities; absent digits and abnormalities of hands, feet, arms or legs; extremity edema; asymmetry of facial expression and involuntary movement; extremity weakness during activities of daily living such as walking, sitting, rising, writing or dressing; movements that precipitate pain

II. General range of motion (ROM): see description of ROM in Appendix 14-A
   A. Note
      1. Any deviation of limitation
      2. Joint instability (dislocation or subluxation)
      3. Joint stiffness or fixation (ankylosis)
      4. Joint swelling, heat, or tenderness
      5. Bogginess and bone enlargement
      6. Muscle tone and strength, skin condition, subcutaneous tissue, muscle size and shape
      7. Palpate for crepitus or a grating sensation

III. Specific ROM (head to toe assessment)
   A. Head and neck
      1. Palpate jaw or temporomandibular joint for tenderness or swelling; check ROM as client opens mouth
      2. Inspect neck for symmetry and form and size
      3. Palpate cervical spine muscle and trapezius for tenderness
      4. Assess neck ROM: the following degree guide is for formal ROM; make adjustments for clients with arthritis or fracture and elderly persons
         a. Flexion (45 degrees): ask client to touch chin to chest
         b. Extension (55 degrees): ask client to put head back
         c. Lateral flexion (40 degrees): ask client to touch ear to corresponding shoulder
         d. Rotation (70 degrees): ask client to turn head to left, then to right
   B. Trunk (client stands, if possible)
      1. Inspect posterior for exaggerated C- or S-shaped lateral curvature (scoliosis), exaggerated curvature of thoracic spine (kyphosis), and exaggerated curvature of lumbar spine (lordosis); Fig. 14-2 illustrates asymmetry found with scoliosis
      2. Observe differences in height of shoulders or iliac crest
      3. Palpate paravertebral muscles for tenderness
      4. Assess spine ROM
         a. Forward flexion (75-90 degrees): ask client to touch toes while bending from the waist and note rounding of lumbar concavity
         b. Extension (30 degrees): ask client to lean back from pelvis
         c. Lateral flexion (35 degrees): ask client to lean to each side
         d. Rotation (30 degrees): ask client to turn shoulders to the right and then to the left
      5. Inspect anterior and posterior aspects of trunk
         a. Compare right side to left
         b. Compare proximal to distal for symmetry and weakness
   C. Shoulder girdle and arms
      1. Observe for swelling; atrophy; altered shape, size, or form
      2. Palpate sternoclavicular joint, the acromioclavicular joint, and the shoulder joint for tenderness
      3. Assess ROM
         a. Extension (50 degrees): ask client to swing both arms back as if reaching back for something
         b. Forward flexion (180 degrees): ask client to raise arms above head
         c. Internal and external rotation (90 degrees)
            · Internal: ask client to place hands behind in the small of the back
            · External: ask client to place hands behind the neck with elbows out to the side
         d. Adduction (50 degrees): ask client to reach the right hand to the left hand while crossing extended arms in front of the body; reverse the process for the shoulder
         e. Abduction (180 degrees): ask the client to bring the arms away from the body as far as possible
      4. Inspect elbow while flexed at 70 degrees; palpate the olecranon process and grooves with the

Continued

◆

NURSING ASSESSMENT OF MOVEMENT—cont'd

lateral epicondyle for tenderness, swelling, or nodules

5. Assess elbow ROM (0 degrees extension to 160 degrees flexion): ask client to bend and straighten the arms at the elbow; Fig. 14-3 illustrates use of a goniometer to measure the angle at the elbow joint

6. Inspect the radioulnar joint

7. Assess supination (palms up) and pronation (palms down and ROM 90 degrees)

D. Hands and wrists

1. Inspect for swelling, redness, nodules, deformity, atrophy or fasciculations (involuntary twitchings of isolated bundles of muscle fibers)

2. Palpate joints for tenderness, swelling, bogginess, or enlargement

3. Assess ROM of hands and digits: ask client to spread the fingers of each hand and make a fist with the thumb across the knuckles
   a. Extension (70 degrees)
   b. Flexion (0 degrees)
   c. Radial deviation (20 degrees)
   d. Ulnar deviation (55 degrees)
   e. Metacarpophalangeal joint: hyperextension (30 degrees), flexion (90 degrees)
   f. Proximal interphalangeal joint: extension (0 degrees/neutral), flexion (120 degrees)

E. Hips: Ask client to stand, if possible

1. Observe form and asymmetry of iliac crest

2. Palpate for crepitus, nodules, or atrophy

3. Assess ROM of hip: client is supine flexion (90 degrees) with knees straight—ask client to raise each leg separately with knee straight, then with knee bent
   a. Flexion (120 degrees) with knee flexed
   b. Hyperextension (15 degrees): have client prone and ask client to lift each leg separately off surface
   c. Adduction (30 degrees): ask client to cross the right leg over the left leg and vice versa
   d. Abduction (45 degrees): ask client to slide the leg toward the outer edge of bed
   e. Internal rotation (40 degrees): ask client to bend the knee and hip and gently pull the knee laterally and the hip will rotate externally

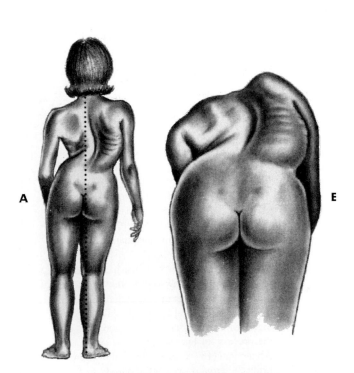

Fig. 14-2 Abnormal spinal curvatures associated with scoliosis. (From *Mosby's Clinical Nursing,* 3rd ed. by Thompson, 1993, St. Louis: Mosby–Year Book. Copyright 1993 by Mosby–Year Book. Reprinted by permission.)

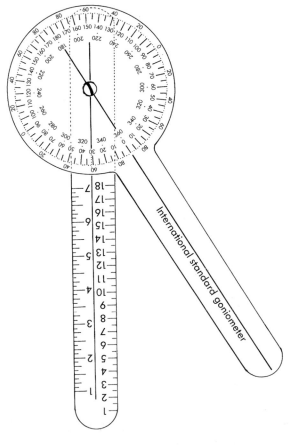

Fig. 14-3 A goniometer is used to assess the angle of flexion of a joint.

NURSING ASSESSMENT OF MOVEMENT—cont'd

    f. External rotation (45 degrees): ask client to bend the knee and hip and gently push the knee medially and the hip will rotate internally

F. Knees
1. Observe for changes in form, shape, or size; atrophy of quadriceps or loss of usual hollows around the patella
2. Palpate the suprapatellar pouch and over the tibiofemoral joint for thickening, bogginess, tenderness, or fluid
3. Palpate the popliteal space
4. Test for bulge sign using fluid and ballottement of a floating patella; refer to Fig. 14-4 for illustration of the ballottement technique
    a. Bulge sign test
      • Use the ball of the hand to milk the medial aspect of the knee firmly upward two or three times and displace any fluid
      • Tap the knee just behind the lateral margin of the patella and watch for a bulge of returning fluid in the hollow medial area of the patella
      • Grasp the thigh above the patella with one hand, forcing fluid out of the suprapatellar space; with fingers of the other hand, push the patella sharply against the femur
5. Assess ROM
    a. Hyperextension (15 degrees): ask client to straighten knee
    b. Flexion (130 degrees): ask client to flex the hip and lift the lower leg off the bed

G. Legs and calf
1. Measure thigh and calf for baseline recording
2. Observe for any changes in size; Record in centimeters as measured at the same location on the leg

3. Test circulation in feet and ankles; assess popliteal and femoral pulses; if compression stockings are used, assess proper application and fit
4. Note whether client is receiving anticoagulant drugs

H. Ankle and feet
1. Observe for altered shape, size, or form; for swelling, nodules, corns, calluses, or bunions
2. Palpate Achilles tendon, anterior ankle surface, and the metatarsophalangeal joint
3. Assess ROM
    a. Dorsiflexion (20 degrees): ask client to point toes up
    b. Plantar flexion (45 degrees): ask client to point toes down
    c. Inversion (30 degrees): client turns sole inward while nurse stabilizes the ankle
    d. Eversion (20 degrees): client turns sole outward while nurse stabilizes the ankle
    e. Metatarsophalangeal joints: ask client to ball up toes and release them

I. Muscle tone and strength
1. Observe tone, flaccidity, spasticity (increased tone), rigidity (inability to relax either flexor or extensor muscles)
2. Note equal or unequal strength on both sides of the body and in proximal and distal positions
3. Assess relative strength by applying resistance to client's movement attempts during ROM
4. Assess the upper extremities by asking client to grasp and squeeze the nurse's hands; note differences or sameness on the right and left side; scales for grading muscle strength often are characterized as described in Table 14-6 on p. 237.

J. Deep tendon reflexes
1. Position client comfortably so that the muscle to be tested is mildly stretched

Continued.

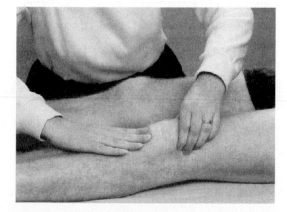

Fig. 14-4 Procedure for ballottement examination of the knee. (From *Orthopedic Disorders* by Mourad 1991, St. Louis: Mosby–Year Book. Copyright 1991 by Mosby–Year Book. Reprinted by permission.)

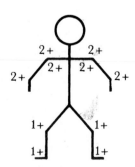

Fig. 14-5 Recording of deep tendon reflex response. (From *Neurological Disorders* by Chipps, 1992, St. Louis: Mosby–Year Book. Copyright 1992 by Mosby–Year Book. Reprinted by permission.)

---

2. Use a reflex hammer to strike the tendon briskly—which, in turn, produces a sudden tendon stretch
3. Major reflexes include the following
   a. Biceps: reflects cervical functions between C5-C6
   b. Triceps: reflects cervical segments C6-C8
   c. Brachioradial: reflects cervical cord functions C5-C6
   d. Patellar: reflects L2-L4 functioning
   e. Achilles: reflects S1-S2 functioning
4. Grade reflex from 0-4+; compare right and left side and upper and lower extremities; hyperactive reflexes are associated with spastic muscle tone and hypoactive reflexes are associated with flaccid muscle tone; Fig. 14-5 illustrates deep tendon reflex sites and Table 14-7 provides a scale of responses for scoring 0-4 results of deep tendon reflex testing

K. Proprioceptive and position sense
1. Upper extremity: hold client's thumb between the nurse's thumb and index finger; move thumb up and down and ask client to correctly identify the position of the thumb with eyes closed; if unable to identify the thumb position, other joints of the upper extremity such as the wrist, elbow, and shoulder may be tested
2. Lower extremity: repeat procedure as with toe; if impairment is noted, proceed to the ankle, knee, and hip

L. Balance coordination: use appropriate safety precautions
1. Observe independent and assisted movements in and out of bed, transfer, and during ambulation
2. Observe sitting balance while in bed or wheelchair: note whether client slumps or sways to either side
3. Observe standing balance: note swaying, reeling, or taking backward steps

4. Perform Romberg test: ask client to stand with feet together, arms stretched in front, and eyes closed; with cerebellar disease, a person falls to the affected side
5. Perform finger to nose test and heel to shin test
6. Perform various types of rapidly alternating movements, such as touching the thumb rapidly to each finger or pronating and supinating hands rapidly

M. Gait
1. Observe balance, arm sways, inability to negotiate turns, and actual gait patterns; typical gait patterns associated with conditions are
   a. Hemiplegia: a stiff gait; knee flexion is diminished on the affected side; hip circumscribes floor with toes scraping the floor; the affected arm does not swing forward as the opposite foot is advanced
   b. Parkinson's disease: a festinating gait; rhythmic arm swinging is diminished; there is hesitation on initiation of ambulation and steps are small, shifting, and shuffling; client may have difficulty initiating gait manifested as marching in place, or with halting once in motion
   c. Cerebellar problems or posterior column problems; ataxic gaits with broad-base stance and staggering, unsteady gait; difficulty with turns
   d. Multiple sclerosis: a scissors gait; bilateral spastic paralysis of the legs, typified by slow steps
   e. Alpha motor neuron (lower motor problem): a steppage gait making clients appear to be walking up stairs
   f. Progressive neuromuscular disease: a waddling gait may appear

---

MOVEMENT DYSFUNCTION IN SELECTED CLINICAL PROBLEMS

Each clinical problem carries its own set of signs and symptoms, treatment goals, and movement therapy modalities. Major clinical problems having unique movement dysfunction include clients with rheumatoid arthritis (RA), amputations, strokes, multiple sclerosis (MS), Parkinson's disease, traumatic head injury, or spinal cord injury. The following discussion considers how movement therapy is involved in each of the clinical entities.

Rheumatoid Arthritis

RA is a major subclassification within the category of diffuse tissue diseases including juvenile arthritis, systemic lupus erythematosus, progressive systemic sclerosis or scleroderma, polymyositis, and dermatomyositis. Signs and symptoms of RA include morning stiffness, pain on motion

or tenderness in at least one joint, swelling of a joint(s), and subcutaneous nodules over bony prominences. Figure 14-6, **A** and **B**, illustrates alterations occurring in the hand with RA (Fig. 14-6, **A**) compared with changes due to osteoarthritis (Fig. 14-6, **B**). The person may have roentgenographic changes, a positive test for rheumatoid factor in the serum, and synovial histopathology.

RA is classified as:

Class I. The person has complete functional capacity with the ability to carry on all usual duties.

Class II. The person has functional capacity adequate to conduct normal activities despite the impairment from discomfort or limited mobility in one or more joints.

Class III. The person has functional capacity to perform only a few or none of the duties of a job or self-care.

Class IV. The person is generally dependent or incapacitated in bed or ambulating via wheelchair.

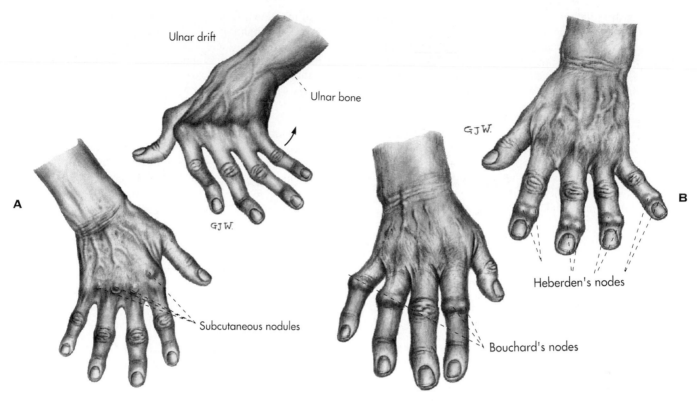

Fig. 14-6   **A,** Joint involvement with rheumatoid arthritis. **B,** Osteoarthritis. Herberden's nodes and Bouchard's nodes. (From *Orthopedic Disorders* by Mourad, 1991, St. Louis: Mosby–Year Book. Copyright 1991 by Mosby–Year Book. Reprinted by permission.)

Table 14-6   Muscle function and strength scales

Grade	Scale	% Function	Muscle level assessment
5	Normal	100 or full	Full ROM against gravity with full resistance
4	Good	75	Full ROM against gravity with some resistance
3	Fair	50	Full ROM with gravity
2	Poor	25	Passive movement, full ROM
1	Trace	10	Slight contractility, no movement
0	Zero	0 or none	No contractility

Adapted from *Neurologic Disorders. Mosby's Clinical Nursing Series.* Chipps, Clanin, & Campbell, 1992. St. Louis: Mosby–Year Book. p. 32. Copyright 1992 by Mosby–Year Book.

Table 14-7   Scale of responses used to score deep tendon reflexes

Grade	Deep tendon reflex response
0	No response
1+	Sluggish or diminished
2+	Active or expected response
3+	More brisk than expected, slightly hyperactive
4+	Brisk, hyperactive, with intermittent or transient clonus

From *Mosby's Guide to Physical Examination, ed 2,* by H.M. Seidel, 1991, St. Louis: Mosby–Year Book. Copyright 1991 by Mosby–Year Book.

♦ Nursing goals. Overall nursing rehabilitation goals are specific according to stage of inflammation. With acute-stage inflammation, the primary goal is to reduce the pain and inflammation by resting the affected joints and applying pain relief modalities. Other goals are to maintain range of motion (ROM), strength, and endurance and to maintain independence in activities of daily living (ADL). In the subacute stage of inflammation, efforts are directed toward increasing ROM, strength, and endurance and regaining independence in ADL. Once the chronic stage is reached, rehabilitative goals include independent resumptions of previous levels of ADL including work.

Amputation

Levels of amputation are referred to by site as upper extremity or lower extremity, the latter usually above the knee or below the knee; however, amputations may be performed at any level in the upper or lower extremities. The postoperative program is usually divided into two phases: the preprosthetic phase and the prosthetic phase. Careful individualized assessment is an important preprosthetic activity. A child can expect to have multiple evaluations and changes in prostheses as growth and development dictate. Data regarding the condition of the residual limb strength of the affected extremity, joint ROM, condition of the nonaffected limb, and the client's psychological status are important considerations.

Many persons report an experience with a phantom limb sensation or with body image disturbance. Others may reject the idea of a prosthesis; some of these persons eventually change their minds and become successful with prosthetic use. Prostheses are made to mirror the shape of the other leg or arm, tinted to match natural skin shade, have numerous options for shoes, and may be virtually undetectable under clothing.

In the immediate postoperative period, many clients are fitted with a rigid dressing or temporary prosthesis. When an elastic wrap or shrinker is used, proper wrapping of the residual limb is essential. Figure 14-7 demonstrates wrapping procedure essential for maintaining circulation, skin integrity, and shaping of the residual limb. Another early goal of movement therapy is to prevent contractures of the adjacent joints by proper positioning. The residual limb is not allowed to roll inward or outward or rest in improper alignment; with below-the-knee amputation, the residual knee joint is not bent nor is the leg allowed to dangle independently.

An individualized exercise program includes strengthening and coordinating activities. Early amputation programs usually include crutch walking techniques for the person with lower extremity amputation and wheelchair activities for those with bilateral lower extremity amputations. Individuals who are not fitted with a prosthesis need to become independent in crutch walking or wheelchair mobility. A client may be taught how to manage a fall and regain standing position as safely as possible. Those who will be active in the community benefit from practice in their environment encountering daily obstacles or barriers. Summer camps and programs in schools have proven to be successful means for teaching and socializing children who have prostheses.

Persons with upper extremity amputations are trained in ways to manage activities for self-care and daily living, use of assistive devices, techniques for work or hobbies, and operation of adaptive equipment or electronic units. Each client is individually assessed and evaluated according to lifestyle, potential of the residual limb and musculature, and preferences before an upper body prosthesis is decided. A number of motor control and upper body control prostheses are available to suit individual needs and abilities.

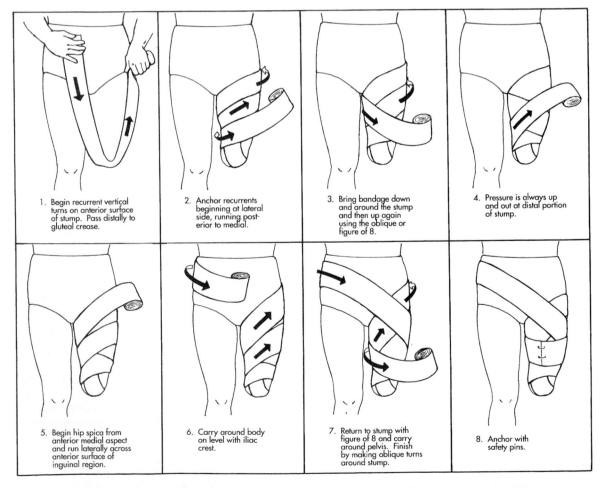

1. Begin recurrent vertical turns on anterior surface of stump. Pass distally to gluteal crease.

2. Anchor recurrents beginning at lateral side, running posterior to medial.

3. Bring bandage down and around the stump and then up again using the oblique or figure of 8.

4. Pressure is always up and out at distal portion of stump.

5. Begin hip spica from anterior medial aspect and run laterally across anterior surface of inguinal region.

6. Carry around body on level with iliac crest.

7. Return to stump with figure of 8 and carry around pelvis. Finish by making oblique turns around stump.

8. Anchor with safety pins.

Fig. 14-7 Method of wrapping to help shape the stump after above-the-knee amputation. (From *Orthopedic Disorders* by Mourad, 1991, St. Louis: Mosby–Year Book. Copyright 1991 by Mosby–Year Book. Reprinted by permission.)

Cerebrovascular Accident

A CVA, or stroke, results from a restricted blood supply to the brain causing cell damage and impaired neurologic function. Motor deficits are characterized by plegia or paresis on the side of the body opposite the site of the brain lesion. The most common causes of stroke are a thrombus, an embolus, a hemorrhage secondary to an aneurysm, or congenital problem. Common anatomic areas of vascular occlusion are the anterior cerebral artery, the middle cerebral artery, the posterior cerebral artery, the internal carotid artery and the vertebral-basilar artery.

Bobath (1978) describes three stages of recovery following stroke: an initial flaccid stage with no voluntary movement, replaced by the stage of spasticity and mass patterns of movement called synergies, and the stage of relative recovery wherein spasticity declines and advanced movement patterns are possible. Recovery stages are sequential, and many clients reach plateaus at any stage.

The person who has had a stroke may exhibit the following:

✦ Upper extremity flexion problems
Scapular retraction, elevation or hyperextension
Shoulder abduction and external rotation
Elbow flexion
Forearm supination
Wrist and finger flexion

✦ Lower extremity flexion problems
Hip flexion, abduction, and external rotation
Knee flexion
Ankle dorsiflexion
Toe dorsiflexion

✦ Other movement problems
Altered postural reflexes
Ataxia and altered gait
ADL impairments
Speech or language impairments
Altered perceptual abilities
Altered behavior

✦ Increased risk for
Contractures and deformities
Deep venous thrombosis (DVT)
Pain
Altered urinary and bowel function
Shoulder dysfunction

Many of these conditions are preventable. The gait of the person becomes altered in response to impairments of sensation, perception, mobility, and motor control. Movement therapy begins as soon as the client is medically stable, usually within 25 to 36 hours.

✦ **Goals following stroke**

General movement therapy goals include the following:
1. Minimizing tonal abnormalities
2. Maintaining ROM
3. Improving respiration and circulatory function
4. Mobilizing the person in early functional activities involving bed mobility, sitting, standing, and transfers
5. Preventing disuse problems
6. Promoting awareness of the hemiplegic side
7. Improving trunk control, sitting and standing balance
8. Maximizing self-care activities

In motor relearning following stroke, visual guidance and demonstration are useful in gaining a client's active participation to use the affected side. Encourage the person to "feel the movement" and learn to distinguish a purposeful movement from an unintended or counterproductive one. Movement therapy includes oromotor activities, tone reduction, motor control learning, trunk and postural control, upper and lower extremity control, balance, and ambulation training. Biofeedback (electromyographic feedback) and isokinetic devices, such as the Kinetron, may improve motor function for a client in mid-to-late recovery stages. Early and progressive stroke rehabilitation has demonstrated that a client can return home, re-enter the community, and have a good quality of life.

Multiple Sclerosis

Multiple sclerosis (MS) is characterized by demyelinating lesions known as plaques that are dispersed throughout the central nervous system white matter. Demyelinization occurs and impairs neural transmission. Ultimately the myelin sheath is replaced by fibrous scarring (gliosis). Since these plaques may occur anywhere, the symptoms vary among individuals, creating an unpredictable disease with sporadic occurrences of symptoms over many years.

Four phases have been described for MS. During the benign phase the individual usually experiences little or no disability. In the exacerbating-remitting phase a seemingly sudden onset of symptoms may be followed by partial to complete remission. However, during the remitting-progressive phase the symptoms do not remit completely. Finally, the progressive phase occurs as the disease leads to severe disability.

Movement dysfunction depends on the locations of the lesions. There may be muscle weakness ranging from mild paresis to total paralysis or weakness due to disuse atrophy. Spasticity may occur due to demyelinating lesions in the pyramidal tracts. Fatigue is a common complaint as the individual tires easily and progressively throughout the day. (Chapter 23 contains a prototype for a client with MS who experiences fatigue.)

Classic cerebellar disturbances are dysmetria, an inability to fix ROM; dysdiadochokinesia, the inability to perform rapidly alternating movements; and ataxia, uncoordinated movement. Ataxia is evident when a client walks with a staggering, wide-based pattern using poor foot placement and slow, uncoordinated progression of reciprocal lower extremity movement. Nonmovement problems associated with MS include visual disturbances, altered communication, altered bladder and bowel functions, cognitive and behavioral disturbances, and psychosocial stressors.

Parkinson's Disease

Parkinson's disease is a chronic, progressive disease of the nervous system involving the basal ganglia, resulting in disturbances of tone, abnormal posture, and involuntary movements due to deficiency of the neurotransmitter dopamine. Three classic motor signs are rigidity, an increased resistance to passive motion which affects striated muscle;

bradykinesia, difficulty in starting movement and slowness with paucity of movement; and tremor, an involuntary rhythmic action with alternating bursts of movement in antagonistic muscle groups.

Persons with Parkinson's disease have altered postural fixation, usually a flexed or stooped posture that occurs when flexor and adductor muscles become more contracted and postural reflexes are diminished. Clients characteristically walk with a slow and shuffling gait. Persistent posturing of a forward head and trunk results in a festinant gait pattern. Although a client takes multiple short steps to avoid falling, eventually the gait becomes an accelerating propulsive gait pattern with a retropulsive gait or backward accelerating one. Related motor problems include a masklike facies, drooling, sialorrhea, and dysphagia.

Traumatic Brain Injury

Traumatic brain injury may cause focal or diffuse brain damage. A frequent delayed complication is epilepsy. Depending on the severity of the problem, prolonged bed rest and inactivity can lead to a large group of complications affecting movement. Among these problems are muscle atrophy, contractures, osteoporosis, heterotrophic ossification, decubitus ulcers, edema, infections, thrombophlebitis or DVT (Herzog, 1993), and urinary tract infections.

Recovery from brain injury is variable and complex. Findings from research are leading to improved understanding and changes in practice with this group of clients. Currently most movement recovery is thought to occur within the first 6 months following the injury. Short-term goals of movement are geared to improving specific areas of abilities such as strength, coordination, ROM, balance, and posture—as well as mobility and safety. Treatment of persons with brain injury is highly individualized, depending on the nature of cardiopulmonary, integumentary, musculoskeletal, or neurologic functioning.

Movement therapy is directed toward improving function. To this end, clients are encouraged to perform functional movements similar to the way they were performed before injury, since individuals tend to respond best to activities that have been learned well enough to become automatic. An approach that sequences activities according to the progression of normal motor skill development is a key therapeutic strategy. Appropriate sequencing of activities cannot be overly emphasized when teaching clients, families, other support persons, or caregivers. These clients have long-term goals related to movement therapy that extend into their home and community settings, where community-based programs are important resources.

Spinal Cord Injury

Spinal cord injury is typically noted as quadriplegia or paraplegia, partial or complete, and according to the level of the spinal cord where the lesion or injury occurred. With a complete lesion no sensory or motor function exists below the level of the lesion, whereas an incomplete lesions may permit some sensory or motor function below the level of the lesion. Those who have Brown-Séquard syndrome with a hemisection of the spinal cord demonstrate asymmetric clinical features. Loss of function occurs on the ipsilateral (same) side as the lesion clinically manifested by

loss of sensation, decreased reflexes, lack of superficial reflexes, clonus, and Babinski's sign due to lateral column damage. Proprioceptive, anesthesia, and vibratory sense losses occur as a result of dorsal column damage, whereas damage to the spinothalamic tracts on the contralateral (opposite) side affects pain and temperature.

Immediately following spinal cord injury a period of areflexia, or spinal shock, is characterized by flaccidity, absence of all reflex activity, and loss of sensation below the level of the lesion. After the spinal shock phase, specific motor and sensory impairments occur according to specific features of the lesion such as the neurologic level, completeness of the lesion, symmetry of the lesion, and presence or absence of sacral sparing or root escape. Movement therapy begins with bed and mat activities and extends into wheelchair management or orthotic prescription and ambulatory training. Each program of movement therapy is highly individualized. Clients may experience a multitude of problems that ultimately affect their movement including:

- Impaired temperature control
- Respiratory involvement
- Spasticity
- Bowel and bladder dysfunction
- Pressure areas
- Automatic dysreflexia (hyperreflexia)
- Postural hypotension
- Osteoporosis
- Contractures
- Thrombophlebitis or DVT
- Painful sensations (dysesthesia)

Newly Emerging Syndromes and Diseases

Over the past decade patterns of chronic disabling disorders have emerged either as sequelae to conditions or as newly recognized diseases. Whether emerging conditions are a trend due to persons experiencing sequelae because they are living longer and surviving disease or injury, or because of improved detection, or due to truly new nemeses is unknown. Post-polio syndrome is an example. Persons who survived encounters with acute poliomyelitis half a century ago are at risk for pain, fatigue, and muscle weakness including impaired respiratory muscle function. These complications are complicated further by changes expected to occur as these clients grow older. Post-polio syndrome is a challenge for rehabilitation nurses, especially in the community-based models of care for assistance with ADL and mechanical ventilation (Macdonald, Gift, Bell, & Soeken, 1993).

Lyme disease, on the other hand, has been recognized only since 1975 as an infectious disease with varying symptoms and potentially chronic complications. Although the disease is prevalent in geographic areas of the U.S. East Coast, it has been identified worldwide. Early symptoms range from headache and polyarthritis to carditis or encephalitis. When resistant to treatment, undiagnosed, or reemerging, the disease produces muscle weakness, paralysis, and various neurologic manifestations such as impaired coordination, cognitive and learning problems, altered sleep-rest patterns, and fatigue. Pain related to muscle and joint tenderness and immobility due to arthritic symptoms are examples of altered movement for these clients. The uncertainty and changing nature of the disease contribute to psychosocial concerns; some clients have disrupted education or vocation plans.

♦ Guillain-Barré Syndrome

This somewhat mysterious syndrome has been known for years and occurs worldwide; however, the etiology remains unclear. A recent nonspecific infection is thought to precede many cases, and the syndrome affects all ages and both genders. Widespread inflammation leading to demyelination of either ascending or descending nerves in the peripheral nervous system account for the loss of function. Although symptoms vary, flaccid paralysis typically begins in the lower extremities and progresses cephalocaudally and symmetrically, often involving respiratory failure as early as 48 hours after onset. Sensory losses may occur as well as motor impairment. Nursing care during this time is crucial to later functional abilities. After several months persons begin to recover function, often completely, in nearly the same sequence as they lost function. Currently researchers are questioning whether there is a sequela, similar to post-polio syndrome, for Guillain-Barré syndrome.

NURSING DIAGNOSES FOR MOBILITY

Nursing diagnoses for clients with altered or impaired movement or mobility include the following:

1. Impaired Physical Mobility of the Upper Extremities related to muscle weakness, paralysis, joint swelling or pain, degeneration of bone and muscle, involuntary movement, or absence of an extremity
2. Impaired Physical Mobility of the Lower Extremities related to insufficient knowledge about the prosthesis, noncompliance with the care plan, lack of support by a family member, insufficient funds to attend therapy, or lack of transportation to therapy
3. Impaired Balance and Coordination related to truncal instability, muscle weakness, paralysis, prolonged bed rest, and lost or diminished vision
4. Dysfunctional Gait Pattern related to muscle weakness, paralysis, incoordination, involuntary movements, fracture of an extremity, lack of knowledge, fear, and dependence

GOALS

Unique and specific goals are based on a client's entire situation and lifestyle. The following potential goals may be mutually established and agreed upon among clients, families, community-based caregivers, and rehabilitation team members:

1. Prevent complications associated with decreased or absent movement
2. Increase muscle strength and mobility
3. Maintain and increase independence in activities requiring motor performance
4. Prevent injury during activity
5. Use assistive devices correctly and consistently, if appropriate
6. Adjust and adapt to altered mobility
7. Participate in social and occupational activities
8. Understand specific interventions related to impaired physical mobility

REHABILITATION NURSING INTERVENTIONS

When a client becomes immobilized or bedbound, a nurse's responsibility for preventive intervention is to maintain the person's potential for eventual mobilization. Potential complications of immobility and nursing interventions to prevent these complications are described in the following section.

Rehabilitation nursing interventions to assist the client in maximizing potential for mobilization include the following:

- ♦ Supporting the body in anatomically correct and functional positions
- ♦ Using mechanical or positioning devices properly
- ♦ Turning according to a regularly set schedule
- ♦ Teaching therapeutic exercise programs for maintaining joint mobility and muscle tone
- ♦ Teaching transfer activities
- ♦ Teaching preambulation and ambulation programs
- ♦ Teaching wheelchair activities
- ♦ Transferring responsibility for prevention and maintenance to client and family

Prevention of Complications Associated with Immobilization

Although bed rest was a common prescription to treat all sorts of diseases and conditions throughout history, it is no longer a panacea for ills. Rest in bed is still used to prevent further damage when normal demands exceed the body's ability to respond. For instance, when the heart cannot provide the blood volume or force for the body to perform daily activities or when the alveoli cannot diffuse adequate oxygen to meet demands of the body cells (pneumonia). Bed rest benefits short-term treatment of musculoskeletal problems such as result from trauma, degenerative disorders, rheumatologic diseases, infection, or congenital disorders.

When a person is unable to move part or all of the body because of disease, injury, or treatment method, a number of complications can occur in a short time. Olson (1967), in a classic article, described the hazardous effects of immobility on every system in the body while noting basic nursing interventions to prevent these hazards. More recently Rubin (1988) described the physiologic effects of bed rest. After only 3 days of bed rest, plasma and calcium are lost, less gastric juice is secreted, less blood flows through the calves, and glucose tolerance is impaired.

Changes in the cardiovascular system have been ascribed to immobility including orthostatic hypotension, increased workload for the heart, and thrombus formation. Preventive measures are passive and active ROM exercises, isometric exercises, and self-care activities. Immobilized persons are taught to avoid holding their breath when moving in bed and avoid the Valsalva maneuver. One of the most effective measures to change the intravascular pressure and provide a stimulus to the neural reflexes of the blood vessels is to change a client's position from horizontal to vertical either by raising the head of the bed or sitting the person upright in a chair, if permissible. Other ways to decrease the workload of the heart are to prevent constipation and support the client in a sitting or squatting position for defecation.

Immobility results in decreased respiratory movement,

decreased movement of secretions, and disturbed oxygen–carbon dioxide balance. For preventive intervention a client's respirations are observed for quality, depth, moisture, work, auxiliary muscle use at abdomen or neck, and any cognitive or neurologic signs such as restlessness or forgetfulness. A client who is dependent in care is turned regularly and encouraged to cough and sigh to facilitate adequate oxygen–carbon dioxide exchange and expel secretions. Chest clapping and postural drainage of all lobes of a client's lungs may help loosen secretions. The nurse teaches a client to use abdominal muscles, diaphragm, and intercostal muscles when performing regular deep breathing and coughing exercises (Murray, Mollinger, Sepic, & Gardner, 1983).

Immobilization accelerates catabolic activity, resulting in a rapid breakdown of cells and a protein deficiency. The consequent negative nitrogen balance can lead to anorexia, further contributing to existing malnutrition and significantly prolonging the disease process. Therefore discover a client's food preferences and provide small, frequent feedings, which are usually more appealing. Supplemental protein may be required. In addition the stress of bed rest may lead to continued stimulation of the parasympathetic nervous system, producing such symptoms as dyspepsia, gastric stasis, distention, anorexia, diarrhea, or constipation. Through use of tension-reducing interventions, the nurse may be able to help alleviate these symptoms. Stool softeners and exercises to strengthen weak abdominal muscles help prevent constipation (Murray et al., 1983).

Bed rest also can result in osteoporosis, contractures, and pressure areas. Exercises and close attention to body position and alignment, skin condition, diet supplemented as necessary to meet nutritional needs, and patient and family education can help prevent these complications (Murray et al., 1983). Immobility may permit urinary tract stones and urinary tract infection. The nurse assesses changes that occur in the production of hormones, sleeping patterns, the immune system, and psychosocial equilibrium. Consequently no client can remain immobile any longer than absolutely necessary. Although it still is not known how often turning is required to prevent some of these complications, it is known that the every 2-hour rule may not be adequate prevention for some persons (Rough, Hocomb, & Wilson, 1988).

Therapeutic Positioning

The client who is bedbound benefits from careful assessment of therapeutic positioning by the nurse. Variables influencing how frequently a client has a change of position include comfort, amount of spontaneous movement, edema, loss of sensation, overall physical and mental status, and time. Clients who experience discomfort after 30 to 60 minutes of lying prone then need to be repositioned, whereas those who are able to shift their weight every 20 to 30 minutes and move independently may change total position every 2 to 4 hours. Loss of sensation, paralysis, coma, and edema are indications for position changes every 2 hours or more frequently, since the client is unable to inform the nurse of discomfort or pain and since edematous, paralyzed tissue is more sensitive to pressure than normal tissue. Persons with progressive diseases with immobility may rely on frequent position changes to prevent pressure areas. (Chapter 15 provides detailed information about processes related to skin integrity.)

Time of day may influence how frequently a client is repositioned. For instance, when a client's overall condition permits, positioning every 4 hours during the night may be desirable to promote a more normal and restful sleep. A turning and positioning schedule posted at the bedside reinforces teaching for client and family, provides initiative for position changes, transfers responsibility to client and family, and stimulates feedback from all parties. While positioning and turning the client, a nurse has excellent opportunity to teach the individual and family about positioning, have them demonstrate procedures, and eventually have them share the responsibility in preparing for discharge.

✦ Basic positions

The basic positions are supine (back-lying), lateral (side-lying), prone (abdomen-lying) (Fig. 14-8), and semiprone (Murray et al., 1983). Because seemingly small positioning details may greatly impact a client's mobility outcome, positions are described in the following section as well as illustrated.

Supine position. To position a client in the supine position, the nurse assists the client to lay on the back (Fig. 14-8, *A*), providing a small flat pillow to support the head, neck, and upper shoulders. The arms are positioned along the person's sides in a neutral position, with elbows extended and palms downward. The position of the upper extremity may be varied by abducting the shoulder slightly with a small pillow or pad and then elevating the forearm and hand.

Other upper extremity positions include full abduction of the shoulder with extension of the elbow and wrist or full abduction of the shoulder with a 90-degree elbow flexion and the arm and hand positioned upward or downward. The hips are extended and supported in place by a trochanter roll. Avoid placing pressure on the back of the legs, which may damage blood vessels, resulting in phlebitis. The knees are extended or slightly flexed, but too great a degree of flexion at the knee may lead to flexion contracture with impairment of posture and gait. The feet are positioned to form a right angle with the leg. There are contradictions about how to prevent contracture formation resulting in foot-drop, but usually some type of device is used to maintain the desired angle of flexion such as adjustable footboards, firmly folded blankets or pillows, resting leg splints with footplates, or high-top sneakers. Precautions in using these devices are in the section on positioning aids in this chapter.

Lateral position. To place a client in the lateral position, the nurse assists the individual to lay on the side (Fig. 14-8, *B*) and provides a firm pillow to support the head and neck. The lower arm is positioned at the side with the uppermost arm supported by a pillow to prevent pressure on the chest. The upper leg is flexed at the hip and knee and positioned on a pillow in front of the lower leg to minimize pressure on the lower leg. Another pillow may be used behind the back to maintain this side-lying position.

For the individual who has had a stroke, the side-lying positioning incorporates the Bobath Neurodevelopmental Approach and promotes a client's lying on the affected side as tolerated. From this position the client begins to estab-

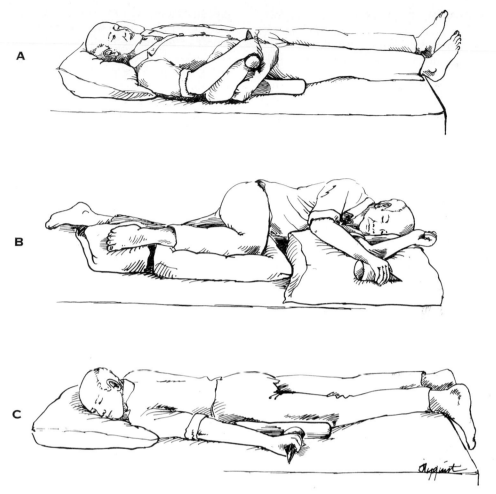

Fig. 14-8   **A,** Supine position with trochanter roll to prevent external rotation of the hips. **B,** Lateral position with hand cone to prevent flexion contracture of the hand. **C,** Prone position with trochanter roll and hand cone.

lish weight-bearing and lengthens the trunk, which later helps to counteract altered posture while sitting and standing. Positioning the person on the affected side may stimulate improved muscle tone through weight-bearing and prepare the individual for the bilateral weight-bearing necessary to move up in bed, move on and off the bedpan, and to stand.

Generally a person lying in bed places the bottom shoulder slightly ahead of the rest of the body while arranging the hip, knee, and shoulder in some degree of flexion. When positioning the individual who has had a stroke in the side-lying position on the affected side, the head is placed in a neutral position, the lower shoulder brought forward with the arm extended and the palm facing up, and the hips and knees flexed. In this position on the unaffected side, the shoulder is placed away from the spastic pattern associated with in hemiplegic posture. A towel or small pillow placed under the trunk at waist level helps elongate the affected side (Olson, 1967).

Prone position. Before placing a client in a prone position, the nurse reviews the record and assesses the person for any possible contraindications, such as increasing intra-

cranial pressure or cardiopulmonary distress. The nurse assists the person to lay on the abdomen (Fig. 14-8, *C*). The head is turned to one side, which facilitates breathing and drainage of oral secretions. A small pillow may be placed under the head for comfort and another between the chest and the umbilicus to relieve pressure on the chest or breasts. Hips and knees are extended and supported on pillows. The feet and toes are supported by another pillow or are positioned between the edge of the mattress and the bed frame to prevent pressure areas. In the prone position a client may feel most comfortable with arms flexed over the head or extended along the body in a neutral position.

Semiprone position. The client is in the semiprone position when resting on the side with the uppermost arm and leg placed farther forward.

Sitting position. All clients sit with their feet placed flat on the floor and the hips well back in the seat, with weight distributed evenly over the hips. Measure the depth, width, and height of the chair for sitting position and to help a client avoid leaning to one side or the other of the chair. Pillows can be used if the chair seat is too wide or too deep to allow the hip and knees to be placed at right angles. Use a small stool for the feet if the height of the chair seat does not allow the client to place the feet flat on the floor or use wheelchair pedals. When clients sit up in bed or in a chair, instruct them to avoid positions that encourage the development of spastic patterns. The affected shoulder is placed forward with a pillow for support if needed; the affected arm may be placed on a table at a comfortable height or in a wheelchair armrest to achieve this position (Murray et al., 1983).

✦ Positioning aids

To maintain correct body alignment, the use of various positioning aids is sometimes necessary. In general, positioning aids may be developed from materials on the nursing unit, from the person's home, or purchased from hospital supply companies. Other aids such as splints may be prescribed by the physiatrist and designed and fitted by the orthotist or occupational therapist. Even the most customized piece of equipment can cause pressure areas or can impair circulation if not applied correctly. To prevent pressure or development of ischemic areas, the nurse checks and removes the equipment every 2 to 4 hours unless ordered otherwise by the physician.

Pillows. Pillows can be used to position, stabilize, and support or provide a bridge beneath a pressure area. Alternatives to pillows include rolled or folded towels, bath blankets, and foam squares covered with washable material. Check contents since some persons have allergies to materials used to stuff pillows or similar items.

Trochanter rolls. A bath blanket or flannel sheet blanket can be used to make a trochanter roll when a commercial trochanter roll is not available or is an added expense. This roll is used to prevent outward rotation of the hip when the client is in a supine position. The blanket is folded lengthwise into thirds and positioned beneath the client's hips from the top of the iliac crest to approximately 6 inches above the knee. It should be rolled under toward the client so that a roll is formed along the outer aspect of the thigh. Figure 14-8, *A, B,* and *C,* illustrates placement of a trochanter roll.

Foot supports. The alternatives to a footboard mentioned previously include blanket-covered boxes, resting leg splints, or high-top sneakers. (Chapter 15 contains additional information and illustrations of booties and other footgear.) With each of these aids, the nurse checks for pressure areas and ischemia. The nurse also exercises the feet according to the client's capabilities to maintain muscle tone, muscle strength, and joint range. If the legs and feet are spastic, positioning against a footboard may produce an undesirable increase in the tendency of the feet to plantar flex. High-top tennis shoes stimulate the top of the foot as well as the sole and assist in achieving a more beneficial outcome.

Hand rolls. One of nursing's time-honored treatments for positioning the hand in a slightly flexed position was the rolled washcloth or soft rubber ball. If a client has normal muscle tone and voluntary movement, no harm will come of this practice. However, the person with a spastic hand may experience overstimulation of the palmar surface, which in turn can increase flexion synergy, resulting in flexion contracture of the hand and wrist. (Mathiowetz, Bold-

ing, and Trombey, 1983) suggested the use of a firm cone, maintained in position by a strip of elastic over the dorsal aspect of the hand. The cone is believed to provide constant pressure over the entire flexor surface of the fingers and to put pressure on the insertions of the spastic wrist and finger flexors. Pressure on these areas is believed to have an inhibitory effect on the long flexors of the hand.

Jamieson and Dayhoff (1980) studied the use of a hard cone on 11 individuals with hemiplegia and flexor hypertonicity of the upper extremity. All measurements of extension of the finger, opposition of the finger to the thumb, pinch strength, and grip strength were taken with the wrist in the neutral and flexed position. They found that flexor hypertonicity of the fingers and wrist decreased significantly after the hard cone was used for 4 weeks, although only slight changes in function occurred. Their findings were similar to findings of an earlier small study of three adults with hemiplegia in whom the greatest improvement occurred after 6 weeks, when the wrist was placed in a flexed position only (Dayhoff, 1975).

Splints. Disagreement exists regarding whether splinting spastic extremities facilitates or inhibits spasticity. Many occupational therapists splint only those persons who have moderate to severe spasticity. A study by Mathiowetz, Bolding, and Trombly (1983) addressed the immediate effects of positioning devices on the normal and spastic hand. They studied the use of the volar resting splint (Fig. 14-9), a foam finger spreader, which is based on Bobath's belief that abduction facilitates extension of the fingers and reduces flexor spasticity of the whole arm, a firm cone, and no device on the normal and spastic hand as measured by electromyography. Their sample was small (n = 8 persons and n = 4 persons with hemiplegia); however, the findings suggest further examination of these devices is in order. In the

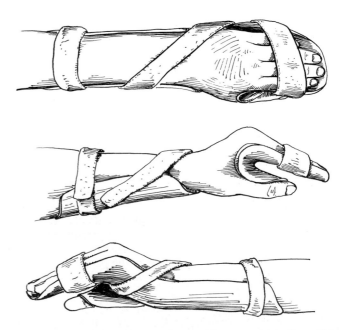

Fig. 14-9 Volar resting splint provides support to the wrist, thumb, and fingers, maintaining them in position of extension.

persons with hemiplegia the electrical activity of the muscles before and after grasp was not significantly reduced while wearing the volar splint, finger spreader, or hand cone, suggesting that a decrease in spasticity does not necessarily occur when these devices are used. In addition, the volar splint appeared to increase electrical activity during application of the splint and during the grasping period. If an increase in electrical activity is undesirable in a spastic hand, then use of a volar splint would be contraindicated when grasping or performing a comparable activity (Marsolais & Kobetic, 1983). The results did not contraindicate the use of a volar splint while a client was resting.

Mills (1984) examined the use of bivalve splints to control postural defects caused by spasticity in eight subjects with spastic extremities manifested by ankle, wrist, or elbow flexion contracture. She concluded that no significant change occurred in the spastic muscles as measured by electromyography during splinted and nonsplinted periods. She reported that some individuals experience an increase in electrical activity while splinted. A consistent approach by the rehabilitation team is necessary when using positioning devices for the spastic hand and arm. The client's individual responses to the device, as well as further research findings, provide the nurse and other team members with the information necessary to determine the best possible approach.

Abductor wedge or pillow. An abductor pillow is a triangular wedge-shaped positioning aid made of heavy foam material. This wedge is used specifically for clients following total hip replacement (THR) for the purpose of maintaining the legs in abduction position needed to keep the prothesis positioned in the joint and until the muscles, soft tissues, and incisions around the hip prostheses heal. Two sets of Velcro straps are positioned to hold the legs to the wedge pillow. Many clients wear a knee immobilizer to control flexion of the knee to the hip on the prosthesis side. Following THR a client must not exceed a 90-degree angle between the knee and hip, which requires attention for seating as recovery continues. Clients frequently have elastic wraps or antiembolism stockings on the legs to promote circulation and prevent edema. These clients will be taught therapeutic exercises and are assessed for weight-bearing ability, obesity as a detriment to weight-bearing, muscle tone and strength, DVT, skin integrity, osteoporosis, seating including home or workplace, and signs of infection or delayed wound healing. Since many older clients receive THR surgery, complications associated with other chronic or disabling conditions, such as RA or diabetes, cannot be ignored during rehabilitation. Positioning schedules that are arranged to take daily activities, socialization, and client preferences into account may empower a client who is otherwise immobilized. Figure 14-10 illustrates an abduction pillow wedge following THR surgery.

◆ Maintaining stability with positioning

Specialized turning frames and mechanized beds enable nurses to change a client's position safely and efficiently when a person must retain spinal stability following severe trauma and/or surgery. Among these devices are Stryker wedge frames, CircOlectric beds, Roto Rest, and airfluidized beds discussed in the following section. In addition to positioning as discussed earlier, bracing or orthotics, and traction may be used to assure stabilization. A client may enter rehabilitation while wearing a halo brace; with surgically placed internal rods, such as Harrington or Leuke rods; with dual brace and traction stabilizers, or with intermittent in-bed traction. With these stabilizers, pin sites are cleansed and inspected regularly throughout the day and a full set of equipment, usually wrenches, accompany the client. For example, wrenches are needed to loosen bolts to remove the front of a halo vest in an emergency. Some halo vests have special "slip" releases for CPR emergencies.

Stryker wedge frame. The Stryker wedge frame is a long-standing aid for prone and supine positioning. Literally "sandwiched" between two padded canvas stretchers, a client is rotated manually from prone to supine, or vice versa. A client always is notified before turning begins. In one smooth movement a client is in a lateral position only during the act of turning, thus reducing variation in positioning. The frame is equipped with safety straps, arm supports, and side rails; the uppermost canvas is usually removed after each turning. The Stryker frame has been used with clients who have spinal cord injury, plastic surgery, and pressure areas, among others. The frame is limited to individuals who weigh less than 200 pounds. A client on the frame has limited visibility to either stare up at the ceiling or look down at the floor, depending on the rotation. Some clients experience fear or apprehension during the manual rotation; and some, especially those in cervical traction, fear injury should a caregiver neglect to secure frames, straps, or nuts and bolts on the frame. Safe and proper use is a clear issue with the Stryker frame.

Mechanical beds

1. *CircOlectric bed.*

   The CircOlectric bed also places a client between a lower mattress and an upper stretcher for turning, all gliding on two circular frames. Positions from supine to prone, those allowing for standing, sitting, and Trendelenburg's position are possible. Again, a client may question the large frame with accessories such as arm support brackets, restraining straps, an overbed table, a mirror assembly, an anterior arm sling, a head halter-collar combination, and a spreader bar. When turning a client from supine to prone or vice versa, the person becomes upright to experience weight-bearing as well as postural changes—both desirable in preventing osteoporosis and hypotension. However, the CircOlectric bed may not be suitable for those who are not weight-bearing or who respond poorly to changes from flat to erect positions, such as those with hypotension or following a high cervical cord injury. Persons who may benefit from the CircOlectric bed include those who have experienced multiple trauma, burns, and reconstructive surgery. The nurse is responsible for assuring safe operation of the bed frame during and after turning.

2. *Roto Rest.* The most recent mechanical adjunct to positioning in kinetic therapy is the Roto Rest, used to deliver kinetic therapy. This oscillating bed turns a client continuously at an interval of every 3.5 minutes over a range of 124 degrees, but can be stopped at any point for nursing or medical care. So gradual is the turning

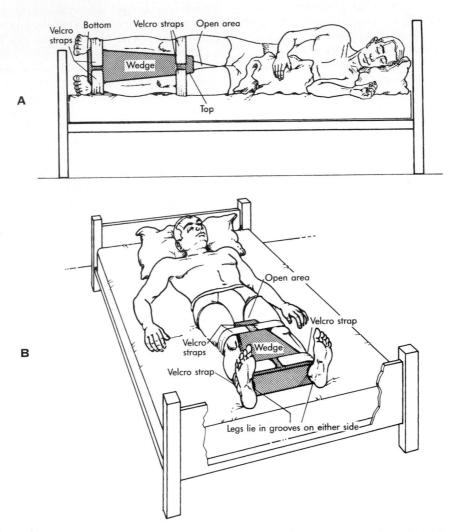

Fig. 14-10   **A,** A client who has a hip fracture or hip replacement surgery is positioned on his uninvolved side. His affected hip is slightly flexed. A foam wedge (or pillows) is used to keep his legs apart and abduct the hip joints. Note the 90-degree angle limit of flexion at the hip. **B,** The same client viewed from the front illustrates the use of the foam wedge (or pillows) between his knees and legs. These supports keep the hip joints abducted. The top or affected knee must be supported firmly and steadily. It must not fall off the wedge. His knees must not be allowed to touch one another. (From *Rehabilitation/Restorative Care* by S.P. Hoeman, 1990, St. Louis: Mosby–Year Book. Copyright 1990 by Mosby–Year Book. Reprinted by permission.)

that an individual does not experience dizziness or discomfort. The Roto Rest conforms to the person with knee and shoulder braces and close-fitting pads placed against the body and extremities. It also minimizes the complications of immobility such as hypostatic pneumonia, pulmonary emboli, constipation, and pressure areas. The table has been used successfully with clients who have experienced multiple trauma, respiratory disorders, severe burns, paralysis, coma, and pressure areas. A few persons report claustrophobia as a result of the pads and braces; however, reports of pain are usually related to improper positioning (Milazzo & Rash, 1982).

3. *Air-fluidized bed.* Air-fluidized beds such as the Clinitron and Kinair are designed specifically for support while reducing pressure on the skin and permitting unimpeded blood flow when persons are repositioned every 3 to 4 hours. The Clinitron bed consists of a loosely fitting polyester filter sheet covering a tank of 1,500 pounds of tiny, sterile glass beads. Warm pressurized air from a blower lifts the beads, floating a client on a dry, fluid medium. Body exudates pass through the filter sheet and fall to the bottom. Since the glass beads are silicone-coated soda lime, the high pH decreases bacterial growth.

The Kinair bed supports a person comfortably on a fabric cushion. Compared with standard hospital beds, this air-fluidized bed decreases pressure against the heel by 60 mm Hg, the sacrum by 19 mm Hg, the scapula by 14 mm Hg, the trochanter by 47 mm Hg, and the occiput by 39 mm Hg. Potential problems with air-fluidized beds are dehydration, related to increased fluid loss from the skin and the respiratory tract; pulmonary congestion, since coughing is ineffective unless the fluidization is turned off; and skin irritation, if microsphere leakage occurs through a tear in the sheet (Rubin, 1988). Clients using an air-fluidized bed report decreased pain and increased comfort and rest and use less pain medication.

Therapeutic Exercise

Regular exercise is an important intervention for the person with impaired physical mobility. (Appendix 14-A provides a review of passive, active, and functional ROM.) Before a client is considered medically stable to begin an active physical or occupational therapy program, the nurse implements a program of exercise based on the person's overall condition. The intent is to prevent contractures or atrophy and maintain muscle tone, strength, and function. Safety is a consideration for any mobility or therapeutic exercise program. For instance, joint damage is possible with passive or active ROM, especially if sensation to the extremity has been impaired. Exercises use isotonic contractions, producing movement of joint and muscle, or isometric contractions, shortening muscle fibers without apparent movement of the limb or joint. The nurse's goals are to teach the exercise program to both client and family or caregiver and encourage active participation; demonstrate the exercise program; lead client and family through practice, observe client and family redemonstrate the exercises, and delegate responsibility for the exercise program to client and family as an activity of daily living.

Although passive ROM has been a cornerstone of nursing care, recent research findings question how widespread it is applied in practice. Do rehabilitation nurses know and practice ROM with clients in facility and community? In another study Clough and Maurin (1983) hypothesized that ROM exercises increase spasticity and flexion contractures in persons with upper motor neuron damage by facilitating flexor activity when muscle fibers are quickly stretched and maintained in the maximum range. In lieu of ROM exercises, they used vibration of extensor muscle groups. Vibration reportedly facilitated extensor muscle contraction while inhibiting contraction of the flexor muscle. Results indicated that vibration plus other methods of neurophysiologic treatment significantly increased ROM at the fingers and wrist, decreasing contractures in clients with CVAs. An unexpected finding was that ROM exercises appeared more effective in decreasing contractures of the shoulder.

◆ Active exercise

In teaching a client to perform active ROM with extremities affected by disability, the nurse takes into account the general principles of teaching and learning including motivation, readiness, attention span, and educational level. In general, clients find exercises easier to learn when they are demonstrated first and supplemented by a written form with diagrams. Redemonstration of the exercise to the nurse helps assure accuracy and effectiveness. As with other forms of exercise, persons with similar disabilities may be grouped during the day for "range" exercises, or a client and family member may exercise together. A cable or online facility television station, a videotape of ROM exercises, or programs of simple bed exercises may encourage and stimulate participation.

ROM modifications for persons with specific impairments, such as hemiplegia or paraplegia, incorporate methods of aiding movement of extremities using the unaffected extremities. For example, a client laces the fingers of the unaffected hand through those of the affected hand for support to exercise; raising one arm above the shoulder supports and raises the other; and flexing and extending the unaffected arm at the elbow assists reciprocal action in the other. To move the legs through ROM, a client may combine the unaffected arm and leg, depending on strength and balance. With paraplegia a person may exercise the legs and feet while sitting in bed because the bed assists in maintaining balance and supports the legs and feet.

◆ Isometric exercises

Isometric exercises shorten muscle fibers without movement of limbs or joints and thus require voluntary participation. The nurse teaches a client how to perform the activity, then monitors and evaluates the results of the exercise. Sometimes referred to as muscle-setting exercises, the most common isometric exercises are abdominal-setting, quadriceps-setting, and gluteal-setting exercises. For abdomen-setting, place one hand on the individual's abdomen while the person tenses the abdominal muscle. The muscle is contracted and held for 10 seconds, then released. Remind clients to maintain a normal respiratory pattern during the exercise, especially those who have had myocardial infarctions or brain injuries. For quadriceps-setting, a client contracts the long muscles in the thighs; for gluteal-setting, the buttocks are "pinched together." Other muscle groups such as the perineal, biceps, and triceps muscles may be contracted isometrically.

Another type of isometric exercise contracts a muscle group against an object—for instance, pushing or plantar flexing the feet against a footboard to prevent circulatory stasis. This isometric exercise is resistive, since the footboard provides resistance to the activity of the muscles of the legs and feet. To maintain normal cardiovascular function, the exercise is limited to contractions of less than 10 seconds (Ahrens, Kinney, & Carter, 1983).

Energy expenditure is an exercise consideration. Hathaway and Geden (1983) compared energy expenditure for clients during three leg exercise programs (active, passive, and isometric) with energy expenditure in a control group (rest). Oxygen consumption and heart rate were found to be comparable and significantly more demanding in isometric and active programs than either passive exercise or rest.

◆ Adjunct measures: biofeedback and electrical stimulation

Biofeedback and/or electrical stimulation may maintain or increase muscle strength and tone. Research findings based on healthy subjects suggest that transcutaneous electrical stimulation alone can strengthen skeletal muscle and may have applicability to those with immobility or impairment. Other findings indicate biofeedback with isometric exercise produces greater gains in muscle strength than isometric exercise alone. A physical therapist evaluation determines whether a client may benefit from electrical stimulation or biofeedback.

◆ Activities in bed

Activities for the individual who is completely bed-bound can be divided into turning and moving up and down. When a client is totally dependent, the nursing staff or family members have to perform the work of moving. Those who are partially able to help may receive some assistance or use adaptive equipment, whereas persons without physical limitations are encouraged to move independently in bed. Use as well as knowledge of proper body mechanics is essential for clients and staff who move a person who is dependent. To move this client in, out, or around the bed, the bed is raised to a comfortable working height at approximately hip level, which coincides with the nurse's center of gravity. If the bed cannot be raised, consider placing the bed legs or frame securely on blocks to the proper height. Lock the bed if on casters, or brace it against a wall, so movement off the blocks is not possible. This allows the nurse to stand with knees slightly flexed and legs positioned apart in a wide base of support. The large muscles of the legs and buttocks, rather than the small muscles of the back, are used to move the client. As the nurse moves, weight is transferred from one leg to the other in the direction of movement.

Turning. In turning a client to the side, stand on the side of the bed toward which the individual is to be turned. The client's arms are positioned on the abdomen, and the farther leg is crossed over the near leg at the ankle (except if contraindicated as with THR). The nurse stands with knees slightly bent, one leg forward and the other back. One hand is positioned beneath the client's far shoulder and the other

hand beneath the hips on the far side. Using a smooth complete motion, the nurse transfers weight from the forward leg to the back leg, thereby moving the client to a side-lying position.

A client who has hemiplegia or paresis may learn to bridge with the hips, a movement used to get on a bedpan. The nurse bends the person's knees, instructing the client to place the unaffected foot over the affected one to stabilize it, places a hand on top of the client's affected knee to move it down toward the feet, and places the other hand under the affected hip to direct the lifting movement of the hips (Borgman & Passarella, 1991). Pressure exerted over the knee causes the hip to rise automatically. (Chapter 12 contains self-care and ADL illustrations for dressing techniques that are related movements [e.g., bridging].)

Moving up in the bed. In moving the client who is dependent toward the top or bottom of the bed, two caregivers are more energy efficient than a single person. The method of moving may depend on the client's weight and breadth. For a person within the average weight range, two persons can efficiently effect the move. Using the hands as levers, with elbows bent, one caregiver slides the arms under the client's upper back. One caregiver's arm is positioned under the shoulders, the other arm under the waist. The other caregiver supports the client's lower back, positioning one arm at the client's waist, the other below the client's hips. Both caregivers stand at the same side of the bed and mentally "divide" responsibility for moving a portion of the client's height and weight. Using their arms as levers, one caregiver supports the client under the shoulders and under the waist, while the other supports under the waist and at the hips. Each caregiver stands with knees slightly flexed and one foot forward. At a given count both caregivers transfer weight from the forward leg to the back leg. The client is moved in one smooth continuous motion to the edge of the bed, with care being taken to prevent friction or shearing of the skin.

A single caregiver can follow the same principles as for two persons. It may be easier with one caregiver to move the client in "thirds," a section at a time. The caregiver would begin by moving the client's head and shoulders, then the waist and hips, and finally the legs and feet. Safety for client and caregiver and proper body mechanics are essential.

The client with hemiplegia or paresis following a stroke can be assisted to the side of the bed using the Bobath Neurodevelopmental Approach. The client is instructed in sequential steps to

1. Clasp hands and stretch them forward
2. Bend the knees
3. Turn the head and look in the direction of the turn
4. Swing the extended arms to the side of the turn
5. Let the knees follow to complete the turn (Borgman & Passarella, 1991)

Encouraging client participation in movement. When a client is able to assist in activities in bed, the nurse encourages participation and provides instruction. To turn to the side of the bed, the client is taught pull up on the siderail with either upper extremity. When siderails are not available, a client is taught to place an immobilized arm on the abdomen so that it is not "left behind" during the turn, or to position the arm carefully when turning onto the affected side. The affected leg is positioned over the other ankle to make the task of turning simpler and ensure the leg is in alignment. If one or both legs are mobile, then a client can facilitate turning by pushing in the direction of the turn with the sole of the foot. The nurse emphasizes that the sole of the foot, rather than the heel, is used to prevent damage to the skin.

To move up toward the head of the bed, the person grasps the siderails, pulls up with the arms, and pushes the soles of both feet down into the mattress, which thrusts the body upward in bed. The head of the bed or a trapeze suspended on a Balkan frame or overbed frame is useful for a client to pull up on for bedpan positioning or while the bed is being made. A physical therapist evaluates a client's ability to use a trapeze and teaches exercises that can be performed in the bed to strengthen the upper extremities.

Activities out of bed. Activity out of bed may be a nursing prescription for persons who are completely dependent, as well as for those who require some assistance. (Refer to Appendix 14-B) Generally a client is moved out of bed to a chair or wheelchair to provide a change in physical position and minimize the effects of immobility, as well as for a change in surroundings. Before sitting in a chair, the client spends time in Fowler's position and is supervised to dangle the legs from the edge of the bed until adjusted to sitting posture. Assess readiness to sit in a chair; monitor vital signs, balance, alertness, and level of comfort before the client moves from high Fowler's position or dangling. Assess circulation to lower extremities with the legs dangling and apply compression or antiembolism stockings or elastic bandages before activity out of bed and to prevent venous stasis. Place the legs and feet fully supported on an elevated wheelchair footrest or on a stool to reduce edema and venous stasis.

Transferring a Person Who is Dependent

Transferring a person who is dependent from bed to a chair requires mechanical devices or trained personnel using lift transfers or pivot transfers, which are described in the following section. Once in the chair, monitor a client's sitting posture and weight shifts.

Mechanical devices. The most commonly used mechanical device is the pneumatic lift—namely, the Hoyer lift. A client is positioned on a one- or two-piece sling connected by chains to a crossbar on the lift. Pumping the hydraulic mechanism, the lift carries the client in a seated position off the bed. Because the lift is stable with a broad base of support and is adjustable, it may be possible to wheel the person while suspended in the lift sling from the bed to a chair or commode. As the pressure is released slowly from the hydraulic pump, the client descends into the seat. Depending on the person's size and impairment, one, two, or three caregivers may be required to transfer the client safely to a chair. The lift slings may be left in place beneath the person until he or she returns to bed or may be removed for use with others. Turn hooks on the slings away from the client to prevent injury and line the sling for hygiene.

Lift transfer. Two caregivers can transfer clients who are of average weight from the bed to a chair. The bed surface is elevated slightly higher than the chair. One nurse stands at the head of the bed and uses both arms to reach under the client's arms, using opposite hands to grasp the client's wrists. The other caregiver supports the client's legs and feet. Using proper body mechanics, the caregivers lift the client out of bed on a predetermined count and glide the client into the chair. When a client is heavier than average, four caregivers use a sturdy lift sheet, one at each of the person's shoulders and one at each of the knees. At the predetermined count, the caregivers use the lift sheet to slide the client above the surface of the bed and then into the seat.

Pivot transfer. When weight-bearing is not contraindicated, a client who is dependent can be pivot transferred from bed to the chair. In a pivot transfer the person is brought to a sitting position on the side of the bed. The client's arms are positioned around the nurse's neck and shoulder with the nurse's arms passing under the client's arms to support the lower back. The nurse then flexes the knees and thighs and rocks back and forth with the client to gain momentum. When both client and nurse are ready, the nurse shifts weight from the forward leg to the back leg, lifting the client off the bed and turning the client toward the chair. The nurse shifts weight from the back leg to the forward leg, bending at the hip and knee as the client is lowered into the chair.

Positioning in the chair. The nurse evaluates the seated posture of a client, ideally a straight, slightly relaxed back, hips and knees flexed at 90 degrees, and feet flat on the floor. If the chair is too high, use a footstool but evaluate alignment and any pressure on the legs. Pillows placed at either side prevent a client from leaning toward one side when a chair is too wide. A pillow at the back prevents "slumping" should a chair be too deep. When a chair is too low, the hips and knees are flexed more acutely than is desirable, predisposing contractures. A foam pad or pillow placed under the client before transfer to the chair may alleviate the problem. Clients (and family) are taught to change position three times each hour while sitting in a chair. The client shifts weight by leaning forward, to the right, or to the left.

✦ **Assisting a Client to Transfer.** Clients who are partially dependent can increase their independence by using several techniques to transfer from one place to another. Techniques described in the following section are for a person with paraplegia, for a person with hemiplegia, and for using a transfer board. The nurse encourages client participation, teaches sequential steps for each technique, is available for assistance, and assures a safe environment and technique such as transfer belts or other safety devices.

Transfer with paraplegia. The person who has paraplegia or limited mobility below the waist, such as with bilateral lower extremity amputation, can use the following transfer. The chair is placed perpendicular to the bed at the middle of the bed. Bed casters are locked, commode or wheelchair wheels are locked, and footrests are removed. The person rises to sit, then uses upper extremity strength to turn the trunk and legs in line with the chair. With the person's back seated nearest the seat of the chair, the person reaches backward with both arms to grasp the armrests and moves the hips and legs from the bed backward into the seat of the chair. As the chair is moved away from the bed, the client lowers the legs carefully (Fig. 14-11). When proficlient, a client may use a push up and side-to-side transfer.

Transfer board. A transfer board assists mobility for the client who has limited function of the lower extremities. Several styles of transfer boards are available, some promoting a client's ability to "lift and bounce" across the board, but the principle is the same. Although often referred to as sliding, a client does not slide literally on the transfer board, an action that would lead to impaired skin integrity. Wheelchair or chair placement at a 45-degree angle alongside the bed is essential for a smooth transfer. Figure 14-12 illustrates positioning of equipment. Lock brakes or casters

and remove any armrests, as possible. Ideally the bed and chair are the same height. Place the transfer board bridging the chair and the bed; a client needs a clear path to avoid the wheel when moving to a wheelchair.

The client wears a transfer belt as needed for safety and for the caregiver to grasp when offering assistance. With assistance the client leans to position a portion of the transfer board under the buttocks, then sits and regains balance. Using the upper extremities, the client performs a series of "little push-ups" across the board. Those with a great deal of upper body strength may pull themselves toward the far

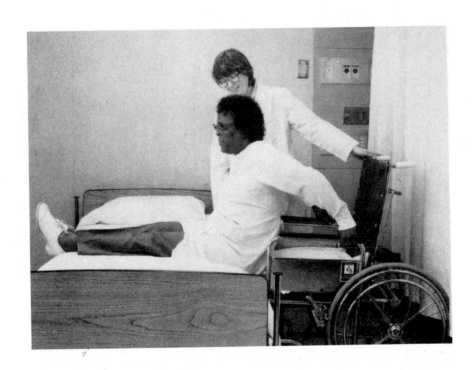

Fig. 14-11 This technique enables a client with good balance and upper extremity muscle strength to transfer independently.

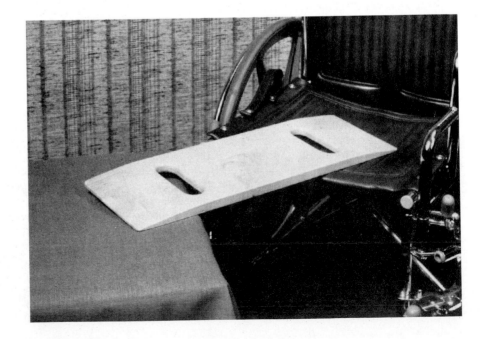

Fig. 14-12 A transfer board may be used to assist clients to move from one seat to another. Position of the wheelchair, bed, and transfer board are basic to a successful move. (From *Rehabilitation/Restorative Care* by S.P. Hoeman, 1990, St. Louis: Mosby–Year Book. Copyright 1990 by Bissell Healthcare Corporation/Fred Sammons, Inc. Reprinted by permission.)

armrest of the chair, but skin friction and shearing must be prevented. Either way, the hips and lower extremities are moved over the transfer board and into the chair. The client tilts the other way and removes the board.

A transfer board may be used to facilitate movement between many seating areas; the chair and tub, the chair and toilet, the chair and car, and so forth. Generally the physical therapy department initiates upper extremity strengthening and the training necessary for the client to begin to use this method of transfer. The nurse reinforces instruction received in physical therapy and provides encouragement as this type of transfer is integrated into daily activities and maximum independence is gained in the home and community.

Transfer for a client with hemiplegia. The person with less muscle strength and/or sensation on one side of the body, such as the person with hemiplegia, can learn to transfer independently in many situations. Most sources advocate that the chair or locked wheelchair be placed at a slight angle to the bed on the client's unaffected side. The client comes to a sitting position on the side of the bed by using the unaffected hand to position the other hand across the abdomen. The client slides the unaffected foot under the other ankle, then moves both legs over the side of the bed on the client's unaffected side. The client assists by grasping the edge of the mattress while pushing with elbow and forearm against the bed to gain a half-sitting position. After moving one hand to the rear, the client pushes to a full sitting position. Now the client is ready to transfer to the chair. Keeping the feet beneath the body and leaning forward, the individual places the unaffected arm near the edge of the bed and pushes to a standing position. Then the client regains balance and steadiness. The unaffected hand is moved to the farther armrest of the chair as the client pivot-turns with weight on the unaffected foot, turning toward the chair, then when over the seat, lowers to a sitting position.

When incorporating the Bobath Neurodevelopmental approach, the chair is placed at an angle to the bed on the client's affected side. The chair is locked and the armrest closest to the bed is removed. The person is assisted to the side of the bed, and the feet are positioned flat on the floor with the heels under or slightly behind the knees. The client is assisted to clasp the hands and extend the arms, leaning forward until the head and trunk are in position over the feet. The nurse then leans over the client's back and assists the client in moving the hips. The nurse rocks back, shifting the weight to the back foot, and pivots while turning the client's hips toward the chair, affected side first. Then the nurse shifts weight forward and client is lowered gently to the chair or other seating (Borgman & Passarella, 1991).

Ambulation/Gait Training

Goal setting and attainment for functional independence in ambulation is a team effort in which the client is an active participant. Generally a physical therapist works with the client to propose an ambulation plan that is reinforced on the nursing unit, in occupational therapy, in the home, or in a community-based setting. A plan may include isometric and therapeutic exercises designed to prepare the muscles used in walking, provide practice in maintaining sitting and standing balance, gain ability for passive standing with adaptive equipment, and select adaptive equipment and assistive devices used with specific gain training techniques.

✦ Preambulation

The exercise program to prepare muscles for standing and walking is initiated early while a client is bedbound. Isometric exercises such as those described earlier in this chapter are implemented for the purpose of strengthening muscles of the lower extremities; muscles of the trunk, including the gluteal and abdominal muscles; and muscles of the upper extremities. The nurse reinforces instruction from physical therapy and encourages a client and family to become involved and work with the program. Other therapeutic exercises that are performed in bed as preparatory to walking are modified sit-ups in the supine position and modified push-ups in the prone position. The nurse monitors a client's cardiovascular response to these and other exercise programs.

✦ Sitting balance

A client develops sitting balance at the side of the bed. Using the least assistance needed, the client sits with the feet resting firmly on the floor or supported by a footstool. The nurse or therapist monitors a client for safety as the person follows instructions to raise the arms left, right, forward, and upward. A client who is able to perform these maneuvers without a loss of balance has sitting balance sufficient to participate in an ambulation program. If walking with crutches is the outcome goal of the ambulation program, the client is taught to perform sitting push-ups, using both upper extremities to support the entire body weight, while sitting in a locked wheelchair or very sturdy armchair.

✦ Standing balance

The client is taught to come to a standing position and practices this activity until it is performed safely. Basically the client is reminded to slide to the edge of the sitting surface, keeping the feet back under the body. The client is taught to push down with the legs and arms while leaning the trunk forward to come to a standing position. Some persons require assistance to achieve a standing position, which enables them to be trained to use assistive equipment to compensate for plegia or disability. Standing requires practice beginning with standing next to a stable support until an erect position and trunk balance can be maintained while moving the extremities. During these activities a client guards against injury, especially preventing falls. Elderly persons may experience impaired balance following altered arm movement, changes in gait patterns, or increased body sway. Activities such as passive rocking in a rocking chair have been suggested as possible methods to increase vestibular stimulation, thereby improving balance.

✦ Passive standing activities

Passive standing activities may precede transfer activities and standing activities. Passive standing is prescribed to prepare the cardiovascular system to adjust to the change in circulatory demands between the recumbent and erect positions. A variety of assistive devices or equipment is available to support a client in passive standing.

Tilt table. A tilt table is a common unit used for passive standing, generally in a physical therapy department. The client is transferred to a tilt table while in the supine position; when the feet rest on a foot support, the body is secured to the table with safety straps. Once a baseline blood pressure and pulse are taken and recorded, the tilt table is elevated slowly to a 15- to 20-degree angle. Thereafter the degree of tilt is increased by 5- to 10-degree increments until the client is able to tolerate a standing position for 10 to 30 minutes. The client is monitored during tilt table activities for blood pressure, pulse, dependent edema of the lower extremities, skin mottling, and sensations of faintness, dizziness, or headache. A client who has been bedbound for a prolonged period or who has a poor cardiovascular response may use elastic wraps, elastic stockings, or an abdominal binder in preparation for tilt table activities. Squires (1983) found the following advantages in using electrically powered tilt tables to achieve standing with elderly persons: relief of gluteal pressure, maintenance of postural reflexes, enhanced bladder and bowel function, unimpeded chest expansion, and psychological motivation to participate in an ambulation program.

Standing frame. A standing frame or table also may be used for passive standing activities. When using standing frames or tables, a client adjusts to transfer from a sitting position to immediate upright standing without the gradual increase in degree of erect position, as with the tilt table. Standing frames or tables have stabilizers, either padded supports at the knees and abdomen or actual countertop or tabletop surfaces. Posterior stabilizers include heel cups, knee stabilizers, and pelvic or gluteal supports. A client using a standing frame or table is able to enjoy the physiologic and psychological rewards of an erect position, while increasing standing balance and freeing the upper extremities for occupational therapy exercises or diversional activities.

Children in pediatric programs may use standing tables to practice being upright, to provide visualization and stimulation, as a means to enhance learning or perform activities, and to promote inclusion with peers. Specially sized standing frames are available for children.

The physical therapist evaluates a client's functional ability to ambulate, prescribes assistive equipment most appropriate for the specific disability and most acceptable to self-image, and initiates teaching and training of both client and family toward accomplishing their desired goal. In the community rehabilitation nurses continue work with community agencies and clients in these areas.

✦ Use of assistive equipment

The type of assistive equipment selected often depends on the client's physical limitations. Crutches are appropriate for individuals with full use and sufficient strength of upper extremities who have limited lower extremity function because of amputation, fracture, paraparesis, or paraplegia. Broad-based canes or tripod or quad-footed canes are appropriate for patients who have weakness or paralysis of one side of the body, including those who have had strokes. Walkers are chosen for those persons who have generalized weakness in both upper and lower extremities and are used with older persons who have generalized arthritis, hip fracture, or neuromuscular diseases.

The physical therapist measures a client relative to each piece of assistive equipment, tailoring equipment to client height, weight, and specific needs. For this reason, assistive equipment such as crutches, canes, and walkers are not able to be shared. In teaching a client to ambulate with any assistive equipment, the following points are covered:

✦ Care of the equipment or device
✦ How to come to a standing position
✦ "Actual" gait training
✦ How to maneuver stairs or curbs
✦ How to return to a sitting position
✦ What to do after a fall, such as coming to a sitting or erect position

Crutch walking. A physical therapist measures a client for crutches; in the community a nurse may perform the measurement. Crutches are measured to allow the client's elbow to flex at 30 degrees while holding the crutch handgrip. Crutch length is the measurement of the distance from 2 inches below the axilla to a mark placed 2 inches out and 6 inches ahead of the tip of the shoe. The nurse and therapist stress and reinforce the fact that a person's weight is supported on the handgrip, never under the axillae.

Depending on an individual client's abilities, the physical therapist prescribes a four-point alternate, two-point, or swing gait with the crutch. The four-point alternative gait is commonly used for persons with limited muscle strength or questionable balance. A very stable and safe gait pattern, the four-point gait is also a slow means of ambulation. The person begins in a crutch stance, elbows slightly flexed and crutch tips placed on the floor 6 inches out from the side of the shoe and 6 inches away from the shoe toes. The crutch axillary bar rests 2 inches below the axilla and is pressed against the chest for lateral stability. The four-point gait pattern is

✦ Left crutch
✦ Right leg
✦ Right crutch
✦ Left leg
✦ Repeat until the destination is reached

The two-point gait more closely resembles a walking gait pattern. Although more rapid than a four-point gait, the two-point gait requires better balance since only two points of contact occur with the floor at any given time. The client begins the gait from the standard crutch stance, then shifts weight to advance the right leg and left crutch simultaneously, follows through with the left leg and right crutch, and continues the pattern to destination.

Swing gaits are used for persons who are unable to bear weight on a lower extremity, such as following hip or leg fracture or amputation. Swing gaits vary from a slow but stable swing-to or step-to gait to a rapid but more complex swing-through gait.

In the step-to gait a client begins in the standard crutch stance, placing no weight on the affected extremity. Both crutches are lifted and moved ahead as a unit whenever the client bears weight on the unaffected extremity, then weight is shifted onto the crutches. The client steps up to the crutches and repeats the step-to gait process. In the step-through or swing-through gait, the client begins in a standard crutch stance. Again both crutches are moved 4 to 6 inches ahead as a single unit as the client supports weight on the unaffected extremity. This time, when the client shifts weight onto the crutches, the unaffected leg is "swung through" to set down in advance of the other leg, landing ahead of the crutches. The process is repeated until the person ambulates the desired distance.

Ambulation with a cane. Canes are available in many styles with features appropriate for specific client needs and lifestyles. For instance, a straight cane makes a single point of contact with the floor whereas quad-footed or tripod canes provide broader bases of support but are bulkier to handle (Fig. 14-13). A person's cane length is equal to the distance between the greater trochanter and the floor. A properly measured cane enables a client to stand with elbows slightly flexed when the cane tip is set on the floor about 6 inches to the side of the foot (Deathe, Hayes, & Winter, 1993). To walk with a cane, the client stands placing weight on both feet and on the hand holding the cane.

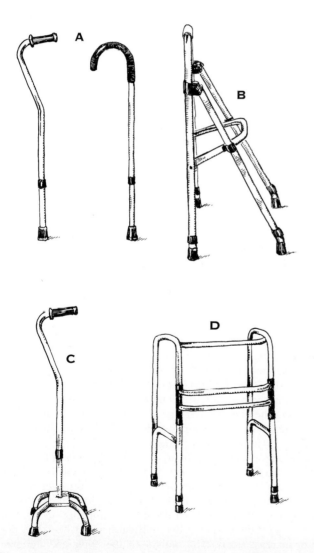

Fig. 14-13 Assistive devices for ambulation. **A,** Straight canes. **B,** Pickup walker. **C,** Quad cane. **D,** Standard walker.

The cane is held on the unaffected side; initially there is a tendency for clients to place the cane on the affected side. The client advances the cane 4 to 6 inches, moves the affected leg up to the cane, supports weight on the affected leg and the cane, then continues by moving the other leg past the cane; this process is repeated for the desired distance. The nurse monitors the client's posture and body alignment and assures the client practices in areas typical of daily living.

A client with hemiplegia may wear a short leg orthosis for the affected lower extremity. Since this brace is attached to the shoe and extends to just below the knee, a client can use it as an aid when raising the toes off the floor during walking, when striking the heel back to the floor, and in preventing the ankle from turning inward during ambulation. The client's standing balance and ambulation activities also may be improved by wearing a sling on the affected arm. A sling keeps the weight of the affected arm close to the body, thereby improving balance and preventing accidental injury or dislocation of the arm. Slings must be properly applied and worn; they are tailored to meet specific client needs by the occupational therapist.

The construction of a sling varies, but traditionally is a one- or two-piece support for the arm, with straps or webbing that distribute weight of the arm across the upper trunk. Dynamic slings are fashioned of elastic, dental dam, or tourniquet hosing, which gives resistance to the triceps as it contracts and provides a quick stretch to the triceps as the arm snaps back up in response to the sling's elasticity (Marsolais & Kobetic, 1983). In addition to providing support, a sling may increase ROM at the shoulder.

Ambulation with a walker. Walkers vary according to structure and purpose. A client able to maintain balance and lift the walker can use one of the lightweight, adjustable, pickup walkers. Reciprocal walkers are suitable for those who might lose their balance and fall backward when lifting a regular walker. Rolling walkers, with or without a seat, are energy efficient; however, the instability of rolling walkers prohibits some clients from using them. A client is measured for a walker as for a cane described previously (Deathe, et al., 1993).

The gait pattern with the pickup walker is to advance the walker, step forward with each leg in turn, keep steps equal, assure balance, and repeat with advancing the walker. An alternate gait is to advance the pickup walker, step with the right foot, advance the walker, step with the left foot, and continue the pattern. Remind clients not to step while the walker is off the floor (Fig. 14-13).

Lower limb bracing. A person with paraplegia may be a candidate for functional ambulation. Long leg orthotics combined with crutches or a walker and the Orlau Swivel Walker are assistive devices for ambulation. Although controversial, electrical stimulation also is used to promote functional ambulation.

Long leg braces, or knee-ankle-foot orthoses, provide stabilizers at the knee, ankle, and foot, making ambulation possible with the assistance of crutches or a walker. Research findings indicate, however, that persons with paraplegia who wear knee-ankle-foot orthoses expend 5 to 13 times as much energy during ambulation as other persons (McClary, 1983).

The Orlau Swivel Walker (Orthotic Research and Locomotor Assessment Unit) consists of a rigid, stable steel frame. The client is held upright in the frame by a thoracic band, a sacral band, and a knee clamp; footplates are sloped upward and outward. The walker moves forward as the client shifts weight from one side to the other. The Orlau Swivel Walker has advantages of increased stability and easy mobility, without depending on the upper extremities for support. However, it provides a very slow method of mobility. Research indicates that this is the least efficient method metabolically when compared with knee-ankle-foot orthoses and wheelchair mobility (Sanchez, Bussey, & Petorak, 1983).

Research using electrical stimulation as an ambulatory aid following paraplegia has dealt with limited groups to date. A four-channel stimulator enables a client with paraplegia to sit, stand, and walk. Equipment and procedures need refinement and further research testing before the stimulator can be used widely (Bajd, Kralj, Turk, Benko, & Sega, 1983; Marsolais and Kobetic, 1983).

Lower limb prosthesis. Although the person with an amputation is mobile with a walker or crutches, a prosthesis provides more stable and acceptable ambulation. In some instances a rigid plaster dressing and pylon may be applied immediately after the amputation. Immediate postsurgical fitting permits the person to participate in transfer and ambulation activities very soon after surgery. However, these persons, as well as those with traditional postoperative treatment, must wait until shrinkage subsides in the residual limb before being fitted with a permanent prosthesis.

A physiatrist prescribes a prosthesis specific for each client, which is then constructed by a prosthetist. Basically the lower limb prosthesis for a person with an above-the-knee amputation consists of a socket, joints at the hip and knee, a suspension system, and a foot and ankle. Specialized cushioned feet and unique knee joints, such as for athletic activities, and computer-assisted design and computer-assisted manufacture (CAD-CAM) represent only a few of the innovations in prosthetics. Because of the diversity of the components available, the prescription and construction are complicated. The suspension system, for instance, may involve a suction system, pelvic band, waist belt, and leather thigh corset.

For some with above-the-knee amputations, one prosthesis style incorporates a hydraulic cylinder to coordinate gait at the hip and knee, which allows a client to walk at several speeds and sustain a quality gain through successive swing and stance phases (Laughman, Youdas, & Garrett, 1983; Mills, 1984). A client is taught to avoid the habit of a pelvic tilt while standing and during ambulation.

The prosthesis should be functional while appearing as natural as possible. Prosthetic design takes the following into account:

+ Length and condition of the residual limb
+ Size of the client's foot
+ Client's general status
+ Client's age, weight, agility, and endurance
+ Client's lifestyle, social goals, and vocation
+ Cosmetic considerations, including skin tone
+ Financial status and payment coverage
+ Individual motivation and family support

Once fitted with the prosthesis, a client continues gait training using a four-point or swing gait; many persons become able to maneuver independently while wearing the prosthesis.

The nurse teaches the client and family to inspect the surgical site and residual limb daily for redness, abrasions, or irritation. Instruction stresses hygiene, gentle care, preventing of edema, positioning to prevent contractures, and care of prosthetic stockings and the prosthetic limb. (Chapter 12 contains information about care of prosthetic stockings and illustrations for donning and doffing a lower extremity prosthesis.) All persons are cautioned to consult a prosthetist to assess or make any mechanical alterations or adjustments as well as for regular maintenance.

Wheelchair Mobility

When used 9 hours a day, the average life-span of a wheelchair in the United States is about 2 years; moreover only 49% to 79% of wheelchairs are used with longevity in mind (Kamm, Thelen, & Jensen, 1990). In many countries around the world, wheelchairs are a scarce commodity with little regard to fit or condition. Architectural barriers, village or countryside terrain, social construction of disability, and cost are a few of the factors that restrict wheelchairs for eligible persons in many countries. As a result persons have restricted access, impaired socialization, and reduced independence and opportunity for self-support. In a few countries persons with disabling conditions have established cottage industries for constructing wheelchairs. Although significantly less sophisticated than the multiple varieties and prescriptions available from manufacturers in the United States and other industrialized countries, these locally constructed wheelchairs are transportation and available.

✦ Wheelchair modifications

Wheelchairs are as diverse as the persons who use them. The prescription for a wheelchair often lists specific recommendations for modifications for a client's needs. Wheelchair height and width are based on the client's physical dimensions, with a goal of proper seated posture for the person when sitting in the wheelchair (Mattingly, 1993). The back and seat of a wheelchair can be modified to accommodate antipressure devices and additional positioning supports. High-back, reclining-back, and other backs are available on wheelchairs for persons who need head and neck support or who tolerate the erect seated position poorly. In a client's initial transfer activities out of bed, the nurse may provide a wheelchair that flattens out completely, enabling the client to perform a simple sliding transfer into the chair. The wheelchair back is then elevated and the client moves into a seated position.

Folding wheelchairs, many with detachable armrests and legrests to facilitate transfers, are transported easily. Clients who have upper body strength may load their own wheelchairs into a car. Cars may be fitted with hand controls enabling persons who pass a driver's examination to operate their own vehicle. As a rule modifications in wheelchair design increase costs. The weight of the chair and the size and type of tires are considerations when a client is traveling within or outside the home. Generally, heavier chairs with tires of more durable construction are better suited to the outdoors; those with lightweight frames, high-quality bearings, and tubular tires may be designed specifically for racing.

Manual hand controls, as well as electronic touch and breath control, can be used to propel a wheelchair. Energy-efficient methods of manual propulsion, such as arm cranks and handrims, are topics of research (Seymour, Knapp, Anderson, & Kerney, 1982). A client may have increased self-image when able to use the hands, rather than the chin, for propelling the wheelchair. With quadriplegia, clients may develop better balance when using hand controls since a manually operated chair does not require a control box, which some persons tend to lean on for support (Mayerson & Milano, 1984).

✦ Psychological aspects

Although some clients may feel a threat to self-esteem when dependent on a wheelchair for mobility, the increased access and conservation of energy allows more and diverse activities that may outweigh the psychological need to ambulate. A study involving elderly persons following bilateral below-the-knee amputations found the clients preferred wheelchair mobility to ambulation on prostheses, since oxygen use and heart rate during ambulation were significantly higher during ambulation (Dubrow, Witt, Kadaba, Reyes, & Cochran, 1983). Competitive sports, such as wheelchair racing or basketball, promote physical, emotional, and social rehabilitation (Lucca & Recchiuti, 1983).

✦ Prescription criteria

Traditionally rehabilitation nurses evaluated clients and prepared "wheelchair prescriptions." Today under ideal circumstances, wheelchair design and use may be evaluated by a team: physical and occupational therapists, rehabilitation engineer, physiatrist, rehabilitation nurse, social worker, and psychologist. (Chapter 9 lists particular means for home and community assessment, and Chapter 5 contains information about access per the ADA.) In any country consult the consumers of wheelchair products for their evaluations.

Criteria for wheelchair prescription as the primary mode of mobility include the following:
- ✦ Energy expenditure and conservation
- ✦ Cost
- ✦ Physiologic factors
- ✦ Cosmetic and psychosocial factors
- ✦ Occupational and educational goals

The rehabilitation nurse and team members teach the client and family how to
- ✦ Transfer to and from the wheelchair, checking dependent body areas for signs of pressure
- ✦ Change position and shift weight while seated in the wheelchair
- ✦ Perform wheelchair maintenance
- ✦ Propel the wheelchair safely and reliably

In the community accessibility is an issue. It is essential to know the environment where the wheelchair will be used—for example, doorways and room dimensions are measured, as are exits and entrances, ramp placement; building access and levels of living area, method of transportation to and from living areas, feasibility of transfer from the wheelchair into a traditional motor vehicle, requirements of specialized or modified vans, and emergency services on call are considered.

SUMMARY

Movement science is a complex field of study involving many disciplines including rehabilitation nursing. Rehabilitation nurses working with clients and their families in the community will need to possess a theoretic knowledge of movement, as well as the structure and function of muscles, joints, bones, and nerves. A complete assessment of the musculoskeletal and nervous systems enables the nurse to formulate nursing diagnoses and set realistic goals with clients that complement the interventions of other members of the rehabilitation team. Educating a client and family about reasons for and methods of optimizing mobility increases the probability of follow-through, maintenance of optimal independence, effective coping, and adjustment, and prevention of further disability or complications.

◆

CASE STUDY
A MOVEMENT PRACTICE PROTOTYPE: CARE OF THE PATIENT WITH A TRAUMATIC BRAIN INJURY

Nursing diagnosis: Impaired physical mobility

Related factors	Nursing intervention	Outcome
Location of brain injury and CNS involvement	**ASSESSMENT**	Patient will
Peripheral neuromuscular impairment	Movement ability	Develop optimal mobility
Decreased strength and endurance	Physical endurance	Develop optimal endurance
Perceptual and cognitive impairment	Cognitive and perceptual deficits	Participate in movement therapy
Memory loss	Emotional response	Practice safe movement patterns
Inability to follow directions	Behavioral response	
Distractibility	Age-specific ability	
Short attention span	Need for devices	
Disorderliness		
Lack of common sense	**PLANNING**	
Inappropriate behavior	Coordinate interdisciplinary care	
Depression	Use common philosophic approaches	
Anxiety	Coordinate care with patient and family	
Motivation		
Age	**IMPLEMENTATION**	
Preexisting physical and mental conditions	Explain movement therapy	
	Involve patient and family	
	Reinforce abilities	
	Coordinate total body movement	
	Use repetitive teaching	
	Use demonstrations	
	Use return demonstrations	
	Provide necessary movement aids/devices	
	Provide safe environment	
	EVALUATION	
	Evaluate daily progress	
	Adapt movement therapy as necessary	

REFERENCES

Ahrens, W.D., Kinney, M.R., & Carter, R. (1983). The effect of antistasis footboard exercises on selected measures of exertion. Heart Lung *12*, 366-371.

Akeson W.H., Ing, D.A., Abel, M.F., Gorfin, S.R., & Woo, S.L-Y. (1987). Effects of immobilization upon joints. *Clinical Orthopaedics and Related Research, 219*, 28-37.

Anderson, M.E. (1993). The role of the cerebellum in motor control and motor learning. *Physical Medicine and Rehabilitation Clinics of North America, 4*, 623-636.

Bajd, T., Kralj, A., Turk, R., Benko, H., & Sega, J. (1983). Use of four-channel electrical stimulator as an ambulatory aid for paraplegic patients. *Physical Therapy, 63*, 1116-1120.

Bartlett, D. & Piper, M. (1994). Mother's difficulty in assessing the motor development of their infants born preterm with implications for intervention. *Pediatric Physical Therapy, 6*, 55-59.

Bates, B. (1994). *A guide to physical examination and history taking* (6th ed.). Philadelphia: J.B. Lippincott.

Bernstein, N. (1967). *Coordination and regulation of movements.* New York: Pergamon Press, Inc.

Bobath, B. (1978). *Adult hemiplegia: Evaluation and treatment* (2nd ed.). London: Heinemann Medical.

Borgman, M.F., & Passarella, P.M. (1991). Nursing care of the stroke patient using Bobath principles: An approach to altered movement. *Nursing Clinics of North America, 26*, 1019-1035.

Brazelton, T.B. (1984). *Neonatal behavioral assessment scale, 2nd ed.* Philadelphia: J.B. Lippincott.

Cerny, K. (1983). A clinical method of quantitative gait analysis: Suggestion from the field. *Physical Therapy, 63*, 1125-1126.

Chandler, L.S., Andrew, M.S., Swanson, M.W. (1980). Movement assessment of infants: A manual. Rolling Bay, WA: Rolling Bay Press.

Clarkson, B. (1983). Absorbent paper method for recording foot placement during gait: Suggestion from the field. *Physical Therapy, 63*, 345-346.

Clough, D.H., & Maurin, J.T. (1983). ROM versus NRx. *Journal of Gerontology Nursing, 9*, 278-286.

Congressional Research Service, Library of Congress. (1989). *Digest of data on persons with disabilities.* Washington, DC: Mathematica Policy Research.

Creason, N.S., Pogue, N.J., Nelson, A.A., & Hoyt, C.A. (1985). Validating the nursing diagnosis of impaired physical mobility. *Nursing Clinics North America, 20*, 669-683.

Dayhoff, N.E. (1975). Rethinking stroke: Soft or hard devices to position hands? *American Journal of Nursing, 75*, 1142-1144.

Deathe, A.B., Hayes, K.C., & Winter, D.A. (1993). The biomechanics of canes, crutches, and walkers. *Critical Reviews in Physical and Rehabilitation Medicine, 5*, 15-29.

de Leon, D., Moskowitz, C.B., & Stewart, C. (1991). Proposed guidelines for videotaping individuals with movement disorders. *Journal of Neuroscience Nursing. 23*, 191-193.

Demarest, C.B. (1983). Using prosthetics to aid independence. *Patient Care, 17*, 45-47, 50, 55-56.

Doheny, M. (1993). Mental practice: an alternative approach to teaching motor skills. *Journal of Nursing Education, 32*, 260-264.

Dubow, L.L., Witt, P.L., Kadaba, M.P., Reyes, R., & Cochran, G. VanB. (1983). Oxygen consumption of elderly persons with bilateral BKA: ambulation versus wheelchair propulsion. *Archives of Physical Medicine and Rehabilitation, 64*, 255-259.

Ducan, P.W., Chandler, J., Studenski, S., Hughes, B.S., & Prescott, B. (1993). How does the physiological component of balance affect mobility in elderly men? *Archives of Physical Medicine and Rehabilitation, 74*, 1343-1349.

Fiorentino, M.R. (1973). *Reflex testing methods for evaluating CNS development.* Springfield, IL: Charles C. Thomas, Publisher.

Glick, O.J. (1992). Interventions related to activity and movement. *Nursing Clinics of North America, 27*, 541-568.

Gordon, M. (1993). *Nursing diagnosis: Process and application* (2nd ed.). New York: McGraw-Hill.

Grimes, J., & Iannopollo, E. *Health assessment in nursing practice.* Monterey, CA: Wadsworth Publishing Company.

Hathaway, D., & Geden, E.A. (1983). Energy expenditure during leg exercise programs. *Nursing Research, 32*, 147-150.

Herzog, J.A. (1993). Deep vein thrombosis in the rehabilitative client: Diagnostic tools, prevention, and treatment modalities. *Rehabilitation Nursing, 18*, 8-11.

Hoeman, S.P. (1990). *Rehabilitation/restorative care in the community.* St. Louis: Mosby–Year Book.

Kotake, T., Dohi, N. (1993). An analysis of sit-to-stand movements. *Archives of Physical Medicine and Rehabilitation, 74*, 1095-1099.

Jamieson, S., & Dayhoff, N.E. (1980). A hard hand-positioning device to decrease wrist and finger hypertonicity: A sensorimotor approach for the patient with nonprogressive brain damage. *Nursing Research, 29*, 285-289.

Kamm, K., Thelen, E., & Jensen, J.L. (1990). A dynamic systems approach to motor development. *Physical Therapy, 70*, 763-775.

Kohn, J., Enders, S., Preston, J. Jr., & Motloch, W. (1983). Provisions of assistive equipment for the handicapped persons. *Archives of Physical Medicine and Rehabilitation, 64*, 378-381.

Laughman, R.K., Youdas, J.W., & Garrett, T.R. (1983). Strength changes in the normal quadriceps femoris muscle as a result of electrical stimulation. *Physical Therapy, 63*, 494-499.

Lew, M.F., & Waters, C.H. (1993). Post-traumatic movement disorders. *Physical Medicine and Rehabilitation: State of the Art, 7*, 519-526.

Lindh, M.H., Johansson, G.A., Hedberg, M., & Grimby, G.L. (1994). Studies on maximal voluntary muscle contraction in patients with fibromyalgia. *Archives of Physical Medicine and Rehabilitation, 75*, 1217-1222.

Lucca, J.A., & Recchiuti, S.J. (1983). Effect of electromyographic biofeedback on an isometric strengthening program. *Physical Therapy, 63*, 200-203.

Macdonald, L.P., Gift, A.G., Bell, R.W., & Soeken, K.L. (1993). Respiratory muscle strength in patients with postpolio syndrome. *Rehabilitation Nursing Research, 2*, 55-60.

Madorsky, J.G.B., & Madorsky, A. (1983). Wheelchair racing: An important modality in acute rehabilitation after paraplegia. *Archives of Physical Medicine and Rehabilitation, 64*, 186-187.

Marsolais, E.B., & Kobetic, R. (1983). Functional walking in paralyzed patients by means of electrical stimulation. *Clinical Orthopaedics and Related Research, 175*, 30-36.

Mason, D.J., & Redeker, N. (1993). Measurement of activity. *Nursing Research, 42*, 87-92.

Mathiowetz, V., Bolding, D.J., & Trombly, C.A. (1983). Immediate effects of positioning devices on the normal and spastic hand measured by electromyography. *American Journal of Occupational Therapy, 37*, 247-254.

Mattingly, D. (1993). Wheelchair selection. *Journal of Orthopedic Nursing, 12*, 11-17.

Mayerson, N.H., & Milano, R.A. (1984). Goniometric measurement reliability in physical medicine. *Archives of Physical Medicine and Rehabilitation, 65*, 92-94.

McClay, I. (1983). Electric wheelchair propulsion using a hand control in C4 quadriplegia. *Physical Therapy, 63*, 221-223.

Mehmert, P.A., & Delaney, C.W. (1991). Validating impaired physical mobility. *Nursing Diagnosis, 2*, 143-154.

Meier, R.H., III. (1994). Upper limb amputee rehabilitation *Physical Medicine and Rehabilitation: State of the Art Reviews, 8*, 165-185.

Merkel, K.D., Miller, N.E., Westbrook, P.R., & Merritt, J.L. (1984). Energy expenditure of paraplegic patients standing and walking with two knee ankle-foot orthoses. *Archives of Physical Medicine and Rehabilitation, 65*, 121-124.

Micheo, W.F., & Lopez, C.E. (1994). Rehabilitation of lower extremity traumatic amputees. *Physical Medicine and Rehabilitation: State of the Art Reviews, 8*, 193-199.

Milazzo, V., & Roush, C. (1982). Kinetic nursing—A new approach to the problems of immobilization. *Journal of Neurosurgical Nursing 14*, 120-124.

Milani-Comparetti, A., & Gidoni, E.A. (1967). Routine developmental examination in normal and retarded children. *Developmental Medical Child Neurology, 9*, 631-638.

Mills, V.M. (1984). Electromyelographic results of inhibitory splinting. *Physical Therapy, 64*, 190-193.

Moskowitz, C. (1991). The American Association of Neuroscience Nurses (AANN) officially recognized an informal group of movement disorder nurses (letter). *Journal of Neuroscience Nursing, 23*, 144.

Mouradian, L.E., & Als, H. (1994). The influence of neonatal intensive care unit caregiving practices in motor functioning and preterm infants. *American Journal of Occupational Therapy, 48*, 527-533.

Murray-Slutsky, C. (1994). Dyspraxia with motor dysfunction. *Rehabilitation Management, 126-128.

Murray, M.P., Mollinger, L.A., Sepic, S.B., & Gardner, G.M. (1983). Gait patterns in patients: A hydraulic swing control versus constant knee components friction. *Archives of Physical Medicine and Rehabilitation, 64*, 339-345.

Noble, L.J., Salcido, R., Walker, M.K., Atchinson, J., & Marshall, R. (1994). Improving functional ability through exercise. *Rehabilitation Nursing Research, 3*, 23-29.

Oldham, J., Tallis, R., Howe, T., & Petterson, T. (1992). Objective assessment of muscle function. *Nursing Standard, 6*, 37-39.

Olson, E.V. (1967). The hazards of immobility. *American Journal of Nursing, 67*, 781-797.

Passarella, P., & Gee, Z. (1987). Starting right after stroke. *American Journal of Nursing, 87*, 802-807.

Paulson, G.W. & others. (1993). Oral and facial movement in the aged. *Journal of Neuroscience Nursing, 25*, 246-248.

Roberts, B., & Fitzpatrick, J. (1983). Improving balance: therapy of movement. *Journal of Gerontology Nursing, 9*, 150-156.

Rose, V. (1992). Understanding motor neuro disease. *Professional Nursing, 7*, 784-786.

Rothstein, J.M., Miller, P.J., & Roettger, R.F. (1983). Goniometric reliability . . . in a clinical setting: Elbow and knee measurements *Physical Therapy, 63,* 1611-1615.

Rough, R.E., Hocomb, J.D., & Wilson, G. (1988). *Basic rehabilitation techniques—A self instructional guide.* Rockville, MD: Aspen.

Rubin, M. (1988). The physiology of bedrest. *American Journal of Nursing, 88,* 50, 55, 57-58.

Rubino, F.A. (1993). Gait disorders in the elderly: distinguishing between normal and dysfunctional gaits. *Postgraduate Medicine, 1,* 185-188, 190, 195-197.

Rush, K.L. & Ovellet, L.L. (1993). Mobility: A concept-analysis. *Journal of Advanced Nursing, 18,* 486-492.

Samuels, M.A. (1989). Making sense of movement disorder. *Emergency Medicine, 15,* 20-24, 29-33.

Sanchez, D.G., Bussey, B., & Petorak, M. (1983). Air fluidized beds revolutionize skin care. *RN, 46,* 46-48.

Schmidt, L.S., Wescott, S.L., & Crowe, T.R. (1993). Interrater reliability of the gross motor scale of the Peabody Developmental Motor Scales with 4 and 5 year old children. *Pediatric Physical Therapy, 5,* 169-175.

Segatore, M. (1991). Determining the interrater reliability of motor power assessment using a spinal cord testing record. *Journal of Neuroscience Nursing, 23,* 220-223.

Seymour, R.J., Knapp, C.F., Anderson, T.R., & Kearney, J.T. (1982). Paraplegic use of Orlau swivel walker: Case report. *Archives of Physical Medicine and Rehabilitation, 63,* 490-494.

Slifer, K.J., Bucholtz, J.D., & Cataldo, M.D. (1994). Behavioral training of motion control in young children undergoing radiation treatment with sedation. *Journal of Pediatric Oncology Nursing, 11,* 35-63.

Smith, P.A., Glaser, R.M., Petrofsky, J.S., Underwood, P.D., Smith, G.B., & Richard, J.J. (1983). Arm crank versus handrim wheelchair propulsion: metabolic and cardiopulmonary responses. *Archives of Physical Medicine and Rehabilitation, 64,* 249-254.

Snyder, M.J. (1988). Movement therapy. *Journal of Neuroscience Nursing, 20,* 373-376.

Squires, A.J. (1983). Using the tilt table for elderly patients. *Physiotherapy, 69,* 150-151.

Steinbrecher, S.M. (1994). The Revised NIOSH Lifting Guidelines. *AAOHN, 42,* 62-66.

Stewart, N.J., McMullen, L.M., & Rubin, L.D. (1994). Movement therapy with depressed inpatients: a randomized multiple single case design. *Archives of Psychiatric Nursing, 8,* 22-29.

Styrcula, L. (1994). Traction basics part I. *Orthopedic Nursing, 13,* 71-74.

Tappen, R.M. (1994). The effect of skill training on functional abilities of nursing home residents with dementia. *Research, Nursing and Health, 17,* 159-165.

Thompson, M.B., & Coppens, N.M. (1994). The effects of guided imagery on anxiety levels and movement of clients undergoing magnetic resonance imaging. *Holistic Nursing Practice, 8,* 59-69.

Topp, R., Mikesky, A., & Bawel, K. (1994). Developing a strength training program for older adults: Planning, programming, and potential outcomes. *Rehabilitation Nursing, 19,* 266-273, 297.

Trombly, C.A. (1989). *Occupational therapy for physical dysfunction.* Baltimore: Williams & Wilkins.

Turner, H., & Hinkle, J. (1987). Motor response study. *Journal of Neuroscience Nursing, 19,* 336-340.

U.S. Public Health Service. Up and around—a booklet to aid the stroke patient in activities of daily living. U.S. Public Health Service Publication No. 1120. Washington, DC: U.S. Government Printing Office.

VanSant, A.F. (1990). Life-span development in functional tasks. *Physical Therapy, 70,* 788-798.

Waters, R.I., Adkins, R.H., Yakura, J.S., & Sie, I. (1994). Motor and sensory recovery following incomplete tetraplegia. *Archives of Physical Medicine and Rehabilitation, 75,* 306-311.

Winstein, C.J., & Knecht, H.G. (1990). Movement science and its relevance to physical therapy. *Physical Therapy, 70,* 759-762.

Woollacott, M.H., & Shumway-Cook, A. (1990). Changes in posture control across the life span—A systems approach. *Physical Therapy, 70,* 799-807.

SUGGESTED READINGS

Appell, H.J. (1986). Skeletal muscle atrophy during immobilization. *International Journal of Sports Medicine, 7,* 1-5.

Bergstrom, D., & Coles, C.H. (1971). *Basic positioning procedures.* Rehabilitation Publication 701, Minneapolis: Sister Kenny Institute.

Bohannon, R.W. (1983). Taping and stabilizing ankles of patients with hemiplegia. *Physical Therapy, 63,* 524-525.

Bohannon, R.W., Thorne, M., & Mierer, A.C. (1983). Shoulder positioning devices for patients with hemiplegia. *Physical Therapy, 63,* 49-50.

Chin, P.L. (1982). Physical techniques in stroke rehabilitation. *Journal of the Royal College of Physicians of London, 16,* 165-169.

Creason, N.S., Pogue, N.J., Nelson, A.A., & Hoyt, CA. (1985). Validating the nursing diagnosis of impaired physical mobility. *Nursing Clinics of North America, 20,* 669-683.

Crockett, J.E. (1982). Power grasp aid to rehabilitation. *Physiotherapy, 68,* 224.

Davies, P., & Ryan, D.W. (1983). Stevens-Johnson syndrome managed in the Clinitron bed, *Intensive Care Medicine, 9,* 87-89.

Getz, P.A., & Blossom, B.M. (1982). Preventing contractures: The little extras that help so much. *Research Nursing, 45,* 44-48.

Hale, S.S., & Stephens, S.E. (1983). Neurological treatment. *Physiotherapy, 69,* 72-75.

Hill, I. (1983). Equipped for the job: Mobile hoists. *Nursing Times, 79,* 24-27.

Hoffman, D., Kusek, N., & Tonjuk, A.M. (1983). Pneumatic lift as an aid to positioning the strength compromised patient. *Physical Therapy, 63,* 969-970.

Hultman, E., & Sjoholm, H. (1982). B/P and HR response to voluntary and nonvoluntary static exercise in man. *Acta Physiologica Scandinavica, 115,* 499-501.

Knapik, J., Knapik, J.J., Wright, J.E., Mawdsky, R.H., & Braun, J. (1983). Isometric, Isotonic, and isokinetic torque variations in four muscle groups through a range of joint motion. *Physical Therapy, 63,* 938-947.

Konikow, N.S. (1985). Alterations in movement: Nursing assessment and implications. *Journal of Neurosurgical Nursing, 17,* 61.

Lainey, C.G., Walmsley, R.P., & Andrew, C.M. (1983). Effectiveness of exercise alone versus exercise plus electrical stimulation in strengthening the quadriceps muscle. *Physiotherapy Canada, 35,* 5.

Lowenthal, D.T., Bharadwaja, K., & Oakes, W.W. (eds.). (1979). *Therapeutics through exercise.* New York: Grune & Stratton.

Malkiewicz, J. (1982). A pragmatic approach to musculoskeletal assessment. *Rehabilitation Nursing, 45,* 56.

McCabe, J.B., & Nolan, D.J. (1986). Comparison of the effectiveness of different cervical immobilization collars. *Annals of Emergency Medicine, 15,* 50.

O'Sullivan, S.B., Cullen, K.E., & Schmitz, T.J. (1981). *Physical rehabilitation: Evaluation and treatment procedures.* Philadelphia: F.A. Davis.

Passarella, P.M., & Lewis, N. (1987). Nursing application of Bobath principles in stroke care. *Journal of Neuroscience Nursing, 19,* 106.

Reddy, M.P. (1986). A guide to early mobilization of bedridden elderly. *Geriatrics, 41,* 59.

Regan, T.J. (1983). Proper use of wheelchairs, *Journal of the American Geriatric Society, 31,* 126.

Scales, J.T., & Lowthian, P.T. (1982). Vapern patient-support system: a new general purpose hospital mattress. *Lancet, 2,* 1150.

Selkurt, E.E. (ed.) (1982). *Basic physiology for the health sciences.* Boston: Little, Brown.

Siegel, I.M., & Silverman, M. (1983). Contoured seating for the wheelchair bound patient with neuromuscular disease. *Physical Therapy, 63,* 1625.

Siegler, S., Selktar, R., & Hyman, W. (1982). Simulation of human gait with the aid of a mechanical model. *Journal of Biomechanics, 15,* 415.

Shelton, M.E., & Guise, E.P. (1982). Variation on pylon for BKA. *Physical Therapy, 62,* 1601.

Soderberg, G.L., & Cook, T.M. (1983). Electromyographic analysis of quadriceps femoris muscle setting and straight lig raising. *Physical Therapy, 63,* 1434.

Sorenson, L., & Ulrich, P.G. (1974). Ambulation guide for nurses. Rehabilitation Publication 707. Minniapolis: Sister Kenny Institute.

Stanton, K.M., Pepping, M., & Brockway, J.A. (1983). Wheelchair transfer training for right cerebral dysfunctions: an interdisciplinary approach. *Archives of Physical Medicine and Rehabilitation, 64*, 276.

Stephens, T.E., & Lattimore, J. (1983). Prescriptive checklist for positioning multihandicapped residential clients. *Physical Therapy, 63*, 1113.

Stern, R.B., & Walley, M. (1983). Functional comparison of upper extremity amputees using myoelectric and conventional prostheses. *Archives of Physical Medicine and Rehabilitation, 64*, 243.

Sullivan, P.E., Markos, P.D., & Minor, M.A.D. (1982). *An integrated approach to therapeutic exercise theory and clinical applications.* Reston, VA: Reston Publishing.

Tiller, J., Stygar, M.K., & Hess, C. (1982). Treatment of functional chronic stooped posture using a training device and behavior therapy. *Physical Therapy, 62*, 1597.

Toth, L. (1983). Spasticity management in spinal cord injury. *Rehabilitation Nursing, 8*, 14.

Walker, J. (1983). Modified strapping of roll sling. *American Journal of Occupational Therapy, 37*, 110.

Warren, M.L. (1984). A comparative study on the presence of the asymmetrical tonic neck reflex in adult hemiplegia. *American Journal of Occupational Therapy, 38*, 386.

Wevers, H.W. (1983). Wheelchair and occupant restraint system for transportion of handicapped passengers. *Archives of Physical Medicine and Rehabilitation, 64*, 374.

Weiss, P.L., & St. Pierre, D. (1983). Upper and lower extremity EMG correlations during normal gait. *Archives of Physical Medicine and Rehabilitation, 64*, 11.

Wilder, P.A., & Sykes, J. (1982). Using an isokinetic exercise machine to improve the gait pattern in a hemiplegic patient. *Physical Therapy, 62*, 1291.

Winter, D.A. (1983). Knee flexion during stance as a determinant of inefficient walking. *Physical Therapy, 63*, 331.

Woodburne, R. (Ed.). (1983). *Essentials of human anatomy* (7th ed.). New York: Oxford University Press.

Yetzer, E.A., Kauffman, G., Sopp, F., & Talley, L. (1994). Development of a patient education program for new amputees. *Rehabilitation Nursing, 19*, 355-358.

✦

Appendix 14-A   Range of motion: Passive, active, and functional

I. Terms: range of motion (ROM): amount of movement present in a joint
   A. Types of ROM
      1. Flexion: bending joint
      2. Extension: straightening joint
      3. Abduction: motion away from midline
      4. Abduction: motion toward midline
      5. Circumduction: circular movement
      6. Internal/external rotation:
      7. Pronation/supination of elbow
      8. Plantar flexion: downward motion of foot at ankle joint
      9. Dorsiflexion: upward motion of foot at ankle joint
      10. Inversion/eversion of ankle
   B. Passive ROM: the nurse moves the extremity in order that full motion occurs at the joint
   C. Active ROM: client uses his muscles to do the moving
   D. Functional activities of ROM: many activities of daily living (ADL) produce full ROM (e.g., rolling over in bed, sitting up, getting dressed); ROM can be done in conjunction with bed bathing, bed positioning, and mobilization activities
   E. Progressive resistive exercises (PRE): muscles begin to work against gravity, enhancing the strength of the muscle
II. General nursing interventions
   A. Explain all activities to client and assure safety
   B. Reinforce all teaching to client and family
   C. Move clients arms and legs gently during ROM and move within client's tolerance and flexibility
   D. Support the extremity above and below the joint being treated
   E. Give passive ROM when client is in the supine position
   F. Perform each exercise 5-10 times during each treatment
   G. Assess the motion of the involved side against the ROM of the uninvolved side
   H. Perform ROM on all extremities if client is immobilized
   I. Use proper body mechanics yourself
III. Specific nursing intervention: upper extremity
   A. Upper extremity ROM: flexion/extension (Fig. 14-14, *A*)
      1. Support the arm at the wrist and elbow
      2. Lift the arm straight over client's head
      3. Rest the arm flat on the bed above the head
      4. Bend client's elbow if there is not enough room for the entire motion
   B. Upper extremity ROM: abduction/adduction (Fig. 14-14, *B*)
      1. Support the arm at the wrist and elbow with client's palm facing his body
      2. Slide the arm sideways away from the body
      3. Allow the arm to roll or turn over when it reaches about a 90-degree angle with the shoulder
      4. Bend client's elbow if there is not enough room for the entire move
   C. Upper extremity: external/internal rotation (Fig. 14-14, *C*)
      1. Support client's hand and shoulder
      2. Bring the arm away from client's side, forming a 90-degree angle with the body
      3. Keep the elbow bent 90 degrees and the arm supported on the bed
      4. Press down on the shoulder toward the bed

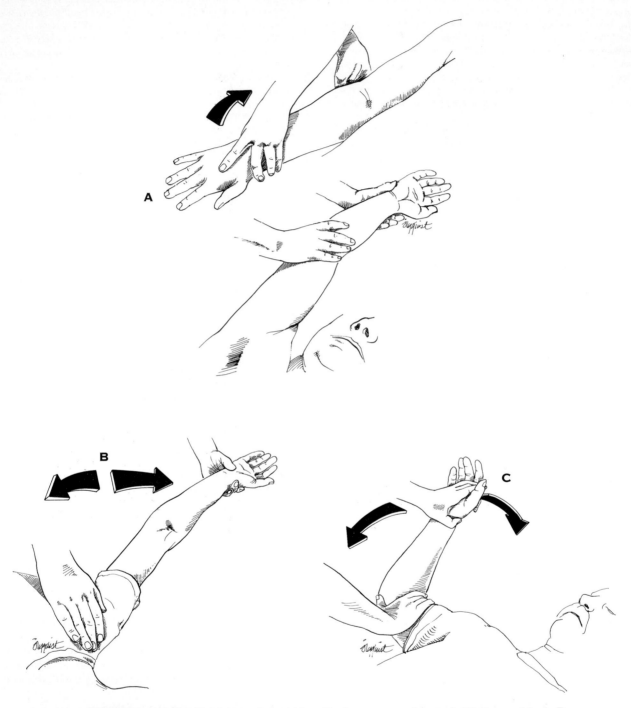

Fig. 14-14   **A,** Shoulder in extended position. Flexion occurs as the arm is lifted up and back. **B,** Sliding the arm toward body produces shoulder adduction. Sliding the arm away from body produces abduction. **C,** As the forearm is brought down, internal rotation occurs at the shoulder joint. As the forearm is brought up and back, external rotation occurs.

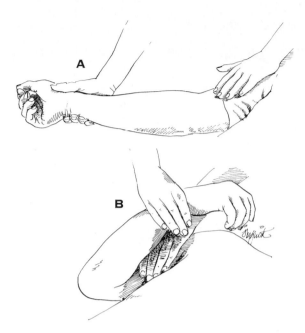

Fig. 14-15 **A,** Elbow extension. **B,** Elbow flexion.

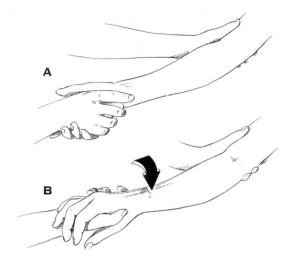

Fig. 14-16 **A,** Forearm in supination. **B,** Rolling the forearm downward places it in pronation.

5. Move client's hand backward until the back of the hand touches the bed
6. Move client's hand forward until the palm touches the bed

D. Upper extremity: elbow flexion/extension (Fig. 14-15)
   1. Support the elbow and wrist
   2. Bend client's arm to touch the hand to the shoulder
   3. Straighten the arm toward the bed

E. Upper extremity: pronate/supinate (Fig. 14-16)
   1. Support the upper arm and wrist
   2. Turn palm of client's hand toward the feet
   3. Turn palm of client's hand upward from the feet

F. Upper extremity: wrist (Fig. 14-17)
   1. Support client's wrist and hand and hold client's fingers in the other hand; bend wrist forward and make a fist
   2. Bend wrist backward and extend fingers; move wrist laterally

G. Upper extremity: finger flexion/extension (Fig. 14-18, *A-C*)
   1. Support client's hand by holding the palm of the hand
   2. Bend all fingers at once
   3. Straighten all fingers at once

H. Upper extremity: thumb abduction (Fig. 14-18, *D*)
   1. Support client's hand by holding the fingers straight with one hand
   2. Pull the thumb away from the palm
   3. Stretch the web space between the thumb and index finger

I. Upper extremity: thumb opposition (Fig. 14-18, *E*)
   1. Support the hand as in thumb abduction
   2. Move the thumb toward the little finger
   3. Move the thumb through a semicircle design

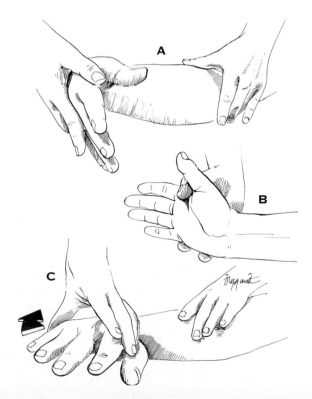

Fig. 14-17 **A,** Flexed wrist. **B,** Extended wrist. **C,** Lateral movement of the wrist produces radial and ulnar deviation.

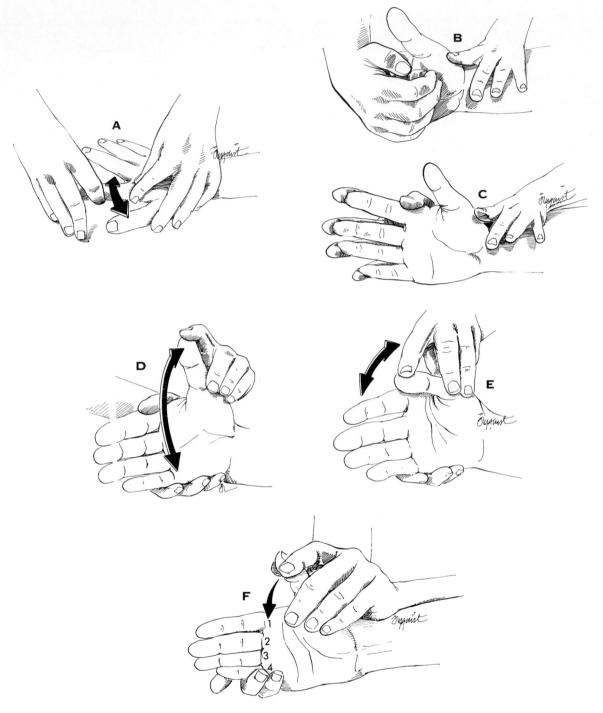

Fig. 14-18   **A,** Fingers abducted away from the midline and adducted toward the midline (of hand). **B,** Fingers flexed as a group into a closed fist. **C,** Finger extension is described as an open fist. **D,** Thumb flexed toward and extended away from the fourth digit. **E,** Thumb abducted and adducted in relation to the other fingers. **F,** Thumb moved in opposition to the base of each of the other four digits.

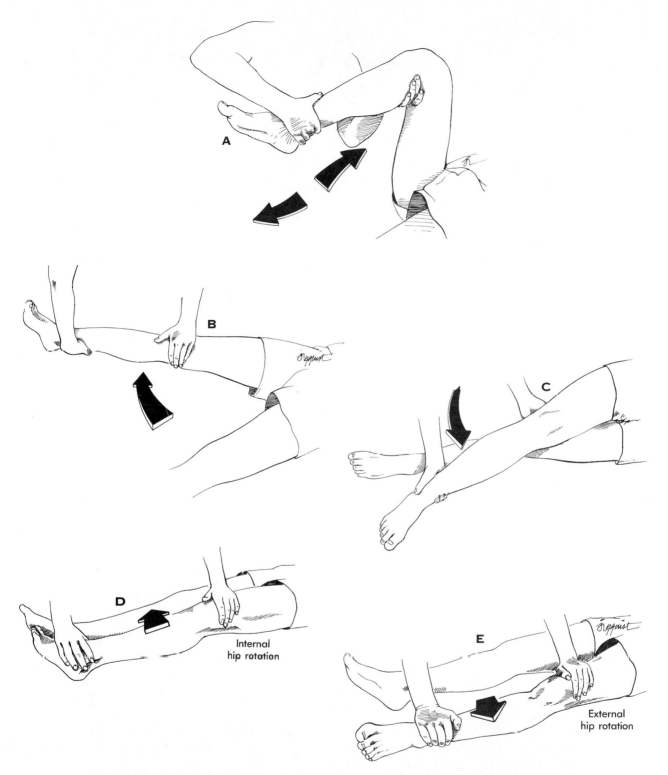

Fig. 14-19   **A,** Caregiver can move the hip in flexion by sliding the leg back. Extension can be produced by sliding the leg forward. **B,** Moving the leg away from the midline of the body abducts the hip. **C,** Moving the leg toward the midline of the body and crossing over it adducts the hip. **D,** Rolling the leg inward causes the hip joint to rotate internally. **E,** Rolling the leg outward causes the hip joint to rotate externally.

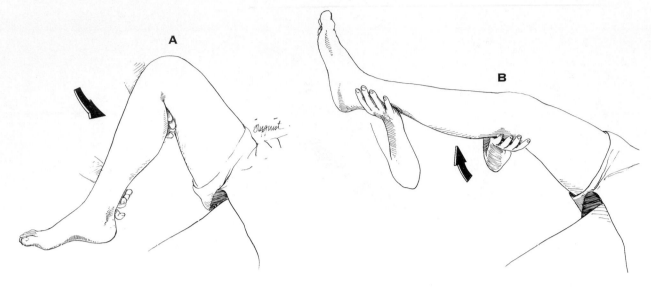

Fig. 14-20   **A,** Knee and hip position of flexion. **B,** Movement of the lower leg upward produces knee extension. The hip also is in extension.

IV. Lower extremity: specific nursing interventions
  A. Lower extremity: hip flexion (Fig. 14-19, *A*)
    1. Support under client's knee and heel
    2. Raise the knee toward the chest
    3. Bend the hip as much as possible
    4. Allow the knee to bend slightly or within client's tolerance
  B. Lower extremity: hip flexion/strength (Fig. 14-19, *B*)
    1. Support under client's knees and heel
    2. Lift client's leg straight and as high as possible
    3. Hold for count of 5
    4. Lower the leg gently
  C. Lower extremity: hip abduction/adduction (Fig. 14-19, *B* and *C*)
    1. Support client's knee and heel, keeping the leg in "toes up" position
    2. Move the leg toward the midline of the body and cross over the other leg
    3. Move the leg toward the other leg
  D. Lower extremity: hip internal and external rotation (Fig. 14-19, *D* and *E*)
    1. Support under client's knee and heel
    2. Bend the hip up to 90 degrees and bend the knee up to 90 degrees
    3. Turn the lower leg toward you, keeping the hip and knee in place
    4. Turn the lower leg away from you, keeping the hip and knee in place
    5. Do not force this motion

  E. Lower extremity: hip internal/external rotation (see Fig. 14-19, *D* and *E*)
    1. Support client's leg by placing your hand on top of client's knee and ankle
    2. Roll the leg inward
    3. Roll the leg outward
  F. Lower extremity: knee flexion/extension (Fig. 14-20)
    1. Support the leg as necessary at the heel and behind the knee
    2. Flex high 90 degrees
    3. Bend and straighten knees (strengthens hamstrings)
  G. Lower extremity: heel cord stretching (Fig. 14-21)
    1. Support client's calf with one hand and press downward on client's leg with the other hand
    2. Pull down on heel
    3. Press your forearm against client's foot, pushing client's foot toward the leg
    4. Hold for count of 5 and relax
  H. Lower extremity: toe flexion/extension (see Fig. 14-9)
    1. Support client's foot
    2. Bend all toes downward
    3. Push all toes backward
  I. Lower extremity: heel inversion/eversion (Fig. 14-22)
    1. Support client's leg bed with one hand and hold the foot with the other hand
    2. Turn foot outward
    3. Turn foot inward

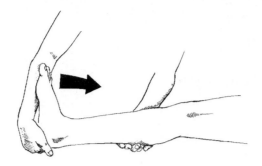

Fig. 14-21   Heel cord stretching involves downward pull on the heel cord and dorsiflexion of the ankle.

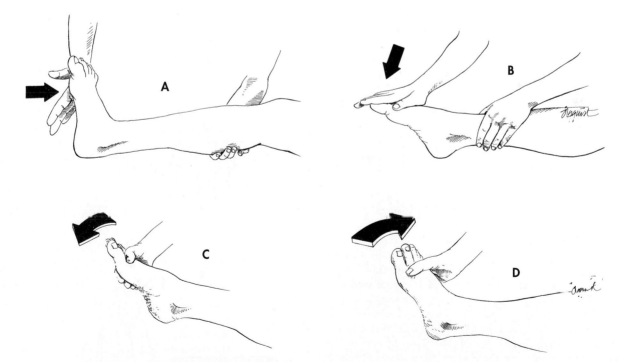

Fig. 14-22   **A,** Pressure with the palm of the hand against the ball of the foot causes ankle dorsiflexion. **B,** Pressure against the top of the foot causes ankle plantar flexion. **C,** Turning the foot inward produces ankle inversion. **D,** Turning the foot outward produces ankle eversion.

Appendix 14-B   Moving exercises (Figs. 14-23–14-26)

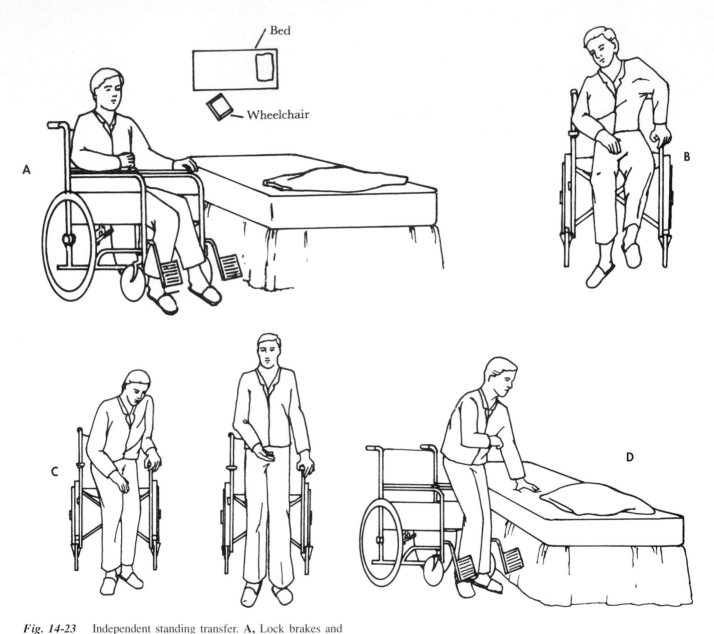

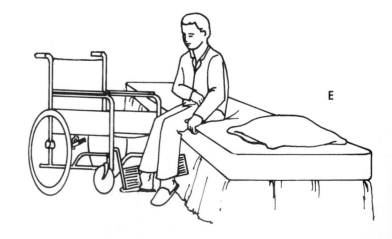

Fig. 14-23   Independent standing transfer. **A,** Lock brakes and lift footrests. Angle the wheelchair close to the bed, facing the head of the bed, preferably on the client's *unaffected* side. Instruct the client to place both feet flat on the floor. **B,** The unaffected foot should be placed directly beneath the wheelchair seat. It will be slightly behind the *affected* foot. The client's *unaffected* hand should be on the armrest and the client should be sitting to the front of the wheelchair seat. **C,** As the client leans forward on the *unaffected* foot and pushes on the armrest, he or she will rise to a standing position. **D,** The client should continue to use the armrest and keep his or her feet slightly apart for safety and balance. If the client is tall, an adjustable height armrest may be needed for the client to stand erect and safely maintain balance. **E,** The client uses his or her *unaffected* arm to balance and support himself or herself on the edge of the bed. The client should be instructed to take short side steps to turn toward the *unaffected* side. When the client's back is perpendicular to the side of the bed, he or she can then sit.

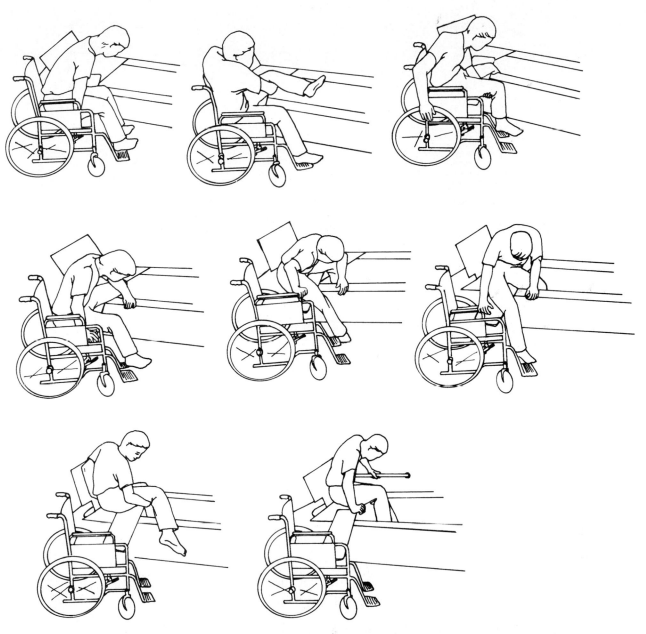

Fig. 14-24   A transfer board may be used to move a client from a wheelchair onto a bathtub seat. Carefully follow directions from the nurse supervisor or physical therapist. Because the client's safety is a priority, a transfer belt may be needed. Practice the transfer under the direction of the nurse supervisor or physical therapist before the client moves to the tub.

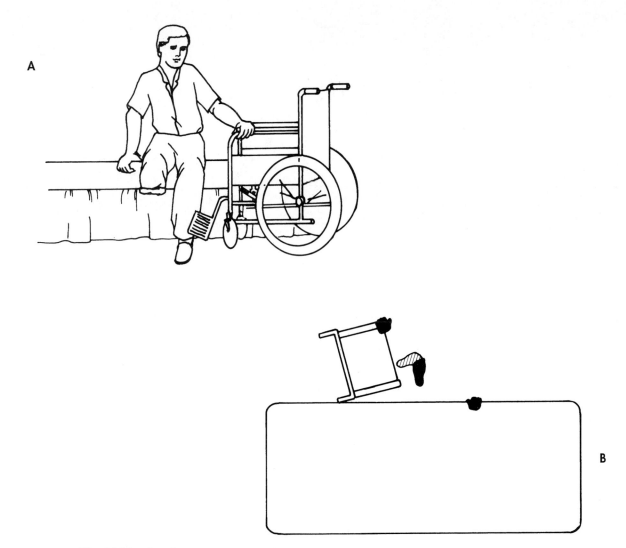

Fig. 14-25 Standing transfers adapted for the person with a lower limb amputation. Lock the brakes or casters and swing away the footrests. The client places their *residual* foot slightly forward to bear most of their body weight. The client then pivots on the *residual* foot and leg to affect a change of position. Placing a hand on the armrest of the wheelchair before the move gives the client the support and balance needed to safely perform the transfer.

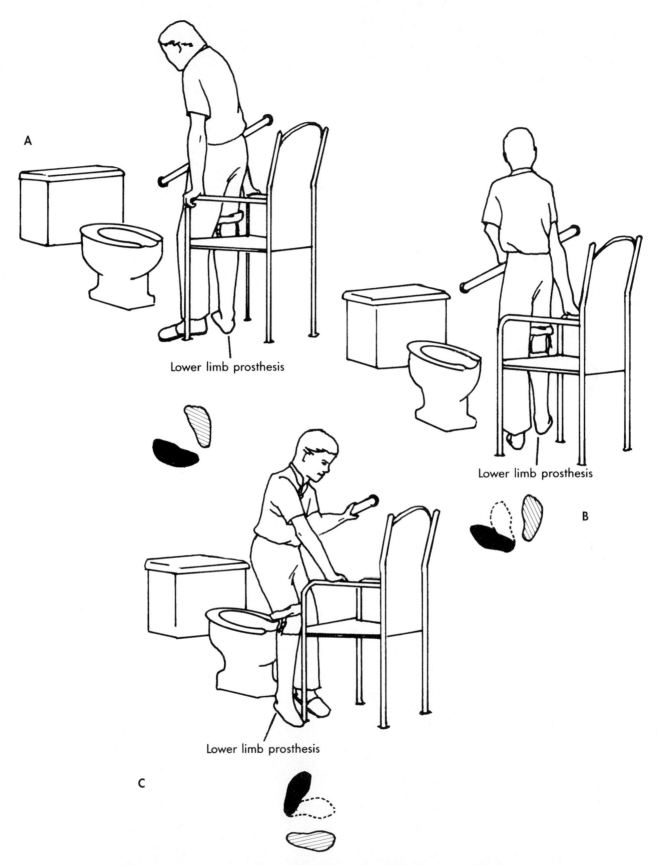

Fig. 14-26 Pivot transfer for the client wearing a lower limb prosthesis. **A,** The client is shown wearing a lower limb prosthesis on the *affected* leg. First, lock any braces or casters; lock the knee of the prosthesis if applicable. **B,** The client will pivot with weight on the *residual* limb (the *unaffected* leg). **C,** The *residual* limb provides the main support and balance for the transfer. Be sure to assist the client as necessary for safety.

III

FUNCTIONAL HEALTH PATTERNS AND REHABILITATION NURSING

15

Skin Integrity

Janet G. LaMantia, MA, RN, CRRN

INTRODUCTION

Maintaining skin integrity and wound management is a major consideration in rehabilitation. Skin acts as a biologic barrier between a person and the environment and also as a psychosocial mediator between a person and society. Failure to maintain skin integrity extends the length of stay in a healthcare facility and interferes with an individual's ability to perform self-care tasks and resume social roles. In some instances loss of skin integrity can be life-threatening. Therefore helping the client maintain and restore skin integrity is a major responsibility of the rehabilitation team. The rehabilitation nurse is the team member primarily responsible for assessing skin and teaching the client and family techniques to assure maintenance of skin integrity from the rehabilitation facility to the home setting.

The rehabilitation nurse is the coordinator of an outcome-driven plan for intact and healed skin. The plan of care is theory based, well researched, and consistently evaluated. The nurse providing the care and coordination of skin and wound care requires a thorough understanding of the normal physiologic processes and the factors that alter them (Bryant, Shannon, Pieper, Braden, & Morris, 1992; Eaglstein, 1986; Rehabilitation Nursing Foundation, 1987). Interventions based on this understanding will enable the rehabilitation nurse to select modalities that are most effective in preventing skin disruption and restoring the wound with the least energy expenditure by clients (Cooper, 1990). The appropriate use of modalities provides for less emotional and monetary cost to client, family, and the system.

ANATOMY AND PHYSIOLOGY

The skin (Fig. 15-1) is composed of two main layers: the epidermis and the dermis, separated by the basement membrane zone (BMZ). Underneath these layers is the hypodermis or superficial fascia (Anthony & Thibodeau, 1983; Habif, 1990; Vidal & Sarrias, 1991).

Epidermis

The epidermis consists of stratified squamous epithelial tissue. Blood vessels do not reach into this outer layer of the skin. The epidermis has five layers: stratum corneum, stratum lucidum, stratum granulosum, stratum spinosum, and stratum germinativum. The stratum corneum—the outermost layer—is composed of dead keratinized cells. These

are the cells lost to daily activities of scratching, bathing, and changing clothes. The basal layer—the stratum germinativum—is the innermost epidermal layer. Cells leaving this layer take 2 to 3 weeks to migrate upward. Melanosomes that contain melanin pigment are located in this layer. Skin color is determined by the size, distribution, and activity of the melanosomes. Exposure to the sun stimulates the melanocytes to produce melanin. Dark-skined individuals have more active melanocytes (Anthony & Thibodeau, 1983; Vidal & Sarrias, 1991).

Dermis

The dermis—the inner thicker layer of the skin—consists of fibrous connective tissue that supports the epidermis. It is tough, elastic, and flexible. Fibroblasts in this layer synthesize and secrete the two main proteins: collagen and elastin. Collagen is the protein that gives the skin its tensile strength. Elastin gives the skin its elastic recoil—the ability of skin to return to its shape (Anthony & Thibodeau, 1983; Vidal & Sarrias, 1991).

Hypodermis

The hypodermis, or superficial fascia, forms the adipose or subcutaneous layer. This layer contains a plexus of blood vessels that gives rise to and supplies the dermal layers. The hypodermis is the anchor to underlying structures (Anthony & Thibodeau, 1983; Solis, Krouskap, Trainer, & Marburger, 1988).

MAJOR SKIN FUNCTIONS (Anthony & Thibodeau, 1983; Vidal & Sarrias, 1991)

Regulation of Body Temperature (Thermoregulation)

Evaporation of moisture on the skin through the sweat glands lowers body temperature. Sweat glands are under control of the nervous system responding to temperature changes and emotional stimulation. Constriction of the blood vessels shunts heat to underlying body organs; dilating the blood vessels causes heat to dissipate by conduction, convection, radiation, and evaporation.

Protection of Underlying Tissue From Injury

Varied thicknesses of the skin protect underlying tissue and organs from mechanical injury. Collagen provides the tensile strength that makes the skin resistant to tears.

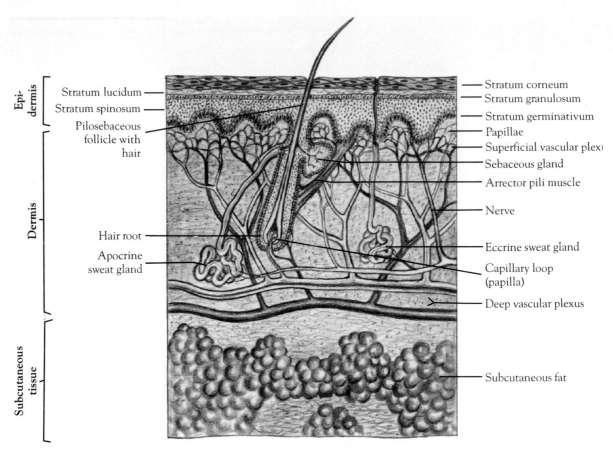

Fig. 15-1 Structures of the skin. (From Thompson JM and others: *Mosby's Clinical Nursing*, 3rd ed., by J.M. Thomson and others, 1993, St. Louis: Mosby–Year Book. Copyright 1993 by Mosby–Year Book. Reprinted by permission.)

Biologic Barrier Protection

The skin prevents passage of harmful microorganisms and chemicals into the body. It provides protection against aqueous, chemical, bacterial, and viral assaults. Sebum secreted by the sebaceous glands provides an acidic coating that retards growth of microorganisms. The oiliness of the sebum gives resistance to aqueous and chemical solutions.

Protection Against Ultraviolet Radiation

Protection against ultraviolet radiation is provided by skin pigmentation. Persons with increased activity of melanocytes are better protected against skin cancer.

Protection Provided by Nerve Receptors

Survival and everyday safety depend on transmission and interpretation of pain, temperature, touch, and pressure sensations received through these nerve receptors. Responses to these sensations protect the body from impending injury.

Metabolism

Vitamin D is produced in the skin when it is exposed to sunlight. Vitamin D assists with calcium and phosphate metabolism and is important to the mineralization of bone and teeth.

Excretion

Salt and water losses through the skin are factors in maintaining fluid and electrolyte balance in the body. Major losses of fluid through burns attests to this.

Expression: Communication

Since the skin contributes to appearance and nonverbal communication, it serves as a means of conveying feelings and projecting body image. The facial skin allows for expression in the form of smiling, frowning, pouting, and grimacing. The physical changes in skin can affect the person from a psychosocial as well as a physical aspect. Disfigurement of the skin affects an individual's feelings about self. Adolescents are particularly sensitive to their appearance and very susceptible to problems of self-esteem when confronted with skin changes (Vidal & Sarrias, 1991). The aging process also influences self-perception and self-esteem. Observers rated women more attractive when they had fewer signs of aging. When women were rated more attractive, independently they rated themselves more positively in terms of looks, physical and mental health, and social life (Krasner, 1991).

IMPAIRED FUNCTION
Factors Altering Skin Function

A number factors can alter the characteristics of the skin: aging, sun exposure, hydration, soaps, and medications (Eaglstein, 1986; Jones & Millman, 1990; Panel for Prediction and Prevention of Pressure Ulcers in Adults, 1992; Vidal & Sarrias, 1991).

♦ **Aging.** The most obvious changes in the aging adult are wrinkling and graying. The loss of underlying tissue results in wrinkling; graying hair is a response to age-related changes in melanocytes. Changes in the skin take place throughout the life-span. At birth our skin and nails are thin, and they thicken over time. At the time of adolescence sebaceous glands increase secretory rates, and hair follicles give rise to the appearance of secondary sexual characteristics. As we age, a number of changes take place that increase the susceptibility to injury and extend time for wound healing:

- ♦ Decreased epidermal turnover (doubles by age 35)
- ♦ Diminished sensory receptors
- ♦ Reduced vitamin D production
- ♦ Decreased inflammatory response
- ♦ Reduced thermoregulatory capacity of skin, resulting from decreasing number of sweat glands
- ♦ Increased capillary fragility
- ♦ Reduced collagen synthesis and neoangiogenesis
- ♦ Slower epithelialization

♦ **Sun exposure.** Ultraviolet rays can accelerate aging of the skin, as well as increase risk of cancer and immunocompetence of the skin.

♦ **Hydration.** A number of factors affect skin hydration including humidity production, amount of sebum, and aging. Decrease in these factors will lead to dryness of the skin with itching and scaling.

♦ **Soaps.** Alkaline soaps reduce the thickness and number of cell layers in the stratum corneum. Excessive use of soaps removes the sebum coating and its antibacterial and antidehydration properties. This can lead to dryness and increased opportunity for infection.

♦ **Medications.** Many classifications of drugs can affect the skin. Corticosteroids interfere with epidermal proliferation. Other medications have photosensitizing effects. The nurse should review drug use for this possibility when skin reactions occur.

♦ **Nutrition.** When healthy skin is altered, provision of a supplemented diet may be necessary to provide necessary nutrients for skin regeneration. Natow established that healing tissue quality depends on protein synthesis, not fat accumulation. Obese clients cannot be thought of as well nourished since fat is poorly vascularized (Natow, 1983).

Wounds and Wound Healing

There are many presentations of skin damage and numerous causes creating the damage. Open or closed wounds of the skin may be caused by blows, cuts, prolonged pressure, and burns from heat, chemicals, or radiation. Invasion of bacteria can lead to infection of these wounds. Stasis dermatitis and ulceration of the lower limbs often are seen as a result of stagnation of blood caused by arteriosclerosis or poor peripheral circulation. In aging persons the skin becomes fragile, particularly on the dorsal surfaces of hands and arms, and is subject to easy bruising and tearing.

Causes of Skin Damage

♦ **Mechanical.** Mechanical injuries result from prolonged pressure, shearing, friction, epidermal stripping, and tearing. A longer and more detailed discussion of the forces of pressure, shear, and friction is presented later in this chapter. Epidermal stripping and skin tears are related to the function of the BMZ or dermal-epidermal junction. Normally the epidermis rests firmly on the dermis with the dermal papillae projecting into the epidermis in a tongue-and-groove fashion. In premature infants this junction is not yet developed, leaving the infant at risk to epidermal stripping. Care also must be exercised with irradiated tissue (Vidal & Sarrias, 1991). With aging the dermal-epidermal junction has reduced collagen and elastin and increased capillary fragility, making the skin more susceptible to injury (Fenske & Lober, 1986; Payne & Martin, 1990). Using corticosteroids also may deplete collagen strength (Payne & Martin, 1990; Vidal & Sarrias, 1991).

Epidermal stripping. Epidermal stripping is the inadvertent removal of the epidermis by mechanical means such as tape removal (Solis et al., 1988). Epidermal stripping refers to the removal of cells of the epidermis by a force of friction. Loss of skin by epidermal stripping is preventable by proper taping techniques, understanding of the problems of aging (as well as immaturity), and of drug and radiation therapies.

Payne describes *skin tears* as a "traumatic injury occurring on the extremities of older adults as a result of shearing and friction forces which separate the epidermis from the dermis " (Patrick, Woods, Craven, Rokosky, & Bruno, 1986). Forces of minor friction or shearing can cause a separation of the epidermis from the dermis at the dermal-epidermal junction. The resulting wounds vary widely in appearance. Skin tears result from such varied traumas as a grasp, dressing, bathing, transfers, and scrapes against objects such as tables and chairs. Risk factors for skin tears include the frail elderly, history of a previous skin tear, senile purpura, and cognitive impairment. The care of these tears follows the principles of wound management, which are discussed later in this chapter. Patients with risk for skin tears need early identification, increased precautions for all activities of daily living, and judicious use of shear and friction protectors (Orem, 1971; Patrick et al., 1986).

♦ **Chemical damage.** Chemical damage to the skin may result from fecal and urinary incontinence, harsh products used to cleanse skin and wounds (e.g., alcohol, povidone-iodine, and antacids), poorly contained damage from acute and chronic wounds, and drainage from percutaneous tubes. Skin irritation also occurs when skin care products are used improperly. Skin care cleansers should be used sparingly and rinsed thoroughly to avoid disruption of the normal acid pH of the skin (Orem, 1971; Vidal & Sarrias, 1991).

♦ **Moisture.** In addition to damage that can occur to skin from chemical irritants such as urine, feces, and wound drainage, there is evidence to support that moisture alone can make the skin more susceptible to injury (Orem, 1971; Young, 1989). When exposed to prolonged moisture, the skin can become macerated and develop a rash (Carlson, King, Kirk, Temple, & Heinemann, 1992; Orem, 1971). Efforts should be made to reduce exposure to prolonged moisture from sweating, urinary and fecal incontinence, and wound drainage. Many materials are available to provide for a dry skin surface while drawing away moisture. Creative use of these products can assist with moisture control in a variety of situations. Moisture barriers (ointments, sealants, solid wafers) also can be used (Orem, 1971; Young, 1989).

✦ **Heat damage.** The skin can be injured due to excess thermal energy or accelerated metabolic activity induced by elevated temperature. Hot water should be avoided for daily cleansing and hygiene. When cleansing the skin, caution should be used to minimize force and friction applied to the skin. The long-standing advice found in many textbooks to massage bony prominences in order to stimulate circulation is to be discarded. Avoid massage over bony prominences. There is no evidence to support the efficacy of this intervention, whereas there is evidence that massage can lead to deep tissue trauma (Orem, 1971).

✦ **Radiation.** Radiation can damage the epidermis, presenting with a loss of accessory structures and atrophy of the skin and scarring. Radiation reduces fibroblasts and destroys the cell nucleus, which can result in wide, shallow, irregularly bordered wounds. The wounds have poorly vascularized beds as well as the skin changes previously noted. These wounds usually require surgical interventions with debridement, skin grafts, and myocutaneous flap procedures (Lindan, 1961; Vidal & Sarrias, 1991). These wounds can appear spontaneously or can be due to slight trauma. Care needs to be directed to assess irradiated skin continually for changes and protect against mechanical and chemical assault in that area.

✦ **Vascular damage.** Many chronic wounds can develop on the lower legs and feet due to vascular origins. Ulcers can occur as a result of venous insufficiency, arterial insufficiency, and neuropathies. Although each produces wounds with unique characteristics (Table 15-1), diagnostic studies often must be employed to identify causation. These wounds require comprehensive management of the disease process as well as wound care (Zackarkow, 1985). (A more detailed discussion of management of circulatory disease, diagnostic aspects, and client supports can be found in Chapter 19.)

Arterial insufficiency. Arterial ulcers are caused by insufficient arterial perfusion to an extremity. These ulcers are not as common as venous ulcers but are more difficult to manage with the complexity of disease processes and complications. The lack of perfusion to the lower extremity creates great difficulty for wound healing. Peripheral vascular disease is the associated disease entity with arterial insufficiency. It involves the arteries, veins, and lymphatics. Symptoms can be treated, but there is no cure for peripheral vascular disease (Zackarkow, 1985).

Venous insufficiency. Venous ulcers result from disorders of the deep venous system. When a disease process alters the flow of blood forward, dysfunction ensues resulting in increased hydrostatic pressure, venous hypotension, leading to dermal ulceration (Vidal & Sarrias, 1991; Zackarkow, 1985). The diseases contributing to venous insufficiency are listed in Table 15-1. Current research indicates venous pressure promotes extravasation of erythrocytes and fibrinogen, leading to a cascade of events that eventually ends in tissue death and dermal ulcers.

Table 15-1   Arterial, venous, and neuropathic ulcers of the lower extremities: a comparison

	Arterial	Neuropathic	Venous
Predisposing factors	Peripheral vascular disease (PVD) Diabetes Advanced age	Peripheral neuropathy	Valve incompetence in perforating veins History of deep vein thrombophlebitis and thrombosis Previous history of ulcer Advanced age Obesity
Location	Between toes or tips of toes Over phalangeal heads Around lateral malleolus Where subjected to trauma or rubbing of footwear	Plantar aspect of foot Over metatarsal heads Under heel	Medial aspect of lower leg and ankle May extend into malleolar area
Characteristics	Even wound margins Gangrene or necrosis Deep, pale wound bed Painful Cellulitis	Painless Even wound margins Deep Cellulitis or underlying osteomyelitis Granular tissue present unless coexisting PVD	Irregular wound margins Superficial (into dermis) Ruddy, granular tissue Usually painless Exudate usually present

Adapted from "Lower Extremity Ulcers" by M. Zink, P. Rousseau, and A.G. Holloway in *Acute and Chronic Wounds: Nursing Management* edited by R. Bryant, 1992, St. Louis: Mosby–Year Book. Copyright 1992 by Mosby–Year Book.

♦ **Diabetic peripheral neuropathy.** A number of factors contribute to dermal ulcers: arterial insufficiency, trauma, and peripheral neuropathy. In peripheral neuropathy clients may have sensory, motor, or autonomic origins or a combination of these. Loss of sensation is the most problematic since it predisposes the foot to trauma and skin breakdown. Motor neuropathies result in muscular atrophies of the foot, leading to bony deformity and gait changes, putting undue stress on the foot, and leading to pressure, shear, and friction problems. Autonomic neuropathies often lead to absence of sweating, which leads to increased heat and drying of skin (Zackarkow, 1985).

Wound Healing

Wounds are healed by a complex series of events. To manage wounds properly, the rehabilitation nurse must understand the process to intervene appropriately at the various stages.

Wounds heal by the process of regeneration or scar formation. The type of closure depends on the type of tissue damage. Regeneration is the restoration of normal tissue structure by the production of undamaged "like" cells (Panel for Prediction and Prevention of Pressure Ulcers in Adults, 1992). Only certain body tissues can regenerate: epithelial, endothelial, and connective tissue. Epidermal, dermal, bone, and muscle tissue can be healed by regeneration. Healing in the muscle and bone by regeneration is impaired by infection, lack of vascularization, or innervation. When these complications are present, the wounds close by scar formation. Scar formation is a process of repair by connective tissue (Patrick et al., 1986; Wysocki & Bryant, 1992).

Classification of Wound Healing

Wound healing can be classified as primary, secondary, and tertiary.

♦ **Primary intention.** Wounds with no tissue loss are closed by primary intention. Examples are wounds where the edges are approximated and closed surgically or with tape. These wounds heal quickly, with minimal scar formation (Clanin, 1989; Doughty, 1992; Patrick et al., 1986).

♦ **Secondary intention.** Wounds with tissue loss close by secondary intention. These wounds have edges that are difficult or impossible to approximate, and heal with scar tissue. Healing time depends on the extent of tissue loss and whether healing is prolonged by infection. Examples of these wounds are burns, abdominal wounds, gastrointestinal ulcers, and pressure ulcers (Clanin, 1989; Doughty, 1992; Panel for Prediction and Prevention of Pressure Ulcers in Adults, 1992).

♦ **Tertiary intention.** Tertiary intention refers to wounds where primary closure is delayed or deliberately left open for drainage and then closed. These wounds have more scar tissue formed than a wound with primary closure but less than secondary closure (Carlson, et al., 1992; Disa, Carlton, & Goldberg, 1991; Norton, McLaren, & Exton Smith, 1975).

Wound Repair

Wound repair is a cascade of physiologic responses initiated by tissue trauma (Doughty, 1992). Wound repair is divided into three phases: defensive, proliferative, and maturation. This process happens interactively, with overlap between the stages (Doughty, 1992; Jones & Millman, 1990).

♦ **Defensive phase.** This phase is the body's first response to injury. There are two stages in this phase: hemostasis and inflammation. The major outcome of this phase is the control of bleeding and a clean wound base.

Hemostasis. Hemostasis results from trauma to tissue disrupting the vascular supply. Released blood contacts collagen to activate coagulation factors, causing an aggregate of platelets. Fibrin clots then form, acting as the initial wound closure (Doughty, 1992). Along with the release of platelets are several growth factors critical to wound healing (Doughty, 1992; Panel for Prediction and Prevention of Pressure Ulcers in Adults, 1992). Hemostasis seems to be the critical factor in initiating the wound-healing process. This may be important to understanding the stagnant nature of chronic nonhealing wounds. Poorly vascularized and often resulting from compromised vascularization, these wounds may lack the necessary stimulus to promote wound healing (Doughty, 1992).

Inflammation. In this stage vasodilation ensues as a result of histamine release. There is increased blood vessel permeability, vasocongestion, and leakage of serous fluid into the surrounding tissue. Leukocytes protect the wound initially from bacterial invasion, and within several days macrophages arrive. Macrophages play an important role throughout the wound-healing process by assisting with wound debridement, producing growth factors, and stimulating collagen synthesis (Doughty, 1992). This defensive phase last 3 to 4 days. The nurse must support the need for the inflammatory process and be aware of problems that might alter it such as steroid therapy or decreased oxygenation. Preventing suppression of inflammation in the first days of a wound's existence will affect the wound's overall quality of healing (Cooper, 1990). The clinical picture of the wound during this phase is red, hot, and edematous.

♦ **Proliferation phase.** The desired outcome of the proliferative phase is to fill the wound defect with connective tissue and cover it with epithelium. There are three major stages to this phase: granulation, contraction, and epithelialization (Panel for Prediction and Prevention of Pressure Ulcers in Adults, 1992).

Granulation. In the process of granulation, neoangiogenesis and collagen synthesis combine to provide a new capillary network and to nourish the collagen tissue filling in the wound bed. These two processes are simultaneous and co-dependent. Neoangiogensis (the production of new blood vessels) is stimulated by hypoxia. Vessels are formed from the wound edges and advance inward, joining at the center of the wound. Collagen synthesis occurs simultaneously in a number of complex events. The fibroblast is the key cell during this phase of healing, rapidly synthesizing collagen and proteoglycans. These two substances together form a "scaffolding" on which the wound repair is made (Cooper, 1990). The collagen fibers develop crosslinks, mature, and provide the tensile strength for the wound and support the migration of the blood vessels (Doughty, 1992). The tissue formed by this process is called granulation tissue. Tiny round projections of connective tissue are noted on the surface of the wound, which appears translucent and red. It is very vascular, fragile, and bleeds easily. As the wound heals, the new vessels will recede (Panel for Prediction and Prevention of Pressure Ulcers in Adults, 1992).

Contraction. Contraction is the reduction of the size of the tissue defect by the inward movement of the tissue and the surrounding skin (Panel for Prediction and Prevention of Pressure Ulcers in Adults, 1992). This is a desirable response since it decreases the size of the wound and with that the healing time. In wounds where there is good mobility of surrounding tissue (e.g., sacral wounds), this occurs easily; however, it is more difficult where tissue is not movable (e.g., bony prominence: trochanteric area) (Eaglstein, 1986; Panel for Prediction and Prevention of Pressure Ulcers in Adults, 1992).

Epithelialization. In this stage, cells of the intact epidermis reproduce and migrate over the defect. In epidermal and dermal wounds, epithelial cells proliferate and cross the wound bed in the first 24 hours. Epidermal tissue is formed at the wound edges and from epidermal tissue. The wound quickly regenerates. In wounds healing by secondary intention, the wounds cannot repair until the wound bed is established. Epithelial cells do not migrate across a dry wound bed. In a dry wound the epidermal cells must tunnel down to a moist level to begin migration. In wounds limited to the epidermis and dermis where scabs are allowed to develop, the epithelial cells first must secrete collagenase to remove scab before epithelial migration. In healing large wounds, epithelialization is limited to about 3 cm from the edges of the wound. Chronic wounds with "rolled" edges will not be able to migrate epithelial cells from the nonpro-

Table 15-2   Influencing factors for wound healing

Decreased tissue perfusion and oxygenation (hypotension, hypovolemia, hypoxia)	Impairs collagen synthesis Decreases epithelial proliferation and migration Reduces tissue resistance to infection
Decreased nutritional status	Impairs inflammatory response Impairs collagen synthesis
Infection	Prolongs inflammatory phase Induces additional tissue destruction Delays collagen synthesis Prevents epithelialization
Hematopoietic abnormalities RBCs ↓ Platelets ↓	Decrease oxygenation of the wound Delay of hemostasis and the cascade of healing events
Aging	Delays inflammatory response Produces capillary fragility Reduces collagen synthesis Slows neoangiogenesis Slows epithelialization
Diabetes	Decreases collagen synthesis Induces leukocyte dysfunction (secondary to hyperglycemia)
Smoking	Decreases oxygen to the wound secondary to coagulation in small blood vessels
Steroids	Inhibit epithelial proliferation Impair inflammatory response Decrease growth factor available for wound healing Increase wound vulnerability to infection Inhibit epithelial proliferation Impair inflammatory response Decrease macrophage activity Increase wound vulnerability to infection
Immunosuppressives	Impair inflammatory process Increase susceptibility to infection Prolong healing process
Radiation	Reduces fibroblast proliferation Inhibits inflammatory response
Sensorimotor dysfunction in affected part	Decreases inflammatory response secondary to decreased vasomotor response
Obesity	Decreases vascularity of adipose tissue Increases tension on wound

Data from "Physiology of Wound Healing" by D. Doughty in *Acute and Chronic Wounds: Nursing Management,* edited by R. Bryant, 1992, St. Louis: Mosby–Year Book, and "Skin and Wound Care: Dressing for Success," by G. Motta, April 1993, Workshop American Healthcare Institute.

liferative edges. These wounds will need surgical intervention to close (Doughty, 1992; Panel for Prediction and Prevention of Pressure Ulcers in Adults, 1992). The proliferative phase lasts from day 3 to 4 to day 21. The nurse supports this phase of wound healing with adequate nutrition, hydration, and oxygenation (Cooper, 1990).

Maturation phase. Maturation is the phase of remodeling. This phase starts when the wound is closed with connective and epithelial tissue. Collagen production stabilizes; fibers organize and increase the tensile strength of tissue (Doughty, 1992; Panel for Prediction and Prevention of Pressure Ulcers in Adults, 1992). Activities during this last phase determine the strength and mobility of scar tissue. If there is an alteration in the remodeling of collagen fibers, contractions or adhesions can occur. The healed tissue will achieve only 80% of previous tissue strength and scars will be less elastic than intact skin. Support for healing during this phase recognizes the decreased strength of tissue; the healing process continues for up to 2 years (Cooper, 1990).

Factors Influencing Wound Healing

Many factors influence wound healing including tissue perfusion, nutritional status, infection, hematopoietic abnormalities, aging, diabetes, smoking, steroid and immunosuppressive therapy, radiation therapy, sensorimotor dysfunc-

Table 15-3 Specific nutritional elements and their effect on wound healing

Decreased protein	Prolongs inflammatory phase Impairs fibroblasts
Increased glucose	Impairs leukocyte function
Vitamin C	Necessary for collagen synthesis Supports integrity of capillary wall
Vitamin A	Counteracts adverse affects of steroids on wound healing Restores local inflammatory response Stimulates epithelial migration
Excessive vitamin A	Exacerbates inflammatory response and damages wound
B complex	Necessary for cross-linkage of collagen fibers
Vitamin E	May protect vitamin A from oxidation during digestion
Iron	Supports oxygen transport Cofactor for collagen synthesis
Copper	Supports cross-linkage of collagen fibers
Zinc	Necessary cofactor for collagen formation and protein synthesis
Calcium	Necessary for remodeling of collagen

Data from "Physiology of Wound Healing" by D. Doughty in *Acute and Chronic Wounds: Nursing Management,* edited by R. Bryant, 1992, St. Louis: Mosby–Year Book; "Skin and Wound Care: Dressing for Success," by G. Motta, April 1993, Workshop American Healthcare Institute; and "Nutritional Assessment and Intervention" by G. Pinchovsky-Devin in *Chronic Wound Care,* edited by D. Kasner, 1990, King of Prussia: Health Management Publications.

tion, and obesity (Doughty, 1992; Konstantides, 1992; Motta, 1993). Children have better capacity for wound repair but have less reserves to combat systemic attack. Factors that are detrimental to wound healing in children include easily upset electrolyte balance, sudden changes in body temperature, and rapid spread of infection (Garvin, 1990). Tables 15-2 and 15-3 summarize the major factors and their impact on wound healing. To aid wound healing, each of these factors must be considered and an appropriate intervention made.

Pressure Ulcers

Pressure ulcers have been challenging societies for centuries (Copeland-Fields & Hoshiko, 1989). In spite of new understanding of causation and wound management, the pressure ulcer problem continues to be a significant healthcare concern. The number of persons affected and costs in terms of life, productivity, and dollars is staggering (Allman et al., 1986; Anderson & Andberg, 1979; Kosiak, 1991). Mortality rates range from 23% to 37% in the hospitalized elderly (Allman et al., 1986). Dollar costs are widely estimated from $2,000 to $30,000 per case (National Pressure Ulcer Advisory Panel [NPUAP], 1989). Pressure ulcers add to a patient's length of stay, extend time for recuperation and return to home and work, and add to the risk of complications (Bryant et al., 1992). Economic downshifting has caused the healthcare system to become cost conscious and result oriented. The pressure ulcer must be viewed as preventable and not a de facto complication of illness and immobility (Copeland-Fields & Hoshiko, 1989). Prevention requires knowledge, commitment, and resources.

✦ Defining the problem

The scope of the pressure ulcer problem is difficult to define with the interchangeable nomenclature used for pressure ulcers, nonuniform standards used to describe pressure ulcers, the multitude of staging systems, and the lack of reporting guidelines (NPUAP, 1989). The comparability of data between populations and institutions is difficult because the data may not always consider the same variables. When stage I ulcers are included in a study, there may be a problem with both overreporting and underreporting. When underreported, it may reflect nonblanchable erythema not being considered a pressure ulcer or it may be missed, especially in individuals with dark skin (Allman, 1989). Underreporting also occurs because facilities equate the presence of pressure ulcers with poor quality of care. Overreporting occurs when vascular or ischemic ulcers or blanchable hyperemia is identified as a stage I pressure ulcer (Allman, 1989; Bryant et al., 1992). With these limitations the epidemiology of a pressure ulcer is reviewed.

✦ Epidemiology

Prevalence is the number or percentage of reported cases at a given point in time. Prevalence requires only one observation and therefore is reported more frequently. In acute settings prevalence is reported from 15% to 18.3% (Maklebust, Mondarx, & Sieggreen, 1986; NPUAP, 1989). The elderly have prevalence rates of 11.6% to 27.5% (Berlowitz & Wilking, 1989; Brandeis, Morris, Nash, & Lipsitz,

1990). Brandeis et al. (1990) conducted a large-scale longitudinal multisite study of the elderly. Prevalence in this group was 17.4%. Of this group with ulcers, 83.4% occurred in the group admitted from hospitals. Brandies et al. compared their study to Berlowitz and Wilking where a 33% prevalence was found and attributed to the difference in increased age, decreased ambulatory status, less continence of bowel and bladder, and a more chronically ill debilitated client (Berlowitz & Wilking, 1989; Brandeis et al., 1990). The prevalence of pressure ulcer in clients with spinal cord injury (SCI) was reported from 25% to 40% (McFarland & McFarland, 1993; Yetzer & Sullivan, 1992; Young & Burns, 1981). Studies of the World War II spinal cord injured had prevalence rates of 57% to 85% (Kosiak, Kubicek, Olson, Danz, & Kottke, 1958). The improvement could be due to better initial management of persons with SCI. Hunter et al. (1992) looked at the rehabilitation population and found a 25% prevalence rate; in this same population the incidence was 0% at the time of the study.

✦ **Incidence.** Incidence refers to the number or percentage of new cases occurring over a given period of follow-up or the rate at which new cases develop. Incidence reports require repeated observations over a period of time within a specific population.

The incidence of pressure ulcers varies widely by population and setting. These studies require more than one observation, and the intervals are in terms of weeks, months, and years. In reports of incidence rates in acute settings, the rates reported varied from 3% to 14% (NPUAP, 1989). Allman et al. (1986) found at least 7.7% of hospitalized patients develop ulcers within 3 weeks of admission. In a study of an oncology community hospital, the incidence rate was 25% (Oot-Giromini et al., 1989). In studies of specific populations, the geriatric and orthopedic groups had rates of 24% (Allman et al., 1986; Oot-Giromini et al., 1989; Yarkony, Roth, Cybulski, & Jaeger, 1992). In spinal cord injured population, the incidence rates show variations from 24% to 59% (Mawson et al., 1988; Munro, 1988; Richardson & Meyer, 1981). Young and Burns (1981) found the incidence rate to be 40% in acute and rehabilitation hospitalization and 30% in each of the 5 follow-up years; higher rates of incidence were found in patients with complete quadriplegia and paraplegia. A higher incidence was reported in quadriplegia than paraplegia during acute and rehabilitation hospitalization but not in follow-up.

In a recent study of 125 spinal cord injuried persons, Carlson et al. (1992) found a 29% incidence for pressure ulcers during acute hospitalization. This rate is slightly higher than Munro's 1940 figure of 24% (Munro, 1940). Carlson et al. attribute this difference to the risk related to increased survival of clients with severe multiple trauma. When compared with more recent studies, the 29% incidence is lower than the incidence reported of up to 59% (Richardson & Meyer, 1981). Carlson et al. (1992) thought this difference could be a function of improvements in prevention or limitations of the various study designs.

✦ **Pressure ulcers: terminology and definition**

Pressure ulcers have long been given multiple interchangeable names to describe the same process: impaired blood supply resulting in damage to the tissue. Some of the terms familiar to nurses include decubitus ulcer, bedsores, and pressure sores. Pressure ulcers can develop anywhere there is unrelieved pressure; it is inaccurate to use terms associating the problem only with lying down (Maklebust, 1987). The term pressure ulcer is more accurate and descriptive. It reflects the etiology of a pressure ulcer—excessive pressure resulting in ischemia and ulceration (Bryant et al., 1992; Maklebust, 1987). The Panel for the Prediction and Prevention of Pressure Ulcers in Adults (1992) defines a pressure ulcer as any lesion caused by unrelieved pressure resulting in the damage of underlying tissue.

✦ **Etiology.** Pressure ulcers develop in response to a number of factors, the most important being pressure (Daniel, Priest, & Wheatley, 1981; Dinsdale, 1974; Kosiak et al., 1958; Kosiak, 1959; Langemo et al., 1991). These factors can be thought of as primary and secondary (Maklebust, 1987). Pressure, shear, and friction are the three major factors. Secondary factors include mobility status, sensorimotor function, nutrition, age, hemopoietic changes, diabetes, circulatory dysfunction, fecal incontinence, medications, and psychosocial issues. Braden and Bergstrom (1987) developed a conceptual schema to organize the etiologic factors in pressure sore formation (Fig. 15-2). The schema divides factors into intrinsic and extrinsic forces and provides a model displaying the interactive nature of pressure ulcer development (Bryant et al., 1992).

✦ **Pressure.** Pressure is the most important factor in pressure ulcer formation. Researchers agree the etiology of pressure ulcers is prolonged, uninterrupted mechanical loading of tissue (Kosiak, 1959; Panel for Prediction and Prevention of Pressure Ulcers in Adults, 1992). There are three aspects: intensity, duration, and tissue tolerance to pressure (Bryant et al., 1992). The critical issue of pressure and its effects on tissue were defined by early researchers. Husain demonstrated that by exerting a force for 2 hours microscopic ischemic changes were produced, and when the same force was applied for 6 hours, total muscle destruction occurred, showing the relationship between time and pressure (International Association for Enterostomal Therapy [IAET], 1991). Kosiak (1959), in experiments with dogs and cats, defined the time-pressure relationships; 70 ml of pressure applied continuously for 2 hours produced pathologic changes. Kosiak also demonstrated the inverse relationship of pressure and time. Intense pressure applied for a short duration can be as damaging as the lower intensity pressures exerted for extended periods (Kosiak et al., 1958; Kosiak, 1959).

Kosiak also determined that tissues can tolerate much higher cyclic pressures than constant pressures. If pressure is relieved intermittently every 3 to 5 minutes, higher pressures can be tolerated (Kosiak, 1959). Pressure needs to be relieved frequently over time as well as reduced over the surface-skin interface. This translates to the clinical practice of weight shifting every few minutes to extend safe sitting times and the use of 2-hour minimum turning times in bed or frequent small position changes in bed to provide pressure relief (Norton et al., 1975; Panel for Prediction and Prevention of Pressure Ulcers in Adults, 1992; Staas & Cioschi, 1991).

The sensitivity of skin to pressure was studied by Daniel et al. (1981); muscle was found to be more sensitive to the

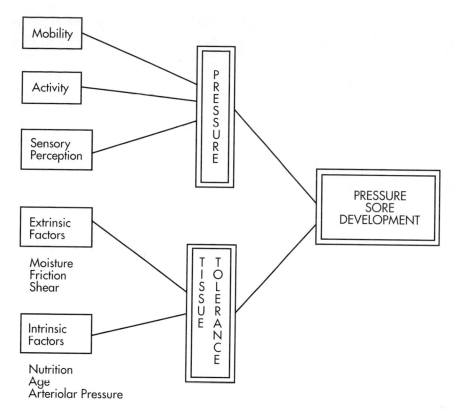

Fig. 15-2 Braden and Bergstrom's conceptual schema of pressure sore risk factors. (From *Rehabilitation Nursing, 14(5)*, Skokie, Il. Reprinted by permission.)

effects of pressure than skin. The concept of tissue tolerance was described by Husain (1953). When muscle is damaged without skin breakdown, a second application of less pressure and less time can result in an ulcer. This is clinically important in the need to relieve pressure at the first sign of skin impairment, blanchable hyperemia, and allow time for tissue recovery.

Pressure is transmitted from the body surface to the underlying bone, and the greatest pressure is over the bone. The pressure is distributed in a conelike fashion, with the base of the cone on the underlying body surface (Fig. 15-3). This information leads to the understanding of why the greatest damage is seen at the muscle layer and not the skin surface. Presentation of ulcers often reflects this, appearing with a small skin defect and large area of undermining below the surface of intact skin.

Kosiak and Lindan determined the amount of pressure human skin is subjected to in supine and sitting positions. In the supine position pressures greatly exceeded 32 mm Hg in the areas under the occiput, spine, sacrum, and heels. Pressure under the buttocks was greater than 70 mm Hg. In the sitting position the ischial tuberosity had pressures exceeding 300 mm Hg (Kosiak, 1959; Lindan, 1961). Earlier research by Landis demonstrated 32 mm Hg to be arteriolar closing pressure and 15 mm Hg to be venous closing pressure. Capillary closing pressure is the minimum pressure needed to collapse the capillary (Landis, 1930). Lindan demonstrated that pressure causes tissue damage by closure of blood vessels, resulting in tissue necrosis (Lindan,

1961). These early capillary blood-flow studies were done in the fingertips of young healthy men. More recent capillary closure studies have shown much lower pressures needed to collapse capillaries in the elderly and debilitated and that these pressures can vary over different sites on the body (Bryant et al., 1992; Garber & Krouskop, 1982; Seiler, Allen, & Stahelin, 1986). There is some difficulty extrapolating this data to the skin–support surface interface pressure. The pressures found by indirect measurements at the skin–support surface interface may not accurately reflect the picture of blood flow through the capillaries (Bryant et al., 1992). Clinically this had led to searching for support surfaces that reduce the skin–support surface pressure below 32 mm Hg. A larger discussion of support surfaces is presented later.

Clinically the facets of pressure—intensity, duration, and tissue tolerance—produce concern for clients with the inability to relieve pressure over a skin surface. Interventions to assist clients with pressure relief for the bed and the wheelchair are presented later in the chapter.

◆ **Shear.** Shear injury occurs when the skin remains stationary and the underlying tissue shifts (Panel for Prediction and Prevention of Pressure Ulcers in Adults, 1992). Shearing forces (Fig. 15-4) are produced when adjacent surfaces slide over one another (Bryant et al., 1992). Reichel found shearing forces caused blood vessels to become angulated, disrupting the perforating arteries of the skin from the supply of the muscle. The typical shear injury presents as a wound with a large amount of undermining (Reichel, 1958).

Common causes of shearing are spasticity, poor sitting posture, poor bed positioning, and sliding rather than lifting. When the head of the bed is elevated above 30 degrees but less than 90 degrees, the client will slide down, producing shearing forces. The sacrum, with attached muscle and fascia, slides down while the skin stays in place as a result of friction forces (Bryant et al., 1992; Vidal & Sarrias, 1991).

✦ **Friction.** Friction occurs when the skin moves against a support surface. In its mildest forms friction produces skin tears, abrasions limited to the epidermal and dermal layers (Bryant et al., 1992; Luckmann & Sorensen, 1980; Panel for Prediction and Prevention of Pressure Ulcers in Adults, 1992). Dinsdale demonstrated friction decreases the amount of external pressure required to produce a pressure sore. In the case where pressure and shear are combined, friction contributes to extensive injury (Dinsdale, 1974; Panel for Prediction and Prevention of Pressure Ulcers in Adults,

1992). Friction occurs when extremities are brushed across a surface. These movements can be inadvertent as in spasticity.

Pathogenesis of Pressure Ulcers

Prolonged pressure in excess of capillary pressure will produce ischemia in the underlying tissue. The blood vessels dilate in response to anoxia, leakage of fluid from the blood vessels causes interstitial edema, and forward flow of blood is impeded. The cells continue to produce metabolic by-products that accumulate since they cannot be transported out secondary to vessel compromise. The amount of damage depends on pressure exerted and tissue involved (Shea, 1975).

Clinical Picture

The progression of tissue changes occurs in response to obstruction of capillary blood flow.

✦ **Reactive hyperemia (blanching hyperemia).** The blood vessels dilate to compensate for periods of anoxia. The skin appears flushed (this may be difficult to note in dark-skinned individuals). When compressed with a fingertip, the area will blanch (turn white) and return to color immediately as the finger is lifted. The area may be cool or warm to touch, and if the client is sensate she may complain of pain. At this stage relief of pressure can reverse tissue damage (Bryant et al., 1992; Luckmann & Sorensen, 1980).

✦ **Nonreactive hyperemia (nonblanching hyperemia).** Vasodilation continues as a response to the anoxia. The skin damage now appears bright red to dark purple. When compressed, the area does not blanch. The area is warm to touch and may feel hard (indurated) or soft and boggy. The tissue damage is not reversible at this stage (Bryant et al., 1992; Luckmann & Sorensen, 1980).

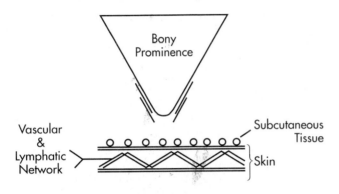

Fig. 15-3 Pressure cone. (From *Pressure Sores in the Elderly* by H. Slater, 1985, Pittsburgh: Synapse Publications. Copyright 1985 by Synapse Publications. Reprinted by permission.)

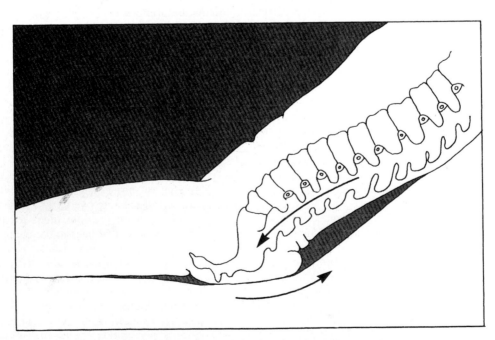

Fig. 15-4 Shearing force. (From *Acute and Chronic Wounds* edited by R.A. Bryant, 1992, St. Louis: Mosby–Year Book. Copyright 1992 by Mosby–Year Book. Reprinted by permission.)

Common Sites of Pressure Ulcers

Pressure ulcers occur most frequently over bony prominences. The most common sites for pressure ulcers (Fig. 15-5) are the sacrum, ischial tuberosity, trochanter, and calcaneus (Shea, 1975). Pressure ulcers will occur anywhere on the body there is compression of soft tissue. The rehabilitation nurse must exercise caution in checking clients with splints, orthoses, and orthopedic immobilizers (e.g., halo jacket). In studies of the SCI population, the sacrum was found to be the most frequent site for severe pressure ulcers (Carlson et al., 1992; Richardson & Meyer, 1981; Yetzer & Sullivan, 1992). This may be in part attributed to factors such as time spent on a spine board or the operating table (Hicks, 1971; Kemp, Keithley, Smith, & Morre-

ale, 1990). As more time is spent in wheelchairs, the pressure ulcer incidence is reflected in increased frequency at the ischial tuberosities and the feet. Carlson et al. found 47% of all ulcers discovered in follow-up were on the foot. The areas on the foot prime to breakdown (Fig. 15-6) are the toes, plantar surfaces at the metatarsal heads, the outer edges of the foot, the heels, and the malleolus of the ankle (Carlson et al., 1992; Knight & Scott, 1990). In a study of children 10 weeks to 13 years, Solis found the occiput to be the site of greatest pressures, changing to the sacrum as the child aged. This is not surprising in consideration of the percentage of body weight the child's head represents. The child's positioning needs must be considered separately from the adult's (Solis et al., 1988).

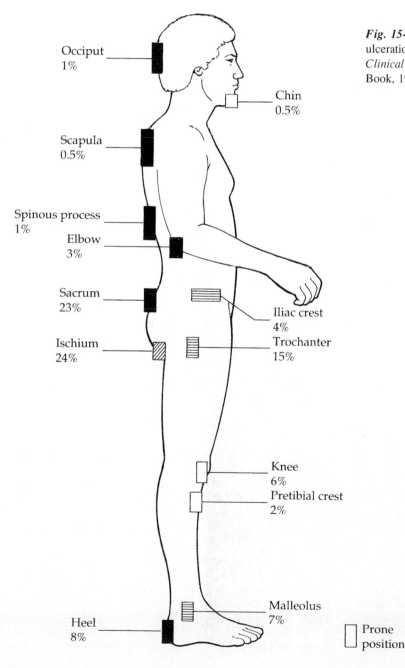

Fig. 15-5 Common sites for pressure ulcers and frequency of ulceration per site. (Data from by J. Agris and M. Spira, 1979, *Clinical Symposia, 31,* p. 2. Artwork Copyright Mosby–Year Book, 1992.)

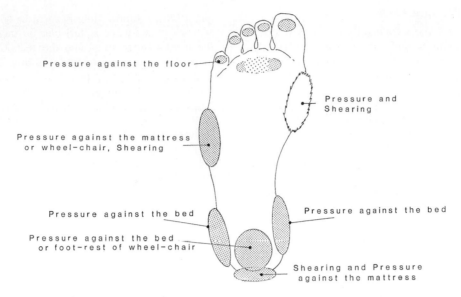

Fig. 15-6 Foot pressure points. (From "Contracture and Pressure Necrosis" by D. Knight and H. Scott, 1990, *Ostomy and Wound Management,* Copyright 1990 by Health Management Publications, Inc. Artwork courtesy *Rehabilitation Nursing,* Skokie, IL.)

Risk Factors: The Secondary Contributing Factors to Pressure Ulcer Development

Gosnell (1989) defines the following risk factors as identifiable intrinsic or extrinsic characteristics that increase a person's susceptibility to forces that induce trauma.

✦ **Immobility.** The inability or decreased ability to change and/or control body position is the most frequently cited factor for risk of pressure ulceration (Braden & Bergstrom, 1987; Gosnell, 1973; Maklebust, 1987; Yarkony, 1987; Norton, 1989; Sieggreen, 1987). Rehabilitation nurses rated this factor as most critical in pressure ulcer development (Copeland-Fields & Hoshiko, 1989).

✦ **Inactivity.** A decreased state of physical activity will predispose a person to pressure ulcers (Braden & Bergstrom, 1987; Gosnell, 1973). The less active, the greater the susceptibility to pressure ulcers. Persons confined to bed and those in wheelchairs are more likely to develop pressure ulcers (Berlowitz & Wilking, 1989). There is a positive relationship between overall health and well-being and increased activity (King & French, 1990; Panel for Prediction and Prevention of Pressure Ulcers in Adults, 1992).

✦ **Nutrition.** Many experts consider nutrition to be an extremely critical factor, second only to immobility in the causation of pressure ulcers (Agarwal, Del Guercio, & Lee, 1985; Allman, 1989; Mulholland, Tui, Wright, Vinci, & Shafiroff, 1943; Pinchocofsky-Devin, 1990). Allman (1989), Stotts (1985), and Pinchocofsky-Devin (1990) all reported low sebum albumin levels were highly associated with pressure ulcer development. In addition to the role of protein and vitamins in wound healing as outlined in Table 15-3, there are specific relationships to causation. Two prospective studies show evidence of poor diet (inadequate calories, protein, and iron) as a causative factor (Bergstrom & Braden, 1992; Panel for Prediction and Prevention of Pressure Ulcers in Adults, 1992). Hypoproteinemia leads to interstitial edema, which impairs the cellular transport of oxygen and nutrients. Vitamin C deficiencies can lead to capillary fragility and an impaired immune system (Alvarez, Rozint, & Wiseman, 1989; Bryant et al., 1992; Luckmann & Sorensen, 1980; Pinchocofsky-Devin, 1990).

✦ **Age.** As discussed previously, several systemic changes occur with age. These changes impair the ability to distribute pressure effectively and vascularize compromised tissue. Compromise to cellular response is greater when the elderly are confronted with several stressors at a time (Jones & Millman, 1990). The elderly are therefore more susceptible to forces of pressure, shear, and friction.

✦ **Moisture/incontinence.** Exposure to urine, stool, perspiration, or wound drainage exposes the client to metabolic wastes and bacterial contaminants. Several researchers have found incontinence to be a major risk factor. Norton showed incontinence to be the most reliable predictor for pressure ulcer formation (Powell, 1989). Allman found fecal incontinence to be more important than urinary incontinence as a predictor (Allman et al., 1989). In addition to the irritating substances in sources of moisture, moisture itself can make the skin more susceptible to injury (Panel for Prediction and Prevention of Pressure Ulcers in Adults, 1992). Prolonged exposure to moisture can cause skin to macerate, develop rash, and become infected—predisposing it to pressure ulcer formation.

✦ **Sensory perception.** Impairment of the ability to detect sensations that indicate a need for position change is rated as a highly critical factor for pressure ulcers. Rehabilitation nurses placed sensory perception third behind immobility and inactivity as a risk very characteristic of clients with pressure ulcers they had seen in their practice (Copeland-Fields & Hoshiko, 1989).

✦ **Smoking.** Lamid, in studying spinal cord injured persons, found smoking to correlate positively with pressure ulcers.

The more the person smoked, the greater his or her incidence of pressure ulcers (Lamid & Ghatit, 1983).

◆ **Elevated temperature.** Researchers have correlated increased body temperature with increased risk of pressure ulceration. Elevated temperature may put increased demands for oxygenation on already compromised tissue (Bryant et al., 1992; Gosnell, 1989).

◆ **Psychosocial.** Psychosocial factors have been found to influence pressure ulcer formation. Anderson and Andberg (1979) found life satisfaction, self-esteem, and practice of responsibility to be significant. In a study of stress resulting from the transfer of elderly persons to a nursing home, Braden (1988) found the prolonged elevation of cortisol placed the person at risk for pressure ulcers. Cortisol may be the trigger for lowered tissue tolerance when stress is present (Bryant et al., 1992; Jones & Millman, 1990). In persons with disabilities a number of psychosocial factors need to be considered: adjustment to disability, family environmental support, vocational opportunity, and financial constraints. Children bring different psychosocial problems to bear on skin integrity: the presence of a supportive parent or caregiver and past experiences with the healthcare system can positively or negatively influence the child's cooperation level. Children fear loss of control, pain, and change in body image. Adolescents have increased stress with perceived alterations in body image, which causes them to question their value as human beings (Garvin, 1990).

Risk factors may be specific to different populations. Incidence is not distributed evenly across all populations. All risk factors are not equal in various populations, and some are higher in certain groups and therefore need to be monitored more closely (Griffin et al., 1991; NPUAP, 1989; Panel for Prediction and Prevention of Pressure Ulcers in Adults, 1992). Versluysen found orthopedic patients may be at a greater risk for pressure sores because of immobility. Patients admitted with fractures had higher risk than patients admitted for elective orthopedic procedures (Versluysen, 1986).

In addition to the obvious factors of decreased mobility, decreased activity, and decreased sensory perception, the spinal cord injured have a number of factors that place them at increased risk for pressure ulcers. Knowledge of these increased risks can help guide prediction and prevention of pressure ulcers.

◆ **Education.** Vidal and Sarrias found lower education level related positively with greater severity of ulcers (Slater, 1985). Carlson et al. (1992) did not find lower education level to be a factor during acute rehabilitation, but it was strongly related at the time of follow-up.

◆ **Level of injury.** Lloyd and Baker (1986) found no relationship between severity of pressure ulcer and level of injury. Young and Burns (1991) saw a higher incidence of pressure ulcer in quadriplegics than in paraplegics during initial hospitalization but not at follow-up. Carlson et al. found that the higher the level of injury during acute care, the greater the incidence of pressure ulcer—but they found no associated significance between increased level of injury and rehabilitation and follow-up phases (Bryant et al., 1992).

◆ **Completeness of injury.** Carlson et al. found a signifi-

cant relationship between complete lesions and increased incidence of pressure ulcers at follow-up. Using the Frankel Scale (indication for presence or absence of sensation and motor activity below injury level), the researchers found the more complete lesion had greater incidence of pressure ulcers during rehabilitation and follow-up. All who developed pressure ulcers in rehabilitation had the highest factor of complete injury on the Frankel Scale (Carlson et al., 1992; Frankel et al., 1969). Of major interest is that no subject who had any preserved function below the level of injury developed a pressure ulcer during rehabilitation and follow-up. It appears that even nonfunctional preserved motor activity reduces risk of pressure ulcer (Carlson et al., 1992).

History of Pressure Ulcers

In what may turn out to be a major predictive factor, Carlson et al. (1992) correlated pressure sores at follow-up with a history of pressure ulcers during initial hospitalization. This is the first citation of this correlation and may assist rehabilitation nurses to focus attention on risk factors.

Nursing Assessment of Skin Integrity and Wounds

The health history obtained before the physical assessment provides insight into past and present skin problems experienced by the client. Information is needed concerning the client's ability to participate in self-care activities to maintain and restore skin integrity. General history questions related to the skin should include the following: client's health concerns about skin, ability to care for skin, current medication, nutritional history, cultural considerations, and held belief system.

Cultural considerations should be included in the interview. The nurse must be sensitive to lifelong held beliefs in order to acknowledge and incorporate them when possible into the daily care. Examples of assessment categories that might elicit important rituals, beliefs, and symbols of care include (1) questions about sleep: the environment, bedroom, coverings, who sleeps with client, bedtime and awakening rituals; (2) personal hygiene questions: "tending" one's body—mouth care, hair, body—and associations with health/illness (e.g., an older person does not interpret a leg sore as a problem but as a mark of aging) (Rempusheski, 1989); and (3) questions about eating: kinds of food, rituals with food, preferences and avoidance of food. Assessment of the client's skin enables the nurse to identify beginning skin problems and evaluate the response to treatment. Specific questions related to the skin and asked when taking the client's history include the following:

◆ Past and present skin problems (lesions, dryness, tumors, prior pressure ulcer)
◆ Changes in skin pigmentation (change in size of moles or dark spots)
◆ Excessive dryness, moisture, or odor
◆ Changes in skin texture
◆ Performance of daily skin inspection
◆ Individual practices of skin care
◆ Frequency of bathing and bathing preferences
◆ Problems obtaining bath equipment or using bathing facilities
◆ Bath and skin care products used (soaps, lotions, and creams)

✦ Sitting time, pressure-relief practice for wheelchair and bed

✦ Types of pressure-reducing and pressure-relieving devices used and methods of treatment of prior pressure ulcers

Questions are asked to identify a knowledge deficit concern safety precautions needed while performing bathing and skin care activities. Inquire for a history of accidents or injuries and safety measures taken to prevent injuries while bathing, transferring from bed to wheelchair, toilet, car, and so on.

After obtaining a history, the nurse inspects and palpates the skin. Observations are made of color, pigmentation, wrinkling, hygiene, lesions, masses, and bites. Any lesion noted should be measured, described, and documented in the client's record. The skin is palpated for texture, dryness, elasticity, and turgor. The extremities are examined for edema, temperature, and pulses. The nurse notes any problems with gait, abnormalities of feet and toes. The presence of spasticity, contractions, or other musculoskeletal problems should be noted.

Bathing provides an excellent opportunity for inspecting the client's skin as well as observing the client's mobility, coordination, gross and fine hand movement, and needs associated with skin care activities. The nurse observes and notes problems with bed positioning. Can the client move limbs or when unassisted are extremities drawn across linens? Can extremities be manipulated independently? Observe the client performing a transfer to the wheelchair and note if sliding and shearing are problematic. Note the posture and seating in the wheelchair and describe any problems noted. Mental and emotional status also are assessed. This assessment assists the nurse to determine the client's ability to perform skin care adequately and safely.

Risk Assessment

The goal of risk assessment is to identify at-risk individuals needing prevention methods and the specific factors placing them at risk. In hospitals geriatric and rehabilitation facilities and the community, risk is not equal across the populations. Instituting costly prevention methods universally is not necessary or a prudent use of resources. Risk Assessment Scales identify which populations are most at risk, allowing resources and efforts to be concentrated on that population. Risk Assessment Scales include factors of immobility, incontinence, nutritional factors such as inadequate dietary intake and impaired nutritional status, and altered level of consciousness (Bergstrom, Braden, Laguzza, & Holman, 1987; Bergstrom, Demuth, & Braden, 1987; Gosnell, 1973; Norton et al., 1975; Panel for Prediction and Prevention of Pressure Ulcers in Adults, 1992). Scoring of individuals should be done on admission and periodically during hospitalization and follow-up. A variety of risk assessment tools are available, but only the Norton and Braden Scales have been tested extensively (Bradeis et al., 1990; Norton et al., 1975). The Braden Scale was tested and validated in critical acute and long-term care settings and has shown high interrater validity (Bergstrom, Demuth, & Braden, 1987; Bryant et al., 1992; Panel for Prediction and Prevention of Pressure Ulcers in Adults, 1992).

Norton Scale

The Norton Scale consists of five factors: physical condition, mental condition, activity, mobility, and incontinence. Each factor is rated 1 to 4; descending score on the scale corresponds with greater risk. The scores range from 5 to 20. Norton determined that a score of 14 indicated onset of risk and a score of 12 and below a high risk of pressure ulcer formation. This scale does not have rater guidelines, and this may lead to interrater reliability problems (Bryant et al., 1992).

Braden Scale

The Braden Scale (see Box, pp. 288-289) consists of six factors: mobility, activity, moisture, sensory perception, nutrition, and friction and shear. The subscales are rated 1 to 4 except for friction and shear, which are rated 1 to 3. A score of 4 to 23 is possible, with 16 or below being considered at risk.

The usefulness of risk assessment tools in the rehabilitation setting is not certain (LaMantia, 1990; Staas & Cioschi, 1991). The sensitivity of the tool may not predict the "more" at-risk rehabilitation client when most will be at high risk with impaired mobility and activity and impaired states of consciousness. Additional risk factors need to be understood, validated, and utilized to increase sensitivity of Risk Assessment Scales for certain groups. For example, a SCI screening tool may include the factor of completeness of injury based on Carlson's work showing a significant relationship between completeness of injury and subsequent pressure ulcer formation. The risk assessment tools are useful in instituting early prevention and focusing care on the highest risk population. Limitations of Risk Assessment Scales include (1) the scales are not proven "predictors" of pressure sores, (2) only registered nurses show reliability in using the scales, and (3) the scales cannot be used as an end in themselves but must be utilized within an encompassing prevention program (Bryant et al., 1992). The Panel for Prediction and Prevention of Pressure Sores developed an algorithm to demonstrate this interaction (Fig. 15-7).

Classification Systems for Pressure Ulcers

Classification systems were developed to more accurately describe the extent of tissue damage. Shea (1975) designed the first scale, which has been widely used in clinical practice. Another widely used scale is the classification published by the IAET (1991). Other scales were developed to meet a specific study need—for example, a grading system for SCI model systems (Yetzer & Sullivan, 1992). Each system is useful but not comparable. Shea's grade 1 is not the same as the IAET's stage 1. In a response to the need for uniformity, the NPUAP (1989) recommends the following system be adopted:

Stage I: nonblanchable erythema of intact skin

Stage II: partial-thickness skin loss; ulcer is superficial; clinically note abrasion, blister, shallow crater

Stage III: full-thickness skin loss; damage with involvement of underlying subcutaneous tissue; superficial to deep fascia

Stage IV: full-thickness skin loss with extensive destruction of tissues deep to the muscle, bone, and support structures

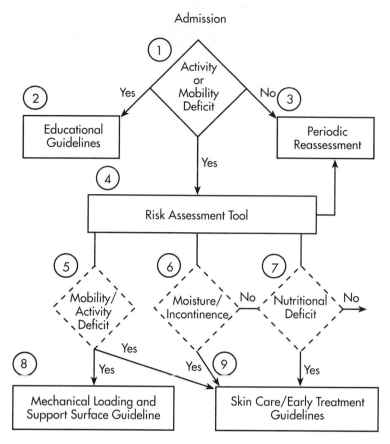

Fig. 15-7 Pressure ulcer prediction and prevention algorithm. (Used with permission from Panel for the Prediction and Prevention of Pressure Ulcers in Adults. Pressure Ulcers in Adults: Prediction and Prevention. Clinical Practice Guideline, number 3. AHCPR Publication Number 92.-0047. Rockville, MD: Agency for Health Care Policy and Research, Public Health Service, U.S. Department of Health and Human Services, May 1992.)

Staging systems have a number of inherent limitations, as follows:

1. Staging depends on gross description of tissue involved (epidermis versus muscle).
2. Accurate staging requires the clinical ability to recognize and differentiate between tissue layers; this aptitude can vary widely between practitioners, as is evidenced by the frequency with which stage I, nonblanchable erythemas, are misread.
3. Reliable staging cannot be done when necrotic tissue is present since necrotic tissue cannot be staged.
4. Healing wounds have tissue that is difficult to classify. Granulation tissue does not fit into the classification schema. Healing of pressure ulcers cannot be "staged" with these descriptors (Bryant et al., 1992; Gray, Salzberg, Petro, & Salisbury, 1990; Motta, 1993).

If a universal system is adopted, staging will give a much needed uniformity to the language of pressure ulcers, increasing the comparability of research studies on prevalence and incidence and the effectiveness of various prevention and wound care modalities (NPUAP, 1989).

◆ **Documentation.** Proper documentation of wounds and ulcers includes the following:

- ◆ Description of anatomic location of wound
- ◆ Wound size and depth in centimeters
- ◆ Staging of wound to include edges (well defined to indistinct)
- ◆ Presence and measurement of undermining (sinus tracts)
- ◆ Linear measurements of sinus tracts
- ◆ Presence or absence of necrotic tissue
- ◆ Absence or presence and amount of exudate of the surrounding skin (e.g., indurated, edematous, red)
- ◆ Description of granulation tissue if present
- ◆ Presence of epithelium at the wound edge (Bates-Jensen, 1990; Cooper, 1992; Luckmann & Sorensen, 1980).

This information is usually collected via a variety of tools from staging protocols to treatment records. Bates-Jensen developed a tool to include all the elements of documentation. A score is assessed by rating all the parameters of the wound and then the score is plotted on the linear scale with one end representing wound degeneration and progressing

---

◆

BRADEN SCALE FOR PREDICTING PRESSURE SORE RISK

PATIENT'S NAME _____   EVALUATOR'S NAME _____

SENSORY PERCEPTION Ability to respond meaningfully to pressure-related discomfort	**1. Completely limited:** Unresponsive (does not moan, flinch, or grasp) to painful stimuli, due to diminished level of consciousness or sedation, *or* limited ability to feel pain over most of body surface.	**2. Very limited:** Responds only to painful stimuli. Cannot communicate discomfort except by moaning or restlessness, *or* has a sensory impairment that limits the ability to feel pain or discomfort over half of body.
MOISTURE Degree to which skin is exposed to moisture	**1. Constantly moist:** Skin is kept moist almost constantly by perspiration, urine, etc. Dampness is detected every time client is moved or turned.	**2. Moist:** Skin is often but not always moist. Linen must be changed at least once a shift.
ACTIVITY Degree of physical activity	**1. Bedfast:** Confined to bed.	**2. Chairfast:** Ability to walk severely limited or nonexistent. Cannot bear own weight and/or must be assisted into chair or wheelchair.
MOBILITY Ability to change and control body position	**1. Completely immobile:** Does not make even slight changes in body or extremity position without assistance.	**2. Very limited:** Makes occasional slight changes in body or extremity position but unable to make frequent or significant changes independently.
NUTRITION Usual food intake pattern	**1. Very poor:** Never eats a complete meal. Rarely eats more than $\frac{1}{3}$ of any food offered. Eats 2 servings or less of protein (meat or dairy products) per day. Takes fluids poorly. Does not take a liquid dietary supplement, *or* is NPO and/or maintained on clear liquids or IV for more than 5 days.	**2. Probably inadequate:** Rarely eats a complete meal and generally eats only about half of any food offered. Protein intake includes only three servings of meat or dairy products per day. Occasionally will take a dietary supplement, *or* receives less than optimum amount of liquid diet or tube feeding.
FRICTION AND SHEAR	**1. Problem:** Requires moderate to maximum assistance in moving. Complete lifting without sliding against sheets is impossible. Frequently slides down in bed or chair, requiring frequent repositioning with maximum assistance. Spasticity, contractures, or agitation leads to almost constant friction.	**2. Potential problem:** Moves feebly or requires minimum assistance. During a move skin probably slides to some extent against sheets, chair, restraints, or other devices. Maintains relatively good position in chair or bed most of the time but occasionally slides down.

NPO, nothing by mouth; IV, intravenously; TPN, total parenteral nutrition.
Source: Barbara Braden and Nancy Bergstrom. Copyright, 1988. Reprinted with permission.

	DATE OF ASSESSMENT				

3. Slightly limited:

Responds to verbal commands but cannot always communicate discomfort or need to be turned,

or

has some sensory impairment that limits ability to feel pain or discomfort in 1 or 2 extremities.

4. No impairment:

Responds to verbal commands. Has no sensory deficit that would limit ability to feel or voice pain or discomfort.

3. Occasionally moist:

Skin is occasionally moist, requiring an extra linen change approximately once a day.

4. Rarely moist:

Skin is usually dry; linen requires changing only at routine intervals.

3. Walks occasionally:

Walks occasionally during day but for very short distances, with or without assistance. Spends majority of each shift in bed or chair.

4. Walks frequently:

Walks outside the room at least twice a day and inside room at least once every 2 hours during waking hours.

3. Slightly limited:

Makes frequent though slight changes in body or extremity position independently.

4. No limitations:

Makes major and frequent changes in position without assistance.

3. Adequate:

Eats over half of most meals. Eats a total of 4 servings of protein (meat, dairy products) each day. Occasionally will refuse a meal but will usually take a supplement if offered,

or

is on a tube feeding or TPN regimen, which probably meets most of nutritional needs.

4. Excellent:

Eats most of every meal. Never refuses a meal. Usually eats a total of 4 or more servings of meat and dairy products. Occasionally eats between meals. Does not require supplementation.

3. No apparent problem:

Moves in bed and in chair independently and has sufficient muscle strength to lift up completely during move. Maintains good position in bed or chair at all times.

TOTAL SCORE

along to tissue health. When multiple scores are plotted with dates, a picture of wound degeneration or generation is seen (Bates-Jensen, 1990).

Tools employed in wound and ulcer measurement and assessment include tape measures, rulers, concentric tracing circles, wound photography, planimetry, three-dimensional wound gauges, and wound molds. The three tools employed clinically are discussed. Other methods of wound measurement have proven to be too costly, inconsistent in measurement, and too complicated and time consuming for clinical use (Cooper, 1992).

✦ **Rulers.** Linear measurements of wounds/ulcers should be taken in centimeters. It helps to use arrows indicating the direction of the wound measurements: north and south (arrow up) and east and west (arrow side) next to the numeric reading—for example, 1.5 cm (arrow up) × 2.5 cm (arrow side) (Bates-Jensen, 1990). Problems encountered with linear measurements include irregular wound edges, which make consistent measurements difficult especially between different raters. When wounds have depth and sinuses, further measurement is needed to give an accurate picture of the wound. Repeated over time, these measurements give a "trend" to the wound repair process (Bates-Jensen, 1990; Cooper, 1992).

✦ **Tracing.** Plastic rulers and concentric circles are available to allow sterile one-time-use tracings of the wound/ulcer surface. Wounds can be difficult to trace depending on location; in addition, the position of the client can change the shape of a wound opening. Tracings can be used successfully to describe a pattern over the time of wound progress (Cooper, 1992; Motta, 1993).

✦ **Photography.** Wound photography with instamatic and delayed exposure can be used to assess and document wound progress. As serial pictures of the wound are collected, the wound status can be evaluated for progress over time. The camera records rough size (this improves if a ruler is placed alongside of the wound), color of the wound, presence of exudate, and the appearance of the surrounding skin. Photographs do not accurately capture depth or color of tissue (Cooper, 1992). Photographs are helpful when there are numerous clinicians evaluating a wound.

Nursing Diagnoses

Data concerning the skin and skin care activities are gathered from the client's health history and physical assessment. Analysis of the data and conclusions about nursing intervention are influenced by current nursing knowledge and past nursing experience. The nursing diagnoses reflect identification of the client's strengths and limitations. Identification of strengths and limitations assists the nurse in determining interventions.

Nursing diagnoses accepted by the North American Nursing Diagnosis Association related to the skin are as follows (McFarland & McFarland, 1993; Rehabilitation Nursing Foundation, 1987):

1. *High risk for skin impairment:* a state in which the individual's skin is at risk of being adversely altered. *Impaired skin integrity:* a state in which the individual's skin is adversely altered. These reflect the inability of the client to take responsibility for performing activities to prevent skin breakdown or restore skin in-

tegrity. Planning is directed toward interventions that encourage maximum client responsibility and performance of activities to maintain or restore skin integrity.

2. *Self-care deficit:* reflects the lack of ability to care for the skin because of impaired motor or cognitive function. The individual may be unable or unwilling to inspect the body for pressure ulcer areas, relieve pressure in the bed or the wheelchair, wash the body or body parts, obtain a water source, or regulate water temperature and flow. Planning should incorporate strategies to assist the individual in performing these tasks with optimum responsibility and minimum assistance.

3. *Activity intolerance:* reflects the inability to carry out activities because of fatigue. Planning should incorporate rest periods as the individual relearns the component steps of these activities and modulates activity based on individual capacity.

4. *Knowledge deficit:* reflects the lack of knowledge regarding skin care. The individual may have never known how to care for the skin properly, or because of the disease condition may have perceptual, motor, or sensory impairments that interfere with the ability to perform these functions adequately. Planning should incorporate strategies that will allow a person to perform these activities as independently as possible.

5. *High risk for injury:* related to sensory or motor deficit or to lack of awareness of skin care practices or environmental hazards. Planning should incorporate use of assistive and adaptive devices and safe practices in the client's and family's performance of bathing and other skin care activities.

Goals

Goals established with the client include provisions for teaching self-care and involvement of the family when self-care is not possible. Nursing judgment concerning self-care of the skin is based on the client's physiologic, psychological, and physical ability (Richardson & Meyer, 1981). The nursing theory postulated by Orem (1971) focuses on self-care as a process whereby individuals contribute to their own health.

Self-care is behavior that evolves from social and cognitive experiences and is learned through interpersonal relationships and culture. Self-care contributes to self-esteem and self-image and is directly affected by self-concept (Orem, 1971).

Generally goals mutually established with the client and family for maintaining skin integrity include plans to

1. Maintain and restore skin integrity
2. Prevent damage to the skin
3. Understand the cause and prevention of pressure ulcers and the rationale for prevention
4. Recognize and intervene on warning signs of skin disruption
5. Establish a management plan recognizing the changes in mobility, activity, and health that the individual will experience over a life-span

Rehabilitation Nursing Interventions

The primary nursing direction is toward prevention. The paradigm for care must encapsulate the hospital to the community and from birth through the aging process. As with most health issues, prevention is the most cost-effective management when compared with the costs of a poor skin outcome. The rehabilitation nurse must plan for interventions that encompass the present setting but will work or have ability to be controlled by the client and caregivers to work with in the home, school, and work settings. The nursing interventions will be arranged to

1. Reduce or eliminate the effects of primary and secondary factors for skin and wound development
2. Optimize the microenvironment
3. Support the client
4. Educate the client and family

The following Box presents examples of specific nursing interventions provided for a client with a nursing diagnoses of high risk for skin impairment.

EXAMPLES OF NURSING DIAGNOSES AND NURSING INTERVENTIONS FOR THE CLIENT WITH HIGH-RISK IMPAIRMENT

High risk for skin impairment

- Assess for the presence of risk factors related to skin breakdown (e.g., poor diet, elderly, steroid therapy)
- Inspect for skin redness, lesions, blisters, swelling, drainage and document
- Relieve pressure by turning, weight shifting, altering turning schedule
- Avoid shearing forces or friction
- Perform skin inspection twice daily
- Control incontinence
- Provide hygiene that maintains clean dry skin
- Teach client and family skin assessment and pressure ulcer prevention
- Avoid massage over bony prominences
- Utilize pressure-reducing device in conjunction with turning schedule
- In collaboration with the physician and nutritionist monitor/assess nutritional parameters: oral/parenteral intake of protein, calories and fluids; albumin and total protein levels

Self-care deficit: bathing/hygiene

- Assess undressing/dressing; checking water temperature; washing self
- Determine level of self-care
- Teach self-care skills
- Provide verbal cues
- Provide adequate time to accomplish self-care activities
- Involve family/caregiver in care
- Collaborate with occupational therapist, physical therapist

Knowledge deficit

- Assess present knowledge of illness/disability; previous self-care behaviors; client/family healthcare beliefs/practices and attitudes; reaction to illness/disability
- Identify potential caregivers and persons(s) who want/need to learn about disability and treatment
- Determine when teaching will be done
- Plan: identify teaching strategies and resources to be used; schedule participation in available health education classes; integrate ethnic, religious values into plan

High risk for injury

- Assess environmental factors; judgment issues
- Eliminate causative factors; modify environment
- Initiate health education; promote positive health behaviors

Specific Nursing Interventions
✦ Risk factors

The rehabilitation nurse first addresses all the risk factors that might affect the quality of a client's skin and wounds. Efforts should be made to minimize these negative effects. Systemic conditions should be monitored—for example, diabetics should have blood glucose levels monitored. Problems with tissue perfusion secondary to hypovolemia, decreased blood pressure, and lack of oxygenation should be handled by providing for compression and elevation of the affected extremities and providing nasal O_2 if needed. Nutrition parameters need to be evaluated and any signs of malnutrition addressed. Multiple studies reported by ACHPR indicate malnutrition is a risk factor for ulcer formation (Fig. 15-8) (Bergstrom, Bennett, Carlson, et al., 1994). The nurse addresses factors interfering with nutrition and offers support—for example, the client may not eat hospital food. The family may be encouraged to bring in favorite foods or supplements may need to be used. A consultation with a nutritionist is recommended for clients at high risk for skin impairment (Konstantides, 1992; Lidowski, 1988). Concern for the effects of lack of activity and immobility on the general health status of the client should be addressed. The client needs a program that will include all aspects of mobility as these will have a general overall impact on improving health status (King & French, 1990; Levin, Simpson, & McDonald, 1989; Panel for Prediction and Prevention of Pressure Ulcers in Adults, 1992).

✦ Hygiene and skin care

Daily activities result in the accumulation of metabolic wastes and contaminants on skin. As discussed previously, these wastes and contaminants can alter skin and reduce tissue capacity to handle pressure. Waste products should be removed promptly using warm, not hot, water and a mild cleansing solution (Bryant et al., 1992; Doughty, 1992; Panel for Prediction and Prevention of Pressure Ulcers in Adults, 1992; Wysocki & Bryant, 1992). Avoid harsh cleansers such as povidone-iodine. Skin will be damaged by the use of harsh cleansers as the natural barriers of sebum and moisture are removed. Elevated water temperature will increase the metabolic activity and demands on skin and tissue. As the client ages, the need for daily baths should be reconsidered. The problems of aging skin will be exacerbated by the unnecessary removal of the natural barrier. Limit hygiene measures to the face, axillae, groin, and genitals using the very mildest of skin cleansers. Other factors that contribute to skin drying are low humidity (less than 40%) and exposure to cold (Panel for Prediction and Prevention of Pressure Ulcers in Adults, 1992). Adequate hydration of the stratum corneum helps protect against mechanical assault. As seen in aging skin, the drier surface results in reduced pliability scaling, and fissuring (Hotter, 1990; Panel for Prediction and Prevention of Pressure Ulcers in Adults, 1992). Moisturizers will protect against the loss of more moisture to air and provide protection. Specific moisturizers have not been shown to be more efficacious than others. The nurse must be familiar with the various products, know the additives, and avoid moisturizers containing irritants (Motta, 1993). Having client rooms in the hospital and home setting set at an increasing humidity level will also decrease the drying impact on skin.

As discussed earlier, moisture can be deleterious to skin. All efforts should be made to control fecal and urinary incontinence with use of bowel and bladder programs. Wound drainage can be contained adequately with proper dressings. Use of incontinence pads that place plastic against skin should be avoided. The nurse should experiment with the newer products that draw moisture away from the skin if incontinence cannot be controlled. Moisture creams also can be used to protect at-risk skin, although research evidence to support this is sparse and the recommendation is based on clinical evidence.

✦ Prevention of pressure

All efforts should be made to relieve and reduce pressure for patients at high risk for skin impairment. From the nursing assessment particular areas of concern are elicited and a comprehensive plan of management to reduce pressure is devised. Pressure reduction encompasses all activities and modalities from bed to wheelchair, transfer activities, clothing fit, and mobility. Each area needs review and intervention if problematic for the client.

✦ Positioning.
Positioning is a concern in the bed as well as the wheelchair. Correct positioning is aimed at distributing the load over a maximum surface area and avoiding weight loading on bony prominences (Krouskop, Noble, Garber, & Spencer, 1983; Krouskop & Garber, 1987). Problems with positioning can be exacerbated by obesity, spasticity, contractures, orthotic devices, traction, and client pain. Generally clients need to be repositioned every 2 hours. This standard was set by Kosiak based on studies reviewed earlier. The Agency for Health Care Policy and Research (AHCPR) recently supported this recommendation (Kosiak, 1959; Panel for Prediction and Prevention of Pressure Ulcers in Adults, 1992). This is a minimum standard, and clients must be assessed individually for skin tolerance to this interval. When interventions and intervals are being increased and introduced, clients' skin at critical areas needs to be checked every hour or more frequently. Bryant suggests that during the first 24 hours of a new interval or introduction of a new modality, a decrease in the dimensions of blanching erythema should be noted, and—for change to be acceptable—no further progression of ischemic signs are seen. Reevaluation of modality or support surface is needed if these parameters are increased.

Changes in position can be accomplished with schedules incorporating all four surfaces with supine, prone, and right and left lateral positioning. A schedule should be developed to monitor time spent in these positions and any problems occurring on a particular surface (Abbruzzese, 1985). If redness and signs of increased pressure are noted in a particular surface, turning to that surface can be eliminated or the time interval can be reduced on that critical surface. A finding of nonblanchable erythema precludes positioning on that surface, and all efforts should be made for pressure relief of that area. The prone position can be accomplished on standard surfaces with bridging techniques (Panel for Prediction and Prevention of Pressure Ulcers in Adults, 1992) or on a standard water mattress without bridging (LaMantia, 1990; Staas & Cioschi, 1991). The side-lying

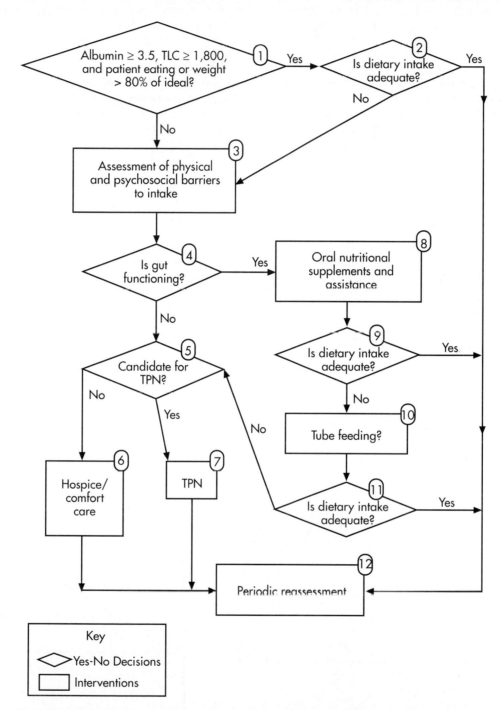

Fig. 15-8 The AHCPR algorithm details recommendations for nutritional assessment and support for the client who has an existing pressure ulcer. TLC = total lymphocyte count; TPN = total parenteral nutrition. (From *Treatment of Pressure Ulcers: Clinical Practice Guidelines, No. 15.* AHCPR Publication 95-0652. December 1994. by N. Bergstrom, M.A. Bennett, C.E. Carlson, et al. Rockville, MD: U.S. Department of Health and Human Services, Agency for Health Care Policy and Research.)

position should avoid direct positioning over the trochanteric area. Studies show higher interface pressure and lower transcutaneous oxygen tension over trochanters when individuals are positioned directly over trochanters (Garber & Krouskop, 1982). Seiler, Allan, and Stahelin (1986) recommend the 30-degree laterally inclined position for side-lying (Fig. 15-9). In addition to these major changes in position, smaller position changes within that rotation can extend time in that position. Studies show conflicting evidence that smaller shifts decrease pressure ulcer incidence, pointing to the area for individual monitoring when this technique is employed (Panel for Prediction and Prevention of Pressure Ulcers in Adults, 1992). Efforts should be made to keep bony prominences from being positioned over another body surface. Use of foam wedges and pillows can accomplish this. The heels have been shown in several studies to be particularly vulnerable to pressure even on pressure-reducing support surfaces (Maklebust, Sieggreen, & Mondoux, 1988; Panel for Prediction and Prevention of Pressure Ulcers in Adults, 1992). Pillows can be used for this purpose, but often an insensate extremity will be inadvertently repositioned off the pillow to the mattress. Pillows are insufficient when spasticity is a concern. A number of pressure-relief devices are available commercially such as sheepskin booties and foam boots. Heel protectors do not appreciably decrease or dissipate pressure. These devices can assist with protection from the trauma of shearing and friction or the bumping that the foot may receive in transfer activity. The device that elevates the foot totally from the support surface is most effective when pressure relief is needed (Pinzur et al., 1991; Yetzer & Sullivan, 1992). Devices that elevate the heel totally are the only recommended devices for pressure relief. Methods used to assist with position changes must be carefully addressed.

Clients need to be taught techniques that decrease the amount of dragging or pulling of the body and extremities across the bed or chair surface. The friction and shearing resulting from poor position changes is extremely injurious to skin and tissue. Transfer boards should be used with a lift and sit method and not to slide clients between surfaces.

Wheelchair positioning should assure maximum support over the available seated area. Footplates should be set at a height that does not transfer weight to the ischium but allows weight to be borne by thighs (Donovan et al., 1988). Clients should have positioners that keep the trunk in alignment but do not cause pressure problems in another location. Position changes in the wheelchair ideally should be done every 15 minutes. Clients with even a major amount of disability can be taught techniques to provide this relief (Fig. 15-10). Clients who cannot do this for themselves or who are learning new techniques need careful monitoring to assure pressure is relieved. Weight shifts can be accomplished with a push-up or side shift. Use a hand check to assess whether there is sufficient space (1 inch or more of uncompressed support surface) between the surface and the weight bearing part of the client's body. Schedules can assist clients to remember shifts. Devices such as beeping chair pads, watches, and timers have not proved too successful as clients found them loud and bothersome (Krouskop & Garber, 1989). Previous criticisms of the ability of devices to know the proper interval at which to signal a weight shift have been studied by researchers. A more user-friendly device utilizes a microprocessor to signal as well as monitor weight shifts. The interesting feature of this research device is the ability to store information and play back data on individual performance (Cumming, Tompkins, Jones, & Margolis, 1986).

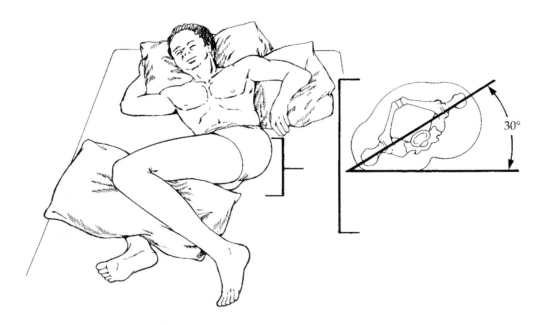

Fig. 15-9 Thirty-degree lateral position at which pressure points are avoided. (From Bryant RA: *Acute and Chronic Wounds* edited by R.A. Bryant, 1992, St. Louis: Mosby–Year Book. Copyright 1992 by Mosby–Year Book. Reprinted by permission.)

✦ Monitoring pressure relief

Systematic skin inspection must be done by clients or nurse every day. These checks should occur at least twice daily. In the morning the skin is checked for any problems with bed positioning and areas for concern during the day. At night all seating position pressure areas are checked. When new tolerances are being tried, clients are started out with a 30-minute sitting times and increased hourly with skin checks after each increment (King & French, 1990; Krouskop & Garber, 1987). Skin checks are done for any area of noted hyperemia. In dark-skinned individuals the hyperemic response may be noted by tactile assessment (Rempusheski, 1989). During this monitoring phase it is essential to critique the current plan of care (Dai & Catanzaro, 1987). Although there is no evidence that systematic, comprehensive, and routine skin inspection decreases the incidence of pressure ulcers, it provides information for designing interventions and standards to evaluate outcomes and make necessary changes based on skin inspection (King & French, 1990; Panel for Prediction and Prevention of Pressure Ulcers in Adults, 1992). The client who has a pressure ulcer on a sitting surface should avoid sitting. If pressure can be relieved, a limited sitting may be allowed (AHCPR, 1994, p. 41). For example, when a client returns from daily therapy for rest, the nurse notes blanchable hyperemia over the right ischium that lasts for the 1-hour rest period. The nurse extends the rest period until the hyperemia resolves, contacts the physical therapist, and consults regarding the quality and sufficiency of the weight shift and the wheelchair cushion. The wheelchair cushion is used to provide an increased base of support for pressure relief and improved sitting posture and mobility. Symmetric postural alignment is important to avoid uneven weight-bearing over the ischium and trochanters to sacrum (Staas & Cioschi, 1991). Pressure relief is only one aspect to the wheelchair cushion. As a device it can provide pressure relief so well that it hinders balance and mobility. Wheelchair cushions are most frequently a compromise between these factors. According to Donovan a wheelchair cushion relieves pressure, distributes weight away from bony prominences, and stabilizes the body for balance and functional position. Wheelchair cushions have similar prop-

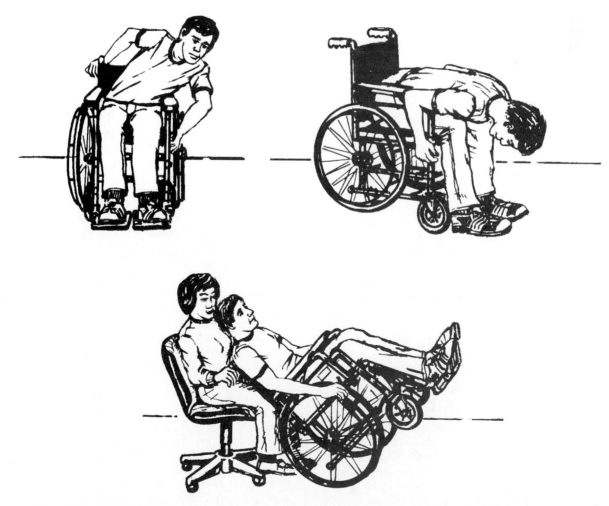

Fig. 15-10 Clients must shift their weight regularly to prevent pressure areas from developing. Weight shifts are simple techniques that help prevent complications with skin integrity. (From *Rehabilitation/Restorative Care in the Community* by S. Hoeman, 1990, St. Louis: Mosby–Year Book. Copyright 1990 by Mosby–Year Book. Reprinted by permission.)

erties to bed support surfaces and the principles in choosing them are similar. Researchers have investigated using lumbar supports to improve the distribution of pressure in the seated position. Shields and Cook (1992) found negligible effect of seated buttock pressures in paraplegics using this device. The wheelchair cushion does not achieve low pressure readings over the ischium. Cushions have been shown to decrease pressures to 40 to 60 mm Hg, but the effort is to distribute weight over the thighs (Garber & Krouskop, 1982). Prescribing the wheelchair cushion takes into account client age, disability/pressure relief need, longevity of cushion, cushion weight, and cushion maintenance and repair costs. Rehabilitation professionals consider the long-term client needs and instruct the client on the proper use of the wheelchair cushion including the warning signs for repair. As client status changes, cushions are reevaluated and changed as necessary.

✦ Support surfaces

Support surfaces reduce interface pressure over the bony prominences by maximizing contact and redistributing weight over a large area (Hicks, 1971; Krouskop et al., 1983). Support surfaces are made to cover a variety of surfaces including beds, chairs, wheelchairs, stretchers, examination tables, and operating room tables.

Numerous investigators have measured the characteristics and properties of support surfaces. The AHCPR reviewed clinical studies that looked at the effects of a variety of pressure-reducing devices and the incidence of pressure ulcers in at-risk patients. When pressure-reducing devices were compared with standard hospital beds, the incidence of pressure ulcers in clients cared for on a standard hospital mattress was much greater. When studies looked at comparisons of two types of pressure-reducing devices, no significant differences in incidence and severity of pressure ulcers was found. There is evidence that pressure-reducing devices can decrease the incidence of pressure ulcers but not that one type of pressure-reducing device is more effective than another to prevent pressure ulcers (Panel for Prediction and Prevention of Pressure Ulcers in Adults, 1992).

Since one support surface is not necessarily superior to another for reducing pressure sores, other considerations are reviewed when selecting one. Conine, Choi, and Lim (1989) suggest "user friendliness" as a guide. Qualities for consideration include the following:

- ✦ Costs: initial, maintenance, replacement
- ✦ Regulations (hospital safety codes)
- ✦ Client pleasing: comfort, stability, temperature, noise, suitability of weight (bed and chair)
- ✦ Caregiver pleasing: difficulty in moving and transferring; frequent need to calibrate and monitor equipment; service and repair availability

The high-tech end of replacement beds usually is retained for the most difficult problems of pressure ulcers, but two recent studies dealt with the area of reduced cost and rapidity of healing as factors for choosing these beds. Strauss et al. (1991) found the cost of home air-fluidized therapy for pressure ulcers was no more costly than alternative therapy and reduced hospitalizations. Ferrell, Osterweil, and Christenson (1993) showed substantial improvement over foam mattresses when using low-air-flow beds for

healing pressure ulcers and demonstrated the rapidity of healing time as compared with a foam mattress. Support surfaces are categorized by their mechanical features. They can be pressure-relieving or pressure-reducing surfaces. Pressure-relief systems consistently keep surface tissue pressure readings below capillary closing pressure. Use of pressure-reducing surfaces results in lower pressures when compared with a standard hospital mattress (Bryant et al., 1992; IAET, 1991). Support surfaces are available as overlays (support surface placed over the hospital mattress), replacement mattresses, and specialty beds. Support surfaces are reviewed for their ability to distribute pressure, avoid humidity buildup, and insulate temperature (Conine et al., 1989). Figure 15-11 illustrates current ACHPR guidelines for management of tissue loads.

Overlays. Used for pressure reduction, overlay systems do not provide complete pressure relief. The higher the density, the increased ability to distribute pressure and allow air circulation (Conine et al., 1989). Clients need to be monitored for individualized pressure relief. When choosing an overlay system consider whether the height of the bed or seat is increased. This may be a concern for both client and caregiver, making assisted or independent transfers more difficult. Caregivers may need a step stool to provide care. Foam overlays should be at least 4 inches in height for bed use. Foam also is popular as a wheelchair cushion. High-density foams can be contoured to meet individual postural needs. However, foam may be hot, increasing skin temperatures and local metabolic needs; foam cannot be washed (removes flammability retardation); foam necessitates the use of a plastic sheet for incontinence, adding concerns about moisture. Examples of commercially available products include Bio Gard, Geo Mat, and Ultra Foam.

Water. Water systems must be checked for proper inflation so that the person floats; they can be underfilled and overfilled. Motion can be a problem; baffle systems on some models control water activity. Additional concerns are weight and puncture problems; also the manufacturer may recommend not raising the head of the bed but others have compartments to allow this. Turning individuals on water surfaces can be more difficult. Temperatures may need heating control. Examples of commercially available products include Rochester modular waterbeds and Tender FLO.

Gel. Gel systems usually are combined with foam. These are easy to clean, low-maintenance systems, are puncture resistant, and do not have the disadvantages of water with motion and difficulty of turning individuals (Bryant et al., 1992). Disadvantages include weight and expense. Mattress weight creates problems for both the caregiver and client. The increased weight for the wheelchair user is of particular concern, as well as the instability created for transfers. Temperature guidelines provided by the manufacturer need to be checked. Some gels get harder in cold temperatures, making them unusable in cold climates (Conine et al., 1989).

Air. Air overlays are divided further into static-air, alternating-air, and low-air-loss systems.

STATIC AIR. Air is forced through interconnected tunnels—bulbous cells—to provide the proper pressure. Static-air systems require skilled monitoring to check for proper inflation (Bryant et al., 1992). Some models allows for cells

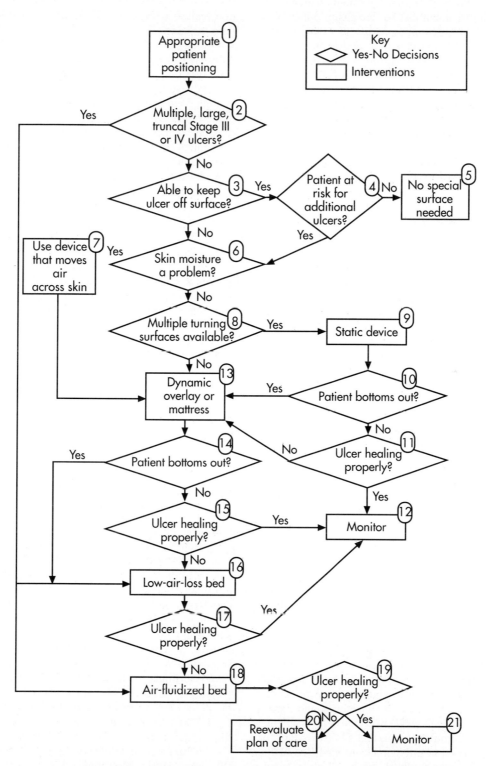

Fig. 15-11   The ACHPR algorithm for management of tissue loads assists the nurse to choose support surfaces that help distribute pressure and reduce friction and shear on the tissue. (From *Treatment of Pressure Ulcers: Clinical Practice Guidelines, No. 15*. AHCPR Publication 95-0652. December 1994. by N. Bergstrom, M.A. Bennett, C.E. Carlson et al. Rockville, MD: U.S. Department of Health and Human Services, Agency for Health Care Policy and Research.)

(bulbs) to be tied off to give pressure relief over designated areas (Conine et al., 1989). These are low-maintenance systems designed for multipatient use but are easily punctured and expensive. Examples of commercially available products include K-soft, Sofcare, Tender Air, and Roho.

ALTERNATING AIR. Air is pumped through interconnecting tunnels with intervals of inflation and deflation. This is promoted as a device to reduce pressure and stimulate circulation. Alternating-air systems have advantages similar to static-air systems with the added client concerns about noise and inflation and deflation (Conine et al., 1989). Commercially available products include Air Flo; Bio Flote and Lapidus.

LOW AIR LOSS. In addition to filling channels with air, low-air-loss systems provide for air movement around the skin. This feature reduces moisture perspiration problems and helps to reduce friction and shear (Bryant et al., 1992). As with the alternating-air overlay, puncture problems and noise are major drawbacks. Commercially available products include Acucair, Biotherapy, and First step plus.

With both static-air and alternating-air cushions, there is the added concern for safe transfers. They do not provide a stable base and are problematic for clients with poor hand and trunk control (Conine et al., 1989). The newer models compensate for this problem with combination products of air and foam.

Replacement mattresses. Replacement mattresses have surface characteristics similar to the overlays but can provide the needed depth to increase density or flotation without the additional height problem of an overlay (Bryant et al., 1992). Examples include Bioguard, Akros Gel and Foam, Maxi Float, Thera Rest, and Ultra Foam.

Specialty beds. The most expensive of support surfaces, specialty beds replace the hospital bed and provide pressure relief as well as decreased shearing, friction, and moisture. High-air-loss, low-air-loss, and kinetic specialty beds are available.

HIGH AIR LOSS. The individual floats on a bed of silicone-coated air-fluidized beads. Pressure relief is not absolute on these beds. Studies have shown pressures over capillary closure in heels (Panel for Prediction and Prevention of Pressure Ulcers in Adults, 1992). Existing pressure ulcers heal faster on these beds and fewer ulcers develop on them (Bryant et al., 1992). High-air-loss beds are extremely helpful to care for clients following skin flap surgery. The flotation provides minimal pressure to tissue at the surgical site and reduces the problems of friction and shear. Concerns for this bed include dehydration, wound drying, increased client and room temperature, and client disorientation (Bryant et al., 1992). The bed can be turned off for procedures and transfers. The height and weight of the bed can be a problem. Examples include Clinitron, Skytron, and Fluid Air Plus.

LOW AIR LOSS. A series of interconnected air-filled bladder pillows frame low-air-loss beds. Each pillow is filled and calibrated for proper inflation and to provide air flow. The head of bed can be elevated and transfers are easier; however, the surface is very slippery. There is decreased shearing and friction, but transfers can be unsafe. Examples include Flexicair, Kinair, and Mediscus.

KINETIC. Kinetic beds provide continuous motion and may be combined with an air-loss feature. These primarily are used as management for multiple problems of immobility usually from trauma. The ability to relive pressure is one feature (Bryant et al., 1992). Examples include Biodine and Roto Rest.

✦ **Wound care.** Failure to address the cause of the wound will result in a nonhealing wound despite appropriate local and systemic treatment (Doughty, 1992). It cannot be stressed enough that topical care supports the wound; the healing comes from removing the cause and addressing systemic concerns. Evolving wound technologies will be addressed when there is interaction between the wound and the topical therapy stimulating healing. Local wound care is based on principles of topical therapy:

1. Cleanse the wound
2. Debride necrotic tissue
3. Treat infection
4. Absorb excess exudate
5. Obliterate "dead space"
6. Maintain moist surface
7. Cover the wound (Doughty, 1992; Motta, 1993)

✦ **Wound cleansing.** Controversy continues about what constitutes proper wound cleansing. Nurses need to be knowledgeable about cleansing solutions, their action on tissues, and the phase of wound healing. In a clean proliferating wound, the goal is to promote the health of cells. Mild commercially available wound cleansers vary from safe to toxic. The AHCPR recommends using normal saline with enough irrigation pressure to enhance wound cleansing without causing trauma to the wound bed (AHCPR, 1994, p. 51). Some researchers feel the wound surface of clean wounds should be left alone, allowing the supportive exudate to heal the wound (Alvarez et al., 1989; Baxter & Rodheaver, 1990). The nurse recognizes the fragile nature of new proliferating tissue and should cleanse only with minimum pressure and mild cleansing agents. Antiseptic cleansers such as povidone-iodine, acetic acid, Dakin's solution, and hydrogen peroxide should not be used because of the harmful effect on healing tissue (Baxter & Rodheaver, 1990; Bergstrom, Bennett, Carlson, et al., 1994; Doughty, 1992).

✦ **Infected wounds.** Wounds are noted to be infected when there are colony counts of more than 100,000 organisms per milliliter. Wounds should be cultured when there is fever, edema, the surrounding wound bed is indurated, and erythema is present. The drainage may be copious and foul smelling. Some wounds are infected with no signs of infection, just chronic nonhealing status. These wounds should have microbial cultures performed. Alvarez et al. (1989) attribute the hypertrophic granulation tissue in these wounds to infection. The nurse obtains aerobic and anaerobic cultures. Topical antimicrobials and antibiotics may be used. Topical antibiotic preparations that are not harmful to the wound include Silvadene, Polysporin, Neosporin, benzoyl peroxide, bacitracin zinc, and J&J First-Aid Cream (Doughty, 1992). Metronidazole will reduce odor in pressure ulcers; however, it must be used in combination with another dressing and will not substitute for systemic antibiotics (Motta, 1993). Wounds can also be cleansed with syringe irrigation using a needle (19 gauge); extreme force is not recommended since healthy tissue will be removed with infected tissue. The traditional wound cleanser previously mentioned will cleanse but also would harm good tissue. The nurse must assess the wound and decide efficacy of the wound cleanser. Povidone-iodine damages granulation tissue and may cause iodine toxicity (Eaglstein, 1986). Acetic acid is effective against *Pseudomonas aeruginosa* but also damages proliferating tissue. Dakin's solution is irritating to granulation tissue as well as surrounding tissue. Although hydrogen peroxide provides mechanical cleansing, it is harmful to new tissue and the air bubbles formed can cause air emboli if introduced into sinus tracts.

◆ **Necrotic wounds.** These wounds need more aggressive cleansing. Debridement can be achieved by mechanical cleansing, sharp debridement and by enzymatic preparation with occlusive dressings. Removal of necrotic tissue will speed along the healing process; the method that can promote healing most quickly without damaging underlying tissue will be the method of choice. Sharp debridement works well when necrotic tissue is delineated clearly and avascular tissue grasped easily. This is contraindicated in clients with adherent necrotic tissue and those with ischemic ulcers (arterial ulcers, diabetic dry gangrene) (Doughty, 1992). Surgical laser debridement now is being employed by surgeons on an outpatient basis. It has superior qualities because of its instant hemostasis and sterilization of the wound. Enzymatic treatment utilizes a number of topical ointments (Travase, Santyl, Elase). For the enzymes to work, the eschar must be removed with a scalpel and the wound kept moist. Manufacturers' recommendations should be followed closely.

◆ **Wound covering.** The wound covering enhances the natural environment as does the skin itself. It provides thermal insulation and protects the wound from bacteria and trauma (Doughty, 1992). The evolving wound research has taught the traditional method of gauze packing—dampened with saline solution allowed to dry slightly and then removed—which removes exudates with good viable tissue. Research for wound healing shows that wounds heal faster with a moist environment, allowing the natural factors in the wound exudate to promote healing of the wound (Alvarez et al., 1989). A variety of wound dressings are available, and research shows the moist environment permitted by dressings heals pressure ulcers more quickly and effectively (Gorse & Messner, 1987). Some studies dispute the cost-effectiveness of hydrocolloid dressings (Xakellis & Chrischilles, 1992). More research is needed to compare dressing choice and wound outcome. The decision for dressing is based on clinical assessment of the wound. The obvious decisions are made about infection, debridement, and presence of sinus tracts. Sinus tracts are a source of bacterial growth. Their "dead space" should be eliminated with light gauze packing. All wounds require moist wound healing; the decision-making process for dressing requires matching wound characteristics with the qualities of a particular dressing. Dressings must be chosen in order to support the wound at various states. If wounds do not progress, review the cause and systemic effects. Plan wound care on a scientific basis. Failure of wounds to improve could be due to infection or systemic problems. New dressing methods

Table 15-4 Wound dressings

Dressing type	Debride	Absorb	Fill dead space	Protect from trauma	Protect from infection	Insulate	Keep moist	Examples
Transparent adhesive	+A			+	+	+	+	OpSite, Bioclusive, Tegaderm, Polyskin, AcuDerm, Blisterfilm, Ensure-it
Hydrocolloid wafer dressings	+A	+		+	+	+	+	DuoDerm, Restore, Intact, Intrasite, Tegasorb, Ultec, Comfeel Ulcer Dressing, Hydrapad, J&J Ulcer Dressing
Semipermeable polyurethane foam		+		+		+	+	Allevyn, Lyofoam, Synthaderm, Epilock
Absorption dressings	+A	+	+	+			+	Bard Absorption Dressing, Hydragran, Sorbsan, Kaltostat, DuoDerm Paste and Granules, Comfeel Ulcus paste and powder, Debrisan
Gauze	+A*	+	+					Gauze dressings, Mesalt
Synthetic barrier dressing		+		+		+	+	Hydron
Gel dressings	+A	+G	+G	+			+	Vigilon, ElastoGel, Intrasite Gel, Geliperm

A, autolytic form; *G*, granulate form.
*If kept moist.
From *Acute and Chronic Wounds*, edited by R. Bryant, 1992, St. Louis: Mosby–Year Book.
Copyright 1992 by Mosby–Year Book.
Reprinted by permission.

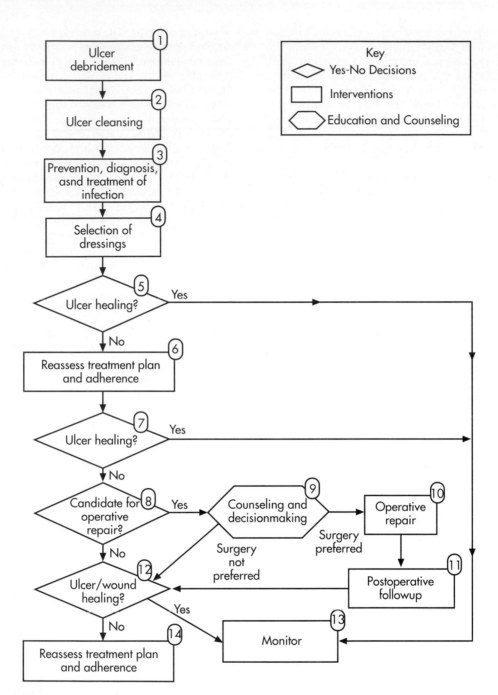

Fig. 15-12 Treatment of pressure ulcers. The AHCPR has prepared guidelines for decision-making in care of pressure ulcers. (From *Treatment of Pressure Ulcers: Clinical Practice Guidelines, No. 15.* AHCPR Publication 95-0652. December 1994. by N. Bergstrom, M.A. Bennett, C.E. Carlson, et al. Rockville, MD: U.S. Department of Health and Human Services, Agency for Health Care Policy and Research.)

might be necessary. Table 15-4 summarizes available dressing and properties, and Fig. 15-12 illustrates decision-making in management of pressure ulcers (Bergstrom, Bennett, Carlson, et al., 1994).

✦ Types of dressings

Thin film (transparent adhesives). Thin-film dressings were the first occlusive dressings devised to insulate, pro-

tect, and maintain the moist wound surface. Exudate can build up under the film, contraindicating its use in wounds of clients with aging friable skin. Films are good choice for dry necrotic wounds requiring debridement. Examples include OpSite and Tegaderm.

Hydrocolloid. Hydrocolloid wafer dressings insulate and protect the moist wound surface and absorb exudate. These are occlusive dressings and do not permit O_2 to diffuse into the wound, which has the hypoxic stimulation that wounds require for healing. Early in their use clinicians worried about collecting exudate and gel formed beneath the embedded in the adhesive wafers with hydroactive particles embedded in the wafers. Now it is understood that occlusion promotes wound healing with growth factors allowed to proliferate beneath the dressing. These dressings are contraindicated for infected wounds and wounds with secretions and large amounts of exudate (Doughty, 1992; Moody et al., 1988). Examples include DuoDerm and Intrasite.

Foam. Foam dressings have nonadherent wafers that are used to promote moist wound healing and provide absorption. These dressings are highly absorptive, remove easily, and their hydrophobic surfaces repel contaminants. They should not be used on wounds with no exudate. Foam dressings are not self-adherent and require an additional taping or another dressing to adhere to skin (Doughty, 1992; Motta, 1993). Examples include Allevym and Lyofoam.

Hydrogel. Available in sheets and granules to pour onto the wound, hydrogel dressings provide a moist wound environment and mild absorption, and can be used to fill in dead space. These dressings are painless and are easy to apply and remove. Care should be taken to keep the dressing from the surrounding skin. Dressing must be covered with secondary dressing. Examples include Vigilon and Intrasite Gel.

Exudate absorbers. Exudate absorbers are powders, or beads, used to absorb exudate and fill in dead space. They maintain a moist wound bed, absorb large amounts of exudate, and can provide a minimum of debridement. This dressing is contraindicated for wounds with dry eschar and wounds without exudate. Examples include Debrisan and Bard Absorption.

Calcium alginates. Calcium alginates occur naturally in seaweed. Although available in the United Kingdom since the late 1940s, they have been slow to be used in the United States (Gensheimer, 1993; Motta, 1989). They absorb exudate, maintain a moist wound surface, and can be used in a variety of wounds from shallow exudative wounds to deep wounds. Calcium alginates are very absorptive and require a topper dressing; they should not be used for nonexudative wounds. Examples include Sorbsan and Kaltostat.

Gauze. The purpose of gauze is to absorb exudate. Gauze support moist wound healing if kept moist. Most often gauze is used to fill large dead spaces or, as ribbons, to pack sinuses. Gauze should be packed lightly to prevent impairment of circulation. Gauze should not be used over healing proliferative wounds or dry eschar.

Synthetic barrier. The purpose of a synthetic barrier is to provide absorption of exudate and maintain a moist wound surface. This dressing forms a paste to conform to the wound bed. The surface of the dressing allows exudate to pass through. It must be used with a secondary dressing or tape and is contraindicated for nonexudative wounds. Example: Hydron.

Topical circulatory stimulants. These agents stimulate circulation.

Lubricating spray. Lubricating sprays are convenient, easy to use, and maintain a moist wound bed. They can be sprayed on gauze to "wet" it before packing the wound. Lubricating sprays require a secondary dressing for absorption. Example: Granulex.

◆ **Evolving wound care modalities.** Research continues on the management of wounds, promising to bring more effective treatments for difficult to heal ulcers. This research is based on wound repair physiology and looks at the interactive nature of wound healing. Major research areas include investigation of growth factors, electrostimulation, and hyperbaric oxygenation (Confer, Frantz, Nemiroff, Junen, Mitchell, & Palmer, 1992). The nurse should keep abreast of this research and become involved in shaping its future relative to wound care. More of the technologies are being used presently as standard therapies but much research is needed.

◆ **Surgical management of pressure ulcers.** When wounds reach stage III to IV, surgical closure becomes an option (Linden & Morris, 1990). Early closure of the wound will decrease loss of fluid and nutrients and improve the client's general health status as well as lead to earlier mobilization and re-entry into social structure (Black & Black, 1987). In planning for surgical intervention, clients should be at optimal nutritional and health status. Clients with a serum albumin level of less than 3 should not be considered. There is a high percentage of failure in young traumatic paraplegics and the frail elderly. Disa et al. (1991) caution that additional prospective study is needed to conclude which patients will benefit most from surgical closure. Surgical closure of chronic pressure ulcers allows clients to be mobilized quickly, return to work, family, and school without the chronic loss of time to bed rest and threatened complications of immobility.

Linden recommends a systematic approach to management of pressure ulcers by stage, employing a comprehensive team approach by the surgeon, nurses, therapists, and nutritionists. When clients have long-term options before surgery and all systemic factors are optimized and spasms controlled, clients need to have proper positioning training and education regarding the procedure and follow-up management. Principles of surgical management include the following:

1. Client is free of infection.
2. The position at surgery mimics the position at which closure will be at greatest tension; when tension is decreased, the flap will have mobility.
3. All contaminated tissue is removed, including bone if it is infected.
4. All scar tissue is removed from the surrounding wound.
5. Incisions should not cross over bony prominences.
6. The defect left from the excision is filled with a rotation flap of muscle (Figs. 15-13 and 15-14).
7. Closed drainage is maintained to prevent seroma formation.
8. All pressure is kept off the area by proper positioning—prone position is popular.
9. Many clients are managed on high-air-loss beds to decrease any tension or stress on the flap or donor sites.
10. Mobility begins after week 3 with careful monitoring (Bryant et al., 1992; Disa et al., 1991).

Additional considerations concern ethical cost issues. Should the wound be closed by surgical methods when, with a fairly predictable model, certain clients will present with another ulcer? Can, or should, care be limited? These is-

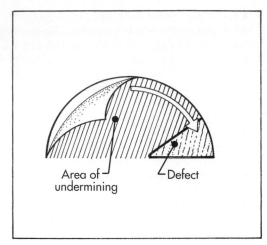
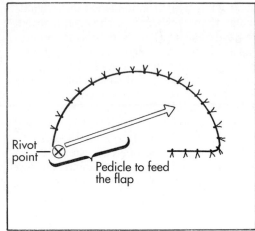

Fig. 15-13 Example of a rotation skin flap. After the removal of a lesion, skin and subcutaneous fat are elevated (undermined) and rotated to cover the defect on a pivot point. The flap is nourished through blood vessels through the pedicle. The arrow on the flap marks the line of greatest tension in the flap. If the skin does not stretch, a skin graft may be needed to cover new defects.

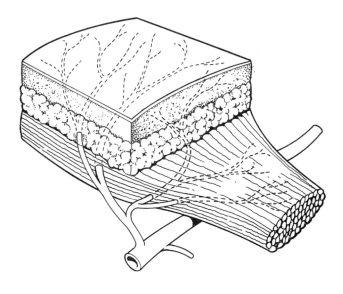

Myocutaneous flap

Fig. 15-14 Example of myocutaneous flaps. Blood vessels from the muscle body nourish the muscle and overlying skin flaps (myocutaneous or musculocutaneous flaps). It is crucial to keep the blood vessels to the muscle intact.

sues are discussed in the literature and additional prospective studies are needed to more accurately predict who might fail, pinpointing reasons and then addressing those concerns (Disa et al., 1992; LaMantia et al., 1987; Petro, 1990).

✦ **Education.** Pressure ulcer prevention is an integral part of rehabilitation practice. The impetus to include all aspects of prevention into a comprehensive program comes from the outcome-driven basis of all healthcare. It provides a paradigm for prevention of pressure ulcers that essentially has been a normal part of rehabilitation practice. The AHCPR

Clinical Practice Guideline—Pressure Ulcers in Adults: Prediction and Prevention—has as an overall goal the reduction of the incidence of pressure ulcers through educational programs (AHCPR, 1994). The AHCPR further recommends the programs be structured, organized, comprehensive, and directed at all levels of healthcare providers, patients, family, and caregivers (Panel for Prediction and Prevention of Pressure Ulcers in Adults, 1992). Rehabilitation nurses have long recognized the importance of this. Recently the geriatric literature presented the success of this comprehensive program with an interdisciplinary approach (Dimant & Francis, 1988; Levine et al., 1989). Involving families and patients in their care is espoused to produce better outcomes (Andberg, Rudolph, & Anderson, 1983; Barnes, 1987). The SCI literature has outcome studies that correlate involvement in care with increased awareness of pressure ulcer risk factors, assessment, and early treatment (Andberg et al., 1983; Krouskop et al., 1983). According to the AHCPR, a comprehensive educational program for professionals and caregivers should include the following:

1. Etiology and risk factors for pressure ulcers
2. Risk assessment tool and its application
3. Skin assessment
4. Demonstration of positioning to decrease risk of tissue breakdown (Alvarez et al., 1989)
5. Instruction on accurate documentation of patient data (Panel for Prediction and Prevention of Pressure Ulcers in Adults, 1992)

In addition to the comprehensive program, programs for clients and families must encompass a piece that addresses the behavioral component. Dai and Catanzaro (1987) studied health beliefs and compliance with skin care. They developed a paradigm for looking at the interaction between individual beliefs, modifying factors, and cues to action (Fig. 15-15). Individuals who believed that they were suspectible to pressures sores were more likely to comply with skin care as were those who perceived the severity of pressure sores. Individual responsibility must be stressed when educating clients (Andberg et al., 1983). Many methods in

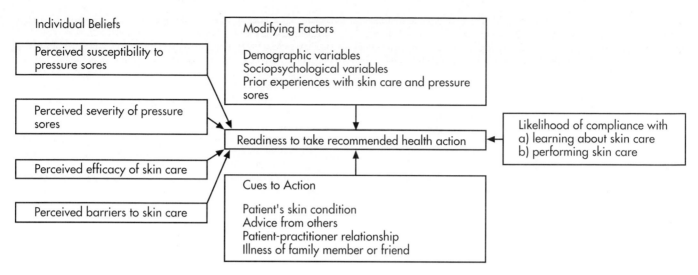

Fig. 15-15 Health beliefs and compliance with skin care (Dai & Catanzaro, 1987).

the literature describe patient education programs from groups to individualized courses and from didactic lecture bases to computer-assisted individual courses. Clients should learn all elements of skin care: nutrition, causes of pressure sores and preventive techniques, safety precautions, management of equipment and supplies, and treatment of any existing sores. Emphasis should be on prevention and early detection.

All education programs should have built-in mechanisms to evaluate the effectiveness of the program—which is to reduce the incidence of pressure ulcers. Ongoing collection of data on a uniform database is critical to evaluating all elements of a program.

SUMMARY

The costs and numbers of people affected has driven national attention to address the issue of pressure ulcers and their prediction, prevention, and treatment. The NPUAP—a multidisciplinary advisory group of leading authorities from the fields of medicine, surgery, nursing, research, gerontology, consumer advocacy, education, and hospital administration—was formed to provide leadership for the prevention of pressure ulcers. The NPUAP held a conference to focus the attention of researchers, clinicians, health policymakers, and financing organizations to answer questions influencing pressure sore research and management. Their work produced a consensus development for pressure ulcer incidence, economics, and risk assessment (NPUAP, 1989). The AHCPR developed a clinical practice guideline for prediction and prevention of pressure sores based on the work of the NPUAP (Panel for Prediction and Prevention of Pressure Ulcers in Adults, 1992). The AHCPR Clinical Practice Guidelines will have a nationwide impact on healthcare policy and practice. The AHCPR guidelines for prediction and prevention have been incorporated into this work. Rehabilitation nurses should be aware of the latest recommendations for treatment when they become available.

The management of wound care was revolutionized in the 1980s. The focus of managing a wound to contain drain-age and decrease infection changed to one of support for the healing of cells and tissues (Cooper, 1990; Doughty, 1992). Initially, management of wounds by moist healing was researched and promoted by the many manufacturers of wound care products. The fact that some literature and many clinicians espouse outdated tissue-damaging treatments speaks to the lack of quality research and the proper dissemination of the current state of the art for wound healing. Rehabilitation nurses must employ consumerism for products with knowledgeable review of research. A more directorial role for nursing is needed in product selection for the individual client and the institution. Nurses should be involved on selection committees in the critical review of products for institutions. Manufacturers always have solicited nursing input for products, and nurses should give their input actively. It is critical that nurses work to promote scientifically based wound care and "debunk" those based solely on tradition (Cooper, 1990).

The holistic care of skin always has been basic to rehabilitation nurses. Combining the art of nursing with the current science will enable nurses to lead in the management of skin and wounds beyond the state of wound care that Cooper (1990) described as the decade of wound, to the decade of healing.

REFERENCES

Abbruzzese, R.S. (1985). Early assessment and prevention of pressure sores. In B.Y. Lee (Ed.), *Chronic ulcers of the skin.* New York: McGraw-Hill.

Agarwal, N., Del Guercio, L.R.M., & Lee, B. (1985). The role of nutrition in the management of pressure sores. In B.Y. Lee (Ed.), *Chronic ulcers of the skin.* New York: McGraw-Hill.

Allman, R.M. (1989). Epidemiology of pressure sores in different populations. *Decubitus, 2,* 30-33.

Allman, R.M., Laprade, C.A., Noel, L.B., Walter, J.M., Moorer, C.A., Dear, M.R., & Smith, C.R. (1986). Pressure sores among hospitalized patients. *Annals of Internal Medicine, 105,* 337-342.

Alvarez, O., Rozint, J., & Wiseman, D. (1989). Moist environment: Matching the dressing to the wound. *1,* 35-51.

Andberg, M., Rudolph, A., & Anderson, T. (1983). Improving skin care through patient and family training. *Topics in Clinical Nursing, 5,* 45-54.

Anderson, T., & Andberg, M. (1979). Psychological factors associated with pressure sores. *Archives of Physical Medicine and Rehabilitation, 60,* 341-346.

Anthony, C.P., & Thibodeau, G.A. (1983). *Textbook of anatomy and physiology* (10th ed.). St. Louis: Mosby–Year Book.

Barnes, S.H. (1987). Patient family education for the patient with a pressure necrosis. *Nursing Clinics of North America, 22,* 463-474.

Bates-Jensen, B. (1990). New pressure ulcer status tool. *Decubitus, 3,* 14-15.

Baxter, C., & Rodheaver, G. (1990). Wound assessment and categorization. In W. Eaglstein, C. Baxter, P. Mertz. (Eds.), *New directions in wound healing.* Princeton, NJ: E.R. Squibb and Sons.

Bergstrom, N., & Braden, B. (1992). A prospective study of pressure sore risk among the institutionalized elderly. *Journal of the American Geriatric Society, 40(8),* 747-758.

Bergstrom, N., Braden, B.J., Laguzza, A., & Holman, V. (1987). The Braden scale for predicting pressure sore risk. *Nursing Research, 36,* 205-210.

Bergstrom, N., Demuth, P.J., & Braden, B.J. (1987). A clinical trial of the Braden scale for predicting pressure sore risk. *Nursing Clinics of North America, 22,* 417-428.

Berlowitz, D.R., & Wilking, S.V.B. (1989). Risk factors for pressure sores. *Journal of the American Geriatric Society, 37,* 1043-1050.

Black, J.M., & Black, S.B. (1987). Surgical management of pressure ulcers. *Nursing Clinics of North America, 22,* 429-438.

Braden, B., & Bergstrom, N. (1987). A conceptual schema for the study of the etiology of pressure sores. *Rehabilitation Nursing, 12,* 8-16.

Braden, B.J. (1988). The relationship between serum cortisol and pressure sore formation among the elderly recently relocated to a nursing home. *Reflections, 14,* 182-186.

Brandeis, G.H., Morris, J.N., Nash, D.J., & Lipsitz, L.A. (1990). The epidemiology and natural history of pressure ulcers in elderly nursing home residents. *JAMA, 264,* 2905-2909.

Bryant, R., Shannon, M.L., Pieper, B., Braden, B., & Morris, D.J. (1992). Pressure ulcers. In R. Bryant (Ed.), *Acute and chronic wounds: Nursing management.* St. Louis: Mosby–Year Book.

Carlson, C.E., King, R.B., Kirk, P.M., Temple, R., & Heinemann, A. (1992). Incidence and correlates of pressure ulcer development after spinal cord injury. *Rehabilitation Nursing Research, 1,* 34-40.

Clanin, N. (1989). *Basic principles of skin and wound management: Independent study module.* Evanston, IL: Rehabilitation Nursing Foundation.

Confer, D.L., Frantz, R.A., Nemiroff, P.M., Junen, A., Mitchell, S., & Palmer, J. (1992). Evolving wound care modalities. In R. Bryant (Ed.), *Acute and chronic wounds: Nursing management.* St. Louis: Mosby–Year Book.

Conine, T.A., Choi, A.K., & Lim, R. (1989). The user friendliness of protective support surfaces in prevention of pressure sores. *Rehabilitation Nursing, 14,* 261-263.

Cooper, D. (1990). Optimizing wound healing a practice within nursing's domain. *Nursing Clinics of North America, 25,* 14-180.

Cooper, D.M. (1992). The wound assessment and evaluation of healing. In R. Bryant (Ed.), *Acute and chronic wounds: Nursing management.* St. Louis: Mosby–Year Book.

Copeland-Fields, L.D., & Hoshiko, B.R. (1989). Clinical validation of Braden and Bergstrom's conceptual schema of pressure sore risk factors. *Rehabilitation Nursing, 14,* 257-260.

Cumming, W.T., Tompkins, W.J., Jones, R.M., & Margolis, S.A. (1986). Microprocessor-based weight shift monitors for paraplegic patients. *Archives Physical Medicine and Rehabilitation, 67,* 172-174.

Dai, Y.T., & Catanzaro, M. (1987). Health beliefs and compliance with a skin care regimen. *Rehabilitation Nursing, 12,* 13-16.

Daniel, R.K., Priest, D.L., & Wheatley, D.C. (1981). Etiologic factors in pressure sores: an experimental model. *Archives of Physical Medicine and Rehabilitation, 62,* 492-498.

Dimant, J., & Francis, M.E. (1988). Pressure sore prevention and management. *Journal of Gerontologic Nursing, 14,* 18-25.

Dinsdale, S.M. (1974). Decubitus ulcers: role of pressure and function in causation. *Archives of Physical Medicine and Rehabilitation, 55,* 146-152.

Disa, J.J., Carlton, J.M., & Goldberg, N.H. (1992). Efficacy of operative cure in pressure sore patients. *Plastic and Reconstructive Surgery, 89,* 272-278.

Donovan, W., Garger, S., Hamilton, S., Krouskop, T., Rodriguez, G., & Stal, S. (1988). Pressure ulcers. In J.A. DeLisa (Ed.), *Rehabilitation medicine: Principles and practices.* Philadelphia: Lippincott.

Doughty, D. (1992). Physiology of wound healing. In R. Bryant (Ed.), *Acute and chronic wounds: Nursing management.* St. Louis: Mosby–Year Book.

Eaglstein, W.H. (1986). Wound healing and aging. *Dermatology Clinics, 4,* 481-484.

Fenske, N.A., & Lober, C.W. (1986). Structural and functional changes of normal aging skin. *Journal American Academy Dermatology, 15,* 571-585.

Ferrell, B.A., Osterweil, D., & Christenson, P. (1993). A randomized trial of low-air-loss beds for treatment of pressure ulcers. *JAMA, 269,* 494-497.

Frankel H.L., Hancock, D.O., Hyslop, G., Melzak, J., Michaelis, L.S., Ungar, G.H., Vernon, J.D., & Walsh, J.J. (1969). The value of postural reduction in the initial management of closed injuries of the spine with paraplegia and tetraplegia. *Paraplegia, 7,* 179-192.

Garber, S.L., & Krouskop, T.A. (1982). Body build and its relationship to pressure distribution in the seated wheelchair patient. *Archives of Physical Medicine and Rehabilitation, 63,* 17-20.

Garvin, G. (1990). Wound healing in pediatrics. *Nursing Clinics of North America, 25,* 181-192.

Gensheimer, D. (1993). A review of calcium alginates. *Ostomy Wound Management, 39,* 34-38.

Gorse, G.J., & Messner, R.L. (1987). Improved pressure sore healing with hydrocolloid dressings. *Archives of Dermatology, 123,* 766-771.

Gosnell, D.J. (1973). An assessment took to identify pressure sores. *Nursing Research, 22,* 55-59.

Gosnell, D.J. (1989). Pressure sore risk assessment: A critique. Part 1: The Gosnell scale. *Decubitus, 2,* 32-33, 36-38, 40.

Gray, B.C., Salzberg, C.A., Petro, J.A., & Salisbury, R.E. (1990). The expanded myocutaneous flap for reconstruction of the difficult pressure sore. *Decubitus, 3,* 17-20.

Griffin, J.W., Toons, R.E., Mendius, R.A., Clifft, J.K., VanderZwaag, R., & El-Zeky, F. (1991). Efficacy of high voltage pulsed current for healing of pressure ulcers in patients with spinal cord injury. *Physical Therapy, 71,* 433-442.

Habif, T.P.L. (1990). *Clinical dermatology: A color guide to diagnosis and therapy* (2nd ed.). St. Louis: Mosby–Year Book.

Hicks, D.J. (1971). An incidence study of pressure sores following surgery. In *ANA Clinical Sessions 1970.* Miami, New York: Appleton-Century-Crofts.

Hotter, A.N. (1990). Wound healing and immunocompromise. *Nursing Clinics of North America, 25,* 193-203.

Hunter, S.M., Cathcart-Silberang T.C., Langemo, D., Olson, B., Hanson, D., Burd, C., & Sauvage, T.R. (1992). Pressure ulcer prevalence and incidence in a rehabilitation hospital. *Rehabilitation Nursing, 17,* 239-242.

Husain, T. (1953). An experimental study of some pressure effects on tissues with reference to the bedsore problems. *Journal of Pathologic Bacteriology, 66,* 347-382.

International Association for Enterostomal Therapy. (1991). *Standards of care for dermal wounds: pressure ulcers* (Revised ed.). Irvine, CA: IAET.

Jones, P., & Millman, A. Wound healing and the aged patient. *Nursing Clinics of North America, 28,* 263-267.

Kemp, M.G., Keithley, J.K., Smith, D.W., & Morreale, B. (1990). Factors that contribute to pressure sores in surgical patients. *Research in Nursing and Health, 13,* 293-301.

King, R.B., & French, E.T. (1990). Procedures to maintain and restore tissue integrity. In *Rehabilitation Institute of Chicago, Division of Nursing Rehabilitation Nursing Procedures Manual.* Rockville, MD: Aspen.

Knight, D., & Scott, H. (1990). Contracture and pressure necrosis. *Ostomy and Wound Management, 30,* 60-62, 65-67.

Knighton, D.R., Cinesi, K., Fiegel, V.D., Schumerth, S., Butler, L., & Cerra, F. (1990). Stimulation of wound repair in chronic, non-healing cutaneous ulcers using platelet derived wound healing formula. *Surgery, Gynecology and Obstetrics, 170,* 56-60.

Konstantides, N.N. (1992). Principles of nutritional support. In R. Bryant (Ed.). *Acute and chronic wounds: Nursing management.* St. Louis: Mosby–Year Book.

Kosiak, M. (1959). Etiology and pathology of ischemic ulcers. *Archives of Physical Medicine and Rehabilitation, 40,* 62-69.

Kosiak, M. (1991). Prevention and rehabilitation of pressure ulcers. *Decubitus, 4,* 60-68.

Kosiak, M., & Kubicek, W.G., Olson, M., Danz, J.N., & Kottke, F.J. (1958). Evaluation of pressure as a factor in the production of ischial ulcers. *Archives of Physical Medicine and Rehabilitation, 39,* 623-629.

Krasner, D. (1991). Resolving the dressing dilemma: Selecting wound dressings by category. *Ostomy Wound Management, 35,* 64-70.

Krouskop, T.A., Noble, P.C., Garber, S.L., & Spencer, W.A. (1983). The effectiveness of preventive management in reducing the occurrence of pressure sores. *Journal of Rehabilitation Research and Development, 20,* 74-83.

Krouskop, T.A., & Garber, S.L. (1987). The role of technology in the prevention of pressure sores. *Ostomy and Wound Management, 16,* 44-54.

Krouskop, T.A. & Garber, S.L. (1989). Interface pressure confusion. *Decubitus, 2,* 8. (Letter.)

LaMantia, J.G., & Hirschwald, J.F., Goodman, C.L., Wooden, V.M., Delisser, O., & Staas, W.E., Jr. (1987). A program design to reduce chronic readmissions for pressure sores. *Rehabilitation Nursing, 12,* 22-25.

LaMantia, J.G. (1990). *Current concepts in skin and wound management. Independent Study Module.* Evanston, IL: Rehabilitation Nursing Foundation.

Lamid, S., & Ghatit, A.Z. (1983). Smoking, spasticity and pressure sores in spinal cord injured patients. *American Journal of Physical Medicine and Rehabilitation, 62,* 300-306.

Landis, E.M. (1930). Micro-injection: Studies of capillary blood pressure in human skin. *Heart, 15,* 209-228.

Langemo, D.K., Olson, B., Hunter, S., Hanson, D., Burd, C., & Cathcart-Silberberg, T. (1991). Incidence and prediction of pressure ulcers in five patient care settings. *Decubitus, 4,* 25-36.

Levine, J.M., Simpson, M., & McDonald, R.J. (1989). Pressure sores: A plan for primary care prevention. *Geriatrics, 44,* 75-76, 83-87, 90.

Lidowski, H. (1988). NAMP: A system for preventing and managing pressure ulcers. *Decubitus, 1,* 28-37.

Lindan, O. (1961). Etiology of decubitus ulcers: an experimental study. *Archives of Physical Medicine and Rehabilitation, 42,* 774-783.

Linder, R.M., & Morris, D. (1990). The surgical management of pressure ulcers: A systematic approach based on staging. *Decubitus, 3,* 32-38.

Lloyd, E.E., & Baker, F. (1986). An examination of variables in spinal cord injury patients with pressure sores. *SCI Nursing, 3,* 219-222.

Luckmann, K., & Sorensen, K. (1980). *Medical surgical nursing—A psychophysiological approach.* Philadelphia: W.B. Saunders.

Maklebust, J. (1987). Pressure ulcers: Etiology and prevention. *Nursing Clinics of North America, 22,* 359-377.

Maklebust, J., Mondoux, L., & Sieggreen, M. (1986). Pressure relief characteristics of various support surfaces used in prevention and treatment of pressure ulcers. *Enterostomal Therapy, 13,* 85-89.

Maklebust, J., Sieggreen, M.Y., & Mondoux, L. Pressure relief capabilities of the Sof-Care bed and the Clinitron bed. *Ostomy/Wound Management, 21,* 32, 36-41.

Mawson, A.R., Biundo, J.J., Neville, P., Linares, H.A., Winchester, Y., & Lopez, A. (1988). Risk factors for early occurring pressure ulcers following spinal cord injury. *American Journal of Physical Medicine and Rehabilitation, 67,* 123-127.

McFarland, G.K., & McFarland, E.A. (1993). *Nursing diagnosis and intervention* (2nd ed.), St. Louis: Mosby–Year Book.

Moody, B.L., Fanale, J.E., Thompson, M., Vaillancourt, D., Symonds, G.J., Jr, Bonasoro, C. (1988). Impact of staff education on pressure sore development in elderly hospitalized patients. *Archives of Internal Medicine, 148,* 2241-2243.

Motta, G. (1993). Skin and wound care: Dressing for success. Workshop American Healthcare Institute, April, Providence.

Motta, G.J. (1989). Calcium alginate topical wound dressings: a new dimension in the cost effective treatment for exudating dermal wounds and pressure sores. *Ostomy Wound Management, 25,* 52-56.

Mulholland, J.H., Tui, C., Wright, A.M., Vinci, V., & Shafiroff, B. (1943). Protein metabolism and bedsores. *Annals of Surgery, 118,* 1015-1023.

Munro, D. (1940). Care of the back following spinal cord injuries. *New England Journal of Medicine, 223,* 391-398.

Munro, H.N. (1988). Aging. In J.M. Kinney, K.N. Jeejeebhoy, G. Hill, & O.E. Owen (Eds.), *Nutrition and metabolism in patient care.* Philadelphia: W.B. Saunders.

National Pressure Ulcer Advisory Panel. (1989). Pressure ulcers prevalence, cost and risk assessment: Consensus development conference statement. *Decubitus, 2,* 24-28.

Natow, A.B. (1983). Nutrition in prevention and treatment of decubitus ulcers. *Topics in Clinical Nursing, 5,* 32-44.

Norton, D. (1989). Calculating the risk: Reflections on the Norton scale. *Decubitus, 2,* 24-31.

Norton, D., McLaren, R., & Exton Smith, A.N. (1975). *An Investigation of geriatric nursing problems in Hospitals.* London: Churchill Livingstone. (Originally published in 1962.)

Oot-Giromini, B., Bidwell, F.C., Heller, N.B., Parks, M.L., Wicks, P., & Williams, P.M. (1989). Evolution of skin care: pressure ulcer prevalence rates pre/post intervention. *Decubitus, 2,* 54-55.

Orem, D.E. (1971). *Nursing concepts of practice.* New York: McGraw-Hill.

Panel for Prediction and Prevention of Pressure Ulcers in Adults. (1992). *Pressure ulcers in adults: Prediction and prevention.* Clinical Practice Guideline, No. 3 AHCPR Pub. No. 92-0047. Rockville, MD: Agency for Health Care Policy and Research, Public Health Service, U.S. Department of Health and Human Services.

Panel for Prediction and Prevention of Pressure Ulcers in Adults (1994). *Pressure ulcers in adults: Prediction and prevention.* Clinical Practice Guideline, No. 3 AHCPR Pub. No. 92-0047. Rockville, MD: Agency For Health Care Policy and Research, Public Health Service, U.S. Department of Health and Human Services.

Patrick, M.L., Woods, S.L., Craven, R.F., Rokosky, J.S., & Bruno, P.M. (1986) *Medical-surgical nursing: Pathophysiological concepts.* Philadelphia: J.B. Lippincott.

Payne, R.L., & Martin, M.L. (1990). The epidemiology and management of skin tears in older adults. *Ostomy Wound Management, 26,* 26-37.

Petro, J.A. (1990). Ethical dilemmas of pressure ulcers. *Decubitus, 3,* 28-31.

Pinchocofsky-Devin, G. (1990). Nutritional assessment and intervention. In D. Krasner (Ed.), *Chronic wound care,* King of Prussia, PA: Health Management Publications.

Pinzur, M.S., Shumacher, D., Reddy, N., Osterman, H., Havey, R., & Patwardin, A. (1991). Preventing heel ulcers: A comparison of prophylactic body support systems. *Archives of Physical Medicine and Rehabilitation, 72,* 508-510.

Powell, J.W. (1989). Increasing acuity of nursing home patients and the prevalence of pressure ulcers: A ten year comparison. *Decubitus, 2,* 56-58.

Rehabilitation Nursing Foundation. (1987). *Rehabilitation nursing: Concepts and practice: A core curriculum* (2nd ed). Evanston, IL: Author. Rehabilitation Nursing Foundation.

Reichel, S.M. (1958). Shearing forces as a factor in decubitus ulcers in paraplegics. *JAMA, 166,* 762-763.

Rempusheski, V. (1989). The role of ethnicity in elder care. *Nursing Clinics of North America, 24,* 717-724.

Richardson, R.R., & Meyer, P.R. (1981). Prevalence and incidence of pressure sores in acute spinal cord injuries. *Paraplegia, 19,* 235-247.

Seiler, W.O., Allen, S., & Stahelin, H.B. (1986). Influence of the 30 degrees laterally inclined position and the "super soft" 3-piece mattress on skin oxygen tension on areas of maximum pressure—Implications for pressure sore prevention. *Gerontology, 32,* 158-166.

Shea, D.J. (1975). Pressure sore classification and management. *Clinical Orthopedics and Related Research, 112,* 89-100.

Shields, R.K., & Cook, T.M. (1992). Lumbar support thickness: Effect on seated buttock pressure in individuals with and without spinal cord injury. *Physical Therapy, 72,* 218-226.

Sieggreen, M.Y. (1987). Healing of physical wounds. *Nursing Clinics of North America, 22,* 439-447.

Slater, H. (1985). *Pressure sores in the elderly.* Pittsburgh: Synapse Publications.

Solis, I., Krouskap, T., Trainer, N., & Marbunger, R., (1988). Supine interface pressure in children. *Archines Physical Medicine and Rehabilitation, 69,* 524-526.

Staas, W.E., Jr., & Cioschi, H.M. (1991). Pressure sores—A multifaceted approach to prevention and treatment. *Western Journal of Medicine, 154,* 539-544.

Stotts, N.A. (1985). Nutritional parameters at hospital admission as predictors of pressure ulcers in surgical patients. *Nursing Research, 34* (Abstract), 383.

Strauss, M., Gong, J., Gary, B., Kalsbeek, W.D., & Spear, S. (1991). The cost of home air fluidized therapy for pressure sores—A randomized controlled trial. *The Journal of Family Practice, 33,* 52-59.

Versluysen, M. (1986). How elderly patients with femoral fracture develop pressure sores in hospital. *British Medical Journal, 292,* 1311-1313.

Vidal, J., & Sarrias, M. (1991). An analysis of the diverse factors concerned with the development of pressure sores in spinal cord injured patients. *Paraplegia, 29,* 261-267.

Wysocki, A.B., & Bryant, R. (1992). Skin. In R. Bryant (Ed), *Acute and chronic wounds: Nursing management.* St. Louis: Mosby–Year Book.

Xakellis, G., & Chrischilles, E.A. (1992). Hydrocolloid versus saline-gauze dressings in treating pressure ulcers: A cost-effectiveness analysis. *Archives of Physical Medicine and Rehabilitation, 73,* 469.

Yarkony, G.M. (1987). Contractures and the immobilized patient. *Ostomy Wound Management, 16,* 64-75.

Yarkony, G.M., Roth, E.J., Cybulski, G.R., Jaeger, R.J. (1992). Neuromuscular stimulation in spinal cord injury. II. Prevention of secondary complications. *Archives of Physical Medicine and Rehabilitation, 73,* 195-200.

Yetzer, E.A., & Sullivan, R.L. (1992). The foot at risk: identification and prevention of skin breakdown. *Rehabilitation Nursing, 17,* 247-251.

Young, J.S., & Burns, P.E. (1981). Pressure sores and the spinal cord injured. *Model Systems; SCI Digest, 3,* 9-18.

Young, L. (1989). Pressure ulcer prevalence and associated patient characteristics in one long term care facility. *Decubitus, 2,* 52.

Zimmer, R.E., Lawson, K.D., & Calvert, C.J. (1986). The effects of wearing diapers on the skin. *Pediatric Dermatology, 3,* 95-101.

Zink, M., Rousseau, P., & Holloway, A.G. (1992). Lower extremity ulcers. In R. Bryant (Ed.), *Acute and chronic wounds: Nursing management.* St. Louis: Mosby–Year Book.

16

Sensory Functions: Hearing, Vision, Taste, and Smell

Elizabeth Forbes, RN, MSN, EdD, FAAN

INTRODUCTION

The nurse's major objective in rehabilitation is to facilitate the restoration and maintenance of independence for individuals including those whose level of function in activities of daily living has been physically and/or emotionally limited due to sensory impairment. At any place along the life-span continuum, sensory impairments will affect communication, which is essential for social interactions and for developing feelings of competency in dealing with the environment. Sensory functions are one area where primary care for persons with disabilities may be erroneously ignored or set secondary to needs associated with the disabling or chronic condition. Communication involves the transmittal of information through writing, reading, listening, touching, observing, scenting, and speaking. Communication occurs between individuals, among groups, and through the media via television, movies, radio, books, magazines, and newspapers. Barriers to receiving and sending messages can result when there are alterations or impairments in seeing or hearing.

Throughout history the eye has been associated with both evil and good: a human glance, the "evil eye," is thought to inflict harm as well as to heal in many cultures. One comes to learn about and appreciate the surrounding environment through the sensory abilities. Aesthetically our vision allows us to feel pleasure when viewing a symphony of colors—for example, a sunset or the changing colors of autumn leaves. Similarly the ears allow us to explore the aural environment, which includes the sounds of the wind, rain, and chirping birds. Vision and hearing stimulate us as we learn about our environment through books, magazines, newspapers, radio, and television. They also serve as a protective mechanism by which we are warned of environmental hazards, whether a flashing red light at a railroad crossing, noxious odor of a gas leak, an uneven sidewalk, or the sirens of an ambulance.

Many sights and sounds may be taken for granted. Consider the changes in your life and your feelings if you could never see the sun set or hear the rain falling on a rooftop. Sights and sounds provide environmental cues, and when they are altered by an impairment, feelings of frustration and social isolation emerge. Altered sensory functions or impairments may be secondary to another chronic condition or result from a disabling disorder, such as hemianopsia following a cerebral vascular accident. Opportunities for primary care and wellness are abundant in rehabilitation. Therefore rehabilitation nursing interventions are needed to assist the client and family in adapting to changes in sensory abilities.

THE EYE
Layers of the Eye

The eyeball, or globe, is composed of three spheres or tunics: (1) the fibrous tunic, which includes the cornea and sclera; (2) the vascular tunic, which includes the iris, ciliary body, and choroid; and (3) the nervous tunic, which includes the retina and retinal pigment epithelium (RPE) (Cohen, 1993).

✦ **The fibrous tunic.** The cornea, the window of the eye, is the major light-focusing surface allowing light to enter the eye in its route to the retina. The cornea is developed fully by 2 years of age. It is a uniquely transparent structure that covers the iris and pupil. (Cohen, 1993). The cornea serves three protective functions: (1) it acts as a physical barrier, (2) it causes tearing and blinking when foreign bodies come into contact with it, and (3) it selectively resists microorganisms and chemicals by virtue of its five different layers (Fig. 16-1).

The sclera, or white part of the eye, comes together with the cornea at a juncture called the limbus. The sclera contains dense bands of parallel, interlacing tissue bundles arranged in a nonuniform pattern creating its opaque color. The rigid sclera protects the inner contents of the eye and allows for variations in intraocular pressure (Cohen, 1993). In children the sclera is thin and appears bluish due to the underlying pigmented structures that are visible through it. With aging, the sclera may appear yellowish due to fat deposits. The optic nerve passes into the eyeball from the posterior opening in the sclera (Burrell, 1992).

✦ **The vascular tunic**

The iris, the colored portion of the eye, surrounds the pupil. It adjusts the pupil size so it can accommodate to brightness and darkness. The pupil dilates in the dark and constricts when there is bright light. There are two muscles in the iris that allow it to change the diameter of the pupil:

(1) the iris sphincter, which encircles the pupil and creates constriction when it contracts and (2) the iris dilator, which extends from the pupil to the iris periphery and creates dilation when it contracts (Cohen, 1993).

The ciliary body is immediately behind the iris and just inside the sclera. Its external layer is a smooth muscle structure called the ciliary muscle and is responsible for altering the shape of the lens. Contraction of the ciliary muscle causes the zonule (tissue strands attached to the lens) to relax. As a result the lens takes on a more spherical shape and optical power increases. When the ciliary muscle relaxes, the zonule becomes taunt and the optical power decreases. This process, called accommodation, focuses the eye. The ciliary muscle is extremely active in children and is deformed easily. Children have powerful ranges of accommodation. With age the ciliary muscle tends to weaken, thereby decreasing the accommodation power of the lens. Presbyopia is the term used when the lens is nonaccommodating and requires the wearing of reading glasses, bifocal lenses, or even trifocal lenses (Stein, Slatt, & Stein, 1988). The choroid contains a rich supply of blood vessels, thus providing nutrition to the outer half of the retina. Anatomically the choroid lies between the sclera and retina (Fig. 16-1). Pressure from the vitreous body holds the choroid in place (Cohen, 1993).

✦ The nervous tunic

The retina, the innermost layer of the eyeball, is predominantly a neuronal layer. It contains all the sensory receptors for the transmission of light and is actually part of the brain (Stein, 1988). The retina resembles a pink net and is barely the thickness of onionskin paper. Nutrients and oxygen are delivered to the retina by the choriocapillaris and the central retinal artery. Interference with this blood supply can lead to damage or death of the retina.

The RPE is the outermost retinal layer of the eye and contacts the choroid. It contains the photoreceptors, the rods and cones, which communicate the light stimulation they receive to the optic nerve fibers. The cones are used to recognize colors and are responsible for fine discrimination and daylight vision, and the rods respond to dim light and are responsible for peripheral vision. The number of cones has been estimated to be 6 million, with rods numbering 125 million (Stein et al., 1988).

The macula lutea, located in the center of the retina, is composed mostly of cones and has a yellowish hue when viewed through an ophthalmoscope because fewer blood vessels feed into this area (Fig. 16-2). The fovea centralis is a small depression in the macula and is the thinnest portion of the retina. Damage to the fovea severely reduces the ability to see directly ahead. The rods are not distributed in the macula but in the periphery of the retina. Damage to the rods results in night blindness; however, the retention of good visual acuity for objects straight ahead remains intact (Stein et al. 1988). Table 16-1 summarizes the layers of the eye.

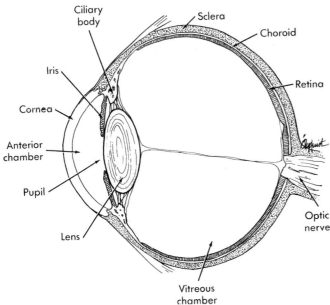

Fig. 16-1   Cross-section of the human eye.

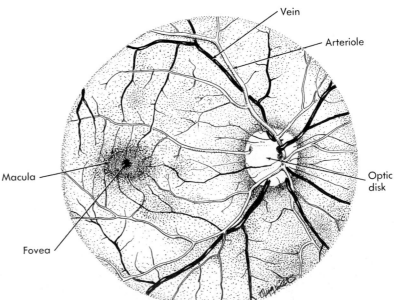

Fig. 16-2   Fundus of the eye showing the optic disc, fovea macula, and blood vessels.

Supporting and Accessory Structures

The supporting and accessory structures of the eye include the eyelids, conjunctiva, lens, anterior and posterior eye cavities, and the lacrimal apparatus. The eyelids and eyelashes protect the eyeball against intrusion of foreign objects. The skin of the eyelid is the thinnest in the body. The lids are loose and elastic, a quality that allows for some swelling to take place without damage occurring. The upper and lower eyelids join at the canthus. The conjunctiva, a mucous membrane, lines each lid and also covers the surface of the eyeball. This transparent structure contributes mucus to the tear film (Hart, 1992).

The lens is a semitransparent structure located behind the iris and is composed primarily of water. No nerves, vessels, or connective tissue are contained in the lens (Apple & Rabb, 1991). The lens brings light rays to a focus on the retina. According to Helmholtz's theory, the ciliary body and choroid are pulled forward toward the lens when the ciliary body contracts. Consequently the lenses bulge for near vision and remain comparatively flat for far vision (Hart, 1992).

The anterior cavity, which is divided into an anterior and a posterior chamber, lies in front of the lens and contains a clear, watery substance called aqueous humor. Aqueous humor maintains pressure inside the eye and bathes and nourishes the iris and the posterior aspect of the cornea. It flows through the anterior chamber, is filtered through the trabeculum, which acts as a sieve, and then passes into the canal of Schlemm. From there, it passes directly into the bloodstream. Vitreous humor, a soft gelatinous material, is contained within the posterior cavity, where it helps to maintain pressure in the eyeball to prevent collapse (Cohen, 1993).

The lacrimal apparatus is composed of the lacrimal glands, lacrimal canals, lacrimal sacs, and nasolacrimal ducts. The lacrimal glands are responsible for tears of emotion, as well as responding to irritants such as dust and odors. These glands are shaped like almonds and are located in the frontal bone of the upper outer margin of each orbit. The lacrimal canals empty into the lacrimal sacs located in a groove of the lacrimal bone. Tears then drain into the nasal cavity through the nasolacrimal ducts. For this reason, a runny nose can often accompany tearing. With a common cold the lacrimal sacs can become so plugged that tears, instead of draining into the nose, overflow from the eyes. Tears not only provide nourishment to the cornea but also help to dilute microorganisms. Tears contain immunoglobulins (IgG and IgE), which inhibit microbial growth (Hart, 1992).

Physiology of the Eye

The eye has often been compared to a camera to illustrate its complex function and structure. The iris acts like a shutter on a camera by controlling the amount of light entering the eye through the pupil. The light rays travel to the retina, which responds similarly to film in a camera. The retina consists of light-sensitive rods and cones among other neurons. Chemical and physical changes take place in the retina and eventually lead to the discharge of electrical impulses. The impulses are conducted along the optic nerve fibers to the occipital lobe of the cortex. Figure 16-3 depicts visual pathways. The brain interprets what has been seen. Figure 16-4 illustrates the vision process in a lateral view.

Nursing Assessment of the Eye

Information about a client's visual status is obtained by gathering both subjective and objective data. Subjective data are obtained when the health history is taken and are based on what the client or family can tell the nurse. None of the assessment steps should be bypassed. If a full and detailed assessment is not conducted, an erroneous diagnosis may be made, entailing inappropriate or unnecessary tests.

Health History

Responses to the following questions can provide a framework for a more in-depth investigation. The health history data base will vary depending on the age of the client. Some questions are age specific for children, adults, and the elderly and are found in the Box on p. 311.

External Eye Examination

The next phase of the assessment elicits objective data through inspection and performance of visual acuity measurements. Inspection, like taking a history, can provide further clues to any visual alteration. The first part of the inspection involves inspecting the exterior of the eye (Table 16-2). When observing both eyes, the rehabilitation nurse should be seated and at eye level with the client. Physical characteristics of both eyes should be similar unless previous surgery or problems has altered one eye.

✦ Eyelids

The position and color of the eyelids should be observed. Normally the color of the eyelids matches the skin color of the face. Observe for edema, redness, crusts and scales, tumors, trauma, and malpositioned lids (e.g., lids that roll out or roll in). Lid edema may indicate the presence of systemic

Table 16-1 Layers of the eye

Layer	Component parts	Characteristics
Outer layer	Sclera, cornea	Serves protective function; acts as physical barrier; selectively resists microorganisms
Middle layer (uvea)	Choroid, ciliary body, iris	Provides nutrition; contains rich blood supply
Innermost layer	Retina, rods, cones	Contains neuronal tissue; communicates light stimulation to optic nerve

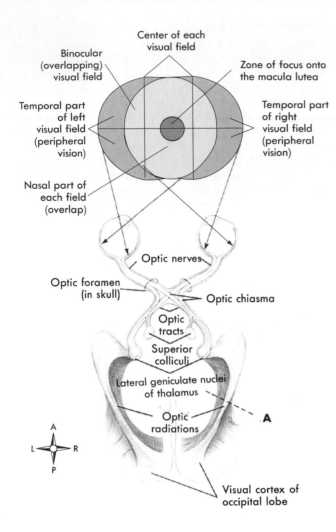

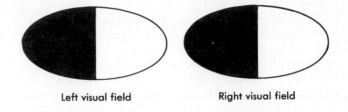

Left visual field   Right visual field

Fig. 16-3 Visual fields and neuronal pathways of the eye. Note the structures that make up each pathway: optic nerve, optic chiasma, the lateral geniculate body of the thalamus, optic radiations, and the visual cortex of the occipital lobe. Fibers from the nasal portion of each retina cross over to the opposite side at the optic chiasma and terminate in the lateral geniculate nuclei. Location of a lesion in the visual pathway determines the resulting visual defect. Damage at point A, for example, would cause blindness in the right nasal and left temporal visual fields, as the ovals beneath indicate. (Trace the visual pathway from point A back to the visual field map to see why this is so.) What would be the effect of pressure on the optic chiasma (e.g., by a pituitary tumor)? Answer: It would produce blindness in both temporal visual fields. Why? because it destroys fibers from the nasal side of both retinas. (From *Anthony's Textbook of Anatomy and Physiology* [14th ed.] by Thibodeau and Patton, 1994, St. Louis: Mosby-Year Book. Copyright 1994 by Mosby-Year Book. Reprinted by permission.)

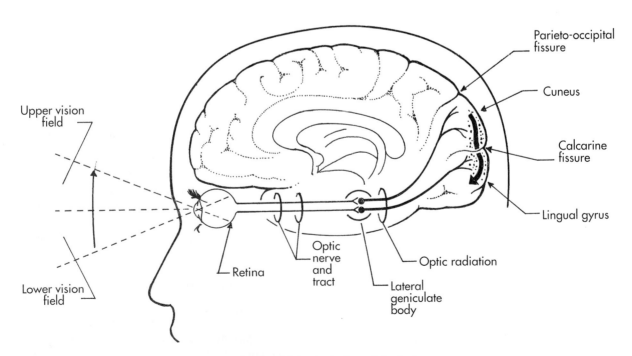

Fig. 16-4 Midsagittal view of the brain.

QUESTIONS FOR OBTAINING A VISUAL HEALTH HISTORY

1. How old are you?
2. What is your occupation?
3. Are you exposed to hazardous substances in your work?
4. Do you wear protective goggles at work?
5. Do you wear glasses or contact lenses? If so, how do they help you?
6. Do you regularly use sunglasses in the summer and winter?
7. Do you squint to see better?
8. Have you noticed any recent change(s) in your ability to see? If so, have these changes affected your activities at home or work?
9. Do you see better out of one eye than the other?
10. Do you have burning, itching, or blurred, double vision? Are your eyelids stuck together when you wake up in the morning?
11. Have you ever experienced sudden loss of vision?
12. Have you noticed swelling around your eyes or tearing or spots before your eyes?
13. Do you experience any discharge from your eyes? (If so, what color and consistency?)
14. Have you noticed any infection or lump on your eyelids?
15. Have you experienced eye pain? If so, How severe is the pain on a scale of 1 to 10, with 10 as the most severe pain?
16. Does light cause pain?
17. When you close your eyes, is your pain reduced?
18. Are you aware of a blind spot? Does it move?
19. Do you see spots? One or many? Do you see showers of spots associated with flashing lights? Is there a veil or curtain across your vision?
20. Are there halos around lights?
21. Have you noticed any difficulty in near or far vision or problems with driving at night? Does glare create problems?
22. Have you been aware of any peripheral vision loss?
23. Have you ever been told that you have cataracts or glaucoma?
24. When was your last eye examination, and by whom was it done?
25. Are you taking any prescription or over-the-counter medication?
26. Do you have any allergies to medicine, food, or any other substance?
27. Do you use prescription or over-the-counter eyedrops or eyewashes regularly? If yes, what do you use and why?
28. Did your mother have rubella or was she exposed to German measles during pregnancy? (This may be related to congenital cataracts or blindness.)
29. Do you have congenital corneal problems?
30. Do you use cosmetics on or near your eyes? Have you had permanent eyeliner applied to your eyes?
31. Is it easy to differentiate colors?
32. Do you have a history of bumping into things or burning yourself?
33. Do you have any blood relatives with any history of eye problems or systemic diseases?
34. Are you a smoker? Are you often in a smoky environment?
35. Do you drink alcohol? At what age did you start drinking? How much do you drink?
36. Do you have any of the following systemic problems: arteriosclerosis, diabetes, thyroid disease, or arthritis?
37. What sports do you play?
38. Does the child recognize colors and letters?
39. Does the child bump into furniture or other things?
40. Does the child need to hold books or papers close to the eyes in order to read?

---

diseases such as heart failure, nephrosis, allergy, or thyroid deficiency. Redness of the margins of the lid could indicate an infection such as hordeolum. Older clients may have redundant tissue on the eyelids. The upper eyelid covers part of the iris but not the pupil, unless a client has ptosis. An ectropion eyelid is everted, exposing the mucous membrane lining the eye and tears may run down the cheeks, since they cannot drain into the nose. When the lower lid is turned in (an entropion eyelid), the lashes can rub against the cornea and lead to a corneal ulcer. Examine the eyelids to determine the rate and smoothness in closing by having the client follow an object in a downward gaze (Lewis & Collier, 1992).

♦ Conjunctiva, sclera, and iris

The color of the conjunctiva and sclera are observed by gently pulling the lower eyelids down with the thumb while the person looks upward. Observe the conjunctiva for color and note the blood vessels against the white sclera background while looking for any nodules or swelling. Paleness in the pink conjunctiva lining may indicate anemia. The thin, transparent conjunctiva covering the anterior surface of the eyeball may become congested or reddened with an infection such as conjunctivitis. The sclera is white in adults but may appear yellowish in the elderly client due to fat deposits; may have a yellowish coloration in persons of African-American heritage; or may appear bluish in children because it is thinner and allows the pigmentation of underlying structures to show through (Brunner & Suddarth, 1989). Otherwise, yellowed or reddened sclera indicates referral for further investigation. In most individuals the iris is the same color in both eyes. A difference in color, heterochromia iris, may or may not be significant. The iris is round and clear (Lewis & Collier, 1992).

Table 16-2 Exterior assessment of the eye

Structure	Expected observations	Variations
Eyelids		
Position	Upper eyelid does not extend	Ptosis: drooping of eyelid
		Ectropion: lower lid turned out
		Entropion: lower lid turned in
Color	Matches skin color	Redness: could indicate infection (e.g., hordeolum; inflammation; chalazion)
Conjunctiva		
Color	Lining of eyelids pink	Paleness: could indicate anemia
	Anterior surface thin and transparent	Congestion/generalized redness: infection (e.g., conjunctivitis)
Sclera		
Color	White	Yellowed/reddened
Iris		
Color	Both eyes same	Heterochromia iridis: difference in color
Shape	Round	Irregular (e.g., iridectomy)
Clarity	Clear	Pus in anterior chamber; could obscure clearness
Pupils		
Size	Varies with color (brown eyes smaller than blue), age (smaller in older adults), and whether nearsighted or farsighted (farsighted smaller)	Unequal in size
Equality	Equal response to light; constriction	Unequal, absent, or sluggish response

✦ **Pupil**

The pupils are examined for size and shape; 5% of the population has unequally sized pupils, which vary from 3 to 7 mm in diameter among individuals, with brown irises being smaller than blue irises, and with age. For instance, infants and elderly persons have a miotic pupil; in childhood the pupil is larger, decreasing in size with increased farsightedness during adulthood (Lewis & Collier, 1992). Individuals with brown eyes have smaller pupils than those with blue eyes. To assess whether a client's pupils react equally to both direct and consensual light, the nurse moves a penlight from the temporal to nasal side of the client's eye while the client focuses on an object straight ahead. The nurse observes whether the pupils constrict at equal speed. Pupillary reaction to accommodation is tested while the client looks into the distance and then at the nurse's finger when held 5 to 10 cm from the bridge of the client's nose. The pupils converge and constrict symmetrically, with slower response in older persons. To test for consensual pupillary response, darken the room while shining a penlight into one pupil and observe for constriction of the opposite pupil. The examined pupil and the other pupil should constrict simultaneously (Stein et al., 1988).

Visual Acuity

The Snellen chart has been used since 1864 as a screening tool for visual acuity for distance. The chart has symbols such as block letters, numbers, animals, or letter Es, which can be used with non-English-speaking persons, illiterate persons, or children. The symbols are placed at various angles on the chart in gradually decreasing sizes. Chil-

dren and elderly persons perform better when instructions are given slowly, clearly, and repeated as necessary. If the client is under stress due to concern about vision or pressured by an examiner's hurried pace, the findings may be distorted.

The Snellen chart is hung on a wall at eye level 20 feet from the person tested. Visual acuity should be tested with and without the client's glasses or contact lenses in place. Each eye is tested separately, first the right eye (OD) and the left eye (OS) and then both eyes (OU). The client is asked to cover one eye while keeping both eyes open and then to read the smallest line that can be seen on the chart. Vision is scored according to the standard of 20/20. The numerator is always 20 to indicate the distance away from the chart, and the denominator is the distance at which a person with normal vision can read the line. Vision of 20/200 means the client sees at 20 feet what a person with normal vision can see at 200 feet. If the client cannot read all the letters on a line, this should be recorded. For instance, if three letters on the fifth line are missed, it is documented as 20/40 − 3, (Catalano, 1992; Ragge & Easty, 1991).

Refer anyone with a visual acuity of less than 20/30 in either eye to an ophthalmologist. In some cases the client may not be able to see the largest letter on the chart (usually the 20/200 letter). If this happens, the nurse should hold up two or three fingers and slowly move toward the person until the number of fingers held up can be identified. This is done to determine what can and cannot be seen and should be recorded as C/F (counting fingers) at the distance when perception occurred (Bates, 1987; Stein et al., 1988).

Many of the Snellen charts have two color bars, one red

and the other green, to help in assessing individuals with color deficits. Congenital color blindness occurs more frequently among males, since it is a recessive trait carried on the X chromosome. Acquired color blindness usually results from diseases of the optic nerve or central retina. The most common form of color blindness involves the red-green hues.

A pinhole test also can be performed if one notices diminished visual acuity. The client should be instructed to hold up a piece of cardboard with a pinhole in the center and read the chart. If vision improves significantly, the acuity problem most likely is caused by refraction (Stein et al., 1988).

Peripheral Vision

Since the Snellen chart measures only central vision, an assessment of peripheral vision is necessary because deficits in this area could indicate glaucoma or a partially detached retina. The confrontation test can be performed by the nurse to provide a rough measurement of peripheral vision. During this test, the client is seated 3 feet from the nurse, asked to close one eye as the nurse closes the same eye, and instructed to focus on the nurse's uncovered eye. The nurse then moves a small object such as a pencil inside and outside the client's visual field until this object is seen. Peripheral vision enables the nurse and client to see the pencil at the same time. Figure 16-5 illustrates visual fields. As previously indicated, this test is not very precise but may be a simple way to detect a client's "blind spot" (Bates, 1994).

Assessment of Internal Eye Structures

The rehabilitation nurse uses an ophthalmoscope to inspect the internal eye lens, noting the red reflex and opacities. In older adults the peripheral wedge-shaped opacities and cobweblike central opacities, "floaters," are common. Internal eye structures are assessed for characteristic changes occurring in the retina that indicate systemic and intracranial disorders such as arteriosclerosis, hypertension, or brain lesions. The ocular fundus, or back portion of the eye's interior, can be examined in a darkened room once a client's pupils are dilated with mydriatic drops in order to expose a view into macula. Often a client with unexplained visual loss is referred to an ophthalmologist. The ophthalmologist may use the following equipment:

1. Ophthalmoscope for magnification
2. Slit lamp to evaluate cataracts and corneal disease
3. Ophthalmometer to measure the curvature of the cornea

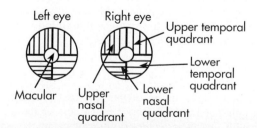

Left eye   Right eye

Upper temporal quadrant

Lower temporal quadrant

Macular   Upper nasal quadrant   Lower nasal quadrant

Fig. 16-5   Map of visual fields.

4. Fluorescent staining to detect abrasions
5. The current instrument, since there have been recent developments in instruments, to measure intraocular pressure for the presence of glaucoma (Intraocular pressure ranges from 12 to 22 mm Hg [Bates, 1991]. The cornea may be prepared for some tests by instilling an anesthetic and dyes.)

VISION CONCERNS AND REHABILITATION NURSING ACROSS THE LIFE-SPAN

A goal of the rehabilitation nurse related to visual function is to educate clients in all aspects of eye therapy and care to prevent unnecessary trauma and diseases. Preventive measures, knowledge of potential dangers to the eye, responsible behaviors, and the importance of seeking prompt medical treatment for any changes in the eye are taught by the nurse. The Box on p. 314 contains health promotion measures.

Refractive Error

Refractive error, a defect of the refracting media of the eye, is the most common visual concern. This defect prevents light rays from converging into a single focus on the retina and is due to irregularities of the corneal curvature, the focusing power of the lens, and the length of the eye. Major symptoms include blurred vision and discomfort. Corrective lenses, including eyeglasses and contact lenses, are required by approximately half of Americans to alleviate this problem. Different types of refractive error are myopia (nearsightedness), hyperopia (farsightedness), astigmatism, and presbyopia (Lewis & Collier, 1992).

Many clients in the rehabilitation facility may wear contact lenses. The nurse may use this as an opportunity for health promotion and caution the client regarding the incorrect wearing of the lenses as an important source of trauma to the eye. Many of the problems that have the potential to cause impaired vision can be avoided with proper instruction on the application of contact lenses.

Strabismus and Amblyopia

Strabismus is an eye deviation and is easily assessed as one eye deviating outward, inward, upward, or downward when the client is fixing on an object. Strabismus is a common symptom of ocular, central nervous system, or general systemic problems and may be paralytic or nonparalytic. This disorder affects approximately 5% of children and requires early medical intervention to prevent development of suppression amblyopia (Luckmann & Sorensen, 1987). Suppression amblyopia reduces vision in one eye and does not respond readily to treatment once the child has reached 6 years of age and the brain has developed severe suppression. Strabismus in elderly clients manifests itself as diplopia or double vision. Thyroid disease, neuromuscular problems of the eye muscles, and cerebral lesions are among the major causes of strabismus in adults (Vaughan & Asbury, 1983).

External Ocular Disease
✦ Infections

Infections of the external eye, including hordeolum (sties), chalazion, blepharitis, herpesvirus type I, herpes zos-

---

PREVENTIVE INTERVENTIONS

- ◆ Maintain appointments with the ophthalmologist.
- ◆ Seek out information on vision changes and major eye diseases that are associated with aging.
- ◆ Investigate any changes or symptoms related to the eye and seek appropriate and prompt medical attention.
- ◆ Participate in vision screenings that are offered at senior citizen centers for older adults and at daycare centers and schools for children.
- ◆ Wear protective eye gear for recreational activities and when working around hot metals or liquids and when welding, cutting, sawing, grinding, or stamping solid materials.
- ◆ Do not rub or touch the eye with dirty hands.
- ◆ Handling fireworks poses a great threat to the vision of the user as well as spectators and their use is not recommended.
- ◆ Wear sunglasses during all seasons of the year and do not look directly into the sun.
- ◆ Use caution when removing lids on containers and especially corks on bottles.
- ◆ Release steam slowly and carefully from ovens, popcorn bags, pots, and autoclaves.
- ◆ Read labels carefully before using over-the-counter and prescription eye medications and preparations.
- ◆ Keep dangerous substances and sharp items out of the reach of children.
- ◆ Avoid childrens' toys with sharp or pointed edges and instruct children not to run or jump with toys in their hands.
- ◆ Instruct children to keep pens and pencils away from the eyes.
- ◆ Have adequate lighting for all activities.
- ◆ Use spray aerosols, such as hair spray, and deodorizers away from the eyes and in the absence of fans or breezes.
- ◆ Pick up rocks, stones, and tree branches before mowing the lawn so they are not hurled out of the rotary blades and into the eyes.
- ◆ When using contact lenses, be sure to follow the doctor's instructions for inserting, removing, and cleaning the lenses.

---

ter, and chlamydial and fungal infections are common across the life-span. Numerous microorganisms can affect the lids and conjunctiva as well as the avascular cornea. Irritation of the cornea, a decrease in tear film, or a decrease in blinking can predispose the client to infectious conditions of the cornea. Fortunately many of the conditions affecting the external eye can be treated on an outpatient basis (Lewis & Collier, 1992).

Clients in rehabilitation programs, living in the community, or attending special sessions may experience eye infections. Health teaching includes the benefits of hand washing as essential to prevent the spread of infection to the other eye, to other clients, and to the nurse. The client is informed about the reasons for recommended procedures including universal precautions, isolation, or medication regimen. For example, when a client uses warm compresses

for the eye, adhering to procedures for disposal of compress material will prevent cross-contamination.

◆ Trauma

Occupational hazards account for a large percent of eye injuries with potential to cause blindness and to require rehabilitation. Childhood injuries or accidents in the home may result in acquired disabling conditions. A small piece of metal from work equipment, or a stone thrown by a child, can penetrate the eyeball, as well as a splash of a caustic substance in the home or at work and can damage vision easily. Clients may be injured in rehabilitation centers, in outpatient treatment areas, or during travel to appointments. In these instances the nurse should be able to perform a quick assessment and take action. Hemorrhage from outside or inside the eyeball indicates that an injury has occurred. Ecchymosis or a black eye from a fist or an object such as a ball may indicate internal damage. Serious injury can be ruled out only by examining the eyes with an ophthalmoscope. Absence of pain does not necessarily mean that damage did not occur. Damage to the surface of the eye is usually painful, whereas damage to the inside of the eye is generally pain free. The individual with altered vision, such as blurring, should be referred to an ophthalmologist for further evaluation.

Chemical burns require prompt treatment to prevent permanent scarring. Regardless of the chemical agent, initial treatment is always the same: prolonged washing of the eyeball for 15 to 20 minutes with large amounts of plain water. After this immediate response, a physician should be contacted (Lewis & Collier, 1992). Place a light patch over both eyes when injury occurs to aid in decreasing ocular movements. Refer a client for immediate medical attention whenever there is concern about foreign objects in the eye. Foreign objects should never be removed or washed out of the eye by the client.

◆ Corneal infections

Inflammation of the cornea (keratitis) is associated with severe pain, marked photophobia, and increased lacrimation and requires the client to seek immediate medical attention. Keratitis is due to bacterial, viral, and fungal microorganisms as well as chemical and mechanical injuries to the epithelium of the cornea. When accompanied with the loss of corneal tissue, a corneal ulcer results. Ulcerations are considered a serious condition because the cornea is such a vital part of vision (Lewis & Collier, 1992).

It is much easier to prevent a corneal ulcer than it is to cure one. Therefore to prevent the occurrence of ulcers, foreign bodies must be removed immediately, and scratches and infections must be treated early. Photophobia can be relieved by wearing dark glasses. Medical management also includes the immediate use of topical antibiotics given every 1 to 2 hours (Brunner & Suddarth, 1989).

Intraocular Diseases
◆ Cataracts

An opacity or clouding of the lens that blocks the passage of light needed for vision is a cataract. A cataract forms slowly with age. The exact etiology of cataract formation is still unknown. Cataracts can result from trauma, such as a foreign body that penetrates the lens, or from exposure to certain poisons, such as naphthalene, an ingredient in mothballs. Symptoms develop gradually and may not be noticed. Clients commonly complain of blurred vision, obliteration of parts of images, double images, decreased perception of color, and distorted images. Other than surgical removal, there presently exists no approved treatment for cataracts (Hart, 1992).

Cataract surgery has increased more than threefold over the last 20 years. There are three basic categories of modern cataract surgery: extracapsular cataract extraction with implantation of an intraocular lens (IOL) in the posterior chamber; small-incision phacoemulsification also with posterior chamber IOL; and intracapsular cataract extraction with implantation of an anterior chamber IOL. During extracapsular extraction, the lens capsule is incised and the lens cortex and nucleus are removed, and the posterior capsule and lens zonule are left in place. Phacoemulsification involves the fragmenting of the lens nucleus with ultrasonic vibrations and aspirating that lens material through an irrigation-aspiration system. The intracapsular approach, a technique used routinely from the 1950s to 1970s, involves removing the entire lens intact. If the cataract is not removed, the client's vision will deteriorate progressively and the enlarging lens may cause increased intraocular pressure, resulting in secondary glaucoma. Clients with a significant cataract in the second eye usually wait several weeks after having the first cataract eye surgery before surgery on the second eye (Paton & Craig, 1990).

These surgical techniques reduce patient risk and the use of IOLs brings about improved vision. With the advent of the IOLs, apraxia (or leaving the eye without a lens) no longer exists. It is estimated that 1.1 million Americans received IOL implants in the United States annually as of 1990 (Apple & Rabb, 1991). In fact, 97% of all clients undergoing surgery for cataracts have intraocular lenses inserted at the time of cataract extraction. Studies still need to be performed to determine the safest, most cost-effective and efficient lens design (Hart, 1992). IOLs do not eliminate the need for cataract glasses or contact lenses but minimize their use (Patton & Craig, 1990).

Virtually all routine cataract operations are performed in an ambulatory surgical center and the nurse has a rehabilitation role in the community setting. Postoperatively the client, family or significant others are instructed on the plan of care and how to implement it. This includes proper care procedures for the eye demonstrated by the clients when they feel comfortable handling self-care skills, and emphasizing the importance of keeping routine postoperative appointments usually scheduled at 1 week, 3 weeks, and 6 to 8 weeks. Because many clients require months to regain their full visual acuity and may not be able to manage their medication regimen, the client's family or significant others should be included in the instruction of medication administration. The client, family, significant others, and rehabilitation nurse should plan for a return visit or home visit to demonstrate correct eye care procedure and administration of medication. Any instructions, directions, or schedules should be written down as these will guide the client and family in the rehabilitation phase and serve as teaching aids related to medication and activity restrictions. Safety precautions need to be observed and the client reoriented to a familiar home environment. Family members are instructed to orient the client to how food is arranged on the plate so the client may be self-sufficient. The client also is instructed not to bend over, strain, lift heavy objects, sneeze, make jerky movements, or read. However, watching TV usually is permitted. If contact lenses are recommended, the client must be instructed on proper insertion and removal of the lenses to avoid undue trauma or injury.

✦ Glaucoma

Glaucoma is the third leading cause of blindness and can slowly damage the eye without any awareness by the person. Glaucoma occurs when there is a buildup of intraocular pressure because of blockage of aqueous humor. This condition can progressively destroy the optic nerve. There are two major forms of glaucoma: open angle and closed angle. In open-angle glaucoma, the most common form, the outflow of aqueous humor is reduced. This form of glaucoma is hereditary and is the most difficult to diagnose. Some early signs of open-angle glaucoma are frequent changes of glasses without any improvement in vision, inability of the eyes to adjust to darkened rooms, loss of side vision, and rainbow-colored rings around lights. Eyedrops (miotics) such as pilocarpine and timolol maleate are usually prescribed for open-angle glaucoma. These work by constricting the pupil and the ciliary muscle, helping to relax and open the outflow channels and reduce pressure. If intraocular pressure is not reduced sufficiently through the administration of eyedrops, surgery is performed (Lewis & Collier, 1992).

As always, the nurse instructs the client on accurate eyedrop administration. Clients needing surgery will require preoperative and postoperative nursing rehabilitation. All procedures to be performed are explained to the client. The nurse gives the client the opportunity to clarify information and to express fears concerning surgery and blindness. Postoperatively, serious consequences can result if the client is not instructed carefully on the proper eye medication administration. Since compliance of medication for chronic conditions is known to be as low as 50%, it is crucial for the rehabilitation nurse to stress strict compliance with medication regimen (Lewis & Collier, 1992). In addition, the client is encouraged to report any vague symptoms indicating increased intraocular pressure such as aching around the eye and change in vision.

Closed-angle glaucoma occurs when the iris is displaced in the periphery of the anterior chamber and blocks the aqueous filtration network. As a result the intraocular pressure rises quickly, causing severe eye pain and even nausea and vomiting. Physiologically the cornea becomes edematous and the pupil dilates. Medical management requires surgery in which part of the iris is removed (iridectomy) (Gaston & Elkington, 1986).

Because closed-angle glaucoma occurs suddenly and is accompanied with severe pain, the client is often frightened. The rehabilitation nurse facilitates communication and addresses any concerns the client may have. The client will not usually need antiglaucoma medications, but the need for follow-up care should be stressed (Lewis & Collier, 1992).

✦ Retinal detachment

The separation of the retina from the choroid is referred to as retinal detachment. Atrophy and damage to the rods and cones can occur because the separation prevents nourishment to the outer portion of the retina. There is no pain associated with retinal detachment, but usually the client complains of blurry vision and sudden flashes of light. Individuals who have had cataract surgery, trauma to the eye, or some form of myopia are at risk for detachment of the retina.

There are two classifications of retinal detachment: rhegmatogenous and nonrhegmatogenous. Rhegmatogenous, which means ruptured in Greek, occurs when holes form in the retina. Nonrhegmatogenous retinal detachment can be caused by the development of fibers within the vitreous. The fibers can adhere to the retina and, when they contract, begin to pull the retina away from its normal attachment. Generally in this case treatment would consist of surgical treatment called a vitrectomy (Brunner & Suddarth, 1989).

Surgical treatment is used to create a scar that seals most holes in the retina. This type of treatment may be accomplished by using photocoagulation, cryosurgery, electrodiathermy, and scleral buckling. About 90% of clients with retinal detachment can be treated successfully. If a client does not seek treatment, further detachment will occur, followed by blindness.

Retinal detachment incapacitates the client suddenly and often causes confusion and apprehension as well as a fear of blindness. Many times the client must leave his business or activity, with little or no time to make plans. The rehabilitation nurse facilitates communication and allows the client to discuss any fears or anxieties. The ophthalmologist may order eye patches to both eyes to decrease stimulation of eye movement, complete bed rest and specific position, whether sitting or lying flat or on one side, before surgery. The rehabilitation nurse can incorporate psychosocial aspects of nursing and enlist the assistance of the family and significant others to encourage the client to adhere to the treatment regimen.

Hemianopsia

Hemianopsia is defective vision or blindness in half of the visual field and usually refers to bilateral defects. It can result from brain damage caused by cerebrovascular disorders, trauma, or tumors.

Hemianopsias are classified as homonymous, bitemporal, and attitudinal. Homonymous hemianopsias are the most common, especially in older persons. Homonymous hemianopsia refers to loss of vision in the temporal field of one eye and the nasal field of the other. A client with a right-sided brain lesion would have a left homonymous hemianopsia with loss of vision in the nasal half of the right eye and the temporal half of the left eye. Figure 16-6 illustrates visual alterations with various hemianopsias. Many times persons with homonymous hemianopsia are unaware of their condition until the deficit is pointed out to them. A more severe visual impairment for reading occurs in a client with a right homonymous hemianopsia, because it is impossible for the client to see the letters or words in advance of the one on which the client is fixating (Brunner & Suddarth, 1989). Bitemporal hemianopsia refers to a defect or loss of the upper or lower half of the visual field, whereas bitemporal hemianopsia refers to a defect in which all or part of each temporal field is depressed.

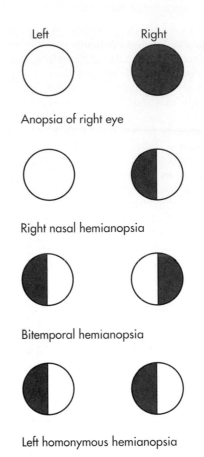

Left   Right

Anopsia of right eye

Right nasal hemianopsia

Bitemporal hemianopsia

Left homonymous hemianopsia

Fig. 16-6   Visual alterations with various hemianopsias.

The rehabilitation nurse can teach the client to position the head and use scanning techniques to increase the visual field, especially for self-care and grooming (Fig. 16-7, *A* and *B*). These clients also must be cautioned about crossing streets since they may not see traffic approaching from the affected side (Luckmann & Sorensen, 1987). The individual should be oriented continually to the environment and always should be approached from the unaffected side. Low-vision aids such as prisms and the bioptic telescope may be helpful for clients with this condition and are listed in optical aids found on page 321.

Effect of Multiple Sclerosis on Vision

Multiple sclerosis (MS) can affect vision. Often persons with this disease describe visual problems as their initial symptoms. These symptoms may include blurred vision, blind spots, (a scotoma: an islandlike gap in the visual field), and diplopia (double vision) in one or both eyes. About 70% of MS clients develop nystagmus. Complete blindness may develop, and some individuals have reported losing total sight in one eye for several hours to several days. The basis for these visual disturbances is optic neuritis (Price & Wilson, 1986). The nurse can give psychological support to the client and family. The nurse encourages the client to see the ophthalmologist regularly and identifies rehabilitation interventions and appropriate visual aids.

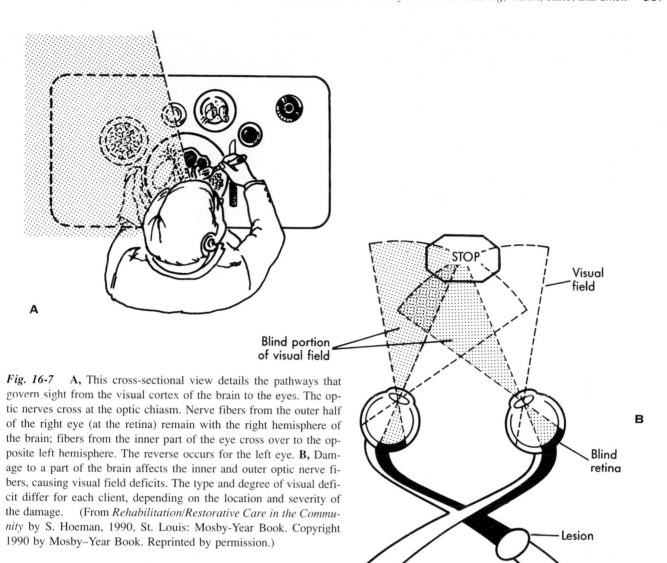

Fig. 16-7 **A,** This cross-sectional view details the pathways that govern sight from the visual cortex of the brain to the eyes. The optic nerves cross at the optic chiasm. Nerve fibers from the outer half of the right eye (at the retina) remain with the right hemisphere of the brain; fibers from the inner part of the eye cross over to the opposite left hemisphere. The reverse occurs for the left eye. **B,** Damage to a part of the brain affects the inner and outer optic nerve fibers, causing visual field deficits. The type and degree of visual deficit differ for each client, depending on the location and severity of the damage.   (From *Rehabilitation/Restorative Care in the Community* by S. Hoeman, 1990, St. Louis: Mosby-Year Book. Copyright 1990 by Mosby–Year Book. Reprinted by permission.)

Effect of Albinism on Vision

About 1 in 16,000 people in the United States in all ethnic and racial groups have albinism. Witkop recognizes 10 different types of oculocutaneous albinism and four types of ocular albinism (Witkop, Ouevedo, Fitzpatrick, & Begudet, 1989). Since almost all types of albinism are transmitted by autosomal recessive inheritance, so that both parents must carry the gene to have a child with albinism, genetic counseling is recommended. Albinism effects the eye in various ways: iris translucency, decreased retinal pigment, foveal hypoplasia, absence of stereo vision, nystagmus, strabismus, and poor visual acuity (Haefemeyer & Knuth, 1991).

The nurse educates clients with albinism on any eye deficits they are experiencing. Driving is also a concern the nurse must address. Assisting clients identify community resources for referral for the proper visual aid to improve driving ability or helping clients plan the most effective use of public transportation are important nursing responsibilities. Since albinism affects the social and emotional functioning of the client as well as the family, the nurse recognizes these as potential problems and facilitates communication to eliminate misconceptions and makes appropriate referrals for information and support. Parents with children diagnosed with albinism should be encouraged to contact the National Organization for Albinism and Hypopigmentation (NOAH) for further support. This organization provides printed information, one-on-one counseling by telephone and in person, newsletters, peer group support in many areas, and national conferences. NOAH also provides information about other resources available such as correspondence courses for parents of visually impaired children, early childhood intervention programs, special education programs, vocations, rehabilitation through state agencies, independent living centers, and other support groups (Haefemeyer & Knuth, 1991).

Eye Prosthesis

An enucleation, the surgical removal of the eyeball, may for cosmetic reasons require a prosthetic eye. An eye pros-

---
◆

MANAGEMENT OF AN EYE PROSTHESIS

REMOVAL

1. Wash hands thoroughly.
2. Line a container with gauze and fill with water to prevent scratching the prosthesis.
3. The client should be in a comfortable position.
4. Remove the prosthesis over a soft surface such as a folded towel to prevent damage if it falls.
5. Use a special small (moistened) suction cup to remove the eye prosthesis. If one is not available, the prostheses may be removed by gently depressing the lower lid, which allows the prosthesis to slide out and down. While the lower lid is depressed, the finger and thumb also may be used to grasp and pull on the prosthesis to break the suction.
6. Place the prosthesis in the container. Wash with mild soap and water and scrub with the thumb and finger. The prosthesis is rinsed carefully under running water. Place it back into the container if it is not to be reinserted.
7. Inspect the edges and surface of the prosthesis for any damaged, rough, or scratched areas. If damages are found, do not reinsert and take the prosthesis to an ocularist for repair. Otherwise the prosthesis should be taken to an ophthalmologist for yearly inspections for damage and for a thorough cleaning.

CLEANING THE EYE SOCKET

1. Irrigate the socket with saline solution from the inner canthus to the outer canthus while pulling down the lower eyelid with the thumb and raising the upper lid with the index finger. Temperature of the saline solution should be lukewarm.
2. Wash around the closed eye and gently dry.
3. Eventually the client will be able to use tap water to clean the socket while washing the face.

REINSERTION

1. Wash your hands.
2. Moisten the prosthesis with saline solution, water, or the recommended ophthalmic solution.
3. Hold the upper lid with your index finger and the lower lid with your thumb. Use the suction cup to hold the prosthesis while inserting it. Remove the suction cup by gently applying a small amount of pressure on the eye while squeezing and removing the suction cup. If you do not have a suction cup, hold the artificial eye in the opposite hand, noting that the top of the prosthesis, which usually is marked, is placed under the upper lid into the socket.
4. Have the client blink to ensure proper insertion.
5. Ask that the client not rub the eye while the prosthesis is in place because rubbing may displace the prosthesis and cause complications (Lewis & Collier, 1987; Luckmann & Sorensen, 1987; Smeltzer & Bare, 1992).

thesis is a hollow or shell-shaped plastic structure painted to match the individual's normal eye. Clients as well as family members may be instructed by the nurse concerning the importance of cleaning the artificial eye for maintaining comfort and assuring its cosmetic appearance. Some clients, such as those with sinus conditions or allergies, may be more sensitive to the prosthesis. Clients with excessive discharge may have to clean their prosthesis daily, whereas those with less discharge may require cleaning only two or three times each week (Burrell, 1992).

The following steps (found in the box at left) for cleaning the prosthetic eye should be reviewed with both the client, family members, and significant others:

Special Considerations for the Client Who is Blind

✦ **Low vision.** Low vision refers to clients who have some usable vision, no matter how little. Clients with low vision are in the middle of the scale between normal vision and blindness. The word "low" indicates that the client's vision is not normal, and the word "vision" indicates that it is not blindness either. Currently 2.4 million Americans have a visual impairment, creating an increasing need to improve the quality and availability of low-vision care and to expand rehabilitation services to persons who are visually impaired (Bailey, 1991). (See vision aids on p. 321.)

The Lighthouse (see Appendix 16-A) traditionally has been a leader in helping visually impaired people maintain their functional independence and in educating health professionals in providing low-vision services. They support experimental research to help understand the mechanisms underlying low vision and the psychosocial outcomes of programs designed to serve the low-vision population. The Lighthouse has presented a framework for shaping research throughout the world (Bailey, 1991). Their research agenda identifying priorities for low-vision research for the 1990s and beyond is found in the Box on p. 319.

✦ **Blindness.** There is no standardized definition for the terms blindness and visual impairment among health professionals specializing in eye care and among the public. Along the continuum of diminished visual capacities, legally blind covers a wide range of definitions developed by legislators in the 1930s and various agencies that support blind and visually impaired citizens. For example, persons who are partially sighted and legally blind are individuals who are legally blind but not functionally blind. Legally blind refers to persons whose visual acuity in their best-corrected better eye is 20/200 or less; or whose visual acuity in their best-corrected better eye is more than 20/200, but with a maximum diameter of visual field that measures 20 degrees or less. Functionally blind persons are individuals who are totally blind or have at the most light projection or light perception (Colenbrander & Fletcher, 1992). The term blindness is reserved for persons who have no usable sight at all, not even light detection in either eye. In the past the individual who was blind was isolated from society through sheltered workshops and segregated educational and rehabilitation agencies—which may have led to society's stereotyping of blind individuals. With the advent of mainstreaming blind children into the school system and the Americans with Disabilities Act, persons who are blind

---

THE LIGHTHOUSE, INC., LOW-VISION RESEARCH AGENDA FOR THE 1990s AND BEYOND

1. Epidemiologic and demographic aspects of vision impairment
2. Development, evaluation, and standardization of assessment tools
3. Processing of visual information with vision impairment
4. Role of the environment in vision impairment
5. Development and evaluation of low-vision devices
6. Effects of multiple impairments on vision disability
7. Assessment and rehabilitation of visually impaired infants and children
8. Psychological and social determinants and consequences of vision disability
9. Evaluation of low-vision services
10. Elucidation of formal structure of vision rehabilitation expertise
11. Development of artificial vision systems

Used with permission from the Lighthouse, Inc., New York, NY.

---

now are integrated into the workplace, colleges, and health professions.

Research has shown that labeling is a factor that hinders adjustment to blindness (Allen, 1989). The labeling of people who are blind affects interpersonal relationships because blind people feel that they are different and that they are treated differently by their sighted counterparts. To minimize the impact of visual impairment and to alter the public's perception of blindness, Allen and Birse (1991) found that the blind use the following strategies: folding the cane out of sight in the presence of others, attempting to walk without a cane, and wearing glasses to disguise the appearance of the eyes.

The nurse advocate is cognizant of the stereotyping of the blind and does not allow interference with meeting the individual needs of the client who is blind. Demonstrating a sincere understanding and acceptance of the client is essential in fostering high individual self-worth. Actively involving a client in all healthcare decision-making will support a therapeutic, caring interpersonal relationship (Allen & Birse, 1991). How well a newly blind person adapts to the situation depends on the individual's personality, developmental stage, attitude, and the attitude of family, friends, and significant others. The nurse's as well as the client's goals are directed toward the development of workable strategies to manage and carry out day-to-day activities effectively. To enhance the person's ability to communicate, navigate, socialize, and take pleasure in the environment, guidelines are provided for health professionals and other individuals in the blind person's life (see the Box on p. 320).

Communication

As stated previously, communication is an important element that requires enhancement for the person who is blind. Items such as writing guides and check-writing guides are available from the American Foundation for the Blind and may be helpful because they allow the visually impaired person to continue to write by hand. Tape recorders can be used to replace letter writing and can provide privacy for personal correspondence. Rehabilitation team members may want to suggest Braille typewriters and Braillewriters, depending on the needs of the individual who is blind. Communication also can be maintained through the use of the telephone by instructing the person who is blind on memorizing the dial or by using Braille or tactile symbols. (See Box on p. 321 for other optical aids for the individual who is blind and for clients with low vision.)

Mobility

Mobility is as important a skill as communication. A long cane or dog guide are common methods of mobility for the person who is blind. Canes are individually prescribed according to the person's height and length of stride to assist in traveling. Canes are light fiberglass or aluminum and approximately half an inch in diameter. Individuals use the wrist to move the cane in front of the body from side to side in an arc to extend the sense of touch by letting them know what lies ahead in their path. However, it requires a great deal of skill to use this technique in bad weather such as snow and thunderstorms, and when tactile and or auditory information is masked. One-to-one mobility instruction enables persons who are blind to travel successfully and maintain their chosen lifestyle (Yeadon & Grayson, 1979).

Some persons who are blind prefer the dog guide to the long cane because of the added protection the dog provides. The dog guide and the person receive special training to work as an effective team. The person who is blind is in control, giving directions such as "right," "left," and "forward" to the dog. The dog will practice intelligent disobedience only in instances where a dangerous command is given such as to cross the street in oncoming traffic. To qualify for a guide dog, the person must be between 16 and 55 years of age, in good health, able to hear, without any remaining vision that would interrupt the dependence on the dog because these dogs require intelligent handling and a regular daily activity program. The guide dog walks on the left-hand side of the blind person and wears a U-shaped harness, which is grasped by the left hand of the master. It is important that sighted people do not distract the dog or try to assist the master physically (Yeadon & Grayson, 1979).

Because of the Americans with Disabilities Act, guide dogs now are permitted to accompany the person who is blind who is admitted into a healthcare facility. Therefore nurses and healthcare personnel need to be oriented regarding interacting with these dogs when persons who are blind are clients in a rehabilitation center or acute care hospital. These healthcare facilities need to develop policies on the proper procedure for meeting the needs of both the person who is blind and the working guide dog. Rehabilitation programs, long-term care facilities, and programs such as adult

---

GUIDELINES TO ASSIST A PERSON WITH VISUAL IMPAIRMENT

1. Do not insist upon helping a person who does not want your help. If you do not know how to help, ask the person with the visual impairment just what kind of assistance is needed. For example, individuals are able to teach others how to assist them in mobility so that they can negotiate doorways, narrow passageways and stairs, and navigate obstacles.

2. When teaching a person with visually impairment, be very clear in verbal explanations because the person cannot watch what is being done as it is described. Therefore let touch and other senses compensate for the lack of vision.

3. Incorporate the same principles of teaching as when teaching a sighted person. Break down tasks into smaller component steps and teach one step at a time. Be sure the person has mastered each step before going on to the next step.

4. Determine whether or not the person has ever had sight. Some people will be able to make use of visual memory and will not be instructed the same way as a person who never had vision.

5. Orient the person to the surroundings and remind visitors to introduce themselves.

6. Maintain personal items such as combs and brushes within easy reach and in the same place or arrangement.

7. Do not reorganize the person's life space (e.g., bedside stand or chair) without permission and orienting the person verbally and physically.

8. Leave doors completely open or completely closed to prevent injury.

9. When speaking to a person with visual impairment, speak directly to the individual use a natural tone of voice, and introduce yourself by stating your name and function. Unless you know that the person has poor hearing, do not shout.

10. Use hand-to-hand contact rather than touching the person on the arm or shoulder, since it allows the person to feel more in control.

11. Allow the individual to be involved in problem-solving, because this activity helps set the tone for rehabilitation.

12. Assist the person in organizing her life space (e.g., teach how to hang clothes by style or color and how to fold money to aid identification).

13. Provide addresses and telephone numbers of agencies and resources for visually impaired persons.

14. Encourage the person to assume good posture and to turn directly toward the individual to whom he is speaking.

15. Attach or sew tactile symbols to clothing and personal items to help identify color and contents.

16. Evaluate and educate the individual to more effectively use the other senses: auditory, kinesthetic, tactile, olfactory, and gustatory.

17. Assist the person in learning to localize and discriminate sounds.

18. Encourage the individual to become involved as soon as possible in self-care practices and personal decision making.

19. Assist the person in learning to detect temperatures and to manipulate objects safely. For example, accurate pouring of a hot beverage can be practiced by placing the palm and fingers of one hand around the cup and hearing and feeling the heat as the hot liquid rises to the desired level.

20. When the person is mastering mealtime activities, such as cutting meat and buttering bread, provide privacy and easily managed foods.

21. Instruct the person to visualize the meal plate as a clock because this can help in communicating about the location of food or other items. For example, the salt shaker is in line with 12 o'clock.

22. When assisting a visually impaired person in walking, walk about a half step ahead of the person, who then grasps the guide's arm lightly but firmly just above the elbow so that the thumb is on the outside and the fingers are on the inside of the arm. Both the guide and the visually impaired person hold their upper arms close to their bodies so that the guide's movements can alert the individual to curbs, turns, and stops.

---

day care programs are developing policies for animals assisting persons with disabilities. Most policies include provisions for readily identifying the animal as an animal helper, specifying restrictions for areas where an animal may not escort or accompany a client; establishing procedures for control, vaccination, and supervision of the animal; limitations for on-site length of time; toileting and feeding animals; and similar provisions.

Rehabilitation Team

Individuals experiencing complex visual problems such as blindness should have the benefit of an interdisciplinary holistic team approach. Examples of members of the team are the rehabilitation nurse, ophthalmologist, occupational therapist, social worker, psychologist, clergy, family, and significant others. The client, family, significant others, and healthcare team work together to identify realistic goals. The expertise of each team member will assist the client to become as independent as possible. The client, family, significant others, and healthcare team develop a plan of care based on the client's goals, preferences, and lifestyle that includes various options and use of optical aids such as Braille instruction, guide dogs, white walking canes, and electronic devices. Outcome criteria also are determined to

AIDS FOR LOW VISION AND BLINDNESS

OPTICAL DEVICES
Magnifiers

- Hand magnifiers improve close vision for reading and writing by increasing the ability to focus on near objects.
- Strong convex lenses possess a short focal distance so reading material can be brought close to the eye.

Distance magnifiers

- Telescopic lenses include binoculars, field glasses, or telescopes for occasional use to magnify objects at a distance.
- Special filters are worn over glasses for light- or glare-sensitive vision.
- Tinted lenses relieve glare intolerance outdoors.
- Prisms improve vision by moving images to a different part of the retina.

NONOPTICAL DEVICES

- Lighting changes can be affected by altering position of existing lamps or shades or altering strength of bulbs to increase contrast between print and background, making details more legible.
- Reading rectangle reduces amount of reflected light from the reading page by showing only a few lines of type at one time.
- Large type includes large-print books and magazines, telephone dials with large numbers, playing cards with large figures.
- Yellow filters decrease fuzzy vision because yellow light improves contrast between dark letters and white paper.
- Marking pens increase client's ability to read her own writing by writing in different widths.

ELECTRONIC DEVICES

- Laser cane detects objects at head level or straight ahead up to 20 feet by emitting a thin beam of infrared light.
- Pathsounder detects objects from waist to top of head by emitting a beam of ultrasound; not used with guide dogs.
- Talking books are provided by the Library of Congress to regional libraries throughout the country.
- Optacon changes print of ordinary material into letter configurations of vibrating reeds that can be read tactually.
- Closed-circuit television and computers magnify printed matter.
- Computer-driven sensing devices improve the mobility needs of individuals with visual impairment by overcoming the limitations of traditional aids.

evaluate the success of nursing and the interdisciplinary team's interventions. The rehabilitation nurse may be instrumental in referring the client for more extensive assistance. Referrals require thought and a complete awareness of the client's needs and goals. For example, the National Eye Institute can provide low-vision aids and information on eye disease to the client, family, and significant others. The re-

habilitation nurse works collaboratively with the interdisciplinary team to ensure the best possible outcomes for the client. Appendix 16-A provides addresses of additional organizations that can provide help to the client.

Diabetic Retinopathy and Vision Loss

Diabetic retinopathy refers to a noninflammatory process in which the eye undergoes vascular changes. Almost all persons with diabetes experience some retinal vascular alterations with increasing longevity. Persons with uncontrolled diabetes or those who have been dependent on insulin for 20 years or more are at higher risk for developing diabetic retinopathy. If complications develop, then blindness can result. More than 50,000 individuals are blind as a result of diabetic retinopathy, and each year there are 8,000 new cases of blindness from this complication (Garcia & Ruiz, 1992). It is the major cause of blindness in the 20- to 74-year-old population and is the second cause of blindness overall (Cryer & Cryer, 1991). Blindness is 25 times more likely to occur in diabetic clients than in nondiabetic clients. The American Academy of Ophthalmology aims to eliminate preventable blindness from diabetes by the year 2000. "Diabetes 2000" also aims to reduce the incidence of legal blindness from diabetes to no more than 4,000 new cases per year (Ghartey, 1990). In addition, diabetic retinopathy was identified as a major health concern to be addressed in Objective 17.4 in Healthy People 2000. Areas identified were improved screening processes to uncover retinopathy earlier and increased awareness of diabetes-related eye problems by the medical community, government, and the public (Garber, 1990).

There are two forms of diabetic retinopathy: proliferative retinopathy and nonproliferative (background) retinopathy. The main difference between the two forms is that proliferative retinopathy is seen most commonly in the insulin-dependent client after 15 to 25 years of having diabetes, whereas diabetic macular degeneration is mainly the condition of the middle-aged and elderly.

Proliferative retinopathy develops in up to 60% of clients with insulin-dependent diabetes mellitus (IDDM) after 25 years of having diabetes. It affects 40% of clients with non-insulin-dependent diabetes mellitus (NIDDM) after having the condition for 20 years and then treating it with insulin. On the contrary, only 20% of non-insulin-dependent diabetics whose treatment entails oral agents and a strict diet develop proliferative retinopathy after 20 years of having the condition. Proliferative retinopathy refers to neovascularization or fibrosis. The new vessels pose a threat if they grow into the vitreous cavity and rupture, causing a vitreous hemorrhage. The proliferative bands or membranes form along the blood vessels. The contraction and pulling of these vessels on the retina causes retinal tears and detachments. The cause of these abnormal blood vessels is unknown. One theory postulates that the retina may be trying to compensate for poor blood perfusion (Crabbe, 1987). The first technique developed to treat proliferative retinopathy by cauterizing and cutting abnormal blood vessels into pieces used focal photocoagulator lasers. A second technique, panretinal photocoagulation, was developed because neovascularization tends to recur. Instead of coagulating abnormal vessels, thousands of laser burns are made over the entire surface of the retina in several sessions over a period of weeks (L'esperance, 1991).

Nonproliferative retinopathy is the most common cause of visual loss in non-insulin-dependent diabetics (Crabbe, 1987). It causes dilation and microaneurysms of the retinal vessels, which can rupture, causing hemorrhage into the retinal layers. If macular edema occurs, then fluorescein angiography is used to determine the potential for return of vision. If the macular capillaries are leaking fluid, then laser treatment may be beneficial. If the capillaries are occluded, vision is unlikely to return.

The Diabetes Control and Complications Trial (DCCT) investigated the progression of diabetic retinopathy since no medical therapy is available to alter the course of this complication effectively. This study demonstrated the effects of tight control and conventional management in delaying the onset and slowing the progression of diabetic retinopathy, nephropathy, and neuropathy in clients with IDDM (Garcia & Ruiz, 1992). The goal of the intensive regimen was to maintain the glycemic status as close to the normal range as safely possible. Other research has evaluated the effect of drugs such as aspirin on diabetic retinopathy. The study identified no contraindications associated with aspirin on the progression or improvement in visual acuity in diabetic retinopathy. It found no reason to withhold aspirin from clients with nonproliferative or proliferative retinopathy who require aspirin for other medical conditions.

Active research regarding different treatment modalities, including drug therapy, is being conducted. For example, ticlopidine hydrochloride is a promising new drug used in a diabetes study to assess its platelet inhibitory properties, which is important in reducing the progression of nonproliferative diabetic retinopathy (Ticlopidine, 1991).

THE EAR
Components of the Ear

The ear is a very complex organ located within and protected by the temporal bone. For ease of discussion, the ear can be divided into three parts: external ear, middle ear, and inner ear (Fig. 16-8).

✦ **External ear.** The two major functions of the external ear include the improvement of the transfer of sound energy to the eardrum and aid in sound localization. The external ear is composed of the auricle (pinna) and external auditory canal. The auricle is composed of cartilage and connective tissue covered by skin and is the portion of the ear that extends from the side of the head. The auditory canal in adults extends approximately 2.5 cm and has a slight S shape. Sebaceous and other glands in the outer half of the canal secrete cerumen (earwax), which has a protective function. In Caucasians and African-Americans, cerumen is moist and sticky, whereas in Asians and Native Americans it is dry or hard. The color can range from creamy pink to brown and black. Hair follicles are also present in the outer half of the canal and may be profuse and coarse, especially in older male clients.

The tympanic membrane (eardrum), which separates the external ear from the middle ear, receives sound waves from the external ear and canal. Normally the tympanic membrane is cone-shaped, shiny, translucent, and pearl-gray and is composed of skin, connective tissue, and mucous membrane. The tympanic membrane is about the size of a pea and is obliquely positioned at the medial end of the canal. Landmarks on the tympanic membrane include the umbo and the cone of light. The umbo is the most retracted part of the membrane. The cone of light refers to the reflection seen on the surface of the membrane if a small penlight is shone into the ear.

✦ **Middle ear.** The middle ear cavity is air filled and transfers airborne sound pressure fluctuations in the external canal to pressure variations in the fluid-filled inner ear. The sound that vibrates the tympanic membrane is transmitted to the cochlea by three small bones or ossicles located directly behind the membrane: the malleus (hammer), the incus (anvil), and the stapes (stirrup). The malleus is the longest bone, and its handle attaches directly to the tympanic membrane. The other end is joined rigidly to the incus so that the two bones move as a unit with the movement of the membrane. The force of this movement is passed to the stapes, a bone partly embedded in the fenestra ovalis (oval window), which forms a flexible entrance to the cochlea. This chain formed by the ossicles receives vibrations from the tympanic membrane and transmits them to the inner ear (Cohen, 1993).

The eustachian tube is another important structure of the middle ear. The eustachian tube opens into the nasopharynx and provides equalization of air pressure between the middle ear and the pharynx. This equalizing mechanism is important when flying at high altitudes or diving under water. The eustachian tube usually is closed but will open when one yawns, swallows, or chews. There is a direct connection between the middle and inner ears. Cranial nerve VII, which controls facial movement, is found within the middle ear. The chorda tympani, a branch of this nerve, supplies taste to the anterior two thirds of the tongue (Reinecke, 1983).

✦ **Inner ear.** The inner ear is a maze formed by a bony labyrinth and a membranous labyrinth. The bony labyrinth is composed of the vestibule, cochlea, and semicircular canals. The vestibule, the organ of balance, makes up the central portion of the bony labyrinth and is bathed in endolymph fluid. The cochlea, a tube coiled around several times, has the appearance of a snail and is divided into three sections: the scala vestibuli (the upper section), the scala media, and the scala tympani (the lower section). Perilymph, a clear fluid, fills both the scala vestibuli and the scala tympani, and endolymph fills the scala media. The cochlea also contains the organ of Corti, the sense organ of hearing. The organ of Corti is composed of approximately 24,000 tiny hair cells bathed in endolymph which become distorted and mechanically bent when sound waves enter the cochlea (Lewis & Collier, 1992). The hair cells are displaced along the length of the cochlea and as they are displaced are transformed into neural activity. The neural impulses travel along to the eighth cranial nerve to the brain to produce the sensation of sound. The three semicircular canals are at right angles to each other. Within each semicircular canal is a membranous semicircular canal. Each canal enlarges into an ampulla, which contains receptors from cranial nerve VIII (the acoustic nerve). Figure 16-9 illustrates cranial nerve insertion in the brain from a baseline view.

The membranous labyrinth is composed of the utricle and

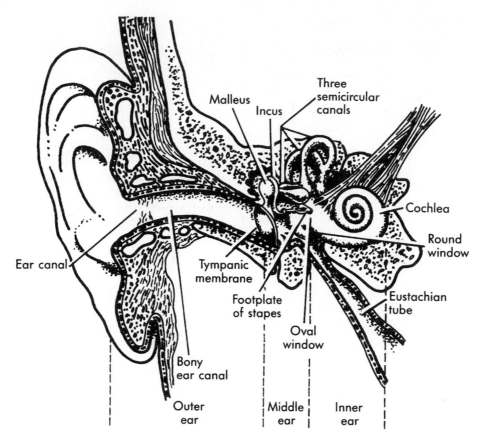

Fig. 16-8 The anatomy of the ear has three main areas: the external auditory area, the middle ear, and the inner ear. Obstructions, including ear wax, in the auditory canal or fluid in the eustachian tube may reduce hearing. The middle ear contains three small bones (the incus, malleus, and stapes) that vibrate to assist in the transmission of sound during normal hearing. The bones may become stabilized by calcified deposits and produce conductive hearing losses. Inner ear deficits often involve sensorineural losses. These may affect a client's balance and produce ringing in the ears as well as hearing loss. (From *Rehabilitation/Restorative Care in the Community* by S. Hoeman, 1990, St. Louis: Mosby-Year Book. Copyright 1990 by Mosby–Year Book. Reprinted by permission.)

saccule. Both the utricle and the saccule are suspended in the vestibule and contain endolymph. A smaller structure, the macula, is located in the utricle and saccule. The macula contains hair cells and otoliths (tiny ear stones). The hair cells project into the endolymph and are responsible in part for maintaining balance. When the position of the head is changed, it causes the otoliths to pull on the hair cells (Kapperud, 1983). Table 16-3 summarizes the structures of the ear and their functions.

Perception of Sound

Sound results from alternating compressions and expansions of air molecules. Air molecules conduct sound waves, which are picked up by the auricles and auditory canal. Sound waves strike the taut tympanic membrane and make it vibrate, which in turn sets the ossicular chain in motion. The chain then vibrates the footplate of the stapes in the oval window, transmitting sound to the liquid in the middle ear. The thousand of tiny hair cells contained within the organ of Corti bend when sound waves enter the cochlea. At

this time sound, which has been a mechanical force, is converted to an electrochemical impulse. This impulse travels to the temporal cortex of the brain via cranial nerve VIII (the acoustic nerve) and then is interpreted as meaningful sound. The hair cells in the cochleal organ of Corti are crucial to hearing. Some of the hair cells are believed to be sensitive to different pitches, whereas others respond to loudness of sounds (Fig. 16-10) (Lewis & Collier, 1992; Riley, 1987).

Nursing Assessment of the Ear

As with visual status, subjective and objective information about hearing status is needed by the nurse so that potential hearing damage can be prevented and appropriate referrals made when hearing problems become apparent. It is often the nurse who detects early subtle clues of alterations in ear health and can assist the client in seeking early intervention so that the probability of permanent disability is reduced. The nurse should perform the assessment in a well-lit, quiet environment free of distractions. It is important

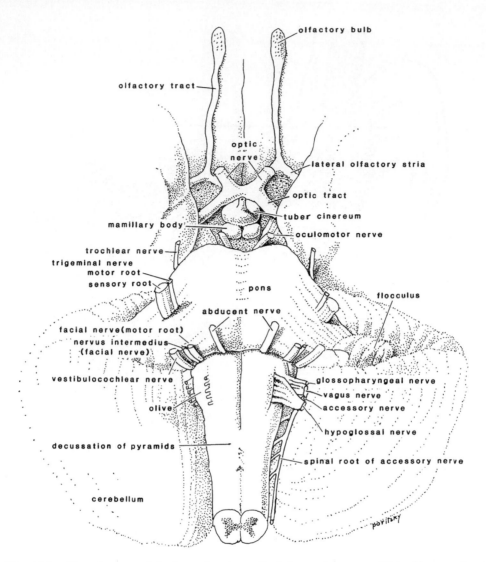

Fig. 16-9   Ventral aspect of the brain showing exit of the cranial nerves. (From *Neuroanatomy* by Poritsky, 1992, St. Louis: Mosby-Year Book. Copyright 1992 by Mosby–Year Book. Reprinted by permission.)

Table 16-3   Structure and functions of the ear

Structural sections	Component parts	Functional attributes
External ear	Auricle	Passageway for sounds
	Auditory canal	Protects organ from microorganisms
Middle ear	Tympanic membrane ossicles; malleus, incus, stapes	Receives and amplifies sound vibrations
	Eustachian tube	Equalizes air pressure between middle ear and pharynx
	Cranial nerve VII (facial)	Controls facial movement
Inner ear	Bony labyrinth: vestibule, cochlea, semicircular canals	Transmission of sound waves; aids balance
	Membranous labyrinth (inside bony labyrinth): utricle, saccule	Aids balance and equilibrium

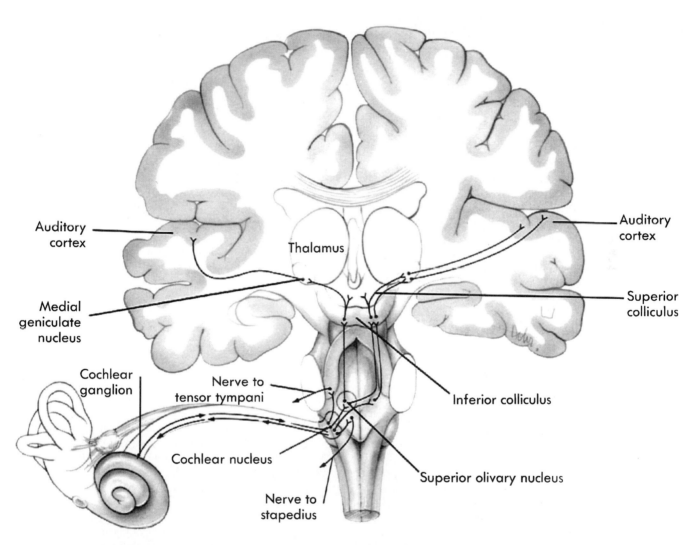

Fig. 16-10   Central nervous system pathways for hearing. Afferent axons from the cochlear ganglion terminate in the cochlear nucleus in the brainstem. Axons from neurons in the cochlear nucleus project to the superior olivary nucleus or to the inferior colliculus. Axons from the inferior colliculus project to the medial geniculate nucleus of the thalamus, and thalamic neurons project to the auditory cortex. Neurons in the superior olivary nucleus send axons to the inferior colliculus, back to the inner ear, or to motor nuclei in the brainstem, which send efferent fibers to the middle ear muscles. (From *Essentials of Anatomy and Physiology* by R.R. Seely, T.D. Stephens, & P.P. Tate, 1991, St. Louis: Mosby–Year Book. Copyright 1991 by Mosby–Year Book.)

for the nurse to face the client and speak slowly in a well-modulated voice. Occasionally assessment of a hearing-impaired client may require written communication or the use of a sign language interpreter.

Health History

Responses to the questions found in the following Box can provide a framework for a more in-depth health investigation and may be used as a guide for data collection. As with the visual health history, the hearing health history database will vary depending on the age of the client; some questions are age specific for children, adults, and older adults.

Persons in our society are often impatient with those who are hearing impaired. They may make jokes about them and sometimes assume that the person who cannot hear well must also be mentally deficient. Detection of hearing problems becomes difficult because individuals are embarrassed and feel stigmatized if they have to wear a hearing aid. Therefore the nurse must be sure to facilitate conversation and help clients feel comfortable when talking about their hearing impairments.

DATA COLLECTION QUESTIONS

1. How old are you?
2. What is your occupation?
3. Have you ever been exposed to dust or dirt or noise at work such as noisy machinery or loud music?
4. In your work do you have to wear protective earplugs?
5. Is your work environment too noisy to carry on a normal conversation?
6. Do you participate in activities such as target practice with a gun, hunting, swimming, scuba diving, skeet shooting, or racket sports that would predispose you to hearing problems?
7. Do you frequently suffer from upper respiratory tract infections (i.e., cold or flu), allergies, sinusitis, or bronchitis?
8. Have you ever had a hearing evaluation? If so, by whom was it done and do you have the results?
9. Do you have any of the following problems with your ears:
   a. Pain (otalgia). In one or both ears? Describe the pain on a scale of 1-5 with 5 being the most severe. Is it present consistently or just when the ear is touched? Does the ear feel blocked?
   b. Discharge (otorrhea). Describe the color, consistency, and the presence of any odor.
   c. Dizziness (vertigo). Is it periodic or persistent? Is it associated with nausea, vomiting, or other symptoms? Do you have to lie down? Do you fall because of it?
   d. Ringing in the ears (tinnitus). In one or both ears? Does it pulsate? Does it make your own voice seem hollow? Is it high pitched or ringing?
   e. Itching.
   f. Fever.
   g. Reduced hearing. In one or both ears?
10. Have you noticed any recent change(s) in your ability to hear? If so, when did you first notice these problems/changes, and have you had them in the past?
11. Can you tell me about the treatment you received for these problems/changes? Was it effective?
12. Do you now or have you in the past used a hearing aid? If so, what has been your response to the aid?
13. Is one or both ears affected?
14. Is the condition improving, staying the same, or getting worse?
15. Do you self-treat the problem/changes, and does it make you feel better or worse?
16. Have these problems/changes affected your activities at home or work, communication or ambulation?
17. Have you ever experienced sudden loss of hearing?
18. Do you ever ask others to repeat themselves? Do you have difficulty following conversations?
19. Do you raise the volume higher than normal when watching television or listening to the radio?
20. Do you have a medical history of surgery for any ear problems?
21. What medications are you currently taking including over-the-counter drugs?
22. In the past have you taken diuretics, streptomycin, quinine, or antibiotics? (The nurse should have a list of ototoxic chemicals and pharmacologic agents that have a negative effect on hearing.)
23. Do you have a family history of hearing loss or ear problems, and what was the age of onset?
24. Describe any ear problems you had as a child.
25. Did you have measles or mumps as a child?
26. During pregnancy, did your mother have rubella or influenza?
27. Have you recently experienced trauma to your head?
28. Do you have any of the following systemic problems: arteriosclerosis, diabetes, or thyroid disease?
29. Have you recently had any facial, dental, or throat surgery?
30. Have you recently traveled by air? Are you planning to do so?
31. Do you put any of the following items into your ears: cotton-tipped applicators, ear-plugs, or earphones?
32. Do you use a Walkman? If yes, what type of headset do you use?
33. Do you have a hard time hearing the teacher or other students talk at school?
34. Do you have to watch people's lips when they talk?
35. Does the child frequently touch, hold, or pull on the ear and complain of an ear ache?

External Ear Examination

Objective data obtained from observing the external ear are the size and shape of the auricle; equality of conformation of both ears; the color of skin; and presence of nodules, swelling, redness, and lesions. In general, the ears lie in close proximity to the head; the surface of the auricle should be smooth. Variations include a lesion, a mass, or a tophus, which is a white, hard nodule. Inspect whether skin color of the external auditory canal is similar to the client's skin color. Redness of the canal may signify an inflammation such as external otitis media. Palpate the auricle and mastoid areas for tenderness and nodules. If grasping the auricle causes pain, acute external otitis is suggested (Smeltzer & Bare, 1992).

Use an otoscope to inspect the ear canal and tympanic membrane. The auditory canal and eardrum should be cleansed gently before the examination to remove accumulated cerumen, particulate matter, pus, and secretions that may impede visualization of the canal and eardrum. Tip the client's head to the opposite shoulder and straighten the client's canal by grasping the auricle and gently pulling upward, backward, and slightly outward. When dealing with children, who may make sudden movements of the head, the thumb and forefinger of the right hand holding the otoscope should be buffered by the examiner's restraining right hand and forearm, which rests firmly on the examining table (Bates & Hoeckelman, 1987). Various instruments are used to inspect the auditory canal and eardrum including an aural speculum, which can be accompanied by either an otoscope or operating microscope to provide further magnification of the eardrum.

The amount and color of cerumen should be noted. Observe the tympanum for color, landmarks, and intactness. When inflammation is present, the membrane may be red or pink; when pus is present, white; when serum is present, yellow or amber; and when there is bleeding, blue. Refer a client who has unexplained perforation or scars, white plaques or flecks (usually indicating old, healed disease), bulging outward of the eardrum (indicating pus in the middle ear), pain, or retracted eardrum (indicating increased pressure in the middle ear) (Luckmann & Sorensen, 1987).

Eustachian Tube Assessment

Symptoms of eustachian tube occlusion include fluid in the middle ear, pressure in the ear, deafness, or tinnitus. The simplest test to assess eustachian tube function is to observe the eardrum while the client does a Valsalva maneuver, if not contraindicated, by gently pinching the nose closed and blowing with the mouth closed. The eardrum moves and the client feels a pressure change in the ear if the eustachian tube is patent. A pneumatic otoscope is used to test patency of the eustachian tube. Indirectly assess patency by exerting pressure on the eardrum and observing its mobility. The eustachian tube is open if the eardrum moves (Luckmann & Sorensen, 1987).

Hearing Acuity

Hearing acuity is assessed in various ways. The nurse can perform a gross assessment to test the client's ability to hear whispered or spoken words or the ticking of a watch. A more precise assessment can be done with special equipment such as an audiometer.

With the masking speech method, the client is prevented from using one ear by having noise produced near that ear. Noise can be produced by crackling paper while the nurse speaks in a whisper. The client is asked to repeat the word or phrase whispered. If the whispered voice is not heard, a normal conversational voice should be used to elicit a response. Normally a whispered voice is heard at a distance of 18 feet and a conversational voice at 40 feet. Masking speech may localize hearing impairment to one ear (Riley, 1987).

The watch tick test is similar to masking speech. A watch is placed 2 to 5 cm from the ear being tested while the opposite ear is masked. This test is easy to administer because it can be done in the client's home. A wristwatch produces a high-frequency sound above the range needed to hear speech. Since loss of hearing often begins with a loss of sensitivity for high frequencies, a defect may be found earlier with this test than with masking.

Tuning forks are designed to produce frequencies that correspond to the musical C scale when they are vibrated. Two tests that require a tuning fork are the Rinne and the Weber tests.

The Rinne test is designed to compare the client's hearing by air conduction and by bone conduction. The base of the vibrating tuning fork is placed on the bone behind the ear (mastoid process). The client is asked to indicate when a tone is heard and when it dissipates. When the tone dissipates, the vibrating tuning fork is brought close to the external auditory canal. Again the client is asked to indicate when a tone is heard and when it disappears. With normal function, the tone should be heard about twice as long by air as by bone conduction. The client with a conductive hearing loss will hear the tone longer behind the ear than at the canal opening since the problem involves the outer or middle ear mechanism (Burrell, 1992).

In the Weber test the stem of the vibrating tuning fork is placed on the midline of the skull to determine whether sound is heard equally in both ears. The client is then asked to indicate in which ear the sound is loudest. Normally the tone is heard equally in both ears. If the tone is lateralized to the poorer ear, then a conductive hearing loss is suspected. In a sensorineural hearing loss, the tone is heard louder in the better ear (Burrell, 1992).

◆ Audiometry

The otologist may refer the client to an audiologist for an audiometric hearing test. Audiometry can be used as both a screening test for hearing acuity as well as a diagnostic test for determining the degree and type of hearing loss (Lewis & Collier, 1992). There are two kinds of audiometric testing: pure-tone audiometry and speech audiometry. With pure-tone audiometry, the sound stimulus is composed of a pure or musical tone. The louder the tone before the client perceives it, the greater the hearing loss. Speech audiometry uses the spoken word to determine the ability to hear and discriminate sounds.

Tones are presented through earphones to each ear, and the client is instructed to signal when she hears the tone and then again when it is no longer heard. Air conduction is measured when the tone is applied directly over the opening of the external auditory canal. When the stimulus is applied to the mastoid, conductive mechanisms of the ear are bypassed and nerve conduction can be tested.

The audiometer is an electrical instrument calibrated so that what is recorded is not the ability to hear but rather hearing loss in the frequencies tested. The hertz (Hz) is the unit for measuring the frequency of sound. Although the normal human ear perceives sounds ranging from 20 to 20,000 Hz, hearing is most sensitive for frequencies between 500 and 4,000 Hz. The decibel (dB) is used to measure the intensity of sound. Hearing loss can be defined as the number of decibels reached before the client hears the sound for each specific frequency. Zero loudness is calibrated for the sound barely heard by the person with normal hearing. A range of 0- to 20-dB loss for a tested frequency is considered normal, whereas a person with a 70- to 89-dB loss for a tested frequency is considered to have a profound loss. Persons with a hearing loss of 30 dB, even though categorized as having a mild loss, will have considerable difficulty in everyday conversation and will be candidates for hearing aids.

✦ Tympanometry

Tympanometry measures eardrum resilience. The eardrum moves because pressures on either side of the eardrum are normally equal. Pressure changes that cause ear problems can be recorded on a tympanogram. Responses of the eardrum are measured as pressure in the external auditory canal changes and complementary movement of the eardrum occurs. This method of assessing hearing acuity is particularly helpful when testing children or other clients that may be unable to give the responses necessary for audiometry (Luckmann & Sorensen, 1987).

Equilibrium Assessment

Labyrinth problems are characterized by dizziness and/or vertigo. Clients often have difficulty describing dizziness, which is a disturbed sense of relationship to space. They may feel a sense of turning or whirling or may even have symptoms that are less clearly defined such as weakness, giddiness, confusion, blankness, or unsteadiness. Vertigo is most often characterized as a sensation of turning or whirling.

By artificially stimulating the semicircular canals through tests such as the Barany test or cold caloric tests, the nurse can assess for dizziness and vertigo. The results from these tests are then compared against normal reactions.

Labyrinth disturbances can also produce nystagmus or a constant involuntary eyeball movement. Labyrinthine nystagmus causes rhythmic eye movement such as slow eye movement in one direction followed by rapid compensatory movement in the opposite direction (Luckmann & Sorensen, 1987).

The result of labyrinth stimulation is past-pointing, falling, or nystagmus. When testing for past-pointing, sit facing the client, whose arms are extended. The nurse's left arm is extended to meet the client's right arm. The client's index fingers are placed on the index fingers of the nurse. With eyes closed, the client raises both arms over the head simultaneously and returns them to the original position, touching the nurse's fingers. If the client "misses" or past-points your fingers, labyrinth stimulation is indicated (Burrell, 1992).

To test for falling, the client stands with his feet together, eyes closed, and arms at the sides. Normally the client will remain still or sway slightly. When there is labyrinth stimulation, the client may sway significantly or even fall (Romberg's sign). The nurse must be prepared to catch or steady a falling person. Past-pointing and falling always occur toward the side of damage (Burrell, 1992; Luckman & Sorensen, 1987).

If a client experiences nystagmus, past-pointing, and falling, there is a problem with equilibrium. Severe reactions to labyrinth stimulation include dizziness, vertigo, nausea, and vomiting and indicate the need for detailed testing for a more specific diagnosis.

Major Types of Hearing Impairment

Hearing impairment is the second most common physical disability in the United States, with 15 million Americans experiencing hearing loss in one or both ears (Lewis & Collier, 1987). Hearing impairment, no matter how slight, is considered deafness of some sort and has a direct, negative impact on the individual's ability to communicate with others. All hearing impairments can be categorized into one of seven categories: conduction deafness, sensorineural deafness, central deafness, mixed-type deafness, functional deafness, congenital deafness, and neonatal deafness (Riley, 1987).

Conduction-type deafness occurs when the normal movement of sound vibration is prevented from entering the inner ear. The client perceives sound as distant or faint (decreased sensitivity) but remains relatively clear (normal discrimination). The causes of conductive hearing loss include impacted cerumen, a ruptured tympanic membrane, otitis media, otosclerosis, and previous ear surgery. Clients with conductive hearing loss speak softly and hear best in a noisy environment because people tend to speak louder over the noise. Their speech discrimination and ability to hear on the telephone are good. They may encounter problems hearing when eating crispy or crunchy foods because bone conduction transmits the sounds of chewing to the ear and masks air-conducted sounds. This type of deafness is treatable by medication, surgery (stapedectomy), or amplification of sound in the form of a hearing aid (Burrell, 1992). The rehabilitation nurse may be very supportive to the client and ease the client's fears about total deafness.

Sensorineural deafness (or "nerve deafness" or "perceptive deafness") results from damage to the neural structures of the inner ear or to cranial nerve VIII (the acoustic nerve). A disruption of normal analysis of sound waves and of the transmission of impulses occurs. The cochlear portion of the inner ear or the cochlear division of the acoustic nerve degenerates or forms lesions. Sensorineural deafness can be caused by prolonged exposure to intense noise, presbycusis, meningitis, ototoxic drugs, acoustic neuroma, syphilis, and Ménière's disease. Clients with this type of deafness speak loudly but hear poorly in a noisy environment. Their speech discrimination and ability to hear on the telephone are poor. Unfortunately, with this type of hearing loss, hearing cannot be restored or improved since nerve tissue does not regenerate. Therefore the nurse's major responsibility is to educate clients on preventing the condition. The nurse also can assist the client with sensorineural hearing loss in choosing the optimal hearing aid (Burrell, 1992; Silverstein, Wolfson, & Rosenberb, 1992).

Mixed-type hearing loss, as the name implies, results from damage to both the conductive and nerve mechanisms in the middle and inner ears. Usually the client has reduced speech discrimination, somewhat reduced bone conduction, and unilateral hearing loss. Only the conductive portion of this condition is treatable.

Central deafness results from an abnormality in the auditory system in the brain. Common causes include cerebrovascular accident, encephalitis, stroke, and brain neoplasm. There is a noticeable difference between the client's hearing level and the ability to interpret speech. No treatment or remedy exists for this type of deafness.

Presbycusis is an unexplained condition that occurs in middle or older age. It is a slow progressive loss of hearing and ability to understand speech. The hearing loss is bilateral and symmetric. This sensory impairment condition is more previlant in males. Research indicates that 25% to 50% of the elderly have difficulty hearing, which may be the result of presbycusis (Burrell, 1992; Riley, 1987). In addition, aging contributes to a loss of neurons from the spiral ganglia of the cochlea and a generalized cerebral atrophy that affects hearing. Other factors being investigated include diet and exercise level and exposure to noise and smoking.

There is no organic basis for the apparent hearing loss found in functional deafness. The client's inability to hear is attributed to emotional factors or may have a psychogenic origin. Clients with this condition are treated with psychiatric intervention (Burrell, 1992; Riley, 1987).

Approximately 60% of all hearing impairments are congenital in origin. Congenital deafness is deafness that exists at the time of birth and can be caused by ototoxic drugs, a genetic predisposition, or the pregnant mother's exposure to rubella during the first trimester of pregnancy (Riley, 1987).

Neonatal deafness can be caused from anoxia during birth, Rh incompatibility, trauma at birth, or prematurity. The nurse's major responsibility is to educate parents about the importance of prenatal care for health promotion and prevention of neonatal deafness (Riley 1987).

Alterations in Ear Functions and Rehabilitation Nursing Across the Life-Span
◆ External ear disorders

Deformities. Deformities of the external ear may be the result of trauma and/or congenital malformations. Perichondritis or "cauliflower ears," hematomas, and sebaceous cysts are common deformities that occur as a result of trauma. Congenital malformations include extremely large ears (macrotia), unusually small ears (microtia), bilateral "winged" ears, total absence of pinna (anotia), or absence or closure of the auditory canal (atresia). Such deformities often can be corrected by plastic surgery and or ear prosthesis (Riley, 1987).

The rehabilitation nurse can intervene by referring the cli-

ent to a plastic surgeon and discussing the deformity openly with the client. The nurse also educates the client about preventing injury to the ears. Hematomas should be treated with cold applications or ice packs to prevent their enlargement.

Foreign bodies. Foreign bodies including insects, cotton balls, peas, and other small items may become lodged in the auditory canal, especially in children and in mentally retarded and confused individuals. The client should receive immediate medical attention to identify the type of foreign body present. The physician assesses the ear for perforations of the tympanic membrane before irrigation or instillation of otic drops begins since they would be contraindicated if a perforation exists. Removal of foreign objects and the use of instruments must be done carefully by the physician to avoid damage to the auditory canal or eardrum. If the client has an insect lodged in the auditory canal, shining a flashlight in the ear may attract the insect to the light. A few drops of mineral oil or olive oil also may be used to smother and immobilize the insect. Vegetable foreign bodies such as peas and beans tend to swell, and therefore the ear should not be irrigated. Anesthesia may be required to remove the particle (Burrell, 1992; Riley, 1987). It is important for the nurse to counsel the parents of small children regarding the removal of small objects from a child's surroundings and the avoidance of cleaning the child's ears with cotton-tipped applicators.

The external auditory canal can also become obstructed by a cerumen impaction, which results in reversible conductive hearing loss. This impaction can be caused from abnormal cerumen that remains soft, a large amount of hair at the conchal opening, or impaired or diminished chewing. Clients with a cerumen impaction will usually have dark yellow-brown wax that appears old and dried. They may experience a feeling of fullness, itching, or tinnitus. Clients may attempt to remove hardened wax from the ear by using cotton-tipped applicators or sharp objects such as a hairpin or a fingernail. Therefore they need to be taught that such a practice not only may push the wax in farther but also can injure the canal (Ney, 1993; Burrell, 1992).

One of the most common procedures the nurse is likely to be involved in is an ear irrigation to remove impacted cerumen as well as foreign bodies. Nurses may remove cerumen using a specific protocol. The nurse should carefully clip and remove hairs in the ear canal. The nurse then instills a softening agent, such as mineral oil (twice daily for a couple of days if needed) to soften the wax. A small cotton ball is placed in the external ear canals to protect clothing and linens from drainage of oil or wax. To irrigate the ear canal and remove cerumen, the nurse uses a handheld bulb syringe, a 2- to 4-oz plastic syringe or Water-Pik with an emesis basin held below each ear to collect the solution. Tap water or a solution of 3 oz of 3% hydrogen peroxide in a quart of warmed water is used to irrigate the canal. The adult auricle should be pulled upward and then backward before injecting the solution along the upper wall of the auditory canal. After the canal has been washed out, it should be dried. If this procedure is not successful in removing the wax, the physician probably will have to use an irrigation technique or a curette under direct vision (Ney, 1993; Burrell, 1992).

External otitis. External otitis is a general term applied to inflammatory conditions of the auricle and external auditory canal and includes swimmer's ear, chronic external otitis, noninfectious external otitis, and malignant external otitis. Clients with external otitis will experience itching and pain in a dry scaling auditory canal, watery discharge, intermittent deafness, adenopathy, or fever (Luckmann & Sorensen, 1987).

A nursing goal when dealing with a client with external otitis is to relieve discomfort, reduce swelling in the ear canal and eliminate the infection. The nurse can provide comfort to the client by getting a physician's order for administering aspirin or codeine and for applying warm, moist compresses or heat to the ear. Local interventions also can include combinations of antibiotics and agents to soothe the inflamed membranes. The nurse should instruct the client on the proper treatment of the infection as well as the prevention of external otitis by thoroughly drying the ear after swimming, bathing, or shampooing.

Furunculosis. Furunculosis is a localized form of external otitis that occurs in the outer half of the auditory canal. The glands and hair follicles in this area become infected and form furuncles or boils. The client may experience fever, severe headache, and enlargement of the local lymph nodes. Administration of antibiotics and the application of hot packs usually leads to resolution of the furuncle. Perichondritis or chondritis may result if the furuncle is excised and drained. Therefore it is best to allow the furuncle to localize (point) and then open or resolve by itself (Smeltzer & Bare, 1992). The nurse may instruct the client on the prevention of furunculosis by keeping the auditory canal dry, clean, and free of trauma.

Malignant tumors. Four to eight percent of all skin cancers occur on the external ear. Therefore it is not uncommon for a client to have a malignancy of the external ear and canal, the most common of which are basal cell carcinoma and squamous cell carcinoma. The typical symptoms include a chronic ulcer of the auricle, blood-tinged ear drainage, deep pain, or hearing loss. Treatment is by surgery including wide local excision and skin grafting. If the temporal bone and ear canal are involved, radical mastoidectomy usually is indicated (Lewis & Collier, 1992; Luckmann & Sorensen, 1987).

Since the most common etiology of malignant tumors of the ear is extensive exposure to the sun, nursing management includes teaching the client how to prevent this condition by reducing sun exposure and protecting the skin of the auricle when sun exposure cannot be avoided (Burrell, 1992). The client with a malignant tumor of the external ear will require special handling by the rehabilitation nurse. Most clients associate cancer with death and look to the nurse for support, understanding, and clarification. The nurse should facilitate communication by listening to the client and other family members and allowing them to express any fears or concerns they may have.

✦ Tympanic membrane perforation

The tympanic membrane can be ruptured either by infection (acute or chronic suppurative otitis media) or trauma (skull fracture, compression, burns, or punctures). The nurse should advise the client with a perforated eardrum not to dive, swim, or shower because the introduction of water into the middle ear can cause infections and other complications. The client also should be careful when washing his hair and may be recommended to wear custom-molded earplugs and a bathing cap when swimming or bathing (Riley, 1987).

Since the client with a perforated eardrum is more susceptible to chronic ear infections or conductive hearing loss, surgery may be indicated. The nurse may have the added responsibility to prepare the client psychologically and physically for surgery. The client should be informed of all aspects of the surgery and feel free to openly discuss any misconceptions or concerns she may have. The nurse can educate the client about postoperative expectations, activity, and medication regimen.

✦ Middle ear disorders

Serous (catarrhal) otitis media. Serous otitis media is characterized by an accumulation of sterile fluid (serous or mucoid) in the middle ear which interferes with hearing. This disorder can occur at any age but is most frequently seen in children. The problem can be caused by a number of factors: eustachian tube obstruction, which prevents normal ventilation of the middle ear; retention of exudates resulting from allergies; upper respiratory infection; or acute infection treated by antibiotics. The client with this condition will experience a full or plugged sensation in the ear, hearing loss, and an unnatural reverberation in her voice (Riley, 1987). The middle ear fluid may be very thick and bloody.

Clients may be treated with decongestants and antihistamines, decongestant nasal spray, and exercises including swallowing and gum chewing to open the eustachian tube. The physician may aspirate the fluid with a needle, or a ventilating tube may be used if the condition does not improve within a few days or a week (Lewis & Collier, 1992).

The rehabilitation nurse's major responsibilities when dealing with clients with serous (catarrhal) otitis media include cause finding, examining for hearing loss, providing referral, and instructing the clients in proper health maintenance. If ventilating tubes are placed in the eardrum, clients and parents of children with tubes must be instructed on specific precautions such as not permitting water to enter the ear. The clients should be instructed to wear earplugs (with the addition of Silly Putty) when swimming or washing their hair to ensure that no water enters the ear. Diving also is prohibited due to the increased pressure it places on the tympanic membrane and inner ear mechanisms.

Chronic suppurative (purulent) otitis media. Chronic suppurative otitis media is the result of repeated attacks of otitis media, which causes a permanent perforation of the eardrum. This condition most commonly occurs in clients who had ear problems in early childhood and may be caused by the virulence of the organism or a bacterial resistance to antibiotics. The client with suppurative otitis media experiences purulent discharge, differing degrees of deafness, usually conductive or mixed, and may or may not experience pain (Riley, 1987).

The physician can treat this condition locally by carefully cleansing the ear with cotton, instilling antibiotic drops, or applying antibiotic powder and doing an radiographic study. Further hearing loss and more serious complications may be avoided by performing plastic surgical procedures called tympanoplasties (Riley, 1987).

The rehabilitation nurse may assist with health prevention and in the elimination of the disease and the promotion of optimal hearing. The nurse should instruct the client on medication administration, keeping the area free of debris, and the importance of continual assessment of hearing. If surgery is indicated, the nurse can educate the client on preoperative and postoperative expectations.

Mastoiditis. Mastoiditis is an inflammation of the mastoid cells of the temporal bone resulting from an infection of the middle ear. Clients with this disorder will experience pain and tenderness behind the ear, discharge from the middle ear, and swelling of the mastoid. Usually mastoiditis can be treated successfully with antibiotics and occasionally myringotomy (an incision of the tympanic membrane that allows for drainage) (Smeltzer & Bare, 1992). If drainage does not subside after 2 to 3 weeks, a simple mastoidectomy may be required to remove all infected mastoid cells. If surgery is indicated, the client should be instructed preoperatively on all procedures and postoperatively on what can be expected in terms of the bulky dressing that may be present following surgery, postoperative positioning and movement, and pain relief.

Since the facial nerve that controls the facial muscles may be in close proximity to the mastoid cells, the nurse must assess postoperatively for facial nerve damage by asking the client to smile or wink. If there are signs of damage, the nurse should inform the surgeon immediately so that necessary repairs to the facial nerve can be made (Riley, 1987). When drainage is present, the nurse's major responsibility is to remove epithelial debris and purulent drainage to maintain as clean an area as possible to prevent further infection. The nurse should also observe the drainage for color, odor, amount, and type.

Otosclerosis. Otosclerosis is a genetic disorder characterized by the formation of spongy bone in the capsule of the labyrinth of the ear. The footplate of the stapes in the oval window is fixated by a bony growth and is unable to vibrate. This immobility of the stapes prevents transmission of sound vibration into the inner ear (Burrell, 1992; Riley, 1987). Otosclerosis is twice as likely to occur in women and 10 times more prevalent in Caucasians. It affects approximately 4 million Americans and is probably the most common cause of conductive hearing loss in the United States (Burrell, 1992).

Clients suffering from otosclerosis will frequently give family histories of deafness and have no history of preoperative ear infections (Hawke, Keene, & Alberti, 1990). They complain of slow, progressive hearing loss, first noticed between the ages of 10 and 30. Hearing loss is usually bilateral and therefore the client may speak softly during the health assessment. The condition may be accompanied by mild tinnitus, recurrent attacks of vertigo, and postural imbalance. The ears usually appear normal unless a lesion is active, in which case dilated blood vessels cause increased redness of mucosa, appearing like a reddish blush visible through the tympanic membrane (Schwartze's sign) (Burrell, 1992).

The rehabilitation nurse must reassure the client that treatment is usually successful and that optimal hearing can

be restored. Otosclerosis may be treated by the use of hearing aids, medical management, and surgical treatment, but not all otologic specialists agree concerning the most effective form of treatment. The nurse can consult with a social worker for assistance in identifying community resources for obtaining a hearing aid for the client. The nurse also may instruct the client on the proper oral administration of medication, usually sodium fluoride, calcium, and vitamin D. Surgical treatment is by a stapedectomy in which the otosclerotic stapes is removed and a prosthesis that replaces the conductive mechanism of the stapes ossicle is inserted. The physician discusses with the client the risks of surgery, including complete loss of hearing, persistent vertigo, or both so the client can be fully informed when making a decision regarding treatment. The nurse explains to the client that dizziness, vertigo, and nausea may occur for 2 to 4 days following the surgery. Adherence to proper positioning as ordered by the surgeon should be stressed as well as the importance of not getting out of bed alone and keeping the side rails up due to the possibility of vertigo (Riley, 1987).

✦ Inner ear disorders

The three symptoms that indicate inner ear disorders include vertigo, sensorineural hearing loss, and tinnitus (Lewis & Collier, 1992).

Labyrinthitis. Labyrinthitis is an inflammation of the labyrinth that may arise from acute or chronic otitis media, an uncomplicated upper respiratory infection, as a complication of labyrinthine surgery, or accompanied by diseases such as pneumonia or influenza. Symptoms include severe vertigo that eventually causes nausea and vomiting. The client also may experience sudden disturbances in equilibrium, nystagmus, photophobia, headache, and anorexia. These symptoms gradually subside in 3 to 6 weeks (Riley, 1987).

The etiology of suppurative labyrinthitis, a severe infection of the inner ear, is unknown although it usually arises from an upper respiratory infection, otitis media, or surgical intervention. The client with this condition eventually will have complete hearing loss and a nonfunctioning labyrinth (Riley, 1987).

Since there is no specific intervention for labyrinthitis except providing relief from symptoms, it is essential for the rehabilitation nurse to reassure the client that she will feel better over time. The nurse should be aware of the type of labyrinthitis the client has, so that if total hearing loss is inevitable the nurse can give the client time to express fears and concerns and to grieve. It is important to support the client and provide personalized care to assist the client in dealing with hearing loss.

Ménière's disease. Ménière's disease stems from a dysfunction of the labyrinth but its exact cause is unknown. It seems that the blood vessels become constricted. The client experiences a triad of symptoms including vertigo (with nausea and vomiting), tinnitus, and unilateral hearing loss. Between attacks of dizziness that may last hours or days and occur several times a year, the client is able to perform activities of daily living normally.

Hearing loss associated with Ménière's disease is a sensorineural type and usually is not incapacitating because the client is still able to hear normally in one ear. Bilateral hearing loss, however, may occur in 10% of those affected.

Abrupt fluctuation of hearing loss can be expected. Sodium intake and/or alcohol and tobacco use is cited as a possible cause of the disease by some authorities. Many forms of treatment have been tried, but a salt-free diet is the best method of controlling the disease (Riley, 1987). Reduction of fluid intake sometimes helps as well as administration of vasodilator drugs or small doses of sedatives. Vertigo can be controlled by administration of the medication ammonium chloride. In severe cases when tinnitus is creating a great deal of distress, a labyrinthectomy may be performed. This operation is used only as a last resort because it destroys the membranous labyrinth and thereby any hearing sensation remaining in the ear (Myerhoff, 1984; Reinecke, 1983).

Regardless of the treatment used, the nurse should provide reassurance and allow for verbalization of feelings regarding the disease. Throughout all phases of the disease, from diagnostic evaluation to medical treatment to surgery, the rehabilitation nurse supports the client both physically and emotionally and educates the client on all aspects of the disease and any procedures to be performed. The nurse should assist the client in determining what precipitates an attack and the feelings experienced before the episode. The client must use care when climbing stairs and should not be permitted to drive a car. The nurse can discuss alternative forms of transportation with the client. If the client refuses to stop driving, the nurse can instruct the client to pull immediately to the side of the road should an attack occur. The nurse should also teach the client to lie down, either on a bed with side rails or on the floor, and to avoid sudden motion when an attack occurs so other injuries are prevented. Furthermore, proper administration of medication should be explained as well as the importance of adherence to a salt-free diet.

Trauma and infection. Sensorineural hearing loss results from injury to the inner ear or the acoustic nerve, or infection. Trauma is most commonly caused by a skull fracture, hemorrhage, thrombosis, or explosive blasts. Temporal bone surgery or intracranial surgery, as well as infection of the cochlea, otitis media, or mastoiditis can also injure the internal ear (Riley, 1987).

One responsibility of the rehabilitation nurse is to teach prevention of trauma and the importance of maintaining optimal health. Medication regimen must be followed strictly and the client should be made aware of the side effects likely to occur. The nurse also stresses the importance of strict asepsis to avoid the introduction of infection.

Hearing Aids

The otologist in conjunction with an audiologist can best determine whether a client would benefit from a hearing aid. A hearing aid is a battery-operated instrument through which sounds are received by a microphone, transformed into electrical signals, amplified, and retransformed into acoustic sounds. Hearing aids make sounds louder but do not improve speech discrimination (Burrell, 1992).

The nurse must inform prospective buyers of hearing aids that a medical evaluation is necessary to assess (1) the etiology of hearing loss, (2) the need for other types of treatment instead of or in conjunction with a hearing aid, and (3) the need for and availability of other aspects of rehabilitation. It will be necessary for the wearer to experiment and adjust the controls for optimal results.

Background noises, mechanical sounds such as a typewriter or vacuum cleaner, and large groups of people who are talking at a social gathering may block the acuity of a hearing aid. Some persons respond by becoming nervous, frustrated, or even disoriented.

Although hearing aids amplify speech, they do not always make speech clear enough for a hearing-impaired client to understand what is being said. Therefore a hearing aid can be used most effectively in conjunction with speech (lip) reading. Speech reading will assist the client in filling in the gaps of those words that might be missed. It is essential for the rehabilitation nurse to direct and refer the client to auditory training when necessary (Burrell, 1992).

Once a hearing aid has been prescribed, the patient and family should be fully educated concerning the benefits and limitations of the device. The nurse should encourage clients to request and thoroughly read instructional brochures that accompany every hearing aid. The client also needs to be supported to continue to wear the hearing aid during the orientation period.

The hearing-impaired client can choose from a variety of hearing aids. The behind-the-ear type of hearing aid is the most common. It works well for slight to severe hearing loss and is preferable when the client has high-frequency loss. The in-the-ear and canal hearing aids are not as powerful, offer fewer variations, and therefore are useful to a smaller population. Seldom recommended are the eyeglass hearing aids with the components attached to the earpiece. This type of aid has a history of service problems. Also, clients who wear their eyeglasses only part time, or who require two or more different kinds of eyeglasses, do not find the eyeglass hearing aids effective. The largest and most powerful type of hearing aid is the body aid. This aid is carried in the pocket and is contained in a case about the size of a pack of cigarettes. It is connected to plastic tubing and an earpiece. The body aid is worn by clients who have severe hearing loss or poor manual dexterity (Burrell, 1992).

The hearing-impaired client who must wear a hearing aid may suffer from a body image disturbance. An external hearing aid draws attention to an otherwise unnoticeable impairment. From a personal perspective the client may feel that the hearing aid is a signal to others for different treatment and that he is not a fully functioning person. The nurse must be prepared to assist the client in dealing with disturbances in body image by facilitating conversation and openly discussing body image disturbances. The client may be encouraged to use assistive devices, teletypewriters, and telephone amplifier devices for the deaf; vibrating lights for the alarm clock, doorbell and smoke alarm; and sound-activated amplifying devices and lights to monitor events in other rooms. The client also may elect to use a special trained hearing ear dog that responds to a ringing telephone, doorbell, and a baby's cry and alerts the hearing-impaired person by running back and forth between the sound and the person.

Cochlear Implants

The cochlear implant is an assistive device for persons with sensorineural hearing loss who are unable to benefit from a hearing aid. It is an auditory prosthesis designed to directly stimulate the auditory nerve and bypass damaged hair cells. The external portion of a cochlear implant is composed of a microphone, microelectric processor, and a transmitter that detects environmental sound, converting it into electrical signals. The signals are then transmitted to the implanted portion consisting of a receiver implanted under the skin above the ear and an electrode wire that is implanted in the cochlea where it stimulates the auditory nerve. Cochlear implantation does not restore normal hearing. Although loud to medium environmental sounds can be heard, speech discrimination is not improved (Burrell, 1992).

Because of the limited availability of approved implantation centers and lack of public awareness of implantation technology, there is a gap of a few years between a client's initial diagnosis of profound deafness and their appearance for evaluation for a cochlear implant. In addition, the fact that implantation costs at least $10,000, which is not covered by insurance or other payment methods, keeps many clients from seeking the treatment they need (Lilly, 1986).

In order to be accepted into an implant program, the client must demonstrate the following:
1. Profound hearing loss
2. Hearing loss occurring after the acquisition of language
3. A trial period using a hearing aid, which results in little or no benefit
4. No medical contraindications for surgery
5. No significant psychological maladjustment as confirmed by interviews and testing
6. A desire to participate in the rehabilitation program (Lilly, 1986)

The rehabilitation nurse has two important responsibilities during the preoperative phase of implantation: preparation of the client and family for preimplantation tympanotomy and preparation of the client to participate in the implantation procedure itself. The nurse prepares the client and family for surgery and educates them preoperatively for this procedure. The client's understanding of the procedure is assessed and questions are answered. The nurse, client, and family member who will be aiding the client during communication attempts with others will want to practice some agreed-upon communication strategies for the operating room.

Postoperatively the nurse and the audiologist are alert during the first activation session of rehabilitation to the clients' reaction to stimulation since information clients receive from their implants differs from what normal-hearing persons hear as sound. Without appropriate preoperative counseling, clients may be disappointed and depressed postoperatively when they realize that the "hearing" they experience is very different from the hearing they had experienced before deafness.

When communicating with a client with severe hearing impairment, the nurse can facilitate understanding by using several strategies identified in the following information.

Strategies for Communicating with a Hearing-Impaired Client

1. When the client is in the hospital, do not rely on intercommunication systems. Go to the client in person and get her attention before speaking if you were not seen entering the room.
2. Face the individual directly during the entire conversation and try to place yourself no more than 8 feet away from the client. Provide adequate lighting so the person can see you clearly and do not cover your mouth or eat, smoke, or chew gum when talking.
3. Tell the client that you would like to be informed when you do not make yourself clear or when you do something that interferes with speech reading.
4. Use nonverbal cues such as facial expressions, hand gestures, writing, or pointing to help convey meaning.
5. Since background noise may make hearing more difficult, provide a quiet environment for the client by turning off televisions and radios and closing windows and doors.
6. State the major topic of discussion first and then elaborate. For example: "Dinner (pause). Do you want beef or chicken?" If necessary rephrase the sentence rather than repeat the same words.
7. Do not drop your voice at the end of sentences. Rather than shouting, speak slowly and distinctly.
8. When necessary, write words that are particularly important or that may be new to the client such as names or medical terminology.
9. The individual's need to rest occasionally must be respected. Because listening is an active process for the hearing-impaired client, fatigue rather than a lack of interest may cause the individual to seek a rest period (Burrell, 1992; Luckmann & Sorensen, 1987).

SMELL AND TASTE

Smell and taste are understood poorly as compared with the previously discussed exteroceptor sensory systems, vision and hearing. The system that controls our sense of smell is called the olfactory system, and the system for the sense of taste is called the gustatory system. These systems are chemoreceptor-exteroceptor sensory systems. Chemoreceptor indicates the nature of the stimulus that stimulates receptor cells, such as the chemical structure of the molecules, whereas exteroceptor refers to the location of the stimulus, which is outside the body. The receptor cells and the central pathways in the brain represent the major differences between the olfactory and gustatory systems (Cohen, 1993).

Smell

Compared with other animals, a human's sense of smell is rather limited and is not relied on as much as other senses. Most people, however, are able to recognize, detect, and decipher a wide variety of odors.

The olfactory receptors are located in the upper part of each nostril in the olfactory epithelium. This surface consists of many free nerve endings embedded in supporting structures and covered by a watery fluid. Nerve endings in the pharynx and the oral cavity contribute to the detection of odors. The presence of cilia, which protrude from the receptor cells, increases the effectiveness of the olfactory epithelium (Cohen, 1993). Efferent axons of the peripheral olfactory sensory cells are unmyelinated and terminate in the olfactory bulb, which is a direct extension of the central nervous system. The olfactory cortex is located in a small region of the anterior portion of the temporal lobe (Estrem & Renner, 1987).

Smells enter the nasal passage in the form of a gas and are absorbed into the mucus covering the olfactory epithelium. They are then diffused to the cilia stimulating the sensitive peripheral olfactory receptors to transmit impulses via the olfactory nerve. These impulses are then transmitted to the cerebrum where interpretation takes place (Bickerton & Small, 1982; Doty & Kimmelman, 1992).

Certain substances can be smelled very easily and, within Western society, have been connected with specific places and activities. A print shop, florist, brewery, bakery, lumberyard, stockyard, farm, and a number of other places can be distinguished by their smells. Smells within the environment elicit either pleasant or unpleasant sensations. Since we cannot recreate smells in our minds as with visual im-

ages or sounds, the sensation of smell is associated with olfactory memories. When we smell something, whether pleasant or unpleasant, we are reminded of the circumstances surrounding the original sensation. An opened can of coffee, a cedar closet, freshly cut grass, and flowers have smells with pleasant associations and make us reminisce about pleasant memories. Poor personal hygiene, infection, and stale whiskey have smells with unpleasant associations. The typical smell of a hospital is often associated with unpleasant memories. Therefore clients may experience unpleasant smells while in the presence of the nurse, which may affect their feelings toward the nurse and rehabilitation.

Taste

Taste and smell are closely interrelated. As foods are eaten, they immediately evaporate and trigger receptor cells in the olfactory epithelium. When our sense of smell is compromised, foods don't taste as they normally do. Taste is also influenced by pain and tactile receptors of the mouth and temperature of ingested substances. Therefore the sense of taste depends on the sensory receptors for taste, smell,

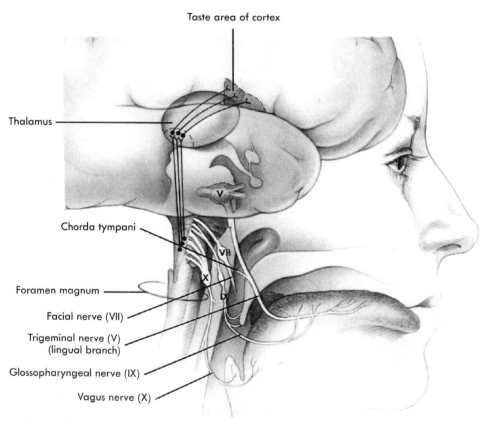

Fig. 16-11 Central nervous system pathways for taste from the facial nerve (anterior two thirds of the tongue), glossopharyngeal nerve (posterior one third of the tongue), and vagus nerve (root of the tongue). The trigeminal nerve is also shown. It carries tactile sensations from the anterior two-thirds of the tongue. The chorda tympani from the facial nerve (carrying taste input) joins the trigeminal nerve. Nerves carrying taste impulses synapse in the ganglion of each nerve, in the nucleus of the tractus solitarius, and in the thalamus before terminating in the taste area of the cortex. (From *Essentials of Anatomy and Physiology* by R.R. Seely, T.D. Stephens, & P.P. Tate, 1991, St. Louis: Mosby–Year Book. Copyright 1991 by Mosby–Year Book.)

pain, texture, and temperature. Upon closer examination, some tastes are found to be odors. For example, vanilla cannot be tasted in the mouth until it can be smelled.

Taste begins with the taste receptors in the taste buds. Each taste bud has approximately 50 receptor cells. Although the number of taste buds can vary more than tenfold among people, it is believed that there are 4,000 to 10,000 taste buds. Taste buds are small cellular areas found in the soft palate, mucous membrane of papillae located in the edges and the upper rear surface of the tongue, pharynx, larynx, and esophagus. The largest number of taste buds are found of the surface of the tongue (Doty & Kimmelman, 1992). Like the receptor cells in the olfactory system, taste bud cells contain cilia that protrude into mucus in the taste pore of the bud. Different chemicals are apparently received by different receptor cells, but their specific interactions are not well understood (Cohen, 1992).

The taste buds' process of innervation is complex. When food dissolves in the saliva, taste bud cells are stimulated and form a chemical substance. Stimulated by this action, afferent nerve fibers then transmit impulses through the facial and glossopharyngeal nerves to the medulla oblongata, where they synapse with ascending tracts. The impulses are then transmitted from the medulla oblongata to the thalamus and cerebrum, where they are interpreted (Fig. 16-11). Cranial nerve VII (facial) innervates the anterior two thirds of the tongue; cranial nerve IX (glossopharyngeal) innervates the posterior third of the tongue and part of the pharynx; and cranial nerve X (vagus) innervates the pharynx and larynx (Gardner, 1975).

Tastes are divided into four basic modalities: sweet, sour, salty, and bitter substances. Sweet tastes are sensed best at the tip of the tongue, bitter at the back part of the tongue, salty at the front and side edges, and sour farther back on each side. Substances with these tastes include sucrose (sweet), sodium chloride (salt), tartaric acid (sour), and quinine sulfate (bitter). Characteristics of taste that greatly influence how these substances are perceived include color, appearance, temperature, texture, flavor, and quality.

Individuals have different taste thresholds, which can vary as much as twentyfold. This may be correlated to the variation in the number of taste buds individuals have. The difference in taste threshold may be genetic and an important factor in determining why different people favor different foods. Beyond age 45 we begin to lose taste buds. Because there is a slow process of regeneration, this may account for the change in food preferences and lack of eating we experience as we become older, since the ability to appreciate the way foods taste is diminished (Cohen, 1993).

There is still much uncertainty concerning the way taste stimuli are coded. Even though the four taste modalities have been established, specific modalities have not been coded by individual taste receptors. Some receptor cells even respond to all four taste modalities. Therefore, even though there are parts of the tongue that respond more strongly to certain taste types, the parts respond, to some extent, to all the others as well (Cohen, 1993).

Although we do recognize tastes that we've experienced previously, tastes cannot be recreated in our minds. We often find ourselves going to great lengths to experience again something that we particularly enjoyed from a certain res-

taurant. Like the sensation of smell, taste sensations also can be associated with unpleasant experiences. We have all at least once become ill after eating a particular food, which thereafter has a distinctively undesirable and unpleasant taste. Interestingly this behavior has been demonstrated to occur during studies using wolves (Cohen, 1993).

Nursing Assessment of Smell and Taste

Observation is the primary method used to assess sensory impairment. Through a sensory assessment, the nurse can obtain valuable information about the client's needs and limitations. The nursing assessment should include attention to the sensations of smell and taste since these senses are easily overlooked. Once the nurse determines that sensory impairment exists, nursing diagnoses can be formulated.

♦ Smell

An evaluation of the client's olfactory status is important, because it may indicate an underlying problem. Unfortunately quantification of olfactory or gustatory impairments has been limited by the absence of precise types of measurement to diagnose these disorders. In addition, a standard vocabulary to assign meaning to odors and tastes is lacking.

Because of the lack of standardized assessment procedures, alterations in olfaction were rarely examined quantitatively. Significant research has been performed in this area, and progress has been made in developing a more detailed clinical description of olfactory disorders. A quantitative assessment of the client's olfactory function is important for a variety of reasons: (1) to determine the validity of the client's complaint, (2) to characterize the nature of the problem, and (3) to develop interventions and treatments and monitor them objectively (Doty & Kimmelman, 1992).

The rehabilitation nurse can discover important information about the client's use of the sense of smell. Some odors are readily discernible such as those from smoking, drinking, and eating highly seasoned food. Certain smells indicate a specific dysfunction such as acetone in diabetic acidosis, stale urine in uremic acidosis, and garlic in arsenic poisoning.

The nurse is concerned with odors characteristic of infections or poor hygiene. Foul body odor or the use of heavy perfumes and deodorants to mask smells should alert the nurse to the need for teaching personal hygiene and self-care. Halitosis, or bad breath, may be the result of poor oral hygiene, which would necessitate dental health teaching and care. Gingival inflammation or stomatitis may be an underlying cause. Upon investigation, odors can be traced to secretions from body orifices and wounds. A nasal malodor may result from pharyngitis or another infection with a postnasal drip. An infected pressure ulcer hidden under old stained dressings will have odors associated with the growth of specific organisms. The client may not be aware of odors given off by the body. Over time, reaction to odor lessens making way for new smells. In Western culture many scents are obscured with the use of deodorants, powders, air fresheners, and perfumes. Once unusual smells are recognized and diagnosed, the sooner treatment can be instituted.

A client who does not respond to odor-producing smells

such as those of flowers and foods may have developed anosmia. Neurologic assessment of cranial nerve I (olfactory), including inspection of the nose, may reveal data about the client's sense of smell not found during the subjective assessment. The client may not be aware of absent or impaired smell unless the loss has been sudden or dramatic.

To test olfaction, nonirritating substances that have distinctive smells such as soap, coffee, tobacco, and alcohol are used. However, ammonia or acetic acid odors are not used, because their pungency can stimulate nerve endings in the mucosa and give a false-positive result. The client may think that she is smelling the testing agent but she is actually tasting dissolved vapors of the substance. Test each nostril separately and ask the client to identify odors while the eyes are closed. Ask the client about the smell of foods; foods are not tasty if one cannot smell them. Nutritional status, healthcare supervision, and support are monitored as an intervention, especially if the cause of the anosmia is unknown.

✦ Taste

Taste is usually not a routine part of a physical examination, and unless a client complains of a related disturbance, it is often not tested. The nurse should palpate and examine the tongue on all sides, assessing for scarring, inflammation, atrophy of papillae, or neoplasm. Sweet, salty, sour, and bitter substances are used for testing taste. The client should be able to recognize these substances on the parts of the tongue used for these tastes if function is normal. This type of test may not be very accurate or reliable since it is difficult to control the area stimulated, and often the volume of stimulus is insufficient to induce a reliable response (Doty & Kimmelman, 1992). Taste sometimes will be tested during tests of cranial nerves, because it involves cranial nerve VII (facial), cranial nerve IX (glossopharyngeal), and cranial nerve X (vagus).

A person's culture determines, to an extent, the development of taste. The use and importance of food provide clues to one's lifestyle. Habits such as drinking coffee, using tobacco, drinking alcohol, and preparing food give insights into the social conduct and economic status of an individual. Observe for changes in a client's ability to taste or lack of response to foods known to elicit strong or distinctive tastes.

Impaired Smell and Taste Sensation
✦ Smell

Olfactory impairments are usually caused by (1) obstruction of access to the olfactory neuroepithelium by inflammation, or rarely, neoplasm; (2) destruction of the olfactory neuroepithelium; and (3) damage to the central olfactory pathways (Doty & Kimmelman, 1992).

The following schema of terms has been used to describe different impairments of smell. The client's complaints and the objective sensory diagnosis can be classified according the schema (Doty & Kimmelman, 1992; Estren & Renner, 1987).

Anosmia: complete loss of the sense of smell; may be unilateral or bilateral

Hyposmia: impairment of smell

Hyperosmia: increased sensitivity to odors

Cacosmia or parosmia: A distorted or perverted sense of smell

Phantosmia: hallucination of smell

Heterosmia: inappropriate inability to distinguish between certain odors

Agnosia: inability to classify or contrast smells, although able to detect odors

Unilateral anosmia and hyposmia may not be noticed by the person affected. People who have a congested upper respiratory tract may have experienced anosmia and may complain of a taste deficit because of the close relationship between these two senses. Anosmia by itself is usually viewed as an annoyance and not as a major health problem (Schiffman, 1983). It becomes a major problem if it interferes with the performance of such occupations as baker, perfume manufacturer, or wine maker.

The single most common cause of olfactory impairment is an upper respiratory tract infection. Some other possible causes of absent or impaired smell include intranasal obstructions such as polyps or neoplasms, acute and chronic sinusitis, rhinitis, injury to the olfactory nerve, intracranial lesions, tumors of the temporal lobe, trauma, infectious meningitis, and abscesses (Wyness, 1985). A decreased sense of smell has been found in persons with viral hepatitis, but this subsided once the illness disappeared (Henkin, 1985). Anosmia also may be congenital or psychogenic in origin. Impairment of the sense of smell may be caused by malfunction of the olfactory receptors (as with the common cold), the olfactory nerve, or the part of the brain concerned with olfaction. Onset of the problem may be acute, as with an inflammatory process or injury, or gradual, as with a slow-growing tumor or poisoning from toxic fumes (Sparks, 1983). The duration of anosmia may be quite short, as seen after some types of head injury, since the olfactory cells can regenerate, or it may be permanent, after more extensive destruction of nerves with massive injuries.

Approximately 7% of smell loss occurs as a result of head injuries (Doty & Kimmelman, 1992). Rehabilitation nurses caring for head trauma patients must be aware of this complication and assess the patient for alterations in olfactory sensation. A frontal lobe contusion may produce anosmia; an occipital blow because of a contrecoup effect when the brain is driven to the opposite side of the skull may also produce this problem. Both of these injuries may cause damage to the olfactory filaments because of shearing, contusion, or tearing as the nerves pass through the cribriform plate. Temporary anosmia may be caused by edema or pressure on the olfactory nerve. The loss of the sense of smell is more likely to be found in persons who have experienced amnesia after injury and in those who have had a fracture of the frontal skull base (Sumner, 1964).

Renal disease, diabetes, and cirrhosis have been associated with olfactory disorders. They also have been found in persons with malnutrition, dietary deficiencies, and autoimmune disorders (Estrem & Renner, 1987). In addition, a number of different drugs, industrial chemicals and pollutants, and tobacco can produce disorders of smell.

Much research has supported the findings that Alzheimer's disease, Korsakoff's psychosis, Huntington's chorea, idiopathic Parkinson's disease, and the parkinsonism-dementia complex of Guam are complicated by alterations in olfaction (Doty, Deems, & Stellar, 1988; Doty et al., 1991; Doty, Reyes, & Gregor, 1987). For example, lesions within the olfactory system are one of the first pathologic changes to occur in Alzheimer's disease (Hyman, Van Horsen, Damasi, & Barnes, 1984).

Medical intervention for the client who has anosmia is directed toward alleviating the source of the problem. Measures may be necessary to decrease intracranial pressure or surgically remove an obstruction. If the cause is unknown or cannot be treated, nursing interventions to assist the individual in making adjustments are needed.

◆ Taste

Many of the same conditions that cause alterations in olfactory function influence taste such as head trauma, zinc deficiency, adrenocortical insufficiency, and viral infections. The use of pharmacologic agents, such as antirheumatic drugs or antiproliferative drugs, is much more likely to cause a disturbance in taste than in smell. In addition, clients with carcinomas are likely to complain of taste loss or distortion (Doty & Kimmelman, 1992).

The following schema of terms has been developed to assist in the classification of the client's complaint:

Ageusia: lack of taste sensation to tastants
Hypogeusia: lessened sensation to tastants
Hypergeusia: heightened taste ability
Dysgeusia: presence of a strange or distorted taste sensation (Doty & Kimmelman, 1992)

True loss of gustatory function is rare. In fact, a number of researchers have reported that less than 1% of head injury patients actually exhibit true taste loss as opposed to more than 7% for loss of olfaction (Doty & Kimmelman, 1992).

Most clients who complain of a loss of taste actually have normal taste function but suffer from abnormal smell function. Most taste abnormalities are in fact disorders of the sense of smell, such as experienced with the common cold (Schiffman, 1987). The loss of taste may be restricted to one portion of the tongue or to areas innervated by one of the cranial nerves. If taste is present in the remainder of the tongue, this disorder may go unnoticed. An individual will experience a loss of taste over the anterior two thirds of the tongue with a diseased facial nerve, such as in mastoid canal lesions. Since a branch of the facial nerve passes through the middle ear on its way to innervate the front two thirds of the tongue, middle ear disease or surgery may be complicated by partial ageusia (Cohen, 1993).

Taste sensation also is influenced by hormones as demonstrated in pregnancy and in menstruation (Westerman & Gilbert, 1985). There also are taste changes in diabetes mellitus believed to be caused by neutrality (Abbasi, 1981). Taste acuity increases in adrenal cortical insufficiency but reverts to normal with steroid therapy (Henkin, Gill, & Bartter, 1963). Central nervous system tumors and pontine cerebrovascular accidents can affect the taste centers in the brain and the major relay tracts to the peripheral end organs (Goto, Yamamoto, Kaneko, & Tomita, 1983).

Rehabilitation Nursing Interventions

Once a nursing diagnosis has been made, nursing interventions for the client with impaired smell and taste sensa-

tion are planned. The nursing interventions for impaired sensation are many and varied. Often the nurse must experiment to find the intervention most appropriate for a particular client.

◆ Impaired smell

Nursing interventions for altered olfactory sensation include provisions for the detection of spoiled and extremely spicy foods. The client should be instructed to inspect food visually for spoilage and to read food labels for the expiration date. Foods should be discarded when the expiration date passes. Spices should be restricted. If possible, an electric stove should be used for cooking, since a gas leak may go unnoticed. The client should be cautioned to remain in the kitchen when food is cooking. Smoke detectors should be hung in the house. Follow-up healthcare supervision and support should be arranged if there are unresolved problems. The nurse should stress the importance of practicing good oral hygiene especially when eating foods seasoned with garlic and onions. In addition, total personal hygiene should be monitored closely since the client may be unable to sense odors resulting from poor hygiene.

◆ Impaired taste

The client's nutritional status is assessed and monitored. Plans are made to improve nutritional state and prevent nutritional problems. Nursing interventions include (1) teaching the client to use other senses to compensate for the loss of taste by preparing food in an attractive and appealing manner; (2) considering the client's likes, dislikes, customs, and special diet requirements; and (3) providing pleasant, neat surroundings free of disturbing sights and odors. Health teaching should include explanations of the importance of a balanced diet. The client should be encouraged to use flavorings such as lemon juice and spices such as mint, cinnamon, and basil to help improve the taste and aroma of food.

It is not uncommon for elderly clients to suffer from anorexia since the loss of taste of favorite foods decreases their desire to eat. Therefore the nurse may collaborate with the dietician to ensure that the nutritional status of the client remains stable for his height and weight. The nurse and dietician working together, sharing their client assessment data, will provide a team effort to meet the individual client's nutritional needs and plan strategies to overcome nutritional deficits.

Summary

Both the olfactory and gustatory systems subtly affect our likes and dislikes. These effects are very powerful, although not always rational or conscious. These systems are essential for our survival by monitoring what we ingest and by signaling us when dangerous situations arise such as fires. Therefore the nurse must remember that the smells and tastes clients experience during their first visit can have a subtle but powerful influence on their desire to return to the healthcare setting. By simply keeping the environment free of unpleasant odors—and nurses being cognizant of odors from their perfume and/or aftershave lotion and by using a breath freshener after smoking—the client will have pleasant associations with the healthcare setting, therapy sessions, and rehabilitation.

CASE STUDY I

The case study method has been used as the first step in the research process to investigate or observe an individual, group, institution, or culture (Polit & Hungler, 1987). It is especially appropriate for investigation of clinical nursing problems. The case study method will address holistic nursing care and the utilization of an interdisciplinary team to address complex client-centered clinical problems.

PERSONAL HISTORY

The client, B.F., is a 38-year-old Caucasian female who lives with her husband and 16-year-old daughter. B.F. has had IDDM for 28 years. She attends the Catholic Church regularly; however, she has curtailed socializing with her husband and friends. B.F. is a secretary at a mortgage company. Three years ago she was diagnosed as having proliferative diabetic retinopathy. Since diagnosis she has had several laser therapy treatments to help maintain her vision. However, due to the progression of the diabetic retinopathy, she now has been diagnosed as having low vision even though B.F. has been very compliant with the medical regimen recommended by her physician.

NURSING ASSESSMENT

The assessment data may be organized around functional health patterns (discussed earlier) and the section on the assessment of the eye found on page 307. These may be used as a guide to organize the assessment of B.F.'s diabetic retinopathy and develop her plan of care. B.F. already has been examined by her nurse and ophthalmologist. The ophthalmologist examined her eyes through dilated pupils with the direct ophthalmoscope, indirect ophthalmoscope, and a slit lamp biomicroscope with a contact lens system to view the retina stereoscopically. In addition, fluorescein angiography, ultrasonography, and electroretinography are three other procedures that enabled the physician to see the characteristic lesions and internal structures of B.F.'s eyes as well as aiding in choosing the optimal course of action (Garcia & Ruiz, 1992). The nurse did a complete health assessment of B.F. These data and input from B.F. regarding her goals are the basis for the following care plan.

NURSING DIAGNOSIS

Diagnosis number one

Visual alterations related to diabetes mellitus and diabetic retinopathy as evidenced by decreasing visual acuity.

GOALS

1. Over the next year B.F. will continue to visit her ophthalmologist every 4 months to monitor her eyes for further visual deterioration and complications.
2. Over the year B.F. will maintain a safe home environment for optimal functional level.
3. Over the year B.F. will be educated on all low-vision services available to her.
4. Over the next 3 months BF will be introduced to and instructed in the use of optical/nonoptical aids to maintain her functional independence.

NURSING INTERVENTIONS

The holistic rehabilitation nursing care plan for B.F. encompasses vocational, educational, and leisure skills with the emphasis of treatment centering on meeting the special needs and

goals of B.F. The nurse educates B.F. on all aspects of diabetic retinopathy and the importance of regular and frequent ophthalmic examinations. The nurse instructs B.F. on recognizing early indications of developing visual changes and encourages her to seek prompt medical evaluation and intervention if any changes occur.

The nurse performs a home assessment to ensure B.F.'s safety. During this time the nurse notes the complexity of the home environment for the low-vision and psychomotor functioning of B.F. The nurse determines safety problem areas such as the two flights of steps B.F. must negotiate in her homemaking responsibilities, inadequate light fixtures throughout the house, and a tendency toward clutter. The nurse discusses these potential problems with B.F., her husband, and daughter with various options to solve them. For example, the nurse recommends that fluorescent orange markings be placed along the edge of each step so that B.F. can access the staircase readily with ease and safety. In addition, B.F. is instructed in using a special diabetic insulin syringe to accommodate for her low vision. B.F.'s early adaptation to her environment will facilitate adjustment to vision loss and give her a feeling of control and independence. B.F. has worked hard at creating some appearance of a normal lifestyle for herself. To assist B.F. and her family to live as normally as possible despite the symptoms and the effects of her disease, the services of the occupational therapist are employed. The nurse is instrumental in providing B.F. with the self-care skills needed to adapt to the new challenges in life and to maximize her independence, health, and dignity.

The nurse introduces B.F. to the American Foundation for the Blind, which maintains a directory of low-vision clinics within B.F.'s geographic area that will complement the nurse's intervention, assist B.F. in adapting to her sight impairment, and enable her to function at an optimal level. Among other things these clinics will provide B.F. with appropriate optical aids on a trial basis and will provide training for their use. (See the box, p. 321 for optical and nonoptical visual aids.)

Another option is for the nurse to refer B.F. to various low-vision services found in medical centers, optometric and rehabilitation centers, and to optometrists and ophthalmologists in private practice who provide low-vision services.

In the rehabilitation nursing model, the active participation of B.F. and her family is very important. The client, B.F., needs to take the active role, adapt, learn, and adjust to her vision loss. The nurse, for example, can give B.F. a magnifier or another visual aid; however, B.F. is the one who must use the aid for reading. The nurse's role is to provide the tools, health education, and guidance. In the rehabilitation nursing model, visual aids are recommended and their use can be demonstrated and taught, but the decision to use them is up to B.F.

EVALUATION

At the 1-year interval B.F. has visited her ophthalmologist three times. B.F. is able to verbalize sensory impairments and recognizes the importance of prompt medical evaluation and intervention. Furthermore, B.F. is able to verbalize and understand her condition and its treatment. B.F. has made appropriate adjustments to her home environment to ensure safety and high functioning ability. She has a working knowledge of all low-vision services available to her. B.F. readily uses a visual aid for reading.

CASE STUDY I—cont'd

Diagnosis number two

Self-esteem disturbance related to low vision as evidenced by social isolation.

GOALS

1. Within the next 3 months B.F. will improve her self-esteem.
2. Within 2 weeks B.F.'s husband and daughter will be more supportive and encouraging and understand the disease process.
3. Over the next 3 months B.F. will receive support through a therapeutic relationship within and outside her family.
4. Over the next 3 months B.F. will exhibit less self-imposed isolation from her friends and family.
5. Within 3 months B.F. will discontinue her fear of losing her job and respect of her family due to her low vision.
6. After 3 months B.F. will report feeling good about herself.

NURSING INTERVENTIONS

The nurse assesses B.F.'s degree of acceptance of vision loss in terms of her high risk for physical and psychological dependence. The nurse assists B.F. to achieve her age-specific developmental tasks so that her vision loss does not impact on the developmental process and prohibit her from proceeding to the next developmental stage. Counseling to prepare for vision changes will facilitate B.F.'s early acceptance and adjustment to her vision loss. Often the client with diabetic retinopathy will deny the existence of the disability and withdraw from society. Since B.F. is experiencing this type of denial, the nurse must assist and motivate B.F. to develop an interest in her environment and social networks. B.F. feels isolated because of her vision loss, and talking with other diabetic clients who are experiencing a similar situation can be therapeutic. B.F. would benefit a great deal from sharing her problems and feelings with others and receiving mutual support and understanding from others with similar difficulties. This will help to prevent her from feeling socially isolated. The rehabilitation nurse can establish a diabetic retinopathy self-help group to provide B.F. with information, education, and social activities.

In addition, the nurse will educate B.F.'s husband and daughter regarding the disease process and the importance of their continued support and understanding when B.F. is feeling isolated. The nurse will make arrangements for B.F. to get medical assistance to determine the optimal low-vision aid that will improve visual performance, make the most effective use of B.F.'s sight, and assist B.F. in performing her job responsibilities. The nurse also will encourage B.F. to develop a plan to educate her employer regarding her condition and the successful use of visual aids in job performance. This will help relieve B.F.'s fear of losing her job. In order to maintain B.F.'s quality job performance, the nurse consults the interdisciplinary team and utilizes the expertise of the social worker, psychologist, occupational therapist, clergy, and the state office for vocational rehabilitation services.

EVALUATION

At the end of 3 months B.F. reports higher self-esteem and verbalizes a positive outlook about herself and her job. B.F. also expresses a realistic view and acceptance of herself and identifies her strengths and herself as a capable person. She is able to verbalize, acknowledge, and discuss her feelings concerning low vision with the nurse, family members, support group, and lastly her employer. She is able to set realistic goals for active participation in social situations. B.F. can verbalize assurance that her family and nurse are available for assistance/support when needed.

Diagnosis number three

Ineffective individual coping and stress alterations related to anxiety/depression due to her fear of future blindness.

GOALS

1. Over 3 months B.F. will be able to identify new coping behaviors for dealing with anxieties and fears.
2. After 3 months B.F. will show less physical or behavioral evidence of stress.
3. During the 3 months new relationships will be developed to assist B.F. in dealing with her stress.

NURSING INTERVENTIONS

Low vision represents a major stressful life event for B.F. involving psychological, social, cultural, and interpersonal dimensions. Many researchers have equated vision loss, whether partial or complete, with the loss of a loved one (Carroll, 1961; Emerson, 1981; Gallagher, 1991). As B.F. attempts to cope with her vision loss, she is going through the stages of the grieving process. B.F. is exhibiting anxiety and shock and is undergoing a period of mourning and depression. These two phases are a necessary and integral part of the grieving process, and the nurse does not inhibit B.F. from experiencing them. B.F. needs to work through all phases of the grieving process in order to progress to the final stage of acceptance.

The nurse facilitates B.F.'s adaptation to changes in activities of daily living due to her diabetic retinopathy and helps B.F. develop effective coping mechanisms for dealing with everyday demands. The nurse develops a trusting relationship with B.F. and encourages her to talk about what is happening at this time and what has occurred to cause her feelings of anxiety and depression. Relaxation techniques such as deep abdominal breathing and progressive relaxation are demonstrated by the nurse and then practiced by B.F. to help her reduce her stress level. The nurse corrects any misconceptions B.F. has about the long-term effects of her diabetic retinopathy by providing factual information. As B.F. is a practicing Catholic, the nurse assists her in coping and reducing stress by facilitating B.F.'s expression of spirituality by listening to her and praying and reading religious materials with her. Again, attending support group meetings and discussing fears and anxiety with family members and friends will help B.F. deal with her stress. The nurse consults with the psychologist, who provides B.F. with additional skills for coping and reducing anxiety.

EVALUATION

After 3 months B.F. is able to verbalize coping mechanisms for dealing effectively with stress and anxiety. She routinely uses the stress reduction techniques of deep abdominal breathing and progressive relaxation. She also verbalizes awareness of her own coping and problem-solving abilities.

After 3 months B.F. states she feels less "stressed out."

After 3 months B.F. identifies the nurse, psychologist, support group, and family members as resources during difficult times.

CASE STUDY II

PERSONAL HISTORY

The client is a 56-year-old Caucasian male, M.T., married with three adult married children. M.T. is the associate dean at a large university on the East Coast. M.T. has experienced two episodes of severe sudden hearing loss. The first episode occurred when he was a teenager in conjunction with the removal of a benign brain tumor. The second episode occurred 1 month ago during root canal surgery. Since this second episode M.T. has no residual hearing and has been on short-term disability from the university.

NURSING ASSESSMENT

The nursing assessment focuses on the area of evaluation of the hearing loss problem and its implications for the aural rehabilitation needs of M.T. and how the nurse can assist in fulfilling these needs. The data collected are organized around the functional health patterns and the ear assessment questions found on page 323. Since normal conversation will be impossible, M.T. and the nurse will communicate by writing. This will not be a difficult task since M.T. is highly educated with excellent comprehension of English. This, however, may be an important consideration for the nurse who has to communicate with clients whose primary language is American Sign Language (ASL). In this instance the client may become frustrated since ASL differs grammatically from English and an interpreter may be required. If an interpreter is used, the nurse should (1) sit close to the interpreter so the interpreter can speak directly to both you and the client without too much head or eye movement and (2) look at the client while speaking directly to her; speak slowly; make sure the interpreter is able to keep up with you; and have the interpreter tell you if you are speaking too fast or if a rest period is necessary.

The nurse must be sure to ask M.T. how his hearing loss has affected his life. The answers to these questions will assist the rehabilitation nurse in appreciating M.T.'s problems more thoroughly, in planning therapy and counseling sessions, and in identifying members of the interdisciplinary team for referral and consultation. Any questions asked of M.T. that result in a "yes" or "no" answer should be double checked for accuracy of the answer. M.T. may indicate yes as an answer to what he perceives as the question when in actuality the nurse is asking something totally different.

The nurse performs an inspection and palpation of the external ear and uses the otoscope to examine the tympanic membrane. The Weber and Rinne tests also are performed. The nurse reviews the results of M.T.'s audiometric testing, paying particular attention to the speech audiometry that evaluates M.T.'s ability to hear and understand the spoken word. The nurse assesses the communication abilities of M.T. as well as the psychological characteristics and any potential associated physical limitation that may influence M.T.'s rehabilitation. These data will be used to develop a rehabilitation care plan for M.T.

Several approaches for aural rehabilitation have been identified in the literature. Tyler, Tye-Murray, and Gantz (1991) divide aural rehabilitation into two areas: evaluation and remediation. The evaluation component addresses communication function and psychological, vocational, educational, and physical limitations as a result of hearing loss. The remediation component addresses psychosocial, instrument, and instruction/orientation needs. Alpiner concludes that the ideal method of re-

habilitation is a combination of three approaches: (1) a traditional approach involving auditory training, lip-reading, and speech conversation; (2) a progressive approach involving a counseling-oriented, problem-solving and information-giving methodology where the client takes an active role; and (3) a community method—involving family, friends, work environment, and support groups—which provides resources and hearing services to assist people with hearing impairments (Alpiner & McCarthy, 1987).

NURSING DIAGNOSIS

Diagnosis number one

Impaired verbal communication related to hearing loss as evidenced by feelings of inadequacy and fear of the unknown.

GOALS

1. Over the year M.T. will receive aural rehabilitation in the form of speech-reading and sign language.
2. Over the year M.T.'s feelings of inadequacy and fear of the unknown will be diminished through education and counseling by various members of the interdisciplinary team.

NURSING INTERVENTIONS

An interdisciplinary team approach is implemented in the aural rehabilitation of M.T. with the major goal being to promote M.T.'s ability to communicate effectively. A team meeting is held with the otologist, nurse, psychologist, social worker, speech therapist, and M.T. and his wife. M.T. expresses his major concerns regarding communication with his family, friends, and colleagues. The inferior position the lack of communication has placed him in and his fear of the unknown are explored with the holistic interdisciplinary team. The physician explains to M.T. the etiology of his condition and the unfavorable prognosis and answers questions from M.T. and his wife. Mutual goals of M.T. and the team are identified and include participation of all the team members.

The nurse's major responsibility is to be the team leader and coordinate all functions and activities of the interdisciplinary team as M.T.'s case manager. The nurse serves as an advocate and role model for M.T. by accepting him and demonstrating effective communication techniques. The nurse is a liaison between M.T., his wife and family and educates them regarding hearing loss and the most effective way of interacting with M.T. M.T. and his wife and family will be assisted by the nurse in coping with lifestyle changes resulting from the hearing loss. Furthermore, the nurse will encourage the continuation of verbalization of feelings to control and minimize stressful situations. The nurse also will encourage M.T. to ask for assistance when needed. Emotional support will be available from the nurse for M.T. and his wife and family.

The psychologist will work with M.T. on skill building, acceptance, understanding, and expectations to reduce his feelings of inadequacy and fear of the unknown. M.T. will go through the stages of the grieving process as he comes to final acceptance of his hearing loss. The sensory deprivation represented by hearing loss will cause concomitant problems for M.T. M.T.'s invisible handicap of hearing loss is distinct from other types of handicaps such as blindness, cerebral palsy, or cleft palate, which are readily recognizable. He may, however, experience emotions such as feeling less masculine, which may

---

CASE STUDY II—cont'd

interfere with his personality adjustment. Therefore the psychologist will provide counseling and address the psychological and emotional problems during M.T.'s period of adjustment.

The social worker will work with M.T. and his wife to address his social, economic, environmental, and personal needs. The social worker is concerned with M.T.'s ability to accomplish his developmental tasks and his ability to earn a living, function independently, and continue to contribute to society. It is also the responsibility of the social worker to refer M.T. to the vocation rehabilitation counselor, who will assist M.T. in reaching his continued employment goals. The social worker will give M.T. and his wife a pamphlet with a list of professional and community services that are available for hearing-impaired people in their community.

The speech therapist will assist M.T. and his wife with his communication strategy training. This will include three components: sign language, finger-spelling, and speech-reading. These components will serve as a means for M.T. to communicate with other people and will require much training and practice. It will be beneficial for M.T.'s wife and children to participate in the training program to facilitate the family's interaction with M.T. and understanding and adjustment to M.T.'s hearing loss. The speech therapist refers the family to a community education program that teaches all the communication skills they will need to learn. M.T.'s speech therapist also supports the family during their communication training period.

Sign language aids communication by using configurations of the hands and body to convey words, phrases, or concepts. Finger spelling, a manual alphabet in which conversation is spelled out letter by letter, uses finger positions of one hand to represent letters and numbers. ASL (or Ameslan) is the most commonly used sign language in the United States. Speech-reading, also known as lip-reading, will require M.T. to learn to watch the movements of the lips and facial expressions to discriminate meaning. Sign language and other cues by the speaker may be used in conjunction with speech-reading to express the message more clearly (Burrell, 1992).

EVALUATION

At the 1-year interval M.T. has a working knowledge of sign language, speech-reading, and finger spelling. M.T. is able to readily communicate with his wife and family using sign language, speech-reading, and finger spelling. His wife and family feel comfortable to readily use sign language and finger spelling when communicating with M.T.

At the 1-year interval M.T.'s feelings of inadequacy have diminished and he has been fully educated on his hearing loss, reducing his fear of the unknown. He is able to communicate and discuss his hearing loss.

Diagnosis number two

High risk for social isolation related to hearing loss as evidenced by withdrawl into one's own world.

GOALS

1. Within the next 3 months M.T. will join and regularly attend a family aural rehabilitation program to continue to improve his visual speech perception skills.
2. Within 4 months M.T. will adjust to his change in hearing and life status through the use of assistive devices.
3. Over the next 4 months M.T. will maintain contact with his social and physical environments.

4. At the end of 4 months and over the year, M.T. will experience support from his wife and family and a strong acceptance of his communication handicap.
5. At the end of 6 months M.T. will be able to return to his position as associate dean at the university.

NURSING INTERVENTIONS

When a person cannot take part in conversation because of hearing loss, it is only natural to withdraw into one's own world to avoid embarrassment or frustration when words in sentences are not grasped. Hearing-impaired persons may even become suspicious, feeling that others are laughing or talking about them. Suspiciousness can lead to paranoia and even greater social isolation. It is important for the rehabilitation nurse to understand that social isolation is likely to occur when clients have alterations in hearing so that a proper diagnosis and referrals can be made.

The nurse assesses M.T.'s degree of acceptance of hearing loss in terms of his potential for self-imposed isolation. The data indicate that M.T. is not receiving enough emotional support from his wife and adult children. The nurse explores with M.T. the benefits of talking with other hearing-impaired individuals and the therapeutic value of support groups. Participation in a support group will enable M.T. to expand his environment and social network and improve his visual speech perception skills.

Since M.T. has expressed the need for additional support from his family, the nurse assesses the strengths and weaknesses of the family unit and identifies with the client goals and activities for educating and counseling individual family members. The nurse and M.T. decide that M.T.'s wife, family, and friends should be integrated into the support group so that they can further understand his disability and provide the support he needs. It will be beneficial for M.T.'s family to interact with other families whose members are hearing impaired. They can find support in interacting with others and learn how they have dealt with some of the problems they have encountered. The family members are given an opportunity to have their personal concerns addressed by the nurse and qualified professionals if needed. This will assist M.T. in maintaining his social and physical networks.

To help put a plan in action for M.T.'s return to the university, the nurse evaluates the resources available at the university for hearing-impaired students that also may be utilized by M.T. The nurse discusses with M.T. the rich resources available at the university including a speech therapy department and an active program for hearing disabled students that can be extended to assist M.T. in effectively carrying out his duties as associate dean.

In addition, the nurse introduces M.T. and his family to consumer groups that have emerged to address the special concerns related to community services for the hearing impaired. Consumer group meetings, newsletters and other publications will provide M.T. and his family with important information regarding hearing loss and professional community services.

The nurse educates M.T. and his family on the various assistive devices available to the hearing impaired. These devices will extend M.T.'s other senses such as sight and touch and make him feel less isolated from his environment. Alerting devices placed on the doorbell, alarm clock, or smoke alarms will signal M.T., through flashing lights or vibration, that something is happening. Telecommunication devices for the deaf (TDDs)

Continued.

♦

CASE STUDY II—cont'd

are small machines that resemble typewriters attached to a regular telephone. The person using a TDD must be calling a person with a similar device. The message to be communicated is typed on the machine's keyboard and displayed on the screen of the TDD at the other end of the telephone line, or on paper if that TDD is connected to a printer (Dattalo, 1992). M.T. can utilize closed-captioned television programming, which will allow him to see dialogue written as script across the bottom of the screen. The hearing ear dog, which is sensitive to certain noises such as the telephone, the doorbell, or a baby's cry can further extend M.T.'s senses. Upon hearing a sound, the dog will run back and forth between M.T. and the sound (Burrell, 1992). The nurse must be sure to include the family in the education regarding assistive devices so that each member will benefit from the information provided on the selection, purchase, and use of assistive devices.

EVALUATION

At the 3-month interval M.T. is an active member of an aural rehabilitation program. At the 4-month interval and throughout the year, M.T.'s family continues to actively support his interest in improving his communication skills. All of his family members participate in the family aural rehabilitation support group and are able to verbalize an understanding of hearing loss and the importance of family support.

M.T. has maintained contact with his social and physical environments through increased family and social interaction and through the use of assistive devices.

At the 4-month interval M.T. has adjusted to his change in hearing and life status by selecting and actively using assistive devices. At the 6-month interval M.T. returns to work after developing an action plan with the nurse, university administration, speech therapy department, and the director of the disabilities department of the university.

The importance of taste and smell is recognized by the fact that the first U.S. clinical research center devoted to the senses of taste and smell was established in 1980 as a result of funding from the National Institute of Neurological Disorders and Stroke. Additional funding was secured from the National Institute of Aging (NIA) and the National Institute on Deafness and other Communication Disorders. The center's three primary goals are (1) to provide clinical evaluation, treatment, and counseling for patients experiencing taste and smell disorders; (2) to provide the facilities and an intellectual focus for research in both basic and applied aspects of chemoreception; and (3) to provide training for undergraduate and graduate students and doctoral level scientists and other interested medical personnel in both basic and applied aspects of chemoreception science (Smell & Taste Center, 1991).

Over 2000 patients have been referred to the center for evaluation, and over 7000 persons have taken the University of Pennsylvania Smell Identification test. Databases for detailed statistical analysis by such items as sensory complaint, documented smell and/or taste dysfunction, diagnostic category, and systemic disease status are stored at the center. Undergraduate students and medical students from universities nationwide have direct experience in its research activities, annual seminar series, and bimonthly journal club. In 1991 the center hosted the largest international meeting ever held on chemical communication, with 22 countries represented (Smell & Taste Center, 1991). The center has contributed to the current state of the art in the care and treatment of chemical communication.

The previous information and case studies discussed in this chapter prepare the rehabilitation nurse with a knowledge base of how sensory-perceptual alterations affect the client's quality of life and independence. Sensory-perceptual alterations encompass the anatomy and physiology, nursing assessment, intervention, and evaluation of four subcategories: visual, auditory, gustatory and olfactory. The nursing rehabilitation focus is to increase, adjust, or manage the environment to meet the individual needs of the client. This will include the facilitation, restoration, and maintenance of independence for clients whose level of function in activities of daily living has been physically and/or emotionally limited due to sensory-perceptual alterations that affect their written, verbal, and chemical communication. The critical elements of the plan of care include utilizing a holistic interdisciplinary team approach to assist the client with sensory-perceptual and chemical communication problems, setting realistic mutual goals, and promoting safe independence. The rehabilitation nurse links these elements to the appropriate community and the family/significant other is integrated into the rehabilitation process in the most efficient and effective manner to address maximizing the client's independence and quality of life.

REFERENCES

Abbasi, A.A. (1981). Diabetes: Diagnostic and therapeutic significance of taste impairment. *Geriatrics, 36,* 73-78.

Allen, M.N. (1989). The meaning of visual impairment to visually impaired adults. *Journal of Advanced Nursing, 14,* 640-646.

Allen, M., & Birse, E. (1991). Stigma and blindness. *Journal of Ophthalmic Nursing and Technology, 10,* 147-152.

Alpiner, J.G., & McCarthy, P.A. (1987). *Rehabilitative audiology: for children and adults.* Baltimore: Williams & Wilkins.

Apple, D.J., & Rabb, M.F. (1991). *Ocular pathology: Clinical applications and self-assessment* (4th ed.). St. Louis: Mosby–Year Book.

Bailey, I. (1991). Improving care of the low-vision patient. In A. Arditi, A.M. Laties, & B. Silverstone (Eds.), *Vision into the future: Toward a low-vision research agenda* (Psart Tenth-Anniversary Scientific Symposium Report) (pp. 36-38). New York: The Lighthouse Inc.

Bates, B. (1994). *A guide to physical examination and history taking* (6th ed.). Philadelphia: J B. Lippincott.

Bickerton, J., & Small, J. (1982). *Neurology for nurses.* Baltimore: University Park Press.

Brunner, L.S., & Suddarth, D.S. (1989). *Textbook of medical-surgical nursing* (6th ed.), Philadelphia: J. B. Lippincott.

Burrell, L.O. (1992). *Adult nursing in hospital and community settings.* Norwalk, CT: Appleton & Lange.

Carroll, T. (1961). *Blindness: What it is, what it does, and how to live with it.* Boston: Little Brown & Company.

Catalano, R.A. (1992). *Ocular emergencies.* Philadelphia: W. B. Saunders.

Cohen, H. (1993). *Neuroscience for rehabilitation.* Philadelphia: J.B. Lippincott.

Colenbrander, A., & Fletcher, D.C. (1992). Low vision rehabilitation: Basic concepts and terms. Part 1. *Journal of Ophthalmic Nursing and Technology, 11,* 5-9.

Crabbe, M.J. (1987). *Diabetic complications: Scientific and clinical aspects.* Edinburgh: Churchill Livingstone.

Cryer, T.H., & Cryer, K.S. (1991). A view of diabetic retinopathy. *Journal of the American Academy of Physician Assistants, 4,* 327-332.

Dattalo, P. (1992). An evaluation of an area-wide message relay program: National implications for telephone system access. *Journal of Rehabilitation, 58,*50-55.

Doty, R.L., & Kimmelman, C.P. (1992). Smell and taste and their disorders. In A.K. Asbury, G.M. McKhann, & W.I. McDonald (Eds.), *Diseases of the nervous system* (2nd ed., pp. 465-478). Philadelphia: W.B. Saunders.

Doty, R.L., Reyes, P.F., & Gregor, T. (1987). Presence of both odor identification and detection deficits in Alzheimer's disease. *Brain Research Bulletin, 18,* 597-600.

Doty, R.L., Deems, D.A., & Stellar, S. (1988). Olfactory dysfunction in Parkinson's disease: A general deficit unrelated to neurologic signs, disease stage, or disease duration. *Neurology, 38,* 1237-1244.

Doty, R.L., Perl, D.P., Steele, J.C., Chen, K.M., Pierce, J.D., Reyes, P., & Kurland, L.T. (1991). Odor identification deficit of the parkinsonium-dementia complex of Guam: Equivalence to that of Alzheimer's and idiopathic Parkinson's disease. *Neurology, 41*(Suppl. 2), 77-80.

Emerson, D.L. (1981). Facing loss of vision: The response of adults to visual impairment. *Visual Impairment and Blind, 75,* 41-45.

Estrem, S.A., & Renner, G. (1987). Disorders of smell and taste. *Otolaryngologic Clinics of North America, 20;* 133-147.

Gallagher, C.M. (1991). The young adult with recent vision loss: A pilot case study. *Insight: The Journal of the American Society of Ophthalmic Registered Nurses, 16,* 8-14.

Garber, N. (1990). Health promotion and disease prevention in ophthalmology. *Journal of Ophthalmic Nursing and Technology, 9,* 193-198.

Garcia, C.A., & Ruiz, R.S. (1992). Ocular complications of diabetes. *Clinical Symposia, 44,* 2–32.

Gardner, E. (1975). *Fundamentals of neurology.* Philadelphia: W.B. Saunders.

Gaston, H., & Elkington, A.R. (1986). *Ophthalmology for nurses.* Dover, NJ: Croom Helm.

Ghartey, K.N. (1990). The importance of early detection of diabetic retinopathy. *Journal of Ophthalmic Nursing and Technology, 9,* 193-198.

Goto, N., Yamamoto, T., Kameko, M., & Tomita, H. (1983). Primary pontine hemorrhage and gustatory disturbance: Clinicoanatomic study. *Stroke, 14,* 507-511.

Haefemeyer, J.W., & Knuth, J.L. (1991). Albinism. *Journal of Ophthalmic Nursing and Technology, 10,* 55-62.

Hart, W.M. (1992). *Adler's physiology of the eye: clinical applications* (9th ed.). St. Louis: Mosby–Year Book.

Hawke, M., Keene, M., & Alberti, P.W. (1990). *Clinical otoscopy: An introduction to ear diseases.* (2nd ed.). Edinburgh: Churchill Livingstone.

Henkin, R.I. (1985). Olfaction in human disease. In G.M. English (Ed.), *Otolaryngology* (Vol. 2). Philadelphia: J.B. Lippincott.

Henkin, R.I., Gill, J.R., Jr., & Bartter, F.J. (1963). The role of adreno cortical steroids and serum sodium concentrate. Studies on taste threshold in normal man and patients with adrenal cortical insufficiency: *Journal of Clinical Investigation, 42,* 727-735.

Hyman, B.T., Van Horsen, H.W., Damasi, A.R., & Barnes, C.L. (1984). Alzheimer's disease: cell-specific pathology isolates the hippocampal formation. *Science, 225,* 1168-1170.

Kapperud, M.J. (1983). *The aging eye: A guide for nurses.* Minneapolis: The Minnesota Society for the Prevention of Blindness and Preservation of Hearing.

L'esperance, F.A., Jr. (1991). The role of lasers in the management of glaucoma and diabetic retinopathy. In A. Arditi, A.M. Laties, & B. Silverstone (Eds.), *Vision into the future: Toward a low-vision research agenda* (Psart Tenth-Anniversary Scientific Symposium Report) (pp. 36-38). New York: The Lighthouse.

Lewis, S.M., & Collier, I.C. (1992). *Medical-surgical nursing: Assessment and management of clinical problems* (3rd ed.). New York: Mosby–Year Book.

Lilly, L.F. (1986). Cochlear implants: The second generation. *Preoperative Nursing Quarterly 2,* 8-25.

Luckmann, J., & Sorensen, K.C. (1993). *Medical-surgical nursing: A psychophysiologic approach* (4th ed.), Philadelphia: W. B. Saunders.

Myerhoff, W.L. (1984). *Diagnosis and management of hearing loss.* Philadelphia: W.B. Saunders.

Ney, D.F. (1993). Cerumen impaction, ear hygiene practices and hearing acuity. *Geriatric Nursing, 14,* 70-73.

Paton, D., & Craig, J.A. (1990). Management of cataracts. *Clinical Symposia, 42,* 2-32.

Polit, D. & Hungler, B. (1995). *Nursing research: Principles and methods* (5th ed.). Philadelphia: J.B. Lippincott.

Price, S.A., & Wilson, L.C. (1986). *Pathophysiology: Clinical concepts of disease processes* (3rd ed.). New York: McGraw-Hill.

Ragge, N.K., & Easty, D.L. (1991). *Immediate eye care.* St Louis: Mosby–Year Book.

Reinecke, R.D. (1983). Loss of vision: eye pain. In R.S. Blacklow (Ed.), *MacBryde's signs and symptoms,* 85-100. New York: J.B. Lippincott.

Riley, M.A. (1987). *Nursing care of the client with ear, nose, and throat disorders.* New York: Springer.

Schiffman, S.S. (1987). Diagnosis and treatment of smell and taste disorders [editorial] *Western Journal of Medicine, 146,* 471-473.

Silverstein, H., Wolfson, R.J., & Rosenberb, S. (1992). Diagnosis and management of hearing loss. *Clinical Symposia, 44,* 2-32.

Smell and Taste Center. (1991). Neffworks. Philadelphia: University of Pennsylvania.

Smeltzer, S.C., & Bare, B.G. (1992). *Medical surgical nursing* (7th ed.). Philadelphia: J. B. Lippincott.

Sparks, R.K. (1983). Sensory-perceptual impairments due to anosmia. In M. Snyder (Ed.), *A guide to neurological and neurosurgical nursing,* 429-436. New York: John Wiley & Sons.

Stein, H.A., Slatt, B.J., & Stein, R.M. (1988). *The ophthalmic assistant: Fundamentals and clinical practice* (5th ed.). St. Louis: Mosby–Year Book.

Sumner, D. (1964). Post-traumatic anosmia. *Brain, 90,* 107.

The Trimad Group (1990). Ticlapidine treatment reduces the progression of non-proliferative diabetic retinopathy. *Archives of Ophthalmology, 108,* 1577-1583.

Tyler, R.S., Tye-Murray, N., & Gantz, B.J. (1991). Aural rehabilitation. *Otolaryngologic Clinics of North America, 24,* 429-445.

Vaughan, D., & Asbury, T. (1983). *General ophthalmologic* (10th ed.). Los Altos, CA: Lange Medical.

Westerman, S.T., & Gilbert, L.M. (1985). Mastication, deglutition and taste. In G.M. English (Ed.), *Otolaryngology* (Vol. 3). Philadelphia: Harper & Row.

Witkop, C.J., Jr., Ouevedo, W.C., Jr., Fitzpatrick, T.B., & Begudet, A.L. (1989). Albinism. In C.R. Scriver, R.A. Knin (Eds.), *The metabolic basis of inherited disease* (6th ed., pp. 58-63). New York: McGraw Hill.

Wyness, M.A. (1985). Perceptual dysfunction: Nursing assessment and management. *Journal of Neuroscience Nursing, 17,* 105-110.

Yeadon, A., & Grayson, D. (1979). *Living with impaired vision: An introduction.* New York: American Foundation for the Blind.

✦

Appendix 16-A Resources for hearing-impaired persons and visually impaired persons

American Academy of Otolaryngology/Head and Neck Surgery
1101 Vermont Avenue NW
Suite 302
Washington, DC 20005
(202) 289-4607

American Annals of the Deaf
5034 Wisconsin Avenue NW
Washington, DC 20016
(April issue lists a directory of services and resources available in each state)

American Athletic Association of the Deaf, Inc.
3916 Lantern Drive
Silver Spring, MD 20902

American Speech-Language-Hearing Association
10801 Rockville Pike
Rockville, MD 20852
(301) 897-5700

American Tinnitus Association
P.O. Box 5
Portland, OR 97207
(503) 248-9985

Association for Education of the Deaf (AED)
814 Thayer Avenue
Silver Spring, MD 20910
(301) 585-4363

Association for Persons with Severe Handicaps
7010 Roosevelt Way NE
Seattle, WA 98115

Better Hearing Institute
1430 K Street NW
Washington, DC 20005
(800) 424-8576
(202) 638-2848 (teletypewriter [TTY])

The Deafness Research Foundation
55 East 34th Street
New York, NY 10016
(212) 684-6556

Dial-a-Hearing-Screening-Test
(A general estimation of hearing adequacy done over the telephone)
(800) 222-EARS
(800) 345-EARS (in Pennsylvania)

Gallaudet College (the national college for deaf individuals)
800 Florida Avenue NE
Washington, DC 20002

Helen Keller National Center for Deaf-Blind Youths and Adults
111 Middle Neck Road
Sands Point
Long Island, NY 11050
(516) 994-8900 (voice/TTY)

International Hearing Dog, Inc.
5901 East 89th Avenue
Henderson, CO 80640
(303) 287-3277 (voice/TTY)

National Association for Hearing and Speech Action
10801 Rockville Pike
Rockville, MD 20852
(301) 897-8682

National Association of the Deaf
Suite 301
814 Thayer Avenue
Silver Spring, MD 20910
(301) 587-1788

National Black Association for Speech, Language, and Hearing
P.O. Box 50214
Washington, DC 20004

National Crisis Center for the Deaf
University of Virginia Medical Center—Box 484
Charlottesville, VA 22908
(800) 446-9876 (toll-free TTY)
(800) 552-3723 (in Virginia)
(Offers 24-hour TDD [telephone device for the deaf] and emergency services for sudden illness, injury, poisoning, or fire)

National Hearing Aid Society
20361 Middlebelt Road
Livonia, MI 48152

National Hearing Association
Suite 308
1010 Jorie Boulevard
Oak Brook, IL 60521
(312) 323-7200

National Technical Institute for the Deaf
Rochester Institute of Technology
1 Lomb Memorial Drive
Rochester, NY 14623

Office of Scientific and Health Reports
National Institute of Neurological and Communicative Disorders and Stroke
Building 31, Room 8A-06
National Institutes of Health
Bethesda, MD 20205
(301) 496-5751

National Registry of Interpreters for the Deaf
814 Thayer Avenue
Silver Spring, MD 20910
(301) 588-2406 (voice/TTY)

Self-Help for Hard of Hearing People, Inc. (SHHH)
P.O. Box 34889
Bethesda, MD 20034
(301) 365-3548

Silent News (publication for people with or concerned about hearing impairment)
193 Main Street
Lincoln Park, NJ 07035

Telecommunications for the Deaf, Inc.
814 Thayer Avenue
Silver Spring, MD 20910
(301) 589-3006 (voice/TTY)

RESOURCES FOR VISUALLY IMPAIRED PERSONS

American Academy of Ophthalmology (AAO)
P.O. Box 7424
San Francisco, CA 94120-7424

American Council of the Blind (ACB)
1211 Connecticut Avenue, NW
Washington, DC 20036

American Foundation for the Blind (AFB)
15 West 16th Street
New York, NY 10011

American Optometric Association (AOA)
243 Lindberg Boulevard
St. Louis, MO 63141

American Society of Ophthalmic Registered Nurses (ASORN)
P.O. Box 3030
San Francisco, CA 94119

Better Vision Institute (BVI)
230 Park Avenue
New York, NY 10017

Blind Outdoor Leisure Development (BOLD)
533 East Main Street
Aspen, CO 81611

Braille Institute (BI)
741 North Vermont
Los Angeles, CA 90029

Eye Bank Association of America (EBAA)
6560 Fannin
Houston, TX 77030

Eye Bank for Sight Restoration
210 East 64th Street
New York, NY 10021

Guide Dog Foundation for the Blind (GDFB)
109-19 72nd Avenue
Forest Hills, NY 11375

Guide Dogs for the Blind (GDB)
P.O. Box 1200
San Rafael, CA 94902

Guide Dog Users (GDU)
Box 174, Central Station
Baldwin, NY 11510

Guiding Eyes for the Blind (GEB)
106 East 41st Street
New York, NY 10017

Hadley School for the Blind (HSB)
700 Elm Street
Winnetka, IL 60093

International Guiding Eyes (IGE)
P.O. Box 18
North Hollywood, CA 91603

Leader Dogs for the Blind (LDB)
1039 South Rochester Road
Rochester, MI 48063

Library of Congress
Division for the Blind and Physically Handicapped
Washington, DC 20540

The Lighthouse, Inc.
111 East 59th Street
New York, NY 10022

National Association for Visually Handicapped (NAVH)
305 East 24th Street
New York, NY 10010

National Braille Association (NBA)
654A Goodwin Avenue
Midland Park, NJ 07342

National Federation of the Blind (NFB)
1800 Johnson Street
Baltimore, MD 21230

National Society for the Prevention of Blindness (NSPB)
79 Madison Avenue
New York, NY 10016

New Eyes for the Needy (NEN)
549 Milburn Avenue
Short Hills, NJ 07078

Pilot Guide Dog Foundation (PGDF)
33 East Congress Parkway
Chicago, IL 60605

Recording for the Blind (RFB)
215 East 58th Street
New York, NY 10022

Seeing Eye (SE)
P.O. Box 375 M
Washington Valley Road
Morristown, NJ 07960

17

Eating and Swallowing

Nancy H. Glenn, MSN, RN, CRRN

INTRODUCTION

The process of swallowing (deglutition) begins in utero during the second trimester. When all swallowing mechanisms are functioning properly, we are generally unaware of swallowing once a minute when awake, or nearly 1000 times a day. An adult independently obtains and ingests proper nutrients to maintain health and function. Eating meals occurs during family or social gatherings, celebrations, or events for many cultural groups and has become associated with feelings of sharing, belonging, and friendship. When an individual can no longer secure or ingest nutrients in an efficient or usual manner, a biologic, social, or psychological crisis may occur. Content in this chapter includes patterns of eating and swallowing, factors associated with altered deglutition, diagnostic tests, and nursing process with outcome criteria for persons with impairments of eating or swallowing.

MECHANICS OF EATING

The ability to eat and swallow food and liquids is dependent on position and function of the oropharyngeal cavity, esophagus, cranial nerves, brain, muscles, and limbs. Anatomic structures, physiologic processes of eating and swallowing, and phases of swallowing comprise the mechanics of eating and swallowing discussed in the following material.

Anatomic Structures

The anatomic structures involved in eating and swallowing form the entrance to the alimentary system and include the oral cavity, pharynx, esophagus, larynx, muscles, cranial nerves, and brain. Ingestion of food begins in the oral cavity, which is composed of the lips, cheeks, gums, hard and soft palate, uvula, anterior and posterior faucial arches, palatine tonsils, salivary glands, teeth, mandible, and tongue (Fig. 17-1).

Pharynx

The oral cavity communicates with the pharynx via the oropharyngeal isthmus. The pharynx is a 12- to 14-cm musculomembranous tube extending from the soft palate to the cricoid cartilage where it connects to the esophagus. Three striated constrictor muscles—the superior, medial, and inferior—propel food along the pharynx during swallowing. Fibers of the inferior constrictor muscle attach to the sides of the thyroid cartilage, forming the spaces of the pyriform

sinuses, ending at the cricopharyngeal muscle (Logemann, 1983) (Fig. 17-2), the most inferior structure of the pharynx. At rest, tonic contractions of the cricopharyngeal muscle prevent air from entering the esophagus during respiration and food from refluxing into the esophagus and up to the pharynx. When a bolus of food enters the esophagus during swallowing, the cricopharyngeal muscle relaxes, allowing the food to pass (Cook et al., 1992) (Fig. 17-3).

Esophagus and Larynx

The esophagus is a hollow muscular tube approximately 23 to 25 cm long with a sphincter at each end. The muscles of the upper third of the esophagus are striated; the muscles of the middle third are a mix of both striated and smooth muscle. The lower third, including the lower esophageal sphincter, is smooth muscle. The bolus of food enters the esophagus from the pharynx and is transported to the stomach by the muscular peristaltic action of the esophagus.

The larynx begins at the base of the tongue with the epiglottis. The space formed between the base of the tongue and the sides of the epiglottis is the valleculae, where food may collect either before or after the swallow reflex is triggered. Other structures of the larynx include the aryepiglottic folds and the true and false vocal cords. During deglutition the larynx is elevated, the epiglottis is displaced downward, and the aryepiglottic folds and true and false vocal cards are adducted to protect the top of the trachea (Cook et al., 1992; Groher, 1992; Logemann, 1983).

Extensive innervation is necessary for eating and swallowing. Six cranial nerves (V, VII, IX, X, XI, and XII) and the first three cervical nerves of the spinal cord are involved in eating and swallowing (Table 17-1). In the swallowing process the brain is involved through the cortical swallow center in the prefrontal cortex and the brainstem reticular formation of the medullary swallowing center. The brain interprets, integrates, and coordinates sensory, motor, and reflex information and activity.

Secondary structures involved in eating are the eyes, arms, and legs, which are necessary for a person to remain functionally independent; able to locate, secure, and prepare food and then deliver it to the oral cavity and swallow. The lips assist in locating and securing food; the eyes locate, choose, and assist with preparing food. Visualizing food may stimulate appetite, while the arms and hands perform tasks essential in securing and preparing food. Although few individuals must run to chase their food sources, access to

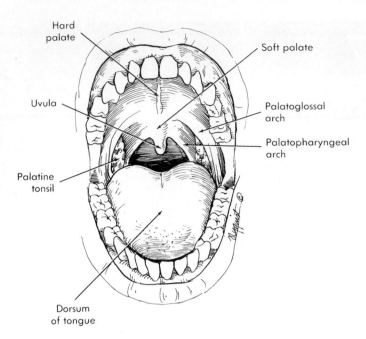

Fig. 17-1 Anatomy of the oral cavity.

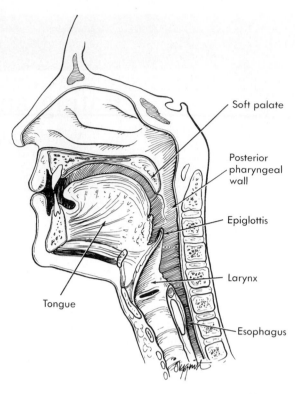

Fig. 17-2 Structures associated with deglutition.

Table 17-1 Cranial nerves used for deglutition

Cranial nerve	Motor (M)/ Sensory (S)	Function
Trigeminal (V)	S	Maxillary, mandibular
	M	Mandibular muscles
Facial (VII)	S	Taste: anterior two thirds of tongue
	M	Submandibular and sublingual salivary glands; facial expression
Glossopharyngeal (IX)	S	Taste: posterior third of tongue; sensation of soft palate and uvula
	M	Stylopharyngeus muscle
Vagus (X)	S	Membrane of larynx and pharynx
Spinal accessory (XI)	M	Muscles: sternocleidomastoid
Hypoglossal (XII)	M	Intrinsic tongue

food supply may be an issue for persons who live alone in the community, for infants and young children, or for those with impaired mobility or cognition.

Physiologic Basis

The physiologic process of eating and swallowing requires the following four stages:

 ✦ Selecting and securing food
 ✦ Preparing food
 ✦ Experiencing the anticipatory motor stage, when food is brought to and placed in the mouth
 ✦ Swallowing

A caregiver may perform the initial two stages of eat-

ing for an individual without evoking serious physiologic consequences. However, social and psychological consequences may result when a person becomes unable to prepare food and self-feed.

The final stage of the eating process is the act of swallowing, which begins once food enters the oral cavity. Swallowing is a complex function accomplished only when activities within the oral cavity, pharynx, larynx, and esophagus are coordinated with interruption of respirations. Afferent, efferent, and central nervous system actions—some of which are volitional and some reflexic—govern the entire swallowing process, which lasts 5 to 10 seconds (Sieberns, 1990).

✦ Oral preparatory phase

The oral preparatory phase is a voluntary phase during which the airway remains open and nasal breathing continues. After food is placed in the mouth, the labial seal holds it in the oral cavity while it is manipulated. The type and amount of manipulation varies with the consistency of the food. Mastication uses rotary and lateral movements of the tongue and mandible to control and manipulate food and upper and lower teeth to crush food.

Mixed with saliva to form a bolus, the food is collected medially on the tongue before the swallow. Soft food may be held on the tongue or between the tongue and hard palate. Liquids are pooled and cupped between the tongue and anterior hard palate until the oral stage begins. Peripheral nerves give feedback about correct positioning of the bolus, as well as prevent injury to the tongue.

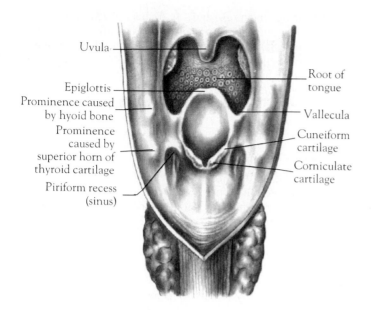

Fig. 17-3 Posterior view of the hypopharynx. (From *Mosby's Clinical Nursing* [3rd ed.] by Thompson, 1993, St. Louis: Mosby–Year Book. Copyright 1993 by Mosby–Year Book. Reprinted by permission.)

Oral Phase

The oral phase, also voluntary, begins as the tongue moves the bolus posterior toward the oropharynx. The bolus sits in a groove created along the center of the tongue until the tongue squeezes the bolus posteriorly toward the oropharynx and against the hard palate. Within a second the bolus passes the anterior faucial arches, completing the oral phase. Cranial nerves V, VII, and XII control this phase (Table 17-1).

Pharyngeal Phase

The most complex part of swallowing is the pharyngeal phase. The person must maintain airway integrity while the bolus moves along the pharynx to the esophagus. Although this phase is reflexic, it must be initiated voluntarily; once initiated it cannot be stopped. The swallowing reflex in most individuals activates when the food bolus comes into contact with the anterior faucial arches. However, sensory receptors that can elicit the swallowing reflex are present in the tongue, epiglottis, and larynx (Logemann, 1983).

Once the swallowing reflex has been initiated, the following events occur: the tongue moves up and back to force the bolus into the upper pharynx; the soft palate elevates to assist in closure of the pharyngeal port to prevent entry of food into the nasal cavity; pharyngeal peristalsis is initiated to carry the bolus past the pharynx by constriction of the pharyngeal constrictors; the lateral walls of the pharynx are drawn up; the larynx is elevated and pulled forward to assist in closure of the larynx; the epiglottis angles down to help protect the airway, and the bolus flows to either side of the epiglottis and down the pyriform sinuses; and the cricopharyngeal sphincter relaxes to permit the bolus to enter the esophagus (Groher, 1992). The impulses travel to the swallowing center in the brainstem via the glossopharyn-

geal nerve. The fifth, seventh, tenth, and twelfth cranial nerves carry the motor impulses that produce the swallowing reflex (Table 17-1). The pharyngeal phase lasts approximately 1 second.

◆ Laryngeal actions

The larynx is protected in part by the downward movement of the epiglottis at an angle of approximately 135 degrees. This moves the laryngeal opening up and forward under the base of the tongue and epiglottis. Laryngeal movement with contraction of the intrinsic laryngeal muscles temporarily decreases the circumference of the laryngeal vestibule. The true and false vocal cords also adduct and the aryepiglottic folds close to provide airway protection (Cook, 1992; Sieberns, 1990).

Esophageal Phase

Swallowing is completed with the esophageal phase, which lasts 8 to 20 seconds. As the bolus enters the esophagus at the cricopharyngeal junction, peristaltic waves respond to the swallow reflex by propelling the bolus down the esophagus. The bolus passes through the gastroesophageal juncture and into the stomach.

◆ Maintaining and protecting airway integrity

Both food and air share the pathways of the pharynx. Consequently, to avoid aspiration while eating, respirations (air flow) must cease during movement of the food bolus through the pharyngeal phase of the swallow. Food is not permitted into the larynx and trachea. The following events maintain and protect the airway during swallowing: respiration is interrupted, the larynx is sealed, and then the larynx is displaced. Regardless of the point in the respiratory cycle at which the swallow occurs, respiration is interrupted when the swallow begins. The central nervous system, in effect, stops the intercostal muscles and diaphragm, interrupting respiration for approximately a half second. Cessation of respiration is not dependent on closure of the larynx.

ASSOCIATED FACTORS

Swallowing is a complex neuromuscular process and many factors can impair its efficiency. Age and neuromuscular impairment and certain structural deficiencies that may alter swallowing are discussed. Research findings increasingly support the contribution of adequate nutrients

---

PHASES OF SWALLOWING

SWALLOWING IS SEPARATED FURTHER INTO THE FOLLOWING FOUR PHASES:

◆ Oral preparatory phase: food is manipulated within the mouth
◆ Oral phase: food bolus is centrally located and pushed posteriorly toward the oropharynx
◆ Pharyngeal phase: bolus is carried by the swallowing reflex through the pharynx
◆ Esophageal phase: peristalsis carries the bolus to the stomach

and appropriate nutrition to improved outcomes in healing, strength, tissue regeneration, and cognitive awareness. Metabolic responses to chronic illnesses, such as pulmonary diseases, and to stresses following trauma are increasingly important areas of concern for rehabilitation nurses. Nutritional status is part of a comprehensive assessment for improving outcome with clients who are at risk for infection, impaired skin integrity, loss of muscle tissue; those who have healing bones or wounds (D'Eramo, Sedlak, Dohney, & Jenkins, 1994); and those who have potential malnutrition due to poor absorption or compromised immunity (De Vito Dabbs, 1993).

Swallowing Changes Across the Life-Span

The fetus begins swallowing in the womb during the twelfth week of gestation. For term infants the sucking reflex, present at birth and throughout the first 7 months, begins the swallow. Swallowing patterns of infants differ from those of adults. An infant's oral cavity is smaller, causing the tongue to fill a greater part of the mouth and to rest more anteriorly. The tongue elevates during sucking and then thrusts the liquid to the posterior oral cavity. The forward sucking movements of the tongue make the intake of even soft solids difficult before the third to fourth month (Groher, 1992). These actions are coordinated with the pharyngeal swallow.

Respirations in the sucking pattern follow in a sequence of expiration and inspiration between swallows. In some term infants, preterm infants, and neurologically compromised infants, feeding apnea may lead to hypoxia or bradycardia.

Changes in mastication and deglutition generally do not occur in normal healthy adults until the eighth decade (Blonsky, Logemann, Boshes, & Fisher, 1975). Changes may include reduced pharyngeal peristalsis with some of the bolus often remaining in the pharynx, decreased size of the opening of the cricopharyngeal sphincter, decreased esophageal peristalsis, and increased esophageal transit time (Cook, 1992; Logemann, 1983; Ozer, 1994). In one study the respiratory cycle was interrupted more often in the inspiratory phase for elderly persons as compared with expiratory-phase interruption in younger persons (Ozer, 1994).

Neuromuscular Impairment

Neuromuscular impairments often affect multiple body systems and may alter stages of swallowing. Major neuromuscular impairments that can affect deglutition are summarized in Table 17-2. The complex innervation of the eating and swallowing process allows multiple variations of impairment to occur, involving minute steps during any one or more stages or phases (Willig, Paulus, Lacau Saint Guily, Béon, & Navarro, 1994). Impairments in the oral preparatory phase frequently result from poor sensation and perception about the quantity and location of the food in the mouth. Impaired motor control of muscles and tongue movement during mastication may leave food improperly chewed or pocketed to the side of the mouth, where the anterior and posterior faucial arches form cavities.

Impaired pharyngeal motility results in a poorly coordinated swallowing reflex. Food then becomes lodged within the valleculae or pyriform sinuses and drains into the trachea, causing aspiration. Aspiration occurs most frequently during the oral phase when the swallowing reflex is delayed and the bolus of food or liquid is allowed to invade the larynx. The most experienced bedside observers do not identify 40% of the individuals who aspirate (Logemann, 1983).

Table 17-2   Neuromuscular diseases associated with poor deglutition

Stages of deglutition	Disease	Characteristics
Oral preparatory	Cerebral palsy	Poor suck reflex
		Inappropriate reflexive behaviors
	Parkinson's disease	Poor mastication
	Multiple sclerosis (when cranial nerve XII is involved)	Foods inadequately chewed
	Amyotrophic lateral sclerosis	Poor tongue control on mobility
	Cerebrovascular accident	
	Huntington's disease	
	Head trauma	
Lingual	Cerebrovascular accident	Delay in swallow reflex
	Huntington's disease	Choking or coughing
	Head trauma	
	Cerebral palsy	
	Parkinson's disease	
	Multiple sclerosis (when cranial nerve IX is involved)	
	Cerebrovascular accident	Lingual hemiparesis
Pharyngeal	Parkinson's disease	Impaired pharyngeal motility and peristalsis
	Poliomyelitis	
	Cerebrovascular accident	Residue remains in valleculae and pyriform sinuses
	Myasthenia gravis	
	Myotonic dystrophy	Aspiration
	Head trauma	
	Amyotrophic lateral sclerosis	

Individuals who have had a cerebrovascular accident may exhibit lingual hemiparesis, which interferes with tongue control and preparation for swallowing.

The child with poor head and trunk control, altered or dependent sitting balance, and impaired swallowing—such as occurs with cerebral palsy—requires special attention to posture, head position, lip and mouth control, eating and swallowing techniques, and feeding environment. This child may retain oral and swallowing reflexes that are expected to disappear in infancy, making risk of aspiration while eating extremely high (Helfrich-Miller, Rector, & Straka, 1986).

Children develop patterns and behaviors associated with eating as part of development. A child with impaired swallowing still needs to be able to experience eating and food-related events appropriate for the culture and age, such as finger foods for toddlers. The same child can be expected to develop food preferences and may use eating as a manipulative tool if too much attention is focused on eating.

Frequently neuromuscular impairments involve more than one stage of swallowing (Glenn, Araya, Jones, & Liljefors, 1993). Robbins, Logemann, and Kirshner (1986) found all participants of their study who had Parkinson's disease "exhibited abnormal oropharyngeal movement patterns and timing during the volitional oral and pharyngeal phases of swallowing." Individuals who have had a cerebrovascular accident or head trauma may have impaired swallowing following the onset or injury; however, speech-language therapy often results in either resolution or improvement of the impairment. Individuals with chronic, progressive diseases such as cerebral palsy, Parkinson's disease, multiple sclerosis, and amyotrophic lateral sclerosis often have progressive difficulty with swallowing.

Anatomic Impairments

Cleft lips and cleft palates—anatomic impairments found in children—require surgical correction. A cleft in the lip may be only a small notch or it may extend to the floor of the nose; cleft palates occur alone or in conjunction with cleft lips. These anatomic impairments may involve only the uvula or may extend through the hard and soft palate, exposing one or both nasal cavities. Until surgical repair is completed, nasal regurgitation complicates the tasks of sucking and swallowing liquids, nutritional intake is compromised during an infant's stage of rapid growth and development, and health status may be affected—all serious consequences to be prevented and avoided.

Severe dysphagia and repeated regurgitation of undigested foods may indicate Zenker's diverticulum, an abnormal pouch arising in the pharyngeal area where food begins to collect. The diverticulum is thought to form secondary to achalasia, or latent relaxation of the cricopharyngeal sphincter (Dobie, 1978). One recent study used manometry and video radiography to find a diminished opening of the cricopharyngeal sphincter and an increase in bolus pressure, indicating that high pressures may contribute to herniation (Cook et al., 1992). Surgery is usually required to correct this dysfunction.

The severity of the eating problem varies with the extent and location of the surgical procedure. Persons who have had radical head and neck surgery often experience impaired swallowing, whereas the first sign of carcinoma of the esophagus is often a difficulty in swallowing. Esophageal cancer tends to develop so quickly that only half of those diagnosed can be considered for surgical repair (Griffin & Tollison, 1980).

FEEDING TUBES

The person with dysphagia who is unable to swallow safely uses alternative means for nutrition. For short-term nutritional intervention, the rehabilitation nurse assesses whether the person has an active gag reflex and gauges the risk for aspiration. The nasogastric method is commonly used by individuals who have some gag reflex provided they are awake and alert. A nasointestinal method is used for an individual without a gag reflex and a history of aspiration. The most serious complication associated with either method is aspiration. Potential for aspiration is lessened when the client is positioned sitting or in bed with the head of the bed elevated at least 45 degrees while eating and for the hour that follows. A surgically placed feeding tube is the method of choice for most long-term assisted nutritional programs, including clients who receive nutritional care at home. The most commonly used tubes are gastrostomy, jejunostomy and esophagostomy; children may have a gastrostomy button. Clients and families are taught to recognize and report signs of complications such as postoperative edema, bleeding, tube dislodgement, peritonitis, aspiration, skin irritations, or diarrhea. A third alternative nutritional method is via percutaneous endoscopic gastrostomy (PEG). Percutaneous gastrostomies can be performed with local anesthesia and result in fewer complications than surgical procedures.

When a client is able to take adequate oral nutrition, the tube is removed. Accurate calorie and nutritional data are indicators as to whether a person can maintain adequate oral intake; however, these must be carefully assessed before the tube is removed. Premature removal and subsequent reinsertion of a feeding tube may add to discomfort for a client, be viewed as regression, or lead to depression for client or family (Ylvisaker & Weinstein, 1989).

NURSING ASSESSMENT

The nursing assessment is central to understanding an individual's eating process and identifying specific deficits. A complete assessment includes a history of difficulties in eating, a measurable review of food and fluid intake, evaluation of laboratory data (D'Eramo, Sedlak, Dohney, & Jenkins, 1994), interpretation of findings from radiology study, and a physical assessment.

Nursing History

The purpose of the nursing history is to establish the present eating patterns of the client and the patterns before the illness or injury, to describe the present difficulties, to determine areas of evaluation for the physical assessment, and to evaluate the client's need for education. The history should focus on the following four broad areas:
   ✦ Ability of the client to obtain and prepare food
   ✦ Adequacy of the diet
   ✦ Difficulties in eating the food
   ✦ Nutritional preferences and habits

Caregivers who obtain and prepare food are part of the history regarding nutritional adequacy of the diet, how food is prepared, personal or ethnic rules about food or eating, when foods are served, and similar data that might affect a client's intake. When a client shops for and prepares food, ask the following questions in the history: How do you get to the store? How frequently do you shop? What storage and preparation facilities are available to you at home? The types of foods selected by the client frequently are determined by these variables.

Answers to the following questions help determine the adequacy of the diet:

+ How much money is available for food on a weekly basis?
+ Do you eat alone regularly?
+ Are meals eaten out? If yes, what are the usual restaurants; what foods are generally ordered?
+ Are any meals provided and brought to the home by someone else?
+ Do you take medications (that may alter nutritional status)?
+ Has a special diet ever been recommended by your physician?
+ How closely do you feel this special diet is followed?
+ Is there a particular type of food used (canned, frozen, ethnic, vegetarian)?
+ Who prepares your food? If you prepare your own food, do you have any difficulty?
+ Are there adequate utensils, safety features, and space for food preparation and storage in your home?
+ Do you feed yourself? If so, do you have any difficulties or are foods modified to help you with eating or drinking? Is any adaptive feeding equipment used?
+ Do you tire easily or become short of breath while eating?
+ Do you sit in any particular position while eating or soon after?
+ What is your actual food intake based on a 3-day diet history?
+ What are cultural or regional preferences?

Economics and access to affordable fresh foods can play an important role in the types of foods available to the client. Convenience or prepared foods may be easier but frequently are more expensive and many contain unwanted fat and salt. Fresh foods may have more nutrient value but are more difficult to prepare and store, and may be more expensive out of season. The social aspect of eating may also encourage nutritional status; persons who eat alone are prone to poor nutrition.

The next phase of the history elicits the client's ability to swallow food effectively. Factors to be considered include the following:

+ Is there a history of aspiration pneumonia?
+ Is there pain with swallowing?
+ Do foods get stuck in the throat?
+ Is there difficulty with swallowing solid or soft foods?
+ Do foods regurgitate nasally?
+ Is there choking or coughing when eating?
+ Is there difficulty with swallowing liquids?
+ Can you sit upright during meals without difficulty?

Obstruction of the pharynx is usually associated with pain and difficulty in swallowing solid foods, whereas a neuromuscular difficulty is associated with more difficulty in swallowing liquids and the presence of nasal regurgitation. The upright sitting position is the most efficient for eating and drinking and allows a more adequate swallow to be performed.

Psychosocial Factors

By the end of the history the nurse should be able to assess the following through conversations with the client:

+ The degree to which loneliness or depression is contributing to a poor nutritional intake
+ The amount of fear the person has regarding eating
+ The degree to which lifelong eating habits are contributing to a poor nutritional intake
+ The degree of willingness and motivation the client has to work in a rehabilitation program

Nutritional status is influenced not only by physical ability to consume food but also by psychological and sociocultural factors as well. In American society many ethnic groups define food choices differently and attach different emotional significance to food. It is important in the assessment to identify these characteristics and to realize that cultural patterns may affect the client's nutritional choices. Additionally food is frequently associated with social events and therefore has significant psychological meaning. Traditional foods for holidays are a good example. As one ages or becomes ill, the lack of significant interactions at meals or lack of other significant social interactions can reduce nutritional intake significantly. It is difficult to change lifelong eating habits, and these can hamper the client's rehabilitation. However, highly motivated clients can frequently overcome these habits and conquer their fear.

Physical Assessment

As part of the nursing assessment it is important to determine the client's ability to understand and follow directions. Poor subjective data form an unreliable basis for the physical assessment of the client's ability to obtain and prepare food, place food in the oral cavity, and swallow food. The physical assessment begins with examination of the head and neck and should include the following:

+ Assess the client's head control while the client is in a seated position.
+ Assess facial symmetry.
+ Inspect the lips for color, symmetry, and moisture. Malignant lesions of the oral cavity may occur on the lips.
+ Is the client drooling, indicating poor control of oral fluids?
+ Ask the client to close the lips tightly. Observe the client's ability to perform this activity.
+ Ask the client to open the mouth; check internal symmetry.
+ Inspect the mucosa of the oral cavity. In dehydration it will appear dry.
+ Inspect the teeth for number and state of repair. Two opposing incisors and two opposing molars are needed to chew adequately.
+ If there are dentures, inspect for proper fit. Ask the

client to remove them (or remove dentures if client is unable to remove them) and inspect the underlying gums.

✦ Test cranial nerve XII (hypoglossal) by inspecting the tongue for irregular movement or asymmetry, both while the tongue is in the mouth and when protruded.

✦ Test cranial nerves IX (glossopharyngeal) and X (vagus) by asking the client to say "ah." The uvula and soft palate should rise. Deviation of the uvula is found with paralysis. When the uvula is touched with a tongue depressor, a gag reflex occurs, indicating intact motor function of the vagus nerve. Although the gag reflex is closely associated with the swallowing reflex, it does not have to be present for the normal swallow to occur.

✦ Inspect the pharynx for color, edema, and ulcerations. This observation includes the anterior and posterior faucial arches and palatine tonsils.

✦ Test cranial nerve V (trigeminal) for strength and symmetry by asking the client to clench the teeth.

✦ Is the client's temperature elevated?

(The examiner palpates the temporomandibular area to determine muscle strength during contraction. The sensory component of the nerve is tested by asking the client to identify sharp and dull sensations on the sides of the face, forehead, and cheeks.)

✦ Test cranial nerve VII (facial) by observing throughout the examination for the presence of tics and unusual movements or asymmetry of the face. Motor function is tested by the client's ability to clench the teeth and smile. The sensory component of this cranial nerve is used to identify sweet (sugar), salt, sour (lemon), and bitter (aspirin) tastes.

✦ Test cranial nerve XI (spinal accessory) by applying hand pressure to the sternocleidomastoid muscle as the person shrugs both shoulders.

✦ If indicated, test the client for the presence of primitive reflex behaviors usually seen only in infants and which, when present in later life, indicate a disturbance of the upper motor neuron system (e.g., following a brain injury). These reflexes include the rooting reflex, stimulated by stroking the lips or corners of the mouth and having the client's head reflexively turn toward the stimulus; the tonic neck reflex, sometimes called the fencing position. The tonic neck reflex is a total body pattern that occurs by turning the head to one side, resulting in extension of the extremities on the face side and flexion of the extremities on the skull side.

✦ Throughout the examination, evaluate the client's voice. Oral and palatal dysfunction are highlighted by dysarthria or hypernasality (Dobie, 1978).

✦ Finally, ask the client to swallow water. Can the client form a seal with the lips? How long does it take to complete the swallow and is a cough reflex present?

✦ Does the client have a moist, wet voice following the swallow of water or does the client frequently clear the throat?

The remainder of the physical examination should focus on the client's ability to eat independently. If the client has difficulty with arm or hand range of motion or coordination, dietary alterations may prepare foods that can be eaten more easily. A description of the difficulty the individual has with feeding is helpful information to use when performing the physical assessment. The following areas should be assessed.

✦ Does the client have sufficient mobility, muscle strength, and control to lift eating utensils from plate to mouth?

✦ Are grip and strength sufficient to hold eating utensils?

✦ Does a tremor or involuntary movement interfere with coordination?

✦ Can the client cut food?

✦ Is the client limited to the use of one hand?

✦ What is the client's visual acuity? Is vision limited (e.g., hemianopsia)?

If the client prepares meals, include the following questions in the history:

✦ Are cooking areas accessible and safe?

✦ Are meals prepared from standing or sitting position? If standing, are any adaptive devices used?

✦ Is there any difficulty with mobility?

✦ Is there sufficient strength and dexterity in the arms and hands to manipulate, open, and prepare foods?

✦ Is there sufficient muscle strength and head control to remain sitting upright for meals?

The nursing history and physical assessment should provide data to describe the client's disability and to form the basis for the nursing diagnoses.

Diagnostic Tests

The most commonly used diagnostic tests for identifying the etiology of dysphagia include the bedside swallow examination, manometry modified barium swallow with videofluoroscopy, and videoendoscopy.

The bedside swallow examination is conducted by the clinician placing two fingers on the thyroid notch between the hyoid bone and larynx. As the client swallows, the clinician should feel the larynx move up and forward. If the larynx does not elevate, the clinician moves the fingers upward to palpate. The purpose is to determine whether the cricopharyngeal sphincter is not opening and the epiglottis is not protecting the airway.

Manometry is a procedure used to obtain information on the pattern of peristaltic pressure waves during deglutition. The client "swallows" pressure-sensitive tubes—which, once in place, measure pressures as the person swallows. Usually the tubes are positioned to measure pressures in the upper esophageal sphincter, the esophagus, and the lower esophageal sphincter. Manometry is used to identify disruptions in the peristaltic waves through the pharynx and esophagus and to diagnosis impairments of the upper or lower esophagus.

The modified barium swallow with videofluoroscopy allows viewing of the oral cavity, laryngopharynx, and cervical esophagus. During the test the person swallows small amounts of a liquid or solid mixed with barium. As the person manipulates the bolus in the oral cavity and swallows, the fluoroscopic study is recorded on videotape. Videotaping of the swallowing study allows clinicians to have repeated viewing and slow-motion analysis.

Compensatory techniques and a client's tolerance for swallowing foods of different consistencies may also be evaluated with this test; however, with repeated testing, clinicians must inform clients about their exposure to some amounts of radiation (Ozer, 1994).

Nasal videoendoscopy is a procedure that uses a fiberoptic nasopharyngoscope to enable a clinician to visually examine a client's palate, pharynx, and larynx. At the same time the clinician is able to assess the sensation in the upper aerodigestive tract, as well as any secretion pooling and the client's ability to swallow.

NURSING DIAGNOSES

Nursing diagnoses that may be used for eating and swallowing problems include the following:

1. Impaired Gas Exchange
2. Aspiration, high risk for
3. Fluid volume deficit
4. Fluid volume deficit, high risk
5. Altered Nutrition; high risk for less than body requirements
6. Altered Nutrition; high risk for more than body requirements
7. Knowledge deficit in proper nutrition, adaptive equipment, or availability of community resources

Physical impairments that reduce the ability to swallow effectively can result in aspiration of food or fluids. The client frequently becomes frustrated and disappointed, further reducing nutritional intake. Clients with a neuromuscular disorder are particularly susceptible to aspiration.

Weight is a key indicator of the degree of difficulty the client may have with eating and should be monitored closely. Whether in the hospital or at home, clients should be weighed at least weekly to monitor weight changes. Clients whose physical disabilities result in reduced activity may gain weight when caloric intake is increased above nutritional and activity requirements. Too often, when physical activity is reduced, eating compensates as an important daily activity, leading to obesity and hampering an active rehabilitation program.

Part of the nursing diagnosis evaluates all the client's medications. The nurse needs to be aware of what medications the client is taking, why, and any alterations in diet that are used. Medications with sedative effects can cause confusion or disorientation, which may affect the client's swallowing abilities. Antispasticity medications may affect swallowing ability by decreasing the strength of the involved muscles. Medications such as diuretics or those that act to decrease secretions can adversely affect swallowing by drying the oral and pharyngeal mucosa and decreasing the saliva necessary to help illicit the swallowing reflex. Other medications that do not directly affect swallowing may affect eating by decreasing appetite.

Finally, clients may have an inadequate nutritional intake because of a knowledge deficit. They may be unaware of what foods and nutrients compose an adequate diet, what adaptive equipment is available for use, or what community resources are available. When dietary plans and menus are offered to persons from differing cultural groups, the nutritional composition of ethnic or regional food selections may be calculated so these foods are included in the plan.

GOALS

Goals established by the nurse and client relate to the nursing diagnoses and are based on information obtained from the client during the nursing assessment, from family members, and home assessment data. Impaired gas exchange may result because of a poor swallowing reflex. The nurse may decrease the episodes of aspiration and choking by improving the swallowing process. Fluid volume deficit, or high risk, means increasing liquid intake either through alternate forms or by more frequent feedings. Liquids are usually the most difficult food to swallow for someone with an inadequate swallowing process. As a result the client may have a great deal of fear when taking liquids. It is important to maximize the safety of the swallowing process and to provide encouragement when the client is taking liquids.

Inadequate caloric intake, particularly of solid foods, necessitates alternate and more frequent feedings. If poor intake is a result of depression, the underlying problem must be addressed. A complete diet history that includes food preferences and the significance of food to the client should be completed to find foods the client might eat. If the client is consuming too many calories, the goal is to reduce caloric intake by substituting reduced-calorie foods. Frequently it is necessary to look for meaningful activities that the client can use to substitute for time previously spent eating.

The goals for the client experiencing difficulty with eating and swallowing may include all or some of the following:

1. Improving or maintaining fluid volume
2. Maintaining adequate nutrition
3. Teaching the client and family
   a. Measures to prevent and alleviate choking
   b. Proper nutrition
   c. Use of adaptive equipment
   d. Availability of community resources to assist in providing adequate nutrition

REHABILITATION NURSING INTERVENTIONS

Once an assessment is completed, nursing diagnoses formulated, and goals established, specific nursing interventions must be considered. If the primary difficulty is a neuromuscular swallowing disorder, interventions are directed to improving the swallowing process. Steps to improve the swallowing process are as follows:

✦ Begin by placing the client in an upright sitting position with the head bent slightly forward. The forward tilt of the head is important to prevent food from hitting the posterior pharyngeal wall before the swallow reflex begins.

✦ If the client has poor head control and the head falls forward, hold the head up by placing the palm of your hand on the client's forehead for support.

✦ Sit down when assisting the client to eat. This action communicates time and willingness to help.

✦ Initially use small amounts of soft food that are easy to swallow (applesauce, purees).

✦ Place a half teaspoonful on the middle to back part of the tongue. However, if the client has tongue or facial paralysis or has had a partial laryngectomy, the correct placement is on the unaffected intact side, not midline.

- ✦ With the spoon, push down on the tongue as you remove the food from the spoon.
- ✦ If swallowing does not occur, remove the spoon from the client's mouth.
- ✦ Instruct the client to move the food around and toward the rear of the mouth.
- ✦ If the swallow comes slowly, press on the tip of the client's head with the palm of your hand. This action will decrease laryngeal tension and facilitate swallowing (Buckley, Addicks, & Maniglia, 1975).
- ✦ Check to see that the client's lips are sealed or the swallowing reflex will not begin. Manually seal the lips together or use a jaw control maneuver to pull the jaws together (Fig. 17-4).
- ✦ If swallowing does not occur, try placing your thumb on the client's chin, moving the chin downward toward the sternum to facilitate the swallow (Buckley et al., 1975).

Liquids

The client with a neuromuscular disorder has more difficulty with liquids than with soft foods due to a lack of tongue control and coordination to form the liquids into a bolus. In these cases liquids may first be placed on a spoon and put on the posterior portion of the tongue. If this procedure does not give the client any difficulty, try using a syringe to place a small amount of liquid posteriorly on the tongue. The syringe technique should be considered a short-term therapeutic intervention and not a long-term option. Before using this intervention, check with state guidelines.

Use of a straw requires the complex functioning of the oral musculature and as a result is less useful for these clients. If the client can drink from a cup, remember that when the glass is less than half full, it becomes necessary to tilt the head back to drink. This position increases the risk of aspiration and should be avoided. Specially designed cups are available, or a cutaway cup can be made easily by cutting a semicircular portion out of a paper cup. This allows the client to tilt the cup further without tilting his head (Fig. 17-5).

Clients who have difficulty managing liquids eat a modified diet without liquids or a diet using liquids of a specified consistency. Consistency of liquids are classified as thick liquids (e.g., honey), modified liquids (e.g., nectars), or thin liquids (e.g., water). Liquids may be thickened by adding a commercial thickening agent like "Thick It." Refer to the product information for obtaining the proper consistency.

Choking (a protective maneuver for the airway) is frightening for a client but unfortunately may be expected to occur at times in individuals with swallowing difficulties. If coughing and choking can be minimized, fear and anxiety associated with feeding will be decreased. When coughing or choking begins, the nurse instructs the client to flex at the waist or neck if possible. Waist or neck flexion assists in more efficient airway clearance. If food becomes lodged in the larynx and compromises breathing, and the client is unable to speak, the Heimlich maneuver should be used.

Milk and milk products should be avoided, since these tend to form tenacious secretions that are poorly handled. If the client can chew, a textured food may be more desirable. Above all, the nurse should encourage the client and

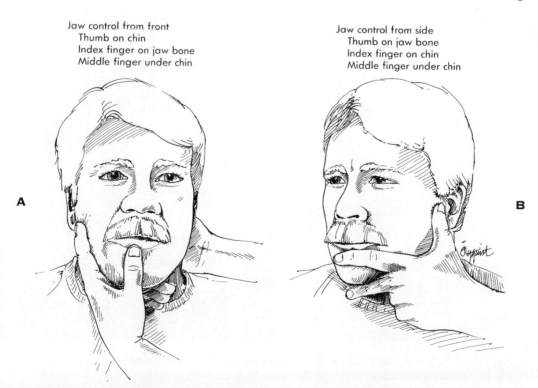

Jaw control from front
  Thumb on chin
  Index finger on jaw bone
  Middle finger under chin

Jaw control from side
  Thumb on jaw bone
  Index finger on chin
  Middle finger under chin

Fig. 17-4   Jaw control from the front (**A**) and side (**B**).

family to keep the diet flexible and reevaluate it often to avoid monotony. For the client who has a self feeding deficit, the nurse can work closely with occupational and physical therapists in muscle strengthening, coordination, and use of adaptive equipment. The nurse's role is to assess intake and implement and reinforce the compensatory techniques and use of adaptive equipment. Examples of adaptive equip-

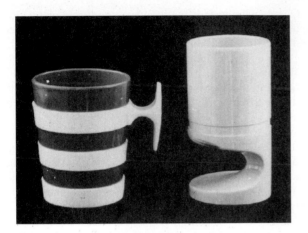

Fig. 17-5   Specially designed cups.

ment include scoop dishes, and plate guards, and silverware modified for easy grasp and effective cutting and eating (Fig. 17-6, *A–D* and Fig. 17-7). Interventions are individualized for each client based on the findings from diagnostic tests so the client, family, and nurse are able to work effectively with the speech/swallowing therapist (Table 17-3 and the swallowing techniques in the Box on p. 358).

Client/Family Education

In addition to understanding the exact nature of the eating deficit, the client and family need to be involved in establishing goals and planning care. Without client and family cooperation, the rehabilitation process will be less effective. The rehabilitation nurse roles include promoting good communication with the family. Throughout the system, between care plan meetings, and elsewhere the nurse is an advocate for the family, explains new treatment approaches, and reports progress (Axelsson, Norberg, & Asplund, 1986). The client and family should demonstrate knowledge of dietary modifications, the hazards of offering "unsafe" food even when requested by the patient, using adaptive equipment if needed, the process for feeding, and performing emergency measures in the event of coughing or choking.

When the client has excessive caloric intake, it is necessary to work with the family and client. For this client, food

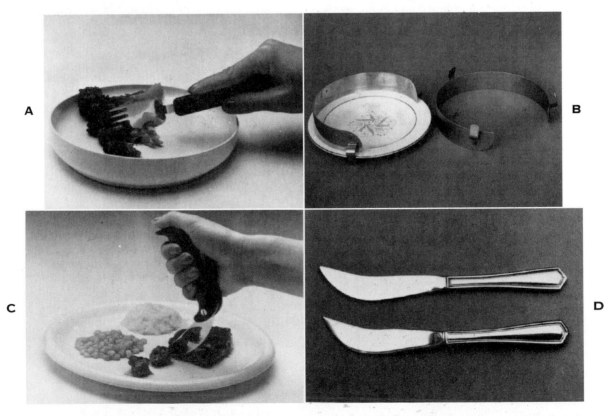

Fig. 17-6   **A,** Scoop dishes and (**B**) dishes with plate guards. **C,** This rounded knife is collapsible. **D,** Utensils with rounded edges can be rocked back and forth to cut food. (From *Rehabilitation/Restorative Care in the Community* by S. Hoeman, 1990, St. Louis: Mosby–Year Book. Copyright 1990 by Mosby–Year Book. Reprinted by permission.)

frequently is substituted for other activities or reinforcements. Family may bring food to the client because it brings pleasure. The nurse can work with the client and family to develop other positive forms of reinforcement, long-term goals for rehabilitation, and help the client to see the consequences of overeating.

REHABILITATION TEAM INTERVENTIONS

Because eating and swallowing disorders are complex, the nurse collaborates with other rehabilitation team professionals. All patients presenting with a neuromuscular disorder should be evaluated for a swallowing impairment as early in the assessment process as possible and referred to the necessary team members. As noted earlier, physical therapy helps improve muscle tone, strength, and coordination. Treatment is directed at improving muscle tone for the primary eating muscles as well as secondary muscles of arms, legs, head, and neck. The occupational therapist performs self-feeding evaluations, recommends and teaches the use of adaptive equipment and exercises to improve hand control and coordination, and offers assistance in food preparation. The therapist also may recommend meaningful activities for the client to engage in during the day as a substitute for eating.

The speech-language pathologist may perform a bedside swallow screening or determine the need for a modified barium swallow. Based on the results of the screening or testing, the speech pathologist designs a program of exercises for the oropharyngeal musculature and identifies what compensatory swallowing techniques are to be used.

The dietitian helps develop a menu plan that meets the nutritional, socioeconomic, and cultural requirements of the client and teaches the proper diet to the client and family.

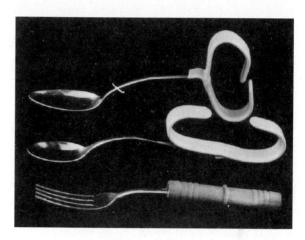

Fig. 17-7 Adapted silverware.

Table 17-3 Compensatory techniques: Postural changes affect how gravity moves food through the pharynx

Position	Benefit	Physiologic disorder
Head down: lowering head so neck is flexed and chin is approximately ¾ of way down toward chest	Widens valleculae; epiglottis covers more of airway, resulting in increased protection and decreased risk of aspiration	Delayed reflex and reduced laryngeal closure
Head back: gently and slowly tossing head back	Moves food more rapidly through the oral cavity	Reduced tongue movement
Head turned toward affected or less functional side	Increases vocal fold adduction; closes pharynx on side to which head is turned, causing bolus to travel down opposite side of pharynx; reduces resting tone	Unilateral pharyngeal dysfunction; reduced laryngeal closures or unilateral laryngeal dysfunction; cricopharyngeal problems
Head tilted to more functional side	Gravity directs food down more functional side of pharynx	Unilateral damage to tongue and pharynx
Supine, lying on one side with head supported	Removes effects of gravity; eliminates postswallow aspiration	Reduced peristalsis; reduced laryngeal elevation
Head turned and chin down	Directs direction of bolus and increases airway protection	Reduced laryngeal closure
Head back and turned	Moves bolus quickly through oral cavity; sets direction of bolus	Decreased tongue function; decreased laryngeal closure; unilateral pharyngeal weakness
Thermal stimulation	Increases sensitivity of swallow reflex but may require 4-6 weeks to note improvement	Decreased oral awareness; delayed pharyngeal swallow
Supraglottic swallow	Increases voluntary airway protection	Decreased laryngeal elevation or closure
Mendelson maneuver	Voluntary increase in laryngeal elevation time and opening of cricopharyngeal sphincter	Decreased laryngeal elevation or opening of cricopharyngeal sphincter

Compiled from "Approaches to Management of Disordered Swallowing" by J.A. Logemann, 1991, *Bailliere's Clinical Gastroenterology, 5*, 269-280.

SWALLOWING TECHNIQUES

THERMAL STIMULATION

- Chill laryngeal mirror in ice for 1 minute.
- With back of mirror lightly touch both sides of mouth 5 times on each side, use short light strokes.
- Have client swallow.
- Repeat a total of 5 times, rechilling mirror between times.
- Repeat 3-4 times a day.

SUPERGLOTTIC SWALLOW (May be Done With or Without Food in the Oral Cavity)

- If using food, place food in mouth.
- Client inhales and holds breath.
- Client swallows while holding breath (cover tracheostomy tube if applicable).
- Client coughs after swallowing without inhaling again.
- Repeat 10 times, 3-4 times a day.

MENDELSON MANEUVER (May be Done With or Without Food in the Oral Cavity)

- Client places hand on larynx.
- Client swallows and feels larynx left to its highest position.
- If using food, client places food in mouth.
- Client swallows and again holds larynx in highest position during the swallow; client then releases hold.
- Repeat 3-6 times, 3-4 times a day.

From "Approaches to Management of Disordered Swallowing" by J.A. Logemann, 1991, *Bailliere's Clinical Gastroenterology, 5,* 269-280.

The nurse conducts a complete history and physical assessment and in-depth self-feeding and swallowing assessments. The nurse also monitors the patient's weight, caloric intake, and laboratory studies for hydration and nutritional status. A primary nursing responsibility is working with the client and family on reinforcement of feeding and swallowing skills and to communicate progress to other team members.

OUTCOME CRITERIA

For the client with a progressive neuromuscular disorder, maintaining the maximum level of independence in eating and attaining adequate nutritional intake are realistic goals. Clients with neuromuscular insults (e.g., cerebrovascular accident, head trauma) may anticipate a return to normal function after an active rehabilitative period but this depends on the extent of the injury. Three months appears to be the critical period in which maximum return of function can be anticipated (Logemann, 1983). Sample measurable outcome criteria that can be used to evaluate treatment results are as follows:

1. Client manipulates utensils for independent eating.
2. Client cuts and prepares foods to be eaten.
3. Client chews without difficulty.
4. Client swallows soft foods without difficulty.
5. Client drinks liquids without difficulty.
6. Client maintains adequate body weight.
7. Client meets nutritional requirements.
8. Client and family describe emergency measures for choking.
9. Client and family describe nutritional requirements.
10. Client and family correctly use adaptive equipment.
11. Client and family are knowledgeable regarding community resources to assist in the provision of adequate nutrition.

For the client who has caloric intake above requirements, the major goal of the treatment program is to reduce caloric intake. Measurable outcome criteria used to evaluate treatment results are as follows:

1. Client and family describe nutritional requirements.
2. Client and family describe how to meet the nutritional requirements of the client.
3. Client and family describe the emotional significance of food to the client.
4. Client consumes the appropriate amount of calories for the physical condition.
5. Client demonstrates gradual weight loss according to the individualized plan.

SUMMARY

Eating and swallowing are essential to an individual's survival physiologically. Psychologically, food and eating are important to feelings of self-worth and community. When one can no longer eat without difficulty, fear is frequently an overriding emotional reaction. It includes not only fear for one's survival and ability to function but fear of or actual loss of significant social interactions. For persons with significant physical disability, excessive food consumption is an emotional response to the loss of function and the decreased need of the body for calories. The nurse is crucial in assisting these individuals and their families and may be the first health-care professional to realize that there is an eating problem. The nurse has the ability to draw in other rehabilitation team members. Patience, understanding, and ability to teach the client and family about this aspect of rehabilitation has many positive rewards and outcomes for the client, family, and nurse.

CASE STUDY

Mrs. R. G. is an elderly widow who moved to the Mid-Atlantic area from Puerto Rico following the death of her husband 6 years ago to live near her two married daughters. She speaks only Spanish and lives alone in a small city apartment located in a culturally diverse community. In addition to having diabetes, she had a stroke 7 months ago and was referred to a rehabilitation center in the next city. She was discharged with only mild residual muscle weakness but persistent dysphagia. Unable to return to her former neighborhood apartment, she lived near the rehabilitation center and was followed by a speech language therapist, a physical therapist, a home health aide, and the rehabilitation nursing consultant from the visiting nurse association. Two immediate goals are to work with Mrs. R. G. to stabilize her nutritional status and to continue the gains she made with swallowing while in the rehabilitation center.

However, Mrs. R. G. has been refusing to eat her meals and appears to be anxious about eating and swallowing. On several occasions, she began shouting and waving her hands when lunch was served, refusing to eat the food or to work with the speech therapist. The physical therapist was a young man who spoke some Spanish in his own home, but Mrs. R. G. would not communicate with him about her concerns other than to tell him, "I had this illness because I am being punished for bad things in my life, and now God has allowed someone, a spirit I think, to place a spell on me."

The home health aide told the nurse that Mrs. R. G.'s daughter was present the next day and translated for Mrs. R. G.; Mrs. R. G. claimed that she was being given food to make her sick, not better. The aide was concerned that Mrs. R. G. was taking medicines she obtained from a relative and using over-the-counter purgatives. The nurse arranged to meet with the daughter and Mrs. R. G. at lunch and to check the medications in the house. After a discussion with the daughter, the nurse met with the interdisciplinary team. A dietician and an espiritisa, a traditional Puerto Rican healer, were invited as consultants. The spiritual healer met privately with Mrs. R. G. and agreed to return the following week. With improved trust and rapport, Mrs. R. G. and the team were able to concentrate on the therapeutic regimen. With proper evaluation and client/family education about common symptoms, swallowing problems can be managed effectively for clients in their home. Presently Mrs. R. G. is on a waiting list for housing in a senior complex in her old neighborhood.

The rehabilitation nurse consultant prepared a staff inservice program based on the discussions with Mrs. R. G.'s daughter and the espiritisa, and this led to mutually agreeable goals and interventions. The staff improved the outcome for Mrs. R. G. by providing culturally sensitive and relevant care. One therapist remarked, "Learning about things that influenced Mrs. R. G.'s care was a bit like unraveling a mystery . . . about why she wouldn't do things. We thought she was being stubborn, or worse, we thought she had undetected residual damage from the stroke; and of course, her diabetes was a concern. I learned a lot about making assumptions and about the importance of cultural values."

For example, Mrs. R. G. would not speak to the young male physical therapist because she was uncomfortable discussing personal information with a man, especially since his family background was Cuban, not Puerto Rican. The importance of finding a translator who is acceptable to the client involves more than a common language. In fact, there is a great deal of diversity among the Spanish language dialects within the many Hispanic/Latino groups in the United States. Furthermore, modesty, privacy, age, and gender issues were extremely sensitive for Mrs. R. G.

Beliefs about spiritual causes of illness, or illness as punishment are commonly held by some Hispanic/Latino persons. Self medication, especially laxatives or purgatives, may be used to rid the body of disease and various herbs are added to teas or foods to replace strength. Mrs. R. G. was at risk for imbalance in the dietary management of her diabetes. Some persons, like Mrs. R. G., believe that there are diseases incurred only by a Puerto Rican and these can be cured only by an espiritisa. Having the traditional healer involved in planning culturally relevant and sensitive care reduced Mrs. R. G.'s stress, improved her perception of her health, and provided essential information to the team.

Dietary differences, including mealtime and food preferences, had not been incorporated into Mrs. R. G.'s nutritional plan. The team discovered that Mrs. R. G. preferred to have four meals a day consisting of a light breakfast, a main meal at lunch, a small supper meal, and another dinner after 8 PM. Mrs. R. G.'s daughter assisted the dietician in preparing the diabetic menus in Spanish and in using foods from Puerto Rican markets in her old neighborhood.

Mrs. R. G. had accused the team of trying to harm her because they had offered her "hot foods for a hot condition." Like many persons from Hispanic cultures (or from Asian cultures, as in the case of those who believe in yin and yang), she believed that a balance among the humoral areas is essential for maintaining health. According to this belief, an illness or disease may have "hot or cold" properties; foods are similarly categorized based on their having "hot or cold" properties, apart from their temperature or nutritional attributes. Thus, offering a "hot" food for a "hot" condition contributes to imbalance and may be perceived as harmful or hazardous to health, such as with Mrs. R. G. An exact list of foods considered "hot" or "cold" is best assembled by each client or family since there are variations among cultural groups. In addition, many persons will respond affirmatively to a health professional's questions regarding their use of medications, adherence to treatments or procedures, and dietary practices. "Yes" may be a polite response, an elusive one, or simply the easiest answer for some persons. Therefore a cross-cultural dietary assessment and evaluation may prevent misunderstandings and build trust.

CROSS-CULTURAL DIETARY ASSESSMENT AND INTERVENTION

✦ Assess individual food preferences, snack or meal patterns, and the symbolic use or meaning of foods, and determine what foods are taboo or inedible for the client and his or her family. Consider the budget available for food.

✦ Assess the client and his or her family for cultural food habits and preferences, available foods or substitutes, and means of food preparation. Consider the time and place of meals and whether eating is accomplished alone or as a social or group event.

✦ Assess lifestyle, socioeconomic, and religious patterns that influence food habits. Evaluate the client's beliefs about the "hot" or "cold" properties of foods, about whether foods should be Kosher, vegetarian, or related to other specific diets, and discover whether there are re-

Continued.

CASE STUDY—cont'd

stricted stimulants, including coffee or tea, or other dietary requirements. Determine if there are beliefs or practices that are used to treat a client's condition from a traditional or cultural treatment perspective (e.g., medicinal food or beverage treatments). Learn whether there are ceremonial or religious observations important to the client and his or her family, such as observing Ramadan, which may influence responses to medication, treatment outcomes, or dietary needs. Enlist traditional healers to participate when possible.

♦ Evaluate how the client's health or specific medical condition is affected by food patterns or habits. Consider ways to incorporate foods and habits that are neutral or not detrimental to health into the therapeutic regimen. Use traditional preferred foods whenever possible. (Kittler & Sucher, 1990).

Courtesy of S.P. Hoeman

REFERENCES

Axelsson, K., Norberg, A., & Asplund, K. (1986). Relearning to eat late after a stroke by systematic nursing intervention: A case report. *Journal of Advanced Nursing, 11*, 5, 553-559.

Bastain, R. (1991). Videoendoscopic education of patients with disphagice: An adjunct to the modified Barium swallow. *Otolaryngology—Head and Neck Surgery, 104*, 339-350.

Blonsky, E., Logemann, J., Boshes, B., & Fisher, H. (1975). Comparison of speech and swallowing function in patients with tremor disorders and in normal geriatric patients: A cinefluorographic study. *Journal of Gerontology, 30*, 299.

Bruckstein, A. (1989). Dysphasia. *American Family Practitioner 39*, 1, 147-156.

Buckley, J., Addicks, C., & Maniglia, J. (1975). Feeding patients with dysphagia. *Nursing Forum, 15*, 1, 69-85.

Cherney, L., & O'Neill, P. (1986). Swallowing disorders and the aged. *Topics in Geriatrics Rehabilitation, 1*, 4, 45-59.

Cook, I., Gabb, M., Panagopoulas, V., Jamieson, G., Dodds, W., Dent, J., & Shearman, D. (1992). Pharyngeal (Zenker's) diverticulum is a disorder of upper esophageal sphincter opening. *Gastroenterology 103*, 1229-1235.

Cook, I. (1992). Normal and disordered swallowing: New insights. *Bailliere's Clinical Gastroenterology, 5*, 2, 245-267.

D'Eramo, A.L., Sedlak, C., Doheny, M.O'B., & Jenkins, M. (1994). Nutritional aspects of the orthopaedic trauma patient. *Orthopedic Nursing, 13*, 13-20.

De Vito Dabbs, A. (1993). Nutrition: An essential component of pulmonary rehabilitation. *Journal of Cardiopulmonary Rehabilitation, 13*, 387-394.

Dobie, R. (1978). Rehabilitation of swallowing disorders. *American Family Physician, 17*, 5, 84-95.

Fisher, S., Painter, M., & Melmoe, G. (1981). Swallowing disorders in infancy. *Pediatric Clinics of North America, 28*, 4, 845-853.

Glenn, N., Araya, T., Jones, K., & Liljefors, J. (1993). A therapist feeding team in the rehabilitation setting. *Holistic Nursing Practice, 7*, 78-81.

Gordon, M. (1993). *Nursing diagnosis: Process and application* (46th ed.). St. Louis: Mosby–Year Book.

Griffin, J., & Tollison, J. (1980). Dysphagia. *American Family Physician, 22*, 154-160.

Groher, M. (1992). *Dysphagia: Diagnosis and management* (3rd ed.). Boston: Butterworth–Heinemann.

Helfrich-Miller, K.R., Rector, K.L., & Straka, J.A. (1986). Dysphagia: Its treatment in the profoundly retarded patient with cerebral palsy. *Archives of Physical Medicine and Rehabilitation, 67, (8)*, 520-525.

Hoeman, S.P. (1989). Cultural assessment in rehabilitation nursing practice. *Nursing Clinics of North America, 24*, 277-289.

Johnson, E.R., McKenzie, S.W., & Sievers, A. (1993). Aspiration pneumonia in stroke. *Archives of Physical Medicine and Rehabilitation, 74*, 973-976.

Kittler, P.G. & Sucher, K.P. (1990). Diet Counseling in a Multicultural Society. *The Diabetes Educator, 16*, 127-130.

Leopold, N., & Kagel, M. (1983). Swallowing. ingestion, and dysphagia: A reappraisal. *Archives of Physical Medicine and Rehabilitation, 64*, 8, 371-373.

Logemann, J.A. (1983). *Evaluation and treatment of swallowing disorders.* San Diego: College Hill Press.

Logemann, J.A. (1991a). *Swallowing disorders II workshop.* Evanston: Northwestern University.

Logemann, J.A. (1991b). Approaches to management of disordered swallowing. *Bailliere's Clinical Gastroenterology, 5*, 269-280.

McCourt, A. (Ed.). (1993). *The specialty practice of rehabilitation nursing a core curriculum* (3rd ed.). Skokie: Rehabilitation Nursing Foundation.

Ozer, M. (1994). *Management of persons with stroke.* St. Louis: Mosby–Year Book.

Reddy, N.P., Canilang, E.P., Sukthankar, S., Gupta, V., Green, P., Suryanarayanan, S., & Palreddy, S. (1992-1993) Biomechanical measurements and classification of dysphagia. Swallowing disorders. *Rehabilitation R & D Progress Reports* (pp. 217-218). Bethesda, MD: National Institutes for Health.

Reynolds, R.P.E. (1993). A simple approach to dysphagia. *Medicine North America, 16*, 788-789, 792-793.

Robbins, J.A., Logemann, J.A., & Kirshner, H.S. (1986). Swallowing and speech production in Parkinson's disease. *Annals of Neurology, 19*, 283-287.

Roueche, J. (1980). *Dysphagia: An assessment and management program for the adult.* Minneapolis: Sister Kenny Institute.

Sieberns, A. (1990). Rehabilitation for swallowing impairment. In F. Kottke & J. Lehmann (Eds.), *Krusen's handbook of physical medicine and rehabilitation* (4th ed.). Philadelphia: W.B. Saunders.

Willig, T.N., Paulus, J., Lacau Saint Guily, J., Beon, C., & Navarro, J. (1994). Swallowing problems in neuromuscular disorders. *Archives of Physical Medicine and Rehabilitation, 75*, 1175-1181.

Wolanin, M., & Phillips, L. (1983). *Confusion: Prevention and care.* St Louis: Mosby–Year Book.

Ylvisaker, M., & Weinstein, M. (1989). Recovery of oral feeding after pediatric head injury. *Journal of Head Trauma Rehabilitation, 4*, 51-63.

18

Respiratory Function and Pulmonary Rehabilitation

Janet L. Larson, PhD, RN
Joyce H. Johnson, PhD, RN
Denise B. Angst, DNSc, RN

INTRODUCTION

Respiratory disability can have a considerable physical, psychosocial, and financial impact on the client, family, and society. The client with a compromised respiratory system presents a complex and difficult problem to the rehabilitation team. To develop an adequate plan of care, the multidimensional nature of impaired breathing must be understood.

From the client's perspective the primary problems are related to breathlessness, a productive cough, fatigue, and intolerance of physical exercise and activities of daily living (ADL). Clients may experience shortness of breath each time they eat or may have difficulty swallowing. The inability to cough or remove secretions may become a problem. Clients with chronic lung disease may experience significant difficulties with fatigue.

From a pathophysiologic perspective the primary problems are related to ineffective airway clearance, ineffective ventilation, or alterations in breathing patterns and ineffective gas exchange. In the rehabilitation setting respiratory problems are most commonly seen in clients with chronic obstructive pulmonary disease (COPD), cystic fibrosis (CF), bronchopulmonary dysplasia (BPD), and persons with neuromuscular disease involving the respiratory muscles.

Consistent early intervention can often alleviate respiratory symptoms and prevent further deterioration. This is best accomplished by a collaborative relationship between the client and rehabilitation team. In the rehabilitation setting the rehabilitation staff assumes responsibility for early diagnosis and treatment of potential and actual respiratory problems, thereby reducing morbidity and mortality. For optimal respiratory health in the home setting, clients must learn to recognize and treat potential and actual respiratory problems in the earliest stages before they become life-threatening. The rehabilitation team plays a vital role in improving the quality of life by teaching clients how to manage their respiratory problems.

This chapter reviews the basic physiologic processes necessary for ventilation and gas exchange. Alterations in ventilation and gas exchange are discussed with emphasis on the respiratory problems experienced by clients in the rehabilitation setting, specifically those with COPD, CF, BPD, and neuromuscular diseases involving the respiratory muscles. Basic assessment of the respiratory system and common respiratory symptoms are presented followed by interventions that can be used in the rehabilitation setting to address problems related to breathing patterns, airway clearance, and gas exchange.

RESPIRATORY PHYSIOLOGY
Structure and Function

The airways are classified as conducting airways and respiratory units. The conducting airways extend from the nose down through the terminal bronchioles and function as conduits for the distribution of gases throughout the lungs (Fig. 18-1). They are not capable of gas exchange. The respiratory units extend from the respiratory bronchioles to the alveoli. The circumference of individual airways decreases with each branching, and the aggregate circumference increases. In the larger airways inspired air moves by bulk flow, but the velocity of air flow decreases as the aggregate circumference of the airways increases. The velocity of air flow is very slow in the smaller airways, and in the alveoli air moves by diffusion of gases.

✦ **Conducting airways.** The nasopharyngeal region extends from the nose to the trachea and functions to warm, humidify, and filter inspired air. The mucosa is well vascularized, enabling inspired air to be heated to body temperature and humidified by the time it reaches the trachea. This region is lined with ciliated columnar epithelium and contains mucus-secreting cells and glands. Large airborne particles are trapped in the mucous layer before they reach the trachea.

The larynx extends from the pharynx to the trachea and includes the vocal cords. The epiglottis, located at the entrance to the larynx, serves as a valve to separate the alimentary tract from the respiratory tract. Closure of the epiglottis protects the airway from aspiration during swallowing and allows for the development of intrathoracic pressure during coughing and the Valsalva maneuver. Sensory fibers in the larynx and tracheobronchial tree are sensitive to chemical and mechanical irritants that stimulate a cough. The cough reflex can be depressed by neurologic dysfunction, unconsciousness, or anesthesia and seems to be less sensitive with age, increasing the risk of infection of the upper respiratory tract. The tracheobronchial region in-

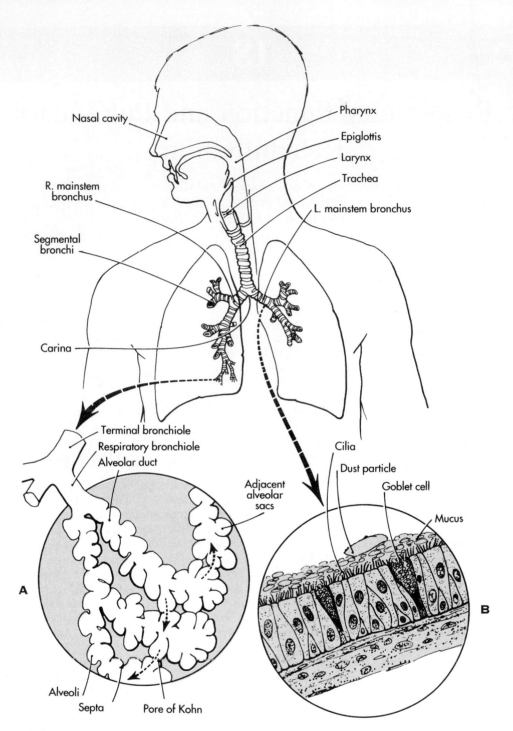

Fig. 18-1 Structures of the respiratory tract. **A,** Pulmonary functional unit. **B,** Ciliated mucous membrane. (From *Pathophysiology: Clinical Concepts of Disease* [4th ed.] by S. Price and L. Wilson, 1992, St. Louis: Mosby–Year Book. Copyright 1992 by Mosby–Year Book. Reprinted by permission.)

cludes the trachea, bronchi, and bronchioles. The tracheo-bronchial region is lined with ciliated epithelial cells, mucus-secreting cells, and mucous glands. Smaller airborne particles are trapped in the mucous layer in this region, and only the smallest particles reach the terminal respiratory units.

The mucus and cilia lining the conducting airways pro-

tect the respiratory system and serve as a major defense mechanism, the mucociliary escalator. The mucous blanket in the airways consists of two layers, a sol layer and a gel layer. The outer gel layer floats on a watery sol layer. The cilia beat within the sol layer at a rapid rate, moving the mucus toward the mouth where it is swallowed. Particles trapped in the mucous layer are moved along with the mucus and ultimately removed from the airways when swallowed. Secretions from the tracheobronchial tree consist of mucus from bronchial mucous glands and goblet cells, tissue fluid transudate, saliva, cellular debris, enzymes, and immunoglobulins. The volume of secretions normally ranges from 10 to 100 ml/day in a normal adult.

✦ **Gas exchange units.** The terminal respiratory unit, or acinus, consists of respiratory bronchioles, alveolar ducts, and alveoli. Alveoli begin to appear as outgrowths of the airways in the smaller bronchioles, increasing in number with each generation.

Alveoli provide an enormous surface area for gas exchange, about the size of a tennis court. The walls of the alveoli are composed of epithelial cells, type I and type II pneumocytes. Type I pneumocytes are large flat cells that serve as a thin barrier to gas exchange. Type II pneumocytes are thicker cells interspersed among the type I pneumocytes. Type II pneumocytes are metabolically active and among other things responsible for secreting surfactant. The outer surface of alveoli are covered by a dense network of pulmonary capillaries. The pulmonary capillary endothelium is composed of a single layer of endothelial cells.

The alveolar epithelial and capillary endothelial cells rest on separate basement membranes. These membranes appear to be fused at some points so that nothing else stands between the endothelial and epithelial cells. The spatial separation of the two basement membranes accommodates some excess fluid without necessarily impairing gas exchange. The interstitium at the alveolar level is continuous with these spaces, and excess fluid normally drains to the lymphatics via this route, protecting the alveolus from edema formation. If fluid accumulates faster than the lymphatics can remove it, pulmonary edema results.

Ventilation

Ventilation is defined as the movement of air into and out of the lungs, and it can be thought of as the pump function of the lungs. The process of ventilation involves the central nervous system, peripheral nervous system, rib cage, and respiratory muscles. The respiratory centers in the brain send messages via the central and peripheral pathways to the respiratory muscles, initiating contraction. The respiratory muscles contract and generate the pressure differences required for air flow.

✦ **Alveolar ventilation**

Minute ventilation includes both dead space ventilation and alveolar ventilation.

$$V_E = V_A + V_{DS}$$

Where V_E refers to minute ventilation, V_A refers to alveolar ventilation, and V_{DS} refers to dead space ventilation. The V_A contributes to gas exchange, whereas V_{DS} does not. In the adult resting V_E is 6 to 8 L/minute, with a tidal volume of 500 ml and respiratory rate of 12 to 16 breaths/minute. The anatomic dead space is composed primarily of the conducting airways, averaging approximately 150 ml in the typical 70-kg male. Anatomic dead space volume remains relatively constant with each breath, whereas alveolar volume changes in direct proportion to tidal volume. If the tidal volume is 500 ml, the alveolar volume is approximately 350

ml. When the tidal volume decreases from 500 to 300 ml, the V_{DS} will remain at 150 ml/breath, but the V_A will decrease to 150 ml/breath. Consequently rapid shallow breathing is inefficient.

The partial pressure of carbon dioxide (Pa_{CO_2}) is used as a clinical indicator of alveolar ventilation. The Pa_{CO_2} rises with alveolar hypoventilation and falls with alveolar hyperventilation. Additionally, severe alveolar hypoventilation can cause hypoxemia.

The V_A is distributed unevenly throughout the lungs with a greater fraction of ventilation flowing to the bases. Regional variations in V_A occur as a result of the vertical gradient of pleural pressure and the effects of gravity on lung tissue. In the upright position more alveoli are open in the apex than in the base of the lung. The lungs are essentially hanging suspended in the thoracic cavity, stretching lung tissue in the apex and compressing lung tissue in the bases. Consequently the alveoli in the apex are partially filled with gas and therefore less compliant, whereas the alveoli in the bases are partially closed and more compliant. Ventilation follows the path of least resistance with a greater fraction going to the bases, particularly in the upright position with normal excursion of the diaphragm.

Mechanics of Breathing

The diaphragm is the primary muscle of inspiration (Fig. 18-2). The diaphragm is innervated by the phrenic nerve arising from spinal cord roots at C3, C4, and C5. It is dome shaped and attaches peripherally to the lower rib cage. When the diaphragm contracts, it pulls downward on the lungs, decreasing intrapleural pressure, intrathoracic pressure, and airway pressure, thereby creating the pressure drop required for inspiratory air flow. Additionally, contraction of the diaphragm pushes downward on the abdominal cavity and increases abdominal pressure. If the abdominal muscles are relaxed, the abdomen will protrude during inspiration.

The parasternal and scalene muscles are active during quiet inspiration. During high levels of ventilation, the accessory muscles of inspiration are active including the external intercostal and sternocleidomastoid muscles. These muscles elevate and stabilize the rib cage to allow for larger tidal volumes.

Normally expiration is a passive process, accomplished by elastic recoil of the lungs. Expiratory muscles are recruited to maintain high levels of ventilation, as is seen during exercise, and they are employed during forced expiratory maneuvers such as a cough. Contraction of the internal intercostal muscles compresses the upper rib cage, increasing intrathoracic pressure and airway pressure, thereby establishing the pressure gradient required for higher expiratory air flows. Similarly contraction of the abdominal muscles compresses the abdominal cavity, pushes the abdominal contents upward against the diaphragm, and increases intrathoracic pressure and airway pressure.

Respiratory muscle strength is influenced by factors that influence strength of the other skeletal muscles. Strength declines in elderly people, in malnourished people, and in sedentary people. Moreover, women have less muscle mass and therefore less functional strength than men.

✦ **Lung compliance.** Lung compliance describes the elas-

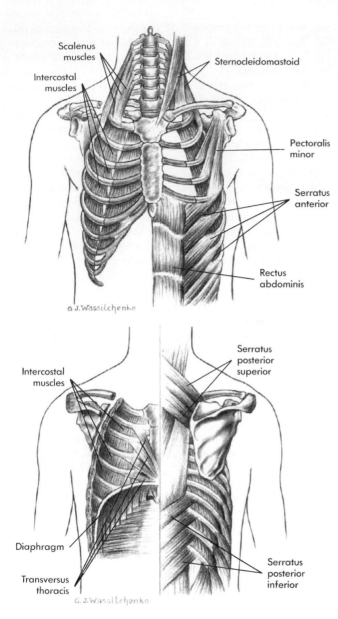

Fig. 18-2 **A & B,** Inspiratory muscles of the chest aid in inspiration and expiration. (From *Respiratory Disorders* by S.F. Wilson & J.F. Thompson, 1990, St. Louis: Mosby–Year Book. Copyright 1990 by Mosby–Year Book. Reprinted by permission.)

tic properties of the lungs. Conceptually, static compliance of the lungs is the change in pressure required to inflate the lungs a given volume. Under normal conditions the pressure-volume characteristics of the lungs are influenced by surfactant. Surfactant reduces the surface tension of alveoli, increasing their compliance and stabilizing them. Without this stabilizing effect there would be a tendency for the smaller alveoli to collapse at low lung volumes during expiration.

Stiff lungs have decreased compliance as seen in pulmonary interstitial fibrosis. The decreased compliance increases the work of breathing required to maintain alveolar ventilation.

✦ **Airway resistance.** Conceptually airway resistance is the pressure required to generate a given air flow. In the airways resistance to flow is inversely related to the diameter of the airways. The diameter of the airways can be decreased by inflammation of the airways, obstruction of the airways, and increased tone of airway smooth muscle. Increased airway resistance increases the work of breathing as seen in clients with COPD, CF, and asthma.

Control of Breathing

Breathing can be modified both involuntarily and voluntarily (Fig. 18-3). Involuntary control of breathing is accomplished primarily through the activity of (1) respiratory centers in the brainstem, (2) peripheral chemoreceptors, (3) central chemoreceptors, and (4) respiratory motor neurons. Voluntary control arises from the cerebral cortex.

✦ **Respiratory centers.** The respiratory centers are composed of interconnected neurons located bilaterally in the reticular substance of the medulla and pons. The basic spontaneous rhythm of breathing is established here. Chemoreceptors, proprioceptors, and the vagus nerve send afferent input to the respiratory centers where the sensory information is coordinated and neural output is initiated via the spinal motor neurons and efferent nerves.

✦ **Central chemoreceptors.** Central chemoreceptors are aggregates of cells in bilateral areas of the medulla that are distinct from respiratory center neurons. They are sensitive to elevations in the H^+ concentration in the surrounding extracellular fluid and respond by increasing the V_E. As the $Paco_2$ rises, CO_2 diffuses across the blood-brain barrier into the cerebrospinal fluid (CSF) where it combines with H_2O to form HCO_3^- and H^+. The CSF has less buffering capacity than the blood; consequently small increases in the partial pressure of carbon dioxide (Pco_2) are associated with greater increases in H^+ concentration. The central chemoreceptors are very sensitive to small changes in $Paco_2$ and are thought to be the major mechanism controlling the ventilatory response to CO_2.

✦ **Peripheral chemoreceptors.** Peripheral chemoreceptors are located at the bifurcation of the common carotid arteries (carotid bodies) and along the aortic arch (aortic bodies). In humans the carotid bodies play a bigger role than the aortic bodies.

The carotid bodies are well vascularized and have a high metabolic rate. Receptors in the carotid bodies and aortic bodies are stimulated by a fall in the partial pressure of oxygen (Po_2), rise in Pco_2, or rise in H^+ concentration in arterial blood. The peripheral chemoreceptors respond to a fall in partial pressure of arterial oxygen (Pao_2) below 60 mm Hg by stimulating the respiratory centers to increase ventilation. In CO_2 narcosis the ventilatory response to CO_2 is blunted, leaving only the hypoxic ventilatory response to stimulate ventilation.

✦ **Pulmonary mechanoreceptors.** Pulmonary mechanoreceptors are sensory receptors within the airways and lungs that transmit signals to the central nervous system through the vagus nerve. Three groups of receptors have been defined: (1) stretch receptors, (2) irritant receptors, and (3) juxtacapillary receptors. Stretch receptors in the smooth muscle of the airway primarily are sensitive to transmural or distending pressure. Irritant receptors line the epithelial

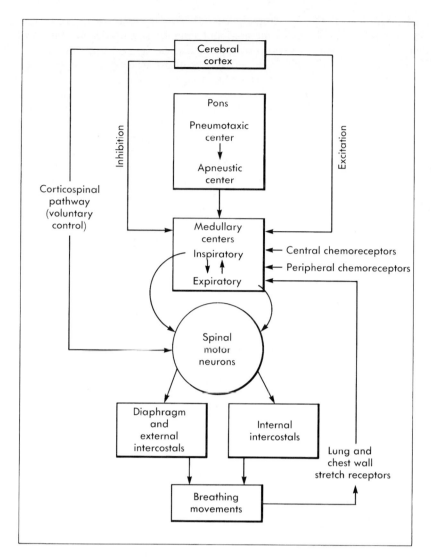

Fig. 18-3 A hypothetical diagram of information flow in the respiratory control system, including some of the inputs that establish respiratory drive. The feedback loops based on the effect of ventilation on blood gas composition are not shown. (From *Human Physiology,* 2nd ed. by D.F. Moffett, S.B. Moffett, and C.L. Schauf, 1993, St. Louis: Mosby–Year Book. Copyright 1993 by Mosby–Year Book. Reprinted by permission.)

layers of the airways and respond to a variety of stimuli, including chemical or mechanical stimulation or rapid inflation of the lungs. These receptors play an important role in defense of the lung by triggering coughing and sneezing and by regulating airway muscle tone and caliber. Juxtacapillary receptors (J-receptors) are located in alveolar walls close to the capillary network. J-receptors consist of the terminal branches of unmyelinated afferent nerve fibers and do not play an active role in normal breathing. Much of the dyspnea and rapid shallow breathing seen in persons with pulmonary congestion or interstitial lung disease may be attributed to activation of J-receptors.

◆ **Cerebral cortex.** Voluntary control of respiration is regulated by the cerebral cortex. Breathing patterns are modified by conscious control for talking, laughing, crying, and swallowing.

The voluntary conducting pathways in the spinal cord are distinct from those involved in involuntary regulation. Fibers from involuntary pathways can be injured while voluntary pathways remain intact and vice versa. Activity of the voluntary control system depends on the state of wakefulness. In central sleep apnea there is dysfunction of the involuntary system but voluntary control is maintained. Apnea occurs during sleep, but normal breathing resumes when the person is awake. Conversely, voluntary control may be impaired while involuntary function is maintained as in a high cervical spinal cord injury. In such a situation the person would respond normally to chemical and reflex stimuli but be unable to perform consciously controlled respiratory maneuvers.

Gas Exchange
◆ **Pulmonary circulation**

The pulmonary vascular system is a low-pressure system that is highly distensible. The mean pulmonary artery pressure is 15 mm Hg as compared with a mean aortic pressure of 100 mm Hg. Systolic and diastolic pressures in the pulmonary artery are 25 mm Hg and 8 mm Hg. The walls of the pulmonary artery are relatively thin with little smooth muscle. The pulmonary vascular system normally contains approximately 1 L of blood with 100 ml in the pulmonary capillary bed. The pulmonary capillary bed is composed of a dense network of short segments of capillaries surrounding the alveoli. The pulmonary capillaries are just large enough to allow red blood cells to pass through in single file, approximately 10 μm in diameter. After spending approximately 0.75 seconds in the pulmonary capillary, arterialized blood is collected in the pulmonary venous system.

The pulmonary vascular bed is a low-resistance system, and under normal conditions the distribution of pulmonary blood flow primarily is influenced passively by posture and exercise. At rest perfusion of the pulmonary capillary bed is greatest in the dependent portions of the lungs. In the upright position perfusion is greatest at the bases of the lungs. When lying on one side, perfusion is greatest in the inferior portion of the dependent lung. This uneven distribution of pulmonary blood flow is caused by hydrostatic pressure differences within the pulmonary vascular system. Because gravity hydrostatic pressures are greater in the dependent regions, distending the vessels and increasing the rate of flow. With mild exercise both the cardiac output and pulmonary blood flow increase, evening out hydrostatic pressures and evening out the distribution of blood flow in the pulmonary vascular bed.

Active vasoconstriction of the pulmonary vascular bed occurs under selected conditions. Regional vasoconstriction occurs in hypoxic areas of the lung, shunting blood flow away from hypoxic alveoli. This response primarily involves the small arterioles. In contrast systemic hypoxemia causes vasoconstriction of the pulmonary arteries and pulmonary hypertension.

The large airways are perfused by the bronchial circulation, which arises from the aorta and empties into the pulmonary veins. The bronchial circulation supplies the tissues of the larger airways, but it is not essential as it is disconnected after a lung transplant.

Gas Transport

♦ Oxygen transport. Most oxygen is transported to the peripheral tissues bound to hemoglobin (Hb), and minimal oxygen is transported as dissolved O_2. The difference in alveolar and pulmonary capillary Po_2 establishes the gradient for the diffusion of O_2 across the alveolar-capillary membrane. The arterial Po_2 in turn drives the binding of oxygen with Hb. The relationship between Po_2 and percent oxyhemoglobin saturation is described by the sigmoid-shaped oxyhemoglobin dissociation curve (Fig. 18-4). Normally the arterial Po_2 is 100 mm Hg and oxyhemoglobin saturation is 97.4%. However, normal Hb is highly saturated with oxygen at a Po_2 of 60 mm Hg; increments above 60 mm Hg do not add appreciably to further oxygen carrying capacity.

♦

NORMAL RANGE FOR ARTERIAL BLOOD GASES

Po_2	80-95 mm Hg
Pco_2	35-45 mm Hg
pH	7.35-7.45
HCO_3^-	21-28 mEq/L

From *Clinical Application of Blood Gases,* 5th ed., by B.A. Shapiro, W.T. Peruzzi, and R. Templin, 1994, St. Louis: Mosby–Year Book. Copyright 1994 by Mosby–Year Book. Reprinted by permission.

If the Po_2 drops below 60 mm Hg, there is an abrupt decrease in oxyhemoglobin saturation and a decrease in oxygen delivery to peripheral tissues.

Content in the box below illustrates the normal range of values for arterial blood gases. Delivery of O_2 to the tissues requires adequate cardiac output and tissue perfusion. As arterialized blood perfuses the tissues, O_2 is unloaded because of the lower Po_2 at the tissue level.

Changes in the relationship between oxyhemoglobin binding and Po_2 are reflected by shifts in the dissociation curve. A right-shifted curve can be caused by an increase in body temperature, increase in Pco_2, decrease in pH, and increase in 2,3-diphosphoglycerate (a product of red blood cell metabolism). A right-shifted curve decreases oxyhemoglobin binding Hb but enhances the release of oxygen at the tissue level. A left-shifted curve can be caused by a decrease in body temperature, decrease in Pco_2, increase in pH, and decrease in 2,3-diphosphoglycerate. A left-shifted curve increases oxyhemoglobin binding but reduces tissue extraction of oxygen. Abnormalities in Hb will also influence oxygen binding.

♦ Carbon dioxide transport. CO_2 is continually produced by cells throughout the body as an end-product of metabolism. The amount of CO_2 produced depends on the metabolic activity and on the dietary source of fuel. Carbon dioxide is transported from the peripheral tissues in three forms: dissolved in plasma, as carbamino compounds, and as bicarbonate. It is eliminated via the lungs, and elimination of CO_2 depends on an adequate level of V_A.

♦ Diffusion

Oxygen diffuses down its concentration gradient from the alveolar gases, across the alveolar-capillary membranes, through the plasma, across the red blood cell membrane, and within the red blood cell to combine with Hb. The rate of diffusion is directly proportional to the alveolar-capillary gradient of Po_2 and the cross-sectional area of the alveolar-

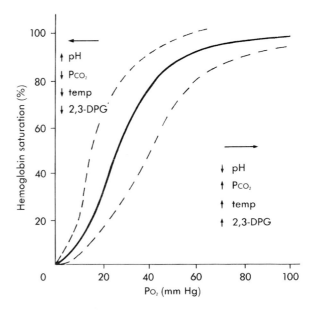

Fig. 18-4 Oxyhemoglobin dissociation curve relating the percentage of Hb saturation and Po_2. Solid line depicts normal curve. Dotted lines represent shift to the left or right.

capillary membrane and inversely proportional to the length of the diffusion path. Theoretically the diffusion capacity can be reduced by destruction of alveolar-capillary surface area as occurs in COPD or by a lengthening of the diffusion path as occurs in interstitial fibrosis. However, multiple factors must be present to impair gas exchange on the basis of a true diffusion defect.

✦ Ventilation-perfusion relationships

The efficiency of gas exchange is dependent on ventilation of the alveoli, perfusion of the pulmonary capillary bed, and the matching of ventilation and perfusion. Uniform distribution of ventilation and perfusion throughout the lungs would be ideal conditions for gas exchange. But in the healthy individual ventilation and perfusion are not evenly distributed throughout the lungs. In the upright position a greater portion of ventilation and perfusion are distributed to the base of the lungs, but the difference is greater for perfusion. Consequently the ventilation-perfusion ratio increases from the base to the apex of the lungs with an average ratio of 0.8, an alveolar Po_2 of 104 mm Hg, and an arterial Po_2 of 100 mm Hg.

ALTERED PHYSIOLOGIC FUNCTIONING

Major alterations in physiologic functioning can be categorized as either alterations in gas exchange or alterations in ventilation. Most chronic lung diseases involve a combination of both, especially in the severe stages of the disease. Clinically clients with chronic lung disease experience a slow progressive worsening of their condition with episodic acute exacerbations secondary to upper and lower respiratory tract infections. When impairment of lung function is mild, the clinical evidence of altered functioning may be apparent only during acute exacerbations. When impairment of lung function is severe, the clinical evidence of altered functioning will be readily visible on a daily basis.

Alterations in Gas Exchange

Alterations in gas exchange are primarily reflected by hypoxemia, decreased Pao_2. Alveolar hypoventilation and abnormalities of diffusion can cause hypoxemia, but the most common cause of hypoxemia is a mismatch of ventilation and perfusion. Chronic problems with gas exchange are described below in five clinical examples of chronic lung disease: COPD, idiopathic pulmonary fibrosis, BPD, and CF. Acute problems with gas exchange occur in clients with respiratory tract infections.

People with severe COPD demonstrate problems with gas exchange. In clients with COPD the development of hypoxemia is primarily related to mismatch of ventilation and perfusion, though diffusion limitations may contribute to hypoxemia. Clients with COPD develop hyperplasia of the mucous glands within the large and central airways, producing excessive secretions. Clients with an emphysematous component develop enlargement of the airspaces secondary to destruction of alveoli and loss of segments of the pulmonary capillary bed. These pathologic changes result in an uneven distribution of ventilation to the alveoli and uneven distribution of perfusion to the pulmonary capillaries, causing hypoxemia. Hypoxemia results when the pulmonary capillaries perfuse unventilated alveoli, dumping unoxygenated blood into the arterial side of the circulation.

Similarly ventilation is wasted by ventilating unperfused alveoli, thereby decreasing the effective V_A and increasing V_{DS}. Clients with hypoxemia develop pulmonary vascular hypertension secondary to hypoxic vasoconstriction of the pulmonary vascular bed. Prolonged pulmonary hypertension ultimately leads to right-sided failure of the heart or cor pulmonale.

It is well established that smoking is the major cause of COPD, though the precise mechanism is not understood (Davis & Novotny, 1989). The risk of COPD is proportional to the overall lifetime exposure to cigarette smoke. Additionally occupational exposure to dust also may contribute to the risk of developing COPD (Becklake, 1989).

Clients with interstitial lung disease experience problems with gas exchange as seen in idiopathic interstitial pulmonary fibrosis. Alveolar-capillary membranes are destroyed by progressive interstitial and intraalveolar fibrosis. These architectural changes cause an uneven distribution of ventilation and perfusion, resulting in a mismatch of ventilation and perfusion. Severe hypoxemia can result.

The etiology of interstitial lung disease includes organic and inorganic dusts, gases, drugs, poisons, radiation, allergic response, and trauma (Fulmer & Katzenstein, 1993). For example, silica dust and antineoplastic drugs commonly cause interstitial lung disease. However, the etiology is unknown for many forms of interstitial lung disease including sarcoidosis, interstitial diseases associated with the collagen-vascular disorders, and idiopathic pulmonary fibrosis.

Characteristic features of BPD include pulmonary edema, airway obstruction, fibrosis, and areas of emphysema alternating with areas of atelectasis (Merritt & Boynton, 1988). Clinically these changes result in ventilation-perfusion mismatch and lead to hypoxemia.

The factors most commonly identified in the development of BPD include premature birth and its inherent lung immaturity, surfactant deficiency, and lung injury caused by mechanical ventilation (barotrauma) and oxygen toxicity (Bancalari & Sosenko, 1990; Boynton, 1988; Hazinski, 1990; Northway, 1992a). The relative contributions of these factors is still widely debated; however, prematurity, and more specifically, low birth weight, is recognized as the most important predictor of BPD (Fiascone, Rhodes, Grandgeorge, & Knapp, 1989; Hazinski, 1990; Northway, 1992b). BPD occurs most commonly in premature infants. Less commonly BPD is observed in term infants with conditions such as pneumonia, meconium aspiration, cyanotic congenital heart disease, and apnea (Merritt & Boynton, 1988).

Acute alterations in gas exchange are observed in clients with respiratory tract infections when the infection results in an area of consolidation in portions of the lung. Hypoxemia results when the pulmonary capillaries perfuse consolidated and atelectatic alveoli. The extent of consolidation and atelectasis will determine the severity of hypoxemia.

Alterations in Ventilation

Alveolar hyperventilation and hypoventilation are clinically defined by the $Paco_2$. Hyperventilation causes the $Paco_2$ to fall below 40 mm Hg, and this is commonly seen in anxious people waiting to have an arterial puncture for measurement of blood gas values. In contrast, alveolar hypoventilation causes the $Paco_2$ to rise above 45 mm Hg, and this is seen in people with severe lung disease and neuromuscular disease. Ventilatory failure is the extreme form of alveolar hypoventilation, characterized by $Paco_2$ above 45 mm Hg and Pao_2 below 60 mm Hg (Roussos, 1993).

Alveolar hypoventilation results from either an inadequate V_E and/or an excessive V_{DS}. Inadequate V_E can be caused by alterations in respiratory mechanics, inadequate ventilatory drive, and respiratory muscle weakness, whereas excessive V_{DS} can be caused by either the mismatch of ventilation and perfusion or by shallow breathing.

Clients with very severe COPD are more likely to experience chronic alveolar hypoventilation as demonstrated by chronic hypercapnia. Hypercapnia is seen most commonly in clients with COPD with a forced expiratory volume in 1 second (FEV_1) of less than 1.0 L, though not all clients with severe air flow obstruction have chronic alveolar hypoventilation (Lane, Howell, & Giblin, 1968). The precise mechanisms for development of alveolar hypoventilation are not well understood in clients with COPD, but evidence points to blunting of the ventilatory response to chemical stimuli such as hypoxia and hypercapnia and/or the development of rapid shallow breathing patterns to reduce the work of breathing and protect against respiratory muscle fatigue (Fleetham, Arnup, & Anthonisen, 1984; Roussos & Macklem, 1982).

Clients with COPD have increased airway resistance, which increases the work of breathing so that the respiratory muscles must generate higher forces to maintain a given level of ventilation. Hyperinflation of the chest wall places the inspiratory muscles at a mechanical disadvantage, reducing their ability to generate the forces required for ventilation. Additionally, nutritional deficits in many clients cause muscle wasting and loss of respiratory muscle mass. These factors predispose clients to respiratory muscle fatigue and rapid shallow breathing, which increases the V_{DS}. In clients with severe COPD, the mismatch of ventilation and perfusion also contributes to the development of alveolar hypoventilation.

Clients with neuromuscular disease develop alveolar hypoventilation secondary to respiratory muscle weakness and decreased compliance of the lungs and chest wall. The primary problem is related to inspiratory muscle weakness and an inability to take a deep breath, leading to a decline in V_E. Secondarily, the reduced vital capacity leads to the development of microatelectasis and increased stiffness of the chest wall, thereby increasing the work of breathing and further contributing to the decline in V_E.

In the early stages of neuromuscular disease, mild respiratory muscle weakness can exist without clinical consequences if the respiratory muscles are capable of meeting ventilatory demands and generating an effective cough. Respiratory muscle fatigue and ventilatory failure will occur when the ventilatory demands exceed the ability of the respiratory muscles.

The extent of respiratory muscle involvement depends on the nature of the pathophysiology and its pattern of progression. In Duchenne's muscular dystrophy the onset of respiratory muscle weakness occurs early in the course of the disease and progresses slowly until death (De Troyer & Pride, 1985; Mier, 1990). In amyotrophic lateral sclerosis

(ALS), respiratory muscle weakness is secondary to denervation atrophy, starting with the abdominal muscles, which are expiratory muscles, and eventually progressing to the inspiratory muscles. In ALS the progression of respiratory muscle weakness is faster than in other neuromuscular diseases. In spinal cord injured persons, the extent of respiratory muscle involvement depends on the level and nature of the injury. Persons with high cervical lesions above C4 typically require mechanical ventilation. Persons with midcervical lesions (C4-C8) experience severe expiratory muscle weakness and/or paralysis and mild inspiratory muscle weakness. Many spinal cord injury lesions are oblique, interrupting innervation to one side of the diaphragm and producing severe diaphragmatic weakness on only one side.

In CF individuals have two abnormal copies of a defective CF gene. In turn, this defective gene codes for a defective or mutant CFTR protein. With a mutant CFTR protein, chloride movement is inhibited, and the balance of sodium, chloride, and water is disrupted in affected cells (Tizzano & Buchwald, 1992). This imbalance results in classic findings in CF; namely, dehydrated secretions and mucous obstruction in the ducts of exocrine glands.

CF affects multiple organ systems to varying degrees in different individuals, but lung disease is the major cause of morbidity and mortality (Boat, Welsh, & Beaudet, 1989; Lloyd-Still, 1983; McMullen, 1991). Generally clients with normal pancreatic function have milder lung disease, and this is thought to be related to improved nutritional status (Tizzano & Buchwald, 1992).

The lung disease in CF results from an ongoing cycle of obstruction, infection, inflammation, and injury. Dehydrated secretions block airway passages. These secretions also contain large amounts of uninhibited proteolytic enzymes, which contribute to tissue injury and impaired mucociliary transport (Zach, 1990). Obstruction leads to endobronchial infection. Two bacteria are primarily responsible for infections in the CF lung; namely, *Staphylococcus aureus* and *Pseudomonas aeruginosa*. Once established, these bacteria will continue to colonize the CF lung. However, clinical improvement is possible with antimicrobial therapies that reduce bacterial colony counts (Boat et al., 1989; Lloyd-Still, 1983; McMullen, 1991).

Chronic obstruction and infection cause progressive deterioration of lung structure and function. Early changes include air trapping, airway inflammation, and peribronchial thickening. These early changes are more prominent in the upper lobes. As lung injury continues, changes become more diffuse with evidence of bronchiectasis, fibrosis, and cyst formation. Restrictive lung disease compounds what began as obstructive lung disease (Boat et al., 1989).

Hypoventilation and hypercapnia also are observed in BPD as a result of ineffective ventilation due to airway damage and obstruction (Bancalari & Gerhardt, 1986; Fiascone et al., 1989; Heldt, 1988). Characteristic interstitial markings or strand densities are evidenced on the chest radiograph (Bancalari, Abdenour, Feller, & Gannon, 1979; Boynton, 1988). Pulmonary function is compromised by increased airway resistance, decreased compliance, increased dead space, and increased airway reactivity (Conte, 1991; Hazinski, 1990; Tepper, 1988).

Clients with neuromuscular disease, COPD, and CF demonstrate respiratory muscle weakness, and they may experience further reductions in respiratory muscle strength during viral infections of the respiratory tract (Mier-Jedrzejowicz, Brophy, & Green, 1988; Poponick, Jacobs, Supinski, & DiMarco, 1992). Additionally viral infections cause increased secretions in the airways and a secondary bacterial infection of the lungs, thereby increasing the work of breathing. Consequently in clients with severe respiratory muscle weakness, the increased work of breathing and reduction in strength may be sufficient to trigger ventilatory failure.

Nursing Assessment

Evaluation of the client with actual or potential pulmonary compromise must include a comprehensive assessment of physiologic as well as biopsychosocial aspects of the problems presented. An individualized approach based on the person's present life situation, perceptions of the problem, concurrent medical conditions, social relationships, and available support systems must be used. The nurse needs this information to identify the care, learning, and emotional needs of clients and their families.

✦ Subjective assessment

Symptoms are the subjective manifestations of disease. Three respiratory symptoms frequently prompt a person to seek medical attention: (1) dyspnea, (2) cough and expectoration, and (3) chest pain. Constitutional symptoms such as fever, weight loss, fatigue, exercise intolerance, and sleep disturbance also may be present, so a total review of body systems should be conducted. For purposes of this text, however, the three respiratory-related complaints frequently most cited are discussed.

Dyspnea. Dyspnea is the sensation of difficulty breathing, usually associated with an increased effort to breathe (Carrieri & Janson-Bjerklie, 1984). Dyspnea manifests itself in many ways and is described by clients in different ways including shortness of breath, difficulty breathing, suffocating, and chest tightness. Dyspnea is the primary symptom for many clients with cardiac and lung disease including COPD, pulmonary fibrosis, asthma, pulmonary hypertension, and congestive heart disease. Additionally dyspnea can be a problem for obese people, pregnant women, and some people with neuromuscular disease (Harver & Mahler, 1990). The intensity of dyspnea does not necessarily correlate with the extent of impairment as some people with severe lung disease report minimal dyspnea, whereas others report intense dyspnea with mild lung disease.

Clinical assessment of dyspnea includes a description of its frequency and intensity. It is useful to ask about the onset of the symptom (acute or chronic), precipitating events, duration, associated symptoms, relieving factors, and identifiable patterns (Carrieri & Janson-Bjerklie, 1986).

In the clinical setting the intensity of dyspnea can be measured with a Borg Category-Ratio Scale for rating of perceived breathlessness, whereby clients rate their dyspnea on a scale from 0 = no dyspnea to 10 = maximal dyspnea (see Box above). The scale is enlarged on an 8.5- by 11-inch sheet of paper, and clients are asked to point to the number on the scale that best describes the intensity of their

---

BORG CATEGORY-RATIO SCALE FOR RATING OF PERCEIVED BREATHLESSNESS

0 Nothing at all
0.5 Very, very slight
1 Very slight
2 Slight
3 Moderate
4 Somewhat severe
5 Severe
6
7 Very severe
8
9
10 Very, very severe (almost maximal)

BREATHLESSNESS SCALES FROM THE ATS-DLD QUESTIONNAIRE

1. Are you troubled by shortness of breath when hurrying on the level or walking up a slight hill?
2. (If yes) Do you have to walk slower than people of your age on the level because of breathlessness?
3. (If yes) Do you ever have to stop for breath when walking at your own pace on the level?
4. (If yes) Do you ever have to stop for breath after walking about 100 yards (or after a few minutes) on the level?
5. (If yes) Are you too breathless to leave the house or breathless on dressing or undressing?

Adapted from "Recommended Respiratory Disease Questionnaires for Use with Adults and Children in Epidemiological Research (Part 2)" by B.G. Ferris, 1978, *American Review of Respiratory Disease, 118,* 7-53.

---

breathlessness. This scale is flexible and can be used to rate the intensity of dyspnea at rest or during physical activity. Different people will use the scale differently, some appearing to be in acute distress while rating their dyspnea as minimal, whereas others will use the full range of the scale reporting maximal dyspnea when they appear to be extremely dyspneic. Consequently with this type of scale, one cannot compare the intensity of dyspnea from one client to the next. But people do tend to use the scale in a consistent manner over time, allowing the clinician to determine if dyspnea is better or worse.

To crudely assess the general intensity of dyspnea, the nurse can use one of the scales that were originally designed for large population studies of lung disease. The breathlessness scale from the Recommended Respiratory Disease Questionnaire (ATS-DLD-78) would be appropriate for this purpose (refer to the box above).

Chronic dyspnea can contribute greatly to functional disability. Adequate breathing becomes a priority need. Activities that produce symptoms or decreased energy are often eliminated, despite the importance they may have had in a person's life. Lifestyles and interests may change accordingly, at great cost to a person in terms of physical, social, and emotional well-being.

Cough. Coughing occurs to clear the airways of secretions and to protect the airways from aspiration and/or inhalation of noxious substances. A cough becomes abnormal when it is persistent, irritating, painful, or productive. It can be acute or chronic, associated with other symptoms (pain, wheezing, dyspnea, syncope), productive or dry, effective or ineffective (unable to clear secretions). All data pertinent to the development of the cough must be obtained. For example, a person may note that the cough followed a recent illness or respiratory tract infection, is exacerbated by seasonal or environmental conditions, or occurs only at a certain time of day. Most persons with a chronic cough notice that it becomes worse when they lie down at night or when they arise in the morning. Persons who cough during or shortly after eating may have a problem with aspiration of food or fluid into the tracheobronchial tree.

Characteristics of the cough including quality, frequency, and alleviating factors must be reviewed. A change in the usual characteristics of a chronic cough also should be investigated. The presence of a cough alone is nonspecific but when associated with other signs and symptoms may suggest a diagnosis.

The production of sputum, including quantity and character, should be assessed. Normally people do not produce noticeable amounts of sputum, but clients with chronic bronchitis expectorate small to moderate amounts of mucoid material each day, often in the morning. The volume is greatly increased with bronchiectasis and CF. A change to thick yellow or green sputum may indicate the onset of an infection in the lower respiratory tract. Some people are predisposed to respiratory tract infections including persons with COPD, bronchiectasis, CF, and spinal cord injury at the midcervical level. In CF sputum is frequently thick, green, and purulent, reflecting *Pseudomonas aeruginosa* infection. Anaerobic bacterial infections may produce foul-smelling sputum.

Hemoptysis generally originates from a problem in the airways, parenchyma, or pulmonary vasculature. The severity varies from blood-streaked sputum, as sometimes seen in chronic bronchitis to frank bleeding, which may accompany pulmonary infarction. Frequently no definite diagnosis can be made. However, the symptom is always worrisome and requires further investigation. A small amount of blood streaking in the sputum is not uncommon in clients with CF, especially in older clients with CF. It is usually self-limiting and does not require intervention.

Chest pain. Chest pain associated with respiratory disease usually occurs secondary to involvement of the parietal pleura, diaphragm, or mediastinum—all of which are extensively innervated with sensory nerve fibers. Lung tissue and visceral pleura do not have these sensory fibers, and as a result significant disease may exist in these areas without producing any pain. Moreover, clients with spinal cord injury at or above the cervical level will not perceive sensations of chest pain.

Nerve endings in the parietal pleura may be stimulated by inflammation or stretching the membrane. Involvement of the pleura may be secondary to an underlying parenchymal lesion in the same area. "Pleuritic" pain may vary in intensity but is often abrupt in onset, becomes worse with inspiration, is well localized, and is generally not relieved by splinting. Diaphragm involvement can cause pain to be referred to the neck and upper shoulder.

Disease in any of the mediastinal structures can cause pain in that area. Pain may be retrosternal or precordial with radiation to the neck or arms or through the back. Causes may be of the following origins: respiratory (tracheobronchitis, pulmonary emboli), cardiovascular (myocardial infarction, dissecting aneurysm), or gastrointestinal (esophageal reflux), and associated symptoms will vary accordingly.

Chest wall pain also may produce considerable distress. It can originate from intercostal or pectoral muscles, ribs, and cartilage or be due to pressure or inflammation along the neural pathway. Usually chest wall pain is described as constant local aching, aggravated by movement and tender to palpation. Complaints of chest pain may be related to coughing paroxysms, and a recent history of trauma or strain should be investigated.

Complaints of chest pain are highly subjective and may be difficult to evaluate. A detailed description—including onset, frequency, duration, and precipitating and relieving factors—must be obtained. Associated factors such as dyspnea, exercise, position change, and emotional environment can help differentiate the cause.

The chronology of presenting respiratory symptoms aids in establishing a nursing diagnosis and developing an appropriate plan of care. Previous medical data and a personal history must be obtained to assess the current situation. Past or concurrent medical problems, present treatment regimens, compliance behaviors, the incidence of respiratory disease, and a complete history of smoking habits should be reviewed. Questions about smoking should include the age at which the habit began, the type and amount of tobacco used (cigarettes, cigar, pipe, snuff, chewing tobacco), current smoking habits, successful and unsuccessful attempts to quit, and reasons for continuing to smoke or for quitting. This information can indicate a readiness for participating in a plan for pulmonary rehabilitation.

Additional information may be elicited, depending on the situation presented at the time of the interview. Evaluation of the psychosocial environment of the client provides essential information in developing an appropriate plan of care.

✦ Objective assessment

Respiratory dysfunction is often the result of other body system impairments, so each new client must have a complete physical examination (Seidel, Ball, Dains, & Benedict, 1991). The focus of this discussion, however, is limited to the basic principles involved in evaluating the respiratory system.

Whenever possible, the client should be seen in a quiet, well-lit room. Examination of the chest involves the techniques of inspection, palpation, percussion, and auscultation. The underlying anatomy of the lungs and thorax must be envisioned at all times during the examination. As each area is assessed, it is always compared with the same region on the other side.

Inspection. Inspection begins during the interview. At this time the nurse observes the client's general appearance, skin color, presence and degree of respiratory distress, character and rate of respirations, quality of voice, pattern of speech, interruptions by coughing or breathlessness, flaring nostrils, use of pursed-lip breathing (PLB), and assumed posture.

Examination of the anterior thorax is best performed with the client supine and the chest exposed. The rib cage should move symmetrically and expand equally as the person breathes. Areas of decreased movement may represent obstruction of air flow, disease of the underlying lung or pleura, splinting part of the chest secondary to pain, or paralysis of the respiratory muscles.

Use of accessory muscles of respiration and retraction or bulging of the interspaces during breathing should be noted. During inspiration, if the abdominal muscles are relaxed, the abdomen will protrude outward. Expiration normally occurs passively as the abdomen returns to the resting position. Paradoxic motion of the abdomen during quiet breathing often indicates abnormal or absent use of the diaphragm as seen in clients with high cervical lesions of the spinal cord.

The shape of the chest is evaluated for pectus excavatum (depression of the lower portion of the sternum) or pectus carinatum (anterior displacement of the sternum, which increases the anteroposterior diameter). The general configuration of the chest is best viewed with the client in a sitting position. The adult thorax normally has an anteroposterior diameter less than the transverse diameter. Advanced age may increase the anteroposterior diameter slightly, and in the client with COPD the increase may be significant.

The thoracic spine is normally straight when viewed posteriorly and has a gentle anterior concave appearance when viewed from the side. The rib cage is also evaluated for deformity. Abnormalities of the rib cage can interfere with chest expansion, causing decreased compliance and reduced lung volume. Common deformities that can lead to a restrictive defect include kyphosis, scoliosis, and kyphoscoliosis. Ankylosing spondylitis causes a straight, immobile spinal column that limits expansion of the chest. Trauma to the chest wall can cause a flail chest, which would appear as a paradoxic movement of a portion of the chest wall.

Cyanosis also is best noted in daylight and best detected in the nail beds and buccal mucosa. Cyanosis reflects severe hypoxemia of arterial blood to a sufficient degree to desaturate Hb. Approximately 5 g/100 ml of reduced Hb must be present to change skin color from the usual pink to blue. For this reason, cyanosis usually is not seen with anemia until hypoxemia is severe, whereas clients with polycythemia may appear cyanotic with less hypoxemia present. The most common cause for cyanosis is generalized hypoxemia (central cyanosis), but hypoxemia also may occur secondary to peripheral vasoconstriction.

Palpation. Palpation is used to evaluate the underlying structure and function of the chest, detect areas of tenderness of crepitation, and assess respiratory excursion. The anterior chest is palpated by placing the hands over the anterolateral aspect of the chest, with the thumbs extended along the costal margins. As the client inhales, the chest should expand equally and symmetrically. Posterior chest excursion is evaluated by grasping the sides of the rib cage and placing the thumbs parallel to the tenth rib. Tenderness noted on palpation should be evaluated; it often indicates a musculoskeletal origin of chest pain. The intercostal spaces should be palpated for the presence of a tumor. Swelling or crepitation must be further investigated.

Fremitus refers to the transmission of voice-generated or vibrating sounds to the surface of the chest. By placing the palmar surface of the hands over comparative areas of the chest as the client speaks, the examiner can determine if there is normal, increased, or decreased fremitus. A variety of chest conditions can alter the transmission of sounds. Decreased transmission can be secondary to weakness of the voice; obstruction of the airway; or the collection of air, fluid, or tissue in the pleural space. Increased density of lung tissue as seen with consolidation or tumor mass increases fremitus if the airway remains patent.

Percussion. Percussion notes are produced by fingers striking the chest and creating a sound and a palpable vibration, helping to evaluate lung tissue underlying the chest wall. Percussion can be performed either directly by tapping areas of the chest with a flexed finger, or indirectly by tapping the distal portion of the interposed middle finger of the opposite hand. Movement of the striking finger should be from the wrist, with a quick direct blow and the lightest touch able to elicit a sound.

Symmetric areas of the chest are percussed systematically from side to side down the chest wall. Bony structures such as the scapulae need not be percussed. Healthy, air-filled lung produces a different sound from fluid-filled lung or solid tissue. The quality ranges from dull to tympanitic. Increased density is accompanied by a loss of resonance and dullness, as seen when percussing over solid organs, areas of consolidation, or fluid-filled spaces. Hyperresonance accompanies an increased accumulation of air such as hyperinflation or pneumothorax.

Diaphragm location and excursion also should be evaluated by percussion. The lower posterior lung fields are percussed down in small increments until a change in sound is heard. The distance between levels of dullness at deep inspiration and deep expiration is compared to evaluate movement of the diaphragm. Normal excursion ranges from 4 to 6 cm. A low-lying diaphragm with limited excursion often accompanies hyperinflation. Diaphragm paralysis, atelectasis, or pleural effusion may be accompanied by elevation of the diaphragm and impaired movement.

Auscultation. Auscultation of the chest allows the examiner to evaluate the quality and intensity of breath sounds and adventitious lung sounds that may indicate a respiratory disorder. Every nurse should be familiar with normal breath sounds so that abnormalities can be noted readily.

Auscultation should be performed in quiet surroundings to block out extraneous environmental noise. The client should be seated in an upright, comfortable position when possible. If weakness or debilitation prohibits this position, the client should be turned from side to side to enable complete examination of all lung fields. Throughout the assessment, the underlying anatomy of the lungs must be considered in order to describe the location of findings correctly.

The diaphragm of the stethoscope generally is used because lung sounds have a high frequency. The bell may be easier to use on very thin or small clients, but it should be placed firmly so that it functions as a diaphragm. The stethoscope always should be placed directly on the chest wall because clothing produces artifact that can interfere considerably with accurate findings.

The client is instructed to breathe somewhat deeper than usual, with the mouth open in a relaxed, unforced manner. Assessment must be systematic. The examiner listens to all lobes on the anterior, posterior, and lateral chest for a complete respiratory cycle in each position and then auscultates from side to side, comparing symmetric areas of the lungs, moving from top to bottom.

Lung sounds are evaluated for location, pitch, intensity, appearance in the respiratory cycle, and distinctive characteristics. The quality of breath sounds varies over different parts of the chest, depending on the proximity of the auscultated site to the large airways.

Vesicular breath sounds are heard over most of the chest and are considered "normal." They have a soft, muffled quality likened to the rustle of trees and the inspiratory component is longer than the expiratory component with a ratio of 3:1. Lung tissue is believed to serve as a filter that changes quality and intensity.

Breath sounds heard over large airways, such as the trachea and major bronchi, are described as "bronchial" and have a hollow, tubular sound. Generally the expiratory component is at least equal to or slightly longer than the inspiratory phase, often with a slight pause between the two.

Bronchovesicular breath sounds are intermediate sound between vesicular and bronchial sounds and can be heard around the upper half of the sternum and in the intrascapular area. Bronchovesicular sounds are more muffled than bronchial breathing, with no pause between inspiration and expiration.

Bronchial and bronchovesicular breath sounds are abnormal if heard in any area other than the normal locations. Breath sounds are transmitted more readily through areas of consolidation than through normal lung parenchyma. For this reason, auscultation over areas of lung consolidation frequently yields bronchial sounds.

Vocal sounds are distorted when transmitted through consolidated portions of the lung. Normally the spoken word sounds soft, muffled, and often barely audible. Over consolidated areas of the lungs, words are heard with increased clarity and intensity. Egophony refers to the transformation of the letter "E" to sound like a nasal "A" over the involved area. Whispered sounds are heard with increased intensity and clarity (whispered pectoriloquy) over consolidated areas of the lung.

Breath sounds will be decreased or absent when the rate of air flow is decreased as seen in persons with increased airway resistance and excessive secretions. Shallow breathing from weakness, obesity, or neuromuscular disorders also will produce diminished breath sounds. Finally, transmission of breath sounds may be diminished by excess subcutaneous fat or pleural effusion.

Adventitious lung sounds are classified as either continuous or discontinuous. Crackles are discontinuous breath sounds of an explosive quality with a low to medium pitch.

Crackles range in quality and intensity from fine to coarse and are heard primarily during inspiration. Crackles are thought to reflect turbulent flow through the airways and the opening sounds in small airways and alveoli. They may or may not clear with coughing. Crackles are commonly heard with pulmonary edema, atelectasis, pneumonia, and interstitial lung disease.

Wheezes are continuous sounds, frequently described as musical. They can be high or low in pitch and can occur during both inspiration and/or expiration. Wheezes are caused by air flow through obstructed airways caused by bronchospasm, secretions, compression, mucosal swelling, and/or a foreign body.

When pleural surfaces become inflamed or roughened, a characteristic sound, a pleural friction rub, can be heard. Often a grating sound or vibration associated with breathing can be heard over the site of discomfort. Many conditions may be associated with a pleural friction rub including pleurisy, tuberculosis, pulmonary infarction, pneumonia, and primary and metastatic carcinoma.

✦ Diagnostic studies

Accurate medical diagnosis of a pulmonary problem usually requires laboratory and radiologic data. Nurses play a major role in client and family education throughout the assessment and ongoing evaluation. Together with other members of the rehabilitation team, the nurse works to establish a complete profile of information on which client care decisions can be based.

Establishing a nursing diagnosis often depends on assessment of the client's functional level. Two common and helpful testing procedures that contribute to the functional assessment of the client with pulmonary problems are pulmonary function tests and arterial blood gas analysis.

Pulmonary function testing provides an objective, noninvasive means of documenting pulmonary impairment. Pulmonary function tests include spirometry to establish the extent of air flow obstruction and lung volumes by body plethysmography or helium dilution to establish the extent of hyperinflation or restrictive lung disease. The most useful of these measurements for the nurse to know are the following:

Vital capacity (VC): maximum amount of air exhaled from the point of maximum inspiration

Forced expiratory volume in 1 second (FEV_1): volume of air exhaled during the first second of a forced vital capacity maneuver

Functional residual capacity (FRC): volume of air remaining in the lungs at the end-expiratory position

Residual volume (RV): volume of air remaining in the lungs after maximum exhalation

Total lung capacity (TLC): volume of air in the lungs after maximum inspiration

Interpretation of results of pulmonary function tests depends on proper performance of the test; the client's ability to understand and perform the maneuvers; equipment; and the use of standards of measurement considering the variations attributed to age, sex, and height. There is a wide range of normal values, and at least three forced expiratory maneuvers should be done with each testing. The results are interpreted in conjunction with available clinical data. Pulmonary function testing can be repeated periodically to document progression of lung disease.

Arterial blood gas values are used to evaluate oxygenation, ventilation, and acid-base balance. Routine arterial blood gases are evaluated for PO_2, PCO_2, and pH. Many persons with pulmonary disease have a complex, mixed picture of abnormalities that can be better understood if periodic monitoring of arterial blood gas values is performed. Blood gas determinations also help determine the need for supplemental O_2, a decision that must be based on objective data.

Pharmacologic Therapy

For patients with COPD the goal of drug therapy is to reduce the work of breathing by decreasing air flow obstruction and decreasing inflammation of the airways. Commonly prescribed drugs are listed in the following Box.

The preceding pharmacologic therapy commonly is prescribed in a stepped approach, according to the order presented in the box below. Clinical response to pharmacologic therapy varies; hence the response to each drug is evaluated before adding another drug to the regimen. If clinical improvements are observed with a drug it is continued, and additional drugs are added only if the clinical response is suboptimal. Initially ipratropium is prescribed for its bronchodilating effects. If optimal treatment is not achieved with ipratropium, one of the inhaled beta$_2$ agonists is added to the regimen and eventually oral theophylline is added if necessary. Inhaled corticosteroids are prescribed routinely for clients with asthma, whereas oral corticosteroids are prescribed during the acute phase of an exacerbation. The dose is tapered and discontinued as soon as possible because of the multiple side effects associated with prolonged use of oral corticosteroids.

Additionally pneumococcal vaccine and revaccination every 6 years is recommended for clients with COPD. Influenza vaccine is recommended on an annual basis. Exacerbations commonly are triggered by viral infections, but broad-spectrum antibiotics are administered to prevent secondary bacterial infections as described later in this chapter.

Inhaled medications are preferred because the same beneficial effects can be obtained with smaller doses than would be required if the medication were given systemically, maximizing therapeutic effects and minimizing potential side effects. Inhaled medications are best administered with a metered dose inhaler (MDI) and spacer device to promote deposition of drugs deep into the airways (Fig. 18-5). When only the MDI is used, approximately 25% to 29% of the drug is deposited in the lungs because the spray hits the back of the throat, depositing much of the drug in the oropharyngeal region (Kim, Eldridge, & Sackner, 1987). The percent deposited in the lung can be increased by timing of inhalation and activation of the MDI, followed by breath holding. However, timing and coordination are difficult for many clients, and spacer devices are available to simplify the required procedure and to improve deposition of the drug. With a spacer device the droplets are suspended in the device long enough for the carrier molecule to evaporate, leaving the smaller molecule of drug to be carried deep into the airways. Spacer devices increase deposition of the drug in the lungs, but they are too difficult for small children to use. Nebulizers are used to administer inhaled medications in small children because they are very simple to use.

For clients with CF respiratory medications generally include antibiotics, bronchodilators, and cromolyn sodium. Broad-spectrum antibiotics are used during exacerbations to treat bacterial infections of the lower respiratory tract. Parenteral and oral antibiotics generally are used for acute exacerbations. Inhaled antibiotics may be used episodically or more continuously to treat chronic infection and improve respiratory status. Bronchodilators and cromolyn sodium

---

♦

PHARMACOLOGIC THERAPY FOR CLIENTS WITH COPD*

Anticholinergic agents (inhaled)
Ipratropium
Beta$_2$ agonist (inhaled)
Terbutaline
Albuterol
Bitolterol
Pirbuterol
Theophylline (oral)
Corticosteroids (inhaled, oral)

*Note: See a pharmacology text for details related to dose and side effects.

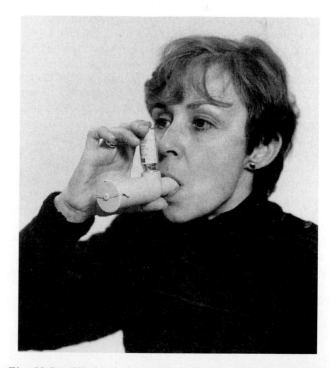

Fig. 18-5 Client using an MDI and spacer device to improve delivery of drugs into the airways. (Courtesy Healthscan Inc., Cedar Grove, NJ.)

are used to treat reactive airway disease. If upper airway problems are present, nasal cromolyn sodium or nasal corticosteroids are used to treat chronic inflammation and nasal polyps. A new mucolytic agent, rhDNase (combinant human deoxyribonuclease), is also currently under investigation for use in CF.

For children with BPD, pharmacologic therapy to enhance respiratory status depends on clinical manifestations. Theophylline is begun in premature infants to control apneic episodes and may be continued for apnea and/or reactive airway disease. Corticosteroids are used in infants to improve respiratory status related to BPD and to facilitate weaning from mechanical ventilation. Corticosteroids also are used intermittently for exacerbations of reactive airway disease. Antibiotics are used during exacerbations, and bronchodilators are prescribed if there is evidence of reactive airway disease. The majority of children with BPD will have some reactive airway disease at some point in the course of their illness, and for many children this reactivity will persist into adolescence and adulthood.

INEFFECTIVE BREATHING PATTERN

Ineffective breathing pattern is defined as the "state in which the individual's inhalation and/or exhalation pattern does not enable adequate ventilation" (Kim, McFarland, & McLane, 1993). Effective breathing requires normal lung and airway structures, a feedback mechanism involving the nervous system structures controlling respiration (peripheral chemoreceptors, central chemoreceptors, and respiratory neurons of the pons and medulla), intact nerve pathways to the muscles of respiration, and the structure of the chest wall. Disorders directly or indirectly involving respiratory centers in the brain result in a variety of ineffective breathing patterns. Patterns of respiration seen include regular-irregular patterns (Cheyne-Stokes respiration) associated with cerebral damage; increased rate and depth (central neurogenic hyperventilation) resulting from damage to brainstem reflex mechanisms of respiration; and increasingly irregular patterns (cluster or ataxic) resulting from damage to the lower brainstem. Improvements in breathing patterns depend primarily on resolution of the underlying pathophysiology of the respiratory centers.

In the rehabilitation setting nurses most commonly address problems related to ineffective breathing patterns as seen in clients with restrictive lung disease and COPD. Clients with restrictive lung disease typically include those with degenerative neuromuscular diseases, spinal cord injury, scoliosis, and interstitial pulmonary fibrosis; clients with obstructive disease include those with emphysema, chronic bronchitis, and CF. In these clients the primary alterations in breathing patterns include an increase in the respiratory rate and decrease in the tidal volume during quiet breathing at rest, placing clients at risk for alveolar hypoventilation and ventilatory failure.

Restrictive Lung Disease

Interruption of neural conduction from respiratory centers in the brain to the muscles of respiration can be seen as shallow breathing in cervical spinal cord lesions and multiple sclerosis. Peripheral neuropathies such as Guillain-Barré syndrome, muscular dystrophy, poliomyelitis, and myasthenia gravis also result in inability to breathe effectively. With increasing weakness and fatigue of the respiratory muscles, clients may develop uncoordinated breathing and alternate between use of the muscles of the chest wall and the diaphragm to breathe. Paradoxic breathing (inward displacement of the abdomen with inspiration) is seen as the diaphragm weakens. Respiratory impairment can be either unilateral or bilateral, temporary or permanent. Paradoxic movement of the abdomen on inspiration becomes especially pronounced in the supine position because the diaphragm cannot fall passively. Disruption of nerve transmission across the myoneural junction also results in the inability to ventilate effectively. Progressive fatigue of the respiratory muscles results in ineffective breathing patterns, causing respiratory failure.

Bony deformities of the chest wall can decrease chest wall compliance and restrict lung expansion, causing rapid and shallow breathing. Scoliosis and ankylosing spondylitis are examples of such conditions.

Chronic Obstructive Pulmonary Disease

During quiet breathing, clients with moderate to severe COPD commonly demonstrate an increased respiratory rate with a normal tidal volume and V_E, even when their lung condition is stable and they are in their best state of health (Loveridge, West, Anthonisen, & Kryger, 1984; Tobin et al., 1983a; Tobin et al., 1983b). During an exacerbation and/or during an episode of respiratory failure, the respiratory rate will further increase and the tidal volume will decrease, producing rapid shallow breathing (Cohen, Zagelbaum, Gross, Roussos, & Macklem, 1982; Gallagher, Hof, & Younes, 1985). The V_E will decrease eventually as the clinical condition deteriorates. The precise mechanisms for altered breathing patterns in individuals with COPD are not well understood.

Assessment

✦ **Subjective.** Dyspnea is the prime subjective complaint of clients with ineffective breathing patterns. Typically this is a subjective feeling that ventilatory requirements are not being met. Dyspnea may occur at rest or be associated only with activity.

✦ **Objective.** A rapid respiratory rate can be observed readily from inspection of the chest; however, normal breathing patterns frequently are interrupted by the process of physical examination, making it difficult to obtain reliable measures of respiratory rate. The most accurate measures of respiratory rate will be obtained through unobtrusive observations conducted while performing an unrelated aspect of care. It is difficult to assess the depth of respirations during a routine physical assessment. A more precise measure of tidal volume could be performed with a simple spirometer, but placing a mouthpiece in the mouth will alter normal breathing patterns. Inductive plethysmography could be used to measure tidal volumes without using a mouthpiece if precise measures were needed. But this equipment typically is not available in the rehabilitation setting, and precise measures of tidal volume generally are not needed unless the client is receiving ventilatory support. The function of breathing patterns is to maintain adequate V_A, hence measures of V_A can be used to document the effectiveness of breathing patterns. The Pa_{CO_2} indirectly measures the adequacy of V_A and thereby provides a reliable indicator of ineffective breathing patterns. An elevation in Pa_{CO_2} reflects alveolar hypoventilation.

Additionally breathing may appear labored with recruitment of the accessory muscles of respiration, PLB, and prolonged expiration. Labored breathing may worsen with low levels of physical activity.

Goals

The primary nursing goals for the client with ineffective breathing pattern are to maximize ventilation and to improve air flow. Client goals include

1. No complaints or reduced complaints of shortness of breath
2. Effective ventilation restored and maintained
3. Reduced anxiety
4. Increased activity levels

Interventions

Nursing management is aimed at maintaining adequate ventilation through relaxation techniques, breathing retraining, respiratory muscle training, mechanical ventilation, and electrical phrenic stimulation.

✦ Relaxation techniques

Dyspnea frequently is associated with high levels of anxiety (Janson-Bjerklie, Carrieri, & Hudes, 1986), especially in clients with COPD (Gift & Cahill, 1990; Gift, Plaut, & Jacox, 1986). Muscle relaxation can be used to reduce the anxiety associated with dyspnea (Gift, Moore, & Soeken, 1992; Renfroe, 1988) (see box below). However, most people will not relax unless provided with a specific technique they believe is effective.

Progressive muscle relaxation is commonly used for pulmonary clients. The box at right provides directions for tensing and relaxing seven muscle groups. By doing so, the client becomes more aware of the differences between ten-

sion and relaxation and perhaps is better able to achieve a relaxed state.

✦ Breathing retraining

Persons with COPD may benefit from breathing retraining techniques such as PLB, abdominal-diaphragmatic breathing, segmental breathing, and glossopharyngeal breathing (GPB). Breathing retraining is designed to (1) assist the client in controlling breathing patterns, (2) promote ventilation through effective breathing patterns, and (3) relieve symptoms of dyspnea.

Pursed-lip breathing. Pursed-lip breathing (PLB) is slow exhalation through partially closed or pursed lips. It is used to control expiration and to facilitate maximum emptying of the alveoli. PLB increases tidal volume and reduces air trapped in lung alveoli. Research confirms that arterial oxygen saturation (Sa_{O_2}) improves by at least 3% to 4% in many clients through use of PLB (Tiep, Burns, Kao, Madison, & Herrera, 1986). Clients with COPD frequently use this technique to gain some control over breathing patterns.

In teaching this technique, the nurse needs to explain to the client that breathing out through pursed lips increases the resistance to outflow at the lips, causing an increase in airway pressure. The small airways remain open longer dur-

---

✦

GENERAL DIRECTIONS FOR RELAXATION

1. Set aside a specific time of the day to relax that is best for you.
2. You are in control of your relaxation program at all times. Do not force yourself to relax.
3. Select a quiet, dimly lit environment with few distractions. Soft, slow music provides a soothing background for relaxation techniques. Instrumental classical arrangements or environmental sounds (e.g., gentle rain) are conducive to relaxation (DiMotto, 1984).
4. Assume a comfortable position with as much support as possible.
5. Loosen all restrictive clothing and remove shoes.
6. When ready, close your eyes and take several slow, deep breaths and exhale through pursed lips.
7. Do not focus on the extent of muscle relaxation at this time.

✦

MUSCLE RELAXATION TECHNIQUE

1. *Right arm.* Hold your arm out straight, tighten your muscles, and make a tight fist. Hold your arm tense for 5 seconds. Relax and let your arm gradually fall to the chair. Feel the muscles from your shoulder to your fingers loosen. To avoid cramps when tensing these muscles or any other muscle do so only to about 75% of your capacity rather than tensing it as hard as you possibly can.
2. *Left arm.* Same as your right arm.
3. *Face.* Close your eyes tightly, furrow your brow, and clench your teeth. Hold your muscles tight for 5 seconds, then relax.
4. *Neck.* Bring your chin down to your chest as tightly as possible for 3 seconds, then relax. Roll your head from side to side in a relaxed manner. Stop when your head assumes a comfortable position.
5. *Shoulder.* Make an exaggerated shoulder shrug and tighten the muscles. Hold the tension for 3 seconds, then relax.
6. *Chest and back.* Before tensing your muscles, slowly take a deep breath and relax. Now take a deep breath and raise and extend your chest and at the same time pull your shoulder blades together. Hold for 3 seconds, then relax.
7. *Right leg.* Extend your leg out in front of you with knee slightly bent. Point your foot and toes back and press down hard against the chair with your thigh. Hold leg tense for 5 seconds. Relax and let leg return to former position. Let tension leave leg until it becomes limp.
8. *Left leg.* Same as your right leg. (Walsh, 1986)

ing exhalation, allowing more air to be exhaled. Exhalation should take two or three times longer than inhalation to effectively empty the lungs of trapped air.

To perform PLB, the client should be instructed to (1) inhale slowly through the nose (with mouth shut) and to pause slightly at the end of inspiration and (2) exhale slowly in a relaxed manner, breathing out through partially closed or pursed lips. Folding the arms across the abdomen while sitting and bending forward while exhaling further aids complete emptying of the lungs.

Abdominal-diaphragmatic breathing. Traditionally abdominal-diaphragmatic exercises have been used in pulmonary rehabilitation to increase efficiency of the respiratory muscles. There have been no studies to date demonstrating the efficacy of abdominal-diaphragmatic breathing, but it is described because it is widely used in many pulmonary rehabilitation programs.

Abdominal-diaphragmatic breathing and PLB should be used together to obtain maximum breathing efficiency. Clients should be told that this breathing exercise is to improve breathing and lung ventilation by reducing the overall work of breathing through making use of the diaphragm rather than the accessory muscles while breathing.

To perform abdominal-diaphragmatic breathing, the client should assume a comfortable, relaxed semisitting or supine position. Ask the client to place one hand over the xiphoid process in the epigastric area of the upper abdomen and the other hand over the apical region of the chest. The client should then be instructed to

1. Relax the abdominal muscles and breathe in slowly through the nose (The hand over the epigastric area should be observed lifting as the abdomen extends and the diaphragm moves downward; the hand over the apical region should remain still.)
2. Hold this breath 1 or 2 seconds before breathing out slowly through pursed lips while contracting the abdominal muscles (This maneuver helps to move the diaphragm upward and empty the lungs.)

The client should be instructed to breathe at a rate of 6 to 10 breaths/minute. Repeat these instructions until the client is able to perform them independently. Focusing the client's attention to feeling the abdomen push against the hand and the lower ribs expanding when inhaling increases the client's awareness of the correct technique. During exhalation attention should be directed toward feeling the abdominal muscles tighten. Clients should be encouraged to practice these exercises 10 to 20 minutes every 4 hours during the day until mastered. If the client has difficulty mastering abdominal-diaphragmatic breathing and does not suffer from orthopnea, and the Trendelenburg position is not contraindicated, place the client in the Trendelenburg position to increase awareness of diaphragmatic movement. After the technique is mastered, a 5-lb weight may be placed on the client's abdomen to further strengthen the abdominal muscles. Eventually the client should be able to use abdominal-diaphragmatic breathing while walking and carrying out ADL (Wilson & Thompson, 1990).

If the client is paralyzed, place your hand on the diaphragm to help focus attention on it, even though the client may not be able to feel your hand. The person who is quadriplegic also may be instructed to rebreathe carbon dioxide to improve deep breathing and stimulate coughing. This therapy is used to prevent atelectasis. A reservoir bag is filled with a mixture of 10% carbon dioxide and 90% oxygen from a prepared tank. The client holds the mouthpiece securely in the mouth and wears a nose clip. The client is instructed to breathe in and out through the mouth until deeper breaths are taken and coughing is stimulated. If the client complains of dizziness or headache, the treatment should be discontinued (Zejdlik, 1991).

Glossopharyngeal breathing. Glossopharyngeal breathing (GPB) or "guppie" breathing, uses the tongue, mouth, and throat to gulp air to the back of the throat and force it into the lungs (Buchanan & Nawoczenski, 1987). It has been used by clients with respiratory muscle paralysis who are ventilator dependent but can tolerate short periods off ventilatory support using this technique. The client must be comfortable on ventilator support and have normal tongue strength before learning GPB. This technique also can be used to increase voice volume for non-ventilator-dependent clients.

✦ Physical conditioning

Physical conditioning emphasizes techniques to maximize the client's functional ability. Dyspnea can be a deterrent to exercise, leading to further deconditioning and curtailment of activities. Exercise conditioning and coordinating breathing with activities can increase levels of functioning. Clients using energy conservation techniques will enhance functional ability by performing activities more slowly, using proper muscle groups and body mechanics, and alternating work with periods of rest.

The rehabilitation team can help the client identify activities that cause the greatest problem and then train the involved muscle groups to enhance muscle strength, coordination, and endurance. Clients with severe COPD report a marked increase in the perception of dyspnea with routine tasks that require arm use, especially those activities associated with unsupported arm elevation (Breslin, 1992). Unsupported arm exercise training has enhanced endurance in COPD clients (Couser, Martinez, & Celli, 1989). A simple and inexpensive unsupported arm training exercise for COPD clients is performing lifts with a lightweight dowel rod from waist to shoulder level (Breslin, 1992). Adding weights to the rods will increase resistance as tolerance increases. Suggesting techniques to provide arm support, such as bracing the arms on a table, may increase the client's ability to perform common arm tasks.

By coordinating breathing with specific activities, the client can take full mechanical advantage of muscle movement to assist breathing during self-care activities. Techniques to reduce dyspnea include (1) inhaling before bending, then exhaling slowly through pursed lips while bending, and then inhaling again while returning to the upright position; (2) moving the arms forward away from the side, or above the head, which elevates the chest and assists with inspiration; and (3) placing the hands on the hips at frequent intervals or moving the arms away from the body on inspiration while performing ADL such as bathing or dressing.

Exercise conditioning increases exercise tolerance and improves the subjective sense of well-being (Swerts,

Kretzers, Terpstra-Lindeman, Verstrappen, & Wouters, 1990). Aerobic exercises will improve aerobic conditioning if the intensity of training is maintained at high levels (Casaburi et al., 1991). Improving aerobic conditioning reduces the ventilatory requirements of exercise, allowing clients to perform a given amount of work with less ventilation. They have greater stamina and interest in life. However, a supervised training program must be continued to maintain the obtained effects.

Many methods have been used to accomplish conditioning including treadmill walking, bicycle ergometry, stair climbing, walking, swimming, and bicycling. Research has shown benefits of regularly participating in less vigorous exercises such as the program of systematic movement set to music sponsored by the American Lung Association (Gift & Austin, 1992). Exercise participants had lower depression and less dyspnea. Some experts believe it is better to condition individuals by walking in corridors and on stairs rather than on treadmills or bicycles because it is more enjoyable (Petty, 1982). Motivation and adherence to exercise can be a problem for some clients, making it important for the nurse to reinforce the importance of exercise training and its effect on respiratory function.

Respiratory Muscle Training. Designed to increase the strength and endurance of the respiratory muscles, respiratory muscle training has been used primarily by clients with COPD. Inspiratory muscle training (IMT) is performed with either an alinear resistive breathing device (Pflex, Healthscan) or a threshold-loaded breathing device (Threshold, Healthscan) (Fig. 18-6). With both devices the client performs IMT by breathing in and out through the device, generating high airway pressures during inspiration and normal airway pressures during expiration. The client must work hard during inspiration and expiration is normal and relaxed.

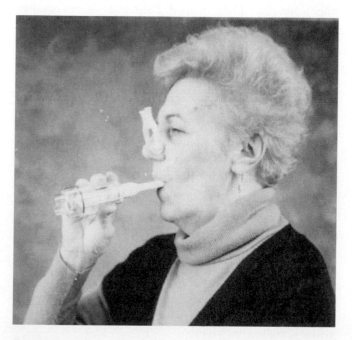

Fig. 18-6 Client using an inspiratory muscle trainer. (Courtesy Healthscan, Inc., Cedar Grove, NJ.)

Alinear resistive breathing devices have a small inspiratory orifice so that clients must generate high inspiratory pressures to maintain ventilation. With the alinear resistive breathing device, IMT is performed by breathing in through the small orifice and breathing out through a larger orifice. If clients use a slow respiratory rate, they can reduce their inspiratory muscle training load; consequently clients must be coached to maintain a preset respiratory rate.

The threshold-loaded inspiratory muscles trainers have a large inspiratory orifice, which is occluded with a spring-loaded poppet valve that can be adjusted to control the airway pressure required to open the valve and allow inspiration. To train with this device, the client generates the preset negative pressure with every inspiration. The inspiratory training load can be carefully controlled with this device, and it is independent of respiratory rate.

Research evidence supports the notion that IMT can be used to improve strength and endurance of the respiratory muscles (Larson, Kim, Sharp, & Larson, 1988; Smith, Cook, Guyatt, Madhavan, & Oxman, 1992). However, it is not clear if improved strength and endurance of the respiratory muscles results in other benefits such as increased exercise tolerance and decreased dyspnea with exertion or improved breathing patterns.

◆ Ventilatory support devices

Noninvasive ventilatory support devices are used to move the chest wall by mechanical means of manually pushing on the stomach, chest, or back. The client must have a chest wall capable of effective movement. Generally these noninvasive devices have been found effective in instances of respiratory muscle paralysis associated with neurologic disease or injury (Bach & Alba, 1990). They are not appropriate for most COPD clients. These devices do not require the use of artificial airways. The two most commonly used ventilatory support devices are the rocking bed and the pneumobelt.

Rocking beds. Rocking beds assist ventilation by using gravity and the pressure of the abdominal contents to alternately apply and remove pressure on the diaphragm. Inhalation is assisted when the client's body is tilted with the head up, the abdominal contents fall, and diaphragm is pulled downward. Exhalation is assisted when the client's body is tilted head down, the abdominal contents push against the diaphragm, and expiration occurs. Rocking beds are simple to operate and maintain and are noninvasive devices. However, many clients cannot tolerate the rocking motion, and it does not control tidal volumes. This device is most appropriate for clients who are bedridden or as a nighttime alternative to a ventilator.

Pneumobelts. Pneumobelts consist of an inflatable rubber bladder inside a corset, which is placed around the client's abdomen. As the bladder inflates, it pushes the abdominal contents up against the diaphragm, assisting expiration. When the bladder deflates, abdominal contents and the diaphragm fall, assisting inhalation. The pneumobelt connects to a positive-pressure generator and usually requires 15 to 50 cm H_2O pressure (Johnson, Giovannoni, & Driscoll, 1986). This device is most effective when the client is upright in a wheelchair. However, clients often find the belt uncomfortable, and it also does not control tidal volumes. A similar device using a metal plate and a compact, lightweight, battery-powered respirator has been developed that fits under a wheelchair lapboard. This system has been used continuously for over 9 months for as long as 9 hours a day.

✦ Mechanical ventilation

Although the care of clients receiving mechanical ventilation is dealt with primarily under acute aspects of respiratory care, some individuals may require long-term mechanical ventilation. These individuals frequently have chronic, underlying lung disease such as emphysema or neurologic impairment such as cervical spinal cord injuries resulting in the inability to breathe. Two commonly used ventilation devices are negative-pressure ventilators (NPVs) and positive-pressure ventilators (PPVs) (Johnson et al., 1986).

Negative-pressure ventilators. NPVs have decreased in popularity since the introduction of PPVs. These devices were used during the 1950s and 1960s to provide mechanical ventilation to victims of poliomyelitis. Cuirass respirators have replaced the iron lung and offer an alternative to the PPVs. Individuals with chronic respiratory or neuromuscular diseases are candidates for this type of ventilator. NPVs effect ventilation through the application of negative pressure around the thorax for inspiration. This creates a pressure gradient inside the thoracic cavity, allowing air to flow into the lungs. The primary disadvantage is that the client must be sealed off in the device. These devices are cumbersome and markedly restrict mobility. One advantage is that no tracheal intubation is required.

Positive-pressure ventilation. PPV is achieved by positive pressure to the airways to promote inspiration; expiration is passive. An artificial airway usually is necessary to connect the ventilator to the client. Mouthpieces, however, can be used if only intermittent ventilation is required. There are two types of PPV devices: pressure-cycled ventilators and volume-cycled ventilators.

Pressure-cycled ventilators inflate an individual's lungs until a predetermined pressure is reached, at which point inspiration ends and expiration begins. With this type of ventilator the volume of air delivered to the client can vary with each inspiration, depending on the compliance of the individual's airways. For example, if an individual is experiencing bronchospasm, the pressure set on the ventilator is reached quickly and only a small volume of air is delivered into the lungs. In contrast, volume-cycled ventilators deliver a fixed predetermined tidal volume of air into the lungs, and the pressure to deliver this volume of air varies, depending on compliance of the lungs and chest wall. There is a safety valve or pressure-limit setting on these ventilators above which the ventilator will no longer continue the inspiratory cycle. This mechanism prevents trauma that could occur if air was forced into the lungs under too high a pressure. Volume-cycled ventilators are preferred for both hospitalized and homebound individuals because a consistent volume of air is delivered to the lungs. The advantages of PPV are the increased accessibility to the client and increased mobility of the client.

Weaning from mechanical ventilation. Clients receiving ventilator assistance require gradual withdrawal or weaning. This gradual process allows time to strengthen existing respiratory muscles in preparation for withdrawal of ventilatory support. The weaning process is often a time of high anxiety for the client. Psychological support, biofeedback with ear oximetry, and use of relaxation techniques have been found to decrease anxiety (Acosta, 1988). The weaning process may be initiated with a vital capacity of at least 800 ml if the client is free of infected secretions and other pulmonary or medical complications.

Three methods of ventilatory support used during the weaning process are a combination of assist-control ventilatory support with use of a T-piece, intermittent mandatory ventilation (IMV) with or without use of a T-piece, and humidified O_2 through a T-piece (Van Sciver & Weaver, 1992). The T-piece is used to provide humidification and oxygen but no ventilatory assistance.

IMV is a primary mode of ventilatory support when weaning clients from ventilators. With IMV clients breathe spontaneously at their own tidal volume and rate. Spontaneous inspiration allows for cardiac output and venous return that are more physiologically normal than with assisted ventilation. IMV allows a smooth transition from controlled to spontaneous ventilation by gradually decreasing the mandatory ventilation rate as clients assume an increasing percentage of the total work of breathing. The diaphragm has to work constantly to maintain adequate ventilation. This method is more appropriate with the COPD client where strengthening of the diaphragmatic muscle is not the primary concern; IMV is not conducive to strengthening the diaphragmatic muscle.

The assist-control method is recommended for situations in which clients are breathing spontaneously but have ventilatory failure due to respiratory muscle weakness resulting from conditions such as spinal cord injury, Guillain-Barré syndrome, and muscular dystrophy. The delivery of a breath is triggered by the inspiratory effort of the client after a preselected time interval. The client initiates her own breathing using respiratory muscles and alters her respiratory rate according to need. If a client fails to initiate breathing after a preselected time interval has elapsed, the ventilator cycles automatically. This method requires little diaphragm effort to trigger the ventilator, and the diaphragm does not have to work at a constant level to provide ventilatory assistance.

With the third method the client is transferred from assisted mechanical ventilation or IMV to humidified O_2 through a T-piece. The time off the ventilator is increased gradually. Initially the client may tolerate weaning for 5 minutes at a time. Both the length and frequency of weaning periods should be increased gradually.

Throughout the weaning process the client must be monitored closely for signs of respiratory distress, restlessness, fatigue, use of accessory muscles, tachycardia, decrease or increase in blood pressure, tachypnea or bradypnea, and somnolence. The use of continuous oximetry to monitor arterial and venous oxygen saturation is helpful. The client should be encouraged in the use of proper breathing techniques, relaxation techniques to decrease anxiety, and assistive coughing techniques.

The goal of the weaning process is to have the client attain complete withdrawal of ventilatory support. However, each client must be evaluated on an individual basis. Some clients may tolerate breathing without the ventilator only during waking hours, whereas others may tolerate weaning for only a shorter period.

Mechanical ventilation in the home. Every effort should be made to choose and modify ventilatory support devices according to the client's and significant other's needs and preferences (Johnson et al., 1986). Ventilators developed for home use are more compact than those used in hospitals (Drayton-Hargrove & Mandzak-McCarron, 1987b) (Fig. 18-7). Some are mounted on motorized wheelchairs. These units are self-contained and self-powered. A sufficient supply of oxygen and suction equipment are included to allow for mobility up to 3 hours. Home ventilators can be driven by electrical power, batteries, or gas.

In choosing home ventilator equipment, consideration should be given to the home environment, long-term home care commitment by the individual and family, financial considerations, and home support services. The physical environment of the home should allow for effective and efficient operation of the equipment. Consideration should be given to the amount of time spent by the client in each area of the house or out of the house. These areas need to be evaluated for electrical requirements, maneuverability of the client and equipment, safety, and temperature and air control. An emergency call system should be set up to allow the client to summon help when needed. Emergency phone numbers should be readily available. Service agencies such as emergency medical services, electrical company, and phone company should be notified that a ventilator-dependent client is living in the community. Home support services including visiting nurses, home health aides, and respiratory therapists may be required. Respiratory equipment is almost always maintained by the company supplying the ventilator. Although third-party payment is available for home ventilator care, the financial ar-

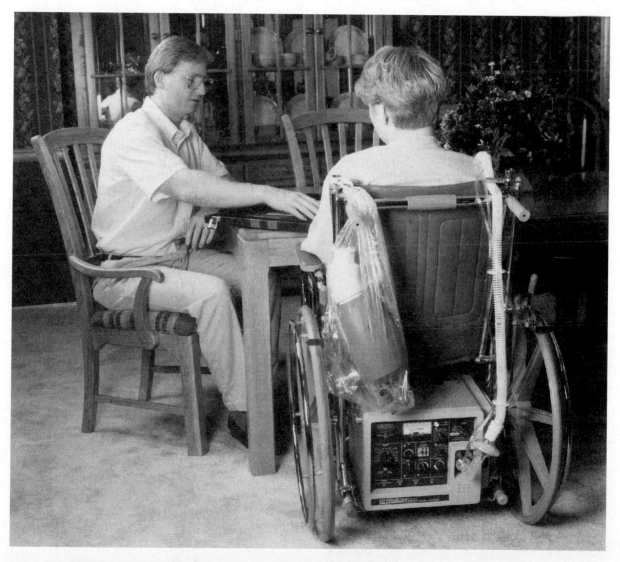

Fig. 18-7   Client in a wheelchair with a portable Puritan Bennett ventilator. (Courtesy Puritan Bennett, Overland Park, KS.)

rangements can be confusing and frustrating. Social workers should be involved to facilitate financial arrangements and reimbursement.

Rehabilitation of ventilator-dependent individuals requires a team approach. Individuals discharged with volume-cycled ventilators must understand ventilator operation and possible mechanical problems. Discharge planning must be a team effort including the nurse, respiratory therapist, physical therapist, speech therapist, social worker, and other team members as necessary (Johnson et al., 1986). A self-inflating resuscitation bag also should be available in case of mechanical failure of the ventilator.

Mechanical ventilation in the home provides certain individuals with an improved quality of life within familiar surroundings. Home care also has been shown to be more cost-effective than institutional care (Bach, Alba, & Holland, 1992). Home care ventilator clients and their families require frequent evaluation of how they are managing physically and psychologically.

Clients requiring long-term mechanical ventilation pose a special nutritional problem. Abdominal distention can occur because of aspiration of air into the stomach. Aspiration of food into the lungs of intubated clients can result. Cuffed tracheostomy tubes should be kept inflated during meals and for 1 to 2 hours after meals to prevent aspiration. Adequate nutritional intake is important in these individuals. It has been shown that semistarvation in clients receiving ventilation therapy can lead to a diminished hypoxic drive, especial in clients with COPD. A diminished hypoxic drive can precipitate respiratory failure (Openbrier & Covey, 1987).

Upper airway mechanics differ between sleep and wakefulness. This may affect air leak around uncuffed tracheostomies. In 9 or 11 children with uncuffed tracheostomies and on volume-controlled ventilators were found to be inadequately ventilated during sleep. Using pressure-controlled ventilation at night alleviated the problem (Gilgoff, Peng, & Keens, 1992). Increased restlessness, confusion, and seizures may indicate hypoxia and hypercapnia.

✦ Electrophrenic nerve pacing

Electrophrenic nerve pacing provides an alternative to some ventilator-dependent clients with an intact phrenic nerve (Carter, Donovan, Halstead, & Wilkerson, 1987). Pacing of the diaphragm is accomplished through high-frequency stimulation of the phrenic nerve by radio frequency transmissions from an electrode surgically attached to the phrenic nerve. A receiver implanted subcutaneously and attached to the electrode receives transmission through a battery-operated transmitter. The phrenic nerve will fatigue with repetitive high-frequency stimulation. Therefore the phrenic nerve should be rested for as long as it is paced. Tolerance for phrenic nerve stimulation will increase with time. Clients initially may be started with a regimen of 1 hour on and 1 hour off. Gradually a tolerance of up to 8 to 12 hours will be achieved. More recently, continuous bilateral simultaneous low-frequency stimulation has been used successfully (Tibealls, 1991). For clients who prefer full-time pacing, one phrenic nerve can be stimulated and then the other for the next period.

In clients with diaphragmatic paralysis such as high cervical spinal cord injury, a readily available alternative method of ventilation should be available in the event of pacer failure. The batteries in the transmitter should be replaced each day. An emergency call system should be available to the client in the home.

Outcome Criteria

For the client with ineffective breathing pattern, the following outcome criteria are identified. The client will demonstrate an effective breathing pattern as evidenced by

1. Blood gas values within baseline range
2. Rate, rhythm, depth, and pattern of respirations normal for client
3. Statement of a feeling of effortless breathing

INEFFECTIVE AIRWAY CLEARANCE

Ineffective airway clearance is defined as the "state in which an individual is unable to clear secretions or obstructions from the respiratory tract to maintain patency" (Kim et al., 1993). Normally the respiratory system produces a small amount of secretions that are cleared by the mucociliary system as described earlier in this chapter. Excessive secretions are produced by clients with a variety of respiratory conditions including chronic bronchitis, CF, bronchiectasis, and lower respiratory tract infection. Under normal conditions deep breathing and coughing are sufficient to mobilize excessive secretions and clear them from the airways. However, problems arise when the volume of secretions are too large to be accommodated in this manner, when the respiratory muscles too weak to produce effective coughing and deep breathing, and/or when the secretions are so thick they are difficult to mobilize.

To generate an effective cough, clients must have sufficient strength of both inspiratory and expiratory muscles. Inspiratory muscle strength is needed to take a deep breath before the cough, and expiratory muscle strength is needed to generate sufficient force to produce the sudden rise in intrathoracic pressure during the cough.

Some clients with COPD experience daily problems with ineffective airway clearance, whereas others experience episodic problems during exacerbations. Clients with a significant amount of chronic bronchitis produce excessive secretions on a daily basis as evidenced by a productive cough on arising in the morning. They must mobilize secretions and clear their airways on a daily basis to prevent stagnation of secretions and growth of bacteria. Other clients with COPD are at risk for problems with ineffective airway clearance when they contract a viral infection of the respiratory tract. They produce excessive secretions that overwhelm the defense mechanisms, causing a secondary bacterial infection of the lower respiratory tract. The problem can be compounded by the skeletal muscle weakness, specifically respiratory muscle weakness, which is caused by some viral infections (Mier-Jedrzejowicz et al., 1988). Recurring problems with ineffective airway clearance are seen in clients with severe COPD.

Episodic problems with airway clearance are seen in clients with respiratory muscle weakness secondary to neuromuscular disease and midcervical injury of the spinal cord. The respiratory muscles are too weak to produce effective coughing and deep breathing as needed to clear the airways of excessive secretions during a respiratory tract infection. Effects of the virus can further impair respiratory muscle strength. Immobility compounds problems with mobilizing secretions by contributing to shallow breathing and stagnation of secretion.

Assessment

✦ **Subjective.** Clients with ineffective airway clearance may complain of an inability to cough up secretions. They may complain of dyspnea.

✦ **Objective.** Typically, adventitious breath sounds will include coarse crackles, low-pitched wheezes, and high-pitched wheezes. The crackles commonly occur on inspiration but can occur on both inspiration and expiration. Low-pitched wheezes indicate the presence of secretions in the airway and generally clear with coughing. A persistent cough and hypoxemia may be present with ineffective airway clearance.

Goals

The primary nursing goals for the individual with ineffective airway clearance are to establish and maintain airway patency and adequate ventilation. Client goals include

1. Maintaining a patent airway by developing an effective cough
2. Mastering techniques that can assist in producing an effective cough
3. Readily mobilizing secretions for expulsion
4. Maintaining adequate hydration and humidification

Interventions for Clients with Intact Airways

The nurse achieves the preceding goals by augmenting the client's natural defense mechanisms through hydration, nebulization, cough techniques, incentive spirometry, postural drainage, percussion, and vibration. Assessment should identify the factors contributing to ineffective airway clearance, then the following selection of interventions may be considered.

✦ Hydration

Clients should be encouraged to drink adequate amounts of fluid to maintain hydration and to keep mucous membranes moist, facilitating the mobilization of secretions. The intake of fluids should be sufficient to replace fluid losses. It is not necessary to force fluids because excessive fluid intake will be excreted through the urine and will not affect the composition of respiratory secretions (Shim, King, & Williams, 1986). Coffee and tea tend to act as diuretics and should be avoided or not included in the daily fluid intake.

Environmental humidification may be necessary during cold weather. The humidifier should be cleaned on a regular basis to prevent growth of bacteria and fungi within the system.

For clients with a tracheostomy, the heat and moisture exchanger (HME) warms and humidifies inspired gases by recovering humidity from expired gases (Misset, Escuder, Rivara, Leclercq, & Nitenberg, 1991). The device connects directly to the tracheostomy tube. Adult and pediatric sizes are available for inpatient and home use with or without mechanical ventilation. The HME should not be used con-tinuously for periods exceeding 24 hours. In addition, coughing up secretions and suctioning requires disconnecting the HME from the tracheostomy tube. If secretions or mucus adhere to the mesh inside the unit, it should be replaced immediately with a new one. The HME should be used in the home only by clients who can independently remove the humidifier when the mesh becomes obstructed with secretions.

✦ Nebulization

Nebulization is the delivery of water vapor or medication in fine mist droplets that can infiltrate the respiratory system and penetrate deep within the lungs. Variations in the method of nebulization can produce droplets of varying sizes. Generally the smaller the particle, the deeper the penetration into the respiratory tract. Particles of 1 to 5 μm penetrate to the periphery, particles of 5 to 10 μm are deposited in the bronchi, and particles larger than 10 μm are deposited in the upper airway passages. Two types of aerosols are bland and medicated. A bland aerosol contains water or saline solution from a reservoir container; it can be delivered either at room temperature or heated. Bland aerosols benefit selected clients with mucous retention problems; however, no research study supports their routine use (Kersten, 1989).

Hazards associated with nebulization include overhydration and mist as a source of infection. Special precautions in the administration of aerosol mists include educating clients on the proper cleansing of nebulizers to prevent infection. One method of disinfecting nebulizers is to soak immersible parts in a weak vinegar solution two to three times a week and then run the nebulizer for 20 minutes before use to eliminate vinegar fumes.

✦ Coughing

Coughing (see the following box) is an important physiologic mechanism for the removal of secretions from the respiratory tract. Maximal effect from coughing can be achieved through controlled cough or cascade cough (Sexton, 1990). Some individuals with COPD or neuromuscu-

---

INSTRUCTIONS FOR A CONTROLLED COUGH

✦ Sit in a chair or on the edge of the bed with knees flexed and feet supported on the floor or on a footstool with shoulders rotated inward and arms supported by pillows.
✦ Take several deep breaths using PLB.
✦ Maximally inhale so that air reaches distal portions of the lung where mucus is retained.
✦ Lean forward and cough gently several times using the abdominal muscles and not the throat until the lungs have little air remaining.

From "Influence of Head Dependent Position on Lung Volume and Oxygen Saturation in Chronic Airflow Obstruction" by J. Marini, M.L. Tyler, L.D. Hudson, B.S. Davis, & J.S. Huseby, 1984, *American Review of Respiratory Disease, 130,* 689-696. Reprinted with permission.

lar disorders may not be able to perform the cascade cough effectively because of collapsed airways.

Huff coughing. Huff coughing ("open glottis coughing") is another form of the controlled cough designed to clear the airways while conserving energy. Clients cross their arms just below the rib cage, take a deep breath while leaning forward with arms crossed over a pillow, and exhale sharply while whispering the word huff several times. Whispering the word huff prevents closure of the glottis and reduces airway compression during the cough (Hanley & Tyler, 1987). Immediately after the huff, clients relax the shoulders and allow the arms to fall limp at the side. They continue to relax with slow diaphragmatic breathing between coughs.

Quad cough. The quad cough is used for persons with expiratory muscle weakness secondary to a spinal cord injury. The technique is also referred to as the manual cough or diaphragmatic push (Buchanan & Nawoczenski, 1987). The person assisting the client positions their hand below the xiphoid process and pushes quickly on the epigastric area, diagonally inward toward the head, while the client attempts to cough. Quad-assist coughing is similar to the Heimlich maneuver. This motion should be coordinated with the client's attempt to exhale forcefully. Some clients can assist themselves by quickly compressing the abdomen. With the feet positioned on the floor or stool, the client takes a slow, deep breath through the nose and exhales, simultaneously bending forward and pressing the pillow against the abdomen. After several deep breaths and exhalations, the client coughs several times while exhaling and bending forward. Clients with neuromuscular disorders with little or no respiratory muscle function can use GPB to increase VC and improve cough force (Kersten, 1989).

Most clients will appreciate privacy during the coughing procedure as it can be embarrassing. It is embarrassing because many people consider sputum to be disgusting and socially unattractive.

✦ Deep breathing exercises

Deep breathing mobilizes secretions to facilitate airway clearance. Difficulty with deep breathing can be caused by inspiratory muscle weakness as seen in clients with neuromuscular disorders and by pain as seen in clients after surgery or trauma.

Deep breathing is maximized in the upright position as gravity assists in pulling the diaphragm and abdomen downward. In the supine position the abdomen pushes caudally on the diaphragm, increasing the FRC and decreasing the VC, thereby decreasing the client's ability to take a deep breath (Marini, Tyler, Hudson, Davis, & Huseby, 1984).

To perform deep breathing, the client assumes an upright position and takes a prolonged deep inspiration through the nose, holding the breath for at least 3 seconds and then breathing out slowly in a relaxed manner. This maneuver simulates a normal sigh. COPD clients should exhale through pursed lips. An incentive spirometer frequently is used to facilitate lung inflation and provide visual feedback of performance.

✦ Incentive spirometer

The incentive spirometer can be used to provide visual feedback to clients during deep breathing. Visual feedback is based on either inspiratory flow or volume, depending on the type of incentive spirometer (Kersten, 1989). The following Box provides a comparison of the two. Generally, incentive spirometers are inexpensive, disposable, safe, and do not require assistance during therapy. Clients should perform deep breathing three to four times a day, according to their clinical condition.

✦ Chest physiotherapy

Chest physiotherapy is a general term that includes chest percussion, chest vibration, and postural drainage. These techniques can be used independently or in combination to assist in mobilizing secretions. Humidification and bronchodilators can be used before chest physiotherapy to facilitate airway clearance. Chest physiotherapy is effective only for clients producing copious secretions as seen with CF and bronchiectasis (Kirilloff, Owens, Rogers, & Mazzocco, 1985).

Chest percussion. Chest percussion is performed by cupping the hands and striking the targeted area of the chest in a rhythmic fashion (Fig. 18-8). The cupped hand creates an air pocket between the hand and chest, producing a hollow but not a slapping sound on percussion. To avoid fatigue, the wrists should be kept loose and the elbows slightly flexed. Clients usually find percussion to be more comfortable when it is performed over a thin layer of clothing rather than on bare skin. If performed properly, this technique requires only 2 to 3 minutes and should cause the client no discomfort. Chest percussion often is used in conjunction with postural drainage, chest vibration, and coughing tech-

---

TYPES OF INCENTIVE SPIROMETERS

FLOW-DEPENDENT SPIROMETER

Flow-dependent incentive spirometers provide visual feedback when the client inhales at a targeted flow rate. These incentive spirometers do not provide positive feedback for slow deep breaths. The targeted flow rate is preset at the factory and may not be optimal for all clients.

VOLUME-INCENTIVE SPIROMETER

Volume-incentive spirometers provide visual feedback regarding the inspired volume. They are available in both reusable and disposable forms. Care must be taken to prevent the transmission of infection with reusable units.

niques. Percussion should not be performed over the sternum, vertebrae, kidneys, or tender areas and is contraindicated in clients with cardiac conditions, osteoporosis, and pleural effusion.

Chest vibration. Chest vibration usually is performed following percussion. In this technique chest vibrations are transmitted through the chest wall while the client exhales slowly after taking a deep breath. The procedure is performed with arms and shoulders straight and placing flattened hands over the area of the chest to be drained. Vibration is then performed by alternate tensing and contracting using the arm and shoulder muscles and should be continued for the duration of expiration. This maneuver produces fine vibratory movements that are transmitted to the client's chest wall. If a spontaneous cough is not elicited, the client should be instructed to cough following vibration or assisted coughing. Chest vibration can be repeated several times.

Postural drainage. Postural drainage is a technique used to drain pulmonary secretions from the various segments of each lung. The principles of gravity are used to help mobilize secretions to facilitate removal. This procedure has been found to be effective for clients producing copious amounts of secretions such as in CF and bronchiectasis (Kirilloff et al., 1985). Postural drainage with percussion and vibration is probably the most important factor in managing respiratory problems associated with CF in children (Ramsay, 1989; Sexton, 1990). However, postural drainage remains controversial with chronic bronchitis (Kersten, 1989). It has been associated with bronchoconstriction and falls in arterial oxygenation (Sexton, 1990).

Twelve positions are used to drain various lobes and bronchopulmonary segments. Most individuals do not require drainage in each position. The nurse should check radiographic reports to determine which lobe(s) require drainage. Several of the positions require the client's head to be below the trunk. These positions will require modification in clients who cannot tolerate the head down position. The head down position should not be used when increased intracranial pressure is suspected. This position should be used cautiously and only when the uppermost lung segment requires drainage. Clients with hypoxemia, cardiovascular or hemodynamic instability, and marked bronchospasm

should be treated with extreme caution and monitored closely (Tyler, 1982). Oxygen may be administered or increased unless contraindicated in clients with compromised respiratory status.

Before beginning, the nurse should explain the procedure and provide the client with tissues and a sputum cup. The client's chest should be auscultated before and after postural drainage to determine effectiveness of the procedure. Postural drainage should not be carried out immediately preceding or following a meal. Loose-fitting clothes facilitate coughing, deep breathing, and position changes. Bronchodilating medications given by nebulization, if ordered, should be given approximately 15 minutes before beginning postural drainage to facilitate drainage through dilated airways. The client is then assisted to the proper position. Extra pillows will be needed for proper positioning. Postural drainage with clients who have spinal cord injury should be carried out within the limitations of orthopedic alignment and stabilization, type of immobilization bed in use, and client tolerance (Buchanan & Nawoczenski, 1987). The client's respiratory status should be monitored continuously. If the client complains of respiratory difficulty or vital signs become unstable, immediately assist the client to a more upright position. Be prepared to provide supplemental oxygen or ventilatory support if necessary.

Percussion and vibration frequently are carried out in conjunction with postural drainage to help push secretions into the upper airways, where expectoration and suctioning can be accomplished. These measures can be fatiguing for clients, especially if all the lung segments require therapy. A client usually is positioned for 5 to 10 minutes to drain one segment of the lung. In the home postural drainage is accomplished most effectively with another person assisting. Mechanical vibrators are available and are especially helpful to clients who must carry out this procedure alone.

✦ **Discharge planning.** A schedule must be established for performing chest physiotherapy based on the client's needs. This procedure commonly is performed in the morning on arising to remove secretions that have pooled during the night and in the evening before retiring to allow optimum ventilation during sleep. Increased secretions that may accompany a respiratory infection may necessitate performing the procedures more frequently (Sexton, 1990).

Suctioning the Intubated Client

Tracheobronchial suctioning (see the box on p. 384) is necessary to remove secretions when the client cannot clear the airway by coughing or by other noninvasive techniques as previously described. In the rehabilitation setting suctioning is avoided unless absolutely necessary. For clients who require suctioning, clinical indications include the presence of audible secretions and low-pitched wheezes (Kersten, 1989; Knipper, 1984). Unnecessary suctioning can be avoided by using clinical assessment of the chest to determine the need for suctioning rather than a routine schedule for suctioning. Suctioning is most effective when carried out after administering bronchodilators and after mobilizing tracheobronchial secretions with the therapies previously described for airway clearance.

Although a common nursing procedure, tracheobronchial suctioning can produce serious complications. Potential

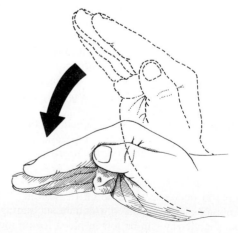

Fig. 18-8 Position of the hand for percussing the chest.

◆

PRINCIPLES OF TRACHEOBRONCHIAL SUCTIONING

GUIDELINE	RATIONALE
Vacuum pressure should read 80-100 mm Hg when the tubing is not occluded.	Excessive suction can cause hypoxemia.
	Higher pressures increase trauma and do not improve removal of secretions.
The external diameter of the catheter should be no more than half the internal diameter of the endotracheal or tracheostomy tube.	Large catheters prevent air from being pulled in around the catheter, thereby increasing the amount of negative pressure applied at the tip of the catheter and promoting atelectasis and hypoxemia.
Lubricate the tip of the catheter with water-soluble lubricant.	Oil-based products are never used when working with respiratory equipment as they can cause pneumonia.
Preoxygenate the client for 30 seconds to 2 minutes, as clinically indicated.	Method and duration of preoxygenation depend on available respiratory equipment, mode of ventilation, and stability of Pao_2. Increasing Fio_2 to 1.0 or 0.40 more than resting Fio_2 is best accompanied by 3-6 hyperinflations.
Quickly advance the catheter until resistance is met. Pull back 1-2 cm and suction intermittently, while slowly withdrawing the catheter. Do not take longer than 10-15 seconds for each suctioning pass.	Do not use continuous suction as it draws the tracheal mucosa into the catheter tip, stripping and traumatizing the mucosa. Avoid poking motions of the catheter.
Postoxygenate and hyperinflate for 1-5 minutes as clinically indicated.	Recovery to baseline Pao_2 takes 1-5 minutes.
Suction the pharynx with the same catheter, if needed. Remember, once you contaminate the catheter with oropharyngeal secretions, use a new sterile catheter and sterile gloves for subsequent tracheobronchial passes.	Some clients have minimal tracheobronchial secretions and large amounts of oropharyngeal secretions. Lung hyperinflations and coughing tend to push secretions up around the cuff and into the pharynx during the procedure.

Adapted with modifications from *Comprehensive Respiratory Nursing* (pp. 684-687) by L.D. Kersten, 1989. Philadelphia: W.B. Saunders. Copyright 1989 by W.B. Saunders. Adapted by permission.

complications of suctioning include hypoxia, atelectasis, bronchoconstriction, hypotension, cardiac arrhythmias, infection, irritation of the mucous membranes, and laryngospasm (Stone & Turner, 1990). Nurse researchers have generated a large body of research examining techniques to minimize the potential complications of suctioning (Preusser et al., 1988; Stone, Bell, & Preusser, 1991). Most studies focused on the effects of hyperoxygenation, hyperinflation, and hyperventilation before and after suctioning to minimize suction-induced hypoxia (Stone & Turner, 1990). Although the combination of hyperoxygenation and hyperinflation are effective in preventing complications for many clients, its efficacy depends on the underlying clinical condition (Riegel & Forshee, 1985). To date there are no definitive research-based guidelines for safe and effective tracheobronchial suctioning.

Suctioning protocols should be modified according to the client's need for suctioning and response to suctioning. Hyperoxygenation and hyperinflation for a few breaths before and after suctioning is recommended (Chulay, 1988; Sexton, 1990). Caution is warranted as suctioning procedures are not well tolerated in clients with increased intracranial pressure and those who are hemodynamically unstable (Rudy, Turner, Baun, Stoke, & Brucia, 1991; Stone, Preusser, Groch, Karl, & Gonyon, 1991).

In the acute and critical care setting, tracheobronchial suctioning of intubated clients is performed as a sterile technique. Lung sounds should be assessed before and after the procedure. Documentation should include the client's response to the procedure as well as the color, consistency, and quantity of secretions obtained.

Tracheobronchial suctioning can be very frightening for intubated clients, but nasotracheal suctioning is more frightening because of the additional discomfort associated with advancing the catheter through the nasal passages to the trachea. For all clients special attention should be given to assessing and reducing anxiety. Before suctioning, fear of the unknown can be attenuated by describing anticipated procedures and their accompanying sensations. During suctioning, anxiety may be reduced by informing clients as you progress from one stage to the next, while preparing them for unpleasant sensations. After suctioning, clients can be reassured by reporting outcomes.

◆ **Nasotracheal suctioning.** Nasotracheal suctioning is performed as an aseptic procedure. The same principles for suctioning are applied with modifications as described in the following box.

The placement of a nasopharyngeal airway can facilitate suctioning and decrease the amount of trauma to the mucous membranes when repeated, frequent suctioning is necessary, but the airway can be left in place for no more than 8 hours. Oral suctioning should not be performed until deep

---

SUCTIONING THE LOWER AIRWAY: THE NONINTUBATED CLIENT

PROCEDURE	RATIONALES AND PRECAUTIONS

1. *Positioning*
  a. Place the client in semi-Fowler's position.
  b. Remove pillow and place head in neutral position.
  c. Choose a patent nares for catheter insertion.
	Promotes general relaxation, oxygenation, and ventilation. Allows the catheter tip to curve anteriorly toward the trachea during catheter advancement. Maintains airway patency as well as client comfort.

2. *Preoxygenation and postoxygenation*
  a. Place an oxygen mask over the mouth, insert a nasal prong in the accessible nostril, or both.
  b. Ask the client to take slow deep breaths during the entire procedure.
  c. Particularly for a client with a borderline low Pao_2, ask another person to assist by holding the oxygen mask to the client's mouth, and holding the client's hand.
	Deep suctioning is a frightening experience. Touching the client or holding the hand provides reassurance and prevents the client from grabbing at the suction catheter during the procedure.

3. *Catheter advancement to the pharynx*
  a. Advance a well-lubricated catheter through the nose inferiorly and medially.
  b. Ask the client to stick out his tongue, as you pass the catheter down the back of the nasopharynx.
	Sticking the tongue out prevents the base of the tongue from falling back toward the posterior pharyngeal wall and narrowing the airway. Also it helps avoid coiling of the catheter in the mouth (a common problem) and greatly facilitates catheter tip advancement past the oropharynx.

c. If catheter advancement into the pharynx stimulates a productive cough, withdraw the catheter and suction intermittently. Do not proceed to tracheal suctioning.	Tracheal suctioning is not necessary, if coughing results in adequate expectoration of mucus.
d. For repeated suctioning, consider insertion of a nasopharyngeal airway. An oral airway may be inserted, if suctioning via the mouth is necessary as in comatose clients.	Avoids trauma to the nose. Oral airway guides the catheter to the hypopharynx.
e. Allow the client to rest 1 to 2 minutes before proceeding to the lower airway.	A brief rest allows the client to relax and prepare psychologically for the rest of the procedure. Also, providing additional reassurance at this time maximizes cooperation.
4. *Catheter advancement into the trachea*	
Traditional blind method	The following method is used when easy tracheal entry is anticipated.
a. Pinch the connecting tubing to eliminate unnecessary suction.	Suction is minimal but may contribute to hypoxemia in clients with borderline low Pao_2.
b. Instruct the client to take a very deep breath in or to cough.	A deep breath or cough opens the glottis.
c. Quickly slide the catheter past the epiglottis and into the trachea until resistance is met or until the client begins to cough vigorously.	Speed and timing are crucial. The catheter will not pass into the trachea unless catheter advancement coincides exactly with the brief opening of the glottis.
Alternative method	
a. Advance the catheter disconnected from the tubing.	Disconnection eliminates suction and allows the client to breathe through and around the suction catheter.
b. Listen at the opening of the air vent for the presence of breath sounds. Check to be sure the client is still deep breathing and not holding his breath.	Presence of breath sounds indicates that the catheter tip is still in the upper airway and the client is not holding his breath. Cessation of breath sounds indicates breath holding or passage of the tip into the esophagus.

Adapted with modifications from *Comprehensive Respiratory Nursing* (pp. 684-687), by L.D. Kersten, 1989, Philadelphia: W.B. Saunders. Copyright 1989 by W.B. Saunders. Adapted by permission.

Continued.

SUCTIONING THE LOWER AIRWAY: THE NONINTUBATED CLIENT—cont'd

PROCEDURE	RATIONALES AND PRECAUTIONS
c. Advance the catheter 1-2 inches during each inspiration. When the tip stimulates a cough, quickly slide the catheter into the trachea.	The glottis is open during inspiration. Remember, timing of catheter advancement with the cough is crucial to successful tracheal entry.
d. Otherwise, advance the tip until breath sounds cease; the tip is entering the esophagus. Withdraw it a few centimeters. Now it is above the epiglottis. Ask the client to cough, while you quickly pass it into the trachea.	
e. Verify tracheal entry by listening briefly for breath sounds before hooking the catheter up to suction.	Breath sounds may be the only reliable sign of tracheal entry in clients without a cough reflex.
5. *Suctioning*	
a. When the catheter tip meets resistance on advancement, pull back 1-2 cm and apply intermittent suction during catheter withdrawal as described above.	
b. Encourage coughing and deep breathing during catheter withdrawal.	
	These techniques help mobilize secretions, increase the amount of mucus aspirated, and decrease need for further suctioning.
6. *Client recovery*	
a. Some clients require complete catheter withdrawal between attempts to avoid hypoxemia and unbearable discomfort. Others tolerate resting with the suction catheter near the epiglottis.	Leaving the catheter near the epiglottis eliminates need for repeated advancements through the upper airway. Also, the catheter is ready for tracheal entry should the client cough spontaneously.

---

nasotracheal suctioning is completed. A metal or plastic (Yankauer) catheter can be used to suction the oral cavity. The client's tolerance of the procedure as well as the color, consistency, and amount of secretions should be documented in the chart.

✦ **Discharge planning.** If nasotracheal suctioning will be required after discharge, the client's caregivers should be instructed in the procedure and potential complications. The client and primary caregivers should be involved early in the rehabilitation process. Initially the nurse should explain the procedure and answer any questions. A mirror may be provided to the client to visualize the procedure and facilitate learning. Certain modifications in the suctioning procedure can be made in the home setting. Although aseptic technique is used in the hospital to prevent nosocomial infections, clean technique can be used in the home. Catheters do not have to be discarded after each use but can be washed in a mild soap solution, rinsed thoroughly, and then boiled for 5 minutes. The catheters are then wrapped in a clean towel, ready for use. The client can make a sterile saline solution by boiling water with salt added and storing the solution in a sealed container. A new supply of sterile water or saline solution should be made daily to avoid bacterial contamination once the receptacle has been opened. The receptacle used for solution storage also should be boiled each time.

Social services can facilitate the purchase or rental of a portable suction machine and other necessary equipment should financial assistance be required. A referral should be made to a home care agency for follow-up care. The home care nurse will be able to evaluate how well the client and significant others are coping and make the necessary modifications in care.

Interventions for Clients with Tracheostomies

For individuals with ineffective airway clearance, tracheostomy tube insertion (Fig. 18-9) may be necessary to (1) relieve airway obstruction, (2) protect the airway from aspiration because of impaired gag reflexes, (3) facilitate the removal of respiratory tract secretions, and (4) provide for mechanical ventilation. Clients often are admitted to rehabilitation facilities with tracheostomies in place. Tracheostomies may be temporary or permanent. Permanent tracheostomies are necessary when a client cannot be weaned from a respirator or cannot effectively cough up secretions.

✦ **Types of tracheostomy tubes**

Commonly used tracheostomy tubes are described in the box on p. 388 (Johnson et al., 1986). In the acute care setting, most tubes are composed of plastic or polyvinyl because they are disposable and lightweight, allow less adherence of secretions, and cause less irritation. They also

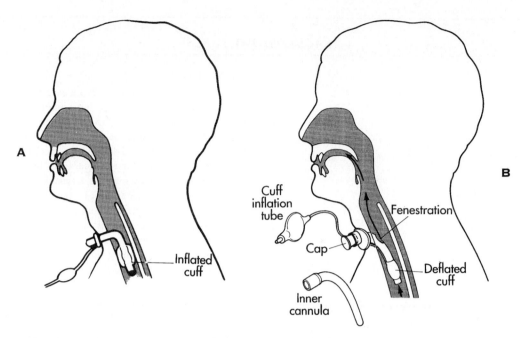

Fig. 18-9   **A,** Placement of tracheostomy tube with inflated cuff. **B,** Fenestrated tracheostomy tube with cuff deflated, inner cannula removed, and tracheostomy tube capped to allow air to pass over the vocal cords. (From *Medical-Surgical Nursing: Assessment and Management of Clinical Problems, 3rd ed.* by S.M. Lewis and I.C. Collier, 1992, St. Louis: Mosby–Year Book. Copyright 1992 by Mosby–Year Book. Reprinted by permission.)

come with or without a cuff. In long-term care settings, plastic tubes are used, but metal and nylon tubes also are used because of their durability. The tracheostomy tube best suited to the client's needs is chosen. Anatomic changes such as growth, development of granulation tissue, or changes in ventilatory needs require ongoing evaluation.

When using a soft cuffed tracheostomy tube, the cuff is deflated when problems arise or once every 2 to 3 days to check for overinflation. Inflation pressures are kept under 25 cm H_2O or over 20 cm H_2O to occlude the trachea, while preventing high-pressure damage to the lateral wall of the trachea. The cuff pressure is monitored three times a day with a manometer without deflating the cuff. The oropharynx is suctioned before deflation to prevent aspiration of pooled secretions above the inflated cuff. Hard cuffs are not recommended because they do not conform to the shape of trachea and therefore require higher pressures to prevent excessive leaking around the cuff. With higher pressures the cuffs press against the lateral wall of the trachea, causing necrosis of the tracheal tissue.

Communication is a problem for intubated clients. The fenestrated tube can be used to facilitate verbal communication as previously described. Additionally a tracheostomy tube with no cuff or deflated cuff can be used as an alternative to the fenestrated tube for clients on mechanical ventilation. If the client is receiving PPV, the ventilator settings can be adjusted to provide higher air flows, allowing air to flow around the tube toward the vocal cords for speaking. The ability to tolerate this procedure will depend on the client's ventilatory stability, strength, and secretion volume (Sexton, 1990). A number of additional communica-

tion aids are available such as the Passy-Muir tracheostomy speaking valve (Drayton-Hargrove & Mandzak-McCarron, 1987a). A speech pathologist should be consulted to evaluate the client's need for additional communication devices.

Tracheostomy buttons can be used by clients who require ventilatory support for only part of the day. The button is used to occlude the tracheostomy and establish normal air flow through the larynx, oral cavity, and nasal passages, allowing the client to speak and to cough. The Kistner tube can be used as a transition before occlusion of the tracheostomy. The Kistner tracheostomy tube has a one-way valve that attaches to the outer cannula and allows air flow in through the tracheostomy during inspiration only (Kersten, 1989). On exhalation air follows the normal route, out through the trachea and upper airways.

◆ Tracheostomy care

Rehabilitation clients with tracheostomies have special care requirements to prevent complications and maintain adequate ventilatory function.

Tracheostomy suctioning. Suctioning principles are applied as previously described. The following differences should be noted. With tracheostomy suctioning, the suction pressure should be reduced to only 60 to 80 mm Hg. The distal tip of the suction catheter is inserted into the tracheostomy until slight resistance is met, with care being taken not to traumatize the airway by pushing forcefully.

With a tracheostomy in place, the humidifying and warming mechanisms of the nose are bypassed. Cold, dry air causes drying of the tracheobronchial mucosa and thicken-

◆

TRACHEOSTOMY TUBES

TYPES	INDICATIONS
Cuffed tube with soft flexible cuff	A soft-cuffed tube is used in mechanically ventilated clients to prevent the leak of air and aspiration of secretions around the tube. Soft cuffs are less likely to cause problems with high pressures on the tracheal wall.
Fenestrated tube	Fenestrated tubes are used during weaning. They have opening(s) or fenestration(s) in the outer cannula so air can flow through the fenestrations to the larynx for speaking (Fig. 18-9). The fenestrations also allow the client to cough and expel secretions through the mouth. The cuff should be deflated before inserting the inner cannula.
Uncuffed plastic and metal tubes	Uncuffed tubes frequently are used for long-term care when the client has a functioning glottis. Metal tubes are rigid and can cause localized tissue irritation and excessive production of mucus.

ing of secretions, and promotes encrustation within the tube. The risk for problems of this nature can be reduced by providing humidity via a tracheostomy collar with a heated jet nebulizer (Manzetti & Hoffman, 1992).

Cannula and stoma care. Cannula and stoma care should be provided every 8 hours according to the institution protocol. Sterile disposable cleaning kits are available. The inner cannula is soaked in hydrogen peroxide, cleansed with a test tube brush and pipe cleaners, and rinsed with saline solution. Be sure the inner cannula is locked securely in place on reinsertion.

The stoma site or area around the tracheostomy tube should be cleansed with hydrogen peroxide to remove secretions. With one hand, hold the tracheostomy tube to lessen its movement and decrease the cough stimulus. Carefully cleanse the area around the stoma site, rinse with saline solution, and replace the tracheostomy dressing. Tracheostomy ties should be changed only with the assistance of another person to hold the tracheostomy firmly in place. If another person is not available, do not remove the soiled ties until the clean ones are tied firmly in place. An extra sterile tracheostomy tube of the same size with its obturator should be immediately available at all times. A sterile hemostat should also be available to hold the stoma open if necessary. Generally reinsertion of a tracheostomy is not difficult if the tracheostomy is more than 72 hours old. The physician should be immediately notified.

◆ **Decannulation.** A tracheostomy tube should remain in place no longer than necessary; delayed complications include tracheal stenosis, tracheoesophageal fistula, and infection. As soon as the client can maintain adequate ventilation and is able to cough and expel secretions, decannulation procedures should be initiated. First, the cuff (if present) is deflated. If cuff deflation is tolerated, the tracheostomy tube can gradually be reduced in size. With the cuff deflated, the tube can be intermittently plugged with a Kistner button or tracheal button. As previously noted, the buttons allow for ready access for suctioning or ventilation, if necessary. The client should be closely monitored at this

time for respiratory distress. This procedure is often stressful for the client. Initially until "plugging" is well tolerated, the nurse should stay with the client to encourage proper breathing technique and provide reassurance. If tracheostomy tube occlusion is tolerated and the client is able to cough and expel secretions, the tube can be removed after 24 to 72 hours. Sometimes the tracheal button is allowed to remain in place, if there is concern that the client may require suctioning. Once the tube is removed, the stoma closes spontaneously in a few days. A sterile gauze should be placed over the stoma until healed. The client needs to be observed closely for any evidence of respiratory distress.

◆ **Discharge planning.** There are instances, however, when a permanent tracheostomy is required—for example, when a client cannot be weaned from a ventilator or cannot effectively cough up secretions. Thus it is necessary to teach the client's caregivers all aspects of tracheostomy care and suctioning. Early participation in care facilitates learning in a relaxed and unhurried manner. Inner cannula care generally is easier and less anxiety producing for the client and primary caregivers to learn.

In the home equipment for cleaning the inner cannula and stoma can be washed and reused. The only purchases are hydrogen peroxide, dressings, and pipe cleaners or a brush to remove secretions from inside the tracheostomy. The primary caregiver should demonstrate and be comfortable with all aspects of tracheostomy care including accidental decannulation. A duplicate sterile tracheostomy tube should be readily available in the home. Clients and primary caregivers need to be taught how to insert a new tracheostomy tube. Emergency telephone numbers should be readily available and visible in the home. The client should also be capable of directing someone in proper tracheostomy care. Proper humidification of the client's air supply is an important discharge concern. A mechanical room humidifier may have to be purchased for the home or a portable source of humidified air or oxygen may have to be supplied. Sometimes wearing a dressing dampened with sterile water over the tracheostomy tube is sufficient. However, the client should be cautioned about the danger of getting water in the tracheostomy. The client should always protect the tracheostomy opening from possible inhalation of foreign substances (e.g., powder, aerosol sprays) and from dry air. The client should be encouraged to drink adequate amounts of fluid to help liquefy secretions.

The client and primary caregiver should be taught to examine the sputum for color, amount, and consistency. Any change in the normal characteristics of the sputum, as well as other signs of a respiratory tract infection (e.g., elevated temperature or increased shortness of breath) should be reported to the physician immediately. Signs of infection around the stoma site (e.g., redness, pain, or purulent drainage) also should be reported. Clients should be told to avoid other individuals with respiratory tract infections, since they are particularly vulnerable to such infections. Good oral hygiene should be stressed because the oropharyngeal area contains many organisms, including anaerobes, which can be aspirated into the lower respiratory tract. Keeping the mouth clean can decrease the number of these organisms and the chance of infection. Family members who smoke should be encouraged to quit. Smoking can irritate the mucous membranes, stimulate production of mucus, impair ciliary function, and increase vulnerability to respiratory tract infections.

It is important to provide the client with a means of communication. An emergency system should be established in the home to allow the client to contact someone if there is an emergency.

Outcome Criteria

For the client with ineffective airway clearance, the following outcome criteria are identified (Siskind, 1989). The client will demonstrate a patent airway as evidenced by

1. Lungs clear to auscultation; no adventitious breath sounds
2. Respiratory rate from 14 to 24 per minute
3. Clear, unobstructed airway
4. Absence of cyanosis; arterial blood gases return to baseline values
5. Absence of dyspnea

IMPAIRED GAS EXCHANGE

Impaired gas exchange is the "state in which an individual experiences an imbalance between oxygen uptake and carbon dioxide elimination at the alveolar-capillary membrane gas exchange area" (Kim et al., 1993). A mismatch in ventilation and perfusion is the most common cause of impaired gas exchange and it is manifested by hypoxemia. Impaired gas exchange is seen in many clients with chronic lung disease including COPD, interstitial lung disease, BPD, and acute infections as described earlier. However, in the pulmonary rehabilitation setting clients with impaired gas exchange most commonly have COPD. In the general rehabilitation setting, impaired gas exchange is seen in clients with severe restrictive lung disease with and without concomitant lower respiratory tract infection as in clients with quadriplegia secondary to spinal cord injury, Guillain-Barré syndrome, and scoliosis.

Assessment

The NANDA (North America Nursing Diagnosis Association) defining characteristics for impaired gas exchange include confusion, somnolence, restlessness, irritability, hypercapnia, and hypoxia (Kim et al., 1993). In general, clinical signs and symptoms of hypoxemia are vague and nonspecific.

✦ **Subjective.** Some clients may complain of feeling anxious, irritable, and restless resulting from decreased oxygen delivery to brain tissues. Dyspnea is also a common complaint.

✦ **Objective.** Impaired gas exchange will be reflected in the arterial blood gas values, measured while breathing room air. The Pao_2 and oxyhemoglobin saturation will be decreased, and the $Paco_2$ may be increased. Changes in oxyhemoglobin saturation can be detected with the pulse oximeter, but significant changes should be verified with measurement of arterial blood gas values.

Goals

The primary nursing goal is that the client will maintain adequate oxygenation without developing complications of oxygen toxicity. Clients will demonstrate adequate gas exchange as evidenced by arterial blood gas values within the normal range for each client. Accompanying changes will include quiet breathing with normal respiratory rate, tidal volume and rhythm, reduced dyspnea, and usual skin color.

INTERVENTIONS FOR CLIENTS WITH IMPAIRED GAS EXCHANGE

The underlying causes of impaired gas exchange may be related to ineffective airway clearance and ineffective breathing pattern as described earlier in this chapter. In most cases clients will have more than one of the related respiratory problems, and a combination of approaches will be warranted—for example, if secretions are excessive and tenacious, nursing interventions related to ineffective airway clearance would be appropriate. In instances where the underlying problem is an ineffective breathing pattern, then interventions to increase breathing effectiveness would be appropriate.

Positioning

Clients with unilateral lung disease should not be positioned routinely from side to side because regional ventilation and perfusion of the lung is affected by gravity. Dependent portions of the lung receive a greater proportion of ventilation and perfusion. In the upright position the bases receive a greater proportion of ventilation and perfusion than the apex. When lying on the side, the dependent lung receives a greater proportion of ventilation and perfusion. Clients with unilateral lung involvement have the highest arterial oxygen levels when they alternate between semi-Fowler's position and lying on the side with the uninvolved lung down for 60 to 90 minutes (Demers, 1987; Gillespie & Rehder, 1987). It is thought that the heart and blood vessels compress the lung more when lying on the left side. Consequently clinical guidelines recommend positioning the client with unilateral lung involvement with the uninvolved side down and positioning the client with bilateral lung involvement at a 90 degree angle with the head elevated 10 to 15 degrees on their right side (Yeaw, 1992).

Respiratory function in spinal cord injured clients also is affected by posture (supine, sitting, and standing). In clients with quadriplegia the forced vital capacity (FVC) fell to 30% to 50% of normal values during sitting and standing (Chen, Lien, & Wu, 1990). In clients with paraplegia the FVC was reduced by 5% to 7% when changing postures from erect to supine. Therefore clients with spinal cord injury should be observed closely during changes in posture, particularly from the supine to upright position.

Oxygen Therapy

Oxygen therapy does not treat the underlying cause of hypoxemia but does decrease the cardiopulmonary workload, allows the client to breathe easier, and reduces the effects of hypoxemia. Oxygen therapy should not be taken lightly as complications may occur as a result of the therapy. Oxygen therapy has a drying effect on respiratory mucosa and therefore should be delivered with humidification. Oxygen toxicity can result if high concentrations of oxygen are maintained for more than 24 hours, although the need for high oxygen concentrations is not common in rehabilitation.

Since clinical signs of hypoxemia may not always be present, the nurse monitors Pao_2 and Sao_2 to determine the need for and evaluation of oxygen therapy. For continuous monitoring, pulse oximetry is preferred to repeated measuring of arterial blood gas values under most conditions. Pulse oximetry is a noninvasive method of measuring Sao_2. The pulse oximeter has a probe that transmits light pulses through capillary beds in the earlobe or finger; the degrees of light absorption through tissue is related to arterial Hb saturation.

The pulse oximeter measures total Hb saturation and does not distinguish between Hb saturation with oxygen and carbon monoxide. This is a problem with heavy smokers, because heavy smoking increases carbon monoxide levels in the blood. A heavy smoker may have a carboxyhemoglobin saturation of 8% and an oxyhemoglobin saturation of 90%, but the pulse oximeter will register 98% Hb saturation. Consequently the pulse oximeter is most useful in monitoring changes in Hb saturation in clients who are not smoking; significant changes should be verified with arterial blood gas values. Small portable pulse oximetry devices are well suited for monitoring clients continuously at rest or during exercise and for use in home settings where documentation for Medicare home oxygen reimbursement may be required (Nelson, Murphy, Bradley, & Durie, 1986).

Candidates for supplemental oxygen therapy are individuals with significant hypoxemia. Critical parameters are (1) Pao_2 of 55 mm Hg or less or Sao_2 of 85% or less at rest; (2) Pao_2 of 55 to 59 mm Hg or Sao_2 of 86% to 89% with evidence of tissue hypoxia, manifested by pulmonary hypertension, cor pulmonale, erythrocytosis, impaired mentation, central nervous system dysfunction at rest; or (3) Pao_2 of 55 mm Hg or less or Sao_2 of 85% or less during exercise or improvement in duration, performance, or capacity for exercise with oxygen (Kersten, 1989). Appropriate oxygen therapy is based on knowledge of the client's arterial blood gas values and pH. Oxygen therapy usually is titrated to maintain a Pao_2 of 70 to 100 mm Hg.

Clients with COPD most frequently require long-term oxygen management. In this group oxygen therapy primarily is initiated to relieve pulmonary hypertension and cor pulmonale, to decrease secondary polycythemia, and to improve mental functioning and exercise tolerance (Fulmer & Snider, 1984; Mitchell, 1992). The efficacy of long-term oxygen therapy is based on the findings of the Nocturnal Oxygen Therapy Trial (NOTT) study (1980) comparing the nocturnal use of oxygen with the use of continuous oxygen. The findings indicated that low-flow oxygen given for 15 hours in a 24-hour period significantly reduces mortality in COPD clients compared with no oxygen; continuous oxygen further decreases mortality by almost twofold compared with nocturnal oxygen. Recent findings over 5 years indicate that long-term oxygen therapy improves the quality of life by improving clients' neuropsychological condition, by increasing their walking distance, and by reducing time spent in the hospital (Petty, 1982; Weitzenblum, Apprill, & Oswald, 1992).

Controlled low-flow oxygen (1 or 2 L) is therefore recommended for part or all of the 24-hour period. An additional 1 L may be provided during exercise or sleep (Petty, 1987). However, the respiratory drive of the client with COPD is stimulated by a need for oxygen. Increasing the concentration of oxygen beyond the recommended limits may result in respiratory depression. Low-flow oxygen should raise the Pao_2 to 60 or 65 mm Hg or the O_2 saturation to 90% to 94%.

◆ **Oxygen delivery systems.** A variety of devices are used for the administration of oxygen. The specific technique chosen depends on the client's clinical condition, concentration of oxygen needed, degree of ventilatory support required, and the client's ability and/or desire to adhere to the therapy.

Low-flow oxygen systems. Low-flow oxygen systems are nasal cannulas or catheters, simple oxygen masks, and partial rebreathing masks. Both high and low oxygen concentrations can be delivered by this system; however, the actual concentration may vary depending on the client's breathing patterns. The advantages of low-flow systems are their ease of administration and client comfort. Oxygen is most frequently delivered through a nasal cannula or mask. The nasal cannula is a simple, effective way to administer low to moderate oxygen concentrations. The client does not have to have oxygen flow interrupted to eat, cough, and perform other activities. One disadvantage is that cannulas can cause nasal irritation, even when the oxygen is humidified. Small amounts of a water-soluble lubricant applied to the nares can reduce or prevent this discomfort (Wilson & Thompson, 1990). The simple oxygen mask is widely used for oxygen therapy and can be combined with humidity for aerosol therapy. For oxygen concentrations of less than 35%, the aerosol can be delivered by compressed air. Its primary disadvantages are that oxygen concentrations can vary depending on how tightly the mask fits the face, the level of respiratory effort, and the need to remove the mask to eat or speak. The partial rebreathing mask consists of a tightly fitting mask connected to a reservoir bag. This mask can deliver oxygen concentrations of approximately 90% to

100%. The oxygen flow rate should be set between 5 and 10 L/minute to prevent the reservoir bag from completely collapsing during inspiration and to provide the system with a continuous oxygen supply. A portion of the client's exhaled gas re-enters the reservoir bag—hence the name, as it fills between breaths. The portion of exhaled gas that enters the bag is the first exhaled from the respiratory tract and therefore has low CO_2 levels. The partial rebreathing mask is primarily used to deliver high concentrations of oxygen for short periods.

T-pieces. T-pieces are used to deliver continuous oxygen through a tracheostomy tube (Mitchell, 1992). The T-piece is a hard plastic tube in the shape of a T. The bottom of the T is attached directly to the tracheostomy tube, and one of the other two ends is attached to the humidified oxygen source; the third end remains open. A tracheostomy mask also may be used to deliver humidified oxygen through a tracheostomy.

Alternate delivery systems. A number of alternate delivery systems are available to conserve oxygen and conceal the nasal prongs and tubing. These systems are most useful for clients using long-term oxygen therapy in the home. Conserving oxygen is especially important for clients because it makes their portable oxygen tanks last longer, enabling them to be away from home for longer periods before the oxygen tank empties. Concealing the nasal prongs improves cosmetic appearances and makes the oxygen less obvious.

Many clients resist the use of 24-hour oxygen therapy, because it symbolizes a worsening of their condition and is inconvenient and bothersome. Adherence may be improved if the client actively participates in selecting the type of oxygen delivery system to be used.

Transtracheal oxygen systems. Transtracheal oxygen systems deliver supplemental oxygen directly into the trachea via a small plastic cannula that is inserted into the trachea at the base of the neck (Hoffman & Wesmiller, 1988). The transtracheal oxygen delivery system is less conspicuous than the standard nasal prongs. A lower flow rate is required because oxygen is delivered directly into the trachea, bypassing part of the anatomic dead space, and oxygen is delivered continuously throughout inspiration and expiration. It also may increase exercise tolerance and reduce dyspnea (Reinke, Hoffman, & Wesmiller, 1992) (Fig. 18-10).

Once the respiratory tract has matured, care of the catheter includes daily removal for cleansing by washing with tap water and antibacterial soap (Hoffman & Wesmiller, 1988). While in place the catheter is irrigated twice a day with normal saline solution to prevent accumulation of mucous balls at the distal end. Mucous balls can build up on the distal end of the catheter, occluding the catheter and causing a buildup of pressure in the tubing. A "pop" when disconnecting the catheter indicates obstruction of oxygen flow.

Reservoir cannula and pulse-dose demand valve device. The reservoir nasal cannula and pulse-dose demand valve device are noninvasive systems that conserve oxygen by restricting flow to the inspiratory phase of ventilation. With the reservoir system, oxygen flows continuously into the reservoir and is inhaled from the reservoir during inspiration. This system is designed with two styles: a pendant device with standard nasal prongs and the reservoir located in a pendant at the neck, or a mustache device (which resembles a mustache) with the reservoir attached directly to the nasal prongs. The pulse-dose demand valve device conserves oxygen by sensing the beginning of inhalation and immediately delivering a bolus of oxygen. Clinical experience with these devices is limited, and the initial cost is higher for the reservoir system (Kersten, 1989). Both systems require some nasal breathing on inspiration and expiration to trigger the device. Clients who are mouth breathers have to use a traditional system at night or the system may not be triggered, resulting in a drop in Sao_2 (Hoffman & Wesmiller, 1988). Special adapted eyeglasses and headbands conceal the nasal prongs for delivery of oxygen.

Supplemental Oxygen Delivery in the Home

There are three methods by which oxygen can be delivered in the home: compressed gas in tanks or cylinders, liquid oxygen in reservoirs, and oxygen concentrators and enrichers (Kersten, 1989; Openbrier, Hoffman, & Wesmiller, 1988).

✦ **Compressed gas.** The most familiar type of supplemental oxygen is compressed gas or tank oxygen. The advantages of this system are delivery of 100% oxygen accurately over the widest possible range of liter-per-minute flow. The disadvantages include the size and weight of tanks and the high pressures generated when oxygen is stored as a compressed gas; in addition, capacity of the tanks is limited. A small E cylinder tank can be attached to a stroller for the ambulatory client. In COPD clients with hypoxic drives who are sensitive to slight changes in oxygen flow, a calibrated flow with ¼-L/minute gradations is recommended. In addition, a back-pressure compensated flowmeter should

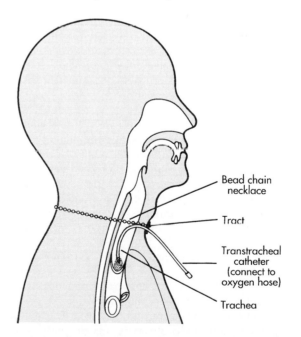

Fig. 18-10 Transtracheal oxygen catheter. (From *Medical-Surgical Nursing: Assessment and Management of Clinical Problems, 3rd ed.* by S.M. Lewis and I.C. Collier, 1992, St. Louis: Mosby–Year Book. Copyright 1992 by Mosby–Year Book. Reprinted by permission.)

be used when long extensions of tubing are used to allow ambulation. This type of flowmeter compensates for increased back pressure in extension tubing and ensures an accurate liter flow delivery of oxygen.

Liquid oxygen. The newest form of oxygen delivery is liquid oxygen. Oxygen is cooled to a liquid −295° C. In its liquid form oxygen can be stored in a smaller space at lower storage pressures. Liquid oxygen can be stored in containers similar to a large thermos bottle. When the outlet valve is opened, the liquid oxygen travels through a series of coils that absorb heat from the atmosphere, converting the liquid oxygen back to gas. The liquid form is preferred by many clients because lightweight portable units (<10 lb) can be easily refilled from the larger reservoir and provide sufficient oxygen for about 8 hours at 2 L/minute (Fig. 18-11). The major disadvantage to liquid oxygen is the cost and the fact that liquid oxygen containers "vent" small amounts of oxygen if not used. Liquid oxygen provides a good solution for clients who are motivated and obliged to walk a great deal (Weitzenblum, 1992).

Oxygen concentrators and enrichers. Oxygen concentrators and enrichers are electrically powered devices that compress room air and pass it through filters to remove nitrogen, water, and carbon dioxide. Oxygen thus is concentrated from the 21% found in the atmosphere to 85% to 90%. The concentration of the oxygen varies with the flow rate. For example, at low-flow rates of 1 to 4 L/minute, the oxygen concentration may be as high as 90%, but at higher flow rates of >5 L/minute, the concentration may be only 82%. These devices are therefore not recommended for restrictive lung disease clients who require high-flow oxygen concentrations. The advantages of oxygen concentrators are that they provide an unlimited supply of oxygen in the home without the worry of refilling. It also is probably the cheapest system for continuous oxygen therapy; however, it does increase the monthly electrical bill. Disadvantages are that the concentrator may be somewhat noisy, and a backup oxygen delivery system is necessary in case of electric power failure. These systems are probably best suited for the bedridden or homebound client.

Implementation for home oxygen use should specify clearly the number of liters per minute, minimal number of hours per day for nocturnal use, and the method of delivery, (e.g., nasal prongs). The need also must be documented for portable oxygen use and conditions for use. For Medicare reimbursement the prescription for oxygen also must include the specific respiratory diagnosis and duration, (e.g., 3 months). Medicare reimbursement covers home oxygen use under the following conditions (Openbrier, Fuoss, & Mall, 1988):

$Pao_2 < 55$ mm Hg or $Sao_2 < 85\%$ or $Pao_2 = 56$ to 69 mm Hg

$Sao_2 = 86\%$ to 89% and client has evidence of one of the following secondary diagnoses:

1. Dependent edema suggests congestive heart failure, or pulmonale on ECG, or erythrocytosis with a hematocrit value over 56%
2. During sleep Pao_2 drops to or below 55 mm Hg, or drops more than 10 mm Hg, or Sao_2 drops to or below 85% or drops more than 5%

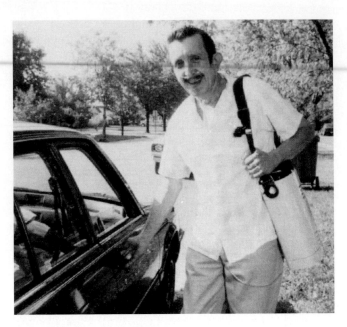

Fig. 18-11 Client getting into his car with portable liquid oxygen. (From *Principles and Practice of Adult Health Nursing* [p. 611] by A.G. Beare and J.L. Myers, 1990, St. Louis: Mosby–Year Book. Copyright 1990 by Mosby–Year Book. Reprinted by permission.)

3. During exercise Pao_2 drops to or below 55 mm Hg, or Sao_2 drops to or below 85%

COPD clients tend to actually reduce the number of hours of oxygen use because they tend to sleep fewer hours, and they dislike the appearance of the oxygen delivery system. Emphasis must be on the use of oxygen to increase functional level rather than as a dependent crutch. Consideration of one of the less conspicuous delivery systems may help feelings of embarrassment. The nurse must reinforce that the full benefits of oxygen therapy may not be fully realized unless the client adheres to the prescribed usage.

Outcome Criteria

For the client with impaired gas exchange, the following outcome criteria are identified. The client will demonstrate adequate gas exchange as evidenced by

1. Normal rate, rhythm, and depth of respirations
2. Usual color of skin and mucus membranes
3. Pao_2 levels at 65 to 80 mm Hg and Sao_2 to 85% or within normal ranges for client
4. Client states breathing is comfortable

Discharge Planning and the Rehabilitation Team

Discharge goals for the client with long-term pulmonary involvement should be established early in the rehabilitation process. Discharge planning is complex and requires involvement of the entire interdisciplinary team. An adult or child may be discharged home on oxygen therapy with or without ventilatory support. An organized and comprehensive plan is essential in assisting the client and primary caregivers to meet physical, emotional, and mental health needs. This process involves assessing specific equipment and supply needs, identifying vendors to procure supplies, and maintaining supplies and equipment in the home. More important the process also involves evaluating the capability of family members to provide the necessary care to meet the client's needs. Consideration also must be given to the needs of caregivers, who must provide care on a continuous basis.

REHABILITATION TEAM MEMBERS, ROLES AND FUNCTIONS

A primary physician, chest specialist, physiatrist, physical therapist, occupational therapist, nutritionist, respiratory therapist, social worker, vocational rehabilitation counselor, and psychologist or psychiatrist may be working with the nurse as members of the pulmonary rehabilitation team. Their roles and functions in working with the client who has impaired respiratory function are described as follows:

Primary physicians or chest specialists: Perform history and physical examination and order diagnostic tests.

Physiatrists: Evaluate clients regarding readiness to engage in vocational rehabilitation based on the results of the physical examination, record review (including radiologic and bacteriologic findings), complete pulmonary function studies, and electrocardiogram.

Occupational therapists: Evaluate clients' ability to perform ADL and develop individualized practical, energy-saving techniques. Occupational therapists evaluate clients' upper extremity strength, sensation, range of joint motion, coordination, cognition, and performance in home activities and teach clients to pace activities properly by monitoring their pulse, coordinating breathing with activity, conserving energy in such maintenance activities as dressing, personal hygiene, and eating and with instrumental activities such as working, socializing, performing household chores, preparing meals, and washing laundry. Occupational therapists also teach relaxation techniques and explain the hazards of air pollution. Progress is measured by observing clients' use of energy conservation measures in all activities, stabilization of pulse rate with activities, and a decrease in dyspnea and fatigue.

Physical therapists: Develop an exercise program designed to diminish dyspnea, improve breathing, and increase endurance. Physical therapists teach the client ways to train the muscles of respiration and facilitate the mechanics of breathing through pursed-lip diaphragmatic breathing. The pulse is monitored during progressive ambulation. The client may be taught postural drainage for home use, manual and mechanical percussion, and vibratory techniques for bronchial toilet, and relaxation techniques.

Nutritionists: Assess eating habits, home or other food preparation facilities, food likes and dislikes, and general nutritional status. Nutritionists teach diet modification, meal planning, principles of cooking, and ways to select food when grocery shopping. In addition, they give general instruction on proper nutrition.

Respiratory therapists: Teach clients to initiate and become competent in the use and care of respiratory equipment including: oxygen equipment, nebulizers and home ventilators.

Social workers: Obtain a social history and identify life roles of the client; reactions and perceptions of the client and family to the disability; and the client's emotional, physical, financial, intellectual, and environmental resources for coping with a disability. Social workers team up with psychologists to provide counseling for anxiety, depression, and other stress responses to illness, hospitalization, and disability. In addition, they provide information and advice about community resources such as attendant care, financial assistance, and legal and vocational aid.

Vocational rehabilitation counselors: Interview clients to establish preliminary psychosocial and vocational assessment. One of the major responsibilities of the rehabilitation program is to evaluate work tolerance and vocational potential of the client who is disabled. The type and amount of work the client can tolerate per day before experiencing discomfort is determined. Any vocational and avocational interests of the client are analyzed to ascertain proclivities. Work history is discussed in great detail and includes the client's employment history, duties and activities, job conditions, salary, ways in which jobs were obtained, and reasons for leaving a job. Clients seem to fall within three groups: (1) those who can return to their previous occupation with no limitations; (2) those who have disability-related conditions that conflict with the activities and conditions of their previous occupations; (3) those who have full work tolerance, usable skills, and the ability to use public transportation but who cannot return to their previous occupations because the activities and conditions involved may jeopardize their health.

Psychologists: Evaluate psychosocial history and reaction to illness and disability and provide counseling to assist clients and their families to adjust better to disability, cope better with illness, and adapt to the situation. Psychologists administer a battery of tests to measure anxiety, depression, somatic focus, and self-esteem. They help clients become more aware of their responses to disability and find solutions to family, economic, and other problems.

Discharge Planning

Discharge planning includes a needs assessment, supply and equipment procurement, home evaluation, and development of care strategies.

✦ Needs assessment

Effective planning first begins with a comprehensive assessment of equipment needs and resources available to the client. The desires of the client, caregivers, and family members should be taken into account. The costs of disposable supplies must be weighed against the time required to clean nondisposable supplies. Sufficient supplies need to be sent home with the client to allow time for procurement of additional supplies from a vendor. A vendor needs to be identified before discharge that will provide the scope and quality of services required by the client. The client's primary nurse is the one who usually determines supplies required for ongoing care and assists in identifying available vendors. Equipment decisions will be made by the physician, respiratory therapist, as well as the occupational and physical therapists. Usually ordering durable medical equipment must be done several weeks before discharge. The selection of a vendor for durable equipment (e.g., a ventilator) should consider the support services provided. The vendor should provide reliable service on a 24-hour-a-day basis. Charges for equipment should be reasonable, and the company should provide for reimbursement from insurance companies and federal agencies.

Counseling clients on equipment needs to accommodate travel for periodic medical evaluations as well as social outings is an important consideration (Kersten, 1989; Openbrier et al., 1988). Equipment needed for travel may include portable ventilator and suction machine, suction catheters and lubricant, portable oxygen or compressed air supply, manual resuscitation bag, and all prescribed medications. Traveling long distances by car is best accommodated by a liquid oxygen or concentrator system. The oxygen concentrator can run off the car battery. If tanks are to be taken along, they should be stored in the trunk and strapped down. Airplane travel will require additional planning. Regulations prohibit the use of portable oxygen systems on airplanes. Pressurized cabins of modern jets maintain an altitude of 5000 to 6000 feet. Clients should be encouraged to check with their physician regarding the safety of airplane travel. Remind clients to arrange for the availability of a portable oxygen tank on arrival at their destination through their oxygen distributor. For many clients travel can be safely undertaken if sufficient plans are made in advance.

Home evaluation. Evaluation of the home environment should be a part of the assessment. One or more home visits by members of the rehabilitation team may be necessary to plan for safety concerns and organizational strategies. Planning for storage of equipment and caregiving space begins early and is completed at discharge. Accessibility of the home to allow the client to move freely from one area to another needs to be determined. Any structural modifications, such as ramps required in the home, should be identified early so modifications will be ready by discharge. A number of safety issues in the home must be addressed before discharge. These include storage of supplies and equipment without obstructing exits or traffic flow, adequate electrical capacity of the home to handle any potential equipment needs, safety issues related to oxygen use, and presence of any children in the home. A plan for emergencies must be identified and in place before discharge. This plan should include all necessary phone numbers and notification of the client's impending discharge provided to the local hospital emergency room, fire department, police department, power company, primary care physician, and equipment vendor.

The non-ventilator-dependent client with COPD also requires home evaluation. Before discharge, the home environment needs to be evaluated so that conditions do not exist that aggravate the condition. For example, irritants and allergens are a primary source of respiratory difficulties—which can be avoided by regular house cleaning, removing any pets from inside the home, avoiding bringing in flowers with strong scents, and avoiding smoke inhalation. The use of a controlled heating and humidifying system with an air filter is recommended.

Care strategies. Most clients requiring long-term ventilator and/or oxygen support require home health care services. The level of care required by the client is an important consideration in the selection of a home health care agency. Some ventilator-dependent clients may require daily home visits or 8 to 16 hours of nursing care, whereas COPD clients may require much less intensive home care. Not all agencies may be equipped or their personnel adequately trained to handle ventilator-dependent clients. Clients receiving Medicare or Medicaid reimbursement must be sure that agencies are approved by these funding sources. Continuity of care must be assured. It is advisable to have the home health nurse identified and participate in the client's care before discharge. A complete health summary and health care plan must be communicated to the home health agency. Arrangements should be made with the home health agency for ongoing evaluation reports of the client's status.

The care demands required by ventilator-dependent clients is physically and emotionally draining on the family. Thomas, Ellison, Howell, and Winters (1992) found that the most important needs identified by family members caring for ventilator-dependent persons in the home were finances, provisions for emergencies, family relationships, and continuity of care. Need for support services ranked highest for caregivers of continuous ventilator-dependent adults and children and caregivers not living in. The handling of emergencies was most important to less experienced caregivers, whereas respite and financial needs ranked highest for full-time and experienced caregivers.

Families and caregivers often require respite from the 24-hour day-to-day care demands. Planning for periodic respite care is an extremely important factor in the client's and family's support network. Identification of respite options should be a part of discharge planning. Unfortunately very few options are available for formal respite care services for ventilator-dependent clients. Another option is to identify and train alternate caregivers that would be willing to relieve family caregivers periodically. Development of respite care options for ventilator-dependent clients and their families is an essential part of discharge planning.

Although the costs of ventilator-dependent care in the home is markedly less than institutional care (Bach et al., 1992; Burr, Guyer, Todres, Abrahams, & Chiada, 1984; Fisher & Prentice, 1982), funding options are limited. The social worker can provide information and assist in obtaining financial assistance. A coordinated well-planned discharge that involves all members of the rehabilitation team is necessary for a successful transition from the rehabilitation setting to the home.

ISSUES, TRENDS, AND NEW DIRECTIONS
Research

Future research should be directed toward establishing a research basis for pulmonary rehabilitation. Many interventions are based on traditional practice rather than on a research basis.

Models of Pulmonary Rehabilitation

Future models of pulmonary rehabilitation could incorporate primary health care within the context of the pulmonary rehabilitation setting. Pulmonary rehabilitation would emphasize health promotion, stressing the client's optimal state of wellness. In this model emphasis would be placed on client self-care behaviors, client independence, and socializing the client to remain active within the community. Pulmonary rehabilitation would be extended from the traditional hospital-based setting to home health care settings and convenient locations within the community. In this model the advanced nurse practitioners would combine the skills of traditional nurse practitioners and clinical nurse specialists, enabling them to provide primary care and assume increased responsibility for coordinating the rehabilitation of individual clients.

Providing primary care within the rehabilitation setting would create new opportunities for advanced practice pulmonary and rehabilitation nurses. In this role the advanced practice nurse would see clients on a regular basis within the structure of a rehabilitation program designed to maintain maximal levels of functioning. The primary population served would include clients with chronic lung disease and neuromuscular conditions affecting respiration as well as clients requiring supplemental oxygen and ventilatory support. Regular monitoring by an advanced practice nurse would allow early detection of potential health problems, facilitating treatment. In this model the advanced practice nurse would assume increased responsibility for the care of individual clients when they were clinically stable and refer them to a physician when they experienced exacerbations. Increased responsibility would include prescribing medications, oxygen therapy, and exercise regimens.

Within the health promotion framework, the advanced practice nurse would address respiratory health-related issues such as smoking cessation and the quality of air in the workplace. This could be accomplished through structured programs and through individual consultation. The nurse would address needs of clients with lung disease by organizing support groups for clients and significant others.

CASE STUDY: BRONCHOPULMONARY DYSPLASIA

Infants with bronchopulmonary dysplasia (BPD) present significant challenges to health care providers, parents, and families. These challenges arise from the problems associated with the disease, and most commonly include problems related to cardiopulmonary status, nutrition and weight gain, fluid balance, and growth and development. In the past, the complexity of these problems required most infants to remain in the hospital for extended periods. Today, with improved home care and follow-up, this hospitalization time has been shortened, reducing the financial, emotional, and developmental costs for affected children and families.

In order to ensure a successful transition to home for both the child and family, discharge planning must begin early and consider the needs and abilities of all persons and services that are to be involved. One critical need for children with BPD is respiratory stability and adequate oxygenation. The following case will be used to illustrate how one prepares for the discharge of an infant with BPD and will focus on the child's respiratory status.

CASE STUDY

Rachel is an 8-month-old girl with BPD. Rachel was born at 30 weeks' gestation, weighing 800 g. She had early evidence of hyaline membrane disease that progressed to classic BPD. She required mechanical ventilation for 4 weeks in the NICU, and since then has remained on supplemental oxygen. One and a half months ago, when she experienced an intercurrent respiratory illness, Rachel was required to return to mechanical ventilation briefly (for 4 days), but since then has been stable without any such further requirements.

Today Rachel receives supplemental oxygen via nasal cannula at a flow rate of 1/2 L/min. She has an oxygen saturation ranging between 90% and 94%, is taking oral feedings fairly well, and is showing slow but steady weight gain. Rachel, her family, and the hospital staff are preparing for Rachel's discharge.

Rachel's family consists of her parents, Joel and Marsha Sardy, and her 3-year-old brother, Sam. The Sardys are of hispanic background, and are bilingual, speaking both Spanish and English. They live in a two-bedroom apartment close to their extended family.

As discharge approaches, both parents are looking forward to Rachel's return home but express some concerns for her safety and for their ability to care for her adequately in their home setting. That Rachel will go home on supplemental oxygen and a cardiorespiratory monitor seems to be their major source of concern.

Goals

The overall goal of care in bronchopulmonary dysplasia is to promote growth and to enhance development. In relation to respiratory care, the goals are to ensure adequate oxygenation to promote growth, and as indicated, to wean from supplemental oxygen in order to enhance mobility and development.

Plan of Care

Patient/Family Problem	Nursing Interventions
Rachel's potential for inadequate oxygenation and respiratory distress	✦ Provide supplemental oxygen as indicated ✦ Monitor Rachel's respiratory status 　✦ Continual monitoring per cardiorespiratory monitor

Continued.

CASE STUDY: BRONCHOPULMONARY DYSPLASIA—cont'd

Plan of Care—cont'd

Patient/Family Problem	Nursing Interventions
Rachel's potential for inadequate oxygenation and respiratory distress—cont'd	✦ Respiratory assessments every 4 hours or as indicated - Oxygen saturation - Respiratory rate - Auscultation - Signs of respiratory distress (i.e., cyanosis, retractions, nasal flaring, wheezing) ✦ Monitor for signs of pulmonary hypertension 　✦ Ensure that an echocardiogram is performed prior to discharge to rule out pulmonary hypertension ✦ Administer bronchodilator therapy as prescribed to prevent bronchospasms and to decrease wheezing, coughing, and accessory muscle use ✦ Perform chest physiotherapy (CPT) as needed to assist clearance of airway secretions ✦ Teach parents how to administer oxygen at home and its storage and importance in Rachel's care 　✦ Explain to parents that over- or under-utilization of oxygen could have significant negative effects on Rachel's health and development 　✦ Explain to parents that there may be periods (i.e., with intercurrent illness or increased activity) where there is increased work of breathing, and an increased level of oxygen support (increased liter flow) may be required 　✦ Provide parents with a written plan that specifies who to contact, and how and when to adjust oxygen support ✦ Teach parents how to administer bronchodilator therapy and to recognize potential side effects ✦ Teach parents how to perform CPT and have the parents demonstrate ✦ Provide parents with a plan of how often to perform CPT in the home setting, and to increase its frequency with evidence of increased secretions, respiratory distress, or intercurrent illness ✦ Explain to parents the importance of home monitoring and how to use such a monitor ✦ Explain to parents that if they fail to use the monitor or fail to respond to an alarm, there may be irreversible consequences for their child ✦ Provide parents with a written plan that specifies the steps to take when the child shows signs of respiratory distress (i.e., how/when to adjust oxygen support, bronchodilator therapy, and other medications, who to contact, and when to bring child to the emergency room) ✦ Require that parents and other caregivers complete an infant CPR course before the child's discharge ✦ Teach the extended family and other caregivers, as well as the parents, about Rachel's status and care needs, as described above
Parental anxiety related to child's impending discharge from the hospital	✦ Explore the individual concerns of Mr. and Mrs. Sardy related to Rachel's impending discharge ✦ Provide parents with information and support ✦ Introduce the Sardys to other parents of children with BPD who have made the transition to home successfully ✦ Contact with other parents can be made in person or by telephone ✦ Introducing them to a family of the same cultural background would be ideal ✦ Provide parents with information on BPD and parent support groups in their community ✦ Teach parents how to care for Rachel's discharge care needs

---

CASE STUDY: BRONCHOPULMONARY DYSPLASIA—cont'd

Plan of Care—cont'd

Patient/Family Problem	***Nursing Interventions***
Parental anxiety related to child's impending discharge from the hospital—cont'd	✦ Familiarize them with Rachel's baseline status and teach them to recognize deviations from normal ✦ Provide them with many opportunities for learning and positive feedback ✦ Encourage parents to ask questions and express their concerns ✦ Have parents perform demonstrations on the techniques/therapies that they learn ✦ Assist parents to identify support persons who could serve as "back-up" caregivers and who could provide parents with some respite ✦ Involve these persons in learning about Rachel and her care prior to discharge ✦ Invite primary caregiver to meet with the care team and family prior to Rachel's discharge to enhance understanding, optimal care, and continuity ✦ Help parents plan for Rachel's environmental needs in the home setting ✦ Safe area for play that will accomodate oxygen delivery system ✦ Safe storage for oxygen ✦ Need for home fire extinguisher(s) ✦ Arrange for visiting nurse follow-up on discharge

---

TEACHING AREAS—BRONCHOPULMONARY DYSPLASIA

- ✦ Baseline of infant (respiratory status, behavior)
- ✦ Signs/symptoms of respiratory and other distress
- ✦ Nutritional/feeding needs and strategies
- ✦ Fluid balance and signs of fluid overload
- ✦ Medications (dosage, route, rationale, and potential side effects)
- ✦ Equipment needs: their use, care, and rationale
  - ✦ Oxygen delivery system
  - ✦ Nasal cannula care and placement
  - ✦ Cardiorespiratory monitor
  - ✦ Nebulized for inhaled medications
  - ✦ Thermometer
  - ✦ Suction devices
- ✦ Emergency care
  - ✦ Written emergency plan
  - ✦ CPR training
  - ✦ Emergency service contact
- ✦ Infection control measures
- ✦ Follow-up care
  - ✦ BPD or NICU follow-up clinic
  - ✦ Primary care follow-up
  - ✦ Subspecialty follow-up
  - ✦ Developmental follow-up and programming

REFERENCES

Acosta, F. (1988). Biofeedback and progressive relaxation in weaning the anxious patient from the ventilatory: A brief report. *Heart and Lung, 17,* 299-301.

Bach, J.R., & Alba, A.S. (1990). Noninvasive options for ventilatory support of the traumatic high level quadriplegic patient. *Chest 98,* 613-619.

Bach, J.R., Intintola, P., Alba, A.S., & Holland, I.E. (1992). The ventilator-assisted individual: Cost analysis of institutionalization vs rehabilitation and in-home management. *Chest, 101,* 26-30.

Bancalari, E., Abdenour, G.E., Feller, R., & Gannon, J. (1979). Bronchopulmonary dysplasia: Clinical presentation. *Journal of Pediatrics, 95,* 819-823.

Bancalari, E., & Gerhardt, T. (1986). Bronchopulmonary dysplasia. *Pediatric Clinics of North America, 33,* 1-23.

Bancalari, E., & Sosenko, I. (1990). Pathogenesis and prevention of neonatal chronic lung disease: Recent developments. *Pediatric Pulmonology, 8,* 109-116.

Becklake, M.R. (1989). Occupational exposures: Evidence for a causal association with chronic obstructive pulmonary disease. *American Review of Respiratory Diseases, 140,* S85-S91.

Boat, T.F., Welsh, J.F., & Beaudet, A.L. (1989). Cystic fibrosis. In C.R. Scriver, J.B. Stanbury, J.B. Wyndaarden, & D.S. Fredrickson (Eds.), *Metabolic basis of inherited disease* (Vol. 2, 6th ed.). New York: McGraw-Hill.

Borg, G., Holmgren, A., & Linblad, I. (1981). Quantitative Evaluation of Chest Pain. *Acta Medica Scandinavica, 644,* 43–45.

Boynton, B.R. (1988). The epidemiology of bronchopulmonary dysplasia. In T.A. Merritt, W.H. Northway, & B.R. Boynton (Eds.), *Bronchopulmonary dysplasia,* Boston: Blackwell Scientific Publications.

Breslin, E.H. (1992). Dyspnea-limited response in chronic obstructive pulmonary disease: Reduced unsupported arm activities. *Rehabilitation Nursing, 17,* 12-20.

Buchanan, L.E., & Nawoczenski, D.A. (1987). *Comprehensive management of spinal cord injury.* Baltimore: Williams & Wilkins.

Burr, B.H., Guyer, B., Todres, I.D., Abrahams, B., & Chiada, T. (1984). Home care for children on respirators. *New England Journal of Medicine, 309,* 1319-1323.

Carrieri, V.K., & Janson-Bjerklie, S. (1986). Strategies patients use to manage the sensation of dyspnea. *Western Journal of Nursing Research, 8,* 284-305.

Carrieri, V.K., & Janson-Bjerklie, S. (1984). The sensation of dyspnea: A review. *Heart and Lung, 13,* 436-447.

Carter, R.E., Donovan, W.H., Halstead, L., & Wilkerson, M.A. (1987). Comparative study of electrophrenic nerve stimulation and mechanical ventilatory support in traumatic spinal cord injury. *Paraplegia, 25,* 86-91.

Casaburi, R., Patessio, A., Ioli, F., Zanabon, S., Donner, C.F., & Wasserman, K. (1991). Reductions in exercise lactic acidosis and ventilation as a result of exercise training in patients with obstructive lung disease. *American Review of Respiratory Disease, 143,* 9-18.

Chen, C.F., Lien, I.N., & Wu, M.C. (1990). Respiratory function in patients with spinal cord injuries: Effects of posture. *Paraplegia, 28,* 81-86.

Chulay, M. (1988). Arterial blood gas changes with a hyperinflation and hyperoxygenation suction intervention in critically ill patients. *Heart and Lung, 17,* 654-661.

Cohen, C.A., Zagelbaum, G., Gross, D., Roussos, C.H., & Macklem, P.T. (1982). Clinical manifestations of inspiratory muscle fatigue. *American Journal of Medicine, 73,* 308-316.

Conte, V.H. (1991). Bronchopulmonary dysplasia. In P.L. Jackson, & J.A. Vessey (Eds.). *Primary care of the child with a chronic condition.* St. Louis: Mosby–Year Book.

Couser, J.I., Martinez, F.J., & Celli, B. (1989). Effect of pulmonary rehabilitation including arm exercise on ventilatory muscle function during arm elevation in patients with chronic airflow obstruction. *American Review of Respiratory Disease, 139,* A332.

Davis, R.M., & Novotny, T.E. (1989). Changes in risk factors. The epidemiology of cigarette smoking and its impact on chronic obstructive pulmonary disease. *American Review of Respiratory Disease, 140,* S82-S4.

Demers, R. (1987). Down with the good lung—usually. *Respiratory Care, 32,* 849-850.

De Troyer, A., & Pride, N.B. (1985). The respiratory system in neuromuscular disorders. In C. Roussos & P.T. Macklem (Eds.), *The thorax, part B.* New York: Marcel Dekker.

DiMotto, J.W. (1984). Relaxation. *American Journal of Nursing, 84,* 754-758.

Drayton-Hargrove, S., & Mandzak-McCarron, K. (1987a). Respiratory rehabilitation: Communication aids for the tracheotomized patient. *Rehabilitation Nursing, 12,* 193-195.

Drayton-Hargrove, S., & Mandzak-McCarron, K. (1987b). Portable ventilation. *Rehabilitation Nursing, 12,* 260-261.

Ferris, B.G. (1978). Recommended respiratory disease questionnaires for use with adults and children in epidemiological research (Part 2). *American Review of Respiratory Disease, 118,* 7-53.

Fiascone, J.M., Rhodes, T.T., Grandgeorge, S.R., & Knapp, M.A. (1989). Bronchopulmonary dysplasia: A review for the pediatrician. *Current Problems in Pediatrics, 19,* 169-227.

Fisher, D.A., & Prentice, W.S. (1982). Feasibility of home care for certain respiratory-dependent restrictive or obstructive lung disease patients. *Chest, 82,* 739-743.

Fleetham, J.A., Arnup, M.E., & Anthonisen, N.R. (1984). Familial aspects of ventilatory control in patients with chronic obstructive pulmonary disease. *American Review of Respiratory Disease, 129,* 3-7.

Fulmer, J.D., & Katzenstein, A.A. (1993). Interstitial lung disease. In R.C. Bone (Ed.), *Pulmonary and Critical Care Medicine* (Vol. 2, M section, Article 1, pp. 1-15). St. Louis: Mosby–Year Book.

Fulmer, J.D., & Snider, G.L. (1984). American College of Chest Physicians—National Heart, Lung, and Blood Institute National Conference on oxygen therapy. *Chest, 86,* 234-246.

Gallagher, C.G., Hof, V.I., & Younes, M. (1985). Effect of inspiratory muscle fatigue on breathing pattern. *Journal of Applied Physiology, 59,* 1152-1158.

Gift, A.G., & Austin, D.J. (1992). The effects of a program of systematic movement on COPD patients. *Rehabilitation Nursing, 17,* 6-10.

Gift, A.G., & Cahill, C. (1990). Psychophysiologic aspects of dyspnea in chronic obstructive pulmonary disease: A pilot study. *Heart and Lung, 19,* 252-257.

Gift, A.G., Moore, T., & Soeken, K. (1992). Relaxation to reduce dyspnea and anxiety in COPD patients. *Nursing Research, 41,* 242-246.

Gift, A.G., Plaut, S.M., & Jacox, A. (1986). Psychologic and physiologic factors related to dyspnea in subjects with chronic obstructive pulmonary disease. *Heart and Lung, 15,* 595-601.

Gilgoff, I.S., Peng, R.C., & Keens, T.G. (1992). Hypoventilation and apnea in children during mechanically assisted ventilation. *Chest, 101,* 1500-1506.

Gillespie, D.J., & Rehder, K. (1987). Body position and ventilation-perfusion relationships in unilateral pulmonary disease. *Chest, 91,* 75-79.

Hanley, M.V., & Tyler, M.L. (1987). Ineffective airway clearance related to airway infection. *Nursing Clinics of North America, 22,* 135-150.

Harver, A., & Mahler, D.A. (1990). The symptom of dyspnea. In D.A. Mahler (Ed.), *Dyspnea* (pp. 1-53). Mount Kisco, NY: Futura Publishing.

Hazinski, T.A. (1990). Bronchopulmonary dysplasia. In V. Chernick (Ed.), *Kendig's disorders of the respiratory tract in children* (pp. 300-320). Philadelphia: W.B. Saunders.

Heldt, G.P. (1988). Pulmonary status of infants and children with bronchopulmonary dysplasia. In T.A. Merritt, W.H. Northway, & B.R. Boynton (Eds.), *Bronchopulmonary dysplasia* (pp. 421-438). Boston: Blackwell Scientific Publications.

Hoffman, L.A., & Wesmiller, S.W. (1988). Home oxygen: Transtracheal and other options. *American Journal of Nursing, 88,* 464-469.

Janson-Bjerklie, S., Carrieri, V.K., & Hudes, M. (1986). The sensations of pulmonary dyspnea. *Nursing Research, 35,* 154-159.

Johnson, D.L., Giovannoni, R.M., & Driscoll, S.A. (Eds.). (1986). *Ventilator-assisted patient care: Planning for hospital discharge and home care.* Rockville, MD: Aspen.

Kersten, L.D. (1989). *Comprehensive respiratory nursing.* Philadelphia: W.B. Saunders.

Kim, C.S., Eldridge, M.A., & Sackner, M.A. (1987). Oropharyngeal deposition and delivery aspects of metered-dose inhaler aerosols. *American Review of Respiratory Disease, 135,* 157-164.

Kim, M.J., McFarland, G.K., & McLane, A.M. (1993). *Pocket guide to nursing diagnoses* (5th ed.). St. Louis: Mosby–Year Book.

Kirilloff, L.H., Owens, G.R., Rogers, R.M., & Mazzocco, M.C. (1985). Does chest physical therapy work? *Chest, 88,* 436-463.

Knipper, J. (1984). Evaluation of adventitious sounds as an indicator of the need for tracheal suctioning. *Heart and Lung, 13,* 292-293.

Lane, D.J., Howell, J.B., & Giblin, B. (1968). Relation between airways obstruction and CO_2 tension in chronic obstructive airways disease. *British Journal of Medicine, 3,* 707-709.

Larson, J.L., Kim, M.J., Sharp, J.T., & Larson, D.A. (1988). Inspiratory muscle training with a pressure threshold breathing device in patients with chronic obstructive pulmonary disease. *American Review of Respiratory Disease, 138,* 689-696.

Lloyd-Still, J.D. (1983). Pulmonary manifestations. In J.D. Lloyd-Still (Ed.), *Textbook of cystic fibrosis.* Boston: John Wright.

Loveridge, B., West, P., Anthonisen, N.R., & Kryger, M.H. (1984). Breathing patterns in patients with chronic obstructive pulmonary disease. *American Review of Respiratory Disease, 130,* 730-733.

Manzetti, J.D., & Hoffman, L.A. (1992). Nursing role in management: Upper respiratory problems. In S.M. Lewis & I.C. Collier (Eds.), *Medical-surgical nursing.* St. Louis. Mosby–Year Book.

Marini, J., Tyler, M.L., Hudson, L.D., Davis, B.S., & Huseby, J.S. (1984). Influence of head dependent position on lung volume and oxygen saturation in chronic airflow obstruction. *American Review of Respiratory Disease, 129,* 101-105.

McMullen, A.H. (1991). Cystic fibrosis. In P.L. Jackson & J.A. Vessey (Eds.), *Primary care of the child with a chronic condition* (pp. 210-228). St. Louis: Mosby–Year Book.

Merritt, T.A., & Boynton, B.R. (1988). Clinical presentation of bronchopulmonary dysplasia. In T.A. Merritt, W.H. Northway, & B.R. Boynton (Eds.), *Bronchopulmonary dysplasia* (pp. 189-190). Boston: Blackwell Scientific Publications.

Mier, A. (1990). Respiratory muscle weakness. *Respiratory Medicine, 84,* 351-359.

Mier-Jedrzejowicz, A., Brophy, C., & Green, M. (1988). Respiratory muscle weakness during upper respiratory tract infections. *American Review of Respiratory Disease, 138,* 5-7.

Misset, B., Escudier, B., Rivara, D., Leclercq, B., & Nitenberg, G. (1991). Heat and moisture exchanger vs heated humidifier during long-term mechanical ventilation: A prospective randomized study. *Chest, 100,* 160-161.

Mitchell, J.T. (1992). Nursing role in management: Lower respiratory problems. In S.M. Lewis, & I.C. Collier (Eds.), *Medical-surgical nursing* (pp. 500-556). St. Louis: Mosby–Year Book.

Nelson, C., Murphy, E., Bradley, J., & Durie, R. (1986). Clinical use of pulse oximetry to determine oxygen prescriptions for patients with hypoxemia. *Respiratory Care, 31,* 673-680.

The Nocturnal Oxygen Therapy Trial (NOTT) (1980). Continuous or nocturnal therapy in hypoxemic chronic obstructive lung disease-a clinical trial. *Annals of Internal Medicine, 93,* 391-398.

Northway, W.H., Jr. (1992a). An introduction to bronchopulmonary dysplasia. *Clinics in Perinatology, 19,* 489-495.

Northway, W.H., Jr. (1992b). Bronchopulmonary dysplasia: Twenty-five years later. *Pediatrics, 89,* 969-973.

Openbrier, D.R., & Covey, M. (1987). Ineffective breathing pattern related to malnutrition. *Nursing Clinics of North America, 22,* 225-247.

Openbrier, D.R., Fuoss, C., & Mall, C.R. (1988). What patients on home oxygen therapy want to know. *American Journal of Nursing, 88,* 198-201.

Openbrier, D.R., Hoffman, L.A., & Wesmiller, S.W. (1988). Home oxygen therapy evaluation and prescription. *American Journal of Nursing, 88,* 192-197.

Petty, T.L. (1982). *Intensive and rehabilitative respiratory care: A practical approach to the management of acute and chronic respiratory failure* (3rd ed.). Philadelphia: Lea & Febiger. 464 pp.

Poponick, J., Jacobs, I., Supinski, G.S., & DiMarci, A.F.. (1992). Effects of upper respiratory tract infections on respiratory muscle strength in patients with neuromuscular disease. *American Review of Respiratory Disease, 145,* A153.

Preusser, B.A., Stone, K.S., Gonyon, D.S., Winningham, M.L., Groch, K.F. & Karl, J.I. (1988). Effects of two methods of preoxygenation on mean arterial pressure, cardiac output, peak airway pressure, and postsuctioning hypoxemia. *Heart and Lung, 17,* 290-299.

Ramsay, J. (1989). *Nursing the child with respiratory problems.* London: Chapman and Hall.

Reinke, L.F., Hoffman, L.A., & Wesmiller, S.W. (1992). Transtracheal oxygen therapy: An alternative delivery approach. *Perspectives in Respiratory Nursing, 3,* 1-5.

Renfroe, K.L. (1988). Effect of progressive relaxation on dyspnea and state anxiety in patients with chronic obstructive pulmonary disease. *Heart and Lung, 17,* 408-413.

Riegel, B., & Forshee, T. (1985). A review and critique of the literature on preoxygenation for endotracheal suctioning. *Heart and Lung, 14,* 507-518.

Roussos, C. (1993). Ventilatory failure. In R.C. Bone (Ed.), *Pulmonary and critical care medicine* (Vol. 3, Section R, Article 2, pp. 1–11). St. Louis: Mosby–Year Book.

Roussos, C., & Macklem, P.T. (1982). The respiratory muscles. *New England Journal of Medicine, 307,* 786-797.

Rudy, E.B., Turner, B.S., Baun, M., Stoke, K.S., & Brucia, J. (1991). Endotracheal suctioning in adults with head injury. *Heart and Lung, 20,* 667-674.

Seidel, H.M., Ball, J.W., Dains, J.E., & Benedict, G.W. (1991). *Mosby's guide to physical examination* (2nd ed.). St. Louis: Mosby–Year Book.

Sexton, D.L. (Ed.). (1990). *Nursing care of the respiratory patient* (pp. 264-305). Norwalk, CT: Appleton & Lange.

Shapiro, B.A., Peruzzi, W.T., & Templin, R. (1994). *Clinical application of blood gases* (5th ed.). St. Louis: Mosby–Year Book.

Shim, C., King, M., & Williams, M.H. (1986). Lack of effect of hydration on sputum production in chronic bronchitis. *American Review of Respiratory Diseases, 133,* A98.

Siskind, M.M. (1989). A standard of care for the nursing diagnosis of ineffective airway clearance. *Heart & Lung, 18,* 477-482.

Smith, K., Cook, D., Guyatt, G.H., Madhavan, J., & Oxman, A.D. (1992). Respiratory muscle training in chronic airflow limitation: A meta-analysis. *American Review of Respiratory Disease, 145,* 533-539.

Stone, K.S., Bell, S.D., & Preusser, B.A. (1991). The effect of repeated endotracheal suctioning on arterial blood pressure. *Applied Nursing Research, 4,* 152-158.

Stone, K.S., Preusser, B.A., Groch, K.F., Karl, J.I., & Gonyon, D.S. (1991). The effect of lung hyperinflation and endotracheal suctioning on cardiopulmonary hemodynamics. *Nursing Research, 40,* 76-80.

Stone, K.S., & Turner, B. (1990). Endotracheal suctioning. *Annual Review of Nursing Research, 8,* 27-49.

Swerts, P.M., Kretzers, L.M., Terpstra-Lindeman, E., Verstappen, F.T., & Wouters, E.F. (1990). Exercise reconditioning in the rehabilitation of patients with chronic obstructive pulmonary disease: A short- and long-term analysis. *Archives of Physical Medicine and Rehabilitation, 71,* 570-573.

Tepper, R.S. (1988). Assessment of pulmonary function in the postneonatal period. In T.A. Merritt, W.H. Northway, & B.R. Boynton (Eds.), *Bronchopulmonary dysplasia.* Boston: Blackwell Scientific Publications.

Thomas, V.M., Ellison, K., Howell, E.V., & Winters, K. (1992). Caring for the person receiving ventilator support at home: Caregivers' needs and involvement. *Heart and Lung, 21,* 180-186.

Tibealls, J. (1991). Diaphragmatic pacing: An alternative to long-term mechanical ventilation. *Anaesthesia and Intensive Care, 19,* 597-601.

Tiep, B.L., Burns, M., Kao, D., Madison, R., & Herrera, J. (1986). Pursed lip breathing training using ear oximetry. *Chest, 90,* 218-221.

Tizzano, E.F., & Buchwald, M. (1992). Cystic fibrosis: Beyond the gene to therapy. *Pediatrics, 120,* 337-349.

Tobin, M.J., Chadha, T.S., Jenouri, G., Birch, S.J., Gazeroglu, H.B., & Sackner, M.A. (1983a). Breathing patterns 1. Normal subjects. *Chest, 84,* 202-205.

Tobin, M.J., Chadha, T.S., Jenouri, G., Birch, S.J., Gazeroglu, H.B., & Sackner, M.A. (1983b). Breathing patterns 2. Diseased subjects. *Chest, 84,* 286-294.

Tyler, M. (1982). Complications of positioning and chest physiotherapy. *Respiratory Care, 27,* 458-456.

Van Sciver, T., & Weaver, T.E. (1992). Nursing role in management: Respiratory failure. In S.M. Lewis & I.C. Collier (Eds.), *Medical-surgical nursing* (pp. 602-648). St. Louis: Mosby–Year Book.

Walsh, R. (1986). Occupational therapy as a part of pulmonary rehabilitation program. *Occupational Ther for the Energy Deficient Patient, 3,* 65-77.

Weitzenblum, E. (1992). Long-term oxygen therapy in chronic obstructive pulmonary disease—usefulness, indications, modes of administration. *Presse-Medicale, 21,* 424-431.

Weitzenblum, E., Apprill, M., & Oswald, M. (1992). Benefit from long-term O_2 therapy in chronic obstructive pulmonary disease patients. *Respiration, 59,* 14-17.

Wilson, S.F., & Thompson, J.M. (1990). *Respiratory disorders.* St. Louis: Mosby–Year Book.

Yeaw, E.M.J. (1992). How position affects oxygenation: Good lung down? *American Journal of Nursing, 92,* 27-29.

Zach, M.S. (1990). Lung disease in cystic fibrosis—An updated concept. *Pediatric Pulmonology, 8,* 188-202.

Zejdlik, C.M. (1991). *Management of spinal cord injury* (2nd ed.). Boston: Jones & Bartlett.

19

Circulatory Function and Cardiac Rehabilitation

Linda Brewer, RN, MSN, ANP
Shirley P. Hoeman, PhD, CRRN, CNAA, CCM

INTRODUCTION

Cardiac rehabilitation nursing is an essential professional discipline within an interdisciplinary specialty—a specialty that is growing in response to needs of an aging population and an increased awareness of the benefits available from cardiac care programs for persons of all ages. Technologic advances, treatment options, early intervention procedures following myocardial infarction (MI), and medications have rescued many lives.

However, in the United States, heart disease remains a major threat to health. Many persons with coronary heart disease are surprisingly young; nearly 2 million are below age 40, another 1.5 million are between 40 and 59 years, and 2.75 million are over age 60 years. Of the 407,000 persons who received coronary bypass surgery in 1991, half were below the age of 55 years (American Heart Association, 1992a). The cost of healthcare services, institutional care, medications, and lost productivity for clients who have cardiovascular disease exceeded $117 billion in 1993 (American Heart Association, 1992b). At the same time the pattern of coronary care has changed and so have treatment philosophies; early hospital discharge is a major force. Supervised programs of exercise, education, and lifestyle changes have improved outcome for clients who have coronary artery disease, MI, and other severe cardiovascular conditions.

Cardiac rehabilitation is defined in this chapter as a continuous process of actively assisting clients who have cardiac disease and their families in an effort to reduce symptoms and achieve optimal health (Wenger & Hellerstein, 1992). This is a dynamic, multidimensional process that involves restoration, attainment, and maintenance of a person's maximum emotional, psychological, physical, sexual, social, and occupational levels (Miller, 1991).

Many clients who enter cardiac rehabilitation programs already have comorbid or disabling conditions. Some develop complications involving additional body systems such as neuromusculoskeletal problems or obstructive vascular impairments in a lower extremity, which must be considered in a plan to improve cardiac function. The interdisciplinary approach and follow-up offered by rehabilitation is an understandable choice for dealing with the complex array of clinical and psychosocial variables associated with these clients and their families.

Some participants in supervised programs would have been rejected as candidates for cardiac rehabilitation programs in the past. Twenty years ago clients were restricted to bed rest with limited activities over several months following an MI. By the early 1970s applicants to participate in hospital-based cardiac rehabilitation programs exceeded the number of programs and trained staff available. In 10 more years community-based cardiac rehabilitation programs and supervised outpatient clinic programs began to serve low-risk clients (Miller, 1991). Researchers continue to investigate client risk factors, client self-help, and program methods. They seek the optimal amount and type of exercise that is safe, the characteristics of clients who will adhere to and benefit from the programs, and relationships between these factors.

CURRENT PROGRAM SERVICES

In the 1990s a cardiac rehabilitation program may be located in a community health setting, a major medical center, or a local hospital. Experiments with self-directed home programs are under way using low-risk clients who live in rural, geographically distant, or other underserved areas (Glick, 1991). The scope, size, goals, and variety of services can be expected to vary among programs. Although clients enter a cardiac rehabilitation program following a cardiac event, prevention is a program cornerstone. Exercise training is a generic ingredient in all programs; however, for clients with severe cardiac disease and who are high risk, programs offering a broad range of services and a full interdisciplinary team are recommended. This chapter provides information that applies to any cardiac rehabilitation program.

Recently several professional and governmental organizations have developed standard competencies for professionals in cardiac rehabilitation (see box, p. 402), which include qualifications specific to each discipline, as well as additional preferred qualifications. A number of leading organizations that have set program standards are listed at the end of this chapter.

Interdisciplinary Team Approach

The minimum cardiac rehabilitation team is composed of a medical director or supervising physician, a program director or coordinator, and a registered professional nurse in

---

CARDIAC REHABILITATION TEAM MEMBERS

Client
Physician
Social worker
Exercise physiologist
Physical therapist
Clergy member
Occupational therapist
Respiratory therapist
Family
Professional registered nurse
Dietitian/nutritionist
Mental health professional
Health educator
Pharmacist
Vocational rehabilitation counselor
Case manager and others, as needed

CORE COMPETENCIES FOR CARDIAC REHABILITATION PROFESSIONALS

Needs assessment
+ Pathophysiology and comorbidity
+ Professional communication
+ Standards of practice
+ Restoration of functional capacity
+ Biopsychosocial
+ Risk factor management
+ Emergency procedures
Goal setting
+ Pathophysiology and comorbidity
+ Professional communication
+ Standards of practice
+ Restoration of functional capacity
+ Biopsychosocial
+ Risk factor management
+ Emergency procedures
Intervention
+ Pathophysiology and comorbidity
+ Professional communication
+ Standards of practice
+ Restoration of functional capacity
Outcome evaluation
+ Pathophysiology and comorbidity
+ Professional communication
+ Standards of practice
+ Restoration of functional capacity
+ Biopsychosocial
+ Risk factor management
+ Emergency procedures

From Core Competencies for Cardiac Rehabilitation Professionals Position Statement of the American Association of Cardiovascular and Pulmonary Rehabilitation by D.R. Southard, C. Certo, P.M. Comoss, N.F. Gordon, W.G. Herbert, E.J. Protas, P. Ribisl, and S.H. Swails, by 1994, *Journal of Cardiopulmonary Rehabilitation, 14,* pp. 87-92. Copyright 1994 by American Association of Cardiovascular & Pulmonary Rehabilitation. Reprinted by permission.

---

instances when the coordinator is an allied health professional other than a nurse (American Association of Cardiovascular and Pulmonary Rehabilitation [AACPR] 1993). Although the nurse's role may vary from program to program, the most consistent role functions are coordination and client and family education, essential activities in all programs. Nursing is viewed as vital to all phases of cardiac rehabilitation in all settings, largely because of the holistically oriented goals inherent in nursing (Jillings, 1988). Ideally professionals will include a cardiologist and a physiatrist with training in cardiac rehabilitation as regular or consulting members and a specialty trained cardiac rehabilitation nurse. A cardiac rehabilitation team may consist of professionals from, but not limited to, those listed in the box above.

Although team members have specialized cardiac knowledge appropriate to their discipline, each professional must understand the role and contribution of the other disciplines. Roles and responsibilities vary across programs (Blocker & Cardus, 1983; Brannon, Foley, Starr, & Black, 1993; Pashkow & Dafoe, 1993). The concept of cross training is valued among members of cardiac rehabilitation teams who regularly share specialty knowledge during team meetings. As a result the team members participate in developing one another's expertise within the specialty and improve outcome for clients (Matheson, Selvester, & Rice, 1975). Regardless of program size, individualized services are one hallmark of quality in a cardiac rehabilitation program— which means the client and family are always active members of the interdisciplinary team (Comoss, Burke, & Swails, 1979).

The success of a cardiac rehabilitation program has been attributed in part to the professional quality of the team members (Pashkow & Dafoe, 1993). Composition of the team will reflect the program philosophy, available resources, client population demand, and administrative policies of the institution or agency (Comoss et al., 1979). Taken together, members of a team of cardiac rehabilitation professionals have advanced practice knowledge about

1. Cardiovascular disease
2. Current intervention strategies
3. Educational goals, methods, and tools
4. Health psychology
5. Nutrition
6. Exercise physiology
7. Emergency procedures (AACPR, 1991)
8. Increasingly a need for knowledge about rehabilitation principles and care for clients with comorbid conditions

An ideally functioning team is characterized by collaborative relationships and collective decision-making, including client and family members. The obvious advantage is full integration of professional expertise and an informed and involved client. However, many teams tend to function as multidisciplinary, rather than interdisciplinary, teams. As a result each member contributes uniquely to a client's cardiac program but all members do not have equal status in decision-making processes. Decisions may not be arrived at jointly and may exclude clients' preferences or ignore their lifestyles. The nurse coordinator who is able to work effectively with each team member to assure continuity and integrated planning is a key to success. (Chapter 2 provides additional discussion of team models for practice.)

Changing Rehabilitation Scene

As changes in the health system reduce hospital length of stay, rehabilitation nurses in facilities and community settings are working with clients who are more acutely ill and who have more complex health problems than in the past. Similarly these same clients have fewer days to accomplish rehabilitation goals in a facility before they move on to community settings. Rehabilitation nurses are being called on to function as case managers and consultants to community programs and to assist with preventing clients from re-entering hospitals.

Cardiac rehabilitation is one of several emerging rehabilitation nursing specialties that deals with clients and settings where increased acuity raises the potential for cardiac and other life-threatening emergencies. Preparation in rehabilitation facilities requires written procedures and equipment to respond to clients' needs and for nurses to be knowledgeable about managing cardiopulmonary emergencies for clients (Calliari & Mark, 1992) and how to implement any advanced directives.

As a result nurses may decide to review critical care and medical-surgical content with current clinical guidelines for practice and to learn how to operate equipment or perform procedures associated with these specialty practices (Gibbons et al., 1992).

Synopsis of Coronary Artery Circulation
✦ Coronary artery perfusion

The following anatomic and physiologic review describes coronary artery perfusion—since impairments are common factors in many cardiac disorders—and contains information that influences nursing assessment and rehabilitation interventions. The epicardial section of the coronary arteries lies on the surface of the heart. Perforator vessels enter the myocardium, delivering blood to the endocardial and subendocardial areas of the myocardium. The subendocardial area is the last area of the heart muscles fed by the coronary arteries. This explains why in an MI, the damage spreads from the endocardial area outward to the epicardial area. The resting coronary blood flow is 5% of the total cardiac output (Guyton, 1990).

Three special factors affecting coronary artery perfusion are (1) cardiac cycle, (2) heart rate, and (3) diastolic intraventricular pressure. These factors must be considered while making all nursing assessments related to the cardiac cycle. In systole the ventricular wall tension greatly limits blood flow through the coronary perforator arteries. Most coronary circulation occurs during ventricular diastole, while the ventricular walls are "relaxing," which allows a significant

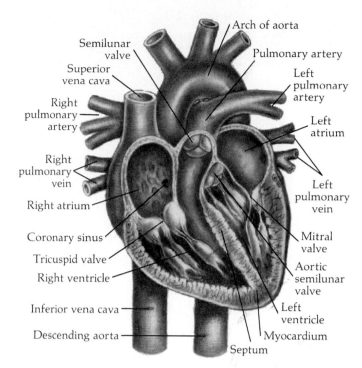

Fig. 19-1 Frontal schematic view of the heart. (From *Mosby's Clinical Nursing,* 3rd ed. by J.M. Thompson, G.K. McFarland, J.E. Hirsch, and S.M. Tucker, 1993, St. Louis: Mosby-Year Book. Copyright 1993 by Mosby-Year Book. Reprinted by permission.)

reduction in ventricular muscle tension (Guyton, 1990). The significant anatomic parts of the heart (Thompson, McFarland, Hirsch, & Tucker, 1993) are illustrated in Fig. 19-1 and distribution of the coronary arteries throughout the heart and great vessels via the coronary arteries (Gravanis, 1993) are illustrated in Fig. 19-2.

✦ Altered coronary artery perfusion

Certain nursing interventions may be appropriate when a nurse assesses a client who has alterations in the coronary artery perfusion. For example, awareness of heart rate is crucial in clients with coronary artery disease. Heart rate dictates the length of diastolic perfusion time for coronary arteries. As the heart rate increases, the diastolic filling time shortens. A client with stable angina has a threshold heart rate in which diastolic filling time shortens to a point where adequate coronary artery perfusion cannot perfuse stenotic arteries. Rest is an efficient and simple intervention to thwart anginal episodes. Rest enables the heart rate to slow, and a slowed heart rate lengthens the diastolic filling time of the coronary arteries (Hall, Meyer, & Hellerstein, 1984).

Conditions associated with higher circulating blood volume, such as congestive heart disease, may cause myocardial ischemia and anginal symptoms when blood flow to subendocardial areas is reduced. Diastolic intraventricular pressure alters perfusion of blood through the perforator arteries. A high diastolic interventricular pressure reduces the blood flow to the subendocardial area. Sublingual nitroglycerine or other nitrates relieve anginal symptoms by causing

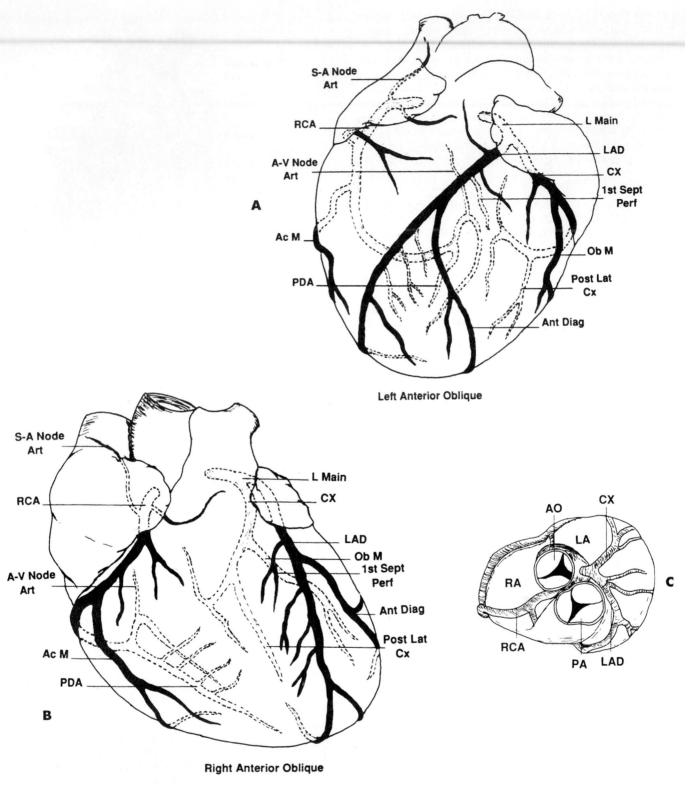

Left Anterior Oblique

Right Anterior Oblique

Fig. 19-2   **A** and **B,** Left and right anterior oblique views of coronary arteries and their distribution. **C,** Cephalad view of coronary artery distribution in relation to the great vessels. S-A, sinoatrial; Art, artery; RCA, right coronary artery; A-V, arterioventricular; AcM, acute marginal; PDA, posterior descending artery; Ant, anterior; Post, posterior; Lat, lateral; Cx, circumflex; ObM, obtuse marginal; Sept, septal; Perf, perforator; LAD, left anterior descending; L, left; Ao, aorta; LA, left atrium; RA, right atrium; PA, pulmonary artery. (From *Cardiovascular Disorders: Pathogenesis and Pathology,* by M.S. Gravanis, 1993, St. Louis: Mosby–Year Book. Copyright 1993 by Mosby-Year Book. Reprinted by permission.)

blood to pool in the extremities, which in turn decreases blood return to the heart and reduces intraventricular diastolic pressure.

Stable angina indicates an unchanging atherosclerotic process in the coronary perfusion. In contrast, unstable angina or preinfarction angina, suggests an active, dynamic atherosclerotic progression. Symptoms of unstable angina appear with less exertion, occur more frequently, and tend not to be relieved as readily as with stable angina. Outcome from unstable angina is unpredictable.

Various symptoms including angina are associated with myocardial ischemia. With atherosclerosis, fixed stenotic lesions develop in the coronary arteries. A lesion that occludes 60% or more of an artery can produce myocardial ischemia and anginal symptoms, which often are precipitated by exertion or emotional (dis)stress, accompanied by increased heart rate. Thus rest is a key intervention once again. At times ischemia of the left ventricle may precipitate transient congestive heart disease. Symptoms of congestive heart failure include dyspnea and paroxysmal nocturnal dyspnea (PND). Elderly clients who develop congestive heart disease classically become fatigued, gain weight due to edema, and develop cough with dyspnea (Jessup, Lakatta, Leier, & Santinga, 1992).

A CARDIAC REHABILITATION PROGRAM
Preliminary Evaluation

A cardiac rehabilitation program begins within a few days following an MI, when a client participates in a predischarge evaluation based on a protocol involving exercise testing. Testing provides one basis for assigning risk to clients to determine their need for further medical treatment, their exercise tolerance and abilities, potential for exercise training, and level of safe exercise with an appropriate level of supervision in a rehabilitation program. Client risk, cardiac drugs and other medications, types of aerobic exercise, parts of the body exercised, and specific therapeutic exercises are all factors in initial prescriptions for exercise training.

The following principles apply to cardiac rehabilitation evaluations:

- ✦ Client and family are active participants in the team.
- ✦ Early evaluations, using exercise testing, are repeated and used to decide activities and medical treatment or medication needs.
- ✦ Individual prescriptions for exercise training are designed to reach optimal level of function.
- ✦ Interdisciplinary assessment, intervention, and evaluation of risk factors; and psychosocial and occupational status are completed and communicated (Miller, 1991).

Phases of Cardiac Rehabilitation Management

Cardiac rehabilitation is a continuous process that commonly is categorized according to phases. Although phases have been numbered 1 through 4 (AACPR, 1992), many programs use the terms inpatient and outpatient to designate phases (Pollack & Schmidt, 1986). Each component or phase of a program needs to be defined and the specific functions described clearly to avoid confusion due to variations among programs (Karam, 1989).

✦ Phase 1: inpatient

Phase 1 is usually a program to limit physical and psychological consequences of the acute cardiac illness for the client who is still hospitalized (Comoss et al., 1979). This phase lasts between 5 days and 2 weeks (Miller, 1991). The major components are risk assessment, early ambulation and physical activity, and education of clients and families. Identifying a client's level of risk not only assures lifesaving measures are available for those with serious conditions but prevents unnecessary restrictions for clients with low risk levels. A treadmill test, described later in this chapter, is a means of evaluating risk and usually is conducted before hospital discharge.

Clients who have uncomplicated cardiac disease, MI, or who have received angioplasty benefit from early ambulation and evaluation because they are discharged quickly and will re-enter the community. Those who survived sudden cardiac death or who have severe cardiac conditions, congestive heart failure, serious ventricular arrhythmias or complex dysrhythmias, left ventricular dysfunction, myocardial ischemia, or certain specific changes with exercise receive intensive monitoring using electrocardiographic telemetry in order to detect problems immediately (ACP, ACC Guidelines, 1986, 1988). These persons and those with contributing factors, such as advanced age, may have become deconditioned as a result of the disease processes and curtailed physical activity or extended immobility.

Progressive physical activity is supervised and performed in a gradual sequence of steps to increase a client's work demand as a means to counter deconditioning, as well as to prevent venous thrombosis or pulmonary emboli. Activities and exercise often improve a client's sense of well-being and control, reduce confusion and depression, and stimulate outlook. Thus within the first 1 to 2 days, clients without medical complications are encouraged to perform grooming and self-care activities, get out of bed for toileting when this requires walking short distances, and perform range-of-motion (ROM) exercises (Miller, 1991).

Throughout the day a client takes several short walks after which the nurse monitors blood pressure, heart rate, and electrocardiogram (ECG) readings for signs of changes that would indicate a reduction of activities. Principles of energy conservation are important considerations as ROM exercises progress from passive to active; eventually 1- to 2-lb weights can be used as resistance. Soon thereafter, warm-up and stretching activities or mild calisthenics are added to ambulation or treadmill work; clients who will encounter stairs at home or work practice climbing and descending stairs.

Clients and families are enabled to participate as members of the team when they receive information, individualized to their needs, as soon as possible following hospitalization and throughout the program. A nursing assessment of stressors and coping is initiated for both client and family, with referral for mental health counseling as needed. Clients and family members may have misconceptions or misunderstandings about the disease trajectory or the benefits from participating in a cardiac rehabilitation program (Moranville-Hunziker, Sagehorn, Conn, Feutz, Hagenhoff, 1994). For instance, some may believe that bypass surgery is a curative procedure that expunges cardiac risk. Health beliefs have been found to be important factors influencing a client's decision and ultimate participation in a cardiac rehabilitation program (Hiatt, Hoenshell-Nelson, & Zimmerman, 1990).

Education in phase 1 includes the following:

+ Empowerment for client and family as team members such as answering questions and concerns, determining learning style and needs, and introducing them to the disease trajectory and anticipated interventions
+ Disease- or condition-specific content such as anatomy and physiology, medical procedures and tests, and purposes of monitoring equipment
+ Specific guidelines or instructions such as activity types and levels, specific exercises, medications, and diet
+ Preparatory information such as about return to work, stress reduction, sexual activity, or lifestyle modifications

+ Phase 2: early outpatient

Clients require close supervision and monitoring during the first 2 to 3 months after discharge. Ideally clients will have access to a supervised cardiac rehabilitation program and then will enroll and attend. This is a phase when clients and families experience the greatest adjustment. They are vulnerable to experience a great deal of anxiety about the type and amounts of activities, develop fears and depressions, misinterpret instructions about medications or regimens, and encounter problems with instituting lifestyle changes such as preparing diets, stopping smoking, or managing stressors. Prescribed exercise programs, discussed further in this chapter, continue to be key interventions for improving functional abilities, controlling weight, and building cardiovascular levels.

On the other hand, this early outpatient phase is the period within which clients experience the highest cardiac mortality rates following hospitalization. Frequent contact, monitoring, and support are essential to assist clients in judging their behaviors and activities and for determining when they have medical complications or emergencies. Many clients return home at low risk and can be monitored effectively by nurses from community-based cardiac rehabilitation programs. At this time a number of models are being tested to serve low-risk clients who live in geographically distant areas or who do not have cardiac rehabilitation programs nearby (Glick, 1991). Strategies for promoting success in phases 2 and 3 include the following:

+ Providing referrals to community agencies or self-help groups for smoking cessation, weight loss or control, or spousal support meetings
+ Providing referrals for professional assistance such as psychosocial or mental health professionals, nutrition counseling or computerized dietary analysis, or professional assistance with comorbid conditions such as diabetes
+ Providing resources to assist with stress reduction and management when appropriate
+ Encouraging accessible activities and events within tolerance levels to promote socialization
+ Generating written health contracts with assigned responsibilities for accomplishing mutually agreed-upon goals (Chapter 13 provides information about how to write a health contract.)
+ Using logs, checklists, calendars, and other record-keeping aids to encourage clients to perform tasks and steps for meeting goals
+ Assessing and intervening with the entire family system and any significant others, not only the client
+ Assuring programs, groups, and referrals are culturally and religiously relevant and sensitive

+ Phase 3: late outpatient

Components of phases 2 and 3 tend to blend for clients who do not have complications; activities may intensify as they continue over a longer period. As a rule clients who were monitored with telemetry during phase 2, but who have achieved goals to this point, continue to be supervised but are no longer monitored with telemetry. By 6 months following hospitalization, clients and families have begun to recognize that exercise, self-monitoring, and lifestyle changes are lifelong goals. At the same time they have been able to reconstruct their lives within the parameters of the client's condition and abilities. For some clients this will mean few changes beyond eliminating detrimental habits and adhering to exercises; others will encounter major adjustments and complications; some will have great difficulties or fail.

A client's motivation to continue the cardiac rehabilitation program and investment in the program are important indicators. Services that are enjoyable, accessible, and acceptable for a client are more likely to be used. Support groups and social activities for clients and families may promote attendance. Some clients find benefits through adjunct therapies as described in Chapter 13.

+ Phase 4: maintenance

The maintenance phase of cardiac rehabilitation is lifelong. Since clients are more clinically stable and knowledgeable about their activity limits, professional supervision is tapered. Activities and exercises are more aggressive, and organized educational programs designed to maintain participation and accomplish lifestyle changes become more important.

Exercise Component of Cardiac Rehabilitation

The exact amount or intensity of physical activity to prevent disease or premature death is unknown (American College of Sports Medicine [ACSM], 1991). However, less physical activity is required to lower the risk of coronary artery disease than is required to optimize cardiopulmonary fitness (Gordon & Scott, 1991). A major physiologic effect of exercise training is improved functional capacity with reduced fatigue, dyspnea, angina, or related symptoms. Overall musculoskeletal condition improves, but the construction of coronary arteries and collateral circulation is not known to be directly affected.

Regular physical activity is known to protect against the progression of many acquired chronic diseases or development of others and assists in maintaining functional abilities (DeBusk, Haskell, Miller, Berra, & Taylor, 1985). Low-intensity exercises, three times a week for 30 minutes plus warm-up and cool-down time, have been found to be more effective in improving functional capacity and endurance than once believed (Pashkow & Dafoe, 1993).

✦ Treadmill Exercise Test

Most persons have become familiar with or performed a "stress test" using a treadmill to categorize their cardiac risk. Following acute MI, clients perform a supervised and monitored treadmill exercise test. Test results are correlated with other factors to form an individualized risk stratification—high, low, or moderate—which is used in the exercise prescription and long-term treatment plan (Pollack & Schmidt, 1986).

The test uses treadmill equipment with recording monitors and with controls to vary the speed and raise the elevation of the exercise surface as the client "walks" to evaluate the level of fitness. The test is conducted at an intensity that is appropriate for the client's physical activity at the time. Predischarge testing is important to determine a home program and activity or work capacity, as well as to minimize a client's anxiety about activity. Repeated testing at certain intervals helps in determining whether the exercise prescription needs to be altered (Fardy, Yanowitz, & Wilson, 1988). For instance, a client's health status, medications, or symptoms may change. Repeated exercise testing at intervals may occur as necessary but is recommended at 6 months and 1 year following the initial testing.

Other modalities for exercise tests include the graded exercise test, stationary cycling, or arm crank ergometry. The arm crank enables clients with lower body paralysis or paresis, such as with paraplegia, to be tested provided they have sufficient upper body strength and function. A variety of modified or adapted equipment and devices have been used in exercise testing of persons with disabilities. Generally these consist of modified bicycles to suit clients' abilities such as a supine model or arm and leg powered model; or equipment attached to existing wheelchairs that connects the equipment to cycles or similar circular modifications. With modifications that rely on the parts of the body with functional abilities to supply crank or cycle power, the exercise workload should not overtax some parts of the body while achieving necessary cardiovascular levels (AACPR, 1991; ACSM, 1991).

✦ Exercise prescription

The exercise component of cardiac rehabilitation is individualized for each client as a means of reaching cardiovascular conditioning goals. This is in effect an exercise prescription. Data collection begins with the client's complete medical history, current health status, medication profile, lifestyle data, and level of fitness based on multiple results from exercise testing including workload, heart rate, and blood pressure, and any signs of dysrhythmia or ischemia. The prescription is a written program or "dosage" for exercise that describes the type or mode of exercise; how often it is to be performed; and the duration, intensity, and rate of progression of intensity (Hall & Meyer, 1988).

Intensity describes the level of demand at which an activity is performed and is tailored to each client's status. Clients are monitored closely for signs or symptoms of myocardial ischemia or ventricular dysrhythmias, or various other criteria (see the following box) for termination of

---

✦

CRITERIA FOR TERMINATION OF EXERCISE SESSION

Fatigue	Dizziness
Dyspnea	Nausea
Nausea	Change in cardiac rhythm

Anginal symptoms

Drop in heart rate >10 beats/minute

Drop in systolic blood pressure >10 mm Hg

Rise in heart rate >20 beats/minute for MI clients (or no. determined with previous exercise testing)

Rise in blood pressure greater than _____ (amount determined with previous exercise testing)

From *Guidelines for Exercise Testing and Prescription*, 4th edition, by the American College of Sports Medicine, 1991, Philadelphia: Lea & Febiger. Copyright 1991 by Williams & Wilkins.

---

the exercise session. The mode of activity describes how the exercise will employ which large muscle groups in sustained and rhythmic activity, most commonly walking. Other appropriate modes include cycling, jogging, rowing, arm ergometry, and aquatic exercises. Duration of exercise refers simply to the length of time an activity is to be performed. Initially exercises are performed at low intensity and should not produce sore muscles or undue fatigue.

The exercise prescription ensures that the exercise session is both beneficial and safe (Fardy et al., 1988); age-related target heart rates are not used as guides for cardiac programs. Guidelines for the prescription are based on results from research, and it is written by a specialist such as an exercise physiologist, who understands the principles and physiology of exercise (AACPR, 1991; ACSM, 1991). Each component of the exercise session is modified further by a client's prognosis of risk (risk stratification factor), which is used to identify clients who may be a higher risk for developing complications during an exercise session. Other guidelines contain information about client selection for exercise and contraindications for exercise. Criteria for terminating an exercise session are listed in the box above.

✦ The exercise session

The exercise session or activity program consists of warm up, conditioning or activity, and cool down (ASCM, 1991). The purpose of a warm up is to prepare muscles and joints for the pending activity, which is exercise. This requires between 5 and 15 minutes of stretching activities and ROM exercises, by which time the resting metabolic rate (1 MET [metabolic equivalent]) has increased to a level necessary for beginning the conditioning segment of the session.

The composition of the conditioning activity is guided by the individualized dosage written in the exercise prescription for frequency, intensity, mode, and duration of exercise, which is approximately 20 to 30 minutes. Although frequencies may be set at several times daily, exercises sessions for outpatient clients generally are set for three to five times a week, since little benefit has been found to be derived from exercises more frequent than five times weekly

(Wenger, 1992b). The 5- to 10-minute cool-down segment of the session is important to prevent exercise-related complications and should not be overlooked.

✦ The MET method

Exercise and activity requirements are described using the MET method. A MET is equivalent to the amount of oxygen an individual requires while standing at rest or 3.5 ml of O_2/kg/minute (ACSM, 1991). Increased expenditure of energy levels results in multiplication of MET values—that is, a 2-MET activity uses oxygen at twice the rate of a 1-MET resting activity, or an 8-MET activity uses oxygen at eight times the resting rate.

The MET method is easy to understand and can be related to both occupational and leisure activities (Table 19-1 and Table 19-2). For example, a client may have ischemic ECG changes at a level of 6 METs on a graded exercise test. Therefore this client's instructions should direct him to perform activities that are below the level of 5 METs. Clients often do not estimate the actual energy requirements (METs) for daily activities or leisurely pursuits. Women routinely have been found to underestimate the energy requirements needed to complete household tasks and thus often work at higher MET levels than recommended soon after an MI (Boogaard, 1984).

✦ Climate for exercise and activity

Ideal climates for exercise are those with less than 65% humidity and temperatures between 40° and 75° F. Exercising under ideal conditions is not always feasible but certainly is preferable for clients who have cardiac conditions. Extremes of heat and humidity are major concerns to health; whenever the humidity exceeds 65%, the metabolic rate required for activities is increased. Excessive heat results in vasodilation, which reduces blood return to the heart, de-creasing the blood pressure and elevating the heart rate. Heat stress may occur in hot air or hot water temperatures and may result in the vasodilatation cycle when a client is using alcohol or nitrates (Brannon et al., 1993).

Clients may choose to modify the environment or alter their exercise time. For example, in hot, humid climates as found in the South, clients may exercise outdoors in the cooler morning or late evenings; during the day they would use an air-conditioned or environmentally controlled indoor space. On the other hand, cold temperatures also increase peripheral resistance and thus a raise the workload of the heart. Clients should consider the fabric and type of clothing worn for exercise so it is appropriate for the weather conditions. For example, covering the mouth and nose with a scarf is effective prevention of cold-induced bronchospasms.

✦ Home-based or unsupervised exercise programs

Clients who are unable to attend or access medically supervised exercise classes may be candidates for home exercise training according to a specific exercise prescription. Under certain conditions clients may be eligible for partial reimbursement for intermittent community health nursing services, therapies, and medical supplies. A large number of community-based providers offer a wide array of health-care services for clients with varying payment options. However, clients and families need to be educated to choose services that will assure a complete assessment followed by ongoing coordination, continuity, and communication with the cardiac rehabilitation program (Niewenhous, 1991).

Modern technology has made home exercise programs more practical by improving communications between a client and the cardiac rehabilitation center. With the availability of telephone, fax, or electronic mail transmissions; transtelephonic ECG recordings; videocassette tape recordings,

Table 19-1   Activities of daily living: household tasks (energy requirements in METs)

1	2	3	4	5	6	7	8
Eat	Dress						
Drive car	←———— Grocery shop ————————→						
Hygiene: sit	Hygiene: stand						
Lie awake	Tub bath	Shower					
Sit		General housework	Paint				
		←———————————————— Sexual intercourse ————→					
	Cook: stand	Mop	←———————— Move furniture ————→				
Walk: 1 mph	2 mph	3 mph	3.5 mph	4 mph			
		Iron		Walk upstairs			
		Hang clothes					
		Dust					
		Make bed			Carry suitcase		
		Wash clothes by machine					
		Clean floors					
Sweep		Clean windows					
		Ride mower	Grass: push power		Grass: hand mower		
	Light gardening	Heavier gardening					
		Polish floor					
			Rake leaves				
		Vacumn					
	Wash dishes		Wash windows		Wash car		

Table 19-2 Activities of recreation/vocation (energy requirements in METs)

1	2	3	4	5	6	7	8	9	10	11	12
	Billards		Volleyball								
Play cards	Do woodwork	Bow?									
Knit	Play musical	Canoe 2.5 mph									
Read	Cycle:	Paint	Do masonry			Chop wood					
Sew	Sew on machine	Instrument	6 mph	8 mph	10 mph ─────→	11 mph	12 mph	13 mph			
Watch TV	Shuffle board	5 mph	──── Folk dance	──── Aerobic dance ────→							
			Ballroom dance	Square dance		Racquetball	Wrestle				
	Fish in boat	Slow dance	Climb ladder	Stream fish		Dig ditch					
			Table tennis ────→			Chop wood					
			Throw Frisbee ────→								
Ride in golf cart		Pull golf cart	Carry golf clubs								
Walk: 1 mph	2 mph	3.5 mph	4 mph		Run	10 mi/minute	11 mi/minute	12 mi/minute			
Desk work	Radio/tv repair		Slow swim			Back stroke	Breast stroke				
	Auto assembly line work										
	Bake		Light carpentry								
Type	Bartend		Tennis:	singles							
	Operate hand tools		Tennis:	doubles							

home educational video, and other electronic telecommunication devices, clients who would otherwise be without services can access a cardiac rehabilitation team (Wenger, 1992a). The nurse as coordinator, educator, advocate, and assessor-evaluator is a key link in communication.

Clients and family members need to be able to demonstrate their knowledge about the individualized exercise prescription, precautions including environmental conditions, signs and symptoms to be reported to the cardiac rehabilitation team, and criteria for terminating exercise. Emergency telephone numbers should be posted near the telephone where family members and other persons in the home can locate them quickly. Emergency response or electronic emergency systems are available in many communities. As additional precautions, clients may wear medical alert bracelets, carry diagnosis and treatment cards, and place a Vial of Life in the refrigerator. Those who have implanted cardiac pacemakers or cardioverter defibrillators should have special information regarding their status and care readily available.

Clients and families need to make arrangements with the primary physician and members of the cardiac rehabilitation team concerning content of any advanced directives or do-not-resuscitate (DNR) orders. The client's situation, preferences, and special needs should be known to members of the local emergency response units, the pharmacist, vendors who supply equipment or goods such as oxygen and backup supplies for electricity or heat, and other similar services or personnel. (Chapter 18 provides information concerning oxygen use and handling.)

Special Considerations

Several subgroups of clients require special considerations when planning exercise testing and formulating exercise prescriptions. Elderly persons have more frequent complications that involve deconditioning and may lead to functional limitations and responses that result in ineffective coping. These clients may require a longer time to achieve training goals; they may benefit from learning and practicing energy conservation measures, using low-impact exercises (especially walking or swimming), having longer warm-up periods, modifying or abstaining from exercise under undesirable climatic conditions, and attending to primary health needs (Anderson, 1991; Kligman & Pepin, 1992; Topp, 1991; Wenger, 1992b).

Clients who have one or more chronic or disabling conditions in addition to cardiac disease require special exercise considerations that will take into account requirements of each specific condition and the combined requirements of all the conditions. For example, increased exercise may alter the MET needs and carbohydrate metabolism for a client with diabetes, creating a change in insulin and/or caloric balance (Gordon, 1993d; Kelleher, 1991; Maynard, 1991). Clients with lower body impairments will need to strengthen the upper body to achieve cardiovascular fitness. Likewise, clients with respiratory disorders (Gordon, 1993b), arthritic conditions (Gordon, 1993a), or chronic fatigue syndrome (Gordon, 1993c), or those who have had a stroke (Gordon, 1993e), and clients who have been recipients of a pacemaker or a heart transplant must be assessed individually (Gordon & Scott, 1991).

Modified exercise routines and/or adapted equipment are needed for those who have altered or impaired function and sensation due to spinal cord injury or amputation or who have hemiplegia (Blocker & Cardus, 1983). However, cardiac rehabilitation teams must use care not to focus only on cardiac management of the disability for these latter clients without attention to the client's one or more chronic conditions and primary care needs.

Rehabilitation nurses examine program plans to meet cardiac goals to assure these do not interfere with other constraints or needs a client may have due to cormorbidity. This entails a holistic assessment with provisions to prevent further complications or disabilities in facilities or community settings. (Chapter 9 provides for additional content on clients re-entering the community.)

Pertinent issues include safety in the home, primary care and health maintenance, pain management, medication regimens that may become complex or costly, rest and energy conservation, recreation and activities, social network, nutritional requirements, religious or cultural dietary preferences, and use of health systems or products from sources other than the cardiac rehabilitation program.

EDUCATION FOR A LIFESTYLE

Clients and families need to be informed and knowledgeable for effective decision-making and problem-solving about lifestyle choices, behaviors, and specific interventions. Clients are taught to understand their risk factors and learn about those lifestyle habits or preferences that may help modify or reduce their coronary risk level. Lifestyle changes are one of the few areas over which a client has direct control. Because lifestyle behaviors are embedded in everyday activities and patterns, as well as having cultural or emotional values, they are difficult to change in the short term and more difficult on a long-term basis. Table 19-3 compares variables related to client and family education with assessment questions (Hall & Meyer, 1988).

Clients may feel as if they have "given up" control over many areas of their lives and find lifestyle preferences a solace. Change requires energy and commitment, which may be emotionally or psychologically overwhelming for them. The key lifestyle changes recommended for clients in a cardiac rehabilitation program are the same as those proposed as preventive measures for others.

Key Areas for Education and Lifestyle Modifications

✦ Control obesity and make dietary changes, especially reducing calorie and fat intake
✦ Institute measures to reduce serum cholesterol levels and improve low-density lipoprotein/high-density lipoprotein (LDL/HDL) ratio; may include medications
✦ Stop cigarette smoking
✦ Reduce or eliminate alcohol intake
✦ Incorporate stress management and measures for effective coping
✦ Develop or maintain a prescribed exercise program

Client-Focused Education

Education is a key function in cardiac rehabilitation programs and a crucial factor in a client's long-term outcome, but the "window of opportunity" to provide education may

Table 19-3 Education—related variables and assessment questions: variables related to education

Variable	Questions
Existing knowledge base	What does the client and family already know?
	What illness-related experiences have the client and family had?
Readiness to learn (motivation)	What priority does the client and family place on learning?
	What questions or comments are being raised?
	What factors may be impeding motivation (denial, anger, depression)?
Learning needs	Does the client and family state these needs specifically?
	Do nurse, client, and family agree on needs and on the resulting plan?
Client and family goals	What goals, if any, does the client and family have in relation to illness, lifestyle changes, or therapeutic regimens?
Client and family energy for learning	Are symptoms present that must be taken into account?
	Can teaching strategies be geared to the energy level?
Presence of support systems	Will others be learning with the client and family?
	Do learning needs of client and family coincide with other support persons?
Time for learning	How much time is available?
	Can a "time line" be designed with the client and family?
Potential for understanding	What factors will influence understanding of the content (educational level, language, presence of sensory dysfunction, amount of anesthetic, medications that depress central nervous system, anxiety level)?
	What resources are available that will promote understanding?

From *Cardiac Rehabilitation Nursing* by C.R. Jillings, 1988, Rockville, MD, Aspen. Copyright 1988 by Aspen. Reprinted by permission.

Table 19-4 Assessment of learner variables in cardiac rehabilitation

Variables	Assessment area
Individual	Demographics
	Developmental stage
	Education
	Prior illness experience
Sociocultural	Culture/ethnicity
	Beliefs about condition
	Social construction or meaning
Illness related	Status of illness
	Stage of intervention
	Anticipated outcome
	Physical limitations
	Social limitations
	Diagnostic activities
Situational	Client/family system
	Extended family/significant others
	Social network or support system
Cardiac status	Specific symptoms and impact
	Diagnostics and treatment
	Therapeutic regimens: diet, exercise, medications
	Illness trajectory

From *Cardiac Rehabilitation Nursing* by C.R. Jillings, 1988, Rockville, MD: Aspen Publications. Copyright 1988 by Aspen. Reprinted by permission.

Many programs are offered in the evening or on Saturday mornings. The content of the program will provide information about the cardiac event, treatments and procedures, lifestyle activities, exercise prescriptions, and medical alerts. Time for participants to raise concerns and ask questions is exceedingly important. As a result clients and families often are able to provide assistance to one another by passing along information or sharing solutions to otherwise troublesome problems, which is an empowering activity.

Although an educational program necessarily contains standardized content and information, the nurse assesses each client and family to identify learner variables that will influence their perspective on learning, identify any barriers to learning, and determine the type and mode most appropriate to be used for this client's educational materials (Table 19-4).

For clients and each family member, it is important to use educational techniques that educate both hemispheres of the brain. The left hemisphere is the analytic side of the brain, which deals with factual information when delivered in a language format. To illustrate, the left hemisphere of the brain is learning when a person makes statements such as, "Tell me about . . ." or "Explain to me . . ." or "I don't understand . . . ." Written materials are examples of tools for right-brain education programs.

In contrast, the right hemisphere is the visual-spatial side of the brain, which prefers to deal with models, drawings, figures, and pictures. The right hemisphere of the brain is learning when a person makes statements such as, "Show me . . ." or "Let me see it . . . ." Diagrams and drawings

be extremely short. The site and format for an educational program can be adapted to meet the available space and group size. For instance, one-on-one interactions, group classes, discussion groups, peer or support groups, and other configurations are conducted in person, via video, or closed-circuit television (Pollack & Schmidt, 1986).

Many programs offer a series of educational sessions conducted by the members of the team. As far as possible, scheduling for educational sessions should be modified so both families and clients are able to attend all sessions.

are methods for educating persons with right brain learning (Boss, 1986). (Chapter 25 on provides additional information in this area.)

The nurse and other team members will be educating clients and families who are coping at different levels and using various coping behaviors. Educational materials are more effective when they meet individual needs. Readability of all educational materials can be tested in order to meet the needs of specific populations (Owen, Johnson, Frost, Porter, & O'Hare, 1993). When selecting educational materials, assess the client and family concerning the following:

+ Diagnosis and health status
+ Education and socioeconomic background
+ Interest in material and mode of presentation
+ Availability of VCR, tape players, or other devices
+ Cultural or religious preferences
+ Literacy level, primary language
+ Visual, auditory, or other sensory impairments
+ Functional abilities
+ Age or developmental factors

Over 21 million persons in the United States are unable to comprehend materials written above the sixth-grade reading level (National Advisory Council on Adult Education, 1986); many are functionally illiterate or speak a primary language other than English. Elderly persons, who account for a large percent of the population who have cardiovascular conditions, also have a 38% rate of illiteracy (National Council on Aging, 1986). Additionally many elderly persons require large print, which is visualized better against a contrasting color. For example, dark letters printed on yellow, light blue, or white paper is easier for them to read (Panchal & Kmetz, 1991).

Educational resources are becoming more sophisticated and readily available. For example, educational materials may include anatomic views of coronary arteries showing blockages of the coronary arteries after the angiograms or pictures that illustrate surgical procedures or complementary product guides from companies that manufacture prosthetic valves and pacemakers. A number of major organizations, such as the American Heart Association, and private vendor or manufacturing companies, have available educational materials, charts, videocassette tapes, handout materials, interactive computer programs, and anatomic models. Preview any prepackaged or "canned" educational materials to individualize the content to meet client goals, match program philosophy, and assure information is current and accurate.

Although clients and family members clearly benefit from a variety of educational materials, select materials based on the assessment of their learning needs and styles. As a rule families prefer simple and illustrated materials that provide complete and informative explanations over highly technical data, unless they request otherwise. Control the temptation to overload them with materials they will never use.

Calendars and other data management tools are inexpensive, portable, and easy to use and interpret. They are useful for recording appointments, class times, reminders for follow-up such as with laboratory test results, and other scheduling matters. The same calendar functions as an activity log. Data records can be maintained to show a profile of a client's changes in weight, daily glucose levels, vital signs or blood pressure, prn medication use, occurrence of symptoms, exercise levels, or similar events. When these logs are analyzed to show patterns of behavior, the results become a powerful teaching tool created by the client.

PSYCHOSOCIAL AND SEXUALITY ISSUES

Many clients recover from a cardiovascular event only to sucumb to depression, anxiety, and other behaviors that prevent them from resuming family and social relationships or returning to a satisfactory and productive life. As survival rates from MI improve, attention to issues surrounding a client's quality of life will become more common (Radtke, 1989).

Quality of life and self-esteem, along with adherence to self-care, medication, and exercise regimens may be deciding factors in a client's continued participation in a cardiac rehabilitation program (Conn, Taylor, & Casey, 1992). Concepts such as quality of life are not easy to measure or evaluate. One group of rehabilitation nurse researchers have used the Perceived Quality-of-Life Scale (PQOL) (Patrick, Danis, Southerland, & Hong, 1988), which has internal consistency reliability to predict participation and outcomes (Conn et al., 1992).

Rukholm and McGirr (1994) have begun to test the reliability and validity of a Quality-of-Life Index (QLI), which has been adapted to specifically measure quality of life for clients who have cardiac problems. The QLI is a 20-item unweighted visual analog scale; clients respond at some point along a line extending between two opposite words. For example, a client may respond to the question "Do you tire easily" by indicating a point on a line between "Not at all" and "A great deal." The QLI also was tested as a instrument for measuring quality of life as an outcome measure following a cardiac rehabilitation program (Rukholm & McGirr, 1994).

Clients may have difficulty maintaining self-esteem as they face changes in their lifestyle and roles (Johnson & Morse, 1990). Depression and anxiety are heightened when a client is unable to return to former activities including work. In a downward spiral, the client assumes a sick role, learns helplessness, and becomes fearful of impending cardiac emergencies, even sudden death. Family members may respond by overly protecting the person or by labeling the client as being overly concerned or having a "cardiac psychosis."

Some clients respond with rebellious behaviors to regain a sense of control or conversely with avoidance and denial by resorting to addictive behaviors, compulsions, and perhaps substance abuse. Clients may develop symptoms of illness secondary to depression such as vague discomfort or pains in the chest, headache, restlessness, insomnia, fatigue, feelings of panic, or altered concentration and memory. (Chapter 13 provides a related discussion.) A comprehensive cardiac rehabilitation program provides for a client's psychosocial needs, as well as for physical training.

Each client and family needs to receive guidance and coaching to cope with the potential psychosocial problems that commonly occur following a cardiac event and often

---

♦

COMMONLY EXPRESSED CONCERNS FOLLOWING A CARDIAC EVENT

WHAT CAN BE EXPECTED FROM A CLIENT REGARDING

Emotions
Symptoms
Medication side effects
Responses to exercise or activity

WHEN CAN A CLIENT RESUME

Sexual activity
Driving a car
Recreational activities or sports
Work-related activities
Housework or laundry

HOW DOES A CLIENT

Manage stress effectively
Exercise safely
Know when to call a physician or emergency responders
Eat properly
Meet financial needs
Modify lifestyle to control risk factors (Karem, 1989)

---

provoke stressful responses. As a group clients and families predictably ask questions about similar concerns (see the box above). Rehabilitation nurses who are aware of these commonly expressed concerns are able to provide anticipatory guidance about specific responses and work through coping responses that enable clients and families to resist or eliminate stressors.

Social and Group Supports

Social networks and social support are two factors that have been found to be valid predictors of outcome following MI. Networking among clients and family members is one way to provide needed psychological support throughout all stages of illness and rehabilitation (Ostergren et al., 1991). Involvement of all family members is imperative because the numbers of family members grow alongside the numbers of clients (Levin, 1987). Family members benefit from networking and sharing experiences whether the client is in a critical care unit or any of the other stages of recovery. Psychosocial issues require the interdisciplinary team to function with awareness and coordinated intervention, with the coordinator ensuring communication among team members (Karam, 1989).

Support groups may be organized or informal; many become very creative, but they exist to meet the needs of the persons who participate in them. For example, separate groups may be organized for spouses, children and parents, or clients in order to present issues or address specific concerns of a group. Some programs organize groups according to diagnostic criteria such as clients with pacemakers,

those with congestive heart disease, clients who receive medical treatment, or those who have surgical interventions.

To be successful, organized groups in a facility meet on an orderly schedule that takes into account other activities or client needs that may interrupt or overrun their gathering time and place. For example, clients may need to meet in a location near a telemetry monitor or with access to emergency equipment. Others may choose a time when family members are not visiting, after physicians' rounds on the unit, or times that will avoid conflict with medication or meal times.

Suggestions for Improving Participation

+ Involve client and family in plan
+ Educate client to make realistic assessments of status; educate family to client's limitations and abilities
+ Refer to counseling program where professionals are knowledgeable about concerns and issues for clients who have had cardiac events; include family counseling
+ Reinforce exercise program
+ Reinforce medication and dietary regimens
+ Reinforce lifestyle modifications
+ Promote activities and programs that enable return to usual lifestyle as much as possible for client
+ Evaluate client and family psychosocial status regularly

Electronic Support Groups

Electronic support groups are flourishing among clients and families who have personal computers with a modem and communications software. Personal computers offer a new form of networking that can extend locally, nationally, or even internationally. Advantages of electronic support groups include the following:

1. Twenty-four–hour access is available.
2. The system can be used from home or facility.
3. Client chooses topics to read and respond to.
4. Client and family are assured privacy, anonymity, and control.
5. A hard copy of all transactions can be printed.
6. Professional personnel are able to exchange information and obtain interactive consultations (Sparks, 1992).

Two resources for locating information about an electronic support group are listed in the box on p. 414.

Return to Work

Many clients who have participated in cardiac rehabilitation programs eventually are able to return to work. Older persons are less likely to return to work than those who are in primary wage-earning years unless there are preexisting medical reasons. Although work and working have high value in the United States, clients and employers may have a sense of fear or confusion about an employee's health status following a cardiovascular incident. As with other behavioral questions, sorting out the complex variables in determining whether a client actually returns to work is not an exact science.

Physical, psychosocial, and medical factors as well as age, access to work, financial situation, and family support are all factors in a client's return to work. Examples of questions a client, family, and employer ask are as follows:

Is the person medically stable and able to return to work?

How soon can work be resumed and at what level of function?

Are other comparable, less strenuous positions available?

Can the same job functions can be performed?

Are there any types of barriers?

Are physical structure or equipment modifications necessary?

How does the environment need to be altered?

Does the person have disability coverage or other financial support?

Does the client/company want the client to return to work?

The cardiac rehabilitation team is prepared to work with a client and family to assess the readiness to return to work and the conditions for doing so. Initially a client completes a treadmill test to identify and calculate the MET level at which she is able to function safely without encountering problems or warning signs. Table 19-2 supplies representative amounts of METs for certain vocational tasks. Some clients will be able to improve their MET score following exercise training for cardiovascular fitness.

It is important for clients to have a realistic evaluation of the ability to perform work and other activities so they do not overextend themselves on the job or restrict themselves needlessly. The client's view of self in the sick role or with learned helplessness is an indicator for a psychosocial assessment, which may reveal a need for counseling before work is attempted.

In some work-hardening programs, a client and team member conduct a detailed workplace assessment documenting activities that would occur during a typical day. They note details of the work style, such as whether a client is sitting at a computer terminal versus climbing or lifting versus standing in an assembly line. The workplace environment and availability of services, such as food choices in the cafeteria and location and accessibility of lavatories are inspected; the client's commute to work and means of transportation are taken during regular commuting hours; and the number of stressful situations and the degree to which the client identifies stressors are noted. The workplace load is calculated in METs, which are compared with the client's exercise test METs level. The MET level, health status, and exercise prescription are important determinants of the client's ability to return to work.

Work hardening is a general term as well as the title for a program that has specific characteristics and goals to determine whether a client returns to work, or under what auspices. The work-hardening program may range from 2 to 8 hours/day. It consists of simulated work-related tasks that may become progressively difficult until the client is able (or unable) to perform the functional tasks as they would be required to do on the job. These tasks are performed under supervision of a trained therapist and in a structured environment.

Other common components of a work-hardening program include functional activities; cardiovascular conditioning; education about proper use of body mechanics to prevent overtaxing, strain, or injury; and a variety of techniques for managing job-related and personal stressors. Assessment of an individual client's ability to return to work and the capacity for a safe expeditous return to workforce is conducted by the full team, using current standards and program guidelines.

Future Directions

The future of cardiac rehabilitation programs includes offering more individualized services to a greater variety of clients and families regardless of their geographic location. The needs of an aging population in an era of shrinking hospital stay are accompanied by social changes in work patterns and lifestyles, electronic technology, and a growing body of research knowledge. Findings from research of highly structured and uniform aspects of cardiac rehabilitation programs need to be translated into programs that are available to all clients who have experienced a cardiac event and their families, not only those who are geographically available (Gattiker, Gains, & Dennis, 1992). Prevention, education for self-care, and lifestyle modification are key components for improved outcomes.

◆ ——
ELECTRONIC SUPPORT GROUP INFORMATION

American Self-Help Clearinghouse
St Clares–Riverside Medical Center
Denville, NJ 07834

New Jersey (800) 367-6274
Elsewhere (201) 625-7101
TDD line (201) 625-9053
Weekdays 9 AM-5 PM EST

◆ ——
CARDIAC REHABILITATION REFERENCE ORGANIZATIONS

American Association of Cardiovascular and Pulmonary Rehabilitation
7611 Elmwood Avenue
Suite 201
Middleton, WI 53562

American College of Sports Medicine
600 Washington Square
Philadelphia, PA 19106-4198

American Heart Association
7272 Greenville Avenue
Dallas, TX 75231-4596

American Nurses Credentialing Center
1101 14th Street NW
Suite 700
Washington, D.C., 20005

✦

CASE STUDY

Mrs. Doe, a 68-year-old widow, suffered an acute anterior MI complicated by congestive heart failure (CHF). She now has an ejection fraction of 30%, no signs or symptoms of CHF, no murmur or gallop, no crackles. She lives 100 miles from the nearest "formal" cardiac rehabilitation program in a rural area with two pets. Her children live out of state. She describes her neighbors as "helpful whenever I call."

A treadmill test before hospital discharge documented her tolerance of 1 to 2 METs. Mrs. Doe has been very active with yard and garden work before her MI. Her risk factors for atherosclerosis include cholesterol 220 (high), HDL 40 (low). She does not use tobacco but has had heavy tobacco smoke exposure until 1.5 years ago, and has non-insulin-dependent diabetes. (NIDDM). She has had a hysterectomy with oophorectomy 10 years ago and is not on estrogen replacement therapy.

CARE PLAN

Educational component

First, what are the client's questions and concerns?

A few facts: 80% clients experiencing an acute MI return to preinfarction activity level; proper education, activities, and follow-up facilitate this return to "normal" lifestyle.

Home health referral is appropriate for continued education, continued assessment, and on-site follow-up. Consult a home health agency that has a formal program for post-MI and CHF clients utilizing specialty nurses and additional disciplines such as physical therapy, dietary, and social worker. Jointly decide roles and responsibilities of "consultant and consultee" of client, who is to continue under the umbrella of formal cardiac rehabilitation. For example, the home health nurse may need to confer with appropriate cardiac rehabilitation personnel regarding an increase in exercise or activity plan.

Regarding MI: definition, cause, healing process, rationale for activity/exercise limitations and recommendations, signs and symptoms to report, awareness of preinfarctional anginal symptoms.

Regarding CHF: definition, cause, factors that lower/raise risk of reoccurrence, signs and symptoms to report, rationale of no-added salt diet, rationale regarding client continuing daily weights and reporting cumulative weight gain of 2 pounds to the home health nurse or MD or cardiac rehabilitation personnel, daily weight rules (approximate same time, same amount of clothing, no weights on carpeted floor and use only on set scale (home health personnel should use client's scales also), importance of early symptom awareness and reporting.

What is to be expected? Emotions, symptoms, medication side effects, responses to exercise and activity. Which to report and to whom.

When can client resume work, sex, driving, recreation (e.g., gardening, club activities), housework (carefully review which MET activities are permitted and project when additional activities may be added to the established schedule).

How does the client exercise and eat properly and safely, manage stress, control risk factors—specifically for this client: lower cholesterol to below 200 and raise HDLs to above 65, investigate estrogen replacement therapy, which also will assist in the elevation of HDLs. Maintain NIDDM status under strict control.

Know when to call physician, home health nurse, or cardiac rehabilitation personnel. Be sure lines of communication are clearly in place among all parties involved.

Exercise and activity: specific information on which activities are allowed and which are not. What type of exercise is best for client's life and routines of daily living? What symptoms indicate client should terminate an activity or exercise? A good rule of thumb is that 30 minutes after an activity or exercise, the client should feel good. If the client is tired after 30 minutes, she probably has overdone it. Usually people push speed of an activity or exercise too fast. Gradually increasing the time of an exercise or activity is preferred before increasing the speed of work.

REFERENCES

American Association of Cardiovascular and Pulmonary Rehabilitation. (1991). *Guidelines for cardiac rehabilitation programs.* Champaign, IL: Human Kinetics.

American Association of Cardiovascular and Pulmonary Rehabilitation. (1993). *Guidelines for pulmonary rehabilitation programs.* Champaign, IL. Human Kinetics.

American College of Sports Medicine. (1991). *Guidelines for exercise testing and prescription* (4th ed.). Philadelphia: Lea and Febiger.

American Heart Association. (1992a). *1992 heart and stroke facts.* Dallas, TX: Author.

American Heart Association. (1992b). *Cardiovascular statistics.* Dallas, TX: Author.

American Heart Association—Georgia Affiliate. (1987). *Guidelines for cardiac rehabilitation programs in Georgia.* Atlanta: Author.

Anderson, J. (1991). Rehabilitating elderly cardiac patients. *Western Journal of Medicine, 154,* 573-578.

Blocker, W.P., & Cardus, D. (1983). *Rehabilitation in ischemic heart disease.* New York: SP Medical and Scientific Books.

Boogaard, M.A.K. (1984). Rehabilitation of the female patient after myocardial infraction. *Nursing Clinics of North America, 19,* 3.

Ross, B.J. (1986). The neuroanatomical and neurophysiological basis of learning. *Journal of Neuroscience Nursing, 18,* 256-264.

Brannon, F.J., Foley, M.W., Starr, J.A., & Black, M.G. (1993). *Cardiopulmonary rehabilitation: Basic theory and application* (2nd ed.). Philadelphia: F.A. Davis.

Calliari, D., & Mark, M.C. (1992). Management of cardiopulmonary arrest in the rehabilitation setting. *Rehabilitation Nursing, 17,* 76-79.

Carnegie, D. (1981). *How to win friends and influence people.* New York: Pocket Books.

Comoss, P.M., Burke, E.A.S., & Swails, S.H. (1979). *Cardiac rehabilitation: A comprehensive nursing approach.* Philadelphia: J.B. Lippincott.

Conn, V.S., Taylor, S.G., & Casey, B. (1992). Cardiac rehabilitation program participation and outcomes after myocardial infarction. *Rehabilitation Nursing, 17,* 58-62.

DeBusk, R.F., Haskell, W.F., Berra, K., & Taylor, C.B. (1985). Medically directed at-home rehabilitation soon after clinically uncomplicated acute myocardial infarction: A new model for patient care. *American Journal of Cardiology, 55,* 251-257.

Fardy, P.S., Yanowitz, F.G., & Wilson, P.K. (1988). *Cardiac rehabilitation, adult fitness and exercise testing.* Philadelphia: Lea and Febiger.

Gattiker, H., Goins, P., & Dennis, C. (1992). *Cardiac rehabilitation. Cur-*

rent status and future directions. *Western Journal of Medicine, 156,* 183-188.

Gibbons, K.B., Govoni, A., Hazel, C., Lewis, M., Pierce, L.L., & Salter, J. (1992). Critical care elements in a rehabilitation nursing course. *Rehabilitation Nursing, 17,* 80-83.

Glick, D.F. (1991). Home care of patients with cardiac disease. In Kinney, M.R., Packa, D.R., Andreoli, K.G., & Zipes, P.P. (Eds.), *Comprehensive cardiac care* (7th ed.). St. Louis: Mosby–Year Book.

Gordon, N.F. (1993a). *Arthritis, your complete exercise guide.* Champaign, IL: Human Kinetics Books.

Gordon, N.F. (1993b). *Breathing disorders, your complete exercise guide.* Champaign, IL: Human Kinetics Books.

Gordon, N.F. (1993c). *Chronic fatigue, your complete exercise guide.* Champaign, IL: Human Kinetics Books.

Gordon, N.F. (1993d). *Diabetes, your complete exercise guide.* Champaign, IL: Human Kinetics Books.

Gordon, N.F. (1993e). *Stroke, your complete exercise guide.* Champaign, IL: Human Kinetics Books.

Gordon, N.F., & Scott, C.B. (1991). The role of exercise in the primary and secondary prevention of coronary artery disease. *Clinics in Sports Medicine, 10,* 87-103.

Gravanis, M.S. (1993). *Cardiovascular disorders: Pathogenesis and pathology.* St. Louis: Mosby–Year Book.

Guyton, A.C. (1990). *Textbook of medical physiology.* Philadelphia: W.B. Saunders.

Hall, L.K., & Meyer, G.C. (1988). *Cardiac rehabilitation: Exercise testing and prescription* (Vol. 2). Champaign, IL: Human Kinetics Books.

Hall, L.K., & Meyer, G.C., & Hellerstein, H.K. (1984). *Cardiac rehabilitation: Exercise testing and prescription.* Champaign, IL: Human Kinetics Books.

Hiatt, A.M., Hoenshell-Nelson, N., & Zimmerman, L. (1990). Factors influencing patient entrance into a cardiac rehabilitation program. *Cardiovascular Nursing, 26,* 25-29.

Jessup, M., Lakatta, E.G., Leier, C.V., & Santinga, J.T. (1992). CHF in the elderly: is it different? *Patient Care 9,* 40-61.

Jillings, C.R. (1988). *Cardiac rehabilitation nursing.* Rockville, MD: Aspen.

Johnson, J., & Morse, J. (1990). Regaining control: The process of adjustment after myocardial infarction. *Heart and Lung, 19,* 126-135.

Karem, C. (1989). *A practical guide to cardiac rehabilitation.* Philadelphia: Aspen.

Kelleher, K. (1991). Prescribing exercise for the adult with diabetes. *Journal to be found, 2,* 163-165.

Kligman, E.W., & Pepin, E. (1992). Prescribing physical activity for older patients. *Geriatrics, 47,* 33-47.

Levin, R.F. (1987). *Heartmates: A survival guide for the cardiac spouse.* New York: Pocket Books.

Matheson, L.N., Selvester, R.H., & Rice, H.E. (1975). The interdisciplinary team in cardiac rehabilitation. *Rehabilitation Literature, 36,* 366-385.

Maynard, T. (1991). Exercise: Part II, translating the exercise prescription. *Diabetes Educator, 17,* 384-395.

Miller, N.H. (1991). Cardiac rehabilitation. In Kinney, M.R., Packa, D.R., Andreoli, K.G., Zipes, P.P. (Eds.), *Comprehensive cardiac care* (7th ed.). St. Louis: Mosby–Year Book.

Moranville-Hunziker, M., Sagehorn, K.K., Conn, V., Feutz, C., & Hagenhoff, B. (1994). Patients' perceptions of learning needs during the first phase of cardiac rehabilitation following coronary artery bypass graft surgery. *Rehabilitation Nursing Research, 2,* 75-80.

National Advisory Council on Adult Education. (1986). *Illiteracy in America: Extent, causes, suggested solutions.* Washington DC: Government Printing Office.

National Council on Aging. (1986). *Literacy education for the elderly.* Washington DC: Author.

Niewenhous, S.S. (1991). Cardiovascular education programs in the home health arena. *Caring, 10,* 34-40.

Ostergren, P.O. Freitag, M., Hanson, B.S., Hedin, E., Isacsson, S.O., Odeberg, H., & Svensson, S.E. (1991). Social network and social support predict improvement of physical working capacity in rehabilitation of patients with first myocardial infarction. *Scandanavian Journal of Social Medicine, 19,* 225-234.

Owen, P., Johnson, E.M., Frost, C.D., Porter, K.A., & O'Hare, E. (1993). Reading, readability, and patient education materials. *Cardiovascular Nursing, 29,* 9-13.

Panchal J., & Kmetz, L. (1991). The puzzle of educating the client with a cardiovascular disorder: making all the pieces fit. *Journal of Home Health Care Practice, 4,* 1-12.

Pashkow, F.J., & Dafoe, W.A. (1993). *Clinical cardiac rehabilitation: A cardiologist's guide.* Baltimore: Williams & Wilkins.

Patrick, D., Danis, M., Southerland, L., & Hong, G. (1988). Quality of life following intensive care. *Journal of General Internal Medicine, 3,* 218-223.

Pollack, M.L., & Schmidt, D.H. (1986). *Heart disease and rehabilitation* (2nd ed.). New York: John Wiley & Sons.

Radtke, K. (1989). Exercise compliance in cardiac rehabilitation. *Rehabilitation Nursing, 14,* 182-186.

Rukholm, E., & McGirr, M. (1994). A quality-of-life index for clients with ischemic heart disease: Establishing reliability and validity. *Rehabilitation Nursing, 19,* 12-16.

Southard, D.R., Certo, C., Comoss, P.M., Gordon, N.F., Herbert, W.G., Protas, E.J., Ribisl, P., & Swails, S. (1994). Core compentencies for cardiac rehabilitation professionals: Position statement of the American Association of Cardiovascular and Pulmonary Rehabilitation. *Journal of Cardiopulmonary Rehabilitation, 14,* 87-92.

Sparks, S.M. (1992). Exploring electronic support groups. *American Journal of Nursing, 92,* 62-65.

Thompson, J.M., McFarland, G.K., Hirsch, J.E., & Tucker, S.M. (1993). *Mosby's Clinical nursing* (3rd ed.). St. Louis: Mosby–Year Book.

Topp, R. (1991). Development of an exercise program for older adults: Pre-exercise testing, exercise prescription and program maintenance. *Nurse Practitioner, 16,* 16-28.

United States Public Health Service. (1982). *Health Care Finance Administration, Comprehensive outpatient rehabilitation survey report facility form* (Section 488.70 Personnel Qualifications), Washington DC.

Wenger, N.K. (1992a). Supervised vs unsupervised exercise training following myocardial infarction and myocardial revascularization procedures. *Annals of the Academy Medicine, 21,* 141-144.

Wenger, N.K. (1992b). Exercise testing and training of the elderly coronary patient. *Chest, 101* Suppl. 5, 3095-3115.

Wenger, N.K. (1994). Rehabilitation of the patient with coronary heart disease. In R.C. Schlant, & R.W. Alexander (Eds.), *Hurst's the heart: Arteries & veins.* New York: McGraw-Hill (pp. 1223-1237).

Wenger, N.K., & Hellerstein, H.K. (1992). *Rehabilitation of the coronary patient* (3rd ed.). New York: Churchill Livingston.

SUGGESTED READING

California Society for Cardiac Rehabilitation. (1988). *Standards for cardiac rehabilitation in California.* Stockton: California Society for Rehabilitation.

Kinney, M.R., Packa, D.R., Andreoli, K.G., & Zipes, P.P. (1991). *Comprehensive cardiac care* (7th ed.). St. Louis: Mosby–Year Book.

Massachusetts Society for Cardiac Rehabilitation. (1988). *Standards for cardiac rehabilitation programs.* Boston: Author.

20

Bladder Elimination and Continence

Marilyn Pires, MS, RN, CRRN

INTRODUCTION

Care of persons with urinary incontinence has long been a priority of rehabilitation nursing practice. A majority of clients who enter a rehabilitation setting are admitted with urinary incontinence. Conversely the majority of persons leaving a rehabilitation setting are continent. The intervening variable has been specific rehabilitation nursing interventions that primarily address the management of incontinence due to neurogenic etiologies and functional incontinence.

Urinary incontinence due to neurogenic etiologies represents a very small percentage of the prevalence of incontinence in the United States. Recent national recognition of the scope of the problem of incontinence represents an opportunity for rehabilitation nurses to expand their practice by developing and participating in continence programs. To do this, rehabilitation nurses must bolster their knowledge base to include an understanding of the non-neurogenic etiologies of urinary incontinence and the appropriate interventions for these types of incontinence.

SCOPE OF THE PROBLEM OF URINARY INCONTINENCE

Urinary incontinence is defined by the International Continence Society as "a condition in which involuntary loss of urine is a social or hygienic problem and is objectively demonstrable" (Bates, Bradley, & Glen, 1979). The Urinary Incontinence Guideline Panel, convened by the Agency for Health Care Policy and Research (AHCPR), defined urinary incontinence as "the involuntary loss of urine which is sufficient to be a problem" (Urinary Incontinence Guideline Panel, 1992b).

Over 10 million adult Americans experience urinary incontinence (National Center for Health Statistics, 1979). The prevalence of urinary incontinence in persons between 15 and 64 years old ranges from 1.5% to 5% in men and 10% to 25% in women (Thomas, Plymat, Blannin, & Meade, 1980). For community-dwelling persons older than 60, the prevalence of urinary incontinence ranges from 15% to 30%, with the prevalence among women twice that of men (Diokno, Brock, Brown, & Herzog, 1986). At least half of the 1.5 million residents of nursing homes are incontinent of urine at least once a day (National Center for Health Statistics, 1979). It is estimated that the annual direct cost of caring for incontinent persons of all ages in the community is $14 billion, and $5 billion in nursing homes (Hu, 1990).

Although urinary incontinence is highly prevalent, many persons do not seek treatment. Adults are expected to maintain control of their urinary elimination. When they become incontinent, people are often embarrassed and ashamed. Many people believe that incontinence is an inevitable consequence of aging with which they must learn to deal. Until recently this was also the perception of many healthcare professionals including nurses. Although changes associated with aging contribute to older persons' susceptibility to incontinence, it is not a normal part of aging. It is now known that incontinence is a symptom and with proper diagnosis and appropriate interventions, most incontinence can be reversed or managed effectively.

Rehabilitation nurses practice in many settings and work with persons across the life-span. Because of this and the intimacy of interactions with clients, rehabilitation nurses are in a unique position to detect unreported bladder dysfunction and to initiate the assessment and interventions needed to offer treatment to persons with urinary incontinence.

NORMAL BLADDER FUNCTION
Anatomy

The urinary tract is composed of the kidneys, ureters, bladder, and urethra. The kidneys filter waste products from the blood and continuously produce urine. The ureters are bilateral muscular tubes that drain urine from the kidneys to the bladder. The ureters enter the posterior surface of the bladder at an oblique angle, which functions as a valve to prevent backflow of urine. The bladder is a reservoir for urine. It is a hollow muscular organ with two parts. The body is made up of the detrusor muscle, which consists of layers of intertwining smooth muscle. The trigone is a small triangular area at the base of the bladder through which the ureters and urethra pass and is contiguous with the bladder neck. The bladder neck is 2 to 3 cm long and is part of the posterior urethra. The muscles in this area form the internal sphincter. The urethra is a tube that carries urine from the bladder out of the body. Beyond the posterior urethra the tube continues through an extension of the deep perineal muscles. This striated muscle is called the rhabdosphincter, which in conjunction with the urogenital diaphragm, makes up the external sphincter mechanism (Wyman, 1988). Figure 20-1 provides a diagram of the anatomy of the lower urinary tract. The external sphincter mechanism is a voluntary skeletal muscle, in contrast to the smooth autonomic muscle of the bladder body and bladder

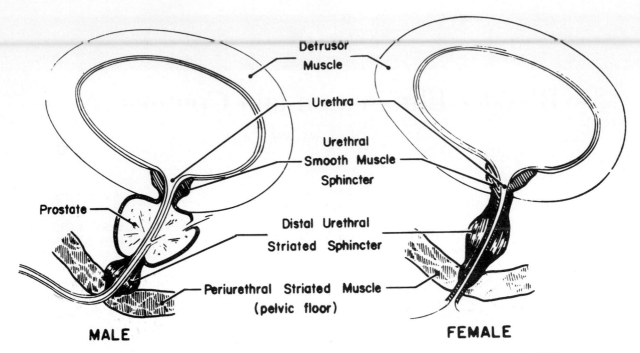

Fig. 20-1 Diagram of the anatomy of the lower urinary tract. (From "The Structure of the Bladder and Urethra in Relation to Function" by J. Gosling, 1979, *Urologic Clinics of North America* *6*, p. 31. Copyright 1979 by W.B. Saunders. Reprinted by permission.)

neck. The external sphincter mechanism is under voluntary control and allows a person to prevent urination even when involuntary mechanisms are attempting to empty the bladder (Guyton, 1991).

Other structures that contribute to continence are the pelvic floor muscles and, in males, the prostate gland. The muscles of the pelvic floor support the bladder. They include the levator ani, pubococcygeus, internal obturator, pyriform and the superficial and deep perineal muscles which make up the urogenital diaphragm. Voluntary contraction of these pelvic muscles results in compression, lengthening, and elevation of the urethra. For example, the voiding stream can be interrupted by voluntary contracting the pubococcygeal muscle. In men the prostate gland is important in maintaining continence. The urethra, which passes through the prostate gland, contains both smooth and striated muscle (Doughty, 1991).

Innervention of the Lower Urinary Tract

The nerve supply of the lower urinary tract includes parasympathetic and sympathetic fibers as well as somatic nerve fibers.

The parasympathetic nerves provide motor stimulation to the bladder, causing bladder contraction via the pelvic nerve. The pelvic nerve exits the spinal cord at S2-4 level. The preganglionic nerves originate in the sacral cord and synapse with the short postganglionic nerves within the bladder wall (Doughty, 1991). Parasympathetic nerves work by releasing the neurotransmitter acetylcholine. Stimulation of parasympathetic fibers causes the ureters to speed up transport of urine from the kidneys to the bladder, causes

the detrusor muscle to contract, thus causing the bladder to empty, and may cause the internal sphincter to open slightly.

The sympathetic nerves mediate the storage of urine in the bladder by stimulating contractions of the bladder neck and proximal urethra. The sympathetic fibers exit the thoracic lumbar cord at the T12-L2 level via the hypogastric nerve. The preganglionic nerves originate in the thoracolumbar cord and synapse with the postganglionic fibers at the inferior mesenteric and hypogastric plexuses. The postganglionic fibers travel from these plexuses to the bladder neck and proximal urethra (Doughty, 1991). Sympathetic nerves work by releasing the neurotransmitter norepinephrine. Stimulation of sympathetic fibers causes the ureters to slow the transport of urine from the kidneys to the bladder and to relax the detrusor muscle (thus facilitating storage of urine) and to constrict the internal sphincter.

Somatic innervation consists of both efferent (motor) and afferent (sensory) fibers. The efferent fibers of the somatic nervous system originate in the anterior horn of the S2-4 segments and travel via the pudendal nerve to the external striated sphincter and the muscles of the pelvic floor. Somatic nerves work by releasing the neurotransmitter acetylcholine. The external sphincter mechanism normally is contracted, supporting bladder storage by preventing leakage of urine. This mechanism, however, can be relaxed at will, allowing urination.

Afferent fibers originate in the bladder and proceed via the pelvic and hypogastric nerves to the posterior horn of the spinal cord. Sensory fibers of the pelvic nerve are stimulated during bladder filling by mechanoreceptors in the detrusor muscle. Messages travel from the bladder to the sa-

Fig. 20-2 Complex reflex arc. (From *Nursing for Continence* by K.F. Jeter, N. Fallen, and C. Norton, 1990, Philadelphia: W.B. Saunders. Copyright 1990 by W.B. Saunders. Reprinted by permission.)

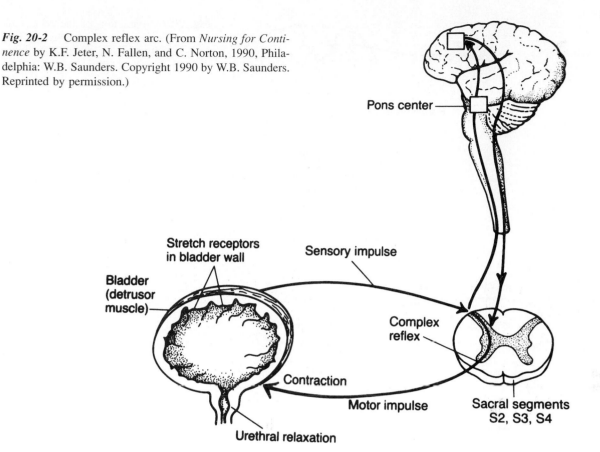

Table 20-1 Neurotransmitters that mediate micturition

Neurotransmitter	Innervation	Neuroreceptor	Location of neuroreceptor	Physiologic effect
Acetylcholine	Somatic	Cholinergic	External sphincter	Bladder storage
Acetylcholine	Parasympathetic	Cholinergic	Bladder base and body	Bladder contraction
Norepinephrine	Sympathetic	Adrenergic	Alpha Bladder base, neck, and proximal urethra	Bladder storage
			Beta Bladder body	Bladder storage

From *Urinary and Fecal Incontinence Nursing Management* by D.B. Doughty, 1991, St. Louis: Mosby–Year Book. Copyright 1991 by Mosby–Year Book. Reprinted by permission.

cral micturition center and stimulate the voiding reflex, while other messages are transmitted to the brain via the spinothalamic tract. Sensation permits voluntary control of the bladder. Table 20-1 lists neurotransmitters that mediate micturation.

Neural Coordination of Micturition

The micturition reflex is mediated by a complex reflex arc (Fig. 20-2). During the micturition reflex, sensory messages pass from the bladder into and through the sacral cord and are coordinated by the pons. The pons coordinates the relaxation of the urethral sphincter with detrusor contraction (Jeter, Faller, & Norton, 1990). The pons is controlled voluntarily by the frontal cortex. If a person does not want to urinate, the frontal micturition center sends inhibitory messages from the frontal cortex through the pons, down the reticulospinal tract to the sacral micturition center and inhibits the motor messages for detrusor contraction and sphincter relaxation (Jeter et al., 1990) (Fig. 20-3). Continence involves active inhibition of the complex reflex arc. There is also direct cortical control of the external sphincter mechanism. Direct corticospinal connections travel from the frontal cortex to the S2-4 segments, then via the pudendal nerve to provide voluntary contraction and relaxation of the external sphincter mechanism (Jeter et al., 1990) (Fig. 20-4).

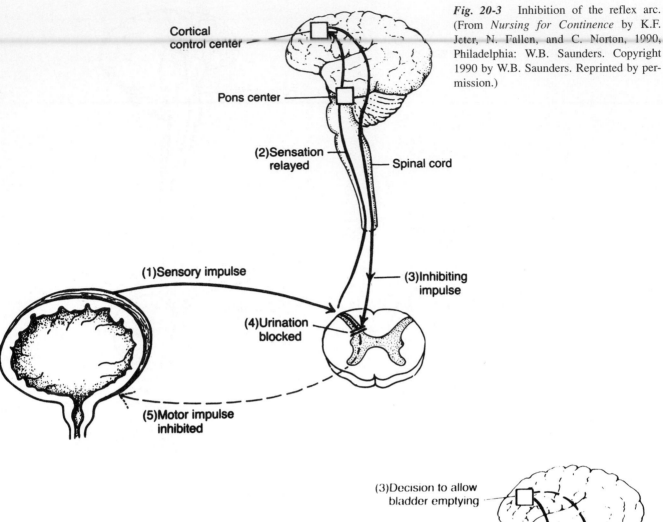

Cortical
control center

Pons center

(2)Sensation
relayed

Spinal cord

(1)Sensory impulse

(3)Inhibiting
impulse

(4)Urination
blocked

(5)Motor impulse
inhibited

Fig. 20-3 Inhibition of the reflex arc. (From *Nursing for Continence* by K.F. Jeter, N. Fallen, and C. Norton, 1990, Philadelphia: W.B. Saunders. Copyright 1990 by W.B. Saunders. Reprinted by permission.)

(3)Decision to allow
bladder emptying

(2)Sensation relayed

(4)Inhibition
ceases

(1)Sensation

(5)Reflex arc
completed

(6)Motor
impulses

Relaxation

Fig. 20-4 Micturition. (From *Nursing for Continence* by J.F. Jeter, N. Fallen, and C. Norton, 1990, Philadelphia: W.B. Saunders. Copyright 1990 by W.B. Saunders. Reprinted by permission.)

Normal Micturition

Normal micturition consists of a filling and storage phase and a contraction and emptying phase. During the filling phase, bladder pressure rises slowly and the normal tone of the urethral sphincters and the pelvic floor muscles maintain continence. When the bladder volume reaches the micturition threshold, usually 200 to 300 ml, the person feels the urge to void and the pressure increases. To remain continent, sympathetic stimulation increases, resulting in contraction of the internal sphincter via alpha-adrenergic reception, which increases urethral resistance. At the same time the sympathetic stimulation suppresses detrusor activity via beta-adrenergic reception. This inhibits bladder contractility (Doughty, 1991). Voluntary contraction of the external sphincter mechanism increases via stimulation of the pudendal nerve. This reaction is known as the guarding reflex and further increases urethral resistance (Siroky & Krane, 1982).

Eventually bladder distention increases sensory afferent stimulation, leading to voluntary coordinated micturition. During the emptying phase voluntary inhibition of somatic stimulation to the striated external sphincter decreases resistance at the urinary outlet. There is a decrease in sympathetic nerve activity, causing unopposed parasympathetic stimulation. This parasympathetic stimulation opens the bladder neck and facilitates bladder contraction. As the detrusor contracts, bladder pressure increases as the bladder neck relaxes, urethral resistance decreases, and normal voiding occurs (Doughty, 1991).

In summary, in order to hold urine during the filling phase, the intraurethral pressure must exceed the intravesical (bladder) pressure. During the emptying phase the intravesical pressure exceeds intraurethral pressure. Continence is maintained as long as the intraurethral pressure remains higher than the intravesical pressure (Wyman, 1988).

This normal voiding pattern can be demonstrated by a simultaneous cystometrogram (CMG), which measures bladder volume and pressure, and electromyogram (EMG), which records electrical activity of the pelvic floor muscles and sphincter (Doughty, 1991). Figure 20-5 provides normal results of a CMG and EMG. The CMG shows low bladder pressure at low bladder volumes. As the bladder fills, the person feels the sensation of fullness and the urge to void. The EMG shows an increase in muscle activity in the pelvic floor and sphincter muscles as the person feels the urge to void. This is the guarding reflex referred to previously. As the micturition threshold is reached, the EMG activity diminishes, and the CMG shows a rapid rise in bladder pressure. These changes are consistent with the contraction of the bladder and appropriate sphincter relaxation associated with normal coordinated voluntary voiding.

Age-Related Factors in Voiding

A newborn baby voids by virtue of the complex reflex arc. As the bladder fills, stretch receptors in the detrusor send sensory messages through the S2-4 segments to the pontine micturition center. When the impulses are strong enough, the reflex arc is completed, motor impulses cause bladder contraction coordinated with urethral sphincter relaxation, and the bladder empties. This filling and emptying cycle is repeated throughout the 24-hour period. At this stage the baby's immature central nervous system cannot consciously appreciate or voluntarily control this cycle. The child is thus incontinent.

Between the ages of 2 and 3 years, continence is acquired due to the combination of two processes: societal expectation and maturation of the central nervous system. By the age of 3 years, most children have the mental and neuromuscular capacity to inhibit the reflex arc to prevent voiding and initiate voluntary voiding appropriately during the day. However, it is common for children up to 5 years old to have periodic accidents during the day and nocturnal enuresis (Doughty, 1991).

At puberty the pelvic genitalia become functional in both boys and girls. In boys the prostate gland grows large enough to assist with ejaculation. The growth of the prostate gland provides support for the pelvic floor and increases urethral resistance. In girls the structures of the pelvic floor mature. The tone of muscles of the pelvic floor and the urethra in women is maintained by stimulating estrogen receptors in those structures. At puberty the release of estrogen increases muscle tone of the pelvic floor and increases urethral resistance.

In the adult male the prostate grows slowly until approximately age 45 years, when growth accelerates. With prostate enlargement, there is increased urethral resistance. Depending on the severity of urethral obstruction, the increased contractility needed to overcome the urethral resistance can cause the bladder to hypertrophy or decompensate, leading to urinary retention (Doughty, 1991).

Women may experience temporary or permanent distortion or trauma to the pelvic floor and urethral anatomy as a result of childbirth. With normal pregnancy and delivery, postpartum exercises and return of normal estrogen levels, the tone of the pelvic floor and the integrity of the lower urinary tract usually will be restored. After menopause women experience a decrease in estrogen levels, causing atrophy of the pelvic floor structures. The urethral mucosa also becomes thin and friable reducing coaptation, thus decreasing urethral resistance and predisposing to infection. Decrease in the tone of the pelvic floor may allow hernia-

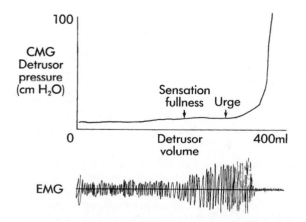

Fig. 20-5 Normal results of CMG and EMG. (From Wheeler JS, Niecestro RM, and Goggin C: J Enterost Ther 15[6]:244, 1988.)

Table 20-2 Common causes of transient urinary incontinence

Potential causes	Comment	Potential causes	Comment
Delirium (confusional state)	In the delirious client incontinence is usually an associated symptom that will abate with proper diagnosis and treatment of the underlying cause of confusion.	**PHARMACEUTICALS**	
		Sedative hypnotics	Benzodiazepines, especially long-acting agents, such as flurazepam and diazepam, may accumulate in elderly patients and cause confusion and secondary incontinence. Alcohol, frequently used as a sedative, can cloud the sensorium, impair mobility, and induce a diuresis, resulting in incontinence.
Infection (symptomatic urinary tract infection)	Dysuria and urgency from symptomatic infection may defeat the older person's ability to reach the toilet in time. Asymptomatic infection, although more common than symptomatic infection, is rarely a cause of incontinence.		
		Diuretics	A brisk diuresis induced by loop diuretics can overwhelm bladder capacity and lead to polyuria, frequency, and urgency, thereby precipitating incontinence in a frail older person. The loop diuretics include furosemide, ethacrynic acid, and bumetanide.
Atrophic urethritis or vaginitis	Atrophic urethritis may present as dysuria, dyspareunia, burning on urination, urgency, agitation (in demented patients), and occasionally as incontinence. Both disorders are readily treated by conjugated estrogen administered either orally (0.3-1.25 mg/day) or locally (2 g or fraction/day).		
		Anticholinergic agents Antihistamines Antidepressants Antipsychotics Disopnamide Opiates Antispasmodics (dicyclomine and Donnatal) Anti-parkinsonian agents (trihexyphenidyl and benztropine mesylate)	Nonprescription (over-the-counter) agents with anticholinergic properties are taken commonly by older patients for insomnia, coryza, pruritus, and vertigo, and many prescription medications also have anticholinergic properties. Anticholinergic side effects include urinary retention with associated urinary frequency and overflow incontinence. Besides anticholinergic actions, antipsychotics such as thioridazine and haloperidol may cause sedation, rigidity, and immobility.
Psychological	Severe depression occasionally may be associated with incontinence but is probably less frequently a cause in older patients.		
Excessive urine production	Excess intake, endocrine conditions that cloud the sensorium and induce a diuresis (e.g., hypercalcemia, hyperglycemia, and diabetes insipidus); expanded volume states such as congestive heart failure, lower extremity venous insufficiency, drug-induced ankle edema (e.g., nifedipine, indomethacin); and low albumen states cause polyuria and can lead to incontinence.	Alpha-adrenergic agents Sympathomimetics (decongestants) Sympatholytics (e.g., prazosin, terazosin, and doxazosin)	Sphincter tone in the proximal urethra can be decreased by alpha antagonists and increased by alpha agonists. An older woman whose urethra is shortened and weakened with age may develop stress incontinence when taking an alpha antagonist for hypertension. An older man with prostate enlargement may develop acute urinary retention and overflow incontinence when taking multicomponent "cold" capsules, which contain alpha agonists and anticholinergic agents, especially if a nasal decongestant and a nonprescription hypnotic antihistamine are added.
Restricted mobility	Limited mobility is an aggravating or precipitating cause of incontinence that frequently can be corrected or improved by treating the underlying condition (e.g., arthritis, poor eyesight, Parkinson's disease, or orthostatic hypotension). A urinal or bedside commode and scheduled toileting often help resolve the incontinence that results from hospitalization and its environmental barriers (e.g., bed rails, restraints, and poor lighting).		
		Calcium-channel blockers	Calcium-channel blockers can reduce smooth muscle contractility in the bladder and occasionally can cause urinary retention and overflow incontinence.
Stool impaction	Clients with stool impaction present with either urge or overflow incontinence and may have fecal incontinence as well. Disimpaction restores continence.		

From *Urinary Incontinence in Adults: Quick Reference Guide for Clinicians* (AHCPR Pub. No. 92-0041) by the Urinary Incontinence Guideline Panel, 1992, Rockville, MD: Agency for Health Care Policy and Research, Public Health Service, U.S. Department of Health and Human Services.

tion of the urinary tract through the supporting structures, decreasing urethral resistance. Postmenopausal women may experience incontinence when bladder pressure surpasses urethral resistance such as during coughing, sneezing, laughing, or exercising (Doughty, 1991).

There are other less clearly understood effects of aging on bladder function. For one, a decrease in bladder capacity makes the urge to void occur more frequently. Older people experience a delayed onset of the desire to void, making it more difficult to further delay voiding. As a result an increase in the residual urine volume raises potential for urinary tract infections. Older people experience an increase in the number of involuntary detrusor contractions, contributing to the symptoms of urgency, frequency, and incontinence. The decrease in urethral and bladder compliance is coupled with lowered maximal urethral closure pressure (Resnick & Yalla, 1985). The elderly also may experience functional changes in vision, mobility, and dexterity, making it difficult to locate and reach the toilet, as well as manage clothing in time to void without being incontinent (Wyman, 1988). All of these problems may be exaggerated by medications such as diuretics, which may increase urgency. Although urinary incontinence should not be accepted as a normal part of aging, these age-related changes predispose older persons to incontinence.

In summary, normal function of the urinary tract and continence are dependent on anatomic integrity of the bladder and urethra, an intact neurologic system that provides voluntary control of micturition, the pattern of urine production, and the physical and mental ability and the psychological willingness of the person to perform tasks associated with toileting (Tanagho, 1990).

Incontinence, then, is a symptom of another problem. A symptomatic approach to the assessment and treatment of incontinence provides opportunities for rehabilitation nursing interventions to improve the quality of life of individuals experiencing incontinence.

TYPES OF INCONTINENCE

For the purpose of this chapter, incontinence is categorized into three basic types: transient, established, and neurogenic. These are somewhat artificial and overlapping classifications; however, these distinctions help to facilitate the discussion of incontinence. Transient or acute incontinence has a precipitous onset. It usually is associated with an acute medical or surgical condition and often resolves when the precipitating condition is addressed. Established, persistent, or chronic incontinence may have a sudden onset precipitated by an acute condition or it may have a gradual onset without a known precipitating cause (Ouslander, 1981). Neurogenic incontinence may have a sudden or progressive onset, depending on the disease or trauma that causes the lesion within the nervous system.

Transient Incontinence

In today's complicated healthcare delivery system, clients are exposed to multiple and interacting factors that can contribute to urinary incontinence. Many of these factors are reversible—for instance, infections, atrophic vaginitis, acute confusional state, immobility, fecal impaction, medical conditions that affect urine production, and medication

side effects. Clients subject to these factors need comprehensive diagnostic evaluation that focuses not only on the lower urinary tract but also on the person's general medical condition and functional status (Urinary Incontinence Guideline Panel, 1992). Table 20-2 lists common causes of transient urinary incontinence.

Established Incontinence

Established incontinence is classified based on the presenting symptoms: stress incontinence, urge incontinence, overflow incontinence, and functional incontinence. Stress incontinence is the involuntary loss of urine when intravesical pressure exceeds intraurethral pressure in the absence of detrusor activity (Bates et al., 1979). Stress incontinence is characterized by sudden loss of small amounts of urine with an increase in intra-abdominal pressure during coughing, sneezing, laughing, lifting, or bending (Jeter et al., 1990) (Fig. 20-6 through Fig. 20-12). Stress incontinence is seen more commonly in women but also may occur in men following prostatectomy (Wyman, 1988).

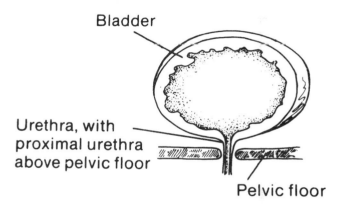

Fig. 20-6 Normal anatomic relationship of the bladder, urethra, and pelvic floor: at rest. (From *Nursing for Continence* by J.F. Jeter, N. Fallen, and C. Norton, 1990, Philadelphia: W.B. Saunders. Copyright 1990 by W.B. Saunders. Reprinted by permission.)

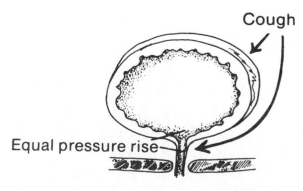

Fig. 20-7 Normal anatomic relationship of the bladder, urethra, and pelvic floor: during a cough. (From *Nursing for Continence* by J.F. Jeter, N. Fallen, and C. Norton, 1990, Philadelphia: W.B. Saunders. Copyright 1990 by W.B. Saunders. Reprinted by permission.)

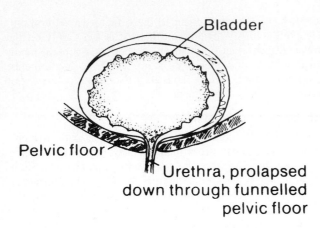

Fig. 20-8 Relationship of the bladder, urethra, and pelvic floor in a woman with stress incontinence: at rest. (From *Nursing for Continence* by K.F. Jeter, N. Fallen, and C. Norton, 1990, Philadelphia: W.B. Saunders. Copyright 1990 by W.B. Saunders. Reprinted by permission.)

Urge incontinence is the involuntary loss of urine associated with a strong urge to void (Bates et al., 1979). Urine is lost in moderate to large amounts. Persons with urge incontinence report that they cannot reach the toilet before leakage occurs. They also report symptoms of urinary frequency and nocturia (Wyman, 1988). Urge incontinence is associated with supratentorial central nervous system lesions. When this is the case, it is referred to as uninhibited bladder (see the neurogenic bladder section). When there is no overt neuropathy, the cause usually is referred to as detrusor instability (Fig. 20-13). The causes may be local irritation of the bladder or simply idiopathic (Jeter et al., 1990).

Overflow incontinence is involuntary loss of urine when the intravesical pressure exceeds the maximum urethral pressure associated with bladder distention, but in the absence of detrusor activity (Bates et al., 1979). Overflow incontinence is characterized by continuous dribbling of small amounts of urine and frequent voiding of small amounts of urine as a result of an overdistended bladder, either because

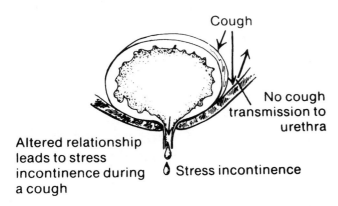

Fig. 20-9 Relationship of the bladder, urethra, and pelvic floor in a woman with stress incontinence: during a cough. (From *Nursing for Continence* by K.F. Jeter, N. Fallen, and C. Norton, 1990, Philadelphia: W.B. Saunders. Copyright 1990 by W.B. Saunders. Reprinted by permission.)

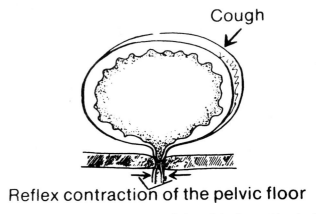

Reflex contraction of the pelvic floor

Fig. 20-11 Normal contraction of the pelvic floor with raised abdominal pressure. (From *Nursing for Continence* by K.F. Jeter, N. Fallen, and C. Norton, 1990, Philadelphia: W.B. Saunders. Copyright 1990 by W.B. Saunders. Reprinted by permission.)

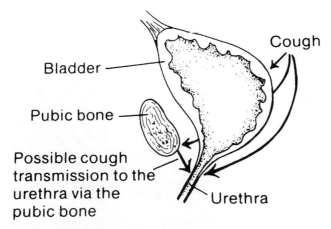

Fig. 20-10 Possible cough transmission to the urethra by way of the pubic bone. (From *Nursing for Continence* by K.F. Jeter, N. Fallen, and C. Norton, 1990, Philadelphia: W.B. Saunders. Copyright 1990 by W.B. Saunders. Reprinted by permission.)

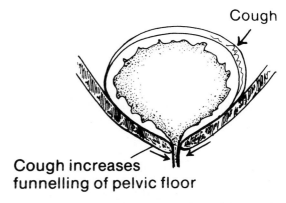

Fig. 20-12 Contraction of the pelvic floor with stress incontinence. (From *Nursing for Continence* by K.F. Jeter, N. Fallen, and C. Norton, 1990, Philadelphia: W.B. Saunders. Copyright 1990 by W.B. Saunders. Reprinted by permission.)

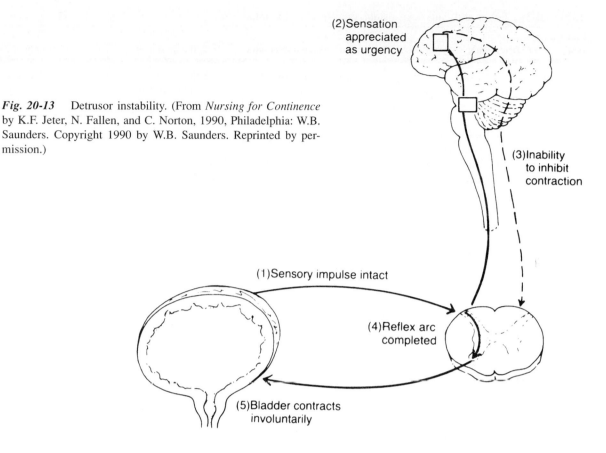

Fig. 20-13 Detrusor instability. (From *Nursing for Continence* by K.F. Jeter, N. Fallen, and C. Norton, 1990, Philadelphia: W.B. Saunders. Copyright 1990 by W.B. Saunders. Reprinted by permission.)

of outlet obstruction (Fig. 20-14) or impaired bladder contractility (Wyman, 1988) (Fig. 20-15). The most common cause of overflow incontinence is prostatic hypertrophy in men.

Functional incontinence is urinary leakage associated with the inability to toilet train due to impairments of cognitive or physical function, psychological unwillingness, or environmental barriers to toilets (Bates et al., 1979). In true functional incontinence, there is normal functioning of the lower urinary tract. Table 20-3 lists types and causes of established urinary incontinence.

Neurogenic Incontinence

Neurogenic bladder dysfunction is the most common form of bladder impairment seen in rehabilitation settings. In the community, rehabilitation nurses are the primary case managers for clients regarding incontinence; in many instances they may advocate for continence issues to be addressed in a client's care plan.

CLASSIFICATION OF NEUROGENIC BLADDER DYSFUNCTION

Neurogenic bladders are classified into five types labeled according to the underlying pathologic process: (1) uninhibited, (2) reflex, (3) autonomous, (4) sensory paralytic, and (5) motor paralytic neurogenic bladders. Most neurogenic bladders represent a combined motor and sensory impairment. For ease of description, the types of neurogenic bladder are described here according to the schema proposed by Lapides and Diokno (1976).

Uninhibited Neurogenic Bladder

The uninhibited neurogenic bladder results from a disruption of the corticoregulatory tract or a malfunction of the supraspinal center that regulates voiding. Figure 20-16 shows areas of the nervous system where damage may occur, and Table 20-4 lists the possible etiologies.

Frequent uninhibited contractions occur, but the bladder usually empties completely, resulting in no residual urine.

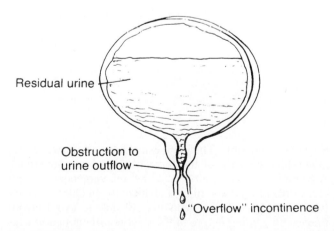

Fig. 20-14 Outflow obstruction. (From *Nursing for Continence* by K.F. Jeter, N. Fallen, and C. Norton, 1990, Philadelphia: W.B. Saunders. Copyright 1990 by W.B. Saunders. Reprinted by permission.)

Table 20-3   Types and causes of established urinary incontinence

Functional type	Description	Associated characteristics	Pathophysiology	Common causes
Stress	Urine leakage associated with a sudden increase in intraabdominal pressure (e.g., as a result of a cough, sneeze, laugh, or exercise); amount of urine loss usually minimal to moderate	Occurs usually in the daytime only; infrequently, nocturnal incontinence may occur	Sphincter incompetence; urethral instability	Pelvic prolapse in women; sphincter weakness or damage (e.g., as a result of a prostatectomy)
Urge	Urine leakage preceded by a strong desire to void; urine loss varies from moderate to large amount	Urinary frequency, nocturia; possible suprapubic discomfort	Detrusor instability	CNS damage secondary to stroke, Alzheimer's disease, brain tumor, or Parkinson's disease; interference with spinal inhibitory pathways secondary to spondylosis or metastasis; local bladder disorders such as bladder cancer, radiation effects, interstitial cystitis, or outlet obstruction
Overflow	Periodic or continuous dribbling of urine resulting from obstruction and/or overdistention of the bladder	Hesitancy, straining to void, weak or interrupted urinary stream; occurs day or night	Outlet obstruction or underactive detrusor	Obstruction, as from prostatic hypertrophy, bladder neck obstruction, or urethral stricture; underactive detrusor, as from myogenic or neurogenic factors (e.g., herniated disk or peripheral neuropathy secondary to diabetes mellitus); anticholinergic/ antispasmodic drugs
Functional	Urine leakage associated with an inability or unwillingness to toilet appropriately because of cognitive or physical impairments, psychological factors, or environmental barriers	May be complicated by other medical problems, iatrogenic illness, or adverse stimuli	Normal bladder and urethral function	Impaired mobility or cognitive status; inaccessible toilets; depression, anger, hostility, or schizophrenia

From "Nursing Assessment of the Incontinent Geriatric Outpatient Population" by J.F. Wyman, 1988, *Nursing Clinics of North America, 23,* 175-176. Copyright 1988 by W.B. Saunders. Reprinted by permission.

The micturition reflex remains intact. Sensation is present as is the bulbocavernosus reflex. A CMG will demonstrate strong, uninhibited contractions as the bladder is filled. The capacity of the bladder is decreased, and involuntary voiding will take place almost as soon as the urge is preceived.

Persons with uninhibited neurogenic bladder frequently complain about the urgency and frequency of urination and nocturia. Once the urge is preceived, they cannot inhibit flow. When the external sphincter is voluntarily contracted, partial control of urination, even with strong voiding contractions, is possible. The intravesical pressure, however, remains high because of the force of detrusor contractions. Anticolinergic medication may be recommended to decrease bladder contractility and increase bladder capacity (Giroux, 1988). These clients may be able to avoid incontinence by voiding before the bladder is full enough to trigger the micturition reflex. Therefore an important part of nursing intervention is scheduled voiding and attention to fluid intake, to anticipate the need to void before the urge becomes too strong.

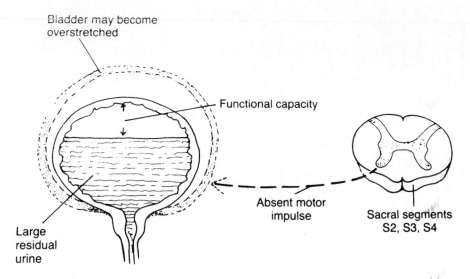

Bladder may become
overstretched

Functional capacity

Absent motor
impulse

Sacral segments
S2, S3, S4

Large
residual
urine

Fig. 20-15 Atonic bladder. (From *Nursing for Continence* by K.F. Jeter, N. Fallen, and C. Norton, 1990, Philadelphia: W.B. Saunders. Copyright 1990 by W.B. Saunders. Reprinted by permission.)

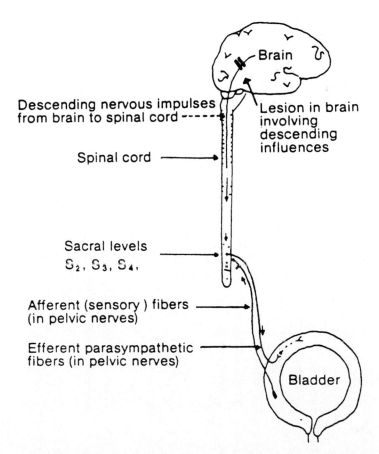

Brain

Descending nervous impulses
from brain to spinal cord

Lesion in brain
involving
descending
influences

Spinal cord

Sacral levels
S_2, S_3, S_4,

Afferent (sensory) fibers
(in pelvic nerves)

Efferent parasympathetic
fibers (in pelvic nerves)

Bladder

Fig. 20-16 Uninhibited neurogenic bladder. (From *Nursing Management of Neurogenic Incontinence* (pp. 11-12, 14) by M. Pires and P. Lockhart-Pretti, 1992, Skokie, IL: Rehabilitation Nursing Foundation. Copyright 1992 by Rehabilitation Nursing Foundation. Reprinted with permission of the Rehabilitation Nursing Foundation, 5700 Old Orchard Road, First Floor, Skokie, IL 60077-1057.)

Table 20-4 Neurogenic bladder dysfunction and management

Dysfunction	Level in neuraxis	Possible etiology	Voluntary control	Saddle sensation	Bulbocavernous reflex	Signs and symptoms	Management
Uninhibited neurogenic	Cortical and subcortical	Newborn child, CVA, MS, cerebral arteriosclerosis, brain tumor, pernicious anemia, trauma	Initiation and/or inhibition diminished	Normal	Normal	Frequency, urgency, urge incontinence, nocturia, decreased bladder capacity	Timed voiding, drugs Male: external collection device (condom type) Female: "padding"
Reflex neurogenic	Spinal cord above conus medullaris	Trauma, tumor, vascular disease, MS, syringomyelia, pernicious anemia	Absent	Absent or Impaired	Hyperactive	Unpredictable voiding: stream starts and stops (may initially appear as areflexic during spinal shock)	Reflex triggering techniques, IC, drugs, surgery
Autonomous (areflex) neurogenic	At conus medullaris or cauda equine	Spina bifida, myelomeningocele, tumor, postoperative radical pelvic surgery, herniated intervertebral disk	Absent	Absent	Absent	Increased bladder capacity, high residual, dribbling incontinence, no bladder contractions, overflow (stress) incontinence with straining or compression	IC, strain (Valsalva maneuver), Credé's method
Motor paralytic	Anterior horn cells or S2, S3, S4 ventral roots	Poliomyelitis, herniated intervertebral disk, trauma, tumor	Absent	Normal	Absent	Voiding similar to clients with symptoms of "prostatism" strain to void, incontinence rare	IC, Valsalva maneuver (strain), Credé's method
Sensory paralytic	S2, S3, S4 dorsal roots or cells of origin or dorsal horns of spinal cord	Diabetes mellitus, tabes dorsalis	Normal initially becomes impaired with chronic overdistention	Absent	Absent	Voids only 1-3 times daily; overflow incontinence rare	Timed voiding, IC

CVA, cerebrovascular accident; MS, multiple sclerosis; IC, intermittent catheterization.
Courtesy of Rancho Los Amigos Medical Center, Downey, CA.

A Special Concern: Spinal Shock

Immediately following spinal injury, the person experiences some degree of spinal shock, a temporary condition of flaccid paralysis and loss of all reflex activity below the level of the lesion. Complete anesthesia and flaccid paralysis are present below the level of the lesion, regardless of the site of damage. The signs of spinal shock mirror the signs of autonomous neurogenic bladder—that is, reflexes are absent; perception of fullness is absent; and the bladder becomes overdistended. Findings from the CMG show a very large bladder capacity, absence of detrusor contractions, and low intravesical pressure. Spinal shock may last from a period of a few weeks to a few months. Signs of resolution vary according to the cord level of the lesion and the type of neurogenic bladder, either reflex or autonomous.

Reflex Neurogenic Bladder

The reflex neurogenic bladder also is referred to as an upper motor neuron, suprasacral, spastic, or central neurogenic bladder. This type of bladder dysfunction occurs when both the sensory and motor tracts of the spinal cord, which send messages between the bladder and the supraspinal center, are disrupted. Figure 20-17 demonstrates where damage may occur, and Table 20-4 contains lists of the possible etiologies.

The reflex arc remains intact, and voiding is involuntary because of the lack of cerebral control and may be incomplete because of uncoordinated bladder contractions. The bulbocavernosus reflex is present and hyperactive. A CMG shows uninhibited contractions with decreased bladder capacity. The detrusor muscle frequently hypertrophies, which can lead to vesicoureteral reflux, hydronephrosis, and permanent renal damage.

The person with reflex neurogenic bladder is unable to sense fullness and is unable to void volitionally; therefore micturition cannot be started or stopped in the normal manner. If the detrusor contraction and external urinary sphincter are coordinated, spontaneous voiding will occur when the micturition reflex arc is stimulated. If the two events are uncoordinated, however, pressure within the bladder wall will increase as the detrusor attempts to contract against the contracted external urinary sphincter. The resulting dysfunction is termed detrusor sphincter dyssynergia (DSD). Com-

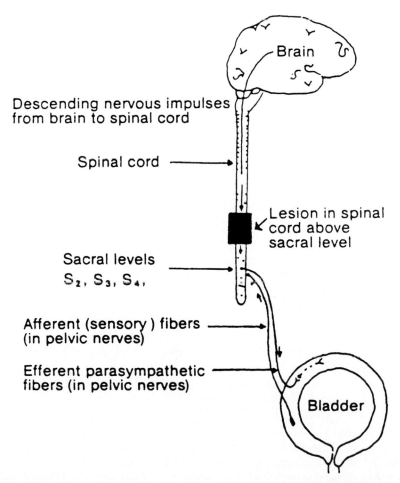

Fig. 20-17 Reflex neurogenic bladder. (From *Nursing Management of Neurogenic Incontinence* (pp. 11-12, 14) by M. Pires and P. Lockhart-Pretti, 1992, Skokie, IL: Rehabilitation Nursing Foundation. Copyright 1992 by Rehabilitation Nursing Foundation. Reprinted with permission of the Rehabilitation Nursing Foundation, 5700 Old Orchard Road, First Floor, Skokie, IL 60077-1057.)

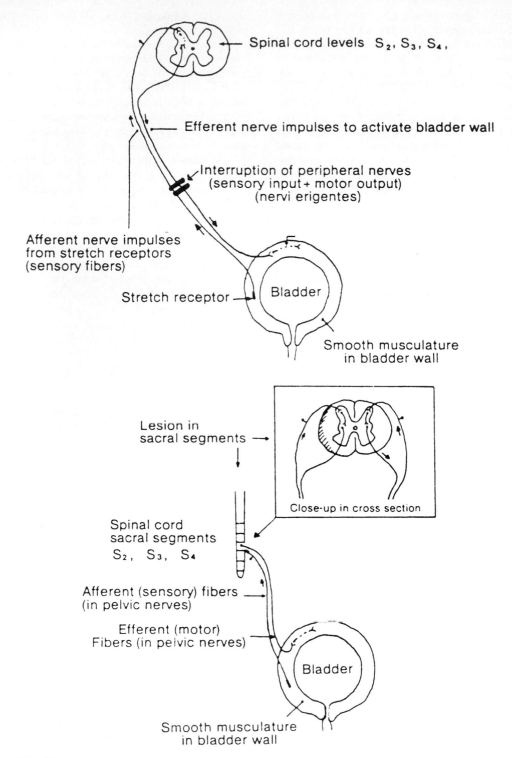

Fig. 20-18 Autonomous (nonreflex) neurogenic bladder. (From *Nursing Management of Neurogenic Incontinence* (pp. 11-12, 14) by M. Pires and P. Lockhart-Pretti, 1992, Skokie, IL: Rehabilitation Nursing Foundation. Copyright 1992 by Rehabilitation Nursing Foundation. Reprinted with permission of the Rehabilitation Nursing Foundation, 5700 Old Orchard Road, First Floor, Skokie, IL 60077-1057.)

bined cystometry and EMG of the external sphincter demonstrates that during detrusor contraction, the periurethreal muscle also contracts. This pattern causes increased resistance to outflow with high intravesical pressure, high residual urine volumes, and poor bladder emptying (Erickson, 1980).

Drugs such as dantrolene sodium (Dantrium), and baclofen (Lioresal) may be valuable in decreasing the spasticity of skeletal muscle, including that of the external sphincter. Anticholinergic medications used in combination with these antispasmotic medications may reduce the voiding pressures enough to allow low-pressure reflex voiding (<40 cm H_2O). This bladder program requires males to use an external condom and leg bag and women to use a system of padding. An alternative for those with good hand function is to increase the anticholinergic medications, allowing the person to stay dry and to empty the bladder by intermittent catheterization every 4 to 6 hours (Giroux, 1988).

Autonomous Neurogenic Bladder

The autonomous neurogenic bladder also is referred to as a lower motor neuron, flaccid, atonic, sacral, or peripheral bladder. It is difficult to determine when spinal shock subsides for a client who has an autonomous neurogenic bladder, because the characteristics are similar. Damage occurs to the cauda equina (lesions involving the reflex arc), disrupting pathways that carry sensory impulses from the bladder to the cord, motor impulses from the spinal cord to the detrusor muscle, and motor impulses from the spinal cord to the external sphincter. Figure 20-18 illustrates areas

where damage may occur, and Table 20-4 lists possible etiologies.

Voiding is involuntary and occurs when the bladder overflows. Peripheral reflexes and the bulbocavernosus reflex are absent or hypoactive. Sensation and motor control also are absent. Findings from a CMG demonstrate the absence of uninhibited contractions, a bladder capacity above normal (600 to 1000 ml), and decreased intravesical pressure; residual urine is present.

As with reflex neurogenic bladder, the client with autonomous neurogenic bladder cannot sense fullness, cannot void volitionally, and therefore cannot start or stop voiding in a normal manner. The bladder can be partially emptied with manual pressure and straining. Two patterns of external sphincter activity may occur: (1) no motor activity or (2) some uncontrollable activity. In the former pattern the client can void while maintaining low intravesical pressure. In both patterns the amount of residual urine depends on how well the individual can expel urine by applying pressure, the tone of smooth muscle and elasticity of the bladder wall, and the amount of muscle resistance offered by the internal and external urinary sphincters. If the bladder cannot be emptied completely when the person performs a Valsalva maneuver or does Credé's method (if permitted), then intermittent catheterization every 6 to 8 hours is the usual management program (Giroux, 1988).

Sensory Paralytic Bladder

The sensory paralytic bladder occurs when the afferent or sensory side of the micturition reflex arc is damaged.

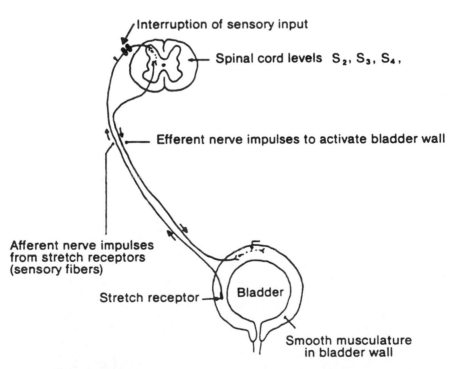

Fig. 20-19 Sensory paralytic bladder. (From *Nursing Management of Neurogenic Incontinence* (pp. 11-12, 14) by M. Pires and P. Lockhart-Pretti, 1992, Skokie, IL: Rehabilitation Nursing Foundation. Copyright 1992 by Rehabilitation Nursing Foundation. Reprinted with permission of the Rehabilitation Nursing Foundation, 5700 Old Orchard Road, First Floor, Skokie, IL 60077-1057.)

This condition is most often seen in persons with diabetes who have sensory neuropathy. Figure 20-19 shows where damage occurs, and Table 20-4 lists the possible etiologies.

The client with sensory paralytic bladder is able to void volitionally, but the sensation of bladder fullness is absent. Findings from the CMG demonstrate the absence of uninhibited contractions with an increased bladder capacity. The presence of residual urine is variable as is the presence of the bulbocavernosus reflex and perineal sensation.

The client senses no fullness, pain, or temperature but is able to initiate voiding unless the bladder has become markedly atonic because of prolonged periods of overdistention. A loss of bladder wall tone may develop because of the large volumes of urine that collect in the bladder between voids. Because persons with sensory paralytic bladder retain motor control, they can avoid incontinence by utilizing a timed voiding program (Giroux, 1988).

Motor Paralytic Bladder

The motor paralytic bladder occurs when the efferent or motor side of the micturition reflex arc is damaged. Figure 20-20 demonstrates areas where damage may occur, and Table 20-4 lists the possible etiologies.

Voluntary control of urination is variable and sensation is normal. The bulbocavernosus reflex is absent. The CMG demonstrates no uninhibited contractions with increased bladder capacity. Residual urine is markedly increased.

Since sensory nerves still are intact, the client will sense fullness. Motor loss, however, will be partial or complete. When the onset of a motor paralytic bladder is slow and left untreated, the detrusor muscle may stretch and lose tone, resulting in large residual urine volumes. The client may complain of difficulties in initiating voiding, decreased force of the urinary stream, and a need to strain to void. These signs and symptoms are from loss of motor function and a decrease in muscle tone. The person may experience overflow incontinence; but distention may be prevented by intermittent catheterization. Persons with motor paralytic bladder may learn to empty the bladder by using a Valsalva maneuver and Credé's method (if permitted) (Giroux, 1988).

NURSING ASSESSMENT

Since urinary incontinence is a symptom and not a condition in itself, the purpose of the urologic nursing assessment is to objectively confirm the incontinence, identify factors contributing to or resulting from incontinence, and to identify persons who may need further evaluation or those who may initiate treatment without further assessment (Urinary Incontinence Guideline Panel, 1992b). Components of the assessment should include history, physical assessment with additional tests, and urinalysis and other laboratory tests.

History

It is important to remember that incontinence carries a social stigma. Not only are many people embarrassed and reluctant to report incontinence, but often they define the problem of incontinence differently. Awareness and sensitivity to the emotional issues clients associate with incon-

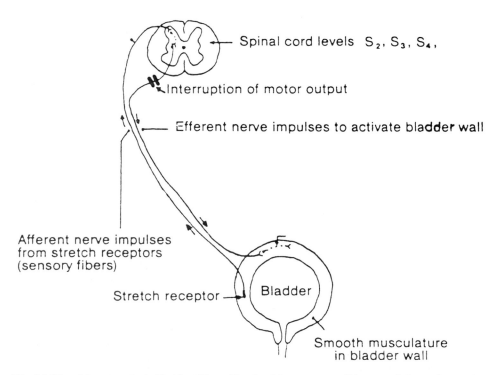

Fig. 20-20   Motor paralytic bladder. (From *Nursing Management of Neurogenic Incontinence* (pp. 11-12, 14) by M. Pires and P. Lockhart-Pretti, 1992, Skokie, IL: Rehabilitation Nursing Foundation. Copyright 1992 by Rehabilitation Nursing Foundation. Reprinted with permission of the Rehabilitation Nursing Foundation, 5700 Old Orchard Road, First Floor, Skokie, IL 60077-1057.)

tinence are crucial. Furthermore, terminology used in the nursing assessment may need to be very pragmatic. Rather than asking, "Are you incontinent?" or "Do you have bladder control difficulties?" it may be more useful to ask, "Do you have trouble making it to the bathroom in time?" or "Do you lose urine (pass water) unexpectedly?" or "Do you wear pads to catch your urine?" (Wyman, 1988). For persons with neurologic impairments, important questions include: "Do you know when you have urinated (passed water)?" and "Can you start or stop your urinary stream"?

The first part of the history focuses on the characteristics of the urinary incontinence in an effort to determine the type (i.e., stress, urge, overflow, neurogenic, functional, or mixed). The characteristics of onset, duration, frequency, and precipitating circumstances of the urinary incontinence are related to the type of incontinence. For instance, urinary leakage that occurs with sneezing, coughing, lifting, bending, laughing, or exercising is suggestive of stress incontinence; whereas leakage that occurs with hand washing or difficulty reaching the bathroom on time is suggestive of urge incontinence. The amount of urine lost with each episode suggests the type of incontinence. A sudden brief spurt of urine may denote stress incontinence; however, a prolonged steady stream is associated with urge incontinence, and continual dribbling is associated with overflow incontinence (Wyman, 1988).

Timing of the incontinence is another variable to note in the history. Usual voiding patterns range from six to eight times during the day and do not exceed two voidings during the night (Abrams, Fenely, & Torrens 1983). Is the incontinence during the daytime only, or is there enuresis?

Other factors to assess include the presence of concomitant fecal incontinence or other alterations in bowel habits, sensation of bladder fullness before or after voiding, ability to delay voiding once the urge is perceived, symptoms of hesitancy or straining to void, dysuria, or hematuria. It also is important to identify how the person manages the incontinence—for instance, with padding, frequent clothing changes, protective garments, or preventive toileting. Has there been an alteration in sexual function as a result of the incontinence or preceding it? Have there been past treatments for incontinence? If so, how successful were they? Has the person had any genitourinary surgery? Review current and past medical problems and any medications used, both prescribed and over-the-counter medications.

✦ Conditions associated with urinary incontinence

In persons with diabetes incontinence may be a result of polyuria or due to a sensory paralytic bladder. Neurologic disorders with neuropathologic lesions in the cortical or subcortical areas, such as cerebrovascular accidents, Parkinson's disease, or traumatic brain injury may lead to uninhibited neurogenic bladder dysfunction, resulting in urge incontinence. Neurologic disorders with neuropathologic lesions in the spinal cord such as multiple sclerosis, spinal cord injury, or tumors cause reflex neurogenic bladder dysfunction. Autonomous neurogenic bladder may be caused by pathology in the lower part of the spinal canal such as disk disease or neurologic lesions of the peripheral nerves (cauda equina). Persons using diuretics may experience incontinence due to a combination of increased urine output and inability to get to the toilet on time.

NURSING HISTORY FOR URINARY INCONTINENCE

Characteristics of incontinence
  Onset and duration
  Frequency
  Timing (day, night, or both)
  Precipitating circumstances (cough, sneeze, laugh, exercise, positional changes, hand washing, other)
  Associated urgency
  Amount of leakage
  Type of loss (spurt or stream, or continuous dribbling)
  Use of pads/protective briefs (number of pads or clothing changes per day)

Toileting patterns
  Diurnal frequency
  Nocturnal frequency

Associated genitourinary symptoms
  Awareness of bladder fullness
  Ability to delay voiding
  Sensation of incomplete bladder emptying
  Dribbling after urination
  Obstructive symptoms (hesitancy, slow or interrupted stream, straining)
  Symptoms of urinary tract infection (dysuria, hematuria)

Genitourinary history
  Childbirth
  Surgery (pelvic or lower urinary tract)
  Recurrent urinary tract infections
  Previous incontinence treatment and results (drugs, pelvic floor exercises, surgery, dilatations)

Relevant medical history
  Acute illness
  Depression
  Diabetes mellitus
  Neurologic disease (e.g., cerebrovascular accident, Parkinson's disease, dementia)
  Cardiovascular disease (e.g., hypertension, congestive heart disease)
  Renal disease
  Bowel disorders (constipation, impaction, fecal incontinence)
  Psychological disorders (depression, mental illness)
  Cancer

Medications (including nonprescription drugs)

Client's/caregiver's perceptions of incontinence
  Perception of cause and severity
  Interference with daily activities
  Expectations for cure

Environmental factors
  Accessible bathrooms
  Distance to bathrooms
  Use of toileting aids

From "Nursing Assessment of the Incontinent Geriatric Outpatient Population" by J.F. Wyman, 1988, *Nursing Clinics of North America, 23,* p. 178-179. Copyright 1988 by W.B. Saunders. Reprinted by permission.

Perceptions of both client and caregiver, or significant others, about the incontinence are important assessments in the history. How does incontinence affect each of their daily lives? What do they expect from the incontinence treatment/management regimen? Are there environmental factors that affect the incontinence such as accessability of the commode or bathroom, lighting, availability of someone to assist with toileting or managing clothing (Wyman, 1988). The box on p. 433 discusses nursing history for urinary incontinence.

Physical Examination

The physical examination includes functional physical and cognitive assessments; examination of the abdomen, the genital/pelvic and rectal areas; and neurologic and general examinations. The functional assessment evaluates a person's mobility and manual dexterity to determine the ability to reach the toilet and to disrobe in time to be continent. A functional assessment of the person's cognitive sta-

tus provides information about the ability to perceive the need to void, to understand how reach and use the toilet or toilet substitute, and to participate in the treatment regimen. The Folstein Mini–Mental State Examination (see Chapter 31) is one tool used in standardizing this portion of the physical examination (Folstein, Folstein, & McHugh, 1975).

The abdominal examination includes inspection of the skin for scars, which may indicate previous surgeries the client has neglected to report. The abdomen is palpated to identify a distended bladder or superpubic masses and the presence of any tenderness.

Male genitals are examined noting the condition of the skin and any swelling, lesions, nodules, or discharge. For women external genitalia are inspected noting the condition of the skin and signs of atrophic vaginitis or monilial infection. A simple pelvic examination performed by inserting one or two lubricated gloved fingers into the vagina can detect the presence of masses, pelvic prolapse, tenderness, or discharge. During the vaginal examination, ask the woman to squeeze around the examiner's fingers to assess her ability to contract the muscles of the pelvic floor and paravaginal muscle tone.

The rectal examination is conducted to test for perineal sensation (Fig. 20-21), sphincter tone with both resting and with active contraction, rectal masses, or fecal impaction. In men the size, consistency, and contour of the prostate is assessed. A bulbocavernosus reflex is attempted during rectal examination for both men and women to determine the status of the sacral reflex arc. This reflex is elicited by squeezing the glans penis or glans clitoris while the examiner's gloved finger is inserted just inside the anus. The examiner notes whether there is anal contraction around the finger and how brisk the contractual response is to the stimulus (Fig. 20-22).

A further neurologic and general examination may detect conditions such as edema, which may contribute to noc-

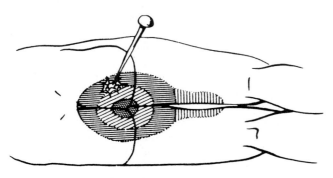

Fig. 20-21 Pinprick test for perineal sensation. (Reprinted with permission of Rancho Los Amigos Medical Center, Downey, CA.)

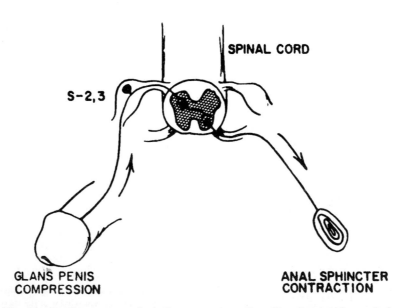

Fig. 20-22 Test for the presence of a bulbocavernosus reflex. (Reprinted with permission of Rancho Los Amigos Medical Center, Downey, CA.)

turia, and neurologic conditions that may contribute to incontinence (Wyman, 1988) (see the following Box).

Urinalysis

Urinalysis is a basic test required to detect conditions that may contribute to urinary incontinence. For instance, hematuria may be a symptom of infection, cancer, or urinary stones; glycosuria and proteinuria indicate further medical workup for diabetes; and pyuria with bacturia suggest infection and a specimen for culture. There is no consensus about the relationship of asymptomatic bacturia and urinary tract infection in nursing home populations and in those

---

✦

PHYSICAL EXAMINATION FOR URINARY INCONTINENCE

Cognitive and affective status
  Mental status
  Mood
  Motivation

Mobility status
  Manual dexterity (ability to disrobe for toileting)
  Gait and balance (walking speed, use of assistive devices)

Neurologic examination
  Focal signs
  Signs of Parkinson's disease

Abdominal examination
  Scars
  Distended bladder
  Suprapubic tenderness
  Mass

Genital examination
  Skin condition
  Signs of infection
  Bulbocavernous reflex
  Women—atrophic vaginitis, pelvic relaxation, or other abnormality

Rectal examination
  Sphincteric tone
  Fecal impaction
  Masses
  Men—prostatic size

Stress test (with full bladder)
  Supine and standing

Other
  Signs of congestive heart failure

From "Nursing Assessment of the Incontinent Geriatric Outpatient Population" by J.F. Wyman, 1988, *Nursing Clinics of North America, 23,* p. 181. Copyright 1988 by W.B. Saunders. Reprinted by permission.

---

with neurogenic bladder dysfunction. However, no correlation has been found associating asymptomatic bacturia with urinary incontinence in noninstitutionalized persons (Boscia, Kabasa, Levinson, Abrutyn, Kaplan, & Kaye, 1986). Until clear data are available about the relationship of asymptomatic bacturia and persons in nursing homes, urinary infection is treated first, even before further diagnostic and treatment are initiated or completed (Ouslander, 1989).

Additional Tests

Two simple tests provide data once the history, physical examination, and urinalysis are completed: estimation of postvoiding residual (PVR) volume and provocative stress testing. Estimation of PVR volume is recommended for all persons with urinary incontinence. Estimation of PVR volume begins with abdominal palpation and percussion and/or a bimanual examination (Urinary Incontinence Guideline Panel, 1992b). Catheterization or pelvic ultrasonography is used when a more precise measurement of PVR volume is needed (Ireton, et al., 1990). However, no clear research is documented in the literature about what are allowable maximum or minimum PVR volumes. The general consensus of the AHCPR Urinary Guideline Panel is that a PVR volume less than 50 ml is considered adequate bladder emptying and over 200 ml is considered inadequate (Urinary Incontinence Guideline Panel, 1992b).

The other simple test, provocative stress testing or direct visualization of incontinence, is performed by having the person relax and cough vigorously while the examiner observes the urethra for loss of urine. If leakage occurs instantaneously, then stress urinary incontinence is suspected. If leakage is delayed or persists after the cough, then urge incontinence or detrusor overactivity is suspected. This test is performed when the client has a full bladder. The person may either stand or recline in the lithotomy position (Urinary Incontinence Guideline Panel, 1992b). As a rule, if the test initially is performed while a client is in the lithotomy position and no leakage occurs, it is repeated with the person standing (Kadar, 1988).

Supplementary Tests

Supplementary tests that may be useful in the evaluation of the person with urinary incontinence include use of a voiding record (Fig. 20-23), evaluation of environmental and social factors, observation of voiding, blood tests, and urine cytologic studies (Urinary Incontinence Guideline Panel, 1992b). A voiding record, or diary, is a tool to determine the frequency, timing, amount of voiding, and other factors associated with urinary incontinence. The person or the caregiver is instructed to document each occurrence in the voiding diary for several days before the incontinence evaluation. These records may provide clues to deciphering the underlying cause of a client's urinary incontinence, as well as setting a baseline to evaluate the efficacy of interventions (Wyman, Choi, Harkins, Wilson, & Fantl, 1988).

Assessing and evaluating environmental and social factors, as mentioned in the history section, are important processes for persons with functional impairments. Environmental factors include the ability to access the toilet

Name: _____   Date: _____

INSTRUCTIONS

Column 1: Place a check next to the time you urinated.

Column 2: Place a check next to the time an incontinent episode, large or small occurred.

Column 3: Place a check next to the time WET PADS were changed.

Column 4: Note the activity that may be associated with the wetting, like sneezing, coughing, lifting something heavy, "couldn't make it to the bathroom", "did not know I had to go".

Time Interval	Column 1 Urinated in Toilet	Column 2 Had an Incontinent Episode	Column 3 Changed Wet Pad	Column 4 Activity Associated With Incontinent Episode
6-8 AM				
8-10 AM				
10-NOON				
12-2 PM				
2-4 PM				
4-6 PM				
6-8 PM				
8-10 PM				
10-MIDNIGHT				
OVERNIGHT				

COMMENTS: _____

_____

Fig. 20-23 Bladder record. (Reprinted with permission and courtesy of Golden Horizons, Inc. Copyright © 1990.)

or toilet substitute. Social factors include living arrangements, social contacts, and caregiver availability (Williams & Gaylord, 1990).

Direct observation of a client's voiding may detect signs of hesitancy or strain, or a slow or interrupted urinary stream. Presence of these symptoms may indicate urinary obstruction or problems with bladder emptying. Ask the person to start and stop the urinary stream to observe volitional control and strength of the pelvic muscles.

Blood tests for blood urea nitrogen (BUN) and creatinine levels are performed for persons with suspected outlet obstruction, noncompliant bladders, or retention. These tests are often part of the routine follow-up in persons with neurogenic bladder dysfunction. In persons with hematuria or recent onset of irritative voiding symptoms in the absence of urinary tract infection, urine cytologic study is completed to screen for malignancy. Urine cytology is also a part of routine follow-up in a person whose bladder dysfunction is managed with an indwelling catheter.

Further Evaluation Using Specialized Diagnostic Tests

The purposes of further specialized diagnostic tests are to identify the cause of urinary incontinence by reproducing leakage during testing; to make a differential diagnosis between causes with similar symptoms, but which require different interventions; to detect functional, neurologic, or anatomic lesions affecting the lower urinary tract; to obtain specific information necessary to choose the appropriate intervention; and to identify risk factors that may affect the outcome of specific treatments (Urinary Incontinence Guideline Panel, 1992b).

These specialized diagnostic tests usually are completed or ordered by qualified specialists including advance practice nurses with knowledge, experience, and interest in the management of urinary incontinence in a specific client population. Specialized diagnostic tests include the following: urodynamic tests, endoscopic tests, and imaging tests of both upper urinary tract and lower urinary tract with and without voiding.

Urodynamic tests are designed to evaluate the anatomic and functional status of the bladder. Uroflowmetry is a visual or electronic measure of the rate of urine flow. When an electronic unit is used, it generates an electric flow curve that displays voiding patterns. Uroflowmetry is used when diagnosing bladder emptying problems but is not useful to distinguish between bladder outlet obstruction and detrusor weakness (Urinary Incontinence Guideline Panel, 1992b) or in diagnosing the types of incontinence specific to women (Diokno, Normelle, Brown, & Herzog, 1990).

Cystometry is a test of detrusor function. Cystometry can be used to assess bladder sensation, capacity, and compliance and to determine the presence and magnitude of both voluntary and involuntary contractions. A filling CMG measures abdominal and rectal pressure simultaneously to differentiate involuntary detrusor contraction from an increase in intraabdominal pressure that occurs when a client strains to void (Pires & Lockart-Pretti, 1992). A voiding CMG or pressure flow study can measure detrusor contractility and detect outlet obstruction when a person is able to void. Another use of the filling CMG is to determine the leak point pressure. That is, the intervesical pressure is measured at the moment fluid leakage begins during urinary straining or involuntary detrusor contraction. This information is useful to determine whether the person has either low or high voiding pressures. Voiding under high pressure may affect the upper urinary tract, especially with reflex neurogenic bladder dysfunction.

Simple cystometry is a test that may become a bladder training procedure as well (see the Box on p. 438). It is performed by using a urethral catheter to fill the bladder by gravity until either an involuntary contraction occurs or until bladder capacity is reached. This test can be conducted at the bedside to answer questions about how the bladder fills. Does the bladder fill appropriately—for example, does the bladder have good compliance, does the pressure in the bladder allow for adequate filling? Results from simple cystometry also can provide answers to questions about how efficiently the bladder stores urine, whether there is sphincter incompetence or detrusor instability, whether the person perceives the urge to void accurately, and whether the person inhibits the urge to urinate. How adequately the bladder is emptied can be assessed by removing the urinary catheter at the "must" urge, then allowing the person to void, then measuring the PVR volume by catheterization.

Urethral pressure profilometry measures resting and dynamic pressures in the urethra. Passive measurements may be used to help identify intrinsic sphincter deficiency. Dynamic measurements may be used to measure the effect of exertion on urethral closure mechanism (Urinary Incontinence Guideline Panel, 1992b). Videourodynamics combines various urodynamic tests with simultaneous fluoroscopy. The ability to observe actions as they occur is helpful in sorting out complex incontinence problems.

EMG is performed on the striated urethral sphincter using needle, wire, or surface electrodes to determine the integrity of and function of its innervation. When CMG and EMG are used together, the results are helpful in diagnosing DSD, which often is seen in reflex neurogenic bladder dysfunction (Blaivas, 1990).

The most useful endoscopic test in evaluating urinary incontinence is cystourethroscopy. This procedure may be helpful in identifying bladder lesions and urethral diverticula, fistulas, strictures, or intrinsic sphincter deficiency (Urinary Incontinence Guideline Panel, 1992b).

Imaging tests sometimes used with persons who have urinary incontinence include upper urinary tract imaging by intravenous pyelogram or, more commonly, ultrasonography of the kidneys. Although these procedures are not routine evaluations of urinary incontinence, they are an important part of routine follow-up in clients with neurogenic bladder dysfunction or those with outlet obstruction who have high bladder pressures. Upper urinary tract imaging can help identify dilation of the ureters and kidney pelvis.

Lower urinary tract imaging with and without voiding is helpful for examining the anatomy of the bladder and the urethra. Nonvoiding cystourethrography can identify mobility or fixation of the bladder neck, funneling of the bladder neck and proximal urethra, and degree of cystocele. The voiding component of the cystourethrogram can identify urethral diverticulum, obstruction, and vesicouretral reflux (Urinary Incontinence Guideline Panel, 1992b). Table 20-5 provides a list of diagnostic test options.

PROCEDURE FOR PERFORMING A BEDSIDE (SIMPLE) CYSTOMETROGRAM

PURPOSE

1. Assess bladder capacity
2. Assess for an indication of detrusor instability
3. Assess for stress incontinence
4. Teach inhibition of the urge sensation

EQUIPMENT

1. IV tubing or cystometrogram set
2. Bottle or bag of sterile water—500-1000 ml
3. Straight urethral catheterization tray

PROCEDURE

1. Verify standing physician's orders.
2. Explain the physician's orders and procedure to client.
3. Before Foley catheterization, set up the IV/cystometry set by placing tubing into bag of sterile water—using sterile technique. Flush tubing with sterile water, removing all air bubbles. Make sure that tip of tubing remains sterile by placing cap back onto tip of tubing.
4. Place the bag of sterile water on an IV pole so that the bag is approximately 2 feet above the client's symphysis pubis.
5. Place the client on the bedpan to measure any leakage during filling.
6. After the client has been catheterized and the flow of urine stops, connect the tip of the IV tubing into the open end of the Foley catheter using sterile techniques.
7. Completely open the valve on the IV tubing to allow the sterile water to flow into the bladder. Note on the record if there is any leakage of fluid around the catheter. If there is a large amount of leakage, discontinue the procedure.
8. Do not instill more than 500 ml of fluid.
9. Tell the client to tell the nurse when he senses the first urge-to-void sensation.
10. When the client senses the first urge to void, shut the valve on the tubing to stop the flow of sterile water into the bladder. Record this amount as the initial (first) urge sensation.
11. Teach the client to take slow, deep breaths to make the urge sensation go away.
12. After the client has been successful in inhibiting this initial urge, open the valve on the tubing to continue the flow of sterile water into the bladder. (Note if there is leakage of fluid around the catheter at 200 ml. If leakage occurs at volumes less than 200 ml, unstable bladder is likely. If 200-300 ml are instilled without leakage, unstable bladder is unlikely.)
13. Tell the client to tell the nurse when he gets the second ("must" or "I can't hold it any more") urge to void.
14. After the client gets the second ("must") urge to void, close the valve on the tubing to stop the flow of sterile water into the bladder. Record this amount as the "must" urge.
15. Again, teach the client to take slow, deep breaths to make the urge go away.
16. After the client has been successful in lessening or inhibiting the urge and it goes away, remove the catheter.
17. With the bladder full, perform a stress maneuver by asking the client to cough forcefully 3 times in the standing position with a pad or tissue near the urethral meatus to collect the urine loss. The nurse also can observe for urine leakage in the supine and standing position. If there is leakage with a cough, estimate the amount (i.e., small, moderate, or large). Stress maneuvers with a full bladder are more sensitive for detecting stress incontinence.
18. Allow the client to empty the bladder into the bedpan or bedside commode, or in the bathroom.

Treatment of Urinary Incontinence

There are three categories of treatment for urinary incontinence: behavioral, pharmacologic, and surgical. The AHCPR Urinary Guidelines Panel suggests that in general the least invasive and least dangerous procedure appropriate for the person should be the first choice. For most types of urinary incontinence, behavioral techniques meet this criteria. However, individual preferences must be respected (Urinary Incontinence Guideline Panel, 1992b). For instance, a person may choose a more invasive treatment for the sake of expediency. When the risks, benefits, and outcomes are understood clearly and the client provides informed consent, the person's wishes may supersede this general guideline.

Treatment categories, notably behavioral techniques, generally fall within the scope of the independent realm of rehabilitation nursing. Pharmacologic and surgical treatments require nurses' collaboration with physicians and reflect the interdependent and dependent realm of nursing practice. It is exciting to consider the possibility of nurses in advanced practice providing the first line of treatment for persons with

Table 20-5 Diagnostic test options according to symptoms, conditions, and associated factors*

Symptom	Condition	Associated factors	Diagnostic test options
Urge	Unstable bladder or detrusor instability	No neurologic deficit	Filling or simple CMG
	Detrusor hyperreflexia, DSD	With neurologic lesion such as stroke, supraspinal cord lesion, multiple sclerosis	Filling or simple CMG, CMG-EMG
	Detrusor hyperactivity with impaired contractility	Elderly; usually also associated with obstructive or stress symptoms	Voiding CMG, videourodynamics
	Urethral instability	With or without neurologic deficit	Filling CMG-EMG, filling CMG-UPP, videourodynamics
Stress	Hypermobility of bladder neck (female)	Pelvic muscle relaxation	Stress test (direct visualization), stress cystourethrogram, dynamic profilometry or leak point pressure, videourodynamics, cystourethroscopy
	Intrinsic sphincter deficiency	Nonneurogenic, traumatic, postoperative (after prostatectomy or antiincontinence surgery), congenital (epispadias)	Same as above
	Neurogenic sphincter deficiency	Neurogenic, sacral, or infrasacral lesion (myelomeningocele)	Same as above
Overflow	Overflow from underactive or acontractile detrusor	Male: prostate gland disease, urethral stricture, neurogenic (low spinal cord lesion, neuropathy, postradical pelvic surgery), idiopathic detrusor failure	EMG, PVR volume, uroflowmetry, voiding CMG (pressure flow), cystourethroscopy
	Overflow from outlet obstruction (female)	Female: antiincontinence surgery, severe pelvic prolapse	Same as above Stress cystourethrogram, videourodynamics

*The diagnostic tests listed here are not recommended for routine use but are options that must be exercised according to the question to be answered. For details on the various tests, see text.
CMG, cystometrogram; EMG, electromyogram; PVR, postvoiding residual; UPP, urethral pressure profilometry; DSD, detrusor sphincter dyssynergia.
From *Urinary Incontinence in Adults: Clinical Practice Guidelines* (AHCPR Pub. No. 92-0038) by the Urinary Incontinence Guideline Panel, 1992, Rockville, MD: Agency for Health Care Policy and Research, Public Health Service, U.S. Department of Health and Human Services.

urinary incontinence. These techniques are discussed in the following sections.

Behavioral Techniques

Although not always considered a behavioral technique, rehabilitation nurses will naturally include bowel management as a primary intervention for persons with urinary incontinence. It is difficult to retrain the bladder until the bowel is retrained. In fact, constipation may be a major contributing factor to urinary incontinence, and restoring regular bowel elimination often alleviates urinary urgency and lack of control (Smith, 1988). An effective method to restore regular bowel elimination is to remove any impaction, increase intake of fiber and fluids, and promote mobility or exercise. A special bowel recipe for constipation has assisted in lowering the incidence of constipation for many clients (Chapter 21).

The behavioral techniques delineated in the AHCPR Urinary Guidelines are low-risk interventions intended to decrease frequency of urinary incontinence in most individu-

als, when techniques are provided by knowledgeable healthcare professionals. These behavioral techniques include bladder training, habit training (timed voiding), prompted voiding, and pelvic floor exercises, which may be enhanced by the use of biofeedback, vaginal cone retention, or electrical stimulation in addition to educating the person or the caregiver and providing positive reinforcement for effort and progress. These techniques are best offered to persons who are motivated to avoid use of protective garments, external devices, or medications or who shun more invasive treatment methods. (Chapter 10 provides information on client education regarding readiness to learn and planning with clients and family or caregivers.) Behavioral techniques have no reported side effects and do not limit future options (Urinary Incontinence Guideline Panel, 1992b).

♦ Bladder retraining

Bladder training, sometimes termed bladder retraining (see the following Box), is defined as a voiding program that uses distraction or relaxation techniques so a client may

◆

PROCEDURE FOR BLADDER RETRAINING

PURPOSE

1. Improve the client's pattern of voiding
2. Restore normal bladder function
3. Teach the client how to redevelop control of his/her voiding

EQUIPMENT

1. Bladder records
2. Bladder retraining teaching tool

PROCEDURE

1. Send the client's bladder records to complete 1 to 2 weeks before the client's evaluation visit.
2. At the time of evaluation, analyze the client's history, symptoms, and bladder records and determine if bladder retraining will be a part of the treatment regimen.
3. Bladder retraining will be initiated if the client is mentally and physically capable of toileting as indicated by the nursing assessment and/or a mini–mental test and if she has frequency, urgency, urge, or functional incontinence. Frequent toileting would be every 3 hours or more often or a schedule that interferes with and limits a person's lifestyle.
4. Always explain the rationale for the instructions in detail.
5. Teach the client to eliminate or reduce from her diet products containing caffeine or NutraSweet.
6. Teach the client to have a daily fluid intake of 48-64 oz of caffeine-free liquids.
7. If the client has nighttime frequency, nocturia, or enuresis, teach the client to stop drinking fluids 2 hours before bedtime or to stop after 6 PM.
8. Teach the client relaxation techniques for inhibiting or diverting the urge sensation.
9. These relaxation techniques can be taught during the bedside CMG as follows:
   · When the client gets the first (initial) urge to void, teach the client to take *slow, deep* breaths through the mouth until the urge sensation lessens or goes away.
   · As the CMG continues, when the client gets the second ("must") urge to void again, instruct the client to take *slow, deep* breaths until the urge sensation disappears.
10. If a bedside CMG is not performed, teach the client to do the following when a strong urge occurs
   · Sit and relax
   · Take slow, deep breaths in and out of the mouth until the urge sensation goes away
   · Concentrate only on the deep breathing until the urge sensation goes away
11. Determine the client's average current voiding pattern from the symptoms and the bladder record.
12. Then increase this interval by 15 minutes at a time, teaching the client to use relaxation techniques if the client gets the urge to void sooner.
13. Teach the client not to empty her bladder before she gets the urge to void.
14. Teach the client first to use relaxation techniques at home—when the client is relaxed and knows that the bathroom is readily accessible—so as to avoid anxiety-producing situations.
15. Gradually increase the client's voiding interval as she meets with success.
16. Also, teach the client to use the relaxation technique for diverting the urge to void in common instances when the urge occurs—for example, the "key in the lock" syndrome. Teach the client that if she gets the urge to void when trying to unlock a door, she should stop and use the relaxation technique.
17. Inform the client that at first these techniques may not work but that she should keep attempting to attain the control that these techniques teach.
18. Teach the client never to rush to the bathroom.
19. Have the client keep bladder records to monitor voiding patterns and to record improvement. The client may not notice significant changes in voiding for 6-8 weeks.
20. Schedule follow-up visits according to the client's needs and reinforce the bladder retraining teaching.
21. Provide encouragement to the client at each visit and do not allow her to get discouraged by setbacks that can occur during a cold or an acute illness, during a menstrual period, or if she becomes anxious or fatigued.

Instructions:
1. Note the time you urinated in the column with the heading "ACTUAL TIME VOIDED."
2. Set the goal time for_____ hours later.
3. Strive for the goal and note in the GOAL column.
4. Note the actual time you void again under the ACTUAL TIME VOIDED column.
5. Reset your GOAL.

ACTUAL TIME VOIDED	GOAL

Fig. 20-24 Goal-oriented bladder record. (Reprinted with permission and courtesy of Golden Horizons, Inc. Copyright © 1986)

consciously inhibit the urge to void. The goal of bladder retraining is to enable the person to resist or inhibit the urge sensation and thus be able to postpone voiding (Smith & Newman, 1992). Three components to bladder retraining are an education program, scheduled voiding, and positive reinforcement. An education program contains information about the physiology and pathophysiology of the lower urinary tract, as well as an educational program for urge control. Bladder training also may be incorporated with a bedside CMG to teach the person how to inhibit the urge to void (Pires & Lockart-Pretti, 1992). The person begins a scheduled voiding pattern, with ideal intervals every 2 to 3 hours, with the exception of sleep time. A goal-oriented bladder record (Fig. 20-24) helps to provide immediate positive feedback to encourage progress to the next interval level. For instance, an initial goal may be to void every 2 hours; using inhibition techniques, the person may progress gradually to 3-hour voiding intervals. Nurses can obtain or create their own relaxation tapes to assist clients who are learning how to relax as a technique for inhibiting the urge to void. Bladder retraining has been used to manage urinary incontinence due to bladder instability; however, recent evidence suggests bladder retraining may be useful in management of stress incontinence (Fantl, Wyman, Harkins, & Hadley, 1990).

Habit training or timed voiding is defined as scheduled toileting on a planned basis. The goal is to keep clients dry by telling them to void at regular intervals. The AHCPR Urinary Guidelines do not make a distinction between habit training and timed voiding; however, rehabilitation nurses have been using the term timed voiding to indicate the practice of toileting a person using a bedpan/urinal, commode, or toilet at regular intervals such as every 2 or 3 hours. Success depends on the caregiver, not the person with incontinence (Pires & Lockart-Pretti, 1992). Within a rehabilitation setting, a timed voiding program is often the precursor to habit training. By observing a person's individual voiding pattern and documenting when voiding occurs in a "voiding diary" or record, the person can be taught to void at predetermined time. By habit training voiding is anticipated and a person often is able to reduce episodes of urinary incontinence. The intent is to match the voiding interval times with the person's natural voiding schedule.

Prompted voiding is defined as a scheduled voiding program that reinforces the person for remaining dry rather than for wetness. The goal is to teach the person responsibility for wetness and toileting behavior. Caregivers learn to give a positive response when the client voids in the toilet or is dry. Three steps are followed. With prompted voiding, a caregiver checks with a client at regular intervals, specifically asking the person to state whether the clothing is wet or dry. Once the person responds, the caregiver offers the prompt to use the toilet. The person who remains dry or voids using the toilet receives praise; one who becomes wet receives a neutral response. Prompted voiding requires a consistent approach by educated caregivers. When properly conducted, prompted voiding has been useful for assisting persons with cognitive impairments and those who reside in nursing home settings.

✦ Pelvic muscle exercises

Pelvic muscle exercises (Fig. 20-25 and Fig. 20-26), also called Kegel exercises, improve urethral resistance through active contraction of the pubococcygeus muscle. Contraction of the pubococcygeal muscle exerts a closing force on the urethra and over time improves muscle support to the pelvic structures and strengthens the voluntary periurethral and pelvic musculature. Components of the pelvic muscle exercises are locating and identifying the correct muscles, engaging in active exercise on a regular basis, and using the muscles to control continence (Pires & Lockart-Pretti, 1992).

The first step in pelvic muscle reeducation is for the client to gain an awareness of the pelvic muscles. This may

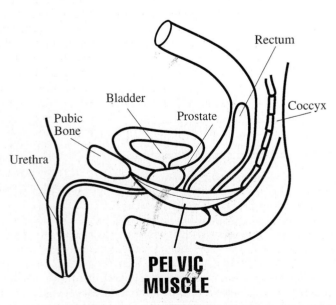

Fig. 20-25 Patient teaching: male pelvis. (Artwork Copyright © 1994 Golden Horizons, Inc.)

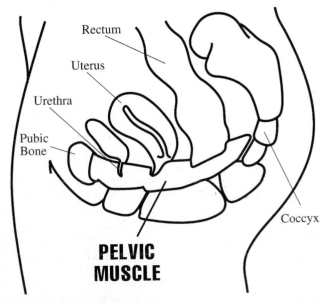

Fig. 20-26 Patient teaching: female pelvis. (Artwork Copyright © 1994 Golden Horizons, Inc.)

require some concentration but is essential to the next step, which is understanding how to manipulate this muscle group in exercises. Pelvic muscle exercises are performed by "drawing in" the perivaginal muscles and the anal sphincter, as if attempting to control urination or defecation but without contracting abdominal, buttock, or inner thigh muscles (Rose, Baigis-Smith, Smith, & Newman, 1990). Even though most people associate Kegel exercises with women, both sexes benefit from improvements in both fecal and urinary incontinence.

Kegel exercises (see the following Box) are performed by holding the muscles in contraction for a count of 10 and then relaxing for a count of 10; repeat for 10 minutes three times daily for a total of 50 to 90 exercises per day. An individual can perform these exercises while in any position; the muscle contractions are not visible to anyone else, require no equipment and thus can be performed in any environment such as work, school, or social gatherings. Pelvic muscle exercises are clearly indicated interventions for women with stress incontinence and have been shown to be effective in reducing incontinence in men following prostatic surgery (Burgio & Engel, 1990) and after multiple surgical repairs in women (Rose et al., 1990).

Many persons have difficulty identifying the correct muscle group in order to benefit from pelvic muscle exercises. Several techniques have been developed to assist persons with urinary incontinence to learn correct pelvic muscle exercises. They include vaginal cones, biofeedback, and electrical stimulation.

Vaginal cones. Vaginal cones may be a useful adjunct to pelvic muscle exercises in women. The woman is given a set of cones that are the same size and shape but increase in weight from 20 to 100 g. The goal of the program is for the woman to be able to retain the weighted cone for 15 minutes, twice a day. The woman starts with the lowest weight and progresses to the next weight when she can retain the lower level weight for 15 minutes. The woman must stand and retain the weight for the exercises to be effective

◆

PATIENT TEACHING: PELVIC MUSCLE (KEGEL) EXERCISES

HOW TO FIND THE PELVIC MUSCLE

To find the muscle, imagine you are at a party and the rich food you have just consumed causes you to have gas. The muscle that you use to hold back gas is the one you want to exercise. Some people find this muscle by voluntarily stopping the stream of urine. If you are a woman, another way to find the muscle is by pulling your rectum, vagina, and urethra up inside. Try to think about the area around the vagina.

EXERCISING THE MUSCLE

Begin by emptying your bladder, then try to relax completely. Tighten this muscle and hold it for a count of 10 or 10 seconds; then relax the muscle completely for a count of 10 or 10 seconds. You should feel a sensation of closing between your legs and lifting of the area around the vagina (in women).

WHEN TO EXERCISE

Do 10 exercises in the morning, 10 in the afternoon, and 15 at night—or else you can exercise for 10 minutes, 3 times a day. Set a timer for 10 minutes, 3 times a day. Initially you may not be able to hold this contraction for the complete count of 10; however, you will build slowly to 10-second contractions over time. The muscle may start to tire after 6 or 8 exercises. If this happens, stop and go back to exercising later.

WHERE TO PRACTICE THESE EXERCISES

These exercises can be practiced anywhere and anytime. Most people seem to prefer exercising lying on their bed or sitting in a chair. Women can try doing these exercises during intercourse. Tighten your pelvic muscles to grip your partner's penis and then relax. Your partner should be able to feel an increase in pressure.

COMMON MISTAKES

Never use your stomach, legs, or buttock muscles. To find out if you also are contracting your stomach muscles, place your hand on your abdomen while you squeeze your pelvic muscle. If you feel your abdomen move, then you also are using these muscles. In time you will learn to practice effortlessly. Eventually work these exercises in as part of your lifestyle; tighten the muscle when you walk, when you sneeze, or when you are on the way to the bathroom.

WHEN WILL I NOTICE A CHANGE?

After 4-6 weeks of constant daily exercise, you will begin to notice fewer urinary accidents, and after 3 months you will see an even bigger difference.

CAN THESE EXERCISES HURT ME?

No! These exercises cannot harm you in any way. Most clients find them relaxing and easy. If you get back pain or stomach pain after you exercise, then you probably are trying too hard and using stomach muscles. Go back and find the pelvic muscle and remember this exercise should feel easy. If you experience headaches, then you also are tensing your chest muscles and probably holding your breath.

From Golden Horizons. Copyright 1986 by Golden Horizons, Inc. Reprinted with permission of Golden Horizons, Inc.

Table 20-6 Drugs used to treat urinary incontinence*

Drug	Mechanism	Uses	Nursing implications
Anticholinergics/spasmodics (propantheline, imipramine, oxybutynin, flavoxate, dicyclomine)	Increase bladder capacity; diminish bladder contractions	Urge incontinence associated with bladder instability	Assess for mental status changes, urinary retention, vision changes, difficulty swallowing or eating, and constipation; monitor blood pressure
Alpha-adrenergic agonists (pseudoephedrine, imipramine, phenylpropanolamine)	Contract the urethral smooth muscle	Stress incontinence associated with sphincter weakness	Assess for mental status changes, weakness, dizziness, difficulty swallowing or eating; monitor blood pressure
Conjugated estrogens (oral, topical)	Increase periurethral blood flow; strengthen periurethral tissues	Stress incontinence associated with sphincter weakness	Assess for vaginal bleeding, genitourinary or abdominal pain, hemorrhagic skin eruptions, and changes in sexual function; monitor blood pressure and weight
Cholinergic agonists (bethanechol)	Promote bladder contraction	Overflow incontinence associated with atonic bladder	Assess for abdominal discomfort, difficulty swallowing, nausea, vomiting, and bowel pattern changes; monitor I&O and blood pressure
Antibiotics (general classification)	Treat bladder infections	Urinary tract infections	General nursing implications for all antibiotics
Oral penicillin	Antibacterial	Urinary tract infections	Read and follow specific information for each medication
Oral cephalosporins	Bactericidal or bacteriostatic	Urinary tract infections	Assess client's allergies/hypersensitivities to antibiotics
Oral tetracyclines	Antibacterial	Urinary tract infections	Obtain a culture and antimicrobial sensitivity test before 1st dose
Oral sulfonamides	Inhibit bacterial growth	Urinary tract infections	Determine client's weight
			Monitor laboratory values
			Assess for allergic reaction
			Assess for overgrowth of nonsensitive organisms
			ASSESS VITAL SIGNS
			Assess appetite
			Assess for dizziness
			Assess bowel pattern
			Monitor I&O
			Assess mental status for changes
			Assess client's sleep/wake patterns
			Assess oral hygiene
			Assess client's ability to ambulate/transfer safely
			Assess renal and hepatic function
			Teach client to avoid sunlight
			Store medication properly
			Check expiration date for medication

*The information in the first three columns is from Ouslander JG: Drug therapy for geriatric incontinence. Clin Geriatr Med 2(4):790, 1986. The information on antibiotics is from Gever L, Robinson J, Rome A, et al: Nurse's Guide to Drugs. Horsham, PA, Intermed Communications, Inc., 1980. I&O, input and output.
From "Nursing Management of Urinary Incontinence in Geriatric Patients" by K. McCormick, A. Scheve, and E. Leahy, 1988, *Nursing Clinics of North America, 23*, p. 238-239. Copyright 1988 by W.B. Saunders. Reprinted by permission.

(Smith & Newman, 1992). The sustained contraction required to retain the weighted cone increases the strength of the pelvic muscles. The weight of the cone is assumed to heighten the proprioceptive feedback to the desired pelvic muscle contraction (Urinary Incontinence Guideline Panel, 1992b).

Biofeedback. Biofeedback is a group of strategies and methodologies that use electronic or mechanical instruments to display information to persons about their neuromuscular activity. The aim of biofeedback in persons with urinary incontinence is to alter bladder dysfunction by teaching the person to change the physiologic responses that affect bladder control (Burgio & Engel, 1990). Methods of biofeedback include the use of surface electrodes, as well as sensors inserted either vaginally or rectally. When the proper muscle contraction is accomplished, this information is displayed so that the client can either hear or see it. Available biofeedback systems range from stationary to portable and include home training devices. Biofeedback is best utilized in conjunction with other behavioral techniques.

Success of biofeedback is dependent largely on the skill of the healthcare provider. The provider must have comprehensive knowledge about evaluation techniques, anatomic and physiologic relationship of symptoms to types of bladder dysfunction, and behavioral principles that guide the procedure. This is an area appropriate for rehabilitation nurses to expand their practice, since a knowledgeable nurse meets and exceeds these criteria (Urinary Incontinence Guideline Panel, 1992b).

Electrical stimulation. Electrical stimulation is a relatively new and as yet unproved technique. It involves stimulation of the pelvic viscera, the pelvic muscles, or nerve supply to these structures. Electrical stimulation has been used to manage bladder and urethral dysfunction in persons with neurologic and non-neurologic impairments. Stimulation of the afferent fibers changes bladder sensation and facilitates storage, whereas stimulation of the detrusor efferent fibers produces bladder contraction (Williams & Gaylord, 1990). Electrical stimulation also has been used to inhibit detrusor overactivity by modifying the sacral micturition reflex arc (Tanagho, 1990).

Pharmacologic treatment of incontinence. The pharmacologic approach to treating incontinence is summarized in Table 20-6 (McCormick, Scheve, & Leahy, 1988). Several medications have been beneficial in treating urinary incontinence. They can be categorized into two main groups: (1) medications for incontinence due to urethral sphincter insufficiency, and (2) medications for incontinence due to detrusor overactivity.

Medications used to treat urethral sphincter insufficiency are alpha-adrenergic agonist agents and estrogen supplementation therapy. Alpha-adrenergic agonist agents increase urethral resistance by stimulation of urethral smooth muscle acting on alpha-adrenergic receptors in the urethra. The recommended medication is phenylpropanolamine (PPA). Estrogen replacement in postmenopausal women may restore urethral mucosal coaptation and increase vascularity, tone, and the alpha-adrenergic response of the urethral muscle, thus increasing bladder outlet resistance and decreasing stress incontinence. Combined alpha-adrenergic agonist and estrogen supplementation therapy may be considered when

initial single medication therapy fails. Imipramine may be helpful in the treatment of mixed stress and urge incontinence (Urinary Incontinence Guideline Panel, 1992b).

Medications used to treat detrusor overactivity are anticholinergic and antispasmodic agents. The purpose of these medications is to relax the bladder and increase bladder capacity. The medications include propantheline, oxybutynin, tricyclic agents, and dicyclomine hydrochoride. Medications not as well documented but considered useful are calcium-channel blocking agents, terodiline and flavoxate (Urinary Incontinence Guideline Panel, 1992b).

Often these medications are used to decrease urinary frequency in patients with urge incontinence or uninhibited bladder. In this situation the PVR volume is checked on instituting or adjusting these medications to ensure that emptying has not been compromised. In persons with reflex bladder who void with high pressures or when bladder emptying is incomplete, anticholinergics may be used as an adjunct to intermittent catheterization with the goals being normalization of bladder pressures and continence between catheterizations.

Intermittent catheterization every 6 hours is the preferred method of management of urinary retention and overflow incontinence that results from autonomous, sensory, or motor paralytic bladder. Although sterile technique commonly is practiced when the client is hospitalized, clean technique generally is considered safe in the home or community environment.

Surgical treatment of urinary incontinence should be considered only after a comprehensive clinical evaluation including an estimation of the surgical risk, confirmation of the diagnosis and the severity, and correlation of anatomic and physiologic findings with the surgery planned and an estimation of the impact of the surgical procedure on the quality of the person's life (Table 20-7) (Urinary Incontinence Guideline Panel, 1992a).

Table 20-7   Surgical management of urinary incontinence

Type of urinary incontinence	Cause	Treatment
Stress	Hypermobility	Retropubic suspension, needle endoscopic suspension
Stress	Intrinsic sphincter deficiency	Sling (mostly female), artificial sphincter, urethral bulking
Urge	Refractory detrusor instability	Augmentation cystoplasty
Overflow	Obstruction	Relieve obstruction
	Nonobstructive	Intermittent catheterization, other

From *Urinary Incontinence in Adults: Quick Reference Guide for Clinicians*. (AHCPR Pub. No. 92-0044) by the Urinary Incontinence Guideline Panel, 1992, Rockville, MD: Agency for Health Care Policy and Research, Public Health Service, U.S. Department of Health and Human Services.

In addition to surgeries listed in Table 20-8, several surgical procedures are available in the care of neurogenic bladder dysfunction. These surgeries are indicated in persons with reflex neurogenic bladder when conservative bladder management has failed to maintain a low-pressure, nonrefluxing system. They include transurethral spincterotomy, augmentation enterocystoplasty, and continent diversion.

Transurethral spincterotomy is a surgery that historically has been useful in management of DSD in males when medications to reduce spasticity of the bladder neck and sphincter have been ineffective and bladder outlet obstruction contributes to high bladder pressures. The indications for transurethreal spincterotomy include DSD, bladder wall trabeculations, persistent high voiding pressure, hydronephrosis, repeated urinary tract infections, vesicoureteral reflux, urolithiasis, and severe autonomic dysreflexia.

The procedure consists of visualizing the posterior urethrea and making an incision at the 12 o'clock position. This procedure permanently opens the sphincter. These men now will void reflexively with low bladder pressures but will require external condom collection devices (Perkash, 1993).

In augmentation enterocystoplasty, a short section of small intestine is detubalized and sutured into place over the bladder, which has been bivalved in the sagittal plane, creating a large low-pressure urinary reservoir. If limited hand function prevents independent urethral catheterization, a continent stoma can be created by bringing an intussuscepted limb of bowel through the anterior abdominal wall and creating a continent stoma, which can be catheterized more easily. Continent diversions generally are reserved for those persons who have undergone prior cystectomy or those with severe urethral dysfunction (Bennett & Bennett, 1993).

There are many subtypes of continent diversions, but they generally consist of creating a neobladder from detubalized small intestine and creating an efferent nipple valve to form the continent stoma, as previously described, and creating an afferent nipple valve to form a nonreflexing attachment for the ureters to pass into the neobladder (Bennett & Bennett, 1993).

SUMMARY

Management of bladder elimination problems is an integral component of rehabilitation nursing practice. As described in this chapter, most incontinence can be remedied. Many of the treatments fall within the independent realm of nursing practice. The incontinence that cannot be cured can be controlled through appropriate management techniques and selection of appropriate products. Nurses are an

---

CASE STUDY

Mr. S. is a 17-year-old with T1 paraplegia secondary to a gunshot wound. Initially he presented in spinal shock, and during his acute care phase, his bladder was managed with an indwelling catheter. He was transferred to a spinal cord injury center 10 days after his injury. An intermittent catheterization program was instituted on an every-4-hour schedule. The rehabilitation nurses did the catheterization for the first few days. They instructed Mr. S. in the technique of intermittent catheterization, using a sterile no-touch catheterization system. He also was instructed in how to regulate his fluid intake. He takes 100 ml/hour for the 12 waking hours of the day and about 400 ml of fluid with each meal. He became independent in self-catheterization after 4 days. Within 10 days of his rehabilitation stay, Mr. S. started to experience lower extremity spasticity and some leaking of urine just before his scheduled catheterization. The appearance of spasticity and some reflex voiding indicated the resolution of spinal shock.

Mr. S. was scheduled for urodynamic testing and his CMG-EMG showed evidence of DSD from uncoordinated bladder and sphincter contractions. The results of his urodynamic studies showed that he was voiding with pressures which exceed 40 cm H_2O. After a discussion with his urologist, he was started on an anticolinergic, oxybutynin cloride (Ditropan) to reduce his detrusor hyperreflexia. Because of his lower extremity spasticity, he had already been placed on baclofen (Lioresal) by his physiatrist. Mr. S.'s nurse explained to him that the oxybutynin chloride will decrease his bladder contractility and lower the pressure in his bladder. He also was told that the baclofen will decrease the spasticity in his external urinary sphincter as well as his lower extremities. Mr. S. was told that he could choose to try to urinate reflexively if low bladder pressures could be maintained. He was told this would require wearing an external condom collection device and a leg bag. His other choice was to increase the dose of the oxybutynin chloride to further reduce bladder contractility. This would mean emptying his bladder every 6 hours by intermittent catheterization, which he would continue to do at home using clean technique. He would remain dry between catheterizations and not require any external devices.

Mr. S. was very concerned about his body image and did not like the idea of using external collection devices. He chose intermittent catheterization and anticolinergic medication. However, Mr. S. had difficulty maintaining a consistent fluid intake and sticking to his catheterization schedule. His intermittent catheterization volumes were over 500 ml at least once a day. After a week of high volumes, Mr. S. experienced a severe pounding headache and was diaphoretic above his level of injury. His nurse took his blood pressure and found that it was 150/90 mm Hg. His usual blood pressure is 100/76 mm Hg. She assisted him with the catheterization and found that his bladder volume was 600 ml. His symptoms resolved as soon as his bladder was empty. Because of his level of injury, Mr. S. is prone to autonomic dysreflexia. He was started on an alpha blocker, prazosin hydrocloride (Minipress), and his nurse worked with him on strategies to maintain his fluid restriction and catheterization schedule. For the remainder of his rehabilitation, Mr. S. remained dry between catheterizations and had no further episodes of dysreflexia.

Mr. S.'s nurse reinforced the need to maintain his fluid restriction and catheterization schedule at home and worked with him on problem-solving techniques such as more frequent catheterizations if more fluid has been taken in. Because of the delicate balance of his bladder with medications, Mr. S. will have repeat urodynamic testing at 3 and 6 months postdischarge. If there are no problems, he will need yearly routine urodynamic testing along with cine or voiding cystourethrography, ultrasonographic scans of the kidney, and a nuclear scan to determine renal plasma flow.

important resource to persons with incontinence in assisting with the selection and management of techniques and products. Other treatments require collaboration with physicians and are within the interdependent scope of nursing practice; however, nursing care is essential to the successful outcomes of the treatments.

REFERENCES

Abrams, P., Feneley, R., & Torrens, M. (1983). *Urodynamics.* New York: Springer-Verlag.

Bates, P., Bradley, W.E., & Glen, E. (1979). The standardization of terminology of lower urinary tract function. *Journal of Urology, 121,* 551-554.

Bell, J., & Hannon, K. (1986). Pathophysiology involved in autonomic dysreflexia. *Journal of Neuroscience Nursing, 18,* 86-88.

Bennett, C.J., & Bennett, J.K. (1993). Augmentation cystoplasty and urinary diversion in patients with spinal cord injury. *Physical Medicine and Rehabilitation Clinics of North America, 4,* 377-389.

Blaivas, J.G. (1990). Diagnostic evaluation of incontinence in patients with neurogenic disorders. *Journal of the American Geriatrics Society, 38,* 306-310.

Boscia, J.A., Kabasa, W.D., Levinson, M.E., Abrutyn, E., Kaplan, A.M., & Kaye, D. (1986). Lack of association between bactururia and symptoms in the elderly. *American Journal of Medicine, 81,* 977-982.

Burgio, K.L., Stutzman, R.E., & Engle, B.T. (1989). Behavioral training for post-prostectomy incontinence. *Journal of Urology, 141,* 303-306.

Burgio, K.L., & Engel, B.T. (1990). Biofeedback-assisted behavioral training for elderly men and women. *Journal of the American Geriatrics Society, 38,* 338-340.

Chui, L., & Bhatt, K. (1983). Autonomic dysreflexia. *Rehabilitation Nursing, 8,* 16-19.

Diokno, A.C., Brock, B.M., Brown, M.B., & Herzog, A.R. (1986). Prevalence of urinary incontinence and other urologic symptoms in the non-institutionalized elderly. *Journal of Urology, 136,* 1022-1025.

Diokno, A.C., Normelle, O.P., Brown, M.B., & Herzog, A.R. (1990). Urodynamic tests for female geriatric urinary incontinence. *Urology, 36,* 431-439.

Doughty, D.B. (1991). *Urinary and fecal incontinence nursing management.* St. Louis: Mosby–Year Book.

Dunn, K.L. (1991). Autonomic dysreflexia: A nursing challenge in the care of the patient with a spinal cord injury. *Journal of Cardiovascular Nursing, 5,* 57-64.

Erickson, R.P. (1980). Autonomic dysreflexia: pathophysiology and medical management. *Archives of Physical Medicine and Rehabilitation, 61,* 431-440.

Fantl, J.A., Wyman, J.F., Harkins, S.W., & Hadley, E.C. (1990). Bladder training in the management of lower urinary tract dysfunction in women: A review. *Journal of the American Geriatrics Society, 38,* 329-332.

Folstein, M.F., Folstein, S.E., & McHugh, P.R. (1975). Mini-mental state, a practical method for grading cognitive state of patients for the clinician. *Journal of Psychiatric Research, 12,* 189-198.

Giroux, J. (1988). Alterations in bladder elimination. In P.H. Mitchell, L.C. Hodges, M. Muwaswe, & S.C.A. Wallack (Eds.), *AANN's neuroscience nursing phenomena and practice.* Norwalk, CT: Appleton & Lange.

Guyton, A. (1991). *Textbook of medical physiology* (8th ed.). Philadelphia: W.B. Saunders.

Hickey, J.V. (1986). *The clinical practice of neurological and neurosurgical nursing.* Philadelphia: J.B. Lippincott.

Hu, T.W. (1990). Impact of urinary incontinence on health-care costs. *Journal of the American Geriatrics Society, 38,* 292-295.

Ireton, R.C., Krieger, J.N., Cardenas, D.D., Williams-Burden, B., Kelly, E., Soucé, T., & Chapman, W.H. (1990). Bladder volume determination using a dedicated portable ultrasound scanner. *Journal of Urology, 143,* 909-911.

Jeter, K.F., Faller, N., & Norton, C. (1990). *Nursing for continence.* Philadelphia: W.B. Saunders.

Kadar, N. (1988). The value of bladder filling in clinical detection of urine loss and selection of patients for urodynamic testing. *British Journal of Obstetrics and Gynaecology, 95,* 698-704.

Kewalramani, L.S. (1980). Autonomic dysreflexia in traumatic myelopathy. *American Journal of Physical Medicine, 59,* 1-21.

Lapides, J., & Diokno, A.C. (1976). Urine transport, storage, and micturition. In J. Lapides (Ed.), *Fundamentals of urology.* Philadelphia: W.B. Saunders.

McCormick, K., Scheve, A., & Leahy, E. (1988). Nursing management of urinary incontinence in geriatric inpatients. *Nursing Clinics of North America, 23,* 231-264.

National Center for Health Statistics. (1979). The national nursing home survey: 1977 summary for the United States. In J.F. Van Nostrand, et al. (Eds.), *Vital health statistics* (DHEW Pub. No. 79-1794) Series 13(43). Washington, DC: Health Resources Administration, U.S. Government Printing Office.

National Institutes of Health. (1988). *Urinary incontinence in adults: National Institutes of Health Consensus Development Conference Statement,* 7(5). Bethesda, MD: U.S. Department of Health and Human Services.

Ouslander, J.G. (1981). Urinary incontinence in the elderly. *Western Journal of Medicine, 135,* 482-491.

Ouslander, J.G. (1989). A symptomatic bactururia and incontinence [Letter]. *Journal of the American Geriatrics Society, 37,* 197-198.

Perkash, I. (1993). Long-term urologic management of the patient with spinal cord injury. *Urologic Clinics of North America, 20,* 423-434.

Pires, M., & Lockart-Pretti, P.A. (1992). Nursing management of neurogenic incontinence: An independent study module. *Rehabilitation Nursing Foundation, 19.*

Resnick, N.M., & Yalla, S.V. (1985). Management of urinary incontinence in the elderly. *New England Journal of Medicine, 313,* 800-805.

Rose, M.A., Baigis-Smith, J., Smith, D.A., & Newman, D.K. (1990). Behavioral management of urinary incontinence in homebound older adults. *Home Healthcare Nurse, 8,* 10-13.

Siroky, M.B., & Krane, R.J. (1982). Neurologic aspects of detrusor-sphincter dyssynergia, with reference to the guarding reflex. *Journal of Urology 127,* 953-957.

Smith, D.A., & Newman, D.K. (Eds.). (1992). Behavioral management of urinary incontinence: an independent study module. *Rehabilitation Nursing Foundation, 10.*

Smith, D.A.J. (1988). Continence restoration in the homebound patient. *Nursing Clinics of North America, 213,* 207-218.

Staskin, D.R. (1986). Age-related physiologic and pathologic changes affecting lower urinary tract function. *Clinics in Geriatric Medicine, 2,* 701-710.

Tanagho, E.A. (1990). Electrical stimulation. *Journal of the American Geriatrics Society, 38,* 352-355.

Thomas, T.M., Plymat, K.R., Blannin, J., & Meade, T.W. (1980). Prevalence of urinary incontinence. *British Medical Journal, 281,* 1243-1245.

Urinary Incontinence Guideline Panel. (1992a). In *Urinary incontinence in adults: Quick reference guide for clinicians* (AHCPR Pub. No. 92-0041). Rockville, MD: Agency for Health Care Policy and Research, Public Health Service, U.S. Department of Health and Human Services.

Urinary Incontinence Guideline Panel. (1992b). *Urinary incontinence in adults: Clinical practice guidelines* (AHCPR Pub. No. 92-0038). Rockville, MD: Agency for Health Care Policy and Research, Public Health Service, U.S. Department of Health and Human Services.

Wheeler, J.S., Niecestro, R.M., & Goggin, C.J. (1988). Urinary incontinence: Diagnosing the Problem. *Journal of Enterostomal Therapy, 15,* 240-246.

Williams, M.E., & Gaylord, S.A. (1990). Role of functional assessment in the evaluation of urinary incontinence: National Institutes of Health Consensus Development Conference on Urinary Incontinence in Adults. Bethesda, MD, October 3-5, 1988. *Journal of the American Geriatrics Society, 38,* 296-299.

Wyman, J.F. (1988). Nursing assessment of the incontinent geriatric outpatient population. *Nursing Clinics of North America, 23,* 169-187.

Wyman, J.F., Choi, S.C., Harkins, S.W., Wilson, M.S., & Fantl, J.A. (1988). The urinary diary in evaluation of incontinent women: A test-retest analysis. *Obstetrics and Gynecology, 71,* 812-817.

✦

Appendix 20-A   American Association of Spinal Cord Injury Nurses: Spinal cord injury guideline for practice Autonomic Dysreflexia

Autonomic dysreflexia is an acute, life-threatening crisis that constitutes a medical emergency for an individual. This condition is seen most often in persons with complete spinal cord lesions at the cervical and high thoracic levels, but has been exhibited in persons with injuries as low as thoracic level T-6. These levels of spinal cord injury are associated with developing neurogenic bladder and bowel. Rehabilitation nurses educate other health professionals, families, and clients to observe signs of an autonomic dysreflexia crisis. Those persons known to have a tendency for incurring this response are taught to report to others when they recognize the conditions or sensations that precipitated a previous autonomic dysreflexia experience (McCourt, 1993; Hoeman, 1990).

Although many clients never experience autonomic dysreflexia, most susceptible persons will manifest symptoms within the first 6 months following injury. A first occurrence of autonomic dysreflexia can take place at any time from 3 weeks to 6 years after the injury. An irritating or noxious stimulus occurring below the level of injury produces an uninhibited sympathetic reflex nervous system response of total body vasoconstriction. The body's normal compensatory mechanisms cannot balance or overcome this response with vasodilatation because the message cannot be transmitted past the level of the spinal lesion. The vagus nerve, however, continues to transmit messages to slow the heart rate. Without intervention, the result is a cycle that leads to seizures, hypertension severe enough to cause cerebrovascular accident, and/or bradycardia continuing into cardiac arrest, then death (Fig. 20-27).

Appendix continues on p. 450.

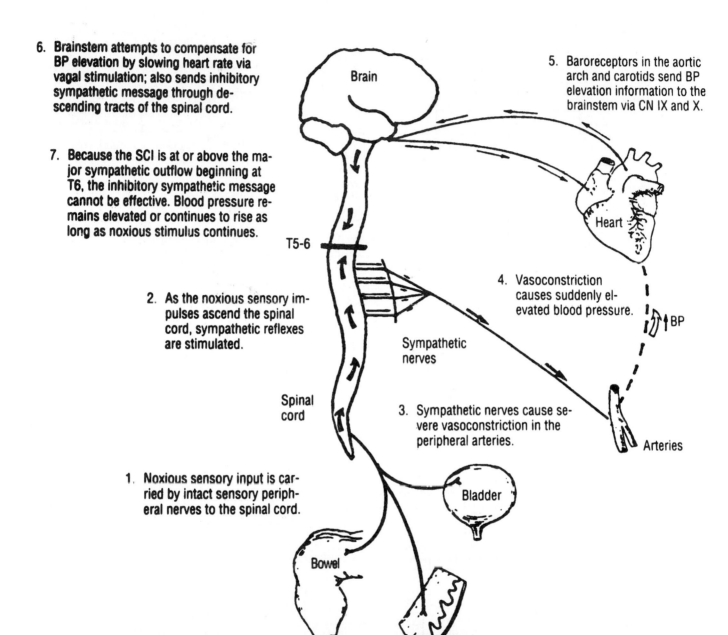

6. Brainstem attempts to compensate for BP elevation by slowing heart rate via vagal stimulation; also sends inhibitory sympathetic message through descending tracts of the spinal cord.

7. Because the SCI is at or above the major sympathetic outflow beginning at T6, the inhibitory sympathetic message cannot be effective. Blood pressure remains elevated or continues to rise as long as noxious stimulus continues.

5. Baroreceptors in the aortic arch and carotids send BP elevation information to the brainstem via CN IX and X.

Brain

T5-6

2. As the noxious sensory impulses ascend the spinal cord, sympathetic reflexes are stimulated.

Heart

4. Vasoconstriction causes suddenly elevated blood pressure.

↑BP

Sympathetic nerves

Spinal cord

3. Sympathetic nerves cause severe vasoconstriction in the peripheral arteries.

Arteries

1. Noxious sensory input is carried by intact sensory peripheral nerves to the spinal cord.

Bladder

Bowel

Skin

Fig. 20-27 Pathophysiology of autonmic dysreflexia. (From "Autonomic Dysreflexia: A Nursing Challenge in the Care of a Patient with a Spinal Cord Injury" by K.L. Dunn, 1991, *The Journal of Cardiovascular Nursing, 5,* p. 58. Copyright 1991 by Aspen Publishers, Inc. Reprinted by permission.)

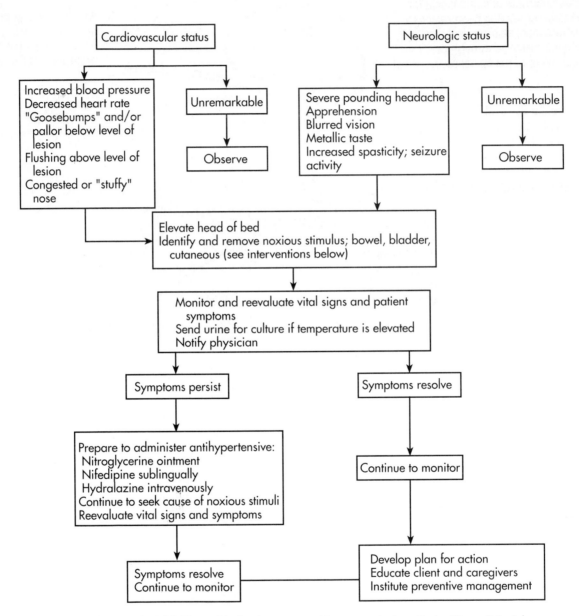

Fig. 20-28 Critical thinking guide for the person with autonomic dysreflexia. (From *Principles and Practice of Adult Health Nursing* by P.T. Beare and J.L. Meyer, 1990, St. Louis: Mosby–Year Book. Copyright 1990 by Mosby–Year Book. Reprinted by permission.)

INDICATORS OF AUTONOMIC DYSREFLEXIA

Severely elevated blood pressure, documented as high as 300/160 (Chui & Bhatt, 1983), associated with a pounding headache that quickly becomes severe

Feelings of anxiety or nervousness, accompanied by sensations of nausea

Sweating above the level of injury, but "goose bumps" and/or pallor below the level of the injury

Flushing with blotched skin on the face and neck

Blurred vision

"Stuffy nose" congestion and a metallic taste in the mouth, cardiac bradycardia and/or respiratory irregularities, increased spasticity, possibly seizure activity.

Figure 20-28 illustrates a critical thinking pathway for early recognition and intervention. Nursing interventions and actions may prevent or resolve autonomic dysreflexia.

The immediate intervention and treatment is to place the person in the full sitting position, provided that the spine is stable to do so. This provides optimal advantage from the natural tendency toward orthostatic hypotension. If possible, place the legs in a dependent position and remove all vascular support devices or clothing. The next step is to identify the noxious stimulus that is triggering the response. Apply an inch of nitropaste to the person's skin to lower or to attempt to control the elevating blood pressure while searching for the stimulus.

Notify the emergency room or designated responder immediately. The person will need to be taken to a local emergency room. A knowledgeable person is assigned to accompany the client as an informed advocate. A vasodilator drug may be used if the stimulus cannot be found and relieved or if the blood pressure continues to be elevated for a time. Drug therapy is less desirable than symptomatic relief because medications may initiate other cycles. For example, with use of a vasodilator, the person is observed carefully for signs of rebound hypotension.

SPECIFIC INTERVENTIONS

Interventions for autonomic dysreflexia can be categorized as actions to remove noxious stimulations from three main sources: urinary, bowel, and sensory.

1. Immediately act to remove sources of noxious *urinary* stimulation. The bladder is checked first, since bladder distension or spasm are major causes.
   ✦ Empty the bladder, draining urine slowly, then insert a new catheter, using a local anesthetic to numb the stimulus

✦ Check patency of the catheter or kinks in tubing
✦ If the catheter is plugged, irrigate with no more than 30 ml normal saline. (With UTI use Pontacaine irrigation.)
✦ If the catheter does not irrigate, remove it immediately and recatheterize the person
✦ If there is no catheter in place, palpate the bladder for distension; if the bladder is distended, immediately insert a catheter. Removing a blocked suprapubic catheter will relieve distension as the urine drains out of the suprapubic orifice.
✦ Evaluate other problems, such as calculi, cystitis, or detrusor sphincter dyssynergia.
✦ Cease procedures, such as cystoscopy or shock lithotripsy

2. Remove sources of noxious *bowel* stimulation
   ✦ Check rectum for fecal impaction. To remove a fecal mass, begin by inserting a topical anesthetic ointment to reduce rectal stimulation or irritating hemorrhoid pain. Gentle digital stimulation usually is sufficient to remove a mass, but the person must be monitored during the process. One person monitors the person's blood pressure while the second person removes the fecal impaction.
   ✦ Reduce bowel distension
   ✦ Cease any procedures in progress, such as enemas

3. Although *sensory* stimulation are implicated in autonomic dysreflexia less commonly than bladder or bowel stimuli, they are the source of some problems.
   ✦ Remove elastic stockings or binders; loosen tight or constricting clothing
   ✦ Relieve pressure on bony prominences or genitalia
   ✦ Check for ingrown toenails, fractures, or pain due to injury
   ✦ Assess for thrombophlebitis or infection
   ✦ Evaluate temperature or environmental changes, such as sunburn or cold weather
   ✦ Evaluate menses for women . . . potential during contractions of labor and delivery
   ✦ Observe a person who has prolonged muscle spasm
   ✦ Observe a person who has congested lungs

In all instances, the client, family, caregivers, and rehabilitation team are to be prepared with a plan of action. Early and on-going the nurse institutes a program of preventive management, readiness for action, and education for family members, the client, and all varieties of caregivers.

21

Bowel Regulation and Elimination

Aloma R. Gender, MSN, RN, CRRN

INTRODUCTION

Bowel elimination is the process by which the body excretes waste products. Undigested dietary matter passes through the gastrointestinal (GI) tract after nutrients and water have been extracted for use by the body. Control of bowel function is a basic human need that is the subject of varying levels of concern throughout a person's life. Children learn early that successful control of bowel function gains them praise and signifies that they are maturing. They learn that control of elimination is valued and that lack of control can be humiliating.

Patterns of elimination change throughout the life-span. Infants from birth to 1 year of age are unable to control their bowels due to lack of neuromuscular maturity. Toddlers are physically ready to control bowel elimination at 18 to 24 months, although cognitive and psychosocial readiness may be achieved later. Daytime control usually occurs at 30 months.

Constipation can be common among preschool and school-aged children due to fevers, dietary changes, or emotional and environmental changes. A characteristic individual elimination pattern usually is established at this time.

As children mature into adolescence and then young and middle-aged adulthood, other developmental tasks become the primary focus and normal bowel function may be given little thought. Bowel patterns may vary, however, due to dietary intake, lifestyle, amount of exercise, and an individual's emotional state. Irregular meals, changing schedules, and increased stress all play a role in elimination.

Bowel function reemerges as an area of concern in the older population, where the main focus tends to be on regularity rather than control. Constipation again often becomes a problem in the over-65 age group due to medications taken for chronic diseases, difficulty chewing due to loss of teeth or poor denture fit, diminished thirst sensation, decreased mobility, and loss of colon and abdominal tone (Berger & Williams, 1992).

When bowel function is compromised, however, by any of various disorders, there may be changed patterns of elimination, and it may become an area of intense concern at any age.

Through time the subject of bowel elimination has been embellished by myths and old wives' tales, advertising, and even medical fads. "Autointoxication from the colon," in the early 1900s, was regarded as a causative factor in a number of diseases of unknown etiology (Brocklehurst, 1980).

It was believed that a process of self-poisoning was occurring by feces coming into contact with the bloodstream in the colon (Ross, 1990). It was taken so seriously that some surgeons performed colectomies for this reason. Many elderly people were brought up during this era and were led to believe that taking laxatives regularly was necessary for good health (Brocklehurst, 1980). Today we continue to hear advertisements promoting products that prevent constipation and imply that a daily bowel movement is necessary. Despite this heightened awareness of bowel function and habits, most people seldom think or talk about the subject unless they are faced with a problem in controlling or regulating function.

The ability to control bowel function may be compromised by a variety of neuromuscular disorders in which the rehabilitation nurse becomes involved. These include multiple sclerosis, stroke, traumatic brain injury, tumor, myelomeningocele, transverse myelitis, diabetes, intervertebral disk disease, polio, and traumatic injury to the spinal cord. Altered bowel function may occur whenever the central nervous system (CNS) has been impaired. When disease or disability results in loss of control of the bowels, incontinence may become as devastating a problem as the disability itself.

Disorders of regularity also cause considerable difficulties for some individuals. Constipation is a problem faced by most persons at one time or another and is especially persistent among the elderly. The two most common causes are improper diet and inactivity. Constipation not only causes discomfort but if neglected it may lead to impaction and possibly bowel obstruction. Diarrhea is the opposite problem from constipation. Causes of diarrhea range from psychosomatic (irritable bowel) origins to infectious (bacterial, viral, or protozoal) agents with hosts of other causes in between such as enzyme deficiency, GI surgery, and drug side effects. Rehabilitation patients with oncology, pulmonary, or pain management problems may be subject to diarrhea or constipation.

Management of impaired bowel function is primarily under the guidance of the rehabilitation nurse.

Control of incontinence and prevention of constipation and diarrhea are possible through an effective bowel program. The development of an effective program requires knowledge of normal and altered bowel physiology as well as an in-depth assessment of bowel function.

NORMAL BOWEL FUNCTION

The primary function of the alimentary tract is to provide the body with a continual supply of water, electrolytes, and nutrients via digestion and absorption. Figure 21-1 illustrates the entire alimentary canal, showing major anatomic differences among its parts. The portion of the tract from the stomach to the anus is the GI tract, but the term is often loosely applied to the entire alimentary tract. Food is stored in the stomach and fecal matter in the descending colon. Digestion of food occurs in the stomach, duodenum, jejunum, and ileum. Absorption occurs in the small intestine and the proximal half of the colon.

A myriad of autoregulatory processes keeps food moving along the GI tract at an appropriate pace—slow enough for digestion and absorption to occur and fast enough to provide the body with nutrients. Food that is neither digested nor absorbed while passing through the GI tract is excreted as feces (defecation). Defecation is a function requiring a complex integration of voluntary and involuntary mechanisms, and any interruption of these mechanisms may result in impaired bowel function.

In this section normal function of the GI tract is discussed in relation to those functions that affect bowel elimination: secretion, innervation, functional movements, and defecation (Guyton, 1991).

Secretion

Secretory glands located throughout the entire GI tract serve two primary functions. First, digestive enzymes are produced from the mouth to the end of the ileum. These secretions are composed of enzymes and electrolytes formed in response to food in the alimentary tract. The quantity secreted in each segment is the amount necessary for proper digestion. Second, mucous glands from the mouth to the anus produce mucus to protect and lubricate the walls of the tract and to ease the passage of food and partially digested products.

Innervation

The GI tract is composed of several layers of smooth muscle fibers. Figure 21-2 illustrates a typical section of the intestinal wall. The smooth muscle fibers of the GI tract are arranged in bundles. In the longitudinal muscle layer, the bundles extend longitudinally down the intestinal tract. The bundles of the circular muscle layer extend around the gut. The muscle fibers within each bundle are electrically connected to each other. Electrical signals can therefore travel readily from one fiber to the next.

The smooth muscle undergoes almost continual but slow electrical activity that produces tonic and rhythmic contractions. The tonic contractions maintain a steady pressure on

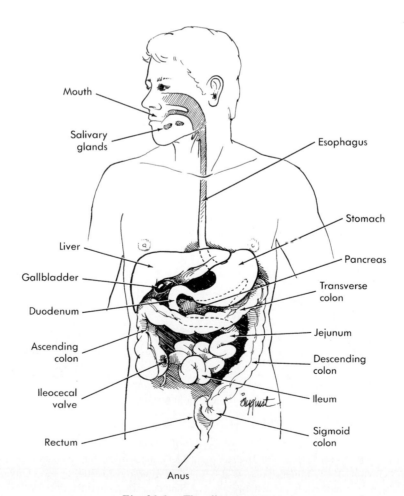

Fig. 21-1 The alimentary tract.

Mouth
Salivary glands
Liver
Gallbladder
Duodenum
Ascending colon
Ileocecal valve
Rectum
Esophagus
Stomach
Pancreas
Transverse colon
Jejunum
Descending colon
Ileum
Sigmoid colon
Anus

the contents of the GI tract. The internal anal sphincter, composed of circular smooth muscle, also is in a state of tonic contraction and thus acts as a safeguard against loss of small amounts of fecal material into the anal canal. The rhythmic contractions are responsible for phasic functions, such as mixing of food and peristalsis (Guyton, 1991).

✦ Intrinsic neural control

In addition to the tonic and rhythmic contractions of the smooth muscle itself, the GI tract has its own nervous system called the enteric nervous system. This system lies entirely in the wall of the gut and begins in the esophagus and extends all the way to the anus. It is composed of two plexuses: (1) the outer or myenteric (motor) plexus located between the longitudinal and circular muscle layers; and (2) the inner layer, which is called Meissner's plexus, or submucosal (sensory) plexus in the submucosa. The myenteric plexus is far more extensive than Meissner's plexus and controls mainly the GI movements. Meissner's plexus controls local intestinal secretion and absorption.

The enteric nervous system allows the gut to continue to function in isolation from its extrinsic nerve supply. However, signals from the brain via the autonomic nervous sys-

tem can alter the degree of activity of the intrinsic nervous system (Guyton, 1991).

✦ Extrinsic neural control

The autonomic nervous system extensively innervates the entire GI tract. Sympathetic and parasympathetic activity may alter the overall activity of the gut or specific parts.

The parasympathetic supply is divided into cranial and sacral divisions. The cranial supply is transmitted almost entirely by the vagus nerve and provides extensive innervation to the esophagus, stomach, pancreas, first half of the large bowel, and to a lesser extent the small bowel. The sacral fibers originate in S2, S3, and S4 segments of the spinal cord and pass through the nervi erigentes to the distal half of the large bowel (Fig. 21-3). The sigmoid, rectal, and anal regions of the large intestine are abundantly supplied with parasympathetic fibers that function to facilitate the defecation reflexes.

The postganglionic neurons of the parasympathetic system are located in the myenteric and submucosal plexuses. Stimulation of the parasympathetic nerves cause increased activity of the entire nervous system.

The sympathetic fibers originate in the spinal cord be-

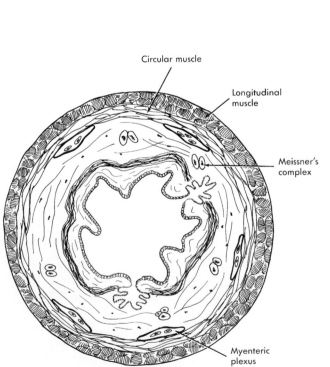

Fig. 21-2   Cross section of the gut. (From *Textbook of Medical Physiology* [p. 689] by A.C. Guyton, 1991, Philadelphia: W.B. Saunders Co. Copyright 1991 by W.B. Saunders. Reprinted by permission.)

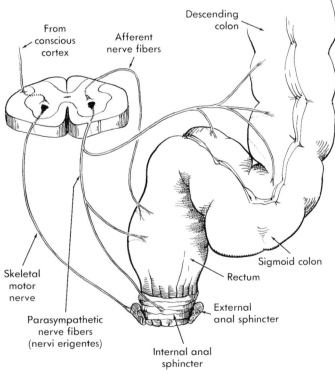

Fig. 21-3   Afferent and efferent pathways of the parasympathetic mechanism for defecation reflex. (From *Textbook of Medical Physiology* [p. 707] by A.C. Guyton, 1991, Philadelphia: W.B. Saunders Co. Copyright 1991 by W.B. Saunders. Reprinted by permission.)

tween spinal cord segments T5 and L2 and innervate essentially all of the GI tract instead of the oral and anal areas like the parasympathetic system. After leaving the cord, the preganglionic fibers enter the sympathetic chains and pass through the chains to the outlying ganglia—that is, celiac ganglia and mesenteric ganglia. The postganglionic neuronal cell bodies are located here, and the postganglionic fibers spread from them along with blood vessels to all parts of the gut.

Stimulation of the sympathetic nervous system generally results in decreased activity of the GI tract, causing effects opposite to parasympathetic stimulation. Strong stimulation of the sympathetic system can totally halt movement of food through the GI tract.

Functional Movements of the GI Tract

The two basic types of movement in the GI tract are mixing and propulsive. Mixing keeps the intestinal contents blended thoroughly at all times during transit. It is caused by contractions of small segments of the gut wall. The basic propulsive movement is referred to as peristalsis. Peristalsis keeps the food moving along the GI tract at an appropriate rate for digestion and absorption. The usual stimulus for peristalsis is distention of a large amount of food collecting at any point in the gut. This distention stimulates the intestinal wall 2 to 3 cm above this point, and a contractile ring appears and initiates a peristaltic movement. To a great extent, however, some mixing and propulsion occur simultaneously.

✦ The oral cavity

The ingestion of food begins in the oral cavity with mastication. Anterior incisors provide strong cutting action on food; the posterior molars provide a grinding action. Proper chewing of food is important for digestion because digestive enzymes act only on the surfaces of the food particles. The rate of digestion is highly dependent on the total surface area exposed to intestinal secretions. Also, grinding into a fine consistency prevents excoriation of the GI tract and increases the ease with which food is emptied from the stomach into the small intestine (Guyton, 1991).

✦ The stomach

The stomach has three motor functions. (1) mixing of food with gastric secretions until it forms chyme, which is

a semifluid mixture; (2) storage of large quantities of food until it can be accommodated by the lower portion of the GI tract; and (3) slow emptying of food into the small intestine at a rate suitable for proper digestion and absorption by the small intestine (Guyton, 1991).

✦ The small intestine

The mixing contractions of the small intestine occur when chyme, is present. The chyme elicits localized, concentric ringlike contractions that are spaced at intervals along the intestine. These areas of segmentation give the intestine the appearance of a chain of sausage (Fig. 21-4). As one set of contractions subsides, another occurs at a different point along the intestine, thus promoting chopping and progressive mixing of the intestinal contents with the secretions of the small intestine. These contractions depend on the myenteric plexus working.

Propulsive or peristaltic activity is a series of waves. These waves are caused by distention and excitation of the stretch receptors in the gut wall, which in turn elicit a local myenteric reflex. The longitudinal muscles contract over a distance followed by a contraction of the circular muscle. The contractile process of peristalsis spreads toward the anus.

Passage of chyme from the pylorus to the ileocecal valve, between the small and large intestine, normally requires 3 to 5 hours. After meals this peristaltic activity is greatly increased, partly because of distention from entry of chyme into the duodenum and partly because distention of the stomach causes a gastrocolic reflex. This reflex occurs when food enters the stomach and stimulates the myenteric plexus to increase peristalsis and secretions in the small intestine. The small intestine (Fig. 21-5) also can increase peristalsis significantly when irritation or overdistention occurs. This mechanism is known as peristaltic rush. The waves travel the entire length of the small intestine in a very short time and can sweep the contents of the small bowel into the colon in a few minutes, thus relieving the small intestine of its irritation or distention.

The ileocecal valve has the principal function of preventing backflow of fecal contents from the colon into the small intestine. The wall of the ileum is thickened near the end immediately preceding the ileocecal valve. This thickened area, known as the ileocecal sphincter, remains mildly constricted at all times and slows the emptying of small intestine contents into the cecum except after meals when the gastrocolic reflex intensifies peristalsis. This resistance to emptying at the ileocecal valve prolongs the stay of intestinal contents and therefore facilitates digestion and absorption. Approximately 1500 ml of chyme empties from the ileum into the cecum every day (Guyton, 1991).

✦ The large intestine

The colon is a tubular structure of muscle lined with mucous membrane extending 5 feet from the ileum to the anal canal. It consists of the following divisions: cecum; ascending, transverse, and descending colon; sigmoid colon; rectum and anus (Fig. 21-1). The two main functions of the colon are to absorb water and electrolytes from the intestinal contents and to store fecal material un-

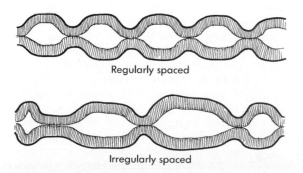

Regularly spaced

Irregularly spaced

Fig. 21-4   Segmentation movements of the small intestine.

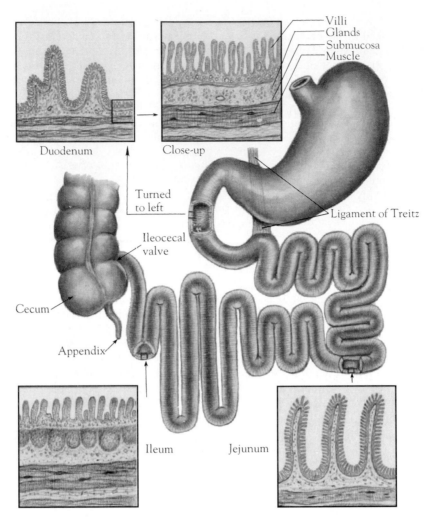

Villi
Glands
Submucosa
Muscle

Duodenum

Close-up

Turned
to left

Ligament of Treitz

Ileocecal
valve

Cecum

Appendix

Ileum

Jejunum

Fig. 21-5   Clinical anatomy of the small intestine. (From *Mosby's clinical nursing,* 3rd ed., by J.M. Thompson, 1993, St. Louis: Mosby–Year Book. Copyright 1993 by Mosby–Year Book. Reprinted by permission.)

til it can be expelled. Very little movement is required for these functions, so movement of the colon is normally sluggish.

Colonic mucus is secreted by the parasympathetic nerves to protect the lining of the colon from acids formed in the feces. The mucus contains large numbers of bicarbonate ions. The mucus also serves as a binding agent to hold the fecal material together. An extreme emotional reaction can cause overstimulation of the parasympathetic nerves and therefore overproduction of mucus, resulting in stringy mucoid stools with little or no feces. The colon absorbs large quantities of water (as much as 2.5 L) in 24 hours. It also absorbs up to 55 mEq of sodium and 23 mEq of chloride daily (Berger & Williams, 1992).

Fecal elimination is accomplished by moving the chyme along the colon and into the rectum and anal canal by muscular actions called (1) haustral shuffling, (2) haustral contractions, and (3) peristalsis. Haustral shuffling moves chyme back and forth and aids in absorption of water.

Haustral contractions (also called segmentation) propel contents along the colon. When one haustra (pouchlike section of colon) is distended completely, it contracts and empties its contents into the next (Berger & Williams, 1992).

Peristalsis in the colon occurs in mass movements. Mass movements propel the feces toward the anus. These movements occur about 15 minutes to 1 hour after a meal and can be the strongest after the first meal of the day. The mass movement occurs when a distended or irritated portion of the colon, most often the transverse or descending colon, constricts, forcing the fecal material en masse down the colon. When the fecal mass has been forced into the rectum, the desire to defecate is felt.

Mass movements are caused in part by stimulation of the gastrocolic and duodenocolic reflexes when the stomach and duodenum are distended, and these movements are transmitted via the myenteric plexus. However, irritation in the colon also can initiate mass movements. For example, a person with ulcerative colitis has mass movements almost all of the time. Temperature changes with ingestion of hot and cold liquids also stimulate mass movements.

✦ Sigmoid colon, rectum, and anal canal

Waste products, now called feces, enter the sigmoid colon and are stored there until just before defecation. The rectum normally is empty of feces until just before defecation. The rectal length in an adult is about 4 to 6 inches. The distal portion is called the anal canal and is 1.5 inches long.

The rectum contains vertical and transverse folds of tissue that help retain the feces. Each verticle fold contains a vein and artery. The veins can become permanently dilated as occurs with hemorrhoidal conditions (Berger & Williams, 1992).

The anal canal contains an internal and external sphincter. The internal sphincter is inside the anus and is a thickened portion of circular muscle surrounding the canal (Zejdlik, 1992). It is involuntarily controlled by the autonomic nervous system. The external sphincter is the visible portion of the anus and is influenced by the internal sphincter and usually is voluntarily controlled. When sensory nerves in the rectum are stimulated by the entrance of the fecal mass, the person becomes aware of the need to defecate.

Defecation

Defecation is influenced by reflexes and voluntary control. The defecation reflex begins when mass movement forces feces into the rectum. This leads to distention of the rectal wall, which in turn initiates afferent signals to the myenteric plexus. Peristaltic waves then begin in the descending colon, sigmoid, and rectum, forcing feces toward the anus. The internal and external anal sphincters relax. These sphincters are normally in a state of tonic contraction to prevent constant dribbling. The internal anal sphincter is composed of smooth muscle, and the external sphincter is composed of striated voluntary muscle controlled by the somatic nervous system. As previously indicated, both autonomic and somatic systems are involved in the act of defecation.

The defecation reflex itself, however, is extremely weak. It needs to be fortified by the sacral segments. When sensory nerve fibers in the rectum are stimulated by the presence of fecal material, signals are transmitted into the sacral portion of the spinal cord (S2-4) and then reflexly back to the descending colon, sigmoid, rectum, and anus by the parasympathetic nerve fibers. These signals intensify the peristaltic waves and convert weak movements into a powerful process.

The afferent signals entering the spinal cord initiate other concurrent activities associated with defecation such as taking a deep breath, closing the glottis, contracting the abdominal muscles (Valsalva maneuver) to force downward on the fecal contents of the colon, and raising the levator muscles around the rectum to aid in expulsion of the feces.

Along with the reflex mechanism, somatic control also is necessary for voluntary defecation to take place. The conscious mind controls the external sphincter and either inhibits its action to allow defecation or further contracts it if it is not convenient to defecate. When contraction of the sphincter is maintained, the defecation reflex dies out, not to return until additional feces enter the rectum. Voluntary inhibition can thus disrupt the normal defecation mechanism. New defecation reflexes may be initiated at a later, more convenient time by taking a deep breath, moving the diaphragm down, and contracting the abdominal muscles to increase abdominal pressure, forcing fecal contents into the rectum and eliciting new reflexes. These reflexes, however, are not as effective as those that arise naturally. Repeatedly ignoring the urge to defecate can result in an abnormally enlarged rectum and loss of rectal sensitivity. The perception of the need to defecate becomes dulled, creating the potential for constipation (Guyton, 1991).

IMPAIRED BOWEL ELIMINATION

Impaired bowel elimination is manifested by incontinence, constipation, and diarrhea. Discussion of each of these conditions follows.

Incontinence

Since the process of voluntary defecation is controlled by the autonomic nervous system (involuntary) and the somatic nervous system (voluntary), when any of these motor and sensory pathways are compromised, voluntary bowel control is altered. Impairment of cerebral control (the awareness of urge and ability to inhibit defecation), anal sphincter control, or anal sphincter sensation results in fecal incontinence.

Damage to the CNS interrupts nervous pathways between the brain, spinal cord, and GI system. A condition referred to as neurogenic bowel can result. There are five categories of neurogenic bowel dysfunction, three of which commonly are seen in rehabilitation practice. These types are uninhibited, reflex, and autonomous neurogenic bowel. Motor paralytic and sensory paralytic neurogenic bowel are seen less frequently. It is important to determine the classification of bowel dysfunction in order to plan an appropriate bowel program for each affected individual.

To differentiate the type of neurogenic bowel dysfunction, certain motor and sensory tests can be performed. To plan successful bowel programs to cope with these dysfunctions, it is necessary to understand the significance of such tests and their use.

Saddle sensation is a perianal sensation elicited in response to a pinprick or light touch. The presence of sensation indicates intact sensory function at the sacral spinal cord level. An awareness of the urge to defecate helps establish bowel control.

The bulbocavernosus reflex is a test performed primarily on clients with spinal cord injuries (SCIs) to determine the presence of an intact reflex arc at the level of the innervation of the bowel, bladder, and genitalia. A positive result indicates the client has an upper motor neuron (above T12), or reflexic injury, and will have reflex activity in these areas. If the client has a lower motor neuron (T12 or below), or areflexic injury, a positive reflex probably will not develop and there will be no reflex activity in the bladder, bowel, or genitalia. The client generally will not have a positive bulbocavernosus reflex while in spinal shock, but it may begin to appear before spinal shock fully subsides (Zejdlik, 1992).

Spinal shock (spinal areflexia) is a transient condition occurring after injury to the spinal cord. There is decreased synaptic excitability of neurons manifested by absence of somatic reflex activity and flaccid paralysis below the level of damage. Hypotension, bladder paralysis, and interference with defecation may occur because of autonomic nervous system involvement, especially in higher level lesions. Spinal shock may last from hours to weeks. A return of reflex activity in a shorter period of time may be expected in persons with incomplete lesions.

The bulbocavernosus reflex may be elicited by inserting a gloved lubricated finger up to the first digit into the client's rectum and gently squeezing the clitoris or glans penis; the nurse observes for a visible contraction of the external anal sphincter and a palpable contraction of the bulbocavernosus and ischiocavernosus muscles. A positive response will be immediate and brisk or slow and weak. Lack of any contraction is a negative result. The test should be done weekly until positive, or until it is determined that the client has a permanent areflexic injury.

The anal reflex (anal wink) is similar to the bulbocavernosus test and may be elicited by a pinprick to the skin adjacent to the external anal sphincter. A visible contraction (or wink) of the sphincter indicates a positive response.

✦ Uninhibited neurogenic bowel (Fig. 21-6)

In cortical and subcortical lesions above the C1 vertebral level, as seen in cerebrovascular accident, multiple sclerosis, and certain types of brain trauma and tumors, bowel function is classified as uninhibited. There is damage to the upper motor neurons located in the cerebral cortex, internal capsule, brainstem, or spinal cord, with sparing of lower motor neurons located in the anterior gray matter throughout the entire length of the spinal cord. Bowel sensation is intact, as is saddle sensation, and the bulbocavernosus reflex and anal reflex are intact or increased.

Sensory impulses travel through the sacral reflex arc to the brain, but the brain is unable to interpret the impulses to defecate. As a result of decreased cerebral awareness of the urge to defecate, there is decreased voluntary control of the anal sphincter. Involuntary elimination occurs when the sacral defecation reflex is activated. Because sensation is not impaired, the incontinence is accompanied by a sense of urgency.

✦ Reflex neurogenic bowel (Fig 21-7)

Reflex neurogenic bowel function (also referred to as automatic) occurs with spinal cord lesions above the T12 to L1 vertebral level. Lesions in this area involve the upper motor neurons and sensory tracts but spare the lower motor neurons. Quadriplegia, high thoracic paraplegia, and multiple sclerosis are associated with this dysfunction. Other possible etiologies include tumor, vascular disease, syringomyelia, and pernicious anemia. In most cases bowel sensation and saddle sensation are diminished or absent, and the bulbocavernosus reflex and anal reflex are increased.

Nerve pathways between the brain and spinal cord are interrupted. This interruption may be complete or incomplete. In a complete and in many incomplete lesions there is no voluntary control of defecation or of the anal sphincter. Fecal incontinence occurs suddenly without warning as part of a mass reflex. The sacral nerve segments of S2-4

are intact, and it is therefore possible to develop a stimulus-response type of bowel control using the mass reflex. The intact spinal reflex are functions when feces accumulate in the rectum and create distention, causing the bowel to empty by reflex. The parasympathetic innervation via the sacral segments of the spinal cord maintains anal sphincter tone so that fecal incontinence between mass reflex emptyings is not a problem.

✦ Autonomous neurogenic bowel (Fig. 21-8)

Autonomous (flaccid or nonreflex) bowel function occurs with spinal cord lesions at or below the T12 to L1 vertebral level. Lesions in this area affect the lower motor neurons and usually are associated with paraplegia, spina bifida, tumor, and intervertebral disk disease. Sensation is diminished to absent, and the bulbocavernosus reflex and anal reflex are absent.

Nerve pathways between the brain and spinal cord are interrupted, but the extent of neural compromise depends on whether the injury is complete or incomplete. As in reflex bowel function, there is neither cerebral control of defecation nor voluntary control of the anal sphincter. Unlike reflex bowel function, however, the lesion directly involves the S2-4 segments, and the activity of the spinal reflex arc is destroyed or unable to be accessed. Therefore, no reflex emptying of the bowel occurs. Additionally both the internal and external anal sphincters lack tone. Since there is little or no resistance to stool in the rectum, fecal incontinence with oozing of stool is frequent.

✦ Motor paralytic bowel

A motor paralytic bowel occurs when there is damage to the anterior horn cells or S2, S3, and S4 ventral roots, such as with poliomyelitis, intervertebral disk disease, trauma, or tumor (Fig. 21-9). Saddle sensation is intact, but the bulbocavernosus reflex and anal reflex are absent. Incontinence is rare except in widespread disease (Cannon, 1981).

✦ Sensory paralytic bowel

Damage to the dorsal roots of S2, S3, and S4 or dorsal horns of the spinal cord results in a sensory paralytic bowel (Fig. 21-10). Diabetes mellitus and tabes dorsalis can cause this type of bowel. Saddle sensation is diminished or absent. The bulbocavernosus reflex and anal reflex may be normal, decreased, or absent. Incontinence is rare except in advanced stages (Cannon, 1981).

✦ Other factors contributing to incontinence

Diseases of peripheral nerves supplying the external anal sphincter may result in fecal incontinence. Bowel problems also may be the result of disease of the anal sphincter or weakness of the diaphragm, the abdominal muscles, or muscles of the pelvic floor.

Bowel incontinence can also occur as a result of the surgical need for an ostomy. Cancer, trauma, or other diseases that will not allow passage of feces through the intestine and anus can necessitate the need for a stoma to be constructed surgically in the abdominal wall. Two types of bowel diversion ostomies are done: ileostomy (opening into the ileum) and colostomy (opening into the ascending, transverse, or descending sigmoid colon) (Fig. 21-11).

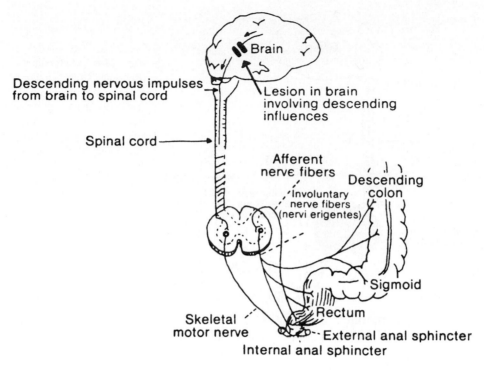

Fig. 21-6   Uninhibited neurogenic bowel. (Reprinted from Nursing Management of Neurogenic Incontinence [pp. 11-12, 14] by M. Pires and P. Lockhart, 1992, Skokie, IL: Rehabilitation Nursing Foundation. Copyright 1992 by Rehabilitation Nursing Foundation, 5700 Old Orchard, First Floor, Skokie, IL, 60077-1057.)

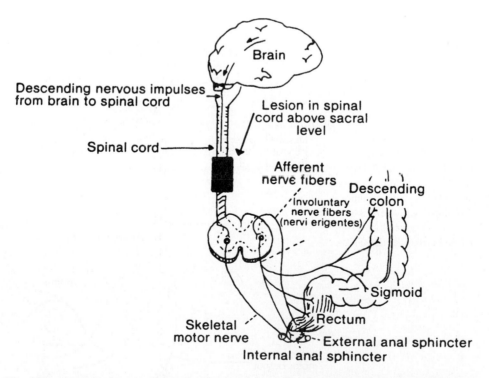

Fig. 21-7   Reflex neurogenic bowel. (Reprinted from Nursing Management of Neurogenic Incontinence [pp. 11-12, 14] by M. Pires and P. Lockhart, 1992, Skokie, IL: Rehabilitation Nursing Foundation. Copyright 1992 by Rehabilitation Nursing Foundation, 5700 Old Orchard, First Floor, Skokie, IL, 60077-1057.)

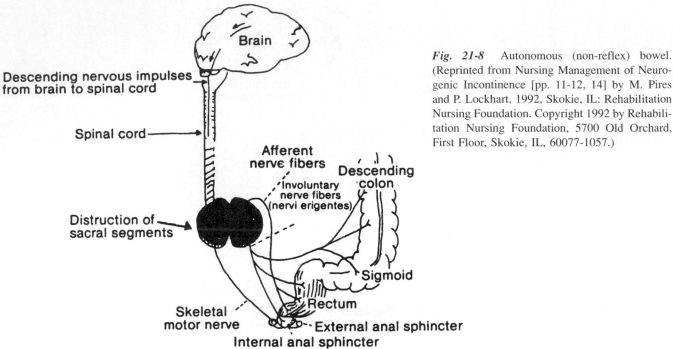

Fig. 21-8 Autonomous (non-reflex) bowel. (Reprinted from Nursing Management of Neurogenic Incontinence [pp. 11-12, 14] by M. Pires and P. Lockhart, 1992, Skokie, IL: Rehabilitation Nursing Foundation. Copyright 1992 by Rehabilitation Nursing Foundation, 5700 Old Orchard, First Floor, Skokie, IL, 60077-1057.)

Fig. 21-9 Motor paralytic bowel. (Reprinted from *Nursing Management of Neurogenic Incontinence* [pp. 11-12, 14] by M. Pires and P. Lockhart, 1992, Skokie, IL: Rehabilitation Nursing Foundation. Copyright 1992 by Rehabilitation Nursing Foundation. Reprinted with permission of the Rehabilitation Nursing Foundation, 5700 Old Orchard Road, First Floor, Skokie, IL 60077-1057.)

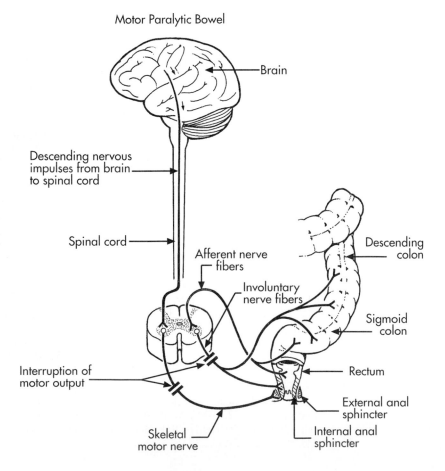

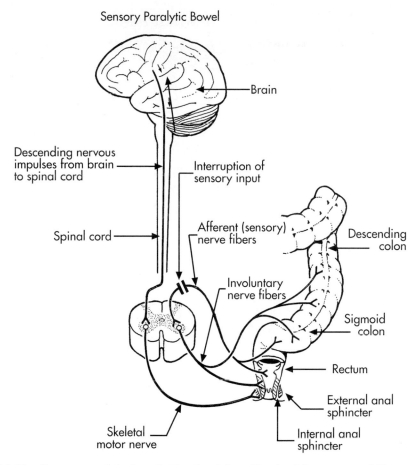

Sensory Paralytic Bowel

Brain

Descending nervous impulses from brain to spinal cord

Interruption of sensory input

Spinal cord

Afferent (sensory) nerve fibers

Descending colon

Involuntary nerve fibers

Sigmoid colon

Rectum

External anal sphincter

Skeletal motor nerve

Internal anal sphincter

Fig. 21-10 Sensory paralytic bowel. (Reprinted from *Nursing Management of Neurogenic Incontinence* [pp. 11-12, 14] by M. Pires and P. Lockhart, 1992, Skokie, IL: Rehabilitation Nursing Foundation. Copyright 1992 by the Rehabilitation Nursing Foundation. Reprinted with permission of the Rehabilitation Nursing Foundation, 5700 Old Orchard Road, First Floor, Skokie, IL 60077-1057.)

The site of the stoma determines the consistency of the stool. Ileostomies result in frequent liquid stools since almost no water has been absorbed. Ascending colostomies also have liquid stools, but transverse colostomies have more solid formed feces, as does the descending and sigmoid colostomy (Berger & Williams, 1992).

Constipation

Constipation is a condition experienced by most persons at some time during life. The term constipation has different subjective meanings to different persons. Some define it as frequency of bowel movements less than it used to be or less than the person thinks it should be; others define it as movements that are difficult and require undue straining. Often both factors are present together. Connell, Hilton, Irvine, Lennard-Jones, and Misiewicz (1965) studied frequency of bowel movements and found that 98% of the population moved their bowels between three times a day and three times a week. Based on this study most experts define constipation as a frequency of defecation of twice a week or less (White & Williams, 1992).

Transit time through the colon can be measured clinically by the radiopaque colonic transit time study. This procedure is carried out by giving the client radiopaque markers in small capsules that are swallowed and then followed with either direct radiographic examination of the abdomen or radiographs of the feces on successive days. A person with normal bowel motility passes 80% of the swallowed markers within 5 days, whereas constipated individuals experience delayed transit time of the markers through the colon. Characteristics or symptoms of constipation are shown in the box on p. 463, left.

◆ Etiology

A variety of factors contribute to constipation. The most frequent cause of constipation in the adult population is irregular bowel habits developed through a lifetime of inhibition of the normal defecation reflexes. Failure to allow defecation to take place when the defecation reflexes are excited or overuse of laxatives to take the place of normal bowel function results in progressively weaker reflexes over a period of time. Consequently the colon becomes atonic.

Immobility also seems to be a crucial factor predisposing to constipation, especially in the older population. It

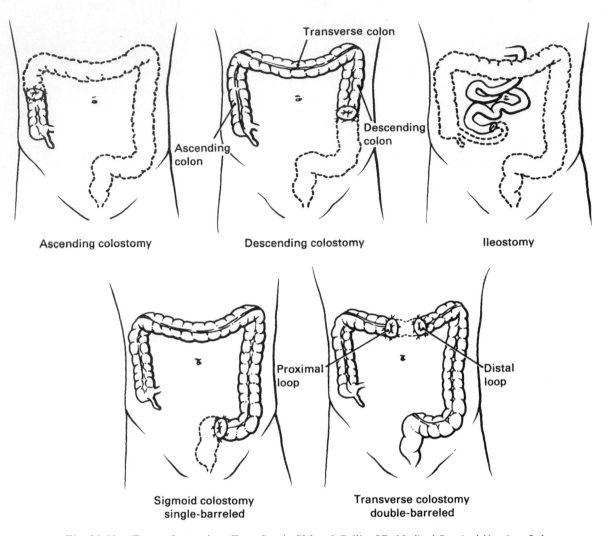

Fig. 21-11 Types of ostomies. (From Lewis SM and Collier IC: *Medical Surgical Nursing,* 3rd ed., by S.M. Lewis and I.C. Collier, 1992, St. Louis: Mosby–Year Book. Copyright 1992 by W.B. Saunders. Reprinted by permission.)

should be noted that the ingestion of food alone does not produce mass movement of the colon in the resting client—physical movement also is important.

The gastrocolic reflex combines with morning physical activity to cause mass propulsive movements, forcing the feces into the rectum. Distention of the rectum then produces the urge to defecate. If the urge is ignored or deliberately inhibited, it passes, and feces may move back from the rectum into the sigmoid colon.

Therefore the immobile person may have two reasons for becoming constipated. First, physical activity to stimulate the mass propulsive movement is lacking, and second, dependence on a nurse to allow the person to respond to the urge to defecate is necessary. If not given the opportunity to respond to that urge at the appropriate time, the urge may pass, and later it may not be possible for the person to defecate.

Constipation also has been linked to dietary habits, specifically a low-residue diet. Many people in the Western world eat highly refined and easy to prepare foods that are low in fiber (Brunton, 1990; Resnick, 1985). Several studies have concluded that the addition of fiber to the diet provides faster passage of digested substances, reduces long transit time, and increases the water content of the stool (Devroede, 1978; Smith, 1990). Mechanisms of this process remain unknown, but shorter transit time in the colon decreases the chance of becoming constipated.

The special recipe suggested by Behm (1985) (see the box on p. 463) assisted clients by lowering the incidence of constipation and reducing the use of laxatives in a study of clients' bowel function while in a nursing home setting (Behm, 1985).

Constipation may be the first symptom of many diseases, such as hypothyroidism, hypercalcemia, and depression. Disorders such as Parkinson's disease, diabetes, or cancer can contribute to constipation (Resnick, 1985). Shortness of breath and weakened abdominal muscles, such as occurs with pulmonary disease, also may affect the expulsion of

---

CHARACTERISTICS OR SYMPTOMS OF CONSTIPATION

- ✦ No stool
- ✦ Decreased frequency of bowel movements (e.g., fewer than 3 times a week)
- ✦ Hard, formed stools
- ✦ Severe flatus
- ✦ Reported feeling of rectal fullness
- ✦ Decreased bowel sounds
- ✦ Distended abdomen
- ✦ Palpable mass in left lower quadrant
- ✦ Headache (in the absence of other causes)
- ✦ Straining and pain on defecation, probably related to hemorrhoids
- ✦ Anorexia
- ✦ Nausea and/or vomiting
- ✦ Diarrhea caused by fecal impaction
- ✦ Generalized fatigue

From "Anticipation and Early Detection Can Reduce Bowel Elimination Complications," by M.O. Hogstel and M. Nelson, 1992, *Geriatric Nursing, 13,* 30. Copyright 1992 by Mosby–Year Book. Reprinted by permission.

BOWEL RECIPE FOR CONSTIPATION

Mix the following ingredients:
1 cup of applesauce
1 cup of unprocessed bran
(which may be purchased at grocery stores or health food stores)
½ cup of 100% prune juice
This mixture will be of a pasty consistency.
Refrigerate mixture in a covered container between uses.
Take 2 tablespoons at bedtime with a glass of fluid.
If constipation is severe, increase this to 2 tablespoons upon rising and at bedtime.

From "A Special Recipe to Banish Constipation" by R. Behm, 1985, *Geriatric Nursing, 6,* pp. 216-217. Reprinted by permission.

---

bowel movements (Ellickson, 1988). Pregnancy can contribute to constipation because of increased progesterone levels, which cause smooth muscle relaxation and slow peristalsis (Berger & Williams, 1992). For children constipation can occur due to emotional upsets, excessive parental concern with toilet training, or a toilet seat that is too high to permit adequate squatting (Benson, 1975).

Some medications also may contribute to constipation. Among these are the following:

1. Analgesics
2. Anticholinergics
3. Anticonvulsants
4. Antidepressants
5. Antiparkinsonism agents
6. Diuretics
7. Opiates
8. Psychotherapeutic agents
9. Iron
10. Muscle relaxants (Brunton, 1990; White & Williams, 1992)

Diarrhea

Diarrhea results from rapid movement of fecal matter through the large intestine. Diarrhea is a too frequent emptying of the bowel with passage of stool in a liquid or very loose form. Normally the colon absorbs water from solid wastes received from the small intestine. When something interferes with that absorption or causes the bowel to secrete rather than absorb liquid, or when something speeds the passage of wastes through the bowel so that there is insufficient time to absorb fluid, diarrhea results.

The greatest hazard of diarrhea is the loss of water and electrolytes needed for normal cell function. Severe dehydration and electrolyte imbalance can cause cardiac arrhythmias, severe hypotension, renal failure, and death, especially in infants and very young children, elderly persons, and persons debilitated by extreme illness. Most of the time, however, diarrhea is not that severe or life-threatening. It may be chronic and recurring or most frequently an acute symptom lasting for only a day or so. In any case diarrhea is a signal that something has disrupted normal function of the GI tract.

✦ Etiology

The major cause of diarrhea is an infection called enteritis, which is caused by bacteria, protozoa, or a virus in the GI tract. The usual sites of this infection are the terminal ileum and the large intestine. Wherever the infection is present, the mucosa of that area of the bowel becomes irritated and increases its rate of secretion. Additionally the motility of the bowel greatly increases. As a result large amounts of fluid are available to wash the infectious agent away, and the strong propulsive movements move the fluid toward expulsion by the anus. Diarrhea, then, is an important mechanism for ridding the intestinal tract of debilitating infections (Guyton, 1991).

Psychosomatic factors also have been linked to diarrhea. Everyone has experienced the cramps and urgency associated with fear, anxiety, or intense excitement just before an important occasion. In general, anger, resentment, embarrassment, and overt or subconscious hostility are associated with hyperemia, engorgement, increased secretion of mucus, and increased motility of the colon. Extreme responses to emotional states may lead to irritable bowel syndrome, characterized by uncoordinated and abnormal motor function, abdominal pain, flatulence, and constipation usually alternating with diarrhea. This syndrome affects some 22 million Americans, with signs and symptoms generally starting between the ages of 20 and 40 years and affecting twice as many women as men.

Irritable bowel syndrome is frequently caused or aggravated by stress, but recent studies have linked it to an intolerance of certain foods such as wheat, corn, dairy products, coffee, tea, and citrus fruits (Jones, McLaughlan,

Shorthouse, Workman, & Hunter, 1982). Persons with irritable bowel syndrome also are unusually prone to migraine headaches and severe menstrual pain, suggesting that they may have a generalized, underlying disorder of the smooth muscles. Lack of fiber in the diet also has been linked to this condition. Signs and symptoms almost always improve when foods high in fiber are added to the diet.

A common but frequently overlooked cause of diarrhea and excessive flatulence may be an insufficiency of the enzyme lactose, which digests milk sugar. Eliminating such foods as milk, cottage cheese, ice cream, and yogurt from the diet for about a week determines if lactose insufficiency is the cause. Lactose insufficiency can often be overcome by pretreating milk with the enzyme or by taking mild digestant tablets just before consuming milk products.

Food allergies, although rare, also may cause diarrhea. In this case severe cramps and other allergic reactions such as hives may accompany severe diarrhea. Some persons develop diarrhea by eating too many bowel-stimulating foods such as prunes, bran, or figs or by drinking too much coffee. Once identified, the diarrhea can be controlled by simply avoiding the offending food.

Diarrhea also may be caused by various drugs. Excessive consumption of certain sugar substitutes such as sorbitol and mannitol found in dietetic foods may cause the problem. Antibiotics often cause diarrhea by killing many bacteria that normally reside in the colon and are responsible for digesting unabsorbed foods passed along from the small bowel. This type of diarrhea ends when the antibiotic therapy is stopped.

NURSING ASSESSMENT

Before any bowel program can be implemented, the nurse must perform a comprehensive assessment of the client. When combined with a knowledge of normal and impaired bowel function, this assessment becomes the foundation for successful management.

To develop a safe, effective bowel program for the particular needs of the individual, there are many factors to be considered:

- ✦ Past bowel routine
- ✦ Physical status
- ✦ Dietary habits
- ✦ Medications
- ✦ Future lifestyle

Past Bowel Routine (Bowel History)

The admission history should elicit a detailed description of the present illness, the perceived bowel problem, bowel function between the time of injury and the present, and past bowel routine. Former bowel habits, including time of and day of evacuation, frequency, and personal habits to stimulate defecation should be reviewed. Prior frequency and use of laxatives or enemas should be determined (Hogstel & Nelson, 1992). The nurse should note when the last bowel movement occurred. Any history of sphincter disturbances, ulcerative colitis, diverticulitis, spastic colon, prolapse, constipation, diarrhea, or hemorrhoids should be noted and explored. Neurologic disease or disability significantly alters lifestyle, and it may not be easy to reestablish former patterns. The nurse must attempt to determine former habits and anticipate future lifestyle to plan an effective, client-centered bowel plan with the client, family, and other team members.

Physical Status

The overall physical condition of the client must be assessed with special notation made of the cause of the disability, the neurologic status, and any other factors that might affect bowel function and ability to participate in a bowel program. The three commonly seen neurogenic bowel dysfunctions discussed previously have specific interventions that are discussed in detail later in this chapter. The level of neural dysfunction of the bowel can be assessed using the motor and sensory tests described previously in the discussion on incontinence. The abdomen should be inspected for distention, visible peristalsis, masses, or bulges. The presence of normal, hyperactive or hypoactive bowel sounds should be auscultated. Percussion should note any unexpected area of dullness, such as over the sigmoid colon, which might indicate a mass. Abdominal palpation is performed to note muscle tone, tenderness, size of organs, and any masses present. A rectal examination is performed to assess sphincter tone and presence and consistency of stool in the rectum (Hogstel & Nelson, 1992). Any rectal excoriations or lesions should be ascertained.

Cognitive and communication ability must be evaluated. Does the client understand the staff when questioned about the need to toilet? Speech and language, visual, or auditory impairments may prevent the client from locating or being able to use the call button and thus from participating fully in a bowel program.

The ability to chew and swallow also must be assessed. The person with a stroke or brain injury may suffer from dysphagia, making chewing and swallowing difficult. Individuals with facial paralysis or who have lost a great deal of weight following their disability may now have ill-fitting dentures that affect their ability to chew food properly.

Ability to turn oneself in bed and transfer from bed to toilet or commode should be assessed and, if necessary, adaptations made to allow the client to perform the bowel program with the greatest degree of independence possible. Ambulation and the ability to perform personal hygiene activities should be assessed as these relate to bowel habits.

Anticipated functional goals must be determined by communication with the rehabilitation team. It may be necessary, for example, to teach family members or attendants to help a person with high quadriplegia, whereas a person with paraplegia may require only assistive devices and equipment. The elderly client may suffer from degenerative joint disease that makes getting to the toilet difficult. The client's ability to manage a bowel routine independently affects planning for the bowel program.

Dietary Habits

The client's diet and appetite should receive careful attention. Assessment of preonset habits should include food preferences, usual meal routine, amount and type of fluid intake, cultural practices, and nutritional adequacy. The sufficiency of the diet for facilitating elimination should then be reviewed. Diets poor in fiber and fluid and high in gas-forming foods, as well as inconsistent diets, must be evaluated and changed because these create problems in regulating routine and consistency of stool. For instance, foods that caused diarrhea, excessive flatus, or constipation before the onset of disability are likely to cause the same response now.

The client's endurance level should be considered when assessing dietary habits. Does the client tire easily and consequently have difficulty completing a large meal? Should small frequent feedings be considered? Is the energy level sufficient to prepare balanced meals while at home, or will "fast foods" dominate the diet? Is there a support system in place at home to assist with food preparation if necessary?

Medications

After disease or disability, the client may be taking many medications. For purposes of establishing a bowel program, the nurse should be aware that those medications fall into two broad categories—those that assist in the bowel program and those that are prescribed for other medical reasons.

To assist with the bowel program, stool softeners and bulk formers often are prescribed. These medications are discussed more specifically later in this chapter. The nurse should determine the effect of the currently prescribed medications in order to plan the bowel program appropriately. For instance, if the client is reporting continuous soft stools throughout the day, the nurse may want to consider increasing the bulk formers within the prescribed range.

Medications prescribed for other medical conditions also must be evaluated, since they may have undesirable side effects (e.g., antibiotics can destroy normal bowel flora and result in diarrhea). Propantheline (Pro-Banthine) and oxybutynin chloride (Ditropan), used in the management of urinary incontinence, can cause constipation.

Future Lifestyle

For any bowel program to be successful, active participation with the client and family on a day-to-day basis is essential. The client's suggestions and preferences should be incorporated into the plan. The nurse should know the individual's mental and physical capabilities when planning a program, so that realistic goals can be established mutually by the nurse and client.

Plans for discharge should be considered from the time of initial assessment. Will the client be attending school or returning to work? An evening program of bowel evacuation may be preferable for someone with morning deadlines. Will assistance be necessary for the client to participate fully in the program? If so, it may be necessary to plan the program for a time when assistance is available. If the plan initiated in the rehabilitation setting cannot be followed at home, it is of little use. The successful plan allows the individual to integrate bowel control conveniently into everyday life.

NURSING DIAGNOSES

From the assessment data the rehabilitation nurse will make an appropriate nursing diagnosis for the client with impaired bowel function. Potential diagnoses are as follows:

1. Bowel Incontinence—uninhibited
2. Bowel Incontinence—reflex neurogenic
3. Bowel Incontinence—areflexic neurogenic
4. Colonic Constipation
5. Diarrhea (Gordon, 1993-1994).

GOALS

Short-term goals are established with the client and may vary according to disability, type of bowel dysfunction, and lifestyle. Goals that may be established are to

1. Achieve control on a regular basis (a bowel movement every 1 to 3 days) at a planned time and place without the need for laxatives or enemas
2. Eliminate or minimize involuntary bowel movements
3. Avoid complications of diarrhea, constipation, and impaction by maintaining adequate nutrition, hydration, and activity (McCourt, 1993)
4. Help the client with an uninhibited neurogenic bowel to plan and regulate bowel elimination at a time when there is likely to be a response
5. Help the client with a reflex neurogenic bowel to stimulate reflex activity that moves feces into the rectum for predictable elimination
6. Assist the client with an autonomous neurogenic bowel to maintain firm stool consistency and keep the distal colon empty

REHABILITATION NURSING INTERVENTIONS

The nurse should be aware that certain factors influence the efficiency of and are common to all bowel programs. In addition, there are specific nursing interventions for bowel management in incontinence, constipation, and diarrhea. The type of neurogenic bowel also influences the development of a bowel management plan.

Basic Components of a Bowel Program

Certain factors are common to all bowel programs. These include a "clean" bowel to start, timing, proper diet and fluid intake, physical exercise, privacy, positioning, and use of medications as indicated.

◆ A "clean" bowel

The bowel must be free from impaction before starting any new bowel program. Manual disimpaction, cleansing enemas, or laxatives may be used to free the bowel from impaction. Laxatives or enemas that may be used are as follows:

1. Milk of magnesia
2. Milk of magnesia with cascara
3. Magnesium citrate
4. Fleet Enema
5. Oil retention enema
6. Bisacodyl enema
7. Soapsuds enema

For children with myelomeningocele who are impacted, Coffman (1986) recommends a cleansing enema of Ringer's lactate solution. Laxatives should be given 8 to 12 hours before the desired results but usually will cause accidents or unplanned times of evacuation.

Once the program is started, no laxatives or enemas should be given unless

1. The client becomes impacted or severely constipated.
2. There is medical necessity, such as bowel preparation for tests or surgery (spinal cord injured clients should have their routine bowel program the night before with manual removal in the morning rather than the usual preparation).

3. It is recommended and determined that this is the best program for the client.

Enemas are not used routinely in bowel programs because of stretch to the colon walls and resultant loss of elasticity. With continued use of enemas, the bowel responds poorly to reflex stimulation, possibly leading to dependence on enemas and laxatives.

✦ Timing

Scheduling the time of day for a bowel program is important for effectiveness. It is also important to accommodate the client's preonset routine in order to fit in with anticipated discharge plans and future lifestyle. Venn, Taft, Carpentier, and Applebaugh (1992) conducted a research study of 46 stroke clients and discovered that when their premorbid time for elimination was used as the scheduled time of day for their bowel training program, a significantly higher number were efficient in establishing effective bowel regimens.

For children and adolescents a regular routine for toileting needs to be planned around school times (Coffman, 1986). For an adult, work hours may need to be considered. For example, defecation may be attempted every morning. However, this schedule may have to be evaluated and modified according to the client's physical condition and response. Some individuals find an every-other-day routine satisfactory; others have good evacuation with a 3-day routine.

A key element is establishing a consistent habit time for elimination. Clinical experience has demonstrated that for prompt bowel response to stimulation (a bowel movement within 30 minutes), the stimulation method must take place at the same hour every time. The gastrocolic reflex also should be used in the bowel routine. After breakfast, lunch, or the evening meal is an ideal time, but a hot cup of coffee or tea or an evening snack also assists in producing the gastrocolic reflex at a more convenient time.

✦ Diet and fluid intake

The client's preonset dietary habits are evaluated before implementing a bowel program. Physical condition is considered, and personal preferences are incorporated as much as possible into the diet. The diet should be high in nutrient value and well balanced, containing a variety of foods from the six basic food groups.

For a successful bowel program, the diet must be high in fiber. Dietary fiber is that part of plant food that traverses the small intestine and is not digested by the endogenous secretions within. The most important function of fiber is to bind water in the intestine in the form of a gel to prevent overabsorption from the large bowel. This action ensures that the fecal content is both bulky and soft and also that its passage through the intestine is not delayed. Delayed transit time of the fecal contents generally results in constipation. Dietary fiber is beneficial in the management of both constipation and diarrhea. Its bulking action helps alleviate diarrhea, and its softening action helps alleviate constipation.

The chief sources of dietary fiber are whole-grain cereals and breads, leafy vegetables, legumes, nuts, and fruits with skins. By simply replacing white bread with whole-grain bread, the fiber content of the diet can be increased greatly. At least five to nine daily servings of vegetables and fruits, two of which should be raw, are recommended. Granola, bran, and wheat germ are excellent sources of fiber and may be easily added to soups, cereals, meatloaf, baked goods, and other foods. Fiber should be introduced into the diet gradually to allow the GI tract time to adapt. Too rapid an increase in the amount of fiber may lead to distressing side effects such as flatulence, distention, or diarrhea.

Unless fluid intake is restricted for medical reasons, clients should drink 2 to 3 quarts of liquid daily to maintain soft stool consistency. Drinking hot coffee, hot water, or prune juice every morning for breakfast is helpful to some persons in initiating a bowel movement. Prunes and prune juice stimulate intestinal motility and therefore act as natural laxatives. Large quantities of prune or other fruit juices, however, may result in loose stools. Setting the table with two or more types of fluid at each meal may increase total intake. Popsicles or ice also may help (Smith, 1988).

✦ Exercise

Physical activity is vital to a successful bowel program. Prolonged bed rest has an adverse effect on bowel motility and tends to cause fecal retention. The client who can be out of bed and involved in physical activities increases muscle tone and has return of bowel function more quickly. In a study of stroke clients, Munchiando and Kendall (1993) discovered that as the number of hours spent in bed increased, the number of days needed to establish a bowel program also increased.

Physical status and type of disability determine exercise capabilities. Encouraging the client to perform activities of daily living (ADL) with minimum assistance from others helps compensate for the decreased activity level as a result of physical disability. Exercise tape may be used to guide activities that can be performed while the client is in a wheelchair (Smith, 1988). When subjected to extended periods of bed rest for medical reasons, the client must be urged to continue to carry out as many activities as possible. Turning in bed, lifting the hips, bathing, performing range of joint motion exercises, and carrying out other self-care activities aid in preventing decreased bowel motility and constipation.

✦ Privacy

The act of elimination, in most cultures, is performed in private. Privacy and modesty are particularly important to clients who are from Mexican-American or Native American heritage (Hoeman, 1989). Privacy facilitates relaxation, which in turn facilitates the act of defecation. Privacy also ensures that embarrassing sounds or odors will not be detected by others. The disabled person in an institution has little privacy. The more dependent the client, the less privacy there is. The individual benefits psychologically when privacy is incorporated into the bowel program. Whenever possible, the nurse should assist the client out of bed and onto a toilet where the bathroom door may be closed. If a portable commode must be used, privacy can be achieved by rolling it into a bathroom or other secluded area.

✦ Positioning

Whenever possible, the client should assume an upright sitting position to defecate. This normal physiologic position allows gravity to assist in peristalsis and stool expulsion. Unless absolutely necessary, bedpans should not be used. They should never be used on anyone who does not have sensation in the buttocks or sacral area. Care should be taken when positioning the client to limit sacral pressure exerted by the bedpan. To limit sacral pressure, the nurse should elevate the head of the bed, support the back and legs with pillows, and bridge the hips and legs as necessary. To avoid excessive pressure and potential skin breakdown, the client should not remain on the bedpan or sit on a toilet or commode for longer than 30 minutes. Five to twenty minutes, however, may be necessary for defecation to occur, and more time must be allowed for the client, if needed (Hogstel & Nelson, 1992). As soon as the client receives medical approval to get out of bed, bedpans should be abandoned. Persons with impaired skin integrity in the buttocks area or who do not have buttock or sacral sensation (i.e., clients with SCI) should evacuate on an incontinence pad in bed. Positioning on the right side after suppository insertion, or for manual removal, aids in elimination due to the position of the descending colon in providing gravity-assisted evacuation.

A squat position with the knees slightly higher than the hips helps to increase abdominal pressure and thus facilitate stool passage. If a raised toilet seat is needed, a footstool can be placed under the feet to raise the knees. For children, feet should be flat on the floor or on a footstool (Smith, 1990). If balance is a problem, armrests and a supportive back should be used (Wald, 1991).

For those persons with weak abdominal muscles, an abdominal binder can be placed to increase abdominal pressure. Bending over at the waist assists the abdominal muscles to push out the stool (Hogstel, 1992). Abdominal massage also may stimulate and hasten the defecation process. Persons with all types of disabilities and ages find it helpful to massage the abdomen in the direction of the bowel from right groin upward, across, and down to the left groin. In addition to abdominal massage, children may be taught to bear down by blowing up a balloon, coughing, or blowing bubbles (Coffman, 1986; Smith, 1990).

♦ Medication and digital stimulation

Suppositories and medications are ordered by a physician. However, protocols may be developed in collaboration with the physician that specify ranges and guidelines so that the nurse can make adjustments according to the individual client's response.

Digital stimulation is a technique used to induce reflex contraction of the colon and relaxation of the anal sphincter muscle (Munchiando & Kendell, 1993), resulting in elimination.

Suppositories and medications. Suppositories are used to initiate reflex emptying of the bowel. To have an optimum effect, the suppository must come in contact with the bowel wall. Before inserting a suppository, the rectum should be checked for stool. If stool is present, enough should be removed to ensure proper placement of the suppository against the bowel wall. The suppository should be stored at room temperature before insertion, because refrigeration delays action and temperatures over 90°F (32.2°C) cause the suppository to melt. Table 21-1 summarizes the three types of suppositories commonly used in rehabilitation settings.

Stool softeners and bulk formers are often prescribed to aid in the establishment of a bowel program. For example, dioctyl sodium sulfosuccinate (Colace), 100 mg, two to three times per day, may be used initially and the dosage adjusted according to the consistency of the stool. When hard stools accompanied by constipation or frequent soft, pasty stools are a problem, bulk-forming laxatives can be given to alter the consistency by making stools soft and bulky. Laxatives should not be prescribed routinely in any bowel routine because of the potential for developing atonic colon. Whenever a mild laxative is needed, senna tablets and granules assist in moving the stool to the lower bowel so that a suppository or digital stimulation can completely empty the bowel. Fecal impaction may require a stronger laxative or enema. The nurse should remember that the terminal goal of any bowel program is continence and control without the need for medication. Should medication be needed, consideration must be given to providing medications that will be covered by the client's insurance carriers on an outpatient basis.

Digital stimulation. To perform digital stimulation, the index finger is gloved, lubricated, and gently inserted ½ to 1 inch into the rectum. To stimulate the inner sphincter to relax, the finger is gently rotated in a clockwise motion against the anal sphincter wall. It may take from 30 seconds to 2 minutes for relaxation of the sphincter to occur. While feces is passing, the rectum is moved gently to one side. When no more stool is expelled, digital stimulation is

Table 21-1 Suppositories

Suppository (strength)	Action	Time when results expected	Disadvantages
Glycerin	Draws fluid from the bowel creating a volume which distends the bowel and initiates reflex peristalsis	Approximately 30 minutes	Abdominal cramping possible
Sodium bicarbonate and potassium bitartrate (CEO-Two)	Activated in water before insertion; suppository releases carbon dioxide, which distends bowel and initiates reflex peristalsis	30-45 minutes	Use of petroleum lubricants negates effectiveness of suppository Abdominal cramping possible
Bisacodyl (Dulcolax)	Contact suppository that stimulates sensory nerve endings in colon and results in reflex peristalsis	15-60 minutes	Abdominal cramping possible

resumed and the process repeated until the bowel is evacuated. The client should be instructed to take slow, deep breaths during this process.

In successful bowel programs, digital stimulation may replace the suppository once a reflex-response defecation pattern is established. However, digital stimulation also may be used to trigger a bowel movement if a suppository has been less than successful. Additionally it may be used to ensure complete emptying of the colon following a bowel movement. In persons with SCI who are susceptible to dysreflexia, dibucaine hydrochloride (Nupercainal) lubricant can be used to lower the incidence of dysreflexia during stimulation.

The Client with Incontinence

Management of bowel incontinence in a rehabilitation setting is an independent nursing function. The physician, however, orders the medication and establishes protocols, whereas the nurse makes the necessary adjustments within the protocols according to the client's circumstances. The nurse must continually evaluate the client's status and alter the bowel program when necessary. Any changes in a bowel program should not be made before at least a 5- to 7-day trial. Only one change should be made at a time. Daily changes in a bowel control program could result in modi-

fying a program blindly without learning the response to the previous bowel program.

Accurate documentation of the results of any bowel program is absolutely vital. Unfortunately management of bowel control for many clients is approached on a trial-and-error basis. The effectiveness of the program can be evaluated only if accurate records are kept (Fig. 21-12).

Uninhibited Neurogenic Bowel

In general, the following measures should be taken in establishing a bowel program for a client with an uninhibited neurogenic bowel:

1. Select the time of day for the bowel program according to past habits and for future convenience.
2. Follow a consistent schedule. Assist client to toilet 30 minutes after meals to take advantage of gastrocolic reflex. Start with a daily program and progress to every other day (Munchiando & Kendall, 1993).
3. Provide a nutritious diet with adequate fiber.
4. Give fluids adequate to stimulate reflex activity and to promote soft stool (2000 to 2400 ml/24 hours unless contraindicated).
5. Begin the program with an empty colon.
6. Obtain a physician's order for stool softeners in the early stages of the program.

Date:							
Suppository = / Type							
Time							
Inserted by:							
Digital stim Time							
Manual removal Time							
Evacuation Time							
Stool Amt.							
Consistency							
Place							
Initials							
Normal evacuation Time							
Amt.							
Consistency							
Place							
Initials							
Accidents Time							
(Chart in red) Place							
Consistency							
Initials							
Accidents Time							
(Chart in red) Place							
Consistency							
Initials							
Enema Time & initials							
Initials R.N., L.V.N.							

Fig. 21-12   Bowel record. Courtesy of San Diego Rehabilitation Institute, CA.

7. Give a daily suppository to initiate the defecation reflex. Venn and associates' (1992) research study suggests that if a spontaneous bowel movement occurs within 4 hours before the scheduled time, the suppository may be held back for that day.

Usually the effects of softeners will not be seen for 3 days. These should be used on a routine rather than an as-needed basis. Softeners that may be used include the following:

1. Docusate sodium (Dialose; usually 1 twice daily)
2. Docusate calcium (Surfak; usually 1 twice daily; good to use if sodium intake is restricted)
3. Dicotyl sodium sulfosuccinate (Colace; usually 1 twice daily; available in liquid form)
4. Dioctyl sodium sulfosuccinate (Doxinate; usually 1 twice daily)

Softeners with a laxative component may be used when additional softening and/or peristaltic stimulus is needed. They should be given approximately 12 hours before desired results and also used on a routine basis. Those that may be used include the following:

1. Docusate sodium and phenolphthalein (Dialose Plus; usually 1 to 2 every day)
2. Casanthranol and docusate sodium (Peri-Colace; usually 1 to 2 every day)
3. Standardized senna concentrate (Senokot; usually 1 to 2 every day)

If combining softeners and softener/laxatives, it is preferable to combine like products (i.e., Dialose with Dialose Plus, Colace with Peri-Colace).

Bisacodyl tablets may be used if all other measures are unsuccessful in preventing constipation or impaction. A maximum of 2 tablets may be given at one time approximately 12 hours before desired results.

Bulk producers may be used for the client who lacks bowel tone, who needs additional softening of the stool, or who has small infrequent stools. They are not appropriate for the impacted client. They may be used to "form up" stools if the client is on a liquid or tube feeding diet or has an "irritable bowel." Those which may be used include the following:

1. Psyllium hydrophilic mucilloid (Metamucil) or psyllium and senna (Perdiem): 1 teaspoon mixed in 200 ml of water or juice and followed by a glass of water
2. "Organic" bulk products of the client's choice, such as alfalfa tablets
3. Calcium polycarbophil (Mitrolan): 1 to 2 tablets chewed one to four times per day

When the client's condition improves so that the diet, fluid intake, and physical activity are well tolerated, these medications may be unnecessary.

Suppositories must be given within a half hour after a meal or hot liquid is taken. Types used are as follows:

1. Biscodyl (usually 1)
2. Glycerin (usually 1)
3. CEO-two (usually 1)

Digital stimulation in place of a suppository is used in some rehabilitation settings. Since clients with uninhibited bowel function have intact sensation, digital stimulation may be painful.

Accurate documentation is necessary to determine progress and to make appropriate changes in the bowel program. Depending on the client's condition, it may take a week or longer to establish a satisfactory pattern. Staff should be alert to verbal and nonverbal efforts by the client to communicate the need to eliminate. In the absence of functional speech, such behavior as restlessness may indicate awareness of rectal sensation. Munchiando and Kendall (1993) discovered that it took longer to establish a bowel program in clients with right-sided hemiplegia, probably due to expressive aphasia and difficulty communicating the urge to defecate. The effectiveness of the program must be evaluated daily and weekly. If a change is needed, only one part of the program is changed at a time. Client and/or family participation in the program and decision-making process is increased gradually. Guidelines for changes in the program to every other day or every third day include the following:

1. Client has small or no results every other day.
2. Client's stool is not hard on daily program.
3. Client is well controlled on every program (i.e., results within 1 hour, no constipation or accidents for at least a week).

By complying with the basic components of a bowel program, continence and control can be achieved by the time of discharge and suppositories and medications discontinued.

Reflex Neurogenic Bowel

During the acute stage of SCI, spinal shock is responsible for tonic paralysis of the GI tract and flaccid tone of the anal sphincter. Manual removal may be used until spinal shock subsides.

In general, the following measures should be taken to establish a bowel program for a client with a reflex neurogenic bowel:

1. Once bowel sounds are present, physical activity increases, and oral fluid and food, including high fiber, is tolerated, administer a suppository daily to trigger reflex elimination. Administration time should be consistent with the establishment of preonset habits and anticipated future lifestyle. The suppository is inserted 15 to 30 minutes ahead of the planned evacuation time (Venn et al., 1992).
2. Once a reliable bowel pattern is observed, suppository administration may be decreased to every other day or every third day as long as the stool consistency remains soft. Be alert for signs of fecal impaction or constipation that may develop with infrequent elimination.
3. Have client evacuate on toilet if possible and bear down if abdominal muscles are strong. The client should lean forward and massage the abdomen in a clockwise manner (Zejdlik, 1992). Digital stimulation may be used alone or in addition to a suppository when the suppository has not produced results within 15 to 20 minutes.
4. Stool softeners and bulk agents may be necessary to assist elimination when abdominal muscles are weak or paralyzed. Harsh cathartics must be avoided. The need for medications should decrease as activity increases (Zejdlik, 1992).

Documentation of progress remains important to detect reliable patterns of elimination and to initiate appropriate changes.

For individuals with spinal cord lesions above the T6 vertebral level (above the splanchnic outflow), autonomic dysreflexia is a potential problem. Autonomic dysreflexia (hyperreflexia) is an abnormal hyperactive reflex activity as a result of an interrupted spinal cord and is set off most often by stimuli arising from a distended bladder, but rectal distention, stimulation, and passage of feces also may precipitate this sympathetic response. This syndrome constitutes a medical emergency that can result in death if not treated promptly. Chapter 20 contains specific information regarding autonomic dysreflexia. Nupercainal ointment applied to the rectum 10 minutes before suppository insertion or digital stimulation is helpful in preventing symptoms in susceptible individuals.

Autonomous Neurogenic Bowel

Management of autonomous neurogenic bowel is difficult. Lower motor neuron loss results in absence of the spinal reflex activity. An atonic bowel with diminished propulsive forces and tone results. A program of suppositories and manual removal can be effective in evacuating stool (Zejdlik, 1992).

In general, the following measures should be taken in establishing a bowel program for the client with an autonomous neurogenic bowel:

1. Develop a stool consistency that is firm yet not hard by providing dietary fiber and using bulk-forming agents such as Metamucil and Citrucel.
2. Have the client evacuate on a toilet and perform the Valsalva maneuver (see the discussion on defecation). Massaging the abdomen and leaning forward will augment the effectiveness of the bowel program.
3. If these measures are not successful, manual removal of the stool with a generously lubricated gloved finger can be performed.
4. After removal of stool from the lower rectum, administer a suppository as high as possible against the rectal wall. This stimulates the colon to empty stool into the rectum for manual removal. When a client is active, any stool in the rectum may be expelled when intraabdominal pressure is increased. Therefore a daily program is recommended (Zejdlik, 1992).
5. Assess stool consistency. Loose stools will leak through a flaccid sphincter. Hard stools are difficult to remove manually and can lead to impaction and atony of the colon over time (Rauen & Aubert, 1992).

Children with neurogenic bowels should follow the same routine as for adults. The goal for a person born with myelomeningocele, for example, is a soft, formed stool on a daily basis at the same time. This can be achieved through a high-fiber diet, adequate water intake, and habit training (Rauen & Aubert, 1992). Stool softeners, suppositories, and digital stimulation also may be needed (Smith, 1990). When suppositories are used, children with neurogenic bowels may need to have the buttocks closed with paper tape after

Table 21-2 Neurogenic bowel dysfunction

Diagnosis	Level of lesion	Possible etiology	Pattern of incontinence	Bowel program
Uninhibited	Brain	Cerebrovascular accident; multiple sclerosis; brain injury	Urgency: Poor awareness of desire to defecate	Consistent habit and time according to premorbid history; physical exercise; high fluid intake; high-fiber foods; stool softener, suppository as needed
Reflex	Spinal cord above T12 to L1 vertebral level	Trauma; tumor; vascular disease; syringomyelia; multiple sclerosis	Infrequent; sudden; unexpected	Consistent habit and time, physical exercise, high fluid intake, high-fiber foods; suppository program, digital stimulation, stool softener as needed
Autonomous	Spinal cord at or below T12 to L1 vertebral level	Trauma, tumor, spina bifida, intervertebral disk	Frequent; may be continuous or induced by exercise or stress	Consistent habit and time, physical exercise continuous, high fluid intake, high-fiber foods and bulk agents as necessary for firm stool consistency; suppository program, Valsalva maneuver, manual removal

suppository insertion to facilitate absorption (Gleeson, 1990).

Table 21-2 provides a summary overview of the types of neurogenic bowel dysfunction previously discussed. A successful bowel routine for the client with incontinence resulting from any type of neurologic bowel dysfunction requires effort and consistency for the client and the nurse.

Ostomies

A bowel program cannot be established with an ileostomy or ascending colostomy. A bag or pouch must therefore be worn at all times. With regular irrigation, a person with a descending and sigmoid colostomy and sometimes a transverse colostomy can regain a regular bowel pattern. Regulating the diet with selected foods at specific times can also lead to a predictable elimination pattern.

The rehabilitation nurse usually works with an enterostomal therapist to establish a routine program including supplies, skin care, and education of the client. Members of the United Ostomy Association are instrumental in visiting clients and explaining how to live with an ostomy (Berger & Williams, 1992).

There is some research being conducted exploring the viability of elective colostomies for people with SCIs in order to aid in preservation of skin integrity, save time for elimination, and thereby facilitate pursuit of vocations and avocations (Saltzstein & Romano, 1990).

The Client with Constipation

Constipation is one of the most common complications in people with neurogenic bowel dysfunction. Interrupted defecation mechanisms can result in a sluggish movement of feces through the bowel (Zejdlik, 1992). To assist the client with constipation in achieving elimination of soft bulky stool on a regular basis, a bowel program based on a comprehensive assessment and database, as previously described, should be developed. Laxatives and enemas should be avoided because the client can develop a dependency on these methods, and they may lead to serious GI disturbances, such as spastic colitis (Brunton, 1990).

If the client's constipation is not related to a pathologic process, then the rehabilitation nurse should proceed to develop the bowel program. Based on the individual's bowel history and assessment, a nursing care plan is developed incorporating diet, fluid intake, exercise, and timing.

✦ Diet and fluid intake

The most important dietary factor when considering constipation is the amount of fiber ingested. Authorities disagree about the amount of dietary fiber that constitutes a high-fiber diet. Six to ten grams of dietary fiber per day have been found to be successful in managing constipation in a majority of subjects (Burkitt & Meisner, 1979; Hull, Greco, & Brooks, 1980). Other sources cite the need for 30 to 40 g (Friedman, 1989). The amount of fiber may need to be individualized according to client need.

In adding fiber to the diet, the rehabilitation nurse must be cognizant of the person's likes and dislikes and especially of ability to chew, since many high-fiber foods require adequate mastication. This consideration is extremely important with persons whose residual deficits affect either the innervation or muscle function of the face, mouth, and throat. If the person is unable to handle high-fiber foods adequately, then supplementing the diet with unprocessed bran or adding bran to cooked vegetables and fruit should be considered.

As stated previously, fiber binds water in the intestine in the form of a gel. This prevents the overabsorption of water in the large intestine and ensures that the feces are bulky and soft. Fiber also adds weight to the stool, speeds up slow passage, and slows down rapid transit (Ellickson, 1988; Wrick, et al., 1983).

The highest source of fiber is minimally processed cereal. Other sources of fiber are legumes such as peas, beans, and millet; root vegetables such as potatoes, parsnips, and carrots; and fruits and leafy vegetables. Bran is one of the most concentrated sources of natural food fiber available. It is the outer layer or covering of the wheat kernel. Miller's bran is the richest source of fiber available, containing 44% dietary fiber (Brunton, 1990).

Fiber should be introduced gradually into the diet to avoid untoward effects such as abdominal discomfort, flatulence, and diarrhea (Brunton, 1990). Bran is considered superior to other bulk laxatives because it is most effective in increasing fecal weight (Iseminger & Hardy, 1982). Bran, however, can bind orally with and reduce the intestinal absorption of many drugs such as cardiac glycosides, salicylates, nitrofurantoin, and coumarin derivatives and therefore should be taken at a separate time (Brunton, 1990).

Adequate fluids are essential to avoid and manage constipation. It is often necessary for the nurse to be creative in assisting the client to meet the necessary fluid intake. The nurse also must be fully aware of all aspects of the client's rehabilitation plan, including bladder rehabilitation and therapy schedules, so as not to jeopardize but rather to enhance and facilitate the comprehensive plan for rehabilitation.

✦ Exercise

Diet alone is not sufficient to alleviate constipation. Physical activity is essential and can be accomplished easily in a rehabilitation setting by incorporating therapy sessions as a means of achieving needed exercise. The nurse needs to realize that movement or physical activity can greatly assist in defecation, and that if the bowel program includes a morning bowel movement after breakfast, the client needs to have sufficient time to attend to the bowel schedule before going to therapy. Episodes of fecal incontinence can be embarrassing and discouraging to an individual trying to cope with a new disability, new body image, and lifestyle change; therefore accidents should be avoided. The activity of ambulating short distances may be sufficient to stimulate defecation.

✦ Timing

The timing of the bowel program should be considered when establishing the therapy schedule. Ignoring the urge to defecate is a major cause of constipation, and the individual should not be given the impression that defecating is less important than any other part of the rehabilitation plan.

✦ **Laxatives**

Laxatives are beneficial in the treatment of acute constipation but are not recommended for chronic problems. Laxatives are divided into three categories including bulk-forming (i.e., Mitrolan), saline and osmotic (i.e., milk of magnesia, glycerin), and stimulant laxatives (i.e., senna, castor oil, bisacodyl) (Brunton, 1990). For more detailed information, the reader should refer to a pharmacology text.

The Client with Diarrhea

When a client experiences diarrhea, an investigation for impaction should first be conducted. If the bowel is impacted, then the basic components of bowel management should be explained and the nursing interventions for the client with constipation should be instituted. If diarrhea is treated without assessing for impaction, then a more complex problem could arise, namely, bowel obstruction.

Diarrhea is managed most easily by treating or eliminating the cause. If it is the result of disease, then the pathologic condition should be managed. As stated previously, if antibiotics are the cause, then other antibiotics should be tried. Yogurt can be beneficial in managing the diarrhea. Foods also may cause diarrhea, and the offending foods should be discovered and eliminated. Some foods are useful in treating diarrhea in children. Bananas, rice, milk products, or applesauce are examples. In the process of juggling the diet, nutritional adequacy should be monitored.

Electrolyte imbalance is a potentially serious problem when diarrhea occurs. The client should drink 2 to 3 quarts of fluid a day and also supplement for fluid lost. Excessive use or an excessive dosage of laxatives can result in diarrhea. In addition, diarrhea can occur in the initial phase of dietary supplementation with bran. The following medications may cause diarrhea as a side effect:

1. Broad-spectrum antibiotics
2. Adrenergic neuron blocking agents (reserpine)
3. Bile acids
4. Quinidine
5. Cholinergic agents and cholinesterase inhibitors
6. Prokinetic agents

If the client experiences incontinence as a result of diarrhea, the nurse should offer assurance and emotional support. The client can become anxious, frustrated, and embarrassed by uncontrollable diarrhea, and the nurse can help the client deal with the situation effectively and positively. Additionally the nurse can assist the individual in avoiding future episodes, thereby alleviating or decreasing anxiety.

Whenever diarrhea or incontinence occurs, the potential for skin breakdown exists. Meticulous perianal hygiene is essential after each episode.

CLIENT AND FAMILY EDUCATION

The details of client education should parallel the individualized bowel program. Education should begin early during hospitalization to give the client sufficient time and opportunity to discover and clarify problems or concerns. The nurse should teach clients about their disability and how it affects bowel control. Anatomy and physiology of the GI tract should be covered. The importance and rationale behind a routine bowel program should include diet, fluid intake, exercise, timing, and positioning. The client's individualized program must be taught and should cover rationale for the program, medication use, purpose, precautions, and how to determine the need to increase or decrease amounts taken at home. The location and positioning for the program and techniques of suppository insertion or digital stimulation must be included. Potential problems that may be encountered with a bowel program should be discussed, and the client should be given problem-solving techniques for diarrhea, constipation, and accidents. They should also be informed when to consult with their physician or rehabilitation nurse. Cultural or familial beliefs regarding bowel movements and/or diet must be discussed, the program adapted to meet their needs, and/or erroneous

---

BOWEL ELIMINATION

Client's name: _____

1. Maintain the diet recommended. Allow for sufficient time for each meal.
2. Schedule a regular time to go to the bathroom.
3. The urge to defecate is a natural process. DO NOT IGNORE IT.
4. Allow sufficient time for defecation.
5. Notify _____ of any change in bowel habits or if there is any change in color, consistency, or regularity of stool.
6. Drink _____ glasses of fluids each day.
7. Do not strain or use excessive effort to defecate.
8. Exercise on a regular basis as recommended.

SPECIAL INSTRUCTIONS: (Include here any schedule of supplemental bran, prune juice, use of suppositories or medication.)

Fig. 21-13 Bowel program.

information corrected. Consistency is an important factor in success. Any variance from the established program could have untoward effects.

During the educational experience, the client should be given reassurance and emotional support as well as information. The client may feel overwhelmed at discharge with all the information presented and anxious at the thought of leaving the security of the rehabilitation setting. It is helpful to give the client an outline or fact sheet that details the instructions and can be used as a reference at home (Fig. 21-13). It often is necessary for the family to be involved, since some clients require assistance with the bowel program at home. It also may be helpful for clients or caregivers to record the date and amount of bowel movements so problems can be anticipated and prevented, such as with an impaction (Hull et al., 1980).

DISCHARGE PLANNING AND FOLLOW-UP

The rehabilitation nurse plays a major role in coordinating the discharge plan and community referrals. Supplies and equipment needs related to the client's bowel program must be considered and arranged well in advance. If a bedside commode will be required, this must be coordinated with the appropriate therapy department for ordering. Clients with SCI may require a suppository inserter in order to be independent in their program. Gloves and lubricant as well as prescriptions for medications need to be arranged.

Each client's needs are different and require different community services, but there are basic considerations when any client with impaired bowel elimination is discharged. The nurse should give attention to the following items:

1. Cost and availability of supplies and equipment needed at home
2. Location of supplier and availability and cost of delivery service
3. Availability of support groups
4. Location of the bathroom in the home
5. Family or agency assistance needed at home to carry out the bowel program

REHABILITATION TEAM INTERVENTIONS

Although the nurse is the primary team member involved in planning and implementing a successful bowel program with the client and family, other members of the interdisciplinary team offer important input for the successful management of impaired bowel elimination. The physician, dietitian, occupational therapist, physical therapist, and speech pathologist collaborate with the nurse to plan interventions based on individual needs.

The physician prescribes treatments and medications and attends to any active medical problems. The dietitian assists the rehabilitation team in meeting the nutritional and fiber needs of the client. The physical therapist assists the client in developing an appropriate exercise program and transfer techniques. The occupational therapist designs adaptive devices to help the individual in managing the bowel program. Also, the occupational therapist and physical therapist perform a home evaluation to determine if any bathroom modifications or adaptive equipment are needed

to carry out the bowel program at home. The speech pathologist assists with helping clients to communicate their needs and, along with the nurse and occupational therapist, assists with feeding and swallowing if a problem is present.

OUTCOME CRITERIA

The following outcome criteria are related to bowel management:

1. In the maintenance and restoration of bowel function and control:
   a. Bowel regularity and continence are restored.
   b. Bowel regularity and continence are maintained.
   c. The client and family (as needed) assume responsibility for the bowel program.
2. In the area of safety, the client and family incorporate safe techniques in managing the bowel program.
3. In the area of education:
   a. The client and family understand the rationale for the bowel program.
   b. The client and family understand causes and prevention of alterations in bowel elimination.
   c. The client and family demonstrate techniques of bowel management.
   d. The client and family are able to problem solve bowel management irregularities.
4. In the area of discharge planning and follow-up:
   a. The client and family use community resources appropriately.
   b. The client and family obtain and utilize needed equipment, supplies, and medication.

FUTURE TRENDS

Control of bowel incontinence and prevention of constipation and diarrhea have been under the purview of the rehabilitation nurse for years. Bowel habits are highly personal, and if not managed effectively can have untoward effects on clients' ability to cope with their disability and to give full effort to the rehabilitation program.

Early research on bowel elimination began in the 1960s. It focused primarily on the effects of enemas versus suppositories in achieving control and decreasing nursing time and hospital costs. These studies demonstrated the superiority of suppositories in terms of client comfort and control.

A paucity of research in the bowel elimination arena exists after this time. The majority of studies have focused on the effects of dietary fiber in preventing constipation and on studying the transit time of food in the GI tract.

Many rehabilitation hospitals and units have their own individual protocols for maintaining bowel control using a variety of techniques, suppositories, medications, and dietary foods and fluids. Little research has been done to prove that one method is better than another. More studies need to be conducted to examine various areas such as what type of suppository works best for a specific diagnosis, which medications are most effective, and when digital stimulation should be used. The nurse is in the best position to initiate future studies in order to validate rehabilitation nursing practice in the area of bowel elimination.

◆

CASE STUDY

ASSESSMENT

R.S. is an Hispanic 55-year-old engineer diagnosed with a right hemisphere cerebrovascular accident. He is married with no children. His wife works as a sales clerk in a bookstore.

Upon admission to the rehabilitation unit, the RN notices weakness in both left upper and lower extremities. R.S. is alert and oriented with some slurred speech. An in-depth history is taken. R.S. denies any past bowel problems. He usually emptied his bowels daily or every other day at 7 AM. Since his stroke 8 days ago, he has been incontinent and has felt a sense of urgency. His last bowel movement was 2 days before admission. Enemas or laxatives have never been used in the past.

Upon physical examination, the nurse noted no abdominal distention, visible peristalsis, masses, or bulges. Normal bowel sounds were auscultated. Percussion and abdominal palpation were normal. A rectal examination revealed a small amount of hard stool. A strong anal reflex was present as was sensation. No rectal excoriations or lesions were present.

R.S. has his own teeth and a bedside swallowing examination conducted by the speech pathologist was normal. R.S. usually drank only coffee on arising, had a sandwich for lunch, and ate a full dinner of Mexican cuisine (usually tortillas, beef, and beans as well as salad). Less than two glasses of fluid, other than coffee, were usually consumed in a day.

R.S. stated he was anxious to improve as quickly as possible in order to return home and to work. His wife concurred with this plan and stated that he needed to be as independent as possible since she also works. Current medications revealed none that would cause a problem with either constipation or diarrhea.

NURSING DIAGNOSIS AND GOALS

A nursing diagnosis of Bowel Incontinence due to uninhibited neurogenic bowel was made. The nurse explained to R.S. and his wife how a stroke can affect bowel function. The long-term goals mutually established with R.S. and his wife were to
1. Achieve control without accidents on the toilet on a daily or every-other-day basis at 7 AM without the need for suppositories or medications
2. Avoid any complications of constipation or diarrhea
3. Demonstrate the techniques of bowel management and assume responsibility for the program
   The short-term goals were to
1. Achieve control without accidents on the toilet daily at 8:30 AM with the use of stool softeners and daily suppositories
2. Avoid any complications of constipation or diarrhea
3. Understand the rationale for the bowel program
4. Understand the causes and prevention of alterations in bowel management

INTERVENTIONS

Interventions for establishing bowel control were established by the nurse in consultation with R.S. and his wife. Since R.S.'s usual time was 7 AM after a cup of coffee, and it was felt that this would still allow him sufficient time to get to work, an AM program was established.

In exploring R.S.'s usual diet, good fiber was present in the salads and beans and tortillas, but fruits and vegetables were low in frequency. The importance of fiber in motility and bulk of the stool was explained to R.S. and his wife. R.S. stated that he believed that eating beans helped his bowels move. The nurse concurred with him and explained the fiber content of beans. A consultation between the nurse and dietitian was made to provide a Mexican diet but increase fruits and vegetables. No additional bran was planned for at this time.

The importance of six to eight glasses of fluid per day was explained and this was recorded as an intervention and also discussed with the dietitian. It was felt that good exercise and mobility would be accomplished through increasing wheelchair endurance, therapy activity, and beginning to perform his own activities of daily living (ADLs).

The RN planned for evacuation to take place on a commode over the toilet in the bathroom where privacy would also be maintained. This would be particularly important with R.S.'s Hispanic background. The commode would permit a safety belt to be applied around R.S. to prevent a fall until it could be determined that no problem existed.

A stool softener (Surfak, 1 twice daily) was initiated along with a bisacodyl suppository every day 30 minutes after breakfast. The RN explained the purposes of each. Since R.S. had not had a bowel movement in 2 days and stool in the rectum was hard, the RN decided to order a bisacodyl tablet, per hospital established protocol, to be given at HS on a one-time basis to clean the bowel.

IMPLEMENTATION AND EVALUATION

The next day R.S. had good results on the bathroom commode after a suppository. R.S. maintained this program for 5 days without accidents. On the sixth day the RN noticed that his stools were becoming too soft. Surfak was decreased to once a day at bedtime after agreement with R.S. On the eighth day R.S. had no results, but on the ninth day a good bowel movement was achieved. Again on the tenth day there were no results. The RN decided to change R.S.'s program to every other day with his concurrence.

On the twelfth day R.S. began to have a bowel movement on his own without the need for a suppository. This occurred again on the fourteenth day. The RN placed his suppository on an as-needed basis "if no bowel movement in 2 days." The rehabilitation team members agreed that he had good safety awareness, so the commode was discontinued and R.S. began using a regular toilet seat.

Fluid intake of six to eight glasses each day was able to be achieved. A planning team conference determined that R.S. would be ready for discharge by the twenty-first day following his admission. He was doing well in ambulation with physical therapy and needed minimum to moderate assistance in ADLs.

TEACHING AND DISCHARGE PLANNING

Teaching continued with R.S. and his wife. The nurse proposed problem-solving situations for both of them. She asked them, for example, what they would do if R.S. didn't have a bowel movement in 3 days once he was home. R.S. replied that he would use a suppository and add more fiber and fluid to his diet.

On the sixteenth day the nurse decided to discontinue the remaining daily Surfak. R.S. remained continent with a daily or every-other-day bowel movement.

On the day of discharge, the RN told R.S. to feel free to call her if any questions or problems arose following discharge. R.S. had been informed where to purchase over-the-counter stool softeners or suppositories if needed. It was also explained that plastic wrap could be used in place of expensive latex gloves for use with suppository insertion, if needed.

REFERENCES

Behm, R. (1985). A special recipe to banish constipation. *Geriatric Nursing, 6,* 216-217.

Benson, J.A. (1975). Simple chronic constipation: Pathophysiology and management. *Postgraduate Medicine, 57,* 55-60.

Berger, K.J., & Williams, M.B. (Eds.). (1992). *Fundamentals of nursing collaborating for optimal health.* Norwalk: Appleton & Lange.

Brocklehurst, J.C. (1980). Disorders of the lower bowel in old age. *Geriatrics, 35,* 47-54.

Brown, M.K., & Everett, I. (1990). Gentler bowel fitness with fiber: A recipe for bowel regularity and cost savings too. *Geriatric Nursing, 11,* 26-27.

Brunton, L.L. (1990). Agents affecting gastrointestinal water flux and motility, digestants, and bile acids. In A.G. Gilman, T.W. Rall, A.S. Nies, & P. Taylor (Eds.), *The pharmacological basis of therapeutics* (8th ed.). New York: Pergmon Press.

Burkitt, D.P., & Meisner, P. (1979). How to manage constipation with high-fiber diet. *Geriatrics, 34,* 33-35, 38-40.

Cannon, B. (1981). Bowel function. In N. Martin, N. Holt, & D. Hicks (Eds.), *Comprehensive rehabilitation nursing.* New York: McGraw-Hill (pp. 223-241).

Coffman, S. (1986). Description of a nursing diagnosis: alteration in bowel elimination related to neurogenic bowel in children with myelomeningocele. *Issues in Comprehensive Pediatric Nursing, 9,* 179-191.

Connell, A.M., Hilton, C., Irvine, C., Lennard-Jones, J.E., & Misiewicz, J.J. (1965). Variation of bowel habit in two population samples. *British Medical Journal 2,* 1095-1099.

Devroede, G. (1978). Dietary fiber, bowel habits, and colonic function. *American Journal of Clinical Nutrition, 31.* S157.

Ellickson, E.B. (1988). Bowel management plan for the homebound elderly. *Journal of Gerontological Nursing, 14,* 16-19, 40-42.

Friedman, G. (1989). Nutritional therapy of irritable bowel syndrome. *Gastroenterology Clinics of North America, 18,* 513-524.

Gleeson, R.M. (1990). Bowel continence for the child with a neurogenic bowel. *Rehabilitation Nursing, 15,* 319-321.

Gordon, M. (1993–1994). *Manual of Nursing Diagnosis.* St. Louis: Mosby–Year Book.

Guyton, A.C. (1991). *Textbook of medical physiology* (8th ed.). Philadelphia: W.B. Saunders.

Hoeman, S.P. (1989). Cultural assessment in rehabilitation nursing practice. *Nursing Clinics of North America, 24,* 277-289.

Hogstel, M.O., & Nelson, M. (1992). Anticipation and early detection can reduce bowel elimination complications. *Geriatric Nursing, 13,* 28-33.

Hull, C., Greco, R., Brooks, D.L. (1980). Alleviation of constipation in the elderly by dietary fiber supplementation. *Journal of American Geriatric Society 28,* 410-414.

Iseminger, M., & Hardy, P. (1982). Bran works! *Geriatric Nursing, 3,* 402-404.

Jones, V.A., McLaughlan, P., Shorthouse, M., Workman, E., & Hunter, J.O. (1982). Food intolerance: A major factor in the pathogenesis of irritable bowel syndrome. *Lancet 2,* 1115-1117.

McCourt, A.E. (Ed.). (1993). *The specialty practice of rehabilitation nursing; A core curriculum* (3rd ed.). Skokie, IL: Rehabilitation Nursing Foundation.

Munchiando, J.F., & Kendall, K. (1993). Comparison of the effectiveness of two bowel programs for CVA patients. *Rehabilitation Nursing, 18,* 168-172.

Rauen, K.K., & Aubert, E.J. (1992). A brighter future for adults who have myelomeningocele—one form of spina bifida: A comprehensive overview of this complex disease. *Orthopaedic Nursing, 11,* 16-27.

Resnick, B. (1985). Constipation: Common but preventable. *Geriatric Nursing, 6,* 213-215.

Ross, D.G. (1990). Constipation among hospitalized elders. *Orthopaedic Nursing, 9,* 73-77.

Ross, D.G. (1993). Subjective data related to altered bowel elimination patterns among hospitalized elder and middle-aged persons. *Orthopedic Nursing, 12,* 25-32.

Saltzstein, R.J., & Romano, J. (1990). The efficacy of colostomy as a bowel management alternative in selected spinal cord injury patients. *Journal of American Paraplegia Society, 13,* 9-13.

Smith, D.A. (1988). Continence restoration in the homebound patient. *Nursing Clinics of North America, 23,* 207-218.

Smith, K.A. (1990). Bowel and bladder management of the child with myelomeningocele in the school setting. *Journal of Pediatric Healthcare, 4(4),* 175-180.

Venn, M.R., Taft, L., Carpentier, I.B., Applebaugh, A. (1992). The influence of timing and suppository use on efficiency and effectiveness of bowel training after a stroke. *Rehabilitation Nursing, 17,* 116-121.

Wald, A. (1991). Approach to the patient with constipation. In T. Yamada (Ed.), *Textbook of gastroenterology* (Vol. 1). New York: J.B. Lippincott (pp. 779-796).

White, M., & Williams, J. (1992). A good start to a full life: Managing continence in children with spina bifida and hydrocephalus. *Professional Nurse, 7,* 474, 476-477.

Wrick, K.L., Robertson, J.B., Van Soest, P.J., Lewis, B.A., Rivers, J.M., Roe, D.A., & Hackler, L.R. (1983). The influence of dietary fiber source on human intestinal transit and stool output. *Journal of Nutrition, 113,* 1464-1479.

Zejdlik, C.P. (1992). *Management of spinal cord injury.* Boston: Jones and Bartlett.

IV

SENSORY AND PSYCHOSOCIAL PATTERNS

22

Impact of Regulatory and Immune Systems

Margaret J. Griffiths, MSN, RN

INTRODUCTION

With respect to physiologic functioning, the human body has several mechanisms to prevent invasion by foreign substances and subsequent development of disease. The skin is the first line of defense; an intact skin tissue serves to protect the internal environment from harmful organisms that flourish in the external environment. If invasion by microorganisms does take place, however, the body responds by activating the inflammatory process to render these agents incapable of altering homeostasis. If this secondary mechanism fails, the body relies on the complexity of the immune response to neutralize or destroy the invading organisms. Key to these safeguards is the mechanism of temperature regulation. This chapter discusses these processes as primary lines of defense in maintaining homeostasis.

TEMPERATURE REGULATION

The maintenance of normal body temperature is vital to life. Normally body temperatures vary from person to person and may range from 96.4° to 100° F (35.8° to 37.8° C). For every degree of elevation in body temperature, the demand for oxygen and nutrients increases; likewise, with a decrease in body temperature, the demand for these elements decreases. Under normal circumstances internal body temperature remains relatively constant. Even in abnormal circumstances a constant body temperature is maintained by the use of internal defense mechanisms and feedback systems.

Mechanisms of Body Temperature Control

The hypothalamus, located in the brain beneath the thalamus, is the center for control of body temperature. It consists of several structures and forms the wall of the third ventricle. The hypothalamus also controls metabolic activities such as maintenance of water balance, glucose levels, and fat metabolism. The temperature control function of the hypothalamus is regulated by neural feedback. Sensitive receptors located in the preoptic area of the anterior hypothalamus maintain body heat equilibrium. Heat-sensitive receptors increase their output as the environmental temperature decreases; cold-sensitive receptors decrease their output when the environmental temperature increases. Heat and cold receptors in the skin transmit impulses by way of the spinal cord to the hypothalamus to help control body temperature. Figure 22-1 illustrates the temperature-regulating mechanism of the hypothalamus.

Shivering

The dorsomedial portion of the posterior hypothalamus is the primary motor center for shivering. This area is inhibited by the preoptic thermostatic area. When the preoptic area is cooled, the normal inhibition of the primary motor area is denervated. The self-excitation mechanism of this area causes it to transmit impulses through the bilateral tracts of the brain to the brainstem and the lateral columns of the spinal cord, increasing tone of the skeletal muscles throughout the body. When the tone increases to a certain level, shivering begins. During shivering, body heat production rises as high as 100% to 200% above normal. The intensity of the shivering response depends on the activity of the anterior hypothalamus and cerebellum. The cerebellum controls the rhythm of the shivering, and tracts in the spinal cord control the frequency. Treatment of shivering is directed at modifying or interfering with the rate of heat loss by warming the body or manipulating the environmental temperature (Holtzclaw, 1990).

Sweating

Overstimulation of the preoptic thermostatic area of the hypothalamus results in sweating. Sweat glands, located in the subcutaneous layer of the skin, can be stimulated, thus causing heat loss by evaporation. Most of these glands are controlled by the sympathetic postganglionic cholinergic division of the autonomic nervous system. Vasodilation of blood vessels occurs when the sympathetic centers of the posterior hypothalamus are inhibited. When internal body temperature falls below 98.6° F (37° C), sympathetic areas located in the posterior hypothalamus send impulses to constrict blood vessels over the entire skin surface. In response to these skin receptors, the preoptic thermostatic area is inhibited and causes sweating to cease. The body's evaporative cooling mechanism is then halted. Sweating begins at precisely 37° C and increases rapidly as the temperature rises. Conversely, sweating ceases when the temperature falls below this level.

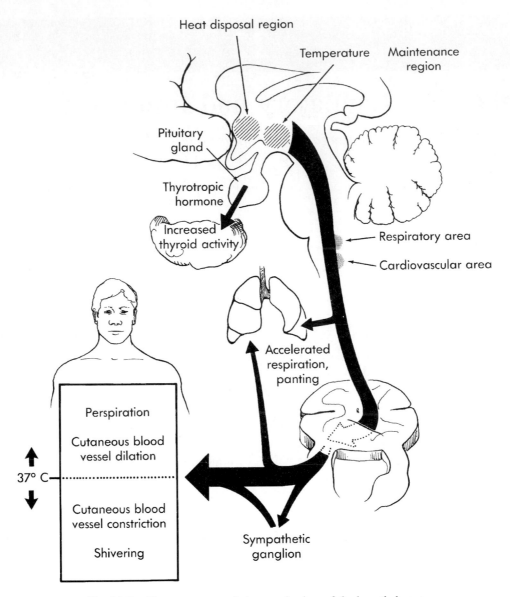

Fig. 22-1   Temperature-regulating mechanism of the hypothalamus.

FACTORS AFFECTING BODY TEMPERATURE

To assess temperature variations and evaluate the significance of changes from normal, the nurse must be aware of the factors that affect body temperature.

Age

In neonates and infants the mechanisms to control body temperature are not fully developed; therefore body temperature may change drastically with changes in the environmental temperature. A newborn loses up to 30% of body heat through the head and needs to have this source of heat loss addressed in order to prevent physiologic problems. When protected from environmental extremes by head caps, for example, the newborn's body temperature is maintained within acceptable limits. Infants and toddlers have a higher metabolic rate, thus resulting in a higher body temperature. Heat production steadily declines as the younger child grows into school age. Temperature regulation is unstable until children reach puberty, and individual differences in body temperature of fractions of degrees are acceptable variations in children (Potter & Perry, 1993). The range of temperature considered to be normal gradually drops as individuals approach older adulthood. At this age level it is not unusual to see oral temperatures of 36° C (96.8° F) accepted as being within normal limits. Older adults are particularly sensitive to temperature extremes because of deterioration in thermoregulation; the thermoreceptors in the hypothalamus may be impaired because of disease, injury, or degenerative changes. Other factors include poor vasomotor control, structural and functional changes in subcutaneous tissue, reduced sweat gland activity, decreased circulation, and reduced metabolism. The elderly, because they have less heat to lose before reaching the hypothermic state, are at particular risk for developing intraoperative hypothermia (Burkle, 1988). The presence of elevated body temperatures also can interfere with absorption of some medications commonly taken by elderly persons. In summary, infants and older adults are most likely to be affected by environmental temperatures because their temperature-regulating mechanisms are less efficient.

Exercise

Muscle activity requires an increased blood supply and an increase in carbohydrate and fat breakdown for more energy. This increased metabolism causes an increase in heat production. Any form of exercise can cause increased heat production and consequently elevate body temperature. Prolonged periods of exercise can increase body temperature to levels considered beyond normal without any underlying pathology. Once the systemic effects of the exercise have been balanced, the temperature returns to normal. Conversely lack of exercise will have an effect on lowering body temperature, particularly in combination with external conditions such as lowered environmental temperature.

Hormone Level

Because of the influence of hormones, women generally experience greater fluctuations in temperature regulation than do men. Women who are ovulating have a body temperature that often rises and falls, but during the time following ovulation the temperature remains elevated until the onset of menstruation. Body temperature changes also occur in women during menopause. Women who have stopped menstruating may experience periods of intense heat and sweating which last for variable periods of time. These alterations in body temperature regulation are thought to be related to the influence of hormones on the vasomotor controls for vasodilation and vasoconstriction. Other essential hormones not related to reproductive function also affect heat production and the basal metabolic rate.

Circadian Rhythms

Temperature is one of the most stable rhythms in humans. However, body temperature generally changes slightly during the course of a day and is an important indicator of health status. Temperature usually is lowest between 2 and 6 AM. During the day hours temperature rises until approximately 8 PM. From this point it then declines to the level found in the early morning hours. At one time daily temperature fluctuations were related to the level of activity the individual pursued during the day. Research, however, has shown that the lowered nighttime body temperature is not necessarily related to inactivity at this time. Subtle variations in temperature patterns exist in each human being; this understanding should be incorporated into any process related to making decisions regarding alteration in body temperatures.

Stress

Physical and emotional stress increase body temperature through hormonal and neural stimulation. With stress the client will experience increased respiratory rate and increased cardiac rate. Emotional states lead to increased metabolic rates, probably caused by the interactions of nervous system stimulation, hormone secretion, and muscle contraction. Increased heat production and a reading of a higher than normal temperature may be obtained without any underlying pathology to serve as an originating factor.

Preexisting Disease

All individuals with diabetes mellitus, cardiovascular disease, and obesity, as well as those individuals who abuse alcohol, are at risk for experiencing elevated body temperatures. In addition, the existence of impaired mental/cognitive functioning may preclude the ability to make sound judgments about environmental conditions and to act appropriately to extremes in environmental conditions.

Environment

Elevated or decreased body temperatures may be caused by environmental factors. The ambient temperature has a direct bearing on the body's ability to maintain temperature balance.

ELEVATED BODY TEMPERATURE

When body temperature elevates, it indicates that the body is responding to some sort of injury. When injury occurs, the hypothalamus is set at a higher level in an attempt to maintain normal body temperature. The resulting fever may have a known or an unknown etiology. In situations where the precipitating factor is a documented infection, fever may be the result of the body's inflammatory response to eradicate the offending organisms. Fever results from the effects of pyrogenic substances secreted by injured cells. The exudate formed in this process contains substances that produce a fever. Pyrogens, which can be endogenous or exogenous, cause the set point of the hypothalamic thermostat to rise and, within hours of the rise, the body temperature becomes elevated. Figure 22-2 illustrates the phases of the febrile episode related to endogenous pyrogen activity on the hypothalamic set point. When fever occurs as part of the disease state, the controlling mechanisms of the hypothalamus fail and the temperature continues to rise unless measures are taken to promote heat loss. Neurogenic fever, caused by injury to the anterior hypothalamus, results when the ability to promote heat loss is impaired. This finding occurs in individuals with severe closed head injuries and basilar skull fractures.

Clients with spinal cord injury often demonstrate a fever that may be related to the interruption of autonomic nervous system communication with the hypothalamus during the acute phase postinjury. When local reflex activity resumes, the severity of this problem subsides. Other known causes of fever are infections, deep vein thrombosis, pulmonary embolus, and drug hypersensitivities. It also is known that some medications such as phenothiazides, anticholinergics, diuretics, and some antihypertensives also can interfere with heat loss. In those situations where the cause of the elevated body temperature cannot be readily identified, research suggests that the underlying cause may be related to malignancies or collagen-vascular diseases.

Hyperthermia

The clinical term given to body temperatures elevated to 106° F (41° C) or above is hyperthermia. Manifestations of hyperthermia include heat cramps, heat exhaustion, and

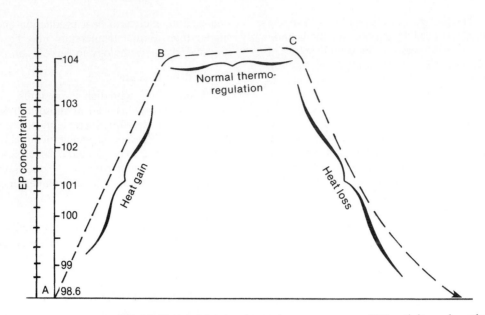

Fig. 22-2 Phases of the febrile episode related to endogenous pyrogen (EP) activity on hypothalamic set point. Dotted line from *A* to *B* indicates chill phase during which warming mechanisms are activated to lessen discrepancy between body temperature and set point; from *B* to *C,* the plateau phase during which discrepancy is alleviated; and from the defervescence phase during which falling EP or accumulated heat mandates heat loss. (From *Basic Pathophysiology: A Holistic Approach, 3rd ed.* by M.W. Groer & M.E. Shekleton, 1990, St. Louis: Mosby–Year Book. Copyright 1990 by Mosby–Year Book. Reprinted by permission.)

heatstroke. Heat cramps—painful muscle spasms triggered by inadequate serum sodium levels—occur in muscles that are used during strenuous activity and may be prevented by allowing for an increased sodium intake. Heat exhaustion is the most common heat-related illness. Sign and symptoms of heat exhaustion include weakness, nausea, and lightheadedness caused by excessive sodium and water loss from heavy sweating. If the underlying fluid and electrolyte deficit is not corrected, heatstroke may result.

Heatstroke is characterized by a body temperature at least 40% above normal and a failure of all body cooling mechanisms. It must be considered a life-threatening condition. The absence of sweating is caused by a failure of or exhaustion of the sweat glands. Signs and symptoms of heatstroke include faintness, dizziness, headache, nausea, rapid pulse, and flushed skin. The affected person may be agitated, confused, stuporous, or comatose. Cerebral and motor dysfunctions that may be evident, such as ataxia and hemiparesis, may be caused by cerebral edema. Clinical findings in the hyperthermic individual include skin that is pale, hot, and dry. Seizures frequently occur when temperature increases to 105° F (40.5° C) and over. Hyperthermia may be preceded by a hypertensive episode, signs of increased intracranial pressure, shivering, quivering, or shaking chill. Figure 22-3 illustrates physiologic responses to heatstroke.

✦ Treatment of hyperthermia

Because of the critical consequences of extreme elevations of temperature on oxygen demands of cerebral tissue, it is imperative to recognize and begin aggressive treatment of hyperthermia immediately. Antipyretics are administered and are effective in most situations in reducing temperature elevations. In cases in which hypothalamic control of temperature is altered, however, the use of antipyretics will have no effect. In these cases other measures to cool body temperature need to be initiated. Cool sponge baths (with or without alcohol), ice bags to areas of abundant blood supply such as the axilla and groin, and cooling blankets are effective measures. The instillation of cool fluids into the gastrointestinal system via lavage or enema cools internal tissues and will promote relatively rapid decreases in elevated temperatures. Measures to control the external environment need to be considered as well. Patients with elevated temperatures should be kept in a cool room where air is circulated freely over the body. Since the underlying premise in using these measures is to promote heat loss through evaporation, the use of heavy clothing and/or blankets is not appropriate while attempting to reduce elevated temperatures. In cases of severe hyperthermia, the use of an automatic cooling blanket is indicated. Cautious monitoring of the client for the effects of rapid cooling is warranted. The goal in using a cooling blanket is to reduce the body temperature as quickly as possible without inducing shivering, since shivering can raise body temperature.

Hyperthermia as a Treatment Option

It is interesting to note that hyperthermia also is used, under controlled circumstances, to treat disease. Recently there has been renewed interest in using this phenomenon as a modality in the treatment of cancer. However, hyperthermia has a long history as a method of treatment. Its

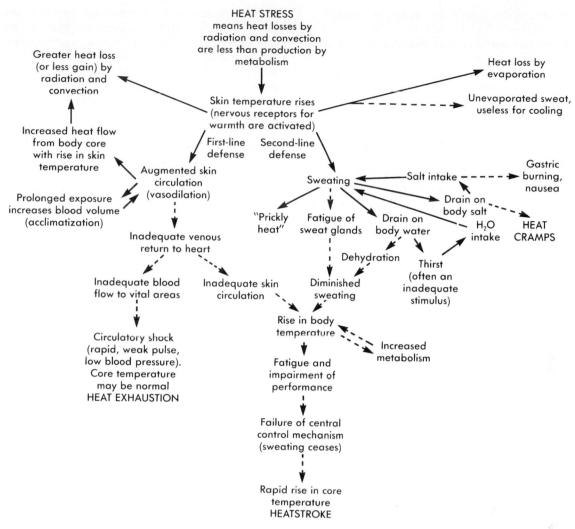

Fig. 22-3 Physiologic responses to heat stress. Solid lines indicate usual response; directions of arrows show cause-and-effect relationships. Broken lines denote events leading to injury. (From *Clinical Nursing: Pathophysiological and Psychosocial Approaches,* 4th ed. by I.L. Beland and J.Y. Passos, 1981, New York: Macmillan. Copyright 1981 by Macmillan. Reprinted by permission.)

medical use is documented in the literature extending back to the time of the ancient Greeks. Hippocrates wrote in 400 BC of heated sticks inserted into tumors of the skin and stated, "The diseases that cannot be cured by medicine, could be cured by surgery. Those that cannot be cured by surgery can be cured by heat, and those that heat does not cure must be considered incurable." The first modern-era scientist to recognize a relationship between hyperthermia and cancer was Busch in 1866 when he noticed a sarcoma of the face cleared after a fever caused by erysipelas. Coley, in 1893, noticed an improvement when fever was induced. In 1898 Westermark used localized heat to produce tumor regression by way of hot water circulated over uterine tumors. In the early 1900s a number of investigators studied the use of heat (generated by electromagnetic frequencies between 0.5 and 100 MHz) as a treatment of malignant and nonmalignant tumors. Although the techniques for hyperthermia delivery and measurement of tissue temperature

were crude, the general conclusions from those works regarding the relationship between time, temperature, and cell killing remain valid today.

The purpose of hyperthermia is to heat the tumor tissue to temperatures of 40° C or higher (about 109° F). Hyperthermia causes a number of effects at the cellular and tissue level that provide the rationale for its use in cancer therapy. When temperatures reach 40° C, there is increased blood flow to the tissue. When the temperature exceeds 41.5° C, cellular cytotoxicity is observed. Cytotoxicity is pronounced at low pH and also in cells that are in the S phase of the cell cycle. Malignant tumors often present these characteristics. That is why heat can have a greater cytotoxic effect in the tumor than in normal tissue. At temperatures above 42.5° C vascular destruction occurs in tumor. Hyperthermia also lowers the resistance of some cancer cells to radiation so that radiation therapy has a greater effect.

Heat is applied to the area of the tumor by using tiny, closed-ended catheters referred to as probes. These are used to house the thermometers or heat antennae during each treatment. An average of three to five probes are placed per tumor site for external heat treatments and are stitched into place. These probes remain in place for the duration of the hyperthermia treatments, which are given one to four times per week and usually last for four to five weeks. Since the probes are closed-ended, the risk for infection is minimal. The probes are removed once the therapy is completed. Hyperthermia usually is a painless procedure using microwaves, ultrasound, or radiofrequency waves to heat a tumor and surrounding tissues. Depending on the composition of the tissues and the volume and depth to be treated, one or several methods of heat delivery may be used in treatment. External heat is administered by placing an applicator, which is soft and pliable, directly in contact with the tumor area. It generally causes little to no discomfort to the client, although some surface heat sensation may be experienced. Interstitial heat is administered by placing microwave heat antennae into the catheter probes. This heat is delivered directly into the tumor where the catheters are placed and is used for larger volume, deep-seated tumor tissue.

Although it cannot cure cancer by itself, hyperthermia can slow the growth of cancer cells, shrink the tumor size, reduce pressure and bleeding, alleviate pain, and generally enhance the quality of life in cancer clients with advanced disease.

Malignant Hyperthermia

The term malignant in this case refers to the rapid progressive nature of the condition, which may become fatal if not promptly recognized and treated. Hyperthermia refers to the rapid rise in body temperature that occurs in operative clients. Malignant hyperthermia is an inherited disorder of abnormal muscle metabolism characterized by an uncontrollable increase in muscle metabolism and heat production in response to stress or certain anesthetics. The exact pathophysiology of malignant hyperthermia is not completely understood but appears to result from an alteration of the calcium-storing properties of the cellular or intracellular muscle cell membrane. Clinical signs of malignant hyperthermia include tachycardia, tachypnea, profuse sweating, and cardiac dysrhythmias. Vasomotor changes and muscle rigidity also may be evident. The only specific treatment for this condition is the administration of a muscle relaxant, along with cessation of the anesthetic agent (Frederick, Rosemann, & Austin, 1990).

DECREASED BODY TEMPERATURE

Hypothermia is the clinical term for body temperature decreased below 35° C (95° F) and occurs when cold persists and heat loss exceeds heat production. The body attempts to compensate for heat loss by shivering. This mechanism of maintaining body temperature usually is adequate when the environmental temperature is not extreme. Hypothermia usually develops gradually and may not be noticed for several hours. Generally, changes in sensorium are early indications of decreasing body temperature. Skin temperatures may decrease gradually to approximately 35° C (95° F),

which will precipitate uncontrolled shivering. It is important to remember that core body temperature—that is, the temperature of vital internal organs—must remain at a relatively constant level to prevent physiologic changes. If body temperature falls to below 34.4° C (94° F), heart and respiratory rates and blood pressure begin to fail and the skin becomes cyanotic. Permanent circulatory and tissue damage may occur. Sustained hypothermia may produce cardiac rhythm abnormalities, compromised respirations, loss of consciousness, and ultimately death (Cox, 1992).

Destructive lesions impairing the function of the hypothalamus also may cause hypothermia through loss of the mechanism that produces shivering and vasoconstriction. Because the fibers for both gain and loss of heat must pass through the hypothalamus to reach the brainstem, large hypothalamic lesions could produce a loss in both responses, causing a poikilothermic state in which the client's temperature matches that of the environment. Causes of hypothermia other than a lesion interrupting hypothalamic or brainstem function are starvation, spinal shock, metabolic or toxic coma, and terminal illness, particularly neurologic disease. Clients most at risk include infants, older adults, and persons debilitated by trauma, stroke, diabetes, drug or alcohol consumption, sepsis, and Raynaud's disease (Buczkowski-Bickmann, 1992). Particular concern must be given to mentally ill or handicapped clients and the homeless because they are unaware of the potential dangers of cold temperatures. Persons who have inadequate clothing and poor diet also are at risk. Additional causes of hypothermia include accidental immersion in cold water or prolonged periods of outdoor exposure to subzero temperatures without adequate clothing or with wet clothing; consumption of alcohol combined with exposure to cold temperatures, resulting in vasodilation and consequent heat loss; and depression of the central nervous system by morphine and barbiturates (Wright, 1991). Age, sex, weight, and physical condition also are factors that affect the response of persons exposed to a cold environment. In addition, a slowed metabolic rate accompanied by a slow pulse, hypotension, oliguria, and atrial arrhythmias can contribute to or exaggerate hypothermia. Hypothermia also can be artificially induced by external or surface cooling, internal or body cavity cooling, or extracorporeal cooling. These procedures are used to decrease oxygen needs of the brain when open heart surgery and neurosurgery are performed. Clinical findings in the hypothermic client include, in addition to a body temperature less than 98.6° F, bradycardia, bradypnea, and decrease in the level of consciousness.

Treatment of Hypothermia

Rewarming can be either passive or core and is the priority treatment for hypothermia. Passive rewarming are those interventions undertaken to rewarm externally, and core rewarming refers to efforts to raise the temperature of the internal body cavity and organs. In the conscious client the goal is to prevent a further decrease in body temperature by removing cold wet clothes and wrapping warm blankets around the individual. Encouraging the intake of hot liquids and increasing the temperature of the environment also are effective passive measures to elevate body temperature. Individuals who are exposed to extremes in low temperatures without adequate protection also may experience frostbite of the hands, feet, and face. The following Box discusses appropriate measures to prevent further tissue damage in this situation.

In cases of severe hypothermia, rewarming of the body core is the immediate priority. Heated oxygen mist is a common therapy used in core rewarming and is a most important adjunct in resuscitating hypothermic individuals. Although by itself it can raise core temperature only 1° C to 2° C/hour and must be supplemented by other modalities, it is safe and easy to use. The transfer of heat from the airway to the mediastinum is rapid, resulting in the return of warmed, well-oxygenated blood from the lungs to the heart. This leads to myocardial warming both through direct heating of the endocardium and through coronary perfusion. Myocardial warming may in turn decrease the risk of ventricular fibrillation (Nelson, 1988). The infusion of warmed intravenous solutions or the use of warm fluids in gastric or peritoneal lavage is successful in contributing to an increase in core temperature. Warmed peritoneal fluids provide rapid rewarming. Although warmed intravenous fluids will very slowly increase core temperature, they, like warm humidified oxygen, are more of an adjunct than a primary means of raising core temperature. The use of cardiopulmonary bypass is also a very effective way to rapidly rewarm the hyperthermic client, and in many institutions partial cardiac bypass is considered the rewarming method of choice, especially if the client also is suffering from cardiac arrest. Heating pads and hyperthermic blankets also are used frequently (Dexter, 1990). Caution must be exercised, however, to initiate core rewarming for the profoundly hypothermic individual before peripheral rewarming is started. With the hypothermic blanket the desired temperature is set and an electronic probe is inserted into the rectum. With the probe so positioned, an automatic thermostat is activated. A client with both heat loss and heat production problems may need to be altered between the cooling and warming mechanisms to maintain a normal range of body tem-

---

✦

EMERGENCY TREATMENT OF FROSTBITE

Hands: tuck into the person's armpits under the coat.
Face: cover with dry, gloved hands until normal color returns.
Feet: slightly elevate feet off cold ground.

✦ Take the person inside or under shelter to increase body temperature.
✦ Put the affected area in warm water (104°-108° F) for 15-30 minutes.
✦ Observe the affected area for change in skin color to pink or bright red. This indicates that thawing is complete.
✦ Small blisters will form on the area and will burst in 4-10 days. Normal tissue forms beneath the scabs. Keep this healing area clean and do not cover with bandages or dressings.
✦ Protect healing area from refreezing or excessive heat.
✦ If joints are affected, exercise them regularly to preserve flexibility (Lavoy, 1985).

---

perature (Danzl & Ghezzi, 1991). Hypothermic clients require electrocardiographic monitoring throughout the warming process. Warming should proceed slowly at approximately 1° to 2° F/hour. If, however, the core temperature is below 31° C, rewarming may need to progress more rapidly because of the severity of the hypothermia and the instability of the myocardium at these temperatures (Cox, 1992). Problems occurring during rewarming may reflect the fact that hypothermia may be hiding a variety of other illnesses such as sepsis, endocrinopathy, drug overdose, head trauma, or acute myocardial infarction (Lawson, 1992). Urinary output, vital signs, and neurologic assessments need to be assessed every 15 minutes until the client's condition has stabilized and rewarming has effected a significant rise in the core body temperature. Clinical signs of neurologic impairment, commonly found in individuals who are profoundly hypothermic, are not necessarily irreversible. All efforts should be undertaken aggressively to begin rewarming for clients who display these signs (Michal, 1989).

SPECIFIC CONDITIONS ACCOMPANIED BY ALTERED BODY TEMPERATURE

Several pathologic states are unique in that they predispose clients to alterations in the body's ability to maintain a temperature within normal limits.

Spinal Cord Injury

After a spinal cord injury, every body system may be involved in attempts to maintain homeostasis. Fever is common in clients who sustain cervical spinal cord injuries. It is thought that disturbed thermoregulatory control in clients with spinal cord injury is caused by loss of autonomic control over vasomotor activity and the sweating mechanism. This problem is particularly prominent in clients with quadriplegia who are unable to maintain a desirable central temperature when not protected from changes in environmental temperatures. After injury, individuals with damage to the spinal cord above the thoracolumbar outflow of the sympathetic nervous system lose function in the hypothalamic thermoregulatory mechanisms. They are unable to internally control temperature below the level of the lesion, mainly because of absence of vasoconstriction, loss of ability to shiver to conserve body heat, and loss of thermoregulatory sweating to dissipate heat. With chronic loss of vasomotor tone and passive vasodilation, body heat tends to be lost continually.

Clients with complete spinal cord lesions sweat only above the level of the lesion. However, those with incomplete lesions can sweat both above and below the level of the lesion. When sweating becomes excessive in persons with lesions above the T6 spinal cord level, autonomic dysreflexia should be suspected, and measures should be instituted to treat this problem. Because controlling body temperature is difficult in clients with high cervical injuries and possible damage to the hypothalamus and brainstem, these individuals must be monitored closely for alterations in body temperature that might be signs of brainstem or medullary dysfunction. Infection, deep vein thrombosis, and emboli are additional common causes of fever in clients with spinal cord injuries.

Head Trauma

The most frequent causes of head trauma are falls, gunshot wounds, and motorcycle accidents, occurring in males between the ages of 15 and 30. The prognosis for these individuals depends on the severity of the injury, the area of the brain involved, and the duration of coma. Hyperthermia during the acute phase of head trauma is an indicator of damage to the hypothalamus or brainstem. Other causes of elevated body temperature are dehydration and infection. When the temperature becomes elevated, metabolic demands increase, producing an increase in the elimination of carbon dioxide to the cells. Carbon dioxide acts as a vasodilator and causes an increase in intracranial pressure. If the client already has increased intracranial pressure, hyperthermia will lead to further damage. When oxygen supply to the cerebral tissue is insufficient, cerebral ischemia develops. Therefore it is imperative to treat hyperthermia in the client with head injury rapidly and effectively.

Cerebrovascular Accidents

A cerebrovascular accident is caused by interruption of blood flow to an area of the brain, resulting in ischemia, necrosis, and often permanent damage to neurons and neural pathways. Among the contributing facts are hypertension, diabetes, obesity, heavy smoking, high cholesterol levels, and sedentary lifestyles. Arteriosclerosis, hardening of the arteries, and atherosclerosis, narrowing of the arteries caused by the accumulation of fatty deposits, commonly are found in clients who have suffered a cerebrovascular accident. Hyperthermia in the acute phase of a cerebrovascular accident can result from damage to the brainstem or hypothalamus. Substantial temperature elevations seen in clients with hemorrhagic stroke or subarachnoid hemorrhage can be caused by blood in the cerebrospinal fluid contributing to hypothalamic dysfunction or the development of aseptic meningitis. Elevated temperatures also can be caused by dehydration and infection.

Multiple Sclerosis

Multiple sclerosis, a disease of the central nervous system, is characterized by plaques forming in the spinal cord, cerebellum, cerebrum, brainstem, and optic nerve. These plaques cause demyelination of the myelin sheaths, subsequently causing destruction of the nerves traveling to the lower limbs, eyes, and to a lesser extent the upper limbs. Although the reason is unknown, there is increased thermosensitivity in clients with demyelinating disease. This is a critical problem, because increased core body temperature exacerbates neurologic symptoms. Thus the use of the "hot bath test" as a diagnostic tool for multiple sclerosis is discouraged.

CLIENT AND FAMILY EDUCATION

A major goal in the rehabilitation of all clients is the prevention of complications and maintenance of functions by client and family. Formal and informal education programs can be used to teach the client about the prevention and treatment of complications occurring with alteration in body temperature. Information about changes in body temperature should be incorporated into educational programs for all clients with cerebrovascular accidents, spinal cord injuries, head trauma, and multiple sclerosis. Community-based educational programs for parents of young children and elderly persons can help prevent hyperthermia and hypothermia in these special age groups. Inpatient programs should stress prevention of infections and fever. For example, the majority of clients with spinal cord injury readmitted to hospitals are admitted because of infected pressure sores, urinary tract infections, respiratory tract infections, and generalized septicemia. With proper education a client and family can learn to prevent these complications and decrease the length and cost of hospitalization. Since clients with altered neurologic sensation have difficulty differentiating hot and cold, they must always be conscious of extremes in temperature. Clients with cerebrovascular accidents and spinal cord injuries must beware of hot stoves, hot water in bathtubs, and overexposure to the sun. These clients can be burned severely in short exposures to the sun. Excessive heat in the form of hot baths also can exacerbate symptoms in clients with multiple sclerosis.

Prevention of hyperthermia can be accomplished in several ways. The elderly are particularly susceptible to the effects of heat, especially if they are hypertensive, diabetic, obese, consume large quantities of alcohol, or have poor dietary habits. Risk factors can be reduced by teaching the client to stay inside or in the shade during the heat of the day and to wear light, loose-fitting clothing and a hat when going outside. The family also should be informed about these precautions. The home can be made cooler by the use of shades and drapes to block the sun, the use of fans or air conditioners if the client can afford them (tax deductible if medically prescribed), and by cooking only during the coolest part of the day. Clients should drink plenty of fluids and limit exercise to cool times of the day. Hypothermia also is preventable. Emphasis should be placed on the fact that the ingestion of alcohol is contraindicated during prolonged exposure to the cold. Clients susceptible to cold, especially the elderly, should pay attention to weather reports, especially wind chill factors. Clothing should be worn in layers, preferably natural fibers that conserve body heat. Any layers that become wet should be removed promptly to prevent heat loss. The home should be heated adequately. With the high cost of home heating fuel, this can be difficult, but community agencies can aid clients in defraying costs. Clients should be cautioned against the use of kerosene space heaters, and wood-burning stoves, or, when there is no other choice but to use these devices, they should be warned of precautions to take. These appliances can be possible fire hazards and have the potential to emit toxic fumes.

REHABILITATION TEAM INTERVENTIONS

All members of the rehabilitation team play a part in assessment and intervention aimed at controlling body temperature. The physiatrist orders diagnostic tests and establishes the medical regimen for the client. It is the responsibility of the other rehabilitation team members to incorporate these orders into their specific treatment plans and into the team plan for rehabilitation. Clients also may need to be referred to additional medical specialists to facilitate their return to optimal functioning. Depending on the unique needs of the client who has experienced an alteration in thermal regulation, continuing care by neurologists, neurosurgeons, orthopedic surgeons, urologists, internists, endocrinologists, and psychiatrists may be warranted. Psychologists can be helpful in assisting the client with adjustment to disability. Many rehabilitation centers offer services to discharged clients and their families. These centers offer peer-group counseling and discussion groups for significant others and parents of clients.

Physical therapists help the client improve mobility, thus preventing the hazards of immobility that can cause fever. Occupational therapists play a part in teaching the client to avoid hot stoves and baths of extreme cold or hot water. Speech/language pathologists help the client in making needs known by improving speech/language function or using alternatives, such as communication boards or electronic vocal cords. Social workers can provide valuable assistance by evaluating the home environment for potential risks for altered temperature recurrence and in obtaining appropriate housing and clothing to reduce the potential for repeated episodes. Social workers also can assist clients in obtaining financial help for climate controls in the automobile and home and in paying heating/cooling costs (Niederpruem, 1989).

The registered nurse assesses the client's function; plans, implements, and evaluates nursing interventions; reinforces the educational programs of all disciplines; and provides emotional support. Once the client is discharged to home, the community health nurse will provide continuing monitoring, as necessary, so that the client's problems can be fully resolved and complications can be prevented. Finally, the pharmacist needs to be considered a vital contributor to the prevention effort. Careful monitoring of medication regimens and the client's response to them is key to preventing repeated episodes of altered temperature due to medication reactions.

THE IMMUNE RESPONSE

In order to understand the mechanisms involved in the development of disease, it is necessary to have an understanding of the immune response—that is, the process by which individuals become resistant to certain illnesses and diseases. The immune system is a defense mechanism that has the capacity to recognize self from nonself, as well as to attack itself, as in autoimmune diseases. The first sign of the immune system in humans appears in the second trimester of pregnancy and does not become fully developed until some time after birth. Although the fetus receives passive immunity from the mother, primarily in the form of immunoglobulins through the placenta, this protection is incomplete because it is dependent on the organisms the mother herself has been exposed to and has produced antibodies against.

The three primary functions of the immune system are (1) defense—that is, resisting microorganisms; (2) homeostasis—that is, removing worn out cellular components; and (3) surveillance—that is, the perception of and destruction of mutant cells. However, in order to fully understand the immune response, it is important to understand the components of the inflammatory response. For this reason, a brief review follows.

The inflammatory response consists of cellular components and processes, each with a unique role in maintaining the balance of homeostasis. The center of the inflammatory response are the leukocytes and their activity. Mononuclear leukocytes (monocytes) are of two types. Monocytes are large and aggressive cells that have the capacity to digest large numbers of bacteria. Lymphocytes, which release antibodies, act in phagocytosis and assist with tissue repair. Mononuclear leukocytes are slower to respond to infection and exert their effect in the later stages of the inflammatory response.

Polymorphonuclear leukocytes (granulocytes) are the first line of defense and mount an immediate and rapid reaction to an infection. Granulocytes, which arise in the bone marrow, are of three types: neutrophils, basophils, and eosinophils. These cells play varying roles in facilitating the body's reaction to an invading organism by secreting substances that decrease the potential for cell clumping and that allow for the start of phagocytosis. Phagocytosis is the process by which engulfment and digestion of particulate matter is accomplished by the neutrophils particularly (for small particulate matter) and by the macrophages. For phagocytosis to take place, there must be recognition of the offending organism, chemotaxis, and ingestion and subsequent intracellular digestion. In summary, the inflammatory response is a process of phagocytosis utilizing macrophages and granulocytes, which is enhanced by the release of vasoactive substances. The inflammatory response also activates the clotting system and increases serum globulins. Phagocytosis and inflammation are considered nonspecific responses but cannot be divorced from the specific response—that is, the immune response.

The Immune System and Response

This chapter contains detailed information concerning the immune system and related pathophysiology because this is the first inclusion of this information in a rehabilitation nursing book and because many rehabilitation practice settings are developing or redefining guidelines in these areas. With respect to normal physiologic functioning, the immune system serves to protect the body from foreign invaders. These invaders might be disease-producing microorganisms or abnormal cells, such as cancer cells. However, the immune system is actually the body's third and slowest line of defense against such invasion. An intact skin provides the first line of defense. The inflammatory response is second, reacting to an invading organism that has gotten beyond the barrier formed by the skin. As previously described, the inflammatory response annihilates or neutralizes harmful organisms primarily through the process of phagocytosis. When this second line of defense is ineffective or fails completely, then the immune response is launched.

Acting much as a surveillance mechanism, the immune system monitors the internal environment for foreign agents. It is a complex system of organs and cells capable of distinguishing self from nonself, remembering previous invaders, and reacting according to needs as they arise. The primary organs of the immune system are the thymus, lymph nodes, spleen, and tonsils. Contributing to the effort of the immune response are lymphoid tissues in nonlymphoid organs and circulating immune cells such as T cells, B cells, and phagocytes (Bullock, 1992).

The organs responsible for effecting the immune response

NURSING ASSESSMENT FOR CLIENTS WITH ALTERATIONS IN TEMPERATURE REGULATION

1. Health perception and health management pattern
   - ✦ Past or present preexisting medical problems
     Chronic illness
     Repeated infections
     Circulatory problems
     Mobility problems
     Neurologic disorders
     Substance abuse
     Medications
     Radiation, chemotherapy, and/or immunosuppressive
       therapy
   - ✦ Recent exposure to infection/communicable disease
   - ✦ Environmental conditions
     Recent exposure to extremes in temperature and/or
       humidity
     Economic status and ability to access needed
       environmental supports
     Home environment
       Adequate ventilation
       Adequate heat
       Adequate shelter
       Appropriate clothing, blankets, etc.

2. Nutritional-Metabolic Pattern
   - ✦ Vital Signs
     Temperature
     Cardiac rate and rhythm
     Respiratory rate and pattern
     Blood pressure
   - ✦ Fluid and electrolyte balance
     Skin turgor
     Integrity of oral mucosa
     Intake and output
     Serum electrolytes
     Nausea/vomiting
   - ✦ Physical Stature
     Nourishment: over or under ideal weight

   - ✦ Nutritional intake
     Pattern and amount of food
     Alcohol ingestion
     Integrity of oral mucosa
   - ✦ Skin integrity
     Color
     Temperature
     Sensation
     Shivering
     Sweating
     Lesions
   - ✦ Laboratory data
     Arterial blood gas levels
     Complete blood cell count
     Clotting studies

3. Elimination pattern
   Intake and output
   Urinalysis
   Diarrhea

4. Activity-exercise pattern
   Fatigue
   Exercise pattern
   Peripheral pulses
     Rate
     Quality

5. Cognitive-perceptual pattern
   - ✦ Pain related to fever
   - ✦ Neurologic status
     Alert and oriented
     Drowsy
     Confused
     Recent memory loss
     Restless
     Comatose
     Fixed, dilated pupils

---

serve varying roles in this process. The primary function of the thymus is the development of lymphocytes; rapid production of lymphocytes occurs in this region from the early years of life through puberty. During embryonic life most lymphocytes develop from stem cells in the bone marrow and travel to the thymus after birth to be marked as T cells. However, there is also evidence that some lymphocytes are actually in the thymus before birth and, along with other cells, migrate and become the spleen and the lymph nodes. During extrauterine life the role of the thymus is to differentiate lymphocytes into various types of T cells. In this process the thymus alters the surface antigens of these cells, which gives them their identity as T cells, a specialized lymphocyte. Mature and differentiated lymphocytes are re-

leased into the bloodstream, and they relocate in peripheral lymph tissue such as lymph nodes, tonsils, intestines, and spleen, where they await a call to action in body defense. The thymus produces a hormone called thymosin, which is thought to be active in the production of lymphocytes and also is under investigation as an agent that stimulates the immune function in some immunodeficiency states. Much like the thymus in T-cell maturation, the bursa equivalent in the bone marrow differentiates lymphocytes into B cells. Once released, these immature B cells migrate to the peripheral lymph tissue where they mature and await the body's need for defense against foreign agents (Hodges, 1992).

The blood is filtered continuously by the lymph system.

EXAMPLES OF NURSING DIAGNOSES RELATED TO PERSONS WITH ALTERATIONS IN THERMAL REGULATION

1. Health perception-health management patterns
   ✦ Health maintenance, altered related to
     Chronic illness
     Substance abuse
     Disease treatment plan
     Medication
   ✦ Infection, high risk for related to
     Recent exposure to infectious/communicable disease
   ✦ Injury, high risk for related to
     Increased body temperature
     Decreased body temperature

2. Nutritional-metabolic pattern
   ✦ Nutrition, altered: more than body requirements related to decreased metabolism
   ✦ Nutrition, altered: less than body requirements related to increased metabolism
   ✦ Fluid volume deficit related to increased metabolism
   ✦ Fluid volume excess related to decreased metabolism
   ✦ Hyperthermia related to
     Central nervous system injury
     Reaction to medication
     Infectious process
     Exposure to elevated temperatures in environment
   ✦ Hypothermia related to
     Inadequate home temperature
     Lack of adequate shelter
     Inappropriate clothing for external environment

3. Elimination pattern
   ✦ Urinary elimination, altered pattern related to excessive sweating

4. Activity-exercise pattern
   ✦ Activity intolerance related to reduced energy stores
   ✦ Impaired gas exchange related to increased oxygen consumption

5. Cognitive-perceptual pattern
   ✦ Pain related to fever
   ✦ Thought processes, altered related to hyperthermia or hypothermia

NURSING INTERVENTIONS

Nursing interventions that are essential in providing care for clients with alterations in temperature include the following:

1. The temperature should be taken every 15-30 minutes while measures are being used to return the temperature to normal baseline. Other vital signs should be monitored as well, since alterations in body temperature can have a profound effect on cardiac and respiratory function. Assessments of skin color and temperature also should be accomplished.
2. Initiate an intravenous (IV) line to provide a route for fluid and medication administration. Carefully maintain IV sites because finding new sites is especially difficult if the client is being cooled.
3. Monitor urinary output hourly. An output greater than 30 ml/hour is needed to ensure renal perfusion.
4. Neurologic assessments should be done hourly. As the client regains consciousness, remember that disorientation may be present as consciousness returns; reorientation and protection from injury are important aspects of nursing management.
5. Initiate temperature management utilizing a hypothermia-hyperthermia blanket device, if appropriate for the client's extremes in temperature. In using these devices, the following guidelines will ensure client safety and comfort.
   ✦ Place one blanket under and one over the client. If only one under the client is used, provide top covers as appropriate for the client's temperature extreme.
   ✦ Protect the heels and the head from direct contact with the surface of the blanket.
   ✦ Elevate male genitalia on a towel to protect them.
   ✦ Insert the temperature probe into the rectum and tape it in place. The connecting tubing is attached to the machine so that the desired body temperature may be dialed and automatically maintained by a thermostat, based on the probe reading of the client's temperature. Calibrate the probe for accuracy with a standard rectal thermometer every 8 hours.

Continued.

EXAMPLES OF NURSING DIAGNOSES RELATED TO PERSONS WITH ALTERATIONS IN THERMAL REGULATION—cont'd

---

✦ Stop the rewarming/cooling effort once the recorded temperature is within 1°-2° of the desired temperature. The temperature will continue to rise/fall somewhat once the blanket is removed. The goal is to prevent the temperature from drifting beyond the desired level.

✦ Continuously monitor the temperature-regulating effort for the client's response. Caution should be taken to prevent a rapid reduction in temperature. The client should not be allowed to shiver. Shivering significantly increases oxygen consumption, metabolic demand, myocardial effort, carbon dioxide production, cutaneous vasoconstriction, and lactic acid production. These responses will produce heat and cause the temperature to rise.

✦ Assess the skin frequently and protect the skin with lotion or oil.

✦ Reposition the client frequently (Flannery, 1992).

6. Administer antipyretics and analgesics as ordered.

OUTCOME CRITERIA FOR INTERVENTIONS UTILIZED IN PROVIDING CARE FOR INDIVIDUALS WITH ALTERED THERMAL REGULATION

1. Body temperature returns to within normal limits.
2. Fluid and electrolyte balance, vital signs, and level of consciousness return to normal.
3. A sense of comfort and rest is attained.
4. Knowledge of causes of extremes in body temperature and of ways to prevent subsequent episodes has been demonstrated.
5. Appropriate environmental resources to prevent alterations in body temperatures have been obtained.

Lymph nodes are distributed throughout the body, and large clusters of lymph nodes are found in the axillae, groin, thorax, abdomen, and neck. The lymph nodes actually serve two purposes for the body. Basically they serve as a series of filters so that all lymph in the lymph vessels is filtered by at least one node. They also act as a filtering system for foreign materials, and they serve as a reservoir for the specialized immunologic T and B cells. Peripherally the serous portion of the bloodstream diffuses from the capillaries into the peripheral lymph channels where it is progressively filtered and then returned to the cardiovascular system. Lymph ducts carry this serous fluid through lymph nodes where is filtered. With many infectious processes these nodes become enlarged as their activity and defense cells proliferate. T cells are most abundant in the lymph nodes, although B cells also can be found (Bullock, 1992).

The spleen is the largest lymphatic organ and serves three functions, only one of which is actually immune related. First, it is a site for the destruction of injured and worn-out red blood cells. Second, it is a reservoir for B cells, although T cells also are found there. Third, it is a storage site for blood. Mucosa-associated lymphoid tissue includes the tonsils, Peyer's patches in the intestines, and the appendix. Aggregates of lymphoid tissue also are found in the respiratory and urogenital tracts. These systems normally are the main portals of entry for microorganisms. Therefore the presence of lymphoid tissue can, through secretory immunoglobulins and other immune factors, prevent entry of these microorganisms into the body. In summary, the ability to produce and maintain an intact immune system requires the effective interaction of the thymus, bursa equivalent, lymph nodes, spleen, and tonsils as well as lymphoid tissue in nonlymphoid organs. Although much of the immune system is in place before birth, ongoing processes of marking and maturation of cells are critical to adequate functioning for nonspecific immune responses and specific antigen-antibody reactions to occur (Bullock, 1992).

Immunity is a normal adaptive response to the external environment. It functions to protect the body from disease by means of both resistance to offending organisms and attack on offending organisms. Immunity can be natural or acquired. Natural immunity is species specific. For example, humans are not susceptible to feline leukemia and cats are not susceptible to acquired immunodeficiency syndrome (AIDS). Natural immunity is innate in that we are born with certain immunities.

Other immunities are acquired after birth through exposure to an antigen, through transference of antibodies by inoculation, or through such body fluids as mother's milk. Acquired immunity can be active or passive. Active immunity is developed on exposure to an antigen during which antibodies are programmed to protect the body from illness with future exposures. These antibodies are specific, often providing lifetime immunity against another attack of the same antigen. Active immunity also can be developed, with lifetime protection, by exposure to a specific antigen through inoculation.

Passive immunity is a temporary immunity involving the transference of antibodies from one individual to another or from some other source to an individual. Passive immunity also can be transferred through vaccination either of antiserum, antitoxin, or gamma globulin. Both active and passive immunity create levels of antibodies circulating in the body.

Antigen and Antigen-Antibody Response

The immune system responds to the invasion of the body by foreign material, referred to as antigens. Some antigens are capable of producing disease, whereas others, which are not disease producing, are recognized as foreign and, therefore, can precipitate an immune reaction. Although the immune system is capable of differentiating self from nonself, it cannot differentiate harmful organisms from nonharmful ones.

In addition to foreign particles being antigenic in nature, it is known that all nucleated cells in the body contain surface antigens, proteins found on the surface of a cell. These proteins distinguish an individual's tissue from tissue of other persons. Surface antigens are genetically determined and are referred to as histocompatibility antigens or human leukocyte antigens.

Immune Responsiveness

Immune responsiveness may be either specific or nonspecific. A specific response requires the recognition of a particular antigen and involves the production and action of a programmed antibody for that antigen. Normally an antibody circulates in the bloodstream until it encounters an appropriate antigen to which it can bind. Such binding results in antigen-antibody complexes or immune complexes. The process of binding is such that antibody binds to particularly conformed antigenic determinant sites on the antigen, effectively preventing the antigen from binding with receptors on the host cells. The overall effect is protection of the host from antigen infection or penetration. An antigen-antibody reaction can result in several consequences to the invading agent. The reaction can cause agglutination or clumping of the cells, neutralization of the antigen toxin, cell lysis or destruction of the antigen, enhanced phagocytosis of the antigen by other cells, or activation of the complement system. A nonspecific response requires only the recognition of the invading organism as being foreign but does not involve any specific antibody. A nonspecific immunologic response might involve the complement system, interferons, and phagocytosis. In order to maintain a total surveillance function, the immune response must be diverse enough to provide protection from foreign agents with a variety of immune responses (Hodges, 1992).

Cells of the Immune Response

At least three types of cells are involved in the immune response to foreign material: the T cell, the B cell, and the macrophage. Each cell carries a distinct responsibility and contributes to the integrity of the body as a whole. Each set of cells has effector cells and memory cells. Effector cells are those that are capable of attacking and destroying a particular antigen. Memory cells are those that are further imprinted with the antigenic code and are responsible for remembering and recognizing that antigen within minutes of a subsequent exposure (Bullock, 1992).

T cells provide a type of immunity called cell-mediated immunity and have a life expectancy of several years. They are marked by the thymus with specific surface antigens that characterize them and distinguish them from B cells. T cells represent approximately 70% to 80% of the total number of lymphocytes and are divided into two types depending on their function: effector or regulatory T cells. Effector T cells affect immunity either directly or indirectly. As an indirect effect, they can produce lymphokines, which are substances that influence the function of inflammatory cells and macrophages. Some effector cells directly attack and destroy antigens. The killer T cell is the specific one that directly causes the death of the antigen. Regulatory cells are of two types: helper T cells (T4 cells), which enhance the action of B lymphocytes, or suppressor T cells, which suppress or inhibit the action of B lymphocytes.

B lymphocytes are the larger of the lymphocyte cells and have a much shorter life-span that T cells. They mature with exposure to an antigen. Immature B cells are stored in the bone marrow, the lymph nodes, and other lymphatic tissue. They also are found circulating in the bloodstream. The B cell is primarily responsible for antibody production. Following exposure to an antigen, mature B cells may be transformed into plasma cells, which then secrete antibodies called immunoglobulins. Each plasma cell (B cell) is specialized to produce only one type of antibody. Several types of antibodies have been identified, and each is active within a given course of events in the immune response. Immunoglobulins have been identified as IgA, IgD, IgE, IgG, or IgM.

The macrophage participates in the immune response by processing the antigen and presenting it in such a way as to increase its recognition and reaction by the T and B cells. By means of phagocytosis, the macrophage ingests and digests the antigen, but in the process the altered antigen is released through the macrophage cell membrane where it attaches to receptor sites on the surface of the macrophage. It is at these receptor sites that the interaction takes place with the invading antigen and the T and B cells. Macrophages are primarily responsible for preparing the antigens and carrying them to the lymph tissue, where the T and B cells reside. The macrophage is a critical factor in the immune response to both the T and B cells and is considered to be the link between the inflammatory response and the specific resistance of antibody production and cell mediation. In fact, it also is thought that a substance produced by effector T cells causes migration and activation of the macrophages. All three of these cell types must work in concert in order to facilitate the functioning of an effective immune response.

Mechanisms of Specific Immunity

The immune system can be described as providing two types of immunity. Humoral immunity is based on the activity and characteristics of the B-cell lymphocytes. Cell-mediated immunity is based on the role of the T-cell lymphocyte. Humoral immunity—the recognition of antigen and the production of specific antibody—occurs with a primary and a secondary response pattern. During the primary response pattern, there is a latency period before the antibody can be detected in the serum. This delay may be as long as 72 hours after exposure to the antigen. This represents the time needed for the antigen to be recognized as nonself and identified specifically, and for antibodies to be formed in response to the particular characteristics of the antigen. The secondary response occurs with subsequent ex-

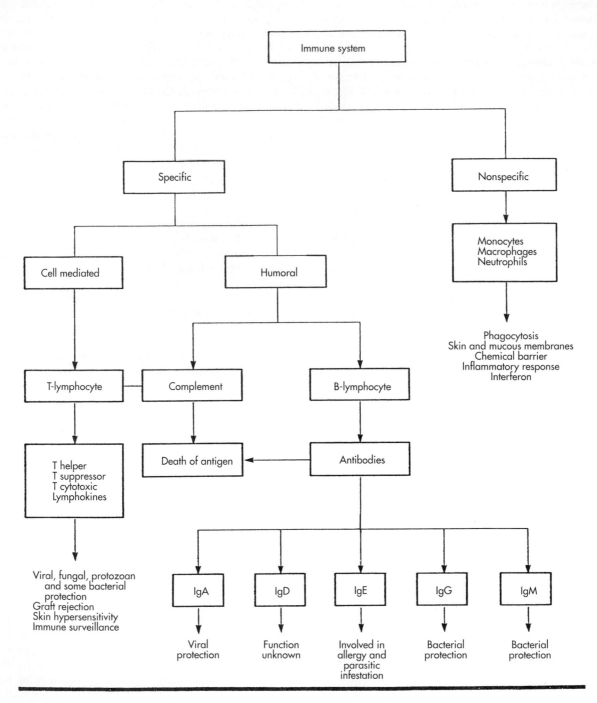

Fig. 22-4 Components of the immune system.

posures to the same antigen. It is during this time that the memory cells of the plasma clones recognize the antigen almost immediately and initiate the immune response with heightened antibody formation.

◆ Cell-mediated (cellular) immunity

Cell-mediated immunity is based on the activity and characteristics of the T cell. During this portion of the immune response, the T cell and the macrophage predominate, creating a direct attack on the invading antigens. Cell-mediated reactions are initiated by the binding of an antigen with an antigen receptor located on the surface of the T cell. This may occur with or without the assistance of the macrophages. The T cells then carry the antigenic message to the lymph nodes where the production of other T cells is encouraged. T-cell immunity provides protection from intercellular organisms (viruses, etc.), cancer cells, and foreign tissue. Therefore the T cell is the mechanism cell that is responsible for much of the rejection phenomenon of transplanted organs and grafts and the development of malignancies. Cell-mediated immunity depends heavily on thymus and lymph node integrity and is influenced strongly by an individual's nutritional state (Hodges, 1992).

◆ Complement

The complement system is an immune mechanism that involves circulating plasma proteins made in the liver that are activated when an antibody couples with its antigen. Once activated, these proteins behave in a way that resembles the blood coagulation cascade in that, once initiated, it progresses through several sequential stages, each contributing to the immune response and resulting in cellular destruction. In addition, activated complement molecules attract macrophages and granulocytes to areas of antigen-antibody reactions. These cells continue the body's defense by devouring the antibody-coated microbes and by

releasing bacterial agents. Complement plays a very important role in the immune response. Destruction of an invading or attacking organism or toxin is not achieved merely by the binding of the antibody and antigens but also requires activation of complement, the arrival of killer T cells, or the attraction of macrophages. The precursors to the complement pathways normally are circulating in the bloodstream. They are activated only by specific agents such as the immunoglobulins. The complement system is instrumental in facilitating phagocytosis by making antigens more susceptible to digestion, lysis of antigen cell membranes, and attraction of phagocytes to the invading antigen (Hodges, 1992).

Mechanisms of Nonspecific Immunity

The nonspecific immune response is initiated solely on the recognition of foreign material being nonself antigens and not on their particular identity and involves the process of phagocytosis and the action of interferons. Interferons have antiviral and antitumor properties and are the first line of defense in the protection of the human organism from viruses and other intercellular invaders such as fungi and parasites. Interferon inhibits the synthesis of viral proteins in their reproduction without inhibiting the host protein synthesis in normal cell reproduction. Interferons are a subfamily of lymphokines originating from effector T cells. Lymphokines are low-molecular-weight proteins with the ability to influence the inflammatory and immune responses to facilitate destruction and removal of foreign cells or toxins. Lymphokines can recruit, hold, and activate other lymphocytes and macrophages to assist in removing the invading antigen. Although interferons are nonspecific for pathogens, they are species specific. Interferons currently are being tested as a treatment modality in certain malignancies.

Phagocytosis is a nonspecific immune mechanism whereby invading foreign materials or injured cells are in-

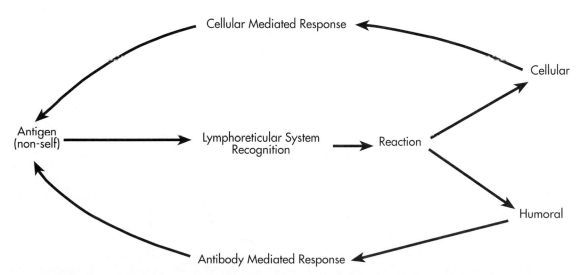

Fig. 22-5 Summary of the immune response. (From *Nursing Care of Infants and Children, 4th ed.* by L.F. Whaley and D.L. Wong, 1991, St. Louis: Mosby–Year Book. Copyright 1991 by Mosby–Year Book. Reprinted by permission.)

gested and destroyed by phagocytic cells. As previously described, both neutrophils and macrophages are instrumental cellular components to the immune mechanism. Phagocytosis involves chemotaxis—the chemical attraction of phagocytic cells to antigens—as well as the engulfing of antigens for the purpose of rendering them harmless. Figures 22-4 and 22-5 illustrate the components of and process for the immune response.

Immunodeficiency

The immune system can be subject to inadequate development, disease, and injury from illness and treatments that can result in deficient immune activity. Such a situation is referred to as a state of immunodeficiency. Regardless of the underlying cause of the immunodeficiency, the cardinal symptoms include recurrent, severe infections often involving unusual organisms. Immunodeficiencies may be classified as primary or secondary. Primary immunodeficiencies are those for which no underlying condition or known cause can be identified. In this situation the cells responsible for mounting an immune response are reduced in number, ineffective in action, or lacking altogether. Most primary states of immunodeficiency are the result of either embryonic abnormality, genetic predisposition, or congenital failure of the system to develop, thus occurring almost exclusively in infants and toddlers. Secondary immunodeficiency states are more common than primary ones and generally occur in adults. They usually are the result of other primary diseases, drug therapies such as corticosteroids and immunosuppressive drugs, or irradiation therapy for malignant disease. Persons with secondary immunodeficiencies are immunosuppressed and are often referred to as immunocompromised hosts. Humans also can become immunodeficient from a direct attack on the immune system by pathogens. When such a situation exists, it is known as acquired immunodeficiency (Bullock & daCunha, 1992).

Factors Affecting the Immune System
✦ Age

The immune response is affected significantly by aging, malnutrition, trauma, and stress. The function of the immune system diminishes with age. T-lymphocyte function and specific antibody responses are particularly depressed, but in contrast there is an increasing pool of antibodies. In the older population the thymus is quite minimal in size and function. T cells, although continuing to be produced and circulated at approximately the same rate, are deteriorating in function, thus impairing cell-mediated immunity. Whereas helper T cells are depressed in number and function, it appears that suppressor T cells are more prevalent and active, which may account for impaired humoral immunity in elderly persons. Elderly persons therefore are less capable of mounting an effective response to pathogens and consequently show increased frequency of disease not found in younger populations. In addition, the incidence of autoimmune diseases also increases with age; this may represent a decreased ability of the antibodies to differentiate between self and nonself.

✦ Nutritional deficiencies

Malnutrition is an additional factor that influences the body's ability to manage pathogen invasion adequately. The basic components of nutritional intake play a major role in the development of, sustainment of, and the integrity of those elements essential for the immune response. Depletion of protein reserves results in atrophy of lymphoid tissues, depression of antibody response, reduction in the number of circulating T cells, and impairment of phagocytic function. The humoral response seems to be less affected by nutritional compromise, although the activity of macrophages and the complement mechanism is depressed. Therefore more frequent manifestations of disease can and do occur in the nutritionally deficient individual. The essential elements, minerals and vitamins, also seem to play a role in the integrity of the immune response (Brunner & Suddarth, 1988; Hodges, 1992).

✦ Stress

Under stress, whether physical or emotional, the body produces larger amounts of cortisol in response to the perceived needs for increased metabolism. Cortisol also directly suppresses the immune system. In particular, the recognition ability of the process to identify foreign matter is impaired and the activity of the T cells is altered. The physiologic and psychological stressors induced during surgical disruption of tissue integrity stimulate cortisol release from the adrenal cortex (Hodges, 1992).

✦ Trauma

In general, trauma suppresses both T- and B-cell function. Research has demonstrated that decreased chemotactic and phagocytic activity and decreased antibody and lymphocyte level result. Both accidental trauma such as burns and intentional trauma as occurs during surgery contribute to these outcomes. Major burns or other factors cause impaired skin integrity and compromise the body's first line of defense. Loss of large amounts of serum with burn injuries depletes the body of essential proteins, including immunoglobulins (Hodges, 1992).

✦ Existence of other diseases

Conditions such as infection, cancer, and other chronic diseases play a role in decreasing the effectiveness of the immune response. Large cancer tumors are able to release antigens into the blood that combine with circulating antibodies and prevent them from attacking tumor cells. Furthermore, tumor cells may possess special blocking factors that coat tumor cells and prevent destruction by killer T cells. Chronic diseases such as multiple sclerosis, in which long-term steroid therapy is the mainstay of treatment, also can precipitate an immunocompromised state. Nursing interventions must have this knowledge as a basis for care planning. Educational efforts need to be directed to ensuring that these clients understand the high risk for infection and have the skills to implement appropriate infection control measures.

The human immunodeficiency virus (HIV) is such a pathogen. In this syndrome there is markedly depressed T-lymphocyte functioning with reduced numbers of T4 cells, impaired killer T-cell capacity, and increased numbers of suppressor T cells. By selectively invading and infecting T cells, the virus damages the very cell whose function it is to orchestrate the identification and destruction of virus as an antigen. Other similarly configured cells also may become infected. Eventually the individual's complement of fully functioning cells becomes depleted. The humoral response in producing antibodies is less affected by HIV, but the induction and regulation of the humoral response may be affected by the lack of T-cell regulators (Brunner & Suddarth, 1988; Bryant-Armstrong, 1988; Luckman & Sorensen, 1987).

The HIV is a retrovirus, carrying genetic information in ribonucleic acid (RNA) rather than in deoxyribonucleic acid (DNA). It infects the T cell by binding to it at the CD4 receptor site and inserting its RNA into the T cell. Through the action of reverse transcriptase, the HIV is able to reprogram the genetic materials of the infected T4 cell. When the T cell is activated to reproduce, its genetic information now is programmed to produce more of the HIV instead of viable and functional T lymphocytes. The newly produced virus can then infect other T4 lymphocytes. Most antiviral drugs now work by inhibiting the action of reverse transcriptase (Cohn, 1989; Hodges, 1992).

HIV, the virus that causes AIDS, is transmitted during sexual contact, through sharing of intravenous needles and other drug paraphernalia, through exposure to infected blood or blood products, and perinatally from mother to newborn. The Centers for Disease Control has developed "Universal Precautions" as recommendations for all professionals who will be (or have a high probability of being) exposed to HIV. Under Universal Precautions, blood and certain body fluids of all clients are considered potentially infectious for HIV, hepatitis B virus (HBV), and other bloodborne pathogens. These guidelines apply specifically to blood, other body fluids containing visible blood, semen and vaginal secretions, and body tissues as well as cerebrospinal, synovial, pleural, peritoneal, pericardial, and amniotic fluids. Universal Precautions are intended to prevent parenteral, mucous membrane, and nonintact skin contact exposure to these substances. Universal Precautions do not apply to feces, nasal secretions, sputum, sweat, tears, urine, and vomitus unless these substances contain visible blood. When in doubt, precautions are in order. Due to an increased potential to exposure to those substances thought to contain HIV, healthcare workers need to be highly cognizant of Universal Precautions and incorporate them *consistently* in caregiving activities whether working in an institution or community setting. In addition, healthcare workers should investigate their institution's or agency's policies regarding bloodborne pathogens and the specific environmental considerations and necessary precautions for invasive procedures that are advised. They also should become familiar with the standards mandated by the Occupational Safety and Health Administration (OSHA). The following Box summarizes the key components of Universal Precautions (Craven & Hirnle, 1992).

As this chapter is being written, new and emerging information about the epidemiology and etiology of HIV infection and AIDS is being discussed. HIV infection is a chronic disease manifesting itself in a variety of ways, with AIDS being considered the most extreme clinical manifestation. In general, the median AIDS-free time is 10 years. There is a small subset of HIV-infected persons that are maintaining normal or near normal CD4 lymphocyte counts for many years. These nonprogressing long-term survivors (NPLTS) currently are being studied to determine their char-

---

UNIVERSAL PRECAUTIONS

✦ Use Universal Precautions with all clients.
✦ Use barriers (gloves, goggles, aprons, masks) appropriately and consistently.
✦ Wash hands and change barriers after exposure to each client.
✦ Needles must not be recapped, broken, sheared, or bent except when no other method is feasible. Sharps must be discarded into labeled, puncture-resistant containers.
✦ Contaminated waste must be placed into leakproof, labeled containers (usually red plastic bags).
✦ Contaminated laundry must be placed in labeled containers. If wet, these containers should be leakproof.
✦ All specimens should be bagged and labeled properly.
✦ Disposable resuscitation equipment should be available at all times.
✦ A private room may be indicated for clients unable to maintain scrupulous hygiene.

---

acteristics that may account for this difference in disease progression.

In the United States the greater majority of AIDS cases occur in homosexual and bisexual men and increasingly in their heterosexual partners; whereas in Africa, South America, and the Caribbean, sexual transmission occurs between men and women. Increasing numbers of past or current intravenous drug abusers also are developing this disease. Other populations with a significant potential to develop AIDS include hemophiliacs, sexual partners of high-risk individuals, and children born to high-risk parents. AIDS is transmitted following heterosexual or homosexual intercourse or through blood and blood products (Bullock & daCunha, 1992).

Three stages of HIV disease can be described. During the period of asymptomatic infection, clients may present with a variety of mild to severe generalized complaints such as persistent generalized lymphadenopathy (PGL), fatigue, diarrhea, as well as a multitude of dermatologic, pulmonary, musculoskeletal, and gastrointestinal conditions.

The acute stage begins when opportunistic infections become evident. Infections and malignancies that develop as a result of immune system dysfunction are referred to as opportunistic infections. Once the individual infected with HIV displays evidence of disease ordinarily not problematic in the general population, an AIDS diagnosis is made. AIDS is a clinical diagnosis, therefore, assigned to individuals who present with opportunistic infections and/or unusual malignancies. These signs are evidence of the failure of the components and processes of the immune response to protect against disease. The chronic stage evolves as ongoing pathologic changes are evident and involve multisystems. The end stage, or terminal stage, presents significant challenges as the management of repeated opportunistic infections, the preservation of self-care and independence, and the coordination of complex nursing care become more difficult.

Clinical manifestations of AIDS generally are related to opportunistic infections preying on an impaired immune system. These diseases include *Pneumocystis carinii* pneumonia (PCP), cytomegalovirus (CMV), toxoplasmosis, and tuberculosis (TB). Neoplasias also occur; as an example, Kaposi's sarcoma presents with purplish, hemorrhagic patches, plaques, and nodules. Anogenital herpes appears with persistent, chronic ulcerations over the penis, vulva, or buttocks. Mouth soreness and dysphagia are caused by candidiasis (Luckman & Sorensen, 1987). Treatment options currently are being aimed at the most susceptible stages in HIV disease. Most antiviral drugs work by inhibiting the action of reverse transcriptase (Cohn, 1989; Hodges, 1992). Zidovudine (AZT) is an example of these agents and generally is the first approach to treatment. However, because the development of drug resistance decreases the effectiveness of single-agent therapy, various drugs and their combinations are being studied, including dideoxyinosine (ddI), dideoxycytidine (ddC)/AZT, D4T, and protease inhibitors.

REHABILITATION PRINCIPLES AND THE PERSON WITH AIDS

Clients with HIV are faced with a number of infections that affect every organ system. The gastrointestinal system is highly vulnerable to the many pathogens that are capable of invading the immunocompromised client, thus creating some of the most frustrating problems for both the client and the nurse (Gallagher, 1993). The physiologic sequelae in the gastrointestinal tract are an important cause of morbidity and mortality. The pathophysiology of intestinal infection is not yet fully understood; however, two main mechanisms have been postulated. The first is reduced intestinal immunity, resulting in chronic opportunistic infections, which themselves cause altered intestinal functioning. The second is that HIV itself affects the intestinal mucosa and causes malfunctioning. The mechanisms for this process are controversial but may result from either direct infection of mucosal epithelial cells or infiltration of the macrophages within the mucosa. In addition, there has been some clinical evidence of degeneration of the intrinsic jejunal autonomic neurons, but the functional significance of such degeneration is not yet known. In short, while it is clear that a variety of HIV processes involve the gastrointestinal tract, the mechanisms of intestinal immune failure are not definitively known (Griffin, 1990).

✦ Nutritional status

The complicated clinical picture presented by persons with AIDS often is exacerbated by compromised nutritional status. Oral and esophageal inflammations cause pain and difficulty with swallowing. Complex medication regimens, with their potential for untoward drug interactions, and the stress of chronic illness contribute to persistent anorexia. Diarrhea, malabsorption, and weight loss frustrate efforts to achieve or maintain adequate nutrition. It is therefore an important and challenging responsibility for nurses to ascertain and implement appropriate interventions to assist persons with HIV to improve their nutritional status, thereby potentially delaying disease progression and significantly contributing to improved quality of life (Keithley & Kohn,

1990). In fact, an epidemiologic study completed by Abrams, Duncan, and Hertz-Picciotto (1993) suggest that the risk of HIV-positive persons developing AIDS can be reduced with the intake of certain micronutrients including iron, vitamin E, and riboflavin. These researchers uncovered a 30% lower risk of AIDS in HIV-positive persons who took multivitamins daily.

It is important for healthcare professionals managing the needs of persons infected with HIV to understand the relationship among nutrition, HIV infection, and the immune system. Progressive weight loss is a major component of the clinical syndrome in persons with HIV infection and AIDS. Weight loss occurs for a variety of reasons, which, when recognized, may be preventable or treatable. Malnutrition occurring with weight loss may adversely affect the function of the immune system and further impair the infected individual's ability to avoid or recover from repeated infections and to effectively manage other stressors (Hoyt & Staats, 1991). Nutritional support in HIV disease is important from early asymptomatic stages through to fully developed AIDS. Asymptomatic HIV-positive persons are advised to have a balanced diet that is adequate in protein, energy, and nutrients. When symptoms develop, weight loss may ensue from reduced food intake, malabsorption, and altered metabolism. Progressive, involuntary weight loss can be the result of a variety of conditions and is common in persons with HIV as the disease progresses. The etiology of this syndrome can include anorexia, conditioned nausea, infection, chronic diarrhea, malabsorption, and poor food availability (O'Brien & Pheifer, 1993). Dietary counseling should be initiated and appropriate home management services provided to relieve symptoms and prevent further weight loss. A team approach to the care of persons with HIV disease is imperative, and close relationships between nurses, dieticians, and other members of the interdisciplinary team are essential to provide more comprehensive care that will help to maintain body mass and self-concept (Law & Baldwin, 1993).

✦ Psychosocial factors

O'Brien and Pheifer (1993) examined physical and psychological problems and needs of persons living with HIV infection using qualitative and quantitative research methods. Psychosocial issues most frequently identified by the study participants were loneliness and disturbed self-concept due to changes in body image and self-esteem. A negative self-concept, however, may predate the diagnosis of HIV/AIDS, which may impact on the person's ability to deal with this additional stressor. The experience of loneliness and the increased need for social supports offer a serious challenge to persons infected with HIV and to their caregivers. This may occur as the result of externally determined factors such as loss of a job or of a relationship, physical limitations, and societal responses, or it may be self-induced isolation caused by a variety of reasons such as apathy or changes in personal appearance. The stigma associated with this diagnosis and the import of disclosure to family and friends is an additional facet of the psychological response that must be considered. The maintenance of appropriate sexual integrity, issues related to home management (the ability to function independently and carry out activities of daily living), impaired communication (often related to involvement of the central nervous system), and spiritual distress frequently were cited as priority psychosocial concerns by the study participants. Hurley and Ungvarski (1994) used a chart review to determine the home healthcare requirements of persons with HIV/AIDS. They reported that the five most common physiologic symptoms were dyspnea, weakness, fatigue and lethargy, pain, and ataxia. Memory deficit, depression, anxiety, impaired judgment, substance abuse, and insomnia were identified as the most frequently occurring psychological symptoms. Other needs reported by persons with HIV/AIDs include assistance with cleaning the home, preparing meals, doing laundry, and shopping.

✦ Fatigue and energy conservation

Although fatigue has been identified as a common complaint of persons with HIV/AIDS, its etiology is unknown. Fatigue often is defined as a generalized malaise and loss of motivation, unrelated to activity and sleep patterns. Specific muscle fatigue has been examined as a possible factor in clients' reports of generalized fatigue (Miller et al., 1991). Initially fatigue does present as a complaint of tiredness. However, in chronic HIV infection, unexplained fatigue is a prominent persistent symptom. Fatigue may be the result of many of the physical and psychosocial (e.g., depression) illness conditions experienced by immunocompromised persons with HIV and may have a profound negative effect on functional level and quality of life (O'Brien & Pheifer, 1993). In addition to complaints of persons with HIV about the draining effects of fatigue, the impact overall looms much larger. The impact on public expenditures may be large. Fatigue may be the overriding symptom that causes persons with HIV infection to discontinue employment. When they are unable to continue to work, they must turn to public support for subsistence. With loss of employment also comes loss of health insurance coverage in almost all cases. These individuals must then rely on public funds for healthcare of their illness, with its prolonged, slowly progressive deterioration (Darko, McCutchan, Kripke, Gillin, & Golshan, 1992).

Perhaps the most common manifestation of HIV infection leading to disability is the lack of endurance. Several factors contribute to this distressing problem: insomnia, nutritional deficits, anemia related to medications, oxygen deficits, as well as the fatigue that accompanies chronic illness. Identification of and correcting or lessening the degree of disturbances in sleep patterns should be one of the primary foci with the goal that the client get adequate sleep and feel well rested. Interventions can include encouraging frequent naps, work and/or social limitations, as well as self-pacing and avoidance of those activities that push the client to his limit. Many patients with AIDS will relate this factor as their priority problem. Although there is no body of clinical evidence to suggest inconclusively the best approach to the rehabilitative management of this problem, many clients can benefit from a mild to moderate program of physical exercise and nutritional support (Levinson & O'Connell, 1991). The key to assisting persons with HIV to live with this problem is to maintain an appropriate balance of activity and rest.

TRAJECTORY OF HIV/AIDS: CARE PRIORITIES

I. Preconversion phase (health promotion)
   Counseling
      Sexual
      Nutritional
      Mental health
      Physical activity
   Education
      Disease progression
      Role of medications
      Need for follow-up care
   Supportive services
      Legal assistance
      HIV/AIDS networks

II. Early conversion phase (acute illness)
   Facilitated access to
      Medical evaluation
      Hospitalized care
      Home care services
      Rehabilitation services
   Education
      Nutrition
      Medication
      Infection control
      Self-care

III. Late conversion phase (chronic illness)
   Activities of daily living
      Personal hygiene
      Energy conservation
      Meal preparation
      Transportation
      Housekeeping
   Residential issues
      Sheltered group housing
      Adult day care
      Episodic social care
      Respite care for family
   Economic concerns
      Continuing employment
      Health insurance
      Medication expenses
      Disability income
      Other entitlements
   Education
      Drug-resistant diseases
      Complex medication regimens
      Nutritional management to deter wasting
      Infection control
      Advanced directives

IV. Terminal phase
   Hospice care
   Bereavement services
   Respite care for family

Adapted from "Home Healthcare Needs of Adults Living with HIV Disease in New York City." by P. Hurky & P. Ungvarski, 1994, *Journal of Association of Nurses in AIDS Care, 5*, 33-40.

✦ Financial impact

As concern about escalating healthcare costs continues to be a significant economic issue, healthcare initiatives that emphasize community care to enhance functional ability in persons with AIDS will become more common. AIDS no longer is considered an acute, fulminating disease but now is studied as a chronic illness with consequences that affect all bodily systems. Many of the chronic musculoskeletal and neurologic problems experienced by the person with AIDS are amenable to rehabilitative care. Rehabilitation professionals will play a central role in enhancing the quality of life for individuals with AIDS, in minimizing their functional dependence, and in lowering healthcare costs (Pizzi, 1989). As more persons with AIDS are retained in community settings throughout the trajectory of their illness, it becomes imperative for nurses to develop expertise in addressing the myriad needs presented by this population of clients. The box on p. 497 highlights priorities for care throughout the course of the illness experience.

It is essential to promote as high a level of independent functioning in the community as possible within the limitations imposed by this chronic disease. Education of the client and the care provider(s) is of paramount importance. The teaching needs for these persons are varied; however, a recurrent theme in preparing for return to the community setting are questions related to the home management of infection risk. Providing the required knowledge base will facilitate discharge and reintegration and will foster the level of confidence and competence these individuals need to achieve a satisfactory quality of life. The following box summarizes guidelines for home management of infection

risk that should be incorporated into the plan of care for the person with AIDS from the first professional contact.

Advancing AIDS involves diffuse and focal central nervous system disorders as well as peripheral neutralities. In fact, AIDS-dementia complex (ADC) or HIV encephalopathy is the presenting feature of AIDS in many cases (Levinson & O'Connell, 1991). Persons diagnosed with ADC may exhibit signs of cognitive, behavioral, and motor disturbances, and each will have a variety of early and late symptoms. A significant number of persons with AIDS eventually develop some degree of cognitive, motor, and/or emotional impairment that responds favorably to counseling and therapeutic interventions such as the use of zidovudine. Figure 22-6 illustrates early signs of cognitive and motor dysfunction commonly demonstrated by persons with AIDS. Later manifestations of central neurologic involvement may include severe memory loss, speech disturbances, and abnormal reflexes and tone. Gait disturbances from an associated myelopathy are common, as are bowel/bladder deficits. Strokes and visual impairment are not uncommon. (Levinson & O'Connell, 1991). Table 22-1 identifies nursing management guidelines that are effective in addressing these chronic problems.

Peripheral involvement may manifest in four distinct clinical patterns of neuropathy including distal sensorimotor polyneuropathy, inflammatory demyelinating polyneuropathy, mononeuropathy multiplex, and progressive polyradiculopathy (Levinson & O'Connell, 1991). These outcomes may be related to progressive disease or to the side effects of medication used to treat the disease. Viruses such as varicella-zoster also may cause neutralities. Persons af-

---

✦

GUIDELINES FOR HOME MANAGEMENT OF INFECTION RISK

- ✦ Wear gloves and other barriers when exposure to blood or body fluids is anticipated or unavoidable.
- ✦ Wash hands thoroughly after providing care and preparing foods.
- ✦ Protect the person with AIDS from pathogens found in raw food by carefully preparing and thoroughly cooking all food products.
- ✦ Use only pasteurized milk.
- ✦ Wash all utensils and surfaces used in food preparation carefully.
- ✦ Carefully wash dishes in hot soapy water either manually or in a dishwasher; however, separate eating utensils are not necessary.
- ✦ Special cleaning techniques and products are not necessary.
- ✦ Clean spills of blood and body fluid with a 1:9 solution of household bleach and water.
- ✦ Launder clothing as usual.
- ✦ Do not share personal hygiene items (e.g., razors).
- ✦ Prevent exposure of the person with AIDS to people with infections.

Table 22-1 Nursing management guidelines

Symptom/problem	Interventions
Forgetfulness	Use calendars
	Keep an appointment book
	Place Post-it notes in conspicuous places
	Make lists: doctor, grocery store, things to check before going out
	Use an alarm clock for medications
	Keep a journal
Decreased concentration	Single task activities
Inattentiveness	Break down large tasks
Distractibility	Do not drive in heavy traffic
	Limit TV
Problems completing multistep tasks	Don't take on new jobs
	Avoid "high-speed" jobs
	Simplify meal preparation
	Plan activities when you feel best (i.e., AM or PM)
Problems with visual perception	Don't drive if vision impaired
	Use verbal directions, not maps
Depression or social withdrawal	Plan regular recreational activities
	Be an active participant
	Rekindle old hobbies
Slowed speech	Allow time to collect thoughts
	Keep talking

fected with neuromuscular complications show wasting of the lower extremities ultimately followed by an extension of wasting to the upper extremities, proximal muscle weakness, and complaints of muscle tenderness. Sensory polyneuropathy is a painful paresthesia that occurs most often on the soles of the feet. The direct cause is unknown but is thought to be a result of HIV infection of the neurons. For persons affected by this process, it is a chronic, disabling condition that requires testing a variety of temporary measures to relieve the pain. Although extremely debilitating, few medical interventions are available to alleviate a client's pain and distress effectively and too often this symptom is ignored. However, amitriptyline, incorporated as an adjunct in the pain management regimen, and capsaicin (Zostrix) cream, applied topically to the painful area, are examples of an appropriate and sensitive approach to this discouraging problem. The box on p. 500 summarizes the more common neurologic manifestations of AIDS and their treatment.

Eventually the physiologic and emotional problems accompanying AIDS will affect the individual's ability to function independently. At this phase in the trajectory of illness, it is appropriate to direct continuing rehabilitation efforts to the support of the caregiver. With little hope for recovery, there comes a feeling of futility or depression for the caregiver. Persons who care for chronically ill individual with AIDS need to be directed to AIDS networks and other group support systems for help in caring for themselves. They also need to be provided with the knowledge base to make informed decisions about care options as the person with AIDS moves into the terminal phase of the illness.

Hospice services are an appropriate option to consider for care at this time. As a general rule, treatment is given only to make the client more comfortable, and active curative measures and invasive diagnostic procedures are not utilized. Hospice programs offer an array of services based on a holistic healthcare philosophy that provides the dying client and the family with comfort, autonomy, and emotional

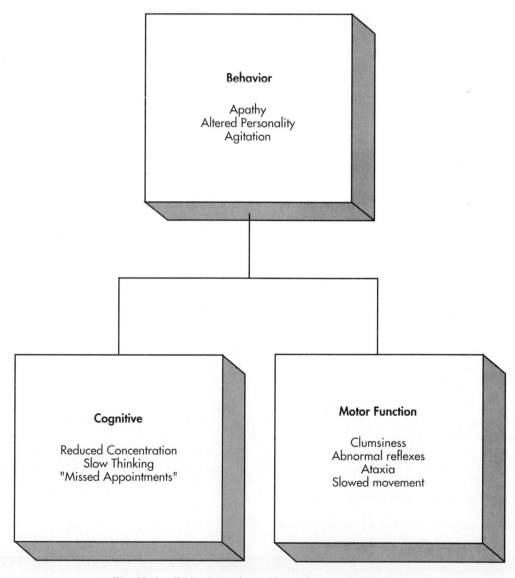

Fig. 22-6 Early signs of cognitive and motor dysfunction.

NEUROLOGIC MANIFESTATIONS ASSOCIATED WITH HIV/AIDS

AIDS-DEMENTIA COMPLEX (ADC)

Frequency in AIDS: 40%-70%

Causes/pathogenesis
- Direct invasion by HIV: In microphages(?), toxic factors(?), autoimmunity(?)

Clinical presentation
- Often subtle
- Memory loss selective for impaired retrieval
- Impaired manipulation of acquired knowledge
- Personality changes: apathy, inertia, irritability
- General slowing of all thought processes
- Later: psychomotor retardation

Clinical progression
- Slow: clients become mute, ataxic, paraplegic, incontinent, have vacant stare

Treatment
- AZT, DDI
- Symptomatic treatment
  Agitation: haloperidol (Haldol)
  Depression: fluoxetine hydrochloride (Prozac)

PERIPHERAL NEUROPATHIES/MYOPATHIES

Frequency in AIDS
- Exact numbers unknown but common in late infection

Cause/Pathogenesis
- Neuropathy
  HIV infection of nerve or dorsal root ganglion: DDI, DDC, D4T
- Myopathy
  HZV, spinal lymphomas, AZT, CMV-spinal cord

Clinical Presentation
- Neuropathy
  Distal and sensory axonal neuropathy
- Myopathy
  Progressive, painless gait disturbance
  Ataxia, spasticity
  Bowel/bladder dysfunction

Clinical Progression
- Slow; if caused by antiretrovirals, will lessen and may disappear when drug is stopped

Treatment
- Neuropathy
  Symptom management: tricyclics and analgesics
- Myopathy
  Symptom management: AZT holiday or stop antiretroviral

TOXOPLASMOSIS

Frequency in AIDS: 5%-15%

Causes/pathogenesis
- *Toxoplasma gondii* (protozoan)
- Reaction of chronic (latent) infection
- Cats: host and reservoir
- Raw or undercooked infected meat

Clinical presentation
- Fever/headache
- Confusion, lethargy
- Diagnosed by CT scan: ring enhancing lesions; definitive brain biopsy

Clinical progression
- Slow; relapses if therapy not followed

Treatment: 4-6 weeks
- Pyrimethamine and sulfadiazine
- Folinic acid (leucovorin)

Maintenance: same

CRYPTOCOCCAL MENINGITIS

Frequency in AIDS: 8%-12%

Causes/pathogenesis
- *Cryptococcus neoformans:* a yeastlike fungus found in
  Pigeon droppings
  Soil
  Fruit and juices
  Unpasteurized milk

Clinical presentation
- Headache
- Nausea, vomiting, malaise
- Fever
- Stiff neck
- Altered mental status
- Diagnosis difficult
  CSF, blood studies
  Radiographic imaging rarely useful

Clinical progression
- Rapid; average survival 16 months

Treatment
- Primary: amphotericin B with/without fluconazole, 5-FU
- Maintenance: fluconazole, amphotericin B if recurrent

HZV, herpes zoster virus; CT, computed tomography; CSF, cerebrospinal fluid; 5-FU, 5-fluorouracil.
Courtesy of Debbie M. Winters, 1992

and physical support. Care is delivered by an interdisciplinary team who coordinate and supervise all hospice services 7 days a week, 24 hours a day. Hospice services may be hospital based or provided in the home setting or in other community-based programs.

CHILDREN WITH AIDS

Although pediatric cases represent only 2% of the total AIDS population, the number is growing rapidly. AIDS is now among the 10 leading causes of death in children (Pizzo, 1990). Initially children infected with HIV tended to be hemophiliacs or the recipients of other blood products. More recently increasing numbers of children who are infected during the perinatal period and adolescents who are infected as a result of high-risk sexual behaviors make up the majority of this population.

Children with perinatally acquired AIDS reflect the largest percentage of cases. These children appear normal at birth but generally develop symptoms within 9 months. This represents a shorter incubation period than adults experience. The damage caused by the virus can be rapid and devastating for infants and children because of their immature immune systems. Failure to thrive, development of recurrent diarrhea, and enlargement of the lymph nodes, liver, and spleen are constitutional symptoms that may go unrecognized early in the disease. Oral candidiasis and diaper dermatitis, chronic nasal discharge, and recurrent otitis media that is unresponsive to the usual therapies also may be present. Frequent bacterial infections are a common complication of HIV disease in children. Treatment must be of a longer duration and is aimed at antibiotic therapy based on the sensitivity of the isolates. The progression of the disease may cause damage and dysfunction to one or multiple organs including the central nervous system, heart, lungs, and gastrointestinal systems. Encephalopathy frequently is manifested and is characterized by delayed developmental milestones, impaired cognition and expressive language, spastic paraparesis, ataxia, and hyperirritability (Whaley & Wong, 1991).

Rehabilitation efforts are directed to minimizing the deficits caused by these progressive neurologic problems, emphasizing the maintenance of existing cognitive skills and facilitating developmental achievement through the use of infant stimulation, and through speech and language therapy. The incorporation of physical and occupational therapy can assist these children to compensate for motor deficits. Rehabilitation programs also need to address problems and issues generated by the demographic profile of these children. The greater majority of perinatally infected children are from socially and economically disadvantaged families. The social structure of these families often is under stress and does not present a framework for the optimal care and management of problems presented by the pediatric client with AIDS. Social services and the use of available community resources are highly appropriate referrals to include in the pediatric rehabilitation plan (Levinson & O'Connell, 1991).

REHABILITATION NURSING ASSESSMENT

Nursing care of the person with AIDS encompasses a knowledge base from the areas of infection control, neurology, oncology, psychiatry, and pediatrics. Clients can sometimes present with only one AIDS-related condition but more often than not find themselves hospitalized with multiple, complicated problems and/or multisystem failure. The person with AIDS commonly succumbs to uncontrollable infection, becoming increasingly debilitated, feverishly ill, and malnourished, and often is in pain. Lymphadenopathy, pulmonary infiltrates, wasting syndrome, and neurologic abnormalities such as dementia, tremors, and encephalitis contribute to the debilitated state. Because the HIV travels from cell to cell rather than circulating in the bloodstream, it is usually not susceptible to circulating antibodies of the body's remaining immune system of B cells. Aside from the specific treatments used to combat opportunistic infections and malignancies in persons with AIDS, there is no effective cure for AIDS at this time. Efforts are directed to preserving and enhancing the immune capabilities of the T cells for as long as possible. Some treatment approaches are mainly symptomatic, and others are highly experimental. The mortality rate for individuals with documented AIDS, once as high as 95% at 2 years, is improving but the rate and extent of change remains to be seen. AIDS is an example of a devastating secondary immunodeficiency that results in increased susceptibility of the client to a variety of infections and rare malignancies. It is the most severe form of a continuum of illnesses associated with HIV infection.

Our existing knowledge base provides an adequate foundation for designing delivery strategies and for planning interventions to meet the complex physiologic and psychosocial needs of the person with HIV/AIDS. Professional nurses, however, have the responsibility to keep fully informed of changes in the epidemiology of and treatment approaches for this disease and to modify their care accordingly. Other issues that will require nursing's attention for the remainder of this century are the need to define critical pathways and initiate case management approaches that will direct holistic, yet cost-effective, care for these patients. Ethical dilemmas will continue to surround the issues of disclosure and the right to confidentiality. As client advocates, nurses must be diligent in their efforts to respect the client's rights without allowing personal fears and viewpoints to interfere.

Society is clamoring for a solution to the AIDS crisis and issues related to funding—both for the most efficacious treatment and ultimately for a cure—which will continue to be volatile professional and societal considerations. Arguments over testing issues have yet to be resolved and bode a difficult future for transmission issues, not only from the perspective of the individual who contracts AIDS but also from that of the healthcare professional who is at increased risk or who unfortunately develops the disease as an outcome of lapse in the practice of Universal Precautions. Finally, one of the evolving issues yet to be fully addressed within the profession is the problem of the nurse who also has HIV/AIDS; this situation has multiple implications for mandatory testing and disclosure. Nursing professionals are well advised to monitor these issues and to take an active role in the definition of professional positions on this issue.

ACKNOWLEDGMENT

The author and editor acknowledge the contributions of Debbie M. Winters, MSN, RN, CRRN, to this chapter.

NURSING ASSESSMENT OF THE CLIENT WITH IMMUNODEFICIENCY

1. Health perception and health management pattern
   - ✦ Past or preexisting medical problems
     Present health status
     Past health status
     Intravenous drug use
     Current medications
   - ✦ Recent exposure to infection/communicable disease
2. Nutritional-metabolic pattern
   - ✦ Vital signs
     Temperature
     Cardiac rate/rhythm
     Respiratory rate and pattern
     Blood pressure
   - ✦ Nutritional intake
     Pattern and amount of food
     Alcohol intake
     Height and weight
     Difficulty swallowing
     Anorexia, nausea, vomiting
   - ✦ Skin integrity
     Skin lesions
       Location
       Size
       Color
       Character
     Anogenital lesions
     Oral lesions
3. Elimination pattern
   - ✦ Diarrhea
     Frequency
     Character
     Color
     Control
   - ✦ Urinary incontinence
4. Activity: exercise pattern
   - ✦ Activity tolerance
     Pattern of activity
     Duration of activity
     Fatigue
       Frequency
       Duration
       Measures to resolve
     Level of independence in self-care activities
   - ✦ Strategies utilized for diversion
   - ✦ Airway clearance
     Cough
     Frequency
     Sputum production
       Character
       Amount
       Odor
       Sputum culture
     PPD response
     Adventitious sounds

   - ✦ Gas exchange
     Skin color
     Arterial blood gas levels
     Shortness of breath
     Dyspnea on exertion
5. Sleep-rest pattern
   - ✦ Nighttime sleep pattern
   - ✦ Daytime naps
     Frequency
     Length
   - ✦ Night sweats
6. Cognitive/perceptual patterns
   - ✦ Hearing
   - ✦ Vision
   - ✦ Alterations in taste, smell
   - ✦ Educational background
     Learning style
     Academic experience
     Identified knowledge deficits
     Informational needs
   - ✦ Pain
     Location
     Duration
     Character
     Pattern
   - ✦ Orientation
7. Self-Perception: Self-concept pattern
   - ✦ Fear about current illness
   - ✦ Anxiety about treatment plan
8. Role-relationship pattern
   - ✦ Current occupational role
   - ✦ Significant others in life
   - ✦ Value of relationships
   - ✦ Living arrangements
   - ✦ Economic stability
   - ✦ Social patterns
9. Sexuality: reproductive pattern
   - ✦ Sexual orientation
   - ✦ Sexual practices
   - ✦ History of venereal disease
10. Coping: stress tolerance pattern
    - ✦ Effective coping strategies used
    - ✦ Support needed for coping
11. Value-belief pattern
    - ✦ Religious preference
    - ✦ Spiritual practices

PPD, purified protein derivative.

CASE STUDY: NURSING CARE PLAN FOR THE CLIENT WITH AIDS

Andrew Gerrity, 36 years old, was into the twelfth day of a 2-week camping and hiking trip with a group of friends to the mountains of Colorado. Andrew led an active life, participated frequently in sports, traveled extensively, was successful in building his career, and was involved in a long-term relationship with his friend, John. Up to the time of his admission to the hospital, he has been in excellent health with only occasional episodes of colds/flu and no injuries of any significance.

Andrew awoke in the middle of the night to find his bed clothing and sleeping bag soaked with perspiration. He was sweating profusely and could tell, even though no thermometer was available, that he was running a fever. Since he had never felt as sick as he felt at that time, he anticipated that this episode was different from his previous illnesses. He became alarmed at his distance from his usual healthcare resources and insisted on going home. Andrew was able to get a flight leaving for Boston that afternoon, flew home and immediately presented at his physician's office with a fever of 104.2° F and a nonproductive cough. He verbalized complaints of dyspnea on exertion and malaise. He was admitted to the hospital with diagnosis R/O (rule out) pneumonia. The admitting orders were as follows: isolation room, if available; routine vital signs; temperature every 4 hours; house diet as tolerated; chest radiograph; routine complete blood cell count (CBC), serum electrolytes and urinalysis; blood cultures ×2; sputum cultures ×3; 2 acetaminophen (Tylenol) tablets every 4 hours as needed for temperature elevated over 100° F; IV: 5% dextrose and normal saline solution at 60 ml/hour.

Nursing assessment at the time of admission showed a well-nourished, alert, and oriented man who was visibly concerned at what was happening to him. Vital signs were as follows: temperature, 104.6° F orally; pulse, 106; respirations, 26 breaths/minute; blood pressure, 132/86 mm Hg. Height and weight were within normal parameters for his age and frame. Pulmonary assessment revealed diffuse crackles at both lung bases. The remainder of the physical examination was unremarkable.

Laboratory and diagnostic data revealed the following:

Na: 130 mEq/L
K: 4.2 mEq/L
Cl: 100 mEq/L
CO_2: 24 mEq/L
BUN: 13 mg/100 ml
Creatinine: 0.8 mg/100 ml
Hemoglobin: 13.6 mg/100 ml
Hematocrit: 34.6 g/100 ml
White blood cell count: 12,000/mm³
Lymphocytes: 64%
Blood culture: negative
Sputum culture: *Pneumocystis carinii*

PRIORITY NURSING DIAGNOSES, INTERVENTIONS, AND OUTCOME CRITERIA AT THIS TIME FOR ANDREW ARE AS FOLLOWS:

1. Hyperthermia related to opportunistic infection as manifested by fever and elevated above 100° F orally.
   ✦ Ensure adequate hydration of at least 100 ml hourly.
   ✦ Monitor temperature of room, and provide adequate ventilation.
   ✦ Instruct client to use as little bed covers as possible until temperature is reduced to at least 100° F orally.
   ✦ Administer 2 acetaminophen tablets every 4 hours while temperature is elevated above 100° F orally.
   ✦ Monitor vital signs every 4 hours.
   ✦ Initiate sponge baths with cool water if temperature remains elevated over 103° F orally for more than 4 hours.
   ✦ Place ice bags at axilla and groin to facilitate reduction in body temperature.
   ✦ Assess for pain related to fever every 4 hours and provide analgesia.

Effective implementation of this plan will be shown by the following:
   ✦ Body temperature is maintained at 100° F orally or below.
   ✦ There is no evidence of pain associated with fever.

2. Knowledge deficit related to progress of illness as manifested by frequent questions and anxiety.
   ✦ Provide client with information about the condition. Answer all questions as fully as possible.
   ✦ Provide frequent contact and emotional support.
   ✦ Encourage client to communicate his questions and concerns to the medical staff.
   ✦ Collaborate with the medical staff on the kinds of information that are being communicated to the client and the ways in which information is shared.
   ✦ Teach the importance of medications and their side effects.
   ✦ Teach the importance of obtaining current and accurate information about AIDS.
   ✦ Teach the importance of regular, follow-up care.
   ✦ Instruct the client to keep a diary of symptoms experienced and treatment(s) prescribed.

Effective implementation of this plan will be shown by the following:
   ✦ Client is able to verbalize his understanding of the progress of his illness and to communicate his need for specific information to the medical staff.
   ✦ Anxiety levels are not interfering with client's ability to function.

To confirm the diagnosis of PCP, Andrew was scheduled for a bronchoscopy, which revealed the presence of this pathogen in the lung tissue. He was informed of his diagnosis and responded with tears and expressions of fear and anxiety.

3. Infection, high risk for transmission related to lack of knowledge about the mechanisms for transmitting the AIDS virus.
   ✦ Provide the necessary facts to dispel the myths regarding AIDS transmission.
   ✦ Initiate health teaching:
      Safe sexual practices.
      Risk of intravenous drug use and sharing needles.
      "Chain of infection" and client's responsibility to attend closely to hygiene.
      Blood is the primary mode of transmission. Exercise caution in the event of any trauma that produces bleeding. Special care must be taken in disposing of any material used to dress a bleeding wound.
      Hand washing is the single most important measure to prevent the spread of infection.
      AIDS virus is not transmitted by insect bites, swimming pools, clothes, eating utensils, toilet seats, or close contact.

Continued.

CASE STUDY: NURSING CARE PLAN FOR THE CLIENT WITH AIDS—CONT'D

AIDS virus has not been demonstrated to be transmitted in urine, feces, saliva, tears or sweat.

✦ Initiate referrals:

Provide client with AIDS hotline (1-800-342-AIDS) for more information.

Contact the infection control nurse to provide additional knowledge about AIDS transmission.

Effective implementation of this plan will be shown by the following:

✦ Client is able to describe the causes of AIDS and factors that contribute to its transmission.

✦ Client is able to describe and demonstrate, if appropriate, practices that reduce the risk of transmission.

Andrew is started on the following medications: sulfamethoxazole and trimethoprim (Bactrim), 1 g IV twice a day, and pyridoxine, 50 mg/day given orally.

His elevated temperature quickly responds to antihyperthermic measures. He is conscientious about hydration and adequate nutritional intake. He responds well to health teaching and is discharged to home after a 14-day hospital stay to continue on sulfamethoxazole and trimethoprim I DS tablet twice a day. He is instructed to return to the doctor in 3 months.

Andrew does well with the prescribed treatment plan. Subsequent follow-up examinations completed at 3, 6, and 9 months postdischarge show no evidence of recurrent infection. His nutritional status is excellent, and he has been able to resume his previous lifestyle. His relationship with John has continued as well. At Andrew's encouragement, John has undergone testing for HIV; no HIV antibodies have been detected in his case.

Eighteen months after his last medical checkup, Andrew begins to notice increasing fatigue and malaise. He is exhausted by just completing his work-related responsibilities and no longer has the stamina to pursue diversional activities. He also has noted a weight loss of 15 lb in the last 3 months. When he begins to develop fevers, night sweats, and a cough productive of thick mucus, he presents to his doctor for treatment and is immediately hospitalized. Significant diagnostic data are a white blood cell (WBC) count of 2000/mm^3, lymphocytes 30%, and T-helper cell count of 230. Chest radiograph reveals diffuse, bilateral infiltrates and the sputum sample is positive for moderate *Mycobacterium tuberculosis*.

Nursing assessment reveals lymphadenitis and oral lesions suggestive of *Candida albicans* infection. Andrews also reports difficulty in eating, especially with foods that are warm/hot in temperature, and in swallowing. He attributes his weight loss to his difficulty with eating. He admits to changing his oral hygiene care to compensate for the soreness he feels in his mouth.

Andrew appears moderately anxious on admission and relates to the nurse, "Getting another infection has been a real concern for me. Now it's happened and I'm afraid I'm never going to be healthy again." Andrew is started on sulfamethoxazole and trimethoprim I DS tablet twice a day; rifabutin 150 mg twice a day given orally; and ciprofloxacin 500 mg every 12 hours.

PRIORITY NURSING DIAGNOSES, INTERVENTIONS, AND OUTCOME CRITERIA FOR ANDREW AT THIS STAGE OF HIS ILLNESS ARE AS FOLLOWS:

1. High Risk for Recurrent Infection related to immunocompromised state as manifested by depressed white blood cell count, lymphocyte ratio, and T-cell count.

✦ Monitor continuously for signs and symptoms of the following additional opportunistic protozoal infections:

PCP: dry, nonproductive cough, fever, increasing dyspnea.

Toxoplasma gondii encephalitis: headache, lethargy, seizures.

Cryptosporidium enteritis: watery diarrhea, nausea, abdominal cramps, increasing malaise.

✦ Monitor continuously for signs and symptoms of the following additional opportunistic viral infections:

Herpes.

CMV.

Shingles.

✦ Monitor continuously for signs and symptoms of the following additional opportunistic fungal infections:

Cryptococcus neoformans meningitis: fever, headaches, blurred vision, stiff neck, confusion.

Emphasize need to report symptoms promptly.

✦ Initiate teaching regarding the following signs and symptoms of infection:

Redness.

Swelling.

Pain, soreness, stiffness, body aches.

Changes in oral mucosa.

Ulcerations, skin breakdown.

Fever.

Increased fatigue, sputum production, or cough.

✦ Teach method of self-assessment for recurrent infections.

✦ Teach importance of meticulous hygiene.

✦ Reinforce knowledge related to the mode of transmission of infectious organisms

✦ Discuss or demonstrate the following techniques to prevent infection:

Hand washing.

Clean home environment.

Proper handling of raw foods.

Stress reduction techniques.

Limiting contact with persons with known infection.

✦ Initiate nutritional teaching and emphasize the role that nutrients play in preventing infection.

✦ Refer to Home Care Department for home management follow-up.

✦ Emphasize the importance of cooperating with continuing, follow-up medical care

Effectiveness of these interventions will be demonstrated by the following:

✦ Client is able to describe the usual modes by which disease is transmitted.

✦ Client is able to describe and demonstrate those techniques and health practices that may provide protection from opportunistic infections.

✦ Client is able to describe the early signs and symptoms of infection.

✦ Client does not display any signs of additional opportunistic infections.

Continued.

CASE STUDY: NURSING CARE PLAN FOR THE CLIENT WITH AIDS—CONT'D

2. Altered Nutrition: less than body requirements related to anorexia, *Candida,* and dysphagia as manifested by weight loss of 15 lb.
   ✦ Initiate plans to treat the underlying cause (e.g., infection, fungus), as possible.
   ✦ Discuss the relationship between nutrition and infection control.
   ✦ Identify food preferences.
   ✦ Identify food intolerances (e.g., fat, lactose).
   ✦ Explain the rationale for daily weights.
   ✦ Initiate calorie counts.
   ✦ Encourage small, frequent feeding of food high in essential nutrients.
   ✦ Discourage snacking behavior.
   ✦ Add dietary supplements (e.g., ADVERA, Ensure) to promote weight gain.
   ✦ Explore the potential for nutritional drug therapy (e.g., Megace) to stimulate appetite.
   ✦ Consult with nutritional therapist to provide foods client will be able to eat and that are to his liking.
   ✦ Allow client to retain control over diet.
   ✦ Offer frequent oral care and suggest anesthetic mouth rinses before meals.
   ✦ Provide encouragement and emotional support.
   ✦ Teach the principles of a balanced diet.
   ✦ Encourage daily vitamin supplements.

   Effectiveness of these interventions will be demonstrated by the following:
   ✦ Client will progress toward ideal body weight.
   ✦ Client is able to discuss the relationship between nutritional intake and maintenance of optimal health status.

3. Oral tissue Integrity, impaired related to opportunistic infection as manifested by oral lesions and complaints of difficulty with eating and swallowing.
   ✦ Modify diet to limit foods high in spice or very hot in temperature.
   ✦ Initiate oral assessments every shift.
   ✦ Encourage frequent, gentle mouth care.
   ✦ Provide mouth rinses to enhance level of comfort and promote healing.
   ✦ Consult with medical staff regarding the efficacy of oral antifungal troches.

   Effectiveness of these interventions will be demonstrated by the following:
   ✦ Client will assume responsibility for oral hygiene.
   ✦ Oral lesions will diminish.
   ✦ Status of oral tissues does not inhibit eating and/or drinking and client relates less discomfort.

4. High Risk for Impaired Skin Integrity related to compromised nutritional state and immobility.
   ✦ Assess skin integrity regularly for lesions, pallor, redness, poor wound healing, and/or evidence of skin breakdown.
   ✦ Monitor any abnormal findings for progression.
   ✦ Implement measures to prevent additional skin breakdown: careful positioning, frequent pattern of turning, reducing potential for shearing injury to skin, gentle skin

massage, and application of moisturizing lotions and/or powders.
   ✦ Keep skin clean and dry and prevent prolonged contact with substances (e.g., diarrhea) that are irritating to the skin.
   ✦ Investigate the feasibility of a reduced-pressure bed.
   ✦ Maintain adequate nutrition and hydration.
   ✦ Encourage client to assume responsibility to change position and maintain skin integrity.
   ✦ Teach the importance of meticulous hygiene.

Effectiveness of these interventions will be demonstrated by the following:
   ✦ Client will assume responsibility for frequent repositioning.
   ✦ Assessment of skin reveals no areas of redness, irritation, or breakdown.
   ✦ Nutritional intake and hydration are maintained at acceptable levels.

Andrew returns to the suburban condominium he shares with John. Over the next few months, he is increasingly affected by bouts of severe nausea and diarrhea and profound fatigue. He is no longer able to work, and although he is able to take advantage of accumulated sick leave at the office where he was employed, he soon will be without income and health benefits. These realities looming in his future cause him to become depressed and generally unable to function. He no longer socializes with friends and has come to rely totally on John for companionship as well as emotional support. When the home care nurse visits, he expresses to her his dissatisfaction with this state of affairs and states that he is afraid that he is going downhill rapidly. "Why has God let this happen to me?"

PRIORITY NURSING DIAGNOSES, INTERVENTIONS, AND OUTCOME CRITERIA FOR ANDREW AT THIS PHASE OF HIS ILLNESS ARE AS FOLLOWS:

1. Fatigue related to advancing disease as manifested by client's inability to work and to participate in meaningful activities.
   ✦ Assess causative or contributing factors.
   ✦ Explain causes of fatigue.
   ✦ Allow for expressions of feelings regarding the effect of fatigue on goals and lifestyle.
   ✦ Assist client to identify energy patterns and the need to schedule activities with care.
   ✦ Assist client to establish priorities.
   ✦ Explain the purpose of pacing and prioritization.
   ✦ Plan for rest between tasks of daily living.
   ✦ Assist client to determine which tasks can be delegated.
   ✦ Teach energy conservation techniques.
   ✦ Initiate referrals to social work to explore the feasibility of home care assistance and supplemental income assistance.

Effectiveness of these interventions will be demonstrated by the following:
   ✦ Client will be able to discuss the cause of fatigue.
   ✦ Client will be able to identify priorities in tasks of daily living.
   ✦ Client will be able to participate in activities that address his intellectual and emotional needs without experiencing fatigue.

Continued.

◆

CASE STUDY: NURSING CARE PLAN FOR THE CLIENT WITH AIDS—CONT'D

2. Social Isolation related to effects of terminal illness as manifested by client's verbal statements of loneliness and dissatisfaction with present life.
   ◆ Discuss community resources available:
     Hospice volunteers.
     AIDS Action "Buddy System."
     AIDS support groups.
   ◆ Provide reading material about AIDS support services.
   ◆ Provide telephone number and name of contact person of local or regional AIDS Action Task Force and initiate referral, if necessary.
   ◆ Identify additional strategies to expand the client's social contact.

   Effectiveness of these interventions is demonstrated by the following:
   ◆ Client will verbalize increased satisfaction with life events.
   ◆ Client will follow through in obtaining AIDS support services.
   ◆ Client's community support network is expanded.

3. Anticipatory grieving related to terminal illness and anticipated premature death as manifested by client's verbal statements.
   ◆ Encourage communication of concerns and losses.
   ◆ Identify and acknowledge client's strengths.
   ◆ Identify community resources that may assist in grief work.
   ◆ Make referrals to community agencies as indicated.

Effectiveness of these interventions will be demonstrated by the following:
◆ Client will identify areas of loss that have occurred or have the potential to occur as a result of the AIDS diagnosis and strategies to cope with the loss(es).

4. Spiritual Distress related to impending death as manifested by client's verbal statements.
   ◆ Encourage communication.
   ◆ Be available and willing to listen actively.
   ◆ Use silence or touch, as appropriate, to communicate understanding and concern.
   ◆ Introduce the concept of life review.
   ◆ Promote quiet, uninterrupted time to explore depth of feelings.
   ◆ Allow expressions of anger.
   ◆ Help client to recognize, discuss, and redirect anger.
   ◆ Offer to contact spiritual leader.
   ◆ Make referral to pastoral care if no spiritual leader is identified.

Effectiveness of these interventions will be demonstrated by the following:
◆ Client freely expresses his feelings and identifies strategies to resolve them.
◆ Client expresses achievement of spiritual comfort.
◆ Client can express acceptance of suffering and death.

REFERENCES

Abrams, B., Duncan, D., & Hertz-Picciotto, I. (1993). A prospective study of dietary intake and acquired immune deficiency syndrome in HIV-seropositive homosexual men. *Journal of Acquired Immune Deficiency Syndrome, 6,* 949-958.

Brunner, L., & Suddarth, D. (1988). *Textbook of medical surgical nursing* (6th ed.). Philadelphia: J.B. Lippincott.

Bryant-Armstrong, T.B. (1988). The pathophysiology of human immunodeficiency virus infections. *Journal of Advanced Medical-Surgical Nursing 1,* 9-20.

Buczkowski-Bickmann, M.K. (1992). Thermoregulation in the neonate and the consequences of hypothermia. *CRNA: The Clinical Forum for Nurse Anesthetists, 3,* 77-82.

Bullock, B. (1992). Normal immunologic response. In B. Bullock & P. Rosendahl (Eds.), *Pathophysiology* (pp. 312-321). Philadelphia: J.B. Lippincott.

Bullock, B., & daCunha, M. (1992). Immune deficiency. In B. Bullock & P. Rosendahl (Eds.), *Pathophysiology.* Philadelphia: J.B. Lippincott.

Burkle, N.L. (1988). Inadvertent hypothermia. *Journal of Gerontological Nursing 14,* 26-30, 36-37.

Cohn, J.A. (1989). Virology, immunology, and natural history of HIV infection. *Journal of Nurse-Midwifery, 34,* 242-252.

Cox, A. (1992). Ventricular dysrhythmia secondary to select environmental hazards. *AACN Clinical Issues in Critical Care Nursing, 3,* 233-242.

Craven, R., & Hirnle, C. (1992). *Fundamentals of nursing.* Philadelphia: J.B. Lippincott.

Danzl, D.F., & Ghezzi, K.T. (1991). Hot tips on handling hypothermia. *Patient Care, 25,* 89-92, 94-96.

Darko, D.F., McCutchan, J.A., Kripke, D.F., Gillin, J.C., & Golshan, S. (1992). Fatigue, sleep disturbance, disability, and indices of progression of HIV infection. *American Journal of Psychiatry, 149,* 514-520.

Dexter, W.W. (1990). Hypothermia. Safe and efficient methods of rewarming the patient. *Postgraduate Medicine, 88,* 55-58, 61-64.

Flannery, J. (1992). Common problems of the nervous system. In L. Burrell (Ed.), *Adult nursing in hospital and community settings* (p. 914). Norwalk, CT: Appleton & Lange.

Frederick, C., Rosemann, D., & Austin, M.J. (1990). Malignant hyperthermia: Nursing diagnosis and care. *Journal of Post-Anesthesia Nursing, 5,* 29-32.

Gallagher, D.M. (1993). Gastrointestinal manifestations of HIV/AIDS. *Critical Care Nursing Clinics of North America, 5,* 121-126.

Griffin, G.E. (1990). Human immunodeficiency virus infection and the intestine. *Baillieres Clinical Gastroenterology, 4,* 657-673.

Hodges, H. (1992). Immunocompetence. In P. Kidd, & K. Wagner (Eds.), *High acuity nursing* (pp. 409-418, 423-427). Norwalk, CT: Appleton & Lange.

Holtzclaw, B.J. (1990). Control of febrile shivering during amphotericin B therapy. *Oncology Nursing Forum, 17,* 521-524.

Hoyt, M., & Staats, J. (1991). Wasting and malnutrition in patients with HIV/AIDS. *Journal of the Association of Nurses in AIDS Care, 2,* 16-28.

Hurley, P., & Ungvarski, P. (1994). Home healthcare needs of adults living with HIV disease/AIDS in New York City. *Journal of Association of Nurses in AIDS Care, 5,* 33-40.

Keithley, J.K., & Kohn, C.L. (1990). Managing nutritional problems in people with AIDS. *Oncology Nursing Forum, 17,* 23-27.

LaVoy, K. (1985). Dealing with hypothermia and frostbite. *RN, 48,* 53-56.

Law, V., & Baldwin, C. (1993). Nutritional support in HIV disease. *Physiotherapy, 79,* 394-399.

Lawson, L.L. (1992). Hypothermia and trauma injury: temperature monitoring and rewarming strategies. *Critical Care Nursing Quarterly, 15,* 21-32.

Levinson, S.F., & O'Connell, P.O. (1991). Rehabilitation dimensions of AIDS: A review. *Archives of Physical Medicine and Rehabilitation, 72,* 690-696.

Luckman, J., & Sorenson, K. (1987). *Medical surgical nursing* (3rd ed.). Philadelphia: W.B. Saunders.

Michal, D. (1989). Nursing management of hypothermia in the multiple-trauma patient. *Journal of Emergency Nursing, 15,* 416-421.

Miller, R.G., Carson, P.J., Moussavi, R.S., Green, A.T., Baker, A.T., & Weiner, M.W. (1991). Fatigue and myalgia in AIDS patients. *Neurology, 41,* 1603-1607.

Nelson, M.S. (1988). Rewarming techniques for hypothermia. *Topics in Emergency Medicine, 10,* 23-29.

O'Brien, M., & Pheifer, W.G. (1993). Physical and psychosocial nursing care for patients with HIV infection. *Nursing Clinics of North America, 28,* 303-316.

Pizzi, M. (1989). Occupational therapy: Creating possibilities for adults with HIV infection, ARC, and AIDS. *AIDS Patient Care, 3,* 18-23.

Pizzo, P.A. (1990). Pediatric AIDS: Problems within problems. *Journal of Infectious Diseases, 161,* 316-325.

Potter, P., & Perry, A. (Eds.). (1993). *Fundamentals of nursing: Concepts, process and practice.* St. Louis: Mosby–Year Book.

Whaley, L.F., & Wong, D.L. (1991). *Nursing care of infants and children.* St Louis: Mosby–Year Book.

Winters, D.M. (1992). Presentation at NJ State Chapter Educational Program for ARN, West Orange, NJ.

Wright, J. (1991). Accidental hypothermia. *Professional Nurse, 6,* 197-199.

23

Sleep, Rest, and Fatigue

Maureen Habel, MA, RN, CRRN

SLEEP

Restorative sleep is an essential component of health, affecting well-being and quality of life (Jensen & Herr, 1993). Numerous studies indicate that a significant number of Americans have serious sleep problems that are both unrecognized or untreated. Additionally, when sleep problems are recognized, lack of knowledge regarding current therapeutic strategies often results in ineffective treatment (Habel, 1993). At the same time compelling evidence continues to mount that demonstrates a causal relationship between poor sleep quality, sleep deprivation and fatigue, impairments in cognitive functioning, decreased productivity, and increased potential for accidental injury. The sequalae of sleep problems are known to increase the probability of human error and fatigue-related accidents, including trauma that results in physical disability (Dement & Mitler, 1993). In 1988 a congressional mandate was given to the National Commission on Sleep Disorders Research to determine the effects of sleep deprivation in American society. The results of this national study showed widespread lack of awareness of the extent of the problem among both the lay public and health professionals. Dement and Mitler (1993) state that the statistics gathered from a number of epidemiologic studies establish unequivocally that sleep deprivation poses tangible risks to society and that these risks are compounded by lack of awareness of the nature, incidence, and significance of sleep disorders and sleep loss.

For rehabilitation nurses the ability of individuals with physical disabilities or chronic illness to obtain sufficient restorative sleep is of specific concern. Many disabling disorders and chronic diseases are associated with sequelae that impact previously satisfactory sleep and rest patterns. Both participation in an active rehabilitation program and lifestyle changes that occur as the result of a disability increase the individual's need for high-quality physical and mental restoration. Because the rehabilitation client faces multiple physical and psychosocial problems, it may be difficult for the client or the nurse to attribute functional decrements to the effects of inadequate or ineffective sleep patterns or to a physiologic process that increases the need for rest. The client may complain of changes in performance or depression without connecting a disruption of previously satisfactory sleep patterns as a potential etiology. The nurse may observe changes in energy level or behavior without recognizing these signs as consequences of impaired sleep patterns. Chennelly (1989) suggests that it is best to assume that every client attempting to cope with physical disability or a new environment is at high risk for sleep problems. Nurses are in an excellent position to evaluate a client's past and present sleep problems, to implement nursing interventions that promote sleep, and to respond to problems associated with sleep disturbances in clients of all ages (Jensen & Herr, 1993). Sleep disruption is a significant and often unrecognized stressor that is compounded when an individual is experiencing other physiologic and psychological stresses. Rehabilitation nurses can play a pivotal role in assisting persons with significant health status changes to reestablish and/or to develop effective sleep patterns.

The Purpose of Sleep

Sleep is a state that is necessary for the restoration of energy and other anabolic processes (Locsin, 1988). Experimental evidence indicates that the processes of cellular growth and renewal are increased during sleep as opposed to waking periods (Chennelly, 1989). Sleep in humans may share a common evolutionary origin similar to hibernation in animals as a way of conserving energy (Biddle & Oaster, 1990). Theories of sleep function have addressed the role of sleep in restoration, protection, and energy conservation. Sleep of both adequate quantity and quality now is viewed as important in maintaining optimal health and well-being (Chennelly, 1989). When sleeplessness occurs, various psychological and physiologic changes take place (Locsin, 1988). The physiologic effects of sleep deprivation include less efficient body temperature regulation, with a fall in body temperature, some changes in cardiovascular and respiratory function, hormonal changes, and a decrease in the control of eye movements such as accommodation and convergence. Psychologically individuals who do not obtain sufficient sleep and rest have been observed to become increasingly aggressive and irritable (Hodgson, 1991). Inadequate sleep potentially impacts the rehabilitation client's ability to achieve desired life goals.

The Process of Sleep

The process of sleep, once seen as a passive activity, now is viewed as an active, complex phenomenon (Kedas, Lux, & Amodeos, 1989). Cycles of wakefulness and sleep are controlled by neurologic systems located in the brainstem, hypothalamus, thalamus, and basal forebrain. These neurologic systems involve complex neuroanatomic, neurophysiologic, and neurochemical mechanisms (Culebras, 1992a). Human sleep is recurrent, spontaneous, reversible, and occurs with eyelids closed (Webb, 1989). Sleep is a phenomenon common to all humans. During sleep we are unable to seek food or to find shelter, and our ability to defend ourselves from danger is markedly reduced (Hodgson, 1991). While asleep, pharyngeal reflexes remain intact; there are specific brain wave manifestations and absence of the goal-directed behavior that characterizes the waking state. There is decreased awareness of the external environment and alerted ego functioning in the form of dreaming. Recall of sleep events ranges from no recollection to vivid recall of mental and motor activities (Biddle & Oaster, 1990).

Sleep is a state of active neurophysiologic functioning that is synchronized with the light-dark cycle of the environment and influenced by complex neurochemical reactions arising from the reticular formation of the brainstem and mediated by a number of neurotransmitters (Culebras, 1992a; Hodgson, 1991). Neurotransmitters currently implicated in sleep and wakefulness include acetylcholine, norepinephrine, serotonin, dopamine, histamine, adenosine, and gaba-aminobutyric acid (GABA) (Biddle & Oaster, 1990). Wakefulness and sleep are antagonistic states controlled by the reticular activating system (RAS) located in the brainstem's reticular formation (Fig. 23-1). Wakefulness is maintained by tonic activity in the RAS and is reinforced by sensory input, with pain and acoustic stimuli having the most pronounced influence. The RAS is a complex pathway containing multiple synapses. The various sensory pathways that relay impulses to the cerebral cortex also send inputs to the RAS. Sensory input to the RAS is devired from

ascending sensory tracts and from the trigeminal, auditory, visual, and olfactory systems (Ganong, 1993). Within the RAS catecholamine and acetylcholine neurons are active during arousal. Neurotransmitters such as epinephrine and histamine contribute to the state of wakefulness, facilitating alertness (Ganong, 1993). During illness the RAS also is stimulated by internal somatic factors including nausea, fever, and dyspnea and by emotional events such as anxiety, depression, and grief. Nurse-initiated activities—medication administration, position changes—and movement, light, and noise in the hospital setting also stimulate the RAS (Richardson, 1994).

Sleep-generating structures are located in the lower brainstem. Through a decrease in sensory input, combined with visceral sensations of warmth and comfort, and influenced by neurotransmitters such as serotonin, sleep-inducing neurons dampen the activity of the RAS, producing relaxation and sleep (Kryger, Roth, & Dement, 1989). In a sleeping state environmental input to the organism is decreased and the critical threshold of electrical activity influencing the RAS fall to a level producing somnolence (Biddle & Oaster, 1990).

Acting in conjunction with neurophysiologic influences on sleep is the influence of a circadian rhythm mediated by the hypothalamus. The term circadian is derived from the Latin "circa dies," meaning "around a day." Circadian rhythms describe alterations in physiology and behavior that occur with regularity over a 24-hour period (Hodgson, 1991; Monk, 1989). Circadian rhythms have been identified in many neuroendocrine, behavioral, and psychophysiologic functions including body temperature, heart rate, and blood pressure. During sleep, for example, body temperature falls but begins to rise several hours before the indi-

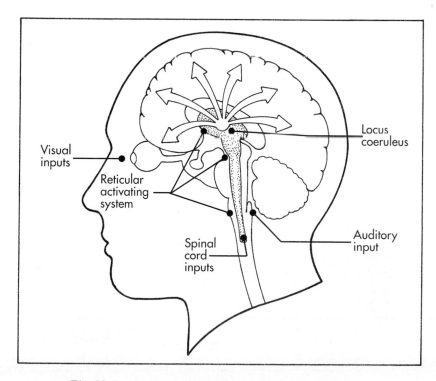

Fig. 23-1   Anatomic relationship of sleep-related structures.

vidual's usual waking time in preparation for optimum functioning (Hodgson, 1991).

The Phases of Sleep

Sleep is characterized by the repetition of distinct phases that cycle several times throughout each sleep period. Sleep in humans has been studied objectively through both direct observation of sleep behaviors and through the process of somnography. The identification of specific stages of sleep is based on the presence of distinctive brain waves, eye movements, and muscle activity as measured through electroencephalography (EEG), electrooculography (EOG), and electromyography (EMG) (Shaver & Giblin, 1989) (Fig. 23-2). Sleep research has confirmed that the various sleep stages, referred to as sleep architecture, represent two vastly different sleep stages based on physiologic differences in each stage (Hodgson, 1991).

Sleep is differentiated into nonrapid eye movement (NREM) sleep or rapid eye movement (REM) sleep. NREM sleep consists of four separate stages. In adults NREM sleep occupies the first part of the sleep cycle, and REM sleep predominates during the last portion of the sleep period. In terms of percentages, NREM sleep comprises approximately 75% of total sleep time and REM sleep accounts for 25% (Biddle & Oaster, 1990). During a normal sleep period, NREM and REM sleep stages cycle at periods of approximately 90 minutes (Fig. 23-3). Stage 1 NREM sleep

is a transitional stage between drowsiness and light sleep. Muscles relax, and the heart rate and respiratory rates decrease. In stage 2 sleep, sleep intensity increases, although the sleeper can be aroused easily. Stages 3 and 4 NREM sleep are the deepest stages of sleep and are classified as slow-wave sleep or delta sleep based on the EEG pattern. Muscles are relaxed but with muscle tone maintained, and vital signs are decreased significantly (Biddle & Oaster, 1990). Human growth hormone is secreted during stage 3 and 4 sleep (Hodgson, 1991). It is also during stage 4 deep sleep that sleepwalking or enuresis is most likely to occur (Biddle & Oaster, 1990). Following stage 4 NREM sleep, the sleeping individual begins an ascent back up through the sleep stages until she enters REM sleep (Reimer, 1989).

REM sleep is characterized by random, rapid, low-voltage EEG waves that closely resemble a waking state (Reimer, 1989). Eye movements are very rapid, vital signs may become irregular, and oxygen consumption increases (Biddle & Oaster, 1990; Reimer, 1989). Cerebral blood flow is increased and sexual arousal occurs. Nearly all dreaming occurs during REM sleep. If awakened during this phase of the sleep cycle, the individual is more likely to recall the content of dreams than during other sleep stages (Hodgson, 1991). Dreaming is considered to be an important function for learning, storage of memory, and psychosocial adaptation to stress. In the same way that stage 4 NREM sleep promotes physical restoration, REM sleep assists with mental and psychological rest and repair (Biddle & Oaster, 1990).

Various terms are used to describe the structure and process of sleep. Sleep patterns describe the amount and timing of sleep over a 24-hour period, including nocturnal sleep and naps. A sleep period is defined as the time from the actual onset of sleep until the time the individual awakens (Webb, 1989). Sleep latency refers to the amount of time that occurs between the intention to sleep and actual sleep. Sleep continuity is a measurement of the length of uninterrupted sleep. Sleep efficiency refers to the percentage of time in bed actually spent sleeping. Sleep pattern reversal describes alterations in sleep patterns characterized by early morning awakening and daytime sleeping with nocturnal wakefulness (Johnson, 1991a). Sleep pattern reversal occurs when the individual has wakeful periods at night and a desire for sleep during daytime hours. An arousal index may be used to measure the number of sleep stage changes from deep sleep to either stage 1 sleep or awakening that last less than 10 seconds/hour (Shaver & Giblin, 1989). Subjective

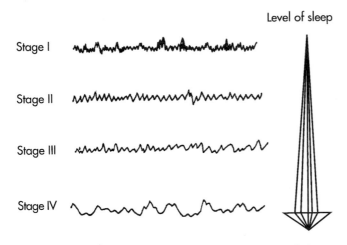

Fig. 23-2 EEG characteristics of the NREM stages of sleep.

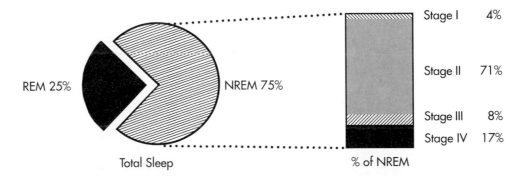

Fig. 23-3 Relative contributions of the sleep stages to total sleep.

measurements of sleep by clients include satisfaction with sleep, perceptions of the soundness of sleep, and reports of feeling rested and alert after the sleep period (Shaver & Giblin, 1989). Statements evaluating sleep often include terms such as "good," "poor," "light," and "tossing and turning."

Classification of Sleep Disorders

Sleep problems can be classified as nocturnal disturbances affecting normal sleep patterns and the undesirable daytime consequences of sleep disturbances (Rosekind, 1992). Most studies place the incidence of insomnia among adults at 30% to 35% of the population; insomnia appears to be widely underdiagnosed and the significance of insomnia as it affects human behavior and performance has been historically underestimated (Rosekind, 1992).

In 1990 the International Classification of Sleep Disorders was revised and updated. The new classification is based on pathophysiologic processes and consists of four major categories: dyssomnias; parasomnias; medical/psychiatric sleep disorders; and proposed sleep disorders, an unspecified category available for future diagnostic classification (see the following box).

General Factors Affecting Sleep

Many substances interfere with an individual's ability to either initiate or to maintain effective sleep. Alcohol, caffeine, and nicotine are the most common substances responsible for sleep disturbances in the general population (Moran & Stoudemire, 1992). Although alcohol has a sedating effect and may assist with sleep onset, it is also associated with multiple sleep awakenings and sleep disruptions (Monane, 1992). Prescription drugs that are associated with insomnia include thyroid hormone, theophylline preparations, cimetidine (Tagamet), phenytoin (Dilantin), levodopa, and diuretics given on a schedule that causes nocturnal diuresis (Monane, 1992). A variety of over-the-counter drugs may also interfere with sleep, particularly those with stimulant properties, such as nasal decongestants and anorexic agents (Moran & Stoudemire, 1992). Many over-the-counter sleep aids contain antihistamines or scopolamine as an active ingredient. These medications may cause delirium due to their anticholinergic effects and may result in excessive sedation in the elderly. Additive effects may also occur if the individual also is taking other anticholinergic or sedating drugs (Moran & Stoudemire, 1992).

Persons who have a significant health status change or are experiencing a stressful life change, including hospitalization or long-term institutional care, face many challenges in achieving normal sleep. Most healthy individuals experience transient sleep problems when sleeping in a new environment (Chennelly, 1989). Attempting to cope with functional losses as a result of disability or chronic illness often produces anxiety, which further impairs adequate sleep and rest (Chennelly, 1989). For persons who are hospitalized, institutional routines often conflict with the person's natural circadian rhythm and sleep routines and may create inadvertent iatrogenic sleep disorders. Individuals experiencing depression often have an early onset of the first REM sleep period and decreased stage 4 sleep (Monane, 1992). Pain can increase the sleep onset period and increase the number of awakenings, thus contributing to the person's

---

♦

CLASSIFICATION OF SLEEP DISORDERS

DYSSOMNIAS

Dyssomnias are subdivided into three subcategories: intrinsic disorders; extrinsic disorders; and circadian rhythm disorders. Intrinsic dyssomnias describe sleep disorders that result in either insomnia or hypersomnia and are the consequence of internal alterations. Examples of intrinsic dyssomnias include psychophysiologic insomnia, and primary sleep disorders (e.g., narcolepsy; obstructive, central, and mixed sleep apneas; and periodic leg movements [nocturnal myoclonus]). Extrinsic dyssomnias include inadequate sleep hygiene, environmental sleep disorders, such as one might experience in sleeping in an unfamiliar situation, and hypnotic dependent sleep disorders. Circadian rhythm disorders are those associated with time zone changes as a result of transmeridian travel (jet lag), shift work sleep disorders, and irregular sleep-wake schedules.

Dyssomnia, or insomnia, caused by either intrinsic or extrinsic factors, is the most common of the sleep disorders. Transient insomnia frequently occurs with minor situational and psychological stressors such as bereavement, minor illness, or changes in environment. Short-term insomnia occurs over weeks and often is experienced in conjunction with acute medical illness or a change in health status. Long-term insomnia, lasting weeks to months or longer, may occur with chronic health problems or as a result of primary sleep disorders.

PARASOMNIAS

Parasomnias are undesirable phenomena that occur predominately during sleep. Sleepwalking, sleep terrors, confusional arousals, nightmares, and sudden infant death syndrome (SIDS) are all classified as parasomnias.

MEDICAL/PSYCHIATRIC SLEEP DISORDERS

Medical/psychiatric sleep disorders are divided into three subcategories. The first category describes sleep problems related to mental disorders such as psychoses, anxiety or panic disorders. The neurologic disorders category includes dementia, Parkinson's disease, and sleep-related epilepsy. The third category refers to sleep problems associated with other medical disorders, including gastroesophageal reflux, peptic ulcer disease and Fibrositis syndrome.

PROPOSED SLEEP DISORDERS

A category reserved for the identification of future sleep disorders.

From "Update on Disorders of Sleep and the Sleep-Wake Cycle" by A. Culebras, 1992, *Psychiatric Clinics of North America, 15,* 469-470. *International Classification of Sleep Disorders: Diagnostic and Coding Manual* (pp. 15-17) by Diagnostic Classification Steering Committee, M.J. Thorpy, Chairman, 1990, Rochester MN: American Sleep Disorders Association.

perception of inadequate rest (Davis-Sharts, 1989). Poor sleep hygiene—extended time in bed, frequent daytime napping, keeping an irregular sleep-wake schedule, and lack of an effective bedtime routine—also is associated with insomnia. A poor sleep environment, either in the hospital or at home, is known to interfere with effective sleep. Noise, ambient temperature, lighting, and sleeping surface are all important components of a sleep environment (Topf, 1992).

Many persons with disabilities and chronic illness, as well as their families and/or caregivers, experience anxiety, irritability, and depression. Sleep deprivation in these individuals may occur not only as a result of nighttime care needs, but may be compounded by other issues such as fear and worry regarding the illness, concerns about treatment and prognosis, or inability to plan for the future (Hodgson, 1991). Persons with medical problems and those caring for them will release increased amounts of corticosteroids and adrenalin in response to increased sympathetic activity, resulting in increased catabolism and sleeplessness (Hodgson, 1991). Chronic sleep disruption and sleep deprivation may impact the rehabilitation process by increasing anxiety, lessening motivation, and interfering with the coping abilities of both the client and caregivers (Hodgson, 1991). Psychological and social factors may contribute markedly to sleep disorders in persons with chronic illness. Studies have demonstrated a higher incidence of sleep problems in clients who have affective disorders compounded by musculoskeletal problems. Positive relationships also have been found among masked depression, insomnia, and daytime sleepiness (Hyppa & Kronholm, 1989).

The sleep of nearly all nursing home residents appears to be quite disturbed. Potential etiologies include extended periods of time in bed, excessive daytime napping, a deterioration of circadian rhythms, noisy environments, sleep apnea, dementia, and concommittant medical problems such as pain and nocturia (Ancoli-Israel, 1989). It is estimated that approximately 23% of those 85 or older reside in long-term care facilities. Institutionalization is an important risk factor for both disordered sleep and for hypnotic administration (Gottlieb, 1990). Multiple psychological, medical, and pharmacologic causes disrupting sleep often are concentrated in the long-term care resident (Monane, 1992).

Sleep Disorders Associated with Specific Disabling Conditions

✦ Post-polio syndrome

Persons with post-polio syndrome (PPS) have an increased risk of developing sleep apnea as a result of both weakening musculature and aging. Sleep apnea occurs when there are periods of breathing cessation during sleep. An increased risk of stroke and cardiovascular disease have been correlated with sleep apnea (Bonnet & Arand, 1989; Jamison & Becker, 1992). In obstructive sleep apnea there are continued paradoxic thoracoabdominal respiratory efforts against an occluded pharyngeal airway. Snoring and choking during sleep are prominent signs of obstructive apnea and are the result of recurrent obstruction of the upper airway (Schwartz & Smith, 1989).

Central apneas are characterized by the complete absence of respiratory muscle efforts. Mixed apneas include components of both obstructive and central apnea. With obstructive sleep apnea, narrowing of the nasopharyngeal dimen-

sions, obesity, and the use of sedating drugs, especially alcohol, are primary contributing factors (Jamison & Becker, 1992). To confirm sleep apnea, a sleep study known as a polysomnogram is performed. The number and length of apneic episodes, sleep stage determination, number of arousals, respiratory effort, heart rate, and percentage of oxygen saturation are measured (O'Donnell, 1992). When treatment is indicated for sleep apnea, a number of general measures are advised including weight loss; avoidance of alcohol, sedatives, and hypnotics; avoidance of the supine sleeping position; and management of any nasal or nasopharyngeal disease or structural abnormalities. Persons with PPS who are experiencing excessive daytime sleepiness, snoring, or disrupted sleep, or who have an unexplained rise in the red blood cell count should be evaluated for the presence of sleep apnea via sleep studies. To keep the airway open during sleep, persons with obstructive apnea may be treated with nasal continuous positive airway pressure (CPAP) or with BiPap (S/T Respironics, Inc., Monroeville, PA), a ventilatory support system with separate inspiratory and expiratory pressures (Stice & Cunningham, 1995). Persons who already have some form of respiratory assistance, such as a rocking bed, may be treated effectively with long-term nasal mechanical ventilation (Steljes, Kryger, Kirk, & Millar, 1990).

✦ Spinal cord injury

Complaints of sleep problems appear to be relatively frequent in those with high spinal cord lesions (Culebras, 1992a). It has been identified that a significant number of persons with high quadriplegia may be at risk for potentially serious nocturnal hypoxic episodes, characterized by severe oxygen desaturation (Flavell, et al., 1992). Several factors predispose persons with cervical spinal injury to sleep-induced respiratory problems including paralysis of the intercostal and abdominal muscles; diaphragmatic weakness if the injury is at or above C5; the sedating effects of antispasmodic drugs, which may result in obstructive or central hypoventilation; and the development of obesity as a result of decreased activity. Obesity in these clients is associated with causing upper airway narrowing, which further increases the stress on weakened respiratory muscles (Culebras, 1992a; Flavell, et al., 1992).

✦ Multiple sclerosis

The demyelinization of axons responsible for motor movements may cause periodic limb movements that result in frequent sleep interruptions in persons with multiple sclerosis (MS). Sleep disturbances in MS also seem to be increased if the client also is affected by depression, fatigue, spasticity, or bladder problems (Clark, 1991).

✦ Rheumatoid arthritis

Pain is a problem that interrupts the sleep of persons with rheumatoid arthritis (RA). Reducing pain through the use of medication, rest, and joint splinting improves the quality of sleep in these clients (Crosby, 1991).

✦ Brain injury

Closed injuries of the head that result in loss of consciousness can cause interruptions of the sleep-wake cycle (Culebras, 1992a). Sleep disturbances, including both problems in initiating and maintaining sleep and excessive somnolence, have been recognized in both adults and children following traumatic brain injury. Sleep abnormalities most often are seen in the first few months postinjury. During the process of recovery from brain injury, the organization of sleep tends to become more normalized as rehabilitation proceeds, with a parallel increase in both cognition and percentage of REM sleep (Culebras, 1992a). There also appears to be a correlation between frequent nocturnal awakenings and daytime behavioral problems (Askenasy & Rahmani, 1988). Other studies have described the problems of brain-injured clients as frequent nighttime awakenings, problems getting back to sleep after arousal, and needing an extended period of time to function at peak efficiency after waking (Reimer, 1989). Some of the medications used to treat the sequelae of brain injury also may disrupt sleep. Phenytoin (Dilantin) and haloperidol (Haldol) both may produce insomnia as a side effect. Although haloperidol is effective in managing agitation, its action also is thought to block dopamine, one of the neurotransmitters involved in sleep (Reimer, 1989). Carbamazepine (Tegretrol) increases slow-wave sleep and decreases nighttime wakefulness.

✦ Pulmonary diseases

Clients with pulmonary diseases may be unable to sleep in a supine position if this position aggravates dyspnea (Chennelly, 1989). The prone position also may be contraindicated as proning inhibits chest wall expansion and inspiratory effort. Sleeping with the head of the bed elevated or in a comfortable chair may be the most effective means of positioning for effective sleep. Reducing anxiety is another essential aspect for sleep effectiveness in pulmonary clients, as rising anxiety increases oxygen consumption and demands increased respiratory effort (Chennelly, 1989).

✦ Alzheimer's disease

Alzheimer's disease (AD) is a progressive deterioration of cortical and subcortical neurons arising from an as yet unknown cause. Common features of AD include reduced ability to maintain attention to external stimuli; restlessness and agitation; perceptual problems in the form of hallucinations, fear, and anger; and sleep pattern disturbances. Sleep frequently is impaired in dementing conditions as a result of neuroanatomic or functional brain abnormalities, which are etiologic factors in these conditions. Progressive dementia, particularly AD, is associated with a deterioration in sleep quality, fragmented and shallow sleep, and a reversal of normal diurnal rhythms (Moran & Stoudemire, 1992). Thus disturbances of sleep and sleep-wake rhythms are common in AD (Vitiello, Bliwise, & Prinz, 1992). AD clients spend a considerable amount of their nighttime hours awake and spend long periods of time sleeping during the day. The daytime sleep is often of poor quality and consists primarily of stage 1 and 2 sleep, which does not compensate for the nighttime losses of slow-wave NREM and REM sleep (Vitiello & Prinz, 1989). These changes in sleep-wake patterns have been observed even at early stages of AD. As the disease progresses, there is a significant loss of REM sleep and a breakdown of normal circadian control of sleep and alertness.

"Sundowning" is a term used to describe the onset of de-

lirium during the evening or night in persons with AD or other dementing disorders. In the acute hospital and long-term care setting, sundowning presents a major client management problem for nursing staff. In the community the combination of sleep disturbances and sundowning places an enormous burden on the caregivers of persons with dementia. Disturbances of sleep, including nighttime insomnia and wandering, often become the determining factor in the decision of families to institutionalize a family member (Vitiello & Prinz, 1989).

✦ Parkinson's disease

Sleep pattern disturbances are common in persons with neurologic problems such as Parkinson's disease. Up to 70% of persons with Parkinson's disease experience sleep problems (Reimer, 1989). Some of the sleep disturbances may be directly related to the pathology associated with the neurologic condition; other symptoms may be due to secondary problems including impaired mobility, pain, and depression (Reimer, 1989). One of the earliest symptoms of Parkinson's disease is declining nocturnal sleep quality. Clients may complain of difficulty initiating sleep but more frequently report fragmented sleep as a result of prolonged multiple awakenings, resulting in daytime sleepiness and fatigue. Parkinsonian tremors abate during sleep but may reappear in association with sleep arousals or body movements during sleep. The effects of antiparkinsonian medications and the loss of body movements while in bed also may be contributing factors to unsatisfactory sleep (Culebras, 1992a). Under normal conditions individuals change positions about 30 times each night, with a position shift approximately every 15 to 20 minutes. These position changes may cause an adjustment in the sleep stage but do not ordinarily involve arousal. However, for the person with profound weakness who needs assistance to effect a position change, position shifts may require complete awakening for the client and the caregiver (Reimer, 1989).

✦ Stroke

After a large hemispheric stroke, there may be a temporary reversal of the sleep-wake rhythm with lethargy during the day and wakefulness and agitation at night. In the course of recovery, clients with stroke recover normative sleep stage patterns (Culebras, 1992a).

✦ Myasthenia gravis

In this disorder of neuromuscular transmission, fatigability may affect the diaphragm and accessory respiratory muscles, with resulting respiratory failure. Sleep complaints in persons with myasthenia gravis include waking in the middle of the night with a sensation of breathlessness, morning headaches, and daytime somnolence (Culebras, 1992a).

Perceptions of Healthcare Professionals

A number of studies indicate that health professionals often pay little attention to the sleep problems experienced by their clients. A study of physician attitudes about sleep in elderly persons revealed that although experienced geriatricians reported sleep problems as a frequent and clinically significant problem for their clients, few used appropriate interventions. Nearly half the physicians did not gather a definitive sleep history, and few diagnosed primary sleep disorders or made referrals to evaluate sleep problems refractory to conventional therapy. Although the hazards of pharmacologic therapy were cited, few physicians in the study used programs that emphasized nonpharmacologic sleep-promoting behaviors (Haponik, 1992). Physicians participating in this study reported that they had little formal training in the area of sleep and often attributed sleep complaints to either the secondary consequences of chronic illness or to the side effects of medications.

Recent publications in the medical literature have focused attention on the importance of physician education in sleep and sleep disorders. The accumulating body of knowledge pointing to the prevalance of sleep disorders in the population at large and the impact of inadequate sleep on mortality, morbidity, and quality of life has resulted in a call to action on the part of physicians (Rosen, Rosekind, Rosevear, Cole, & Dement, 1993). A recently published study of 126 accredited medical schools in the United States found that current medical students receive approximately 2 hours of total education in sleep medicine within the curricula. The study concluded that physician education in sleep and sleep disorders generally is inadequate (Rosen et al., 1993). Another commentary in a prestigious medical journal challenges physicians to legitimize sleep as a human concern and to increase their efforts to acknowledge, diagnose, and treat sleep disorders (Dement & Mitler, 1993).

A study of the frequency of use of nursing diagnoses in rehabilitation nursing practice revealed that the nursing diagnosis of Sleep Pattern Disturbance was used frequently by less than 50% of the study respondents (Sawin & Heard, 1992). A study of critical care nurses by Pulling (1991) disproved the hypothesis that there would be a positive relationship between knowledge about sleep and the initiation of sleep-promoting behaviors. When priority given to sleep, managing an environment conducive to sleep, ability to change the intensive care unit (ICU) environment, and the quantity of client sleep were controlled as variables, the number of nursing interventions aimed at sleep promotion was unrelated to the nurses' knowledge about sleep (Pulling, 1991). Those nurses participating in this study who perceived sleep as a priority for their clients, whatever their knowledge base about sleep, were more likely to initiate sleep-promoting behaviors. Data from this study also suggested that nurses did not keep up to date on nursing knowledge and research in the area of sleep, despite a considerable amount of available information (Pulling, 1991).

Reimer (1989) looked at which nursing interventions were perceived by clients and nurses as facilitating nocturnal sleep in the hospital environment. Clients in this study reported significant differences between home and hospital sleeping patterns. Nurses identified pain as an etiologic factor in sleep pattern disturbances, but indicated less awareness of other concerns cited by clients, including positional discomfort, attached medical equipment, and personal worries about health status and family concerns (Reimer, 1989). Neither clients nor nurses viewed sleep hygiene measures as important interventions despite the fact that clients ranked sleep hygiene within their preferred top 10 interventions. Environmental stimuli (e.g., light, temperature, noise, and bed quality) were cited as disturbing to sleep with consistent frequency. The implications of Reimer's study suggest that nurses could play a major role in helping clients sleep through simple environmental modifications and management.

Beyerman (1987) conducted a chart review of 100 cases in which neither physicians nor nurses made an appropriate diagnosis in regard to sleep pattern disturbance, although 48 of the clients stated during their initial assessment that they had at least one major defining characteristic of sleep pattern disturbance before hospitalization. Beyerman's speculations as to why nurses neglected to diagnose sleep pattern disturbance in their clients was a result of not being taught about sleep pattern disturbance, not valuing its significance, expecting that clients will have sleep problems, not believing they can affect the problem, or being unaware of the problem.

A study by Richardson (1994) looked at sleep pattern disturbances in the critically ill. Richardson's hypothesis was that sleep pattern disturbance in the critically ill adult is underdiagnosed and is treated primarily with medications as a collaborative problem, in part due to the lack of definition of related factors for nursing. The mean sleep time of subjects in this study was 28 minutes. Study results indicated that 100% of subjects experienced severe sleep deprivation; subjects were interrupted much more frequently than predicted; voices and other noises at the nursing station were the primary awakening stimuli; and internal somatic, cognitive, and emotional stimuli were correlated more strongly with waking than anticipated.

Sleep Changes Across the Life-Span

There is a relatively predictable and consistent relationship between age and sleep (Biddle & Oaster, 1990) (Fig. 23-4). Newborns experience 16 to 18 hours of sleep within a 24-hour period. Young children who are hospitalized experience the distress of being separated from their home environment. If falling asleep or nighttime awakenings previously have been associated with comfortable experiences such as being rocked, nursed, or cuddled, the withdrawal of these experiences may add to the distress of young children (Shaver & Giblin, 1989). White, Williams, Alexander, Powell-Cane, and Conlon (1990) studied the effects of a bedtime story on the onset of sleep in hospitalized children. Study findings confirmed a positive relationship between children hearing a recorded bedtime story with a stranger's voice using a theme of family reunion and the onset of sleep.

The aging process is associated with both subjective and objective changes in the quantity and quality of sleep, which affect the individual as a whole (Gottlieb, 1990). Although older persons do not have a decrease in the amount of sleep they require for physical and mental restoration, they experience significant and progressive changes in sleep architecture. EEG and sleep pattern changes that occur with age reflect changes in neurologic and nervous system functioning (Davis-Sharts, 1989). Although there is a wide range of differences among individuals, sleep characteristics in the elderly include a slight shift toward earlier bedtimes and earlier rising times, an increase in sleep awakenings after

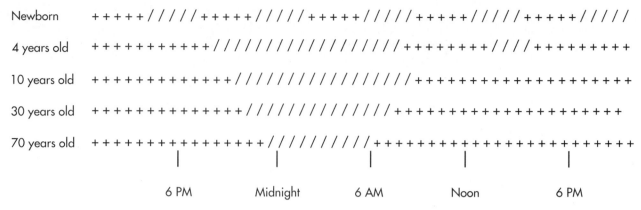

Fig. 23-4   Relative time spent in sleep by age group. //// = sleep; ++ = wake.

onset, and an increase in daytime napping (Webb, 1989). Aging is characterized by decreased slow-wave sleep and an increased incidence of sleep-disordered breathing (Buyesse, Browman, Monk, Reynold, Fasiczka, & Kupfer, 1992). By age 60 it is estimated that stage 3 and 4 sleep has decreased to less than 10%. The lighter stages of sleep, especially stage 1 sleep, are increased as individuals age. Both the amplitude and duration of stage 3 and 4 sleep, the deepest stages of NREM sleep, diminish greatly with advancing age (Monane, 1992) (see Fig. 23-4).

Although the total duration of REM sleep declines with total sleep time, relative proportions of REM sleep appear to be maintained until the eighth and ninth decades of life (Gottlieb, 1990; Johnson, 1991a). Gender differences also appear to be of importance. Elderly women are more likely to express concerns regarding their sleep and are more likely to take hypnotic medications than men; men are more likely to have sleep disorder breathing problems (Gottlieb, 1990).

Nocturnal myoclonus, a phenomenon characterized by frequent, repetitive leg movements during sleep, is correlated strongly with geriatric insomnia (Gottlieb, 1990). These periodic leg movements frequently are followed by arousals from sleep and subsequent reports of inadequate sleep and daytime performance decrements. It is thought that the etiology of periodic leg movements may be a central nervous system (CNS) disorder that results in increased excitability of segmental reflexes (Kovacevic-Ristanovic, Cartwright, & Lloyd, 1991).

Iatrogenic drug-induced insomnia also may present a particular challenge in the elderly. It is estimated that elderly clients take between 5 and 10 prescription medications daily, some of which may interfere with effective sleep (Monane, 1992). Drug absorption, metabolism, distribution, and excretion are all affected by the normal physiologic changes that occur with aging (Jamison & Becker, 1992). Chronic pain syndromes as a result of arthritis, myalgia, and other orthopedic or musculoskeletal problems are more common in the elderly. Such conditions may limit mobility and often are associated with spending increasing amounts of time in bed. The elderly, who sleep more lightly as a result of changes in sleep architecture, are more affected by environmental changes imposed by hospitalization. The

amount of time individuals spend in bed as they age increases from the fourth decade on. Elderly people report spending more time in bed, whether or not they are trying to initiate sleep, and resting or napping during the day; the elderly also are more easily aroused by noise due to their loss of deep-stage sleep (Horne, 1991).

Many older people experience a variety of medical and psychological problems that are associated with sleep pattern disturbances (National Institutes of Health [NIH], 1991). By age 60 the average number of sleep awakenings increases to four to six per night and the average time to sleep onset also increases (Johnson, 1991a). Adverse effects of sleep problems in the elderly include heightened pain awareness and decreased daytime vigilance, a factor that increases the potential for injuries (Johnson, 1991). Ancoli-Israel (1989) found that although elderly subjects described their sleep and daytime functioning as satisfactory, they also reported being sleepier during the day as they grew older. Daytime napping may represent a change in the adult biphasic pattern of sleep in favor of the polyphasic sleep patterns of infancy. It has been suggested that this change, together with boredom and impaired nocturnal sleep, may account for an increase in daytime naps with advancing age (Kedas et al., 1989). Although the exact mechanisms may not yet be evident, it is clear that circadian rhythms change as one gets older and that these changes negatively impact both nocturnal sleep and daytime functioning (Monk, 1989).

Older people do not sleep with the same efficiency as younger adults. These age-related changes occurring with sleep are systematic and generally irreversible (Monk, 1989; Webb, 1989). Because a decline in psychomotor performance normally is seen as a consequence of aging and because there are predictable changes in sleep stage distribution during the aging process, it has been hypothesized that the decrease in performance ability in the elderly is related to increasing sleep fragmentation, decreased slow-wave sleep, and/or decreased ability to maintain sleep (Bonnet & Arand, 1989). The severity of sleep fragmentation has been correlated with the amount of daytime sleepiness, a critical factor in daytime functioning (Gottlieb, 1990). Not only do drug pharmacokinetics and the potential for drug interactions increase with age, but the nature of sleep itself and the incidence of sleep disorders also changes. The combination of altered sleep; sleep pathology; and changes in drug absorption, metabolism, and elimination in elderly persons results in a higher risk of drug-induced insomnia and daytime sleepiness in this age group (Roehrs & Roth, 1989).

Evidence suggests that sleep apnea is prevalent in asymptomatic elderly individuals (Schwartz & Smith, 1989). Health professionals should view an elderly client's report of deterioration in the continuity of sleep and consequent daytime somnolence as a potential sleep disorder (Ancoli-Israel, 1989). Subjective reports by clients or caregivers of poor sleep quality, insomnia, snoring, intellectual deterioration, personality changes, and a decline in daytime alertness should not be taken lightly and should not be assumed to be a normal consequence of aging (Ancoli-Israel, 1989; Schwartz & Smith, 1989).

Nurses can play a pivotal role in counseling elderly clients about the value of a regular bedtime routine. Johnson (1991b) studied the relationship between a bedtime routine and effectiveness of sleep in elderly men and women. The Bedtime Routine Questionnaire used in the study listed activities such as brushing teeth; bathing; combing, curling or washing hair; listening to the radio; watching television; writing; reading; drinking; eating; praying, talking to another person; doing relaxation exercises; having a backrub; and taking bedtime medications. The results of Johnson's study indicated that sleep was least disturbed in elderly men who followed a regular routine. Older women who did not have a bedtime routine reported the most dissatisfaction with sleep patterns. Men in this study tended to include food, drink, television viewing, and walking in their bedtime routines. Women were more likely to engage in hygienic activities or to pray, read, or listen to music. Johnson suggests that as nurses become more cognizant of the sleep pattern changes occurring with aging, they will not view concerns regarding sleep disturbances as unusual.

Nurses are in an important position to recognize predictable changes with aging, to provide advice regarding the value of interventions such as bedtime routines, and to assess significant changes in sleep as potential symptoms of a pathologic sleep disorder such as sleep apnea for which the client should receive an appropriate referral (Johnson, 1991a).

Assessment of Sleep Pattern Disturbance

An organized and comprehensive assessment (see the following box) is the first step in diagnosing an actual or potential sleep pattern disturbance. The initial evaluation of sleep problems can become an important part of nursing evaluation before hospital admission and should be systematically reassessed on an inpatient and outpatient basis. The initial assessment should include a sleep history, observation of both sleeping and waking behaviors, and an environmental assessment (Chennelly, 1989). In performing the assessment, the nurse should consider the fact that each person has unique sleep needs and habits; that to the greatest extent possible, previous sleep routines should be used to reestablish and maintain normal sleep patterns; and that previous sleep requirements are the best indicator of the client's minimum current needs. The stress of illness and/or hospitalization may significantly increase the client's requirements for sleep and rest (Chennelly, 1989).

SLEEP ASSESSMENT

TAKING A SLEEP HISTORY

✦ What is client's usual sleep pattern?

✦ What lifestyle changes or recent events are occurring that interfere with sleep?

✦ What is the primary sleep problem? Difficulty with sleep onset, frequent awakenings during the night, waking earlier or later than desired, waking without feeling rested, feelings of sleepiness during the day, changes in abilities to perform daytime activities?

✦ How is the sleep pattern disturbance affecting other areas of functioning?

✦ What specific bedtime routine or sleep hygiene measures does client normally do to facilitate sleep and rest?

✦ What medications, either prescribed or over the counter, is client currently taking?

✦ Does client consume alcohol before bedtime and/or regularly consume stimulants such as coffee, tea, or caffeinated soft drinks?

PERFORMING AN ENVIRONMENTAL ASSESSMENT

✦ What is the noise and light level in the sleep environment?

✦ Is the temperature and ventilation in the sleeping environment conducive to sleep?

✦ Are there disturbances caused by roommates or other environmental factors such as odors which impair sleep?

✦ Is the bed surface comfortable? Are linens fresh and clean?

Nursing Diagnosis: Sleep Pattern Disturbance

Carpenito (1991) describes sleep pattern disturbance as a state in which the individual experiences or is at risk of experiencing a change in the quality or quantity of his/her rest pattern as related to his/her biologic and emotional needs. Gordon (1991) describes sleep pattern disturbance as a "disruption of sleep time causing discomfort or interference with desired life activities."

Major defining characteristics used for the nursing diagnosis of Sleep Pattern Disturbance include difficulty falling asleep, sleep interruptions, awakening earlier or later than desired, complaints of not feeling rested, changes in daytime performance, and excessive daytime sleepiness (Gordon, 1991). A study by Rossi, et al. looked at the incidence and characteristics of sleep pattern disturbance in clients with cardiac disease (Rossi, Fitzmaurice, Glynn, & Conners, 1987). Defining characteristics in these subjects included, in descending order of frequency, sleep interruption, difficulty falling asleep, not feeling well rested, and early awakening. Ninety-two percent of the subjects reported more than one defining characteristic. Supporting cues include changes in behavior and/or performance and reports by the client, caregivers, or significant others of changes in sleep quantity or quality and physical cues such as listlessness and irritability. Sleep pattern disturbance may be related to knowledge deficit, pain and/or discomfort, sleep interruptions, and impaired mobility (Carpenito, 1991; Gordon, 1991). The rehabilitation nurse should consult with other interdisciplinary colleagues both in making a diagnosis of Sleep Pattern Disturbance and in gaining cooperation for planned interventions.

Desired Outcomes for Interventions for Sleep Pattern Disturbance

Successful nursing interventions, including referrals for therapy, are directed toward achievement of the following outcomes:

- ✦ Client, family, significant others, and/or caregivers will identify factors that help promote effective sleep and rest.
- ✦ Client, family, significant others, and/or caregivers report that the client is able to return to sleep within a short period of time after being awakened for physiologic needs such as repositioning, voiding, or suctioning, or for medication administration or required procedures.
- ✦ Client is free of complications related to hypnotic therapy.
- ✦ Client's daytime performance is not negatively affected by lack of sleep or rest.
- ✦ Within the limits of his or her disability, the client is able to establish a sleep pattern that results in high-quality physical and mental restoration.

Nursing Interventions for Sleep Pattern Disturbance Related to Knowledge Deficit

One of the most important interventions for clients with the nursing diagnosis of Sleep Pattern Disturbance related to knowledge deficit is to provide the individual with sleep hygiene information and to assist the individual to identify, eliminate, and/or manage other factors that interfere with satisfactory sleep. Providing sleep hygiene information includes counseling the client on such issues as the following:

- ✦ Avoiding daytime naps if they interfere with nocturnal sleep
- ✦ Avoiding spending long periods of time in bed without sleeping
- ✦ Keeping a regular sleep-wake schedule
- ✦ Avoiding products known to interfere with sleep onset or maintenance such as caffeine, nicotine, and alcohol
- ✦ Avoiding strenuous exercise close to bedtime
- ✦ Maintaining an appropriate sleep environment with clean bedding, a dark room, a cool temperature and appropriate ventilation, and effective noise control
- ✦ Avoiding going to bed hungry or soon after a large meal
- ✦ Avoiding participation in activities that are emotionally upsetting or excessively stimulating close to bedtime

An intervention as simple as having the family bring in the client's own pillow may make a big difference in providing a comfortable night's sleep (Knapp, 1993). The client and family also should be provided with information regarding the safety of the sleeping environment. Using night lights where appropriate for persons with visual impairments and having an uncluttered path from the bed to the bathroom are important safety considerations (Chennelly, 1989).

Rehabilitation nurses face the challenge of using assessment data regarding previous sleep patterns and replicating these routines to the greatest extent possible within the hospital or institutional environment (Chennelly, 1989). Identifying the client's medication usage pattern is also an important strategy. The nurse should look at both the client's prescription and over-the-counter drugs and advise the client on medication usage and/or management techniques regarding drugs and sleep. Consulting with the client's physician and pharmacist may be helpful at this point. Looking at the impact of the hospital environment on the client's usual bedtime routine is another valuable nursing intervention. Where at all feasible, the environment should flex to match the client's previously satisfactory routine. If clients have not used a bedtime routine, the nurse may advise them on the value of a bedtime routine and provide specific information regarding activities that others use effectively. The nurse also can manage the environment by placing clients with compatible sleep routines together and by placing a client with a sleep problem in an appropriate area where environmental stimuli are reduced (Chennelly, 1989).

Sleep Pattern Disturbance Related to Pain and Discomfort

Effective interventions the nurse can use for the client whose pain or discomfort are interfering with sleep include giving analgesia on a schedule that will ensure maximum effect of the analgesia at the time of sleep onset. For minor discomfort, using positioning, back rubs, nonnarcotic analgesics, and providing time for clients to share their feelings and concerns may be of great assistance.

Assisting clients with pulmonary disease to obtain adequate sleep and rest is a significant challenge for the rehabilitation nurse. In addition to providing an upright position if needed, teaching the client and family to do pulmonary toilet and to take bronchodilators just before bedtime may be of assistance (Chennelly, 1989). Some clients who do not use low-flow oxygen during daytime hours may be of benefit if oxygen is given during the night to compensate for nighttime decreases in pulmonary function. Nursing interventions that can reduce the client's anxiety at bedtime are useful in decreasing respiratory demand. Providing a calm environment and taking time to listen to the client's concerns and fears are important interventions in helping persons with respiratory disorders with sleep problems (Chennelly, 1989).

Sleep Pattern Disturbance Related to Interrupted Sleep

In the hospital or other institutionalized setting, the nurse should take accountability for managing environmental factors, such as light and noise level, over which the client has little control. Noise control is an aspect of care in both hospital and long-term care facilities particularly appropriate for nursing interventions (Walgenbach, 1990). Topf (1992) studied the effects of personal control over hospital noise in a simulated critical care environment. Although the proposed intervention did not facilitate sleep as measured by both subject self-report and polysomnography, the results demonstrated a strong correlation between critical care unit (CCU) sounds and poor sleep. Subjects in simulated noise conditions experienced decreased sleep efficiency, increased problems with sleep latency and sleep continuity, and more sleep interruptions (Topf, 1992).

Specific strategies the nurse can use to assist with interrupted sleep are to have the client void before retiring and to advise on the appropriate dosing of diuretics to avoid nighttime awakening for voiding. If nighttime voiding is unavoidable, a practical intervention is to determine the usual time of awakening so that the staff can plan in advance to assist with toileting. Once the client is awake, the amount of time spent in the deeper phases of NREM sleep decreases. Using a commode at the bedside at night may decrease the amount of time spent out of bed to void and thus decrease the amount of time spent awake (Knapp, 1993). The nurse can also organize procedures during the night to plan for the fewest number of disturbances. Richardson (1994) suggests that nurses intervene by closing doors to client rooms at night; using more desk alarms; clustering interventions within rooms and units; and relieving client internal somatic, cognitive, and emotional stimuli. Clients whose interrupted sleep is caused by excessive spasticity may experience less disruptions if resting splints are applied before sleeping (Chennelly, 1989).

The nurse should ensure that there is a reduction in noise and other environmental distractions that cause sleep arousals in clients and should teach ancillary healthcare workers why such interventions are important. For clients whose interrupted sleep patterns are the result of pathophysiologic alterations in circadian rhythms such as AD, the nurse might advise the family and caregivers to try to minimize the client's daytime napping and to increase daytime activity to consolidate nocturnal sleep. Increasing daytime activity for persons recovering from traumatic brain injury may have a beneficial impact on consolidating nighttime sleep and decreasing nighttime wakefulness and agitation. Teaching clients the importance of proning at night is an important strategy designed to lessen the need for sleep interruptions for pressure relief. Because proning relieves pressure over common areas of skin breakdown, a nighttime proning program can allow for long periods of noninterrupted sleep for both the client and for caregivers.

Sleep Pattern Disturbance Related to Impaired Mobility

The nurse should plan strategies to accomplish position changes with the least time and effort so that the client is not fully aroused from sleep. When awakening a person with spasticity for turning or repositioning, it is important to remember that quick, unanticipated movements provoke a spastic response; arousing the person verbally and moving slowly may allow a position change without causing muscle spasms. For clients with serious neuromuscular disorders such as Parkinson's disease or amyotrophic lateral sclerosis (ALS), a position change at night often results in wakefulness for both the client and the caregiver. Using cre-

---

◆

CRITERIA FOR REFERRAL FOR FURTHER EVALUATION AND TREATMENT

Suggested criteria for referral of a client to a sleep disorders center include chronic insomnia or excessive daytime somnolence, in conjunction with any of the following signs or symptoms:

◆ Failure to respond to customary sleep hygiene and therapy with short-term hypnotic medications
◆ Unacceptable side effects from the controlled and supervised use of hypnotic medications
◆ Potential and/or unconfirmed sleep apnea
◆ Desire for consultation where client has a nursing diagnosis of Sleep Pattern Disturbance that has multiple etiologies or is refractory to therapy (Moran & Stoudemire, 1992)

---

ative strategies such as the use of satin sheets to decrease skin resistance during a position change may be helpful (Reimer, 1989). For persons with muscle tone problems resulting from stroke, planning the last turn of the night on the affected side helps to normalize tone for morning activities (Gee & Passarella, 1985).

The rehabilitation nurse often is positioned to initiate referrals for additional evaluation and treatment of sleep pattern disturbances that are refractory to therapy. Suggested criteria for referral of a client to a sleep disorders center are listed in the box above.

Pharmacologic Treatment of Sleep Problems

Sleep disorder clinicians generally agree that the degree to which sleep disturbances are an etiologic factor in daytime performance determines the need for pharmacologic treatment (Roth & Roehrs, 1992). Hypnotics are prescribed because the improved quantity and quality of sleep resulting from their administration is presumed to lead to improved daytime functioning. The effects of a hypnotic on daytime performance are of particular concern because the drug is given to reverse the daytime performance decrements that result from inadequate sleep. The use of hypnotic medications to promote effective sleep should be viewed as short-term therapy.

Clients should be helped to recognize that the eventual goal of treatment is to achieve normal sleep without medication and that any medication prescribed is part of an overall strategic approach (Walsh & Fillingim, 1990). Despite the problems associated with a pharmacologic approach to sleep disturbances, careful use of hypnotic agents may be included as part of a comprehensive strategy for the rehabilitation client with a sleep pattern disturbance (Chennelly, 1989).

The benzodiazepine hypnotics have been the drugs of choice in the symptomatic treatment of insomnia. Unlike barbiturates, tolerance to the hypnotic effects of the benzodiazepines does not readily occur (Roth & Roehrs, 1992). New drugs that seem to be more selective in influencing

GABA are being introduced. Benzodiazepines bind to GABA receptors, changing the rate of opening of chloride channels. Increased permeability of chloride channels results in reduced neuronal activity, producing sedative, hypnotic, anticonvulsant, and muscle relaxant effects (Culebras, 1992b).

Differences among benzodiazepine drugs occur because of their differing pharmacokinetics including absorption time, duration of action, degree of lipid solubility, and route of metabolism. All of these are important factors which should be considered in deciding on a appropriate agent for a given client (Moran & Stoudemire, 1992). The benzodiazepines are classified as long acting, intermediate acting, and short acting depending on their elimination half-life. Half-life is defined as the period of time in which one half of a drug is excreted from the body. There is a wide range in the half-lives of commonly prescribed hypnotics. Long-acting benzodiazepines are diazepam (Valium), and flurazepam (Dalmane). Intermediate-acting agents include alprazolam (Xanax), estazolam (ProSom), lorazepam (Ativan and others), and temazepam (Restoril). Midazolam (Versed) and triazolam (Halcion) are short-acting benzodiazepines.

The three most common adverse side effects seen with hypnotics are residual sedation, anterograde amnesia, and rebound insomnia. Residual sedation refers to the hypnotic agent's ability to produce sedation extending into the waking period, including associated performance decrements. Anterograde amnesia is experienced when the client is unable to recall events subsequent to the administration of the drug. Rebound amnesia refers to a one to two night sleep that occurs with abrupt discontinuation of hypnotic sedation. The selection of an agent depends on the results desired. A long-acting agent such as flurazepam would be appropriate for individuals with both sleep problems and daytime anxiety if daytime alertness is not critical (Walsh & Fillingim, 1990). Intermediate-acting agents would be most appropriate for persons who do not have problems getting to sleep but have difficulty maintaining sleep. Flurazepam in elderly clients, however, is associated with adverse CNS effects such as confusion, ataxia, and daytime sedation—which may increase the potential for falls and injuries (Monane, 1992). Persons with sleep apnea or a history of snoring are not good candidates for therapy with hypnotic medications as the CNS sedating effects of the hypnotics may exacerbate hypoxemia and sleep disturbances caused by apnea (Walsh, 1990).

Hypnotic drugs are agents intended to increase sleep and decrease alertness (Walsh & Fillingim, 1990). The higher the dose of a hypnotic, the greater the degree of impairment after administration and the longer the duration of the impairment. The lowest effective doses of benzodiazepines are recommended if short-term therapy for insomnia with a hypnotic agent does not place the client at risk. The main uses of low-dose benzodiazepine therapy are to treat intermittent insomnia in the elderly and transient situational insomnia in young and middle-aged adults (Vogel, 1992). The primary advantage of low-dose benzodiazepine therapy is prevention of daytime sedation, anterograde amnesia, and rebound insomnia seen with longer acting agents (Vogel, 1992). In the event of transient insomnia, it is recommended that a small dose of an intermediate-acting agent that does

---

GUIDELINES FOR THE USE OF HYPNOTICS IN THE SHORT-TERM TREATMENT OF SLEEP DISORDERS

♦ Target specific problems to be treated (e.g., sleep onset, sleep maintenance)
♦ Check for interaction of hypnotics with alcohol or other sedating drugs
♦ Check for interactions or possible potentiation of the effects of other medications such as cimetidine, phenytoin, levodopa
♦ Use the lowest effective dose; use half the adult dose in persons over age 65
♦ Monitor side effects
♦ Dispense 20 tablets or less and then provide follow-up (Jamison & Becker, 1992)

---

not interfere with daytime functioning be used for a few nights only (Monane, 1992). For insomnia lasting longer than a few nights, treatment should be directed toward the underlying disorder, with nonpharmacologic approaches being the mainstay of therapy (Monane, 1992).

The box above outlines guidelines for the use of hypnotics in the short-term treatment of sleep disorders.

Nonpharmacologic Treatment of Sleep Disorders

Although treatment of insomnias with hypnotics produces quick symptomatic results, nonpharmacologic cognitive-behavioral therapies produce long-lasting benefits (Bootzin & Perlis, 1992). In addition, nonpharmacologic approaches are the safest approach to managing sleep pattern disturbances in the elderly client (Gottlieb, 1990; Johnson, 1991). Health professionals may not place appropriate value on the use of nonpharmacologic strategies in part because their effectiveness is not immediately apparent (Johnson, 1991).

Providing basic information about sleep and sleep hygiene is a cornerstone of nonpharmacologic therapy (Bootzin & Perlis, 1992). A variety of techniques may be used to improve sleep without the use of hypnotics. Stimulus control techniques are a set of activities that help clients with insomnia establish and maintain a consistent sleep and wake pattern. Strategies used with stimulus-control therapy focus on having the client use the bed and bedroom and cues for sleep and reducing their association with other activities. Specific strategies include lying down to sleep only when drowsy; using the bed and bedroom only for sleeping and sexual activities; getting up and doing other activities when sleep onset is delayed; and avoiding daytime naps, which interfere with nighttime sleep.

Sleep restriction is a method that may be used to help clients consolidate sleep by limiting the amount of time in bed to the actual number of hours of sleep. Chronotherapy is a technique that may be used in circadian rhythm disorders in which the person's sleep-wake cycle is not compatible with the time the individual desires sleep. Using this approach, the person's bedtime is successively moved forward by 3 hours each night until sleep onset coincides with the desired sleep time. Bright light therapy works on the principle that exposure to intensive bright light may be effective in resetting the circadian rhythm. Bright light therapy has potential application for transmeridian travelers, night shift workers, and persons with seasonal affective disorder who live in latitudes where lack of light during winter months produces symptoms of depression.

Progressive relaxation, transcendental meditation, yoga, hypnosis, and biofeedback strategies are all based on the premise that if people can learn to relax at bedtime they will be successful with sleep onset. Holistic approaches such as massage, acupuncture, and homeopathic strategies should be encouraged as legitimate options with few side effects. Cognitive therapy focuses on altering the client's expectations about sleep. The primary goal of cognitive therapy is to change the person's view of the sleep problem from one in which he is a victim of a sleep problem to one in which he is capable of coping with and managing the problem (Bootzin & Perlis, 1992).

Rehabilitation nurses have a critical role to play in assisting clients achieve optimum sleep and rest. Etiologic factors involved in sleep pattern disturbance may result from the disability itself, from the environment, or from a variety or situational issues with which the client must cope. Nursing interventions are aimed primarily toward helping clients reestablish and maintain an acceptable sleep pattern (Chennelly, 1989). In the acute rehabilitation center or long-term institutional setting, nurses have primary control over environmental factors such as noise level, lighting, retiring and rising times, and comfort measures that greatly impact client sleep. In the community setting nurses are in a key position to advise clients, families, and caregivers regarding effective sleep and rest strategies tailored to address the needs of specific individuals in a variety of situations.

The study of the phenomena of sleep by many disciplines has focused on a physiologic approach, with little attention directed to psychosocial and sociocultural factors influencing sleep. Future nursing research studies would be particularly useful in the areas of describing sleep disturbances as they occur in persons with physical disabilities and examining the impact of life transitions, grief, and the stress of both acute and chronic illness on sleep (Shaver & Giblin, 1989). There is limited research on specific intervention strategies to promote sleep and to prevent or modify sleep problems (Jensen & Herr, 1993).

The sleep-promoting interventions that are known to promote sleep with clients of all ages should be incorporated into clinical practice. Reducing pain, decreasing stress, and careful scheduling of institutional routines are essential elements of effective nursing practice. In addition to sleep-promoting nursing interventions, there is an important role for nurses in regard to client education. Teaching clients the importance of establishing bedtime routines and promoting nonpharmacologic methods to promote sleep are key aspects of client and family teaching. Jensen and Herr (1993) state that an important educational intervention is to teach adults about expected changes in sleep patterns with age; knowing what is expected and what is not can alert clients to seek appropriate help in managing sleep disorders. It is critical that nurses continue to assess sleep from the view of the client. As the focus of nursing is on human response, the influence of sleep on health is of great importance to the nursing profession (Jensen & Herr, 1993).

FATIGUE

Most individuals experience fatigue at various times in their lives. For healthy persons feelings of fatigue are temporary phenomena often related to excessive physical activity, a sedentary lifestyle, improper nutrition, an increase in work or social responsibilities, emotional stress, or lack of sleep (Carpenito, 1991). Healthy persons generally experience fatigue as a temporary problem for which relief measures are effective (Tack, 1990a). In many chronic diseases, however, fatigue is a daily experience that affects the whole person. Fatigue is a subjective perception of body sensations characterized by feelings of discomfort, decrements in motor and mental skill functioning, and increased difficulty with task performance. Fatigue is generally an invisible symptom. Within the context of Western cultures, a high energy level is valued. The listlessness and lack of energy that are the concomitants of the fatigue state may be misinterpreted by the client's support system and by healthcare personnel (Hubsky & Sears, 1992).

The Process of Fatigue

Fatigue in persons with disabilities is a common disruptive symptom that may be one of the most difficult aspects of care to manage (Hart, Freel, & Milde, 1990; Voith, Frank, & Pigg, 1989). Activities not tiring to healthy persons can quickly cause symptoms of fatigue in persons with pathologic conditions. Fatigue is considered to be a protective mechanism that prevents injury and sustains physiologic equilibrium by stimulating the need to rest from activity. The fatigue state is different than feeling tired. Tiredness is usually a transient condition that is relieved quickly by rest and/or sleep. Activity intolerance also differs from fatigue in that the person experiencing activity intolerance can be assisted to increase endurance and improve functioning. Persons with chronic fatigue are not expected to return to their previous level of functioning in regard to energy level (Carpenito, 1991).

Fatigue is a specific problem for clients with MS, PPS, and rheumatic disorders. As individuals with physical disabilities age, they may experience increasing problems with fatigue. Nursing interventions can assist the client to maintain and improve energy levels in many situations. When the primary etiologic factors underlying the fatigue state cannot be eliminated, the focus of care is to assist the disabled person and the family to learn fatigue management techniques that conserve energy levels.

The focus of interventions for fatigue occurring in conjunction with a chronic disability should assist clients to function within their limitations with the goal of achieving a balance between feeling as energized as possible and maintaining realistic activity levels to meet felt demands.

Fatigue Associated with Specific Disabling Conditions
✦ Post-polio syndrome (PPS)

Many clients with PPS complain of fatigue, new weakness in muscles that originally were involved in the acute attack of poliomyelitis and those unaffected, muscle and joint pain, and the development of sleep apnea. Studies have indicated that post-polio fatigue peaks in the late morning or early afternoon. Planned rest periods and work simplification techniques are recommended to reduce post-polio fatigue symptoms. Two recent studies have confirmed the value of paced work-rest interval programs as effective methods in reducing fatigue in PPS. (Agre & Rodriguez, 1991; Packer, 1991). A study of activity and PPS fatigue in 12 subjects found that only 5% of daily time was spent resting and only 1% of time was devoted to planning work, suggesting that use of energy conservation techniques is an underused strategy (Packer, 1991).

◆ Multiple Sclerosis (MS)

Complaints of fatigue are common in persons with MS (Hubsky & Sears, 1992). In this progressively demyelinating disease, the loss of myelin—which interferes with nerve impulse conduction—produces changes in sensation and movement and also is thought to contribute to fatigue. One suggested mechanism is that greater energy is required to transmit a nerve impulse along a damaged myelin sheath (McLaughlin, 1986).

Fatigue in MS is chronic, occurs more quickly, and is more severe than normal fatigue. The severity of the fatigue often is not related to other MS symptoms (Hubsky & Sears, 1992). Hubsky and Sears describe four types of fatigue in MS clients: normal fatigue, episodic fatigue, muscular strain, and MS fatigue. Normal fatigue is the type of fatigue experienced by most individuals as a result of exertion and activity. Its onset may be quickened in persons with MS. Episodic fatigue results from hopelessness and/or depression in relation to the disease process. A considerable energy loss may occur from this type of fatigue. Muscular strain, a type of fatigue caused by muscle weakness or nerve fiber fatigue, occurs rapidly in persons with MS. Simple daily activities related to self-care may produce this type of fatigue. MS fatigue, described as a feeling of overwhelming tiredness not related to time of day or activity, is a type of fatigue unique to those with MS (Hubsky & Sears, 1992).

A study by Freal, Kraft, and Coryell (1984) of symptomatic fatigue in MS showed that respondents indicated that their fatigue symptoms included tiredness, a need to rest, and sleepiness. In nearly half of the subjects, fatigue exacerbated their MS symptoms. Ninety percent of the subjects reported that warm environmental temperatures increased their feelings of fatigue (Freal et al., 1984). If spasticity is problematic for the client with MS, antispasmodic drugs may be prescribed; however, the amount of medication needed to suppress spasticity also may increase feelings of fatigue. Use of newer treatments such as the intrathecal administration of antispasmodics may allow control of spasticity without producing sedation in these clients.

◆ Rheumatoid Arthritis (RA)

Fatigue is a commonly reported problem for persons with RA. Although the primary manifestations of RA occur in joints, the systemic nature of RA results in extraarticular symptoms, including fatigue (Tack, 1990). Fatigue has been identified as a client problem in the American Nurses Association and Arthritis Health Professions Nursing Task Force (1983) Outcome Standards for Rheumatology Nursing Practice. Fatigue, pain, and depression are positively correlated in clients with RA (Tack, 1990b). A study by Crosby (1991) found that the three most frequently identified factors associated with fatigue and RA were disease activity, disturbed sleep, and increased physical effort. Crosby suggests that reducing the pain of RA through increased use of rest, splinting, and medications would contribute to better sleep quality, resulting in an improvement in functional ability and a decrease in fatigue levels.

Assessment of Fatigue

Factors that should be considered in the assessment of fatigue include the following:
- History of fatigue: onset, time of day, precipitating factors, fatigue pattern, methods of relief
- Associated signs and symptoms: irritability, desire to sleep, decreased motivation, problems with performance
- Health status: recent illness or chronic disease
- Medications taken and medication usage pattern
- Effects on lifestyle including impact on work, social relationships, role responsibilities (Carpenito, 1991)

Nursing Diagnosis: Fatigue

The nursing diagnosis of Fatigue describes an overwhelming, sustained sense of exhaustion and decreased capacity for physical and mental work (Gordon, 1991). Carpenito (1991) defines fatigue as the self-recognized state in which an individual experiences an overwhelming and sustained feeling of exhaustion and decreased capacity for physical and mental work that is not relieved by rest.

Major defining characteristics of fatigue are verbalization of an unremitting and overwhelming lack of energy and inability to maintain usual routines (Voith et al., 1989). Minor defining characteristics include perceived need for additional energy to accomplish routine tasks, emotional lability, impaired ability to concentrate, increase in physical complaints, decrease in performance, lethargy, listlessness, accident proneness, decrease in libido, and a disinterested attitude toward one's surroundings (Carpenito, 1991; Gordon, 1991; Voith et al., 1989).

Voith et al. (1989) designed a study to validate defining characteristics for the nursing diagnosis of Fatigue. Subjects in this study were 100 nurses caring for clients with rheumatic and cardiac disorders. Respondents identified verbalization of fatigue, inability to maintain customary activity

---

DESIRED OUTCOMES OF NURSING INTERVENTIONS FOR FATIGUE

Client will be able to
- Identify the causes of fatigue
- Express feelings regarding the impact of the fatigue state on life functioning
- Establish daily activity priorities
- Gain increased self-awareness regarding personal factors contributing to fatigue including physiologic, affective, behavioral, cognitive, and environmental issues

level, poor task performance, impaired ability to concentrate, irritability, and an increase in physical complaints as important defining characteristics of fatigue in their clients.

Related factors for the diagnosis of fatigue pertinent to rehabilitation clients include overwhelming psychological or emotional demands; increased energy requirements needed to perform activities of daily living; excessive role demands; discomfort; and altered body chemistry including effects of medications, drug withdrawal, and decreased or increased metabolic energy production (Gordon, 1991). Once the nursing diagnosis of Fatigue is identified, desired outcomes should be planned in collaboration with the client and members of the interdisciplinary team. Suggested desired outcomes of nursing interventions for fatigue are listed in the box on p. 521.

Nursing Interventions

✦ Nursing interventions for fatigue related to the effects of physiologic problems

Fatigue in disorders such as PPS, MS, and RA interfere with self-care and customary daily activities. Suggested interventions include the following:

- ✦ Alternating rest periods with periods of activity (Hubsky & Sears, 1992)
- ✦ Using resting strategies such as napping, reading, listening to music (Freal et al., 1984)
- ✦ Prioritizing essential activities and learning to delegate some tasks to others; client also may benefit from assertiveness training to learn how to carry out desired plans (Voith et al., 1989)
- ✦ Learning and practicing principles of energy conservation such as sitting instead of standing, lying down instead of sitting, working at the most appropriate height, using pockets to carry items instead of a purse (Voith et al., 1989)
- ✦ Pacing activities during the day by planning and organizing activities
- ✦ Consulting with an occupational therapist to design a work simplification program and environmental modification program including issues such as replacing stairs with ramps, installing grab rails, elevation chairs, reducing trips up and down stairs, and organizing kitchen and other work areas
- ✦ Eating small, frequent meals to decrease energy needed for digestion
- ✦ Consulting with a physical therapist to design an individualized exercise program that produces the energizing benefits of mild to moderate exercise without causing further fatigue

✦ Nursing interventions for fatigue related to affective, behavioral, and cognitive problems

Chronic fatigue may result in affective and behavioral responses such as irritability, depression, anxiety, and other symptoms (Hubsky & Sears, 1992). Emotional stress has been associated with both producing fatigue and a result of fatigue (Hart et al., 1990).

Suggested interventions include the following:

- ✦ Using stress management techniques aimed at increasing relaxation and relieving tension (Hubsky & Sears, 1992).

- ✦ Obtaining social support by networking with other individuals facing the same problems may help clients to manage symptoms by benefiting from the experience of others. Support networks organized through the MS Society or the Arthritis Foundation provide important support for both clients and their families.
- ✦ Using a technique such as reframing may be helpful in managing fatigue. Reframing refers to changing the frame of reference of an event with the goal of changing its meaning. As an example, by reframing, the feelings of fatigue could be seen as a positive and valuable protective mechanism rather than as a limitation (Hart et al., 1990).

✦ Nursing interventions for fatigue related to environmental factors:

Suggested interventions include advising the client to manage body and environmental temperatures by adjusting air and water temperatures to avoid fatigue or symptoms of discomfort. Environment influences on a client's fatigue vary. For example, a person with postpolio syndrome may tolerate cold temperatures poorly and experience temporary symptomatic relief from warm water baths. In contrast, a person with MS may report that warm temperatures in baths exacerbate symptoms, while being in an air-conditioned environment may be beneficial for symptom relief.

✦

MINIMIZING FATIGUE BY CONSERVING ENERGY

Levine's nursing Theory of Energy Conservation is useful when one is working with clients who suffer from a great deal of fatigue. Energy is conserved not only by rest, but also by conserving energy expenditures (Levine, 1967). The list below may stimulate ideas about ways to work with each client's capabilities and energy level. Key points are to set mutual goals with clients, families, employers, and others for:

- ✦ **Planning the timing of activities to minimize fatigue**—e.g., organizing hair washing and bathing supplies before the shower and planning to wash one load of clothing every other day, to dust one room at a time, and to run errands at non-peak hours of the day
- ✦ **Redesigning work areas** to obtain maximum ergonomic benefits—e.g., arranging furniture and work spaces to assure proper body alignment and support or installing stove and countertops at wheelchair height
- ✦ **Evaluating and prioritizing work patterns**—e.g., placing frequently used items on an accessible tabletop, keeping cleaning supplies in several rooms, or using a portable telephone; installing household safety devices such as grab bars in the bathroom; and alternating both work load and type of work from day to day
- ✦ **Using assistive devices or adaptive equipment** as personal extenders and using proper body mechanics and techniques to perform self-care activities (Clark, 1991)

Fatigue is a pervasive, protective phenomenon affecting the totality of the individual (Hart et al., 1990). Fatigue is a phenomenon that is both multidimensional and multifactorial. Biologic, psychosocial, and personal factors influence the onset, severity, expression, and perception of the fatigue experience (Tack, 1990). Rehabilitation nurses can provide important interventions through education, support, and referrals to other healthcare professionals to help decrease the disabling effects of fatigue.

CASE STUDY

ASSESSMENT

S.Y. is a 31-year-old married woman who was diagnosed with MS when she was 22. Her husband is a telephone repairperson. They have two children, ages 8 and 5. Until the past year S.Y. had worked full time as an insurance claims adjuster. She has had increasing problems with fatigue, which have begun to impact on her ability to work and to care for her family. Although she had continued to work, she has begun to miss some work days and does not know how long she can continue to work.

S.Y. reports that her fatigue symptoms peak in the early afternoon, at which time she feels so exhausted that napping provides the only relief. Warm weather or exertion as a result of household activities also increases her feelings of exhaustion. S.Y. and her family live in an area of California where summer temperatures often average 90° F. Their house is air conditioned.

She describes her fatigue symptoms as being an overwhelming need to stop, sit down, lie down, or actually sleep to regain any energy. Problems with increasing spasticity have been managed with antispasmodic medication; however, the depressant side effects of her medications have tended to increase her fatigue-related symptoms. Her husband does the major household chores such as laundry and cleaning on his days off. S.Y. expresses some feelings of concern regarding how much she asks her husband to do and is concerned that because of her fatigue she has very little quality time with her husband or children. She also feels strongly about maintaining some independence regarding work and contributing some income to the family.

GOAL SETTING

The nurse works closely with S.Y. and collaborates with other members of the interdisciplinary team in helping S.Y. to establish realistic goals. The nurse begins by listening to the effects of S.Y.'s fatigue on her lifestyle and the quality of her life. Both the nurse and client realize that S.Y. is dealing with a chronic condition and that the goals set today may need to be readjusted in the future. S.Y. would like to establish three goals: to be able to manage her fatigue in a way that allows her to spend quality time with her husband and children, to decrease the amount of work done at home by her husband, and to continue to maintain independence and contribute income to the family.

INTERVENTIONS

The nurse discusses with S.Y. the possibility of her working at home rather than commuting to an office. S.Y. drives 30 minutes to and from the insurance office and reports that driving makes her very tired, especially during the warm months when it takes some time for the car air conditioning to work. She is aware that some individuals in the company have performed work at home using a home computer and a telephone. The ability to perform the majority of her work at home will allow S.Y. to take advantage of rest and activity periods and will automatically save her 1 hour/day by not commuting. A continuing income and the money saved over a period of time through working at home will allow S.Y. and her husband to consider having some household help. Being in an air conditioned environment at home also may alleviate some of S.Y.'s fatigue symptoms. The nurse encourages S.Y. to pursue with her employer available options regarding working at home.

Another area of intervention includes working with S.Y. to be comfortable in delegating some home work tasks to others including her husband, the children, and household assistance, should that be an option she selects. Having chores done around the house by others will allow S.Y. the quality time she wishes to have with her family. The nurse also discusses with S.Y. the need to establish daily activity priorities and to begin to plan an activity-rest program that provides the energy she needs.

The nurse reviews with S.Y. the impact of body temperature on MS symptoms. S.Y. is aware that she needs to avoid hot baths or showers and should avoid exposure to warm temperatures if possible. They also review the importance of S.Y. planning the most strenuous activities in the morning, when her energy level is highest. The nurse teaches S.Y. that exercising muscles not affected by MS may decrease overall fatigue, but that she should stop exercising if she feels tired. The nurse obtains feedback that S.Y. knows that she should avoid very vigorous exercise because it not only increases weakness but also increases core body temperature, setting up a vicious fatigue cycle. They also discuss the effect of antispasmodic medications on S.Y.'s general energy level. The nurse informs S.Y. about the future possibility of an implanted pump to deliver antispasmodic medication at a very low dose intrathecally, should her spasticity continue to increase.

The nurse, in conjunction with occupational and physical therapist colleagues, is able to suggest and/or reinforce the use of many useful home interventions aimed at preserving energy and decreasing fatigue. The box on p. 522 details specific strategies in the areas of cooking, cleaning, shopping, dressing, meal preparation, laundry, desk work, and bathing.

The nurse also talks with S.Y. about the value of becoming involved with the local Multiple Sclerosis Society. The nurse points out the benefits both S.Y. and her family might gain from exposure to other persons who are trying out new ways of dealing with similar problems.

REFERENCES

Agre, J.C., & Rodriguez, A.A. (1991). Intermittent isometric activity: Its effect on muscle fatigue in post-polio subjects. *Archives of Physical Medicine and Rehabilitation, 72,* 971-974.

American Nurses' Association and Arthritis Health Professions Nursing Task Force. (1983). *Outcome standards for rheumatology nursing practice* (Publication MS-12). Kansas City, MO: American Nurses' Association.

Ancoli-Israel, S. (1989). Epidemiology of sleep disorders. *Clinics in Geriatric Medicine, 5,* 347-362.

Askenasy, J.J., & Rahmani, L. (1988). Neuropsycho-social rehabilitation of head injury. *American Journal of Physical Medicine, 66,* 315-327.

Beyerman K. (1987). Etiologies of sleep pattern disturbance in hospitalized patients In A. McLane (Ed.), *Classification of nursing diagnoses: Proceedings of the seventh conference* (pp. 381-394). St. Louis: Mosby–Year Book.

Biddle, C., & Oaster, T.R. (1990). The nature of sleep. *Journal of the American Association of Nurse Anesthetists, 58,* 193-198.

Bonnet, M.H. & Arand, D.L. (1989). Sleep loss in aging. *Clinics in Geriatric Medicine, 5,* 405-420.

Bootzin, R.R., & Perlis, M.L. (1992). Nonpharmacologic treatment of insomnia. *Journal of Clinical Psychiatry, 53*(Suppl.), 29-36.

Buyesse, D., Browman, B.A., Monk, T.H., Reynolds, C.F., Fasiczka, B.A., & Kupfer, D.J. (1992). Napping and 24 hour sleep-wake patterns in healthy elderly and young adults. *Journal of the American Geriatric Society, 40,* 779-786.

Carpenito, L.J. (1991). *Nursing care plans and documentation.* Philadelphia: J.B. Lippincott.

Chenelly, S. (1989). Sleep and rest. In S. Dittmar (Ed.), *Rehabilitation nursing: Process and application* (pp. 227-240). St. Louis: Mosby–Year Book.

Clark, C. (1991). Nursing care for multiple sclerosis. *Orthopaedic Nursing, 10,* 21-32.

Clark, C.M., Fleming, J.A., Oger, J., Klonoff, H., & Paty, D. (1992). Sleep disturbance, depression, and lesion site in patients with multiple sclerosis. *Archives of Neurology, 49,* 641-643.

Crosby, L.J. (1991). Factors which contribute to fatigue associated with rheumatoid arthritis. *Journal of Advanced Nursing, 16,* 974-981.

Culebras, A. (1992a). Neuroanatomic and neurologic correlates of sleep disturbances. *Neurology, 42*(Suppl. 6), 19-27.

Culebras, A. (1992b). Update on disorders of sleep and the sleep-wake cycle. *The Psychiatric Clinics of North America, 15,* 467-489.

Davis-Sharts, J. (1989). The elder and critical care: sleep and mobility issues. *The Nursing Clinics of North America, 24,* 755-767.

Dement, W.C., & Mitler, M.M. (1993). It's time to wake up to the importance of sleep disorders. *Journal of the American Medical Association, 269,* 1548-1549.

Flavell, H., Marshall, R., Thomton, A.T., Clements, P.L., Antic, R., & McEvoy, R.D. (1992). Hypoxia episodes during sleep in high tetraplegia. *Archives of Physical Medicine and Rehabilitation, 73,* 623-627.

Freal, J.E., Kraft, G.H., & Coryell, J.K. (1984). Symptomatic fatigue in multiple sclerosis. *Archives of Physical Medicine and Rehabilitation, 65,* 135-138.

Ganong, W.F. (1993). *Review of medical physiology* (16th ed.). Norwalk, CT: Appleton and Lange.

Gee, Z., & Passarella, P. (1985). *Nursing care of the stroke patient: A therapeutic approach based on Bobath principles.* Pittsburgh: AREN Publications.

Gordon, M. (1991). *Manual of nursing diagnoses.* St. Louis: Mosby–Year Book.

Gottlieb, G.L. (1990). Sleep disorders and their management: Special considerations in the elderly. *The American Journal of Medicine, 88,* 29S-33S.

Habel, M. (1993). Sleep-rest pattern. In A. McCourt, (Ed.), *The speciality practice of rehabilitation nursing: A core curriculum* (3rd ed., pp. 122-130). Skokie, IL: Rehabilitation Nursing Foundation.

Haponik, E.F. (1992). Sleep disturbances of older persons: Physicians attitudes. *Sleep, 15,* 168-172.

Hart, L.K., Freel, M.I., & Milde, F.K. (1990). Fatigue. *Nursing Clinics of North America, 25,* 967-976.

Hodgson, L.A. (1991). Why do we need sleep? relating theory to nursing practice. *Journal of Advanced Nursing, 16,* 1503-1510.

Horne, L.A. (1991). No more wakeful nights: Helping elderly people to sleep properly. *Professional Nurse, 6,* 383-385.

Hubsky, E.P., & Sears, J.H. (1992). Fatigue in multiple sclerosis: Guidelines for nursing care. *Rehabilitation Nursing, 17,* 176-180.

Hyppa, M.T., & Kronholm, E. (1989). Quality of sleep and chronic illness. *Journal of Clinical Epidemiology, 42,* 633-638.

Jamison, A.L., & Becker, P.M. (1992). Management of the 10 most common sleep disorders. *American Family Physician, 45,* 1262-1268.

Jensen, D.P., & Herr, K.A. (1993). Sleeplessness. *Nursing Clinics of North America, 28,* 385-402.

Johnson, J.E. (1991a). A comparative study of the bedtime routines and sleep of older adults. *Journal of Community Health Nursing, 8,* 129-136.

Johnson, J.E. (1991b). Progressive relaxation and the sleep of older non-institutionalized women. *Applied Nursing Research, 4,* 165-170.

Kedas, A., Lux, W., & Amodeos S. A critical review of aging and sleep research. *Western Journal of Nursing Research, 11,* 196-206.

Knapp, M. (1993). Night shift: The restorative sleep specialists. *Journal of Gerontological Nursing, 19,* 38-42.

Kovacevic-Ristanovic, R., Cartwright, R.D., & Lloyd, S. (1991). Nonpharmacologic treatment of periodic leg movements in sleep. *Archives of Physical Medicine and Rehabilitation, 72,* 385-389.

Kryger, M.H., Roth, T., & Dement, W.C. (1989). *Principles and practice of sleep medicine.* Philadelphia: W.B. Saunders.

Levine, M.E. (1967). The four conservation principles of nursing. *Nursing Forum, 6,* 45-59.

Locsin, R.C. (1988). Sleeplessness among the elderly. *Rehabilitation Nursing, 13,* 340-341.

McLaughlin, J. (1986). Multiplying the health potential of the person with multiple sclerosis. *Health Values, 10,* 13-18.

Monane, M. (1992). Insomnia in the elderly. *Journal of Clinical Psychiatry, 53,* 23-27.

Monk, T.M. (1989). Circadian rhythms. *Clinics in Geriatric Medicine, 5,* 347-362.

Moran, M.G., & Stoudemire, A. (1992). Sleep disorders in the medically ill patient. *Journal of Clinical Psychiatry, 53,* 29-36.

National Institutes of Health. (1991). National Institutes of Health Consensus Development Conference statement: The treatment of sleep disorders of elderly people. *Sleep, 14,* 169-175.

O'Donnell, J. (1992). Obstructive sleep apnea syndrome. *Pediatric Nursing, 18,* 174-175.

Packer, T.L. (1991). Activity and post-polio fatigue. *Orthopedics, 14,* 1223-1226.

Pulling, C.A. (1991). The relationship between critical care nurses knowledge about sleep, and the initiation of sleep promoting nursing interventions. *Axon, 13,* 57-62.

Reimer, M. (1989). Sleep pattern disturbances related to neurological dysfunction. *Axon, 10,* 65-68.

Richardson, S. (1994). Sleep pattern disturbance of related factors in the critically ill. Abstract submitted to 10th National Conference on Nursing Diagnosis.

Roehrs, T.A., & Roth, T. (1989). Drugs, sleep disorders and aging. *Clinics in Geriatric Medicine, 5,* 395-404.

Rosekind, M.R. (1992). The epidemiology and occurrence of insomnia. *Journal of Clinical Psychiatry, 53,* 4-6.

Rosen, R.C., Rosekind, M., Rosevear, C., Cole, W.E., & Dement, W.C. (1993). Physician education in sleep and sleep disorders: A national survey of U.S. medical schools. *Sleep, 16,* 249-254.

Rossi, L., Fitzmaurice, J., Glynn, M. & Conners, K. (1987). Validation of the defining characteristics for sleep pattern disturbance. In: McLane,

A. (Ed.), *Classification of Nursing diagnoses: Proceedings of the Seventh Conference*. St. Louis: Mosby–Year Book.

Roth, T., & Roehrs, T.A. (1992). Issues in the use of benzodiazepine hypnotics. *Journal of Clinical Psychiatry, 53* (Suppl. 1), 14-18.

Sawin, K.J., & Heard, L. (1992). Nursing diagnoses used most frequently in rehabilitation nursing practice. *Rehabilitation Nursing, 17,* 256-262.

Schwartz, A.R., & Smith, P.L. (1989). Sleep apnea in the elderly. *Clinics in Geriatric Medicine, 5,* 315-330.

Shaver, J.L., & Giblin, E.C. (1989). Sleep. *Annual Review of Nursing Research, 7,* 71-93.

Stejles, D.G., Kryger, M.H., Kirk, B.W., & Millar, T.W. (1990). Sleep in postpolio syndrome. *Chest, 98,* 133-140.

Stice, K.A., & Cunningham, C.A. (1995). Pulmonary rehabilitation with respiratory complications of postpolio syndrome. *Rehabilitation Nursing, 20,* 37-41.

Tack, B.B. (1990a). Fatigue in rheumatoid arthritis: Conditions, strategies, and consequences. *Arthritis Care and Research, 3,* 65-70.

Tack, B. (1990b). Self-reported fatigue in rheumatoid arthritis—A pilot study. *Arthritis Care and Research, 3,* 154-157.

Thorby, M.J. (1990). *International classification of sleep disorders: Diagnostic and coding manual*. Rochester, MN: American Sleep Disorders Association.

Topf, M. (1992). Effects of personal control over hospital noise on sleep. *Research in Nursing and Health, 15,* 19-28.

Vitiello, M.V., & Prinz, P.N. (1989). Alzheimer's disease: Sleep and wake patterns. *Clinics in Geriatric Medicine, 5,* 289-300.

Vitiello, M.V., Bliwise, D.L., & Prinz, P.N. (1992). Sleep in Alzheimer's disease and the sundown syndrome. *Neurology, 42,* 83-93, 93-94.

Vogel, G. (1992). Clinical uses and advantages of low doses of benzodiazepam hypnotics. *Journal of Clinical Psychiatry, 53,* 19-22.

Voith, A.M., Frank, A.M., & Pigg, J.S. (1989). Nursing diagnosis: fatigue. In R.M. Carrol-Johnson (Ed.), *Classification of nursing diagnoses: Proceedings of the eighth conference* (pp. 453-458). Philadelphia: J.B. Lippincott.

Walgenbach, J.C. (1990). Lullabye and not a good night? *Geriatric Nursing, 11,* 278-289.

Walsh, J.K., & Fillingim, J.M. (1990). Role of hypnotic drugs in general practice. *The American Journal of Medicine, 88,* 345-385.

Webb, W.B. (1989). Age-related changes in sleep. *Clinics in Geriatric Medicine, 5,* 275-287.

White, M.A., Williams, P.O., Alexander, D.J., Powell-Cane G.M., & Conlon, M. (1990). Sleep onset latency and distress in hospitalized children. *Nursing Research, 39,* 134-139.

SUGGESTED READINGS

Aldrich, M.S. (1992). Narcolepsy. *Neurology, 42*(Suppl. 6), 34-43.

Askenasy, J.J. (1993). Sleep in Parkinson's disease. *Acta Neurology Scandanavia, 87,* 167-170.

Becker, P.M., & Jamieson, A.O. (1992). Common sleep disorders in the elderly: diagnosis and treatment. *Geriatrics, 47,* 45-48, 51-52.

Belza, B.L., Henke, C.J., Yelin, E.H., Epstein, W.V., & Gillis, C.L. (1993). Correlates of fatigue in older adults with rheumatoid arthritis. *Nursing Research, 42,* 93-99.

Bliwise, D.L. (1989). Neuropsychological function in sleep. *Clinics in Geriatric Medicine, 5,* 381-394.

Culver, B.H. (1989). Pulmonary responses to sleep. *Respiratory Care, 34,* 510-515.

De Konicnk, J., Lorrain, D., & Gagnon, P. (1992). Sleep positions and position shifts in five age groups: An ontogenic picture. *Sleep, 15,* 143-149.

Edwards, G.B., & Schuring, L.M. (1993). Sleep protocol: A research based nursing practice change. *Critical Care Nurse, 13,* 84-88.

Feijoo, M., & Bilbao, J. (1992). Seizures of sleep onset: Clinical and therapeutical aspects. *Clinical Pharmacology, 15,* 50-55.

Farney, R.J., Walker, J.M., Elnur, J.C., Visconi, V.A., & Ord, R.J. (1992). Transtracheal oxygen, nasal CPAP, and nasal oxygen in five patients with obstructive sleep apnea. *Chest, 101,* 1228-1235.

Gates, D., & Norwessel, N. (1989). Night terrors: Strategies for family coping. *Journal of Pediatric Nursing, 4,* 48-53.

Gorbien, M.J. (1993). When your older patient can't sleep: How to put insomnia to rest. *Geriatrics, 48,* 65-68, 71-72, 75.

Greenblatt, D.J., Harmatz, J.S., Shapiro, L., Engelhardt, N., Gouthro, T.A., & Shader, R.L. (1991). Sensitivity to triazolam in the elderly. *New England Journal of Medicine, 364,* 1691-1698.

Greenblatt, D.J. (1992). Pharmacology of benzodiazepine hypnotics. *Journal of Clinical Psychiatry, 53*(Suppl.), 7-13.

Guilleminault, C., Stoohs, R., & Quera-Salva, M.A. (1992). Sleep-related obstructive and nonobstructive apnea and neurologic disorders. *Neurology, 42*(Suppl. 6), 53-60.

Hock, C.C., Buyesse, D.J., & Reynolds, C.F. (1989). Sleep and depression in late life. *Clinics in Geriatric Medicine, 5,* 259-272.

Johnson, J.E. (1993). Progressive relaxation and the sleep of older men and women. *Journal of Community Health Nursing, 10,* 31-38.

Parsons, C., & Ver Beek, D. (1981). Sleep-awake patterns following cerebral concussion. *Nursing Research, 31,* 260-264.

Quine, L., Wade, K., & Hargreaves, R. (1991). Learning to sleep. *Nursing Times, 82,* 41-43.

Rogers, A.E., & Aldrich, M.S. (1993). The effect of regularly scheduled naps on sleep attacks and excessive daytime sleepiness associated with narcolepsy. *Nursing Research, 42,* 111-117.

Rumble, R., & Morgan, K. (1992). Hypnotics, sleep, and mortality in elderly people. *Journal of the American Geriatric Society, 40,* 787-791.

Wooten, V. (1989). Sleep disorders in geriatric patients. *Clinics in Geriatric Medicine, 8,* 427-439.

24

Sensation, Perception, and Pain

Pamela Muhm Duchene, DNSc, RN, CRRN

INTRODUCTION

Consider for a moment a sunny summer day at the beach. Waves are lapping at the shore, and the smell of salty seawater is in the air. You are lying on the dry, warm sand in a state of absolute relaxation with a cold, big glass of orange drink by your hand. Such an image taps all the senses: visual (the sunny beach), auditory (the lapping waves), olfactory (the smell of salty seawater), tactile (the feel of dry, warm sand), kinesthetic (the state of relaxation), and gustatory (the cold, big orange drink). The way one comprehends and interprets the environment results from sensory input and perception of the input. Interference with sensation and perception may occur with neurologic impairments. When sensory and perceptual functioning are damaged, the way individuals respond to the environment and stimuli may be distorted. Careful assessments, plans of care, and corrective actions can make a difference in the degree to which rehabilitation is successful for individuals with sensory and perceptual deficits.

In this chapter sensory and perceptual function are discussed along with impaired states, assessment, planning, and interventions for sensory and perceptual problems. The sensation and perception of pain is discussed as an example of a sensory and perceptual problem. Finally, a case study of an individual with chronic pain from a work-related injury is presented.

NORMAL SENSORY AND PERCEPTUAL PROCESSES
Sensation

Tactile, kinesthetic, auditory, visual, olfactory and gustatory stimuli are received through sensory receptors in peripheral nerves and ganglia. There are five types of sensory receptors (Table 24-1): mechanoreceptors, thermoreceptors, nocioceptors, chemoreceptors, and photic or electromagnetic receptors. As stated in Table 24-1, nociceptors transmit information resulting in pain perception. However, pain may result from sensory input through other receptors and nerve fibers, since high magnitudes of any stimulus may be perceived as painful (Schmitz, 1988). In addition to peripheral sensory receptors, there are deep sensory receptors in muscles, tendons, and joints, which transmit information on position, tone, and movement. Deep sensory receptors convey information on movement speed, movement direction, and body position in space. The 12 cranial nerves are highly involved in the transmission of sensory information (Erickson & McPhee, 1988). Table 24-2 provides identification of the cranial nerves and their functions. Figure 24-1 illustrates cranial nerve actions. Specifically all cranial nerves but nerves XI (accessory) and XII (hypoglossal) are directly involved in reception and transmission of sensory information. Figure 24-2 details nerve actions.

Sensory input is transmitted through peripheral nerves and ganglia to the parietal lobe of the cerebrum. Alexander Luria, a Russian neuropsychologist, studied brain-behavior relationships and identified a brain functioning model that provides a useful method of conceptualizing sensory and perceptual processes (Rohe, 1988). Luria classifies three functional areas or blocks within the brain that he writes are involved in cognition. The first block contains those areas of the brain responsible for general attentional functions and includes the brainstem and subcortical areas. The reticular activating system (RAS) is part of this system. The RAS influences the entire nervous system through activation or inhibition (Chapter 23). Damage to areas within the first block can impact all other brain functions through limiting the ability to analyze, recall, attend, and respond (Luria, 1980).

The second block contains the brain surface on the sides (temporal aspects) and back (posterior areas). The second block is responsible for information reception, analysis, and storage. Areas within the second block are involved in reception of sensory information including tactile, visual, auditory, and kinesthetic sensations. Luria writes that sensory areas within the second block are divided into three zones. For each sensation, there is a primary zone into which the information is received. In the secondary zone the information is processed and organized, whereas in the tertiary zone information from other areas is combined and consolidated (Luria, 1980).

According to Luria the frontal areas of the brain surface are included in the third block. The major functions of this area are behavior regulation and action determination. The third-block areas assist in determining if actions are in sync with the task. As with the second block, the third block is subdivided into zones. The primary zone (motor cortex) controls motor impulses to peripheral sites. The secondary zone (premotor cortex) assists in programming and organizing motor responses. The tertiary-zone area is responsible for forming intentions, regulating behavior, and verifying actions. In Luria's system sensation and perception are functions of the second block, and cognition is a function of the third block. Effective functioning of the second and third block is dependent on normal functioning of the first block, which controls arousal and attention. Luria's work helps us understand the central nervous system link between brain function and one's behavior (Luria, 1980).

Information is transmitted from the peripheral nerves and ganglia to the dorsal root of the spinal cord. Sensory data travel through either the ascending anterolateral spinothalamic or the dorsal column medial lemniscal tracks. The significance of these tracks in sensation and perception is discussed in greater detail below. Figure 24-3 on p. 530 illustrates the pathway for transmission of light touch.

The anterolateral spinothalamic tract contains pathways that carry nondiscriminative sensations—that is, touch, tickle, itch, pain, and temperature (Schmitz, 1988). The information relayed is not exact with regard to intensity and location of the triggering signal. Mechanoreceptors, nocioceptors, and thermoreceptors activate transmission of impulses through the anterolateral spinothalamic tract. Specifically mechanoreceptors transmit information on touch, tickle, itch, and pressure to the anterolateral segment of the spinal cord, cross to the opposite anterolateral segment, and ascend through the anterior or ventral spinothalamic tract. The tracts terminate throughout the thalamus and lower brainstem. Nocioceptors carry sensations of pain to the spinothalamic tract and cross over and ascend through the lateral spinothalamic and spinoreticular tracts. Thermoreceptors transmit information related to temperature through the lateral spinothalamic tract.

The dorsal column medial lemniscal system conveys impulses on a more precise basis. This system is sensitive to minute differences in intensity and specific localization of impulses. Specialized mechanoreceptors convey information regarding barognosis, kinesthesia, proprioception, vibration, stereognosis, discriminative touch, tactile pressure, two-point discrimination, and graphesthesia. The impulses are relayed through large, rapidly conducting fibers. The fibers enter the dorsal column of the spinal cord and ascend to the medulla, where the impulse crosses to the opposite side and continues to the thalamus through the medial lemnisci (bilateral pathways). The neurons synapse and connect with neurons that project to the sensory cortex.

SPECIAL SENSES

The components of each of the special senses merit discussion due to the frequency with which individuals with chronic illness and disability experience impairments with sensation.

Visual impulses are transmitted along the optic nerve to the occipital lobe. Vision is a sense universally valued; however, individuals tend to underestimate the amount of input received through visual pathways including reading, writing, protection, and enjoyment of nature.

Auditory information is transformed from sound waves to electromechanical impulses through the organ of Corti. Auditory impulses are transmitted through the acoustic nerve, which provides impulses to the thalamus and the temporal lobe of the cerebral cortex. The sense of hearing provides mechanisms for reception of verbal communication and gives individuals feedback on the environment.

Olfactory receptors in the upper nasal cavity area are stimulated by the change from gas to chemicals within the nares. Impulses are transmitted through the olfactory nerve to the temporal lobe of the cerebral cortex. The sense of smell typically is not perceived as a critical sense; however, it is linked closely with the sense of taste and provides information about the environment.

Gustatory impulses are transmitted when food is converted to chemicals within the mouth. Taste buds, containing taste receptors, are stimulated and carry impulses

Table 24-1 Sensory receptors

Type of receptor	Responses
Mechanoreceptor	Transmits information regarding mechanical deformation (e.g., tissue damage) of the area enveloping the receptor; includes cutaneous and deep sensory receptors
Thermoreceptor	Transmits information on temperature change; includes cold and warmth receptors
Nocioceptor	Transmits information resulting in pain perception; includes pain receptors
Chemoreceptor	Transmits information related to chemical substances; includes receptors for taste, smell, arterial oxygen, osmolality, levels of blood carbon dioxide and blood glucose, amino acids, and fatty acids
Photic receptor	Transmits information regarding light; includes visual receptors (rods and cones)

Adapted from "Sensory Assessment" by T. Schmitz, in *Physical Rehabilitation: Assessment and Treatment* (2nd ed.) (pp. 79-92) edited by S. O'Sullivan and T. Schmitz, 1988, Philadelphia: F.A. Davis Company. Copyright 1988 by F.A. Davis. Reprinted by permission.

Table 24-2 Cranial nerves and functions

Cranial nerve	Nerve name	Nerve function
I	Olfactory	Sense of smell
II	Optic	Sense of vision
III	Oculomotor	Visual pathways
IV	Trochlear	Visual pathways
V	Abducens	Visual pathways
VI	Trigeminal	Mastication, facial sensation
VII	Facial	Facial expression, sense of taste, articulation
VIII	Vestibular/auditory	Facial expression, hearing; prevents nystagmus
IX	Glossopharyngeal	Sense of taste, articulation, swallowing
X	Vagus	Sense of taste, articulation, swallowing
XI	Accessory	Sternocleidomastoid and trapezius function
XII	Hypoglossal	Articulation, swallowing

through the facial and glossopharyngeal nerves to the medulla, thalamus, and cerebral cortex.

Somatosensory Impulses

Impulses providing information on touch, temperature, position sense, and pain function differently from the special senses. Impulses relaying tactile stimulation are transmitted from nerve receptors located throughout the skin. Nerve roots are located in all body dermatomes. (Dermatome maps are provided in Fig. 24-4 on p. 531.) As stated previously, tactile impulses are transmitted through the anterior (ventral) spinothalamic tract to the lower brainstem and thalamus, then to the sensory cortex. Figure 24-5 on p. 531 provides a diagram of major motor and sensory path-

ways. A second type of somatosensory impulse, temperature impulses are stimulated by changes in body and environmental temperatures. Similar to tactile receptors, temperature receptors are located throughout the skin. Temperature impulses travel through the lateral spinothalamic tract to the brainstem, thalamus, and cerebral cortex. A third type of somatosensory impulse is proprioception. Information about position sense or proprioception is transmitted from stimulation of sense organs or proprioceptors housed throughout the body in subcutaneous tissues, muscles, tendons, and bones. Proprioceptive impulses travel through the dorsal column medial lemniscal system to the cerebellum and cerebral cortex. A final type of somatosensory impulse is pain, which is discussed later in the chapter.

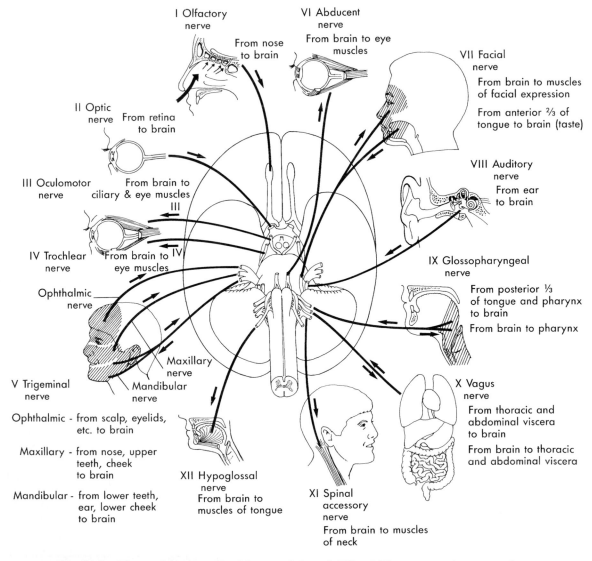

Fig. 24-1   The cranial nerves. Cranial nerves I through VII and XI serve somatic motor and sensory functions. Cranial nerves IX, X, and XII provide motor and sensory input to a variety of integrated regulatory functions.

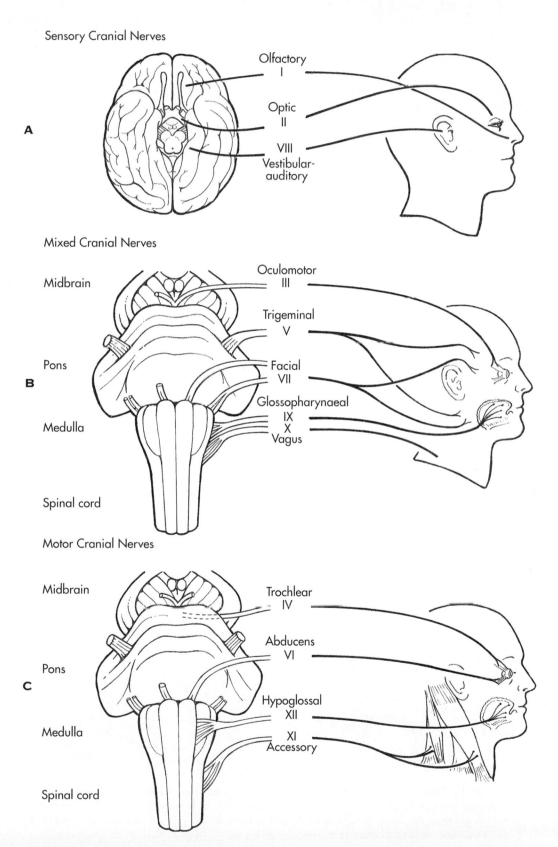

Fig. 24-2 Action of sensory, mixed, and motor cranial nerves. (Courtesy of John Muhm, EdD.)

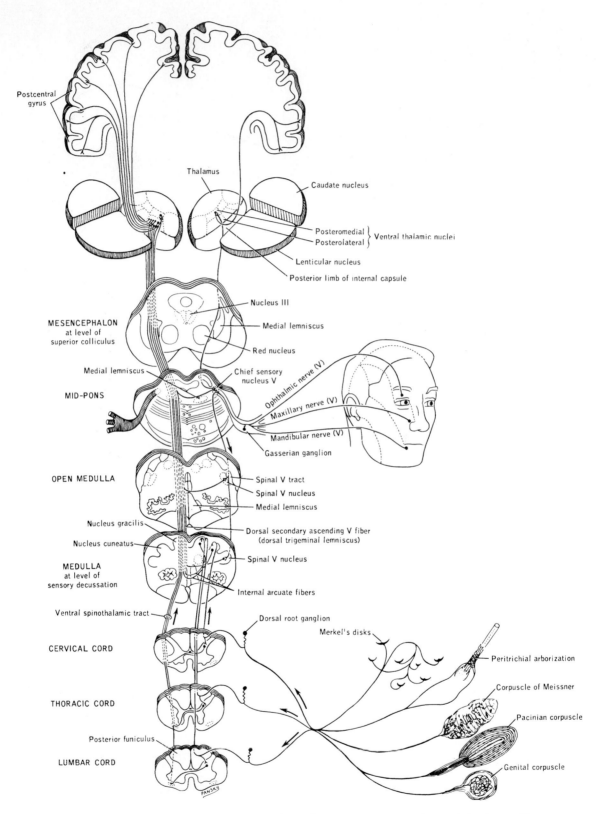

Fig. 24-3 Sensory pathways. The pathway for the transmission of light touch is shown. Note that input from peripheral nerves serving the head and face is at the brainstem level. Touch sensory fibers from the trunk, arms, and legs travel upward in the posterior funiculus and join head and face fibers in the brainstem in the medial lemniscus.

Perception occurs primarily in the parietal lobes of the cerebral cortex. The right and left parietal lobes tend to process different aspects of perception. Perception of verbal input, including reading and writing, tends to occur in the left parietal lobe as does right and left discrimination. The right parietal lobe processes information on space, texture, geography, construction, and body schema.

A highly individualized process, one's perception of stimuli is influenced by past experiences, age, culture, beliefs, education, attitudes, goals, and expectations. Additionally perception is modified through feedback from others and from oneself. Perceptual ability is essential for learning and must be present for successful rehabilitation

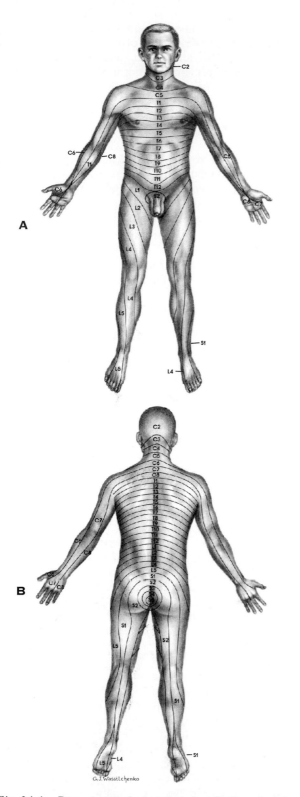

Fig. 24-4 Dermatomes. **A,** Anterior view. **B,** Posterior view.

Perception

The ability to make sense of the environment through the identification, integration, and interpretation of incoming stimuli is perception. It is difficult to consider perception apart from sensation, since perception is the way in which one interprets sensations, making perception and sensation interrelated phenomena (Lamm-Warburg, 1988).

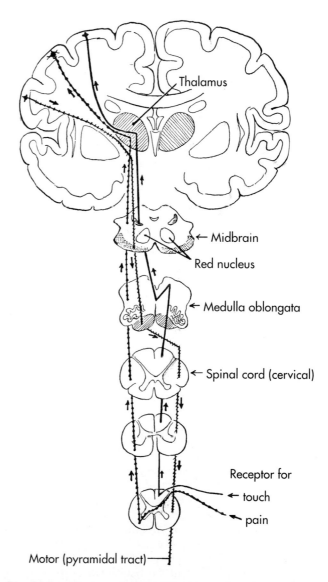

Fig. 24-5 Diagram of the main motor and sensory pathways. The perceptions of touch, passive motion, position, and vibration are transmitted through the posterior tract in the spinal cord through the medial lemniscus in the brainstem to the thalamus and through the internal capsule to the cortex (this pathway is represented by the *solid line*). Pain and temperature sensations are transmitted through the anterolateral tract and lateral lemniscus to the thalamus, then through the internal capsule to the cortex *(dotted lines)*. (Courtesy of John Muhm, EdD.)

of individuals with or without disabilities. For example, in one rehabilitation hospital the number of announcements made through the overhead paging system increased to the point that individuals lost an awareness of the messages. In other words, individuals became desensitized to the paged messages since past experience had indicated that the messages rarely were of any critical significance. Since few within the hospital paid attention to the paging, even when the messages were meant to alarm they went unnoticed. In order to gain attention to the paging system, the administrators needed to break the perception held by most employees that few paged messages were significant. They created a policy that only department directors could be paged, and that all urgent paged messages would be preceded by a bell. The policy was highly successful, and whenever employees heard the bell preceding a paged message, people became prepared for an emergency announcement. Implementation of the policy changed perceptions held regarding paging, and learning occurred.

Pain

Physical pain is a normal sensation that indicates the presence of tissue damage. Pain impulses are transmitted to the substantia gelatinosa within the lateral spinothalamic tract of the spinal cord. The impulses ascend to the thalamus of the brain and to the cerebral cortex. Simultaneously, descending fibers from the cerebral cortex moderate the way in which pain is perceived.

According to Wall (1995), a noted British neurophysiologist, the substantia gelatinosa of the spinal cord is the "gate" of the pain experience. According the Wall's gate control theory of pain, pain impulses are transmitted via small α-delta afferent fibers to the substantia gelatinosa of the spinal cord. Large fibers transmit touch, temperature, and pressure, and travel a similar route to the spinal cord. The gate theory holds that if the large fibers are stimulated simultaneously with the small fibers, the pain impulse will be weakened and perceived to a lower degree. Likewise, if one is experiencing pain, the pain perception may be decreased through stimulating the large fibers through touch, temperature change, or pressure. Simultaneously, the descending fibers from the cerebral cortex decrease the pain perception through distraction and relaxation. Figure 24-6 illustrates the effect of a spinal cord lesion on ascending and descending tracks.

Although pain is a common experience, there are a variety of widely held myths regarding pain perception (McCaffery & Beebe, 1989). It seems that few have objective opinions about another's pain experience. According to McCaffery one common pain myth is that if there is no clear physical reason for pain, it may be due to a psychological or emotional problem. There is little basis for this myth, just as there is little fact in the belief that all pain has a clearly identifiable cause. Actually some individuals have pain without a clear cause, only to learn later the source of the pain experience, and others never learn the actual cause of pain. A second myth is that malingering is common, and individuals will lie about the existence of pain. In fact, there is no basis for validation of this myth. Although some individuals may malinger, it is not a common occurrence. Actually more individuals disclaim the presence of pain when it exists than state they have pain when they do not. An-

other commonly held myth about pain is that individuals in pain always show visible signs of pain that verify the existence of pain. This is not true, since all individuals respond differently to pain. It is not unusual for individuals who have been in pain for long periods to fail to show any emotion, let alone the strong emotion expected to be seen with pain. This trend to fail to demonstrate strong emotion with pain is particularly evident with chronically ill children.

Indeed, until the past two decades, the topic of pain in infancy and childhood was conspicuously absent from the literature or supported by a set of myths. A prevailing notion was that infants and young children with immature neurologic systems could not distinguish pain or realized lesser degrees of pain than did adults. "Growing pains" were just to be outgrown. These ideas, coupled with concern that exposure to pain medication would lead children into addiction, contributed to poor pain management for children. Nurse researchers are credited with instituting many of the changes in this area (McCafferty & Beebe, 1989). However, early studies have centered on acute pain, whereas many children in rehabilitation experience chronic or recurring pain (Hoeman, 1990).

A final myth is that healthcare professionals are the experts about an individual's pain experience—however, no one but the person in pain can say how much pain is being experienced.

The pain experience is highly individualized. People respond to pain based on their culture, their background, and prior ordeals with pain. Culture impacts the way in which the individual responds to pain. In the United States, under Western medicine, we believe that pain is unnecessary and should be treated. An individual who reports having a headache, will be asked if anything has been taken for it. If the person with the headache responds that he has not taken anything for the headache, others will assume that perhaps he deserves to suffer. Another Western expectation of the pain experience is that the afflicted individual will deal with the pain in a quiet, controlled manner. That is, it is not appropriate for an individual in pain to lose control and yell or cry incessantly. The person in pain should not talk about the pain "a lot." In contrast, some cultures, such as some Hispanic groups, consider it proper to display strong emotion with pain. Other groups, such as Scandinavians, consider pain to be character building.

An individual's background also tempers the pain experience. Childbirth is one of the clearest examples of the effect of family background on pain perception. The daughter who heard her mother describe a 40-hour labor involving intolerable pain will dread the onset of labor, anticipating that she, too, will suffer intolerable pain. An additional way in which the pain experience is modified is through prior pain experiences. The individual who suffers from migraine headaches, for example, often recognizes the preceding signs and symptoms and anticipates that the pain experience will equate or surpass prior episodes. Part of the pain experienced with migraine may be due to the fear of impending pain.

Pain is an example of a normal sensation that is perceived uniquely by individuals. The response to pain is both automatic and learned. A child who touches a hot stove will remove her finger automatically and will learn not to touch hot stoves. A similar learned response to perception of other sensations occurs. In addition, individuals learn how to organize and process sensory input. Since we are constantly bombarded with sensory stimulation, we must select to which stimuli we will respond. Individuals adapt to different environments and learn alternative methods of organizing and processing sensory input in those environments. For example, the smell of smoke outside on a fall day is processed as insignificant olfactory stimulation. However, the same smoke smell indoors triggers quite a different re-

sponse. Consider a hospital setting, with all its associated noises, sights, and smells (e.g., paging, footsteps, medication, food carts, alcohol, and cleansers). Although such an environment is not novel to healthcare professionals, it is novel to the individuals we serve. Even individuals with intact neurologic systems may have difficulty organizing and processing the sensory input associated with a hospital setting. When individuals have impaired sensation and perception, their ability to organize and make sense of their environment may be limited severely.

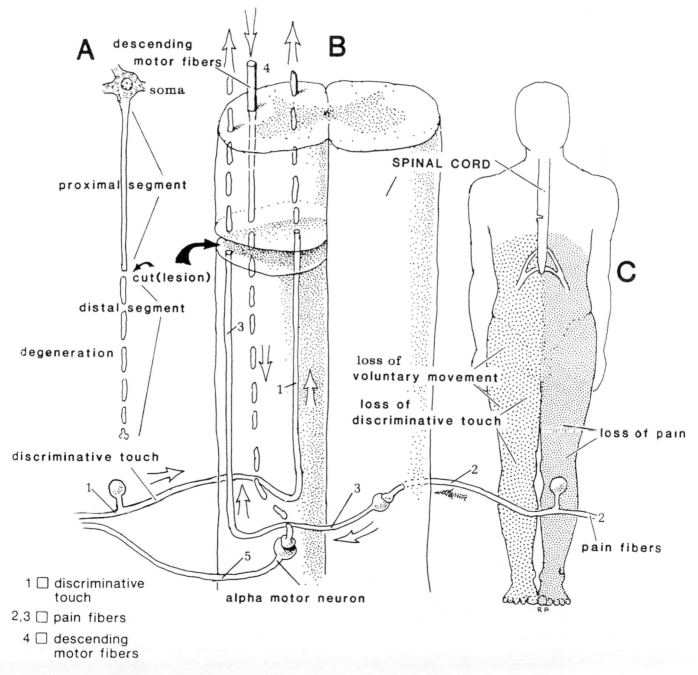

Fig. 24-6 The effect of a spinal cord lesion on ascending or descending tracts. Degeneration of ascending tracts occurs above the lesion; descending tracts will degenerate below the lesion.

IMPAIRED OR ALTERED SENSATION AND PERCEPTION

Deficits in sensation and perception may occur due to a specific disease process or may be related to aging. In general, sensory and perceptual deficits may result in a decline in sensory acuity or in an alteration in sensory stimuli reception, transmission, and integration.

Vision

The most frequent causes of visual impairment are eye injuries, glaucoma, and cataracts. Diabetes may result in retinopathy with severe visual losses. Multiple sclerosis may lead to optic neuritis and blindness. Normal aging results in visual losses also. After the age of 5 years, the lens of the eye becomes gradually less elastic, eventually resulting in decreased accommodation and farsightedness or presbyopia. With age the pupil size decreases and the lens of the eye loses transparency and thickens. As a result more light is needed to compensate. Twice as much light is needed for a 60-year-old individual to see what a 20-year-old can see (Storandt, 1986); however, the development of cataracts may lead the person to avoid bright lights, which cause glare. Adaptation to darkness is more difficult for older individuals. A night light may be needed to ensure that older individuals do not fall when getting up during the night.

Losses in vision are common after stroke and other neurologic problems, but due to other physical problems the visual deficits usually receive little concern. One of the visual problems that commonly presents after a stroke is diplopia or double vision. The individual will see two of everything in the surrounding environment. Added to the perceptual problems that may occur with a stroke, this can be a serious obstacle. The condition can be alleviated in most cases by completing eye exercises (range of motion) and covering alternate eyes (Lamm-Warburg, 1988). Another visual problem that occurs following stroke is hemianopsia or visual field deficits. Individuals with stroke often experience cuts of the visual fields, the most common of which is homonymous hemianopsia; individuals do not see half of the visual field. For example, with a bilateral left visual cut, individuals will see nothing left of their midline. The consequences of this are far reaching. Such individuals may not be able to find the call light located by their left hand, may not eat food items that are placed to the left, or may not notice individuals approaching them from the left. Homonymous hemianopsia is predictive of a difficult rehabilitation course and typically of a higher poststroke mortality rate. Vision, hearing, taste, and smell are discussed in detail in Chapter 16.

Hearing

The most commonly experienced problems with the ears are trauma, infection, Méniére's disease, and otosclerosis. Hearing losses typically occur with age, with the ability to hear high tones lost and the auditory threshold raised. This can impact comprehension of speech, since words containing high-frequency tones (f, g, s, t, z) may become unintelligible (Storandt, 1986).

Significant losses in hearing may occur following damage to the vestibular or auditory nerve (cranial nerve VIII).

Damage to the inner ear or damage to the auditory nerve may result in sensorineural hearing loss. Injuries that prevent or limit the conduction of sound to the inner ear may cause conductive hearing loss.

Taste and Smell

Since the senses of taste and smell are interlinked, individuals experiencing problems with smell tend to perceive problems with taste also. Typically, however, most problems actually are disorders of smell. Problems with taste and smell may occur following upper respiratory infections, renal disease, or neurologic diseases. Intracranial lesions and frontal lobe injuries may cause problems with taste and smell.

Touch

Sensitivity to touch may be lost with aging but typically does not interfere with function. Disorders of the sense of touch may occur with stroke or neurologic injury. The location of problem will vary with the lesion site. Deficits in touch may present as complete loss of tactile sensation (anesthesia), abnormal tactile sensation (paresthesia), decrease in tactile sensation (hypoesthesia), or increase in tactile sensation (hyperesthesia). Significant deficits (anesthesia and paresthesia) may lead to tissue injury, since response to painful stimuli may be impaired. Individuals must be taught to have a continual awareness of the location of the affected extremity or body part.

Temperature

Problems with control of body temperature through the central nervous system may occur with some neurologic lesions and may result in hyperthermia or hypothermia. In general, older adults have a decreased ability to compensate for changes in the temperature of the external environment (Clark & Murray, 1988). Chapter 22 provides information on the impact of the regulatory and immune systems.

Proprioception

Incoordination and ataxia are the common problems occurring with proprioception. A variety of injuries and illnesses may precipitate proprioceptive problems including tabes dorsalis, parietal lobe lesions, severe pernicious anemia, and Brown-Séquard syndrome.

Perceptual Deficits

Perceptual problems commonly are experienced by individuals with brain injuries and lesions. There are seemingly unlimited variations of perceptual problems that may present, several of which are discussed.

Some perceptual deficits present as disorders of *body image or schema*, which may result following brain injury since the ability to integrate and make sense of tactile and proprioceptive input may be impaired. *Somatosognosia* is an unawareness of one's body structure and body parts. It typically occurs with lesions of the dominant parietal lobe and often is associated with right-sided hemiplegia. The individual may have difficulty imitating movements and following directions such as "move your left leg." The individual may have less difficulty responding to simple gestures and instructions identifying specific body parts.

Right and left discrimination is another disorder of body image or schema, which may occur following damage to either the right or left parietal lobe. With this deficit the individual is unable to determine the right or left sides of his own body and will not be able to follow verbal commands that include references to right and left. Correction of right and left discrimination deficit is to exclude mention of right or left in directions but rather give environmental cues or point.

Visual spatial neglect, another disorder of body image or schema, usually occurs after a parietal lobe lesion of the nondominant hemisphere and usually affects awareness of the left side of the body. The individual may be unaware of any stimuli on the affected side, including tactile and environmental stimuli. This disorder creates the potential for serious safety hazards, since the individual is not aware of objects to the left within the environment. While the individual is being taught how to correct the problem, the surroundings needs to be modified to create a safe environment. Therapy revolves around increasing the individual's awareness of the left side of the environment and of her body.

Two additional types of body image or schema disorders are *finger agnosia* and *anosognosia*. With finger agnosia, the individual is unable to identify specific fingers bilaterally. The problem usually results after a lesion to the parietal lobe of the dominant hemisphere and is linked with aphasia. Treatment may involve discriminative touch and pressure to cue the individual in to the fingers. Anosognosia is a serious problem in which individuals deny the presence of paralysis. Usually the parietal lobe of the dominant side is affected. The condition is linked with a poor prognosis, since it is impossible to teach individuals to correct deficits that they do not perceive. Teaching primarily revolves around ensuring a safe environment.

Disorders in spatial relations also are perceptual deficits and may occur following damage to the nondominant hemisphere of the brain and usually are seen in conjunction with left-sided hemiplegia. There are many types of spatial relations problems. *Spatial relations deficits* entail problems in identifying the distance and relationship in space of items. Problems may include an inability to distinguish an item from the background (*figure ground discrimination*), which creates problems in all activities of daily living. For example, it is necessary to be able to distinguish a towel from the wall and a bar of soap from the sink in order to wash one's face. As another example, it is necessary to be able to distinguish a slice of bread from the tablecloth in order to eat. Individuals with this deficit tend to have less difficulty with items that are defined clearly and contrast in color from the background.

Another type of spatial relations problem is *form constancy*, which is difficulty in identifying similarly shaped but distinct objects from one another. For example, an individual with spatial relations problems may not be able to distinguish between a glass and a vase sitting side by side. Likewise, a toothbrush lying near a pencil may be confused. Problems with this deficit can be minimized by controlling the environment and encouraging the individual to feel the objects and to inspect them closely.

Individuals with spatial relations problems may show deficits in other visual spatial areas requiring judgment, for example, with direction, depth, and distance. They may have extensive difficulty using stairs and will need consistent and constant reminders to learn to compensate for the deficits.

An additional category of perceptual deficits is *agnosia*. Individuals with agnosia are unable to identify familiar items with one sense, although the use of an alternative sense may help them recognize the object. For example, an individual may not be able to find her mirror when looking on a table until she actually feels the mirror with her hands. The fork and spoon may be confused until the individual picks up each and recalls the difference. This deficit is corrected by encouraging individuals to use more than a single sense in locating objects. However, correction is not as easy for agnosias involving other senses. For example, with *auditory agnosia* the individual may not recognize familiar nonspeech sounds such as bells, whistles, and car horns. The difference between the telephone ringing and the doorbell may not be distinguishable to the individual.

A final category of perceptual deficit is *apraxia*, in which individuals cannot remember once known movements. Although the individuals have sufficient strength, coordination, and attention to perform the action, they are unable to do so. For example, an individual with *ideational apraxia* may be able to shave, but if he is told to do so, he may not be able to conceptualize the task. If the individual has *ideomotor apraxia*, he may be able to pick up the shaver and shave out of habit. However, if a nurse or therapist tells him to shave, he may be confused as to what to do.

Perceptual deficits often are viewed by family members as indicators of mental confusion. It is essential that they be assisted in understanding the nature of such problems. Through careful assessment of the patterns of behavior and deficits, treatment plans can be designed to correct many of the problems.

Chronic Pain

Although pain is a normal sensation, most people believe they would be better off without it. Just the opposite is true, however, as demonstrated by the devastation of Hansen's disease, or leprosy. One of the key characteristics of Hansen's disease is the destruction of pain receptors resulting in anesthesia. The problem of course is that individuals with Hansen's disease fail to recognize tissue damage in time to prevent serious injury. Yancey (1977) describes an individual with Hansen's disease becoming blind, because the eye surface did not detect irritation, and the individual did not perceive the need to blink, resulting in drying of the eyes. However, just as a complete absence of pain is life-threatening, the unceasing presence of pain also is intolerable. Such is the case with chronic pain syndrome.

Chronic pain is a disorder of sensation that impacts every aspect of an individual's life, family, friends, work, and play. Although there is a wealth of literature on the syndrome, there is no consensus as to why some individuals develop chronic pain syndrome and others with equivalent or even more physically severe injuries do not. One hypothesis is that a pain cycle develops and results in chronic pain syndrome. In response to injury, the individual protects and immobilizes the injured area (e.g., a joint). The immobilization of the area leads to the development of scar tissue around the site and a reduction in synovial fluid production. The joint becomes stiff and difficult to move, leading to increased pain, inflammation, and tendonitis. The individual guards and immobilizes the joint to an even greater degree, with resulting weakness and loss of function. In order to continue guarding the area, the individual develops compensatory mechanisms to "protect" the joint, such as limping and altering the gait. These compensatory mechanisms do not act in the body's favor, and the altered gait leads to back pain, resulting in more extensive guarding of multiple areas. The result is chronic presence of pain without a clear link to a pathophysiologic problem (Keefe & Lefebvre, 1994).

Chronic pain impacts every area of an individual's life (Grennan & Jayson, 1994). Time off from work due to therapy and medical appointments, illness, and loss of function results in poor attendance and difficulty maintaining a job. Complaints about the amount of pain experienced and restrictions of avocational activities lead to limited family and community involvement. Reductions in activity result in weight gain and decreased energy and endurance levels. As more and more money is spent looking for cures, causes, and relief, finances become exhausted. As the pain continues with no relief in sight, depression becomes a way of life. Individuals with chronic pain have little reason to look forward to days filled with more and more pain; less and less function; and constant work, family, and financial problems. Such individuals experience difficulties coping with their pain and may develop addictions to alcohol and narcotics. Eventually they reach the end of the medical therapeutic gamut and are depressed, financially drained, have employment and family problems, and still are in constant pain (Whelan, 1994).

Given the pervasiveness of the problem of chronic pain, it is unlikely that any single modality of intervention will be effective in providing relief from the syndrome. Therefore programs meeting with greatest success provide a variety of interventions and use a comprehensive and multifaceted approach. Comprehensive programs for chronic pain usually involve a variety of disciplines including but not limited to nursing, physical therapy, medicine, occupational therapy, vocational counseling, therapeutic recreation, and psychology.

Just as in other areas of rehabilitation, client education is a cornerstone of treatment for chronic pain. Self-application of local therapies such as ultrasound, transcutaneous electrical stimulation, and hot or cold packs may be of benefit and should be included in client education programs. A second component of client education for chronic pain is instruction in the use of nonpharmacologic methods of pain relief such as biofeedback, relaxation, and self-hypnosis. Clients should be taught the use of work simplification and energy conservation methods but need to be encouraged to increase activity level gradually. The client should receive instructions in posture, body mechanics, and positioning. The program should include an assessment of workplace design and ergonomics.

Chronic Pain across the Lifespan

Individuals in two age groups, the very young and the very old, tend to experience subtle discrimination with respect to chronic pain. Although more than 50 million children in the United States experience chronic pain, there is a paucity of healthcare resources for the child with chronic pain. Healthcare professionals often underestimate the amount of pain experienced by children, and since many children are hesitant to talk to physicians and nurses, their pain may be underreported (Howe, 1993). The second age group in which persons are undertreated for chronic pain is the geriatric group. Many older persons suffer from chronic pain due to chronic illness and disability and assume that it is a normal part of the aging process. Although few children or elderly persons require the comprehensiveness of a chronic pain management program, they will benefit from an open-minded approach toward alleviation and moderation of the pain experienced (Keefe & Williams, 1990).

Common conditions for chronic pain in childhood include juvenile rheumatoid arthritis, sickle cell crises, recurrent headaches, recurrent abdominal pain from a variety of conditions, reflex sympathetic dystrophy syndrome, malignancies, and pain following multiple trauma or amputation. The impact of a child's pain on the family is part of the assessment.

Children with chronic, disabling, or developmental disorders must be assessed within the context of their developmental stage. Two variables contribute to difficulty in assessing pain in children: the expression of pain and the experience of pain. A child's experience and expression of pain will differ with the developmental stage—but more importantly these cannot be equated with adult behaviors or judged using adult terms. A child who has prolonged, chronic pain or whose pain worsens gradually may not be able to distinguish changes in pain intensity or determine duration and location of pain. Children may play or sleep through pain as ways of coping with discomfort. In fact, children may not refer to the pain as pain. A child's self-report of having no pain may not be reliable for a variety of reasons. For instance, some children may not be able to associate pain relief measures with improved comfort; others may assign themselves personal responsibility for the pain or believe they deserve punishment. For these reasons, it often is beneficial to ask a child who or what causes the pain and to describe and explain pain using the child's own words (Hoeman, 1990).

Older persons may try to ignore or bear their pain or conversely may complain about pain. Those who are cognitively intact may not require any adaptations for assessment. However, impaired or altered sensory function, such as vision or hearing, and reduced sensation and perception may alter the pain experience. An older person may deny pain but "guard" movement or positioning, change patterns of ambulation, pace level of activity, or "work around" painful activities without reporting pain. Those with cognitive or communication impairments may become frustrated, angry, or contentious because they cannot express or explain their pain (Toomey & Seville, 1994). Additionally the elderly client may experience chronic but transient pain and describe it as discomfort, aches, or by such colloquial names "old friend" or "rhematiz," thus avoiding the nature of the pain (Hoeman, 1990).

Pain is a multidimensional phenomenon. Even with the use of a comprehensive approach to pain management, the prognosis for individuals with chronic pain is a long and

ELAND COLOR SCALE: DIRECTIONS FOR USE

After discussing with the child several things that have hurt the child in the past

1. Present 8 crayons or markers to the child. Suggested colors are yellow, orange, red, green, blue, purple, brown, and black.
2. Ask the following questions, and after the child has answered, mark the appropriate square on the tool (e.g., severe pain, worst hurt), and put that color away from the others. For convenience, the word *hurt* is used here, but whatever term the child uses should be substituted. Ask the child the following questions:
    ◆ "Of these colors, which color is most like the worst hurt you have ever had (using whatever example the child has given) or the worst hurt anybody could ever have?" Which phrase is chosen will depend on the child's experience and what the child is able to understand. Some children may be able to imagine much worse pain than they have ever had, and other children can understand only what they have experienced. Of course some children may have experienced the worst pain they can imagine.
    ◆ "Which color is almost as much hurt as the worst hurt (or, use example given above, if any) but not quite as bad?"
    ◆ "Which color is like something that hurts just a little?"
    ◆ "Which color is like no hurt at all?"
3. Show the 4 colors (marked boxes, crayons, or markers) to the child in the order he has chosen them, from the color chosen for the worst hurt to the color chosen for no hurt.
4. Ask the child to color the body outlines where he hurts, using the colors he has chosen to show how much it hurts.
5. When the child finishes, ask the child if this is a picture of how he hurts now or how he hurt earlier. Be specific about what earlier means by relating the time to an event (e.g., at lunch or in the playroom).

(Printed with permission of J.M. Eland, who also gives permission for this to be duplicated and used in the care of children with pain.) May be duplicated for use in clinical practice. From *Pain: Clinical Manual for Nursing Practice,* by M. McCaffery and A. Beebe, 1989, St. Louis: Mosby–Year Book. Copyright 1989 by Mosby–Year Book. Reprinted by permission.

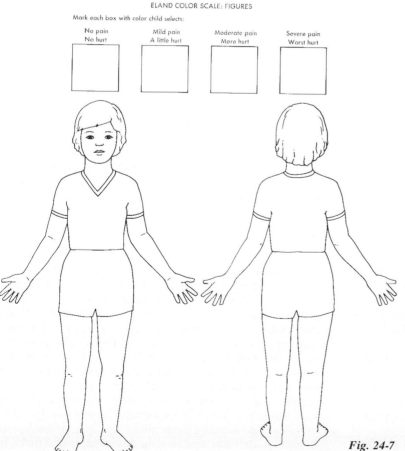

ELAND COLOR SCALE: FIGURES

Mark each box with color child selects:

No pain No hurt	Mild pain A little hurt	Moderate pain More hurt	Severe pain Worst hurt

(Indicate child's use of right and left.)

Fig. 24-7 Eland Color Scale: figures. (Printed with permission of J.M. Eland, who also gives permission for this to be duplicated and used in the care of children with pain.)

Fig. 24-8 Explain to the child that each face is for a person who feels happy because he has no pain (hurt) or sad because he has some or a lot of pain. Face 0 is very happy because he doesn't hurt at all. Face 1 hurts a little bit. Face 2 hurts a little more. Face 3 hurts even more. Face 4 hurts a whole lot, but face 5 hurts as much as you can imagine, although you don't have to be crying to feel this bad. Ask the child to choose the face that best describes how he is feeling.

hard fight for recovery and return to function, without any guarantees that pain will cease.

Malignant Pain

Pain from cancer may occur due to nerve compression, infection, and release of prostaglandins (Cherny & Portenoy, 1994). Unlike chronic pain, the cornerstone of treatment for malignant pain is pharmacologic. The guiding principles of narcotic use for malignant pain are matching dose to client response and giving the medication on a regular and consistent basis rather than on an as-needed basis.

Nonmalignant, Intermittent Pain

Pain that occurs on an irregular but severe basis, such as with sickle cell disease, typically is treated as acute pain. Nonpharmacologic pain relief methods may be of benefit, but the primary mode of treatment is the use of medications to manage the acute episode (Blendis, 1994).

Another type of nonmalignant pain is phantom limb pain, a natural consequence following the loss of a body part (Jensen & Rasmussen, 1994). Typically it does not present problems with therapeutic management, although on occasion individuals experience extreme phantom limb pain. Treatment for severe phantom limb problems usually follows the comprehensive approach used for management of chronic pain (Kamen & Chapis, 1994).

ASSESSMENT OF SENSATION, PERCEPTION, AND PAIN

Sensation

In assessing sensation the nurse evaluates the extent and degree of sensory deficits present. Additionally the client's subjective feelings about the deficit should be evaluated. With regard to vision the nurse inquires about any changes in vision and the use of glasses or contact lenses, while assessing visual acuity through the use of a Snellen chart. The nurse examines the physical appearance of the client's eyes and surrounding areas.

In assessing auditory sensory function, the nurse inspects the external areas around the ear. The Rinne test and the Weber test may be used to differentiate sensorineural hearing loss from conductive hearing deficits. Presence of either type of deficit indicates a need for an audiology referral.

Olfactory function is evaluated through testing each nos-

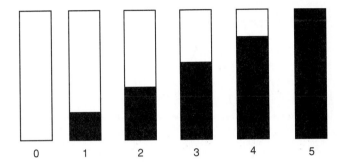

Fig. 24-9 Explain to the child that there are six glasses with different amounts of pain (hurt) in five of them. The empty glass is for no pain. Glass 5 is completely filled with the worst pain imaginable. The glasses in between have from very little to a whole lot of pain. Ask the child to choose the glass that best describes how she is feeling.

tril individually. Substances with distinct but nonirritating odors, such as soap and coffee, are used to detect olfactory deficits. Ordinarily the sense of taste is assessed only when clients complain of problems. Various substances (e.g., salt, sugar, and lemon juice) may be used to check taste.

In areas where deficits are suspected, the nurse assesses the sense of touch with a wisp of cotton. Distal areas are assessed first and proximal areas last. The same pattern may be used to assess temperature sense through using tubes filled with either cold or hot water.

Perception

In contrast to sensory deficits, which tend to be detected readily, perceptual deficits are more difficult to assess. Perceptual problems must be differentiated from sensory deficits, motor problems, disorientation, language barriers, and intellectual and cognitive deficits. A key aspect is comparison with the premorbid perceptual ability. The nurse assesses premorbid and postmorbid behaviors and stimuli response. The degree of compensation possible with adaptive and assistive devices is identified, in addition to the adequacy of the environment. Too much or too little external stimulation may result in transient perceptual problems. Internal factors including medications, hypoxia, or electrolyte imbalance also may lead to transient perceptual deficits. In addition to identification of perceptual deficits, the nurse assesses the functional impact of such deficits. For example, can the client complete activities of daily living or respond to emergencies? The presence of a perceptual deficit is significant only if it remains uncompensated.

Pain

Since there is little correlation between one's physical appearance or facial expressions and degree of pain experienced, assessment of pain depends primarily on subjective reporting. The nurse records the client's pain history including the maximum, minimum, and typical amount of pain experienced. The nurse assesses what the client finds exacerbates the pain and what alleviates the pain. A standardized scale for pain assessment should be used (Coracely, 1995), such as the Visual Analogue Scale or the McGill-Melzack Pain Questionnaire. In addition, with chronic pain the nurse assesses the client's premorbid and postmorbid lifestyle and the impact on lifestyle that the client perceives pain to have had.

A number of assessment tools are available that are designed specifically for assessing pain in children. The Eland Color Scale (Fig. 24-7 and the box on p. 537), which consists of figures on which the child marks the location of pain and indicates intensity of pain with colors, is favored by many nurse clinicians. Other commonly used pediatric assessment scales are the Wong Faces Rating Scale and the Baker Glasses Rating Scale (Whaley & Wong, 1995) (Fig. 24-8 and Fig. 24-9). Children may benefit from art, play, or music therapy as both assessment and intervention techniques. All approaches with children consider the total family system and family participation in child-centered goals (Hoeman, 1990).

NURSING DIAGNOSES

The nursing diagnoses seen with clients with sensory or perceptual deficits vary with the specific problem. The nursing diagnoses commonly seen in individuals with sensory and perceptual problems are listed in the following box.

PLANNING AND GOALS FOR SENSORY AND PERCEPTUAL PROBLEMS

Mutual planning and goal setting are essential with sensory and perceptual problems. The nurse works with the client to determine whether possible adaptive and assistive devices will match the desired lifestyle. If the client or family does not or will not incorporate the use of adaptive devices into the client's lifestyle, determination of equipment is moot.

✦

NURSING DIAGNOSES RELATED TO SENSORY AND PERCEPTUAL PROBLEMS

Uncompensated sensory deficits
Sensory/perceptual alterations (specify: visual, auditory, kinesthetic, gustatory, tactile, and olfactory)
Chronic pain
Intermittent, recurring pain

INTERVENTIONS

Specific interventions for sensory and perceptual problems have been identified earlier in the text, including techniques for relaxation and visualization, or imagery. General approaches to sensory and perceptual problems are presented in this section.

Transfer of Training

The transfer of training approach is based on the belief that learning a skill for one application will carry over to other applications. For example, the practice of scanning for pieces while completing a puzzle can help the client remember to scan the dinner table during meals.

Sensorimotor Approach

With the sensorimotor approach, motor output is controlled, and specific sensory stimulation is offered to influence cerebral sensory organization and processing. Adaptive motor reactions are required in response to carefully controlled sensory stimuli. For instance, the client could be assisted into a standing table for proprioceptive input.

Functional Approach

Probably one of the most commonly employed approaches to sensory and perceptual problems, the functional approach is based on the concept that practicing functional tasks will result in relearning and independence. Methods of compensation and adaptation are incorporated in functional teaching. For example, repeatedly practicing buttoning a shirt with a buttonhook is an example of a functional approach to relearning the skill of buttoning.

Safety Concerns

While the client is relearning functional skills and abilities, the environment must be as safe as possible. For example, the environment around individuals with neglect and homonymous hemianopsia must have essential bedside needs (e.g., telephone, call light, and tissues) on the uninvolved side. While the individual is learning scanning techniques, colored tape may be used to attract attention to items.

EVALUATION

When evaluating the outcomes achieved with the client, the nurse identifies the degree of compensation attained and the ability of the client to function effectively with regard to sensory and perceptual ability. Follow-up of sensory and perceptual problems should be done over several months with the client and family members.

REFERRAL RESOURCES

Depending on the type of deficit experienced, referral to an occupational therapist, physical therapist, speech pathologist, or audiologist may be needed. For problems with chronic pain, a referral to a chronic pain program may be indicated.

ISSUES, TRENDS, AND NEW DIRECTIONS

The use of narcotics for individuals in chronic pain is an area currently under debate. Some advocate that no indi-

---

CASE STUDY

Mike, a 35-year-old long-haul truck driver, experienced a work-related injury while unloading his truck. He arrived at his destination early, and rather than paying for someone to give him assistance or waiting for someone to arrive from the trucking company, he decided to empty the truck. While doing so, Mike states he felt something "pop" in his back and experienced sharp pain radiating from his back down his left leg. He states that he was unable to finish unloading the truck and had to be hospitalized.

A prescription of rest, relaxation, traction, and medications was given to Mike. He remained hospitalized for 2 weeks, and a computerized tomography (CT) scan indicated the presence of a bulging disk in the lower back area. Mike felt better after the hospitalization but was not able to return to trucking owing to the abnormal CT scan and the continued presence of pain. His neurosurgeon explained that the sharp jarring of the truck could result in permanent physical impairment.

As the pain persisted day after day, Mike became more and more inactive. He found that the acetaminophen with codeine tablets no longer worked as well at controlling his pain and discovered that they worked better when taken with a beer.

The Workers' Compensation company hired a private investigator to determine if Mike was "legitimately" functionally impaired. Mike's activity status became more and more sedentary. He spent long hours on the couch in his trailer and tended to gain weight. He was referred for a transcutaneous electrical stimulation unit, which was used constantly, since the medication was working less and less effectively. His consumption of alcohol increased, and he got a prescription for oxycodone and aspirin (Percodan) from a second physician.

Mike's wife reached her breaking point and decided to move out of the trailer. His friends began calling less and less frequently. After 1 year postinjury, Mike found himself taking diazepam (Valium), oxycodone and aspirin, acetaminophen with codeine, and drinking two six-packs of beer a day. His activity level amounted to household activities and short car rides. Once a week he went to a card game with a friend.

The Workers' Compensation company physician referred Mike to a comprehensive pain management program. He was evaluated by a physiatrist who prescribed a program of monitored physical exercise, vocational counseling, medication reduction, nutritional counseling, biofeedback, relaxation training, and psychological counseling. A rehabilitation nurse coordinated the program, serving in the role of an internal case manager, and communicated Mike's progress on a regular basis to the Workers' Compensation representative. After a 2-month program Mike was medication free and consistently used biofeedback and relaxation to control pain. Although he regained much of the physical strength he had lost, he was unable to return to long-haul trucking, since he continued to have abnormal electromyograms. The vocational counselor worked with Mike and he enrolled in college.

Today Mike is working full time as a certified public accountant. He continues to have back pain but manages the problem with relaxation and biofeedback, and on really tough days he uses hot packs. He is considered to be a successful pain program graduate but continues in the pain program support group.

---

vidual in pain be denied substances that can decrease the pain perceived (McCaffery & Beebe, 1989). This perspective has led to the use of continuous morphine pumps for individuals with chronic pain. The traditional perspective on narcotics for treatment of chronic pain is that individuals will develop a tolerance to narcotics and not receive benefit in increased function or alleviation of pain. Since chronic pain does not impact longevity, there seems to be little merit in providing substances to which individuals rapidly become tolerant. While the debate remains unresolved, it is evident that drugs alone will not solve the problem of chronic pain.

REFERENCES

Blendis, L. (1994). Abdominal pain. In P. Wall & R. Melzack (Eds.), *Textbook of pain* (pp. 583-596). New York: Churchill Livingstone.

Cherny, N., & Portenoy, R. (1994). Cancer pain. Principles of assessment and syndromes. In P. Wall & R. Melzack (Eds.), *Textbook of pain* (pp. 787-824). New York: Churchill Livingstone.

Clark, G., & Murray, P. (1988). Rehabilitation of the geriatric patient. In J. DeLisa (Ed.), *Rehabilitation medicine: Principles and practice* (pp. 410-429). Philadelphia: J.B. Lippincott.

Coracely, R. (1995). Studies of pain in normal man. In P. Wall & R. Melzack (Eds.), *Textbook of pain* (pp. 315-336). New York: Churchill Livingstone.

Eland, J.M. (1990). Pain in children. *Nursing Clinics of North America, 25,* 871-884. Philadelphia: W.B. Saunders.

Erickson, R., & McPhee, M. (1988). Clinical evaluation. In J. DeLisa (Ed.), *Rehabilitation medicine: Principles and practice* (pp. 25-65). Philadelphia: J.B. Lippincott.

Grennan, D., & Jayson, M. (1994). Rheumatoid arthritis. In P. Wall & R. Melzack (Eds.), *Textbook of pain* (pp. 397-408). New York: Churchill Livingstone.

Hoeman, S.P. (1990). Chronic pain in childhood. Keynote presentation at Caring for Persons in Pain Workshop, Alvernia College, Reading, PA. October 5.

Howe, C. (1993). A new standard of care for pediatric pain management. *Maternal Child Nursing, 18,* 325-329.

Jensen, T., & Rasmussen, P. (1995). Phantom pain and other phenomena after amputation. In P. Wall & R. Melzack (Eds.), *Textbook of pain* (pp. 651-666). New York: Churchill Livingstone.

Kamen, L.B., & Chapis, G.J. (1994). Phantom limb sensation and phantom pain. *Physical Medicine and Rehabilitation: State of the Art Reviews, 8,* 73-88.

Keefe, F., & Lefebvre, D. (1994). Behavior therapy. In P. Wall & R. Melzack (Eds.), *Textbook of pain* (pp. 1367-1380). New York: Churchill Livingstone.

Keefe, F.J., & Williams, D.A. (1990). A comparison of coping strategies in chronic pain patients in different age groups. *Psychological Aciences, 45,* 161-165.

Lamm-Warburg, C. (1988). Assessment and treatment strategies for perceptual deficits. In S. O'Sullivan & T. Schmitz (Eds.), *Physical rehabilitation: Assessment and treatment* (2nd ed., pp. 79-92). Philadelphia: F.A. Davis.

Luria, A. (1980). *Higher cortical functions in man.* New York: Basic Books.

McCafferty, M., & Beebe, A. (1989). *Pain: Clinical manual for nursing practice*. Philadelphia: Mosby–Year Book.

Rohe, D. (1988). Psychological aspects of rehabilitation. In J. DeLisa (Ed.), *Rehabilitation medicine: Principles and practice* (pp. 66-82). Philadelphia: J.B. Lippincott.

Schmitz, T. (1988). Sensory assessment. In S. O'Sullivan & T. Schmitz (Eds.), *Physical rehabilitation: Assessment and treatment* (2nd ed., pp. 79-92). Philadelphia: F.A. Davis.

Storandt, M. (1986). Psychological aspects of aging. In I. Rossman (Ed.), *Clinical geriatrics* (pp. 606-617). Philadelphia: J.B. Lippincott.

Toomey, T.C., & Seville, J.L. (1994). Assessing functional impairment in elderly patients with chronic pain. *Topics Geriatric Rehabilitation, 10,* 58-66.

Wall, P. (1994). Introduction. In P. Wall & R. Melzack (Eds.), *Textbook of pain* (pp. 1-12). New York: Churchill Livingstone.

Wong, D. (1995). *Nursing care of infants and children* (5th ed.). St. Louis: Mosby–Year Book.

Whelan, K.A. (1994). Case study of a patient with chronic pain. *Rehabilitation Nursing, 19,* 359-360.

Yancey, P. (1977). *Where is God when it hurts?* Grand Rapids, MI: The Zondervan Corporation.

25

Communication: Language and Pragmatics

Barbara J. Boss, PhD, RN, CS
Kay Lewis Abney, PhD, RN, CPNP

INTRODUCTION

Communication is more than talk. Communication is a rich and complex social activity involving linguistic, cognitive, and pragmatic competence. Linguistic competence is the ability to form and use symbols. Language is the symbolic signal system used by a person to communicate with other persons. Effective language involves many processes: development of thoughts to be communicated; selection, formulation, and ordering of words; application of rules of grammar; initiation of muscle movements to produce speech or written output. Speech output also requires control of respiration to produce the required sounds and verbalization. Individuals listen to or look at their language output, evaluate the output, and correct the language when necessary. Language, speech, and writing provide individuals with a well-ordered, rule-bound system of communication. But communication is more than language. Pragmatic competence is the ability to use language appropriately in situational and social contexts and involves all nonlanguage aspects of communication. Cognitive competence is required for communication to be relevant, accurate, and evidence clear thinking. All aspects of communication are active processes, initially learned within the family and deeply influenced by culture.

A working knowledge of the types of communication deficits helps rehabilitation nurses recognize and assess communication deficits experienced by their clients. This is invaluable in planning appropriate therapeutic interventions to assist with communication and helps the nurse appreciate the prognosis for recovery, which is fundamental to facilitating the client and family in their adaptation and coping.

LINGUISTICS

Linguistic or language competence involves the comprehension and transmission of ideas and feelings by use of conventionalized marks and sounds and the sequential ordering of them according to accepted rules of grammar. This competence involves at least three subcompetencies: phonologic competence, semantic competence, and syntactic competence. Phonology is the process of recovering the phonologic formation of a word—that is, ordering the sounds used to form the words (e.g., "wa gon" versus "gon wa"). Semantics refers to the ability to relate a symbol or sign to an object—that is, applying the correct meanings to words. Semantics is the use of nominal words (substantive words). Syntax is the grammatic structure in language production and refers to the rules for interrelating words or ordering statements. Appropriate application of plurality and tense also is involved.

Language Acquisition

Two primary theories of language acquisition postulated by Skinner (1957) and Chomsky (1978) have been challenged in recent years. Skinner advanced the theory that language is learned through reinforcement by the environment when spontaneous sounds of the infant that resemble adult speech are encouraged by the caretaker (family). Chomsky challenged this traditional theory that humans innately possess the capability for language acquisition.

Most recent theoretic explanations of language acquisition are multifactorial. Wexler (1990) proposed innateness/maturational approach to explain linguistic development. Harkness (1990) proposed a cultural model that incorporates the innatist view but also focuses on experiences within cultural context. Zukow (1990) took a socioperceptual/ecologic position founded in the belief that the dynamic structure of the social-interactive environment in which the child develops is central to language acquisition. Dent (1990) argued for a functionalist approach where language development is not rooted in the child or the language environment but rather on perceptual systems that detect language-world relationships and guide attention and action.

Research in the past 30 years has established a genetic, neuroanatomic, and functional basis for many language disorders, and few theorists argue with the contribution of the neural system to language development (Locke, 1992). Recent research on syntactic ability and vocabulary size in 15- to 48-month-old children with unilateral antepartum or perinatal brain injury suggests that both cerebral hemispheres make critical contributions in the earliest stages of language acquisition (Feldman, Holland, Kemp, & Janosky, 1992).

The role of babbling on language development has received recent attention, and research with tracheotomized infants suggests that the audibility of babbling and early language may contribute to later language development (Hill & Singer, 1990; Locke & Pearson, 1990). Locke (1990) asserted that links between babbling and speech support the role of innate factors and central control mechanisms in language development. Neural capabilities provide the child with control over initial speechlike movements and direct attention to salient linguistic patterns (Locke, 1990).

Language development requires the substitution of a series of sounds or marks for objects, persons, and concepts and is similar across racial, cultural, and socioeconomic groups (Adams & Victor, 1989). The first stage of language development is the infantile languageless phase where there is inability to comprehend or to produce language. The newborn initially vocalizes reflexively by crying to indicate discomfort. Cooing emerges around 2 months of age, and the infant experiments with various sounds. Vowel sounds emerge around 2 months of age. As early as 3 to 4 months of age, the consonants "b," "g," "k," and "p" are heard in infant language. Babbling, or repetition of alternating consonant and vowel sounds such as "dadada," begins around 4 months of age. Around 8 months the consonants "d," "t," and "w" appear (Whaley & Wong, 1991). Repetition of heard sounds, or lalling, begins between 6 and 9 months and progresses until intonations approximate adult speech at 1 year. By 12 months of age the infant attends to words.

The second stage of language development is a stage where there is auditory comprehension of language but oral communication is fragmentary, ineffective, and contextually meaningless. Between the age of 12 and 18 months, the toddler begins to use words intentionally and demonstrates behavior that indicates developing understanding of words in context.

By 21 months, however, the child says single words with meaning, evidencing the beginning of the third stage of language development: the use of substantive words, called semantics. Between 18 and 24 months the child's vocabulary grows from 20 to 100 words and consists primarily of free morphemes, the smallest form of sound that possesses meaning (e.g., "go, bye, me, eat"). By 24 months the toddler should be using 2- and 3-word combinations to express needs and ideas (e.g., "me go bye-bye"). Between 2 and 3 years of age, the child's vocabulary expands to approximately 300 words, predominantly nouns and verbs, most of which are intelligible by the end of the third year. By 3 years of age, the child talks in sentences. All vowels should be mastered by 3 years of age. During the third and fourth year, vocabulary expands rapidly from 900 to 1500 words with increasing use of pronouns, adverbs, and adjectives (Schuster & Ashburn, 1986). By 4 years of age the child uses fully intelligible speech. Consonant mastery continues to occur in a hierarchic fashion with "s," "z," "sh," "ch," and "j" being the last sounds to be mastered around age 7 or 8. Consonants "m" and "h" are mastered early, and "w" is substituted for "l" and "r" (e.g., "wice" for "rice" or "wook" for "look"). By 4 to 5 years of age "f" and "v" are mastered, but "r," "l," "s," "z," "sh," "ch," "y," and "th" may still be distorted. By age 6 "r," "l," and "th" are mastered (Whaley & Wong, 1987). By 4 years of age, the child uses fully intelligible speech.

The final stage of language development is the ability to apply the rules of grammar to language, called syntax. Syntax or grammar is the last and highest stage of language development.

Linguistic competence does not appear to decline with

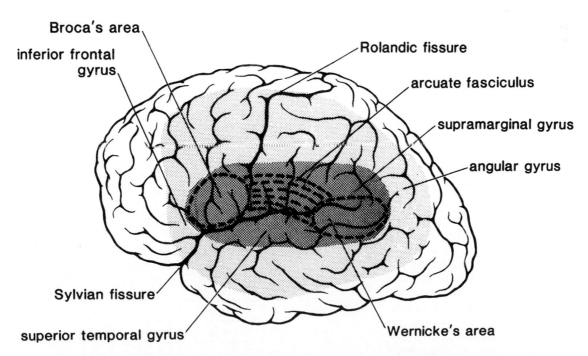

Fig. 25-1 A diagrammatic view of the major cortical language areas of the left hemisphere. (From *Alper and Mancall's Essentials of the Neurologic Examination.* 2nd ed. by E.L. Mancall, 1981, Philadelphia, F.A. Davis. Copyright 1981 by F.A. Davis. Reprinted with permission.)

normal aging. Linguistic disintegration is evidence of a presence of a pathologic process.

Three levels of language production/availability (levels of intention) also are described:

1. Automatic language: the basic level of language output consisting of habitual responses such as prayers, social responses, curses, and songs.
2. Imitation (language heard before): a higher level of language output that requires the person to hear what is said, process the messages, produce the appropriate response, and evaluate the context of the transmission (e.g., repeat after me, "no ifs, ands, or buts").
3. Symbolic language: the highest level of language produced without the benefit of a model, an expression of one's own choice (language of original intention); it involves the use of words with the correct meaning, application of rules for ordering sounds and words, and use of appropriate tense and plurality (e.g.,

"I want to describe for you how my reading difficulty is affecting my life. This has been very hard to deal with.").

Historically, with regard to the neuroanatomic structures involved in language comprehension and production, Geschwind and Levitsky (1968) demonstrated that the posterior part of the upper surface of the left temporal lobe was larger in most persons. The left hemisphere's mediation of language function in nearly all persons regardless of handedness is well accepted today. The primary neuroanatomic structures involved with language competence are Wernicke's area, the angular gyrus, and Broca's area (Fig. 25-1). The angular gyrus at the temporoparietal occipital junction is thought to link the visual impression of an object carried via the primary visual cortex and visual association areas of the occipital and posterior temporal lobes to the spoken word carried via the primary auditory cortex and auditory association areas (Fig. 25-2). After the initial link-

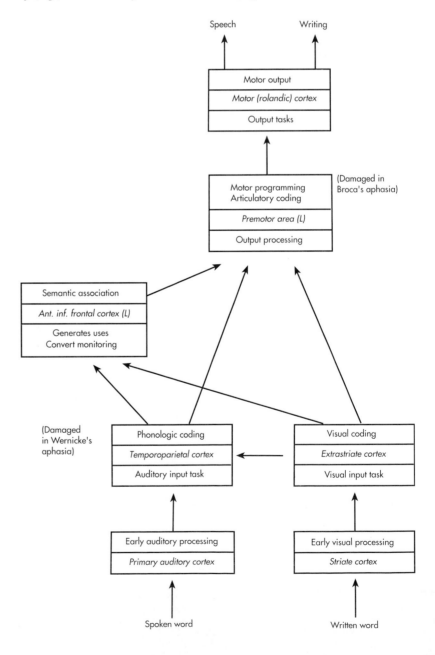

Fig. 25-2   This model represents a fairly simple circuit and shows the relationship between various anatomic structures and functional components of language. At each point the anatomic structure is indicated in italics. The function of the structure is shown below the structure name and the specific language skill is shown above the name. (From "Positron Emission Tomographic Studies of the Cortical anatomy of Single Word Processing" by S.E. Peterson, P.T. Fox, M.I. Posner, M. Minton, and M.E. Raichle, 1988, *Nature, 331;* 588. Reprinted with permission.)

Table 25-1 Clinical features of aphasias

Aphasias	Spontaneous speech	Auditory comprehension	Repetition	Naming	Reading	Writing
Broca's	Nonfluent	Preserved	Impaired	Often impaired	Impaired	Impaired
Wernicke's	Fluent, paraphrasic	Impaired	Impaired	Impaired	Impaired	Impaired
Conduction	Fluent, paraphrasic	Preserved	Impaired	Often impaired	Preserved	Impaired
Global	Nonfluent	Impaired	Impaired	Preserved	Impaired	Impaired
Aphemia (apraxia)	Nonfluent	Preserved	Impaired	Impaired	Preserved	Preserved
Pure word deafness	Fluent	Impaired	Impaired	Preserved	Preserved	Preserved
Transcortical motor	Nonfluent	Preserved	Preserved	Impaired	Preserved	Impaired
Transcortical sensory	Fluent, paraphrasic	Impaired	Preserved	Impaired	Impaired	Impaired
Mixed transcortical	Nonfluent	Impaired	Preserved	Impaired	Impaired	Impaired
Anomic	Fluent	Preserved	Preserved	Impaired	Occasional impairment	Often impaired

Adapted from *Principles of Behavioral neurology* (pp. 202, 210) by M.-M. Mesulam, 1985, Philadelphia: F.A. Davis. Copyright 1985 by F.A. Davis. Adapted by permission.

age is made, when the name is registered by the auditory areas, it is transmitted to Wernicke's area for recognition of the sound pattern of the word. This stimulates the angular gyrus, evoking a visual memory of the seen object.

Linguistic Deficits

Aphasia is the loss or impairment of a previously established capacity for comprehension and/or formulation of language caused by injury to the brain. There is a phonetic, semantic, and/or syntactic disintegration at the production and/or comprehension level of communication. The language dysfunction is manifested by incorrect word sounds, incorrect choice of words, or incorrect grammar. For infants and young children, a linguistic deficit is called a language delay. For older children a linguistic deficit is referred to as a developmental language disorder or a developmental aphasia. The process underlying linguistic deficits in adults or children is not known.

The history of modern aphasiology dates back to Broca (1965), who correlated the clinical picture of clients with the location of the anatomic lesion. This localization approach dominated the field (despite critics who argued that there was only one type of aphasia—a general disturbance of language produced by injury) until after World War I, when a holistic view gained predominance (Marie, 1906). Since the mid-sixties with improved imaging techniques, most researchers and clinicians have returned to a modified localization viewpoint. Therefore one of the useful classification systems for the aphasias based on the neuroanatomic localization of the lesions names the aphasias using anatomic terms (Table 25-1). A linguistic classification of aphasia is given in Table 25-2.

Broca's aphasia reflects a loss of syntax (agrammatism) due to damage in and around Broca's area. The person has impoverished syntax, short utterances, a tendency to delete inflections and other grammatic forms. Contradictory research data related to linguistic deficits have led some aphasiologists to suggest agrammatism represents several different deficits (Goodglass, 1980). Some persons with Broca's aphasia appear to have a disorder of omission of structural

Table 25-2 Linguistic classification of aphasia

Aphasias	Distinguishing features
Syntactic aphasia (loss of grammatic function of language)	Simplified, concrete, often telegraphic speech Little use of connective speech elements Tense and gender may be used improperly Use of substantive words intact
Semantic aphasia (inability to relate the symbol to the object)	Restriction of vocabulary present Circumlocution is dominant Grammatic form may be intact
Pragmatic aphasia (breakdown in regulating function of language; inability to obtain meaning from stimuli and to use such stimuli as a basis for symbol formation)	Disoriented speech with paraphasia, meaningless neologisms Errors in language are not recognized by person
Jargon aphasia (profusion of phonetically disorganized combinations of language elements without understanding of person)	Babbling, noncommunicative speech Reading and writing impaired
Global aphasia (lack of linguistic ability; inability to form verbal symbols for use or in comprehension)	Speechless generally Little response to environmental stimuli Automatic speech and echolalia may be present

form and simplification of the grammatic structure of speech production but retain the ability to understand syntactic relations and to use this understanding to analyze intended sentences. Other persons appear to have a central disorder affecting appreciation of syntactic relations in all modalities (Kean, 1977; Saffran, Schwartz, & Marin, 1980; Zuriff, Caramazza, & Myerson, 1972; Kean, 1985). Still other persons appear to have intact syntactic comprehension; written production is intact and only verbal output is affected (Miceli, Mazzuchi, Menn, & Goodglass, 1983). In addition to the communication deficit, right-sided hemiplegia is present with little use of the right arm and limited use of the right leg. Usually facial apraxia and ideomotor apraxia of the left arm to verbal commands also is present.

In contrast, Wernicke's aphasia represents a semantic problem due to damage to Wernicke's area. The person is unable to understand verbal language. Interestingly understanding axial (truncal, whole body) commands such as "stand up" or "turn around" often is intact. However, extremity commands such as "point to the door" are not understood. Reading comprehension and writing are seriously impaired, although one may be more impaired than the other. Related to language production, the output is fluent—that is, has a normal or above normal number of words per minute. There is ease of language production and normal phase length. Articulation is normal as are melody and inflection qualities. Syntax (grammar) is normal but the semantics abnormal. The words lack specific meaning and little information is communicated. Nonspecific words such as "it," "thing," and "us" are used. There is a tendency to use paraphasia—both verbal or semantic paraphasia—that is, substitution of one word for another (e.g., "The car would spit sweetly down the road." instead of "The car sped swiftly down the road.") and to a lesser extent phonetic or literal paraphasia—that is, a phonetic substitution (e.g., "mesatence is instans" to success instead of "persistence is essential") as well as nonsense or nonexistent words called neologisms (e.g., "lopger" for "plant") (Boss, 1984a). Repetition and naming are impaired. To communicate with this person, one must depend on facial expressions, gestures, pantomime, and tone of voice. In addition to the communication deficit, sensory loss may be present. If a visual field cut is present, it is usually a superior quadrantanopia caused by involvement of the pathway in the temporal lobe. The person may evidence a lack of concern especially early after sustaining the injury. Paranoid behavior more commonly is seen later, following injury.

Conductive aphasia, currently recognized as more common than previously thought, involves a striking repetition problem (Benson, 1979; Green & Howes, 1977). The language output is fluent. Literal paraphasia is more common than verbal paraphasia or neologisms. Naming is impaired mostly due to the literal paraphasia problem. Reading aloud also is impaired. Writing may be less impaired but contains spelling errors, omitted words, and altered letter and word sequencing. Verbal comprehension is relatively intact. The pathology producing conductive aphasia is in the supramarginal gyrus and/or adjacent to the arcuate fasciculus (see Fig. 25-1). With conductive aphasia, paresis or a visual field cut also may be present. A cortical sensory loss involving position sense and stereognosis—that is, the ability to recognize forms of objects by touch—is common.

Pure word deafness manifests as an inability to comprehend verbal language. Repetition also is seriously impaired. Earlier after injury there may be some degree of paraphasia in the person's language production, but the output is fluent. Reading and writing are intact, and ability to name is adequate. A superior quadrantanopia—that is, loss of vision in one-fourth of the visual field—may be present. Pathologically the left auditory association area is isolated from receiving auditory input.

Global (total) aphasia involves a striking inability to understand verbal and written language and to write. Naming and repetition are seriously impaired, and the person is nonfluent. Global aphasia often is accompanied by right-sided hemiplegia. Persistent global aphasia involves damage to a large area of the frontal and parietotemporal language areas.

If repetition is intact despite other language comprehension and/or production deficit, aphasia is termed transcortical aphasia. There are three types of transcortical aphasias. When aphasia resembles Broca's aphasia but repetition is intact, the language disorder is termed transcortical motor aphasia.

Transcortical motor aphasia often is accompanied by hemiplegia. Hemisensory loss and/or visual field loss may be present. The area of damage may be anterior to Broca's area or to the supplementary motor area (SMA) (see Fig. 25-1), and its pathways cause a disconnection of the SMA from Broca's area.

When aphasia resembles Wernicke's aphasia but repetition is intact, the language disorder is called transcortical sensory aphasia. The syndrome often is accompanied by agitation. The area of damage is the border zone of the parietotemporal junction, which is at the end of the arterial supply. Often the middle and lower temporal gyri are damaged also.

When aphasia resembles global aphasia but repetition is intact, the disorder is called mixed transcortical aphasia or isolated speech area. In this rarely occurring aphasia, the person does not speak unless spoken to and then echoes—that is, repeats—what the other person said. The perisylvian language areas are preserved, but there is extensive damage to the surrounding cortical areas. Grossi et al. (1991) offer evidence of right hemisphere involvement. The syndrome has followed head injury and acute carotid occlusion but is most common following hypoxia.

The most common aphasia is anomic aphasia, a phonologic problem involving a word-finding failure. There is an inability to find the correct word in spontaneous speech and writing and when asked to name objects. Many other aphasias resolve into persistent anomic aphasia. Some persons with predominant anomic aphasia also lack comprehension of verbal and written language to some degree and evidence impaired writing especially when fatigued. Severe anomic aphasia of acute onset typically involves damage in the left temporoparietal junction area. Mild anomic aphasia's site of injury may be the left frontal, parietal, or temporal area, a subcortical area, or even a right-sided cortical injury. Anomic aphasia is associated with head injury, Alzheimer's dementia, and space-occupying lesions, as well as metabolic or toxic encephalopathies—although in the latter case, writing usually is more dramatically affected. Four varieties of anomic aphasia are described in Table 25-3.

Language disorders are considered a major developmental disability in children. Concerns about language delay usually emerge around 2 years of age. Global mental retar-

Table 25-3 Syndromes of word-finding impairment (anomia)

WORD-PRODUCTION ANOMIA

Articulatory initiation problem	Failure to name object on request but able to produce name if given a clue
Paraphasic disturbance	Easy initiation of a word but verbal production is so contaminated with literal paraphasia substitutes that response is wrong
Word-evocation anomia	Inability to produce desired name although word is known to person

WORD-SELECTION ANOMIA

	Failure to name object on presentation in any sensory modality but can describe use of object and can select appropriate object when presented for name (pure word-finding problem); cannot think of word

SEMANTIC ANOMIA

	Combination of inability to name object or point to correct object when name is presented (word has lost its symbolic meaning); both comprehension and use of name are disturbed

DISCONNECTION ANOMIA

Modality-specific anomia	Normal naming in all sensory modalities except one
Category-specific anomia	Normal naming except for a given stimulus category (e.g., color)
Callosal anomia	Inability to make or recognize name of unseen object in left hand although may recognize object

dation is the most common cause of delayed language development. Hearing impairments and specific developmental language disorders, called developmental aphasia, may present language delays. Affected children have normal cognition and often develop elaborate gestural communication systems to convey their needs and thoughts. Children with infantile autism in contrast show a global lack of communication and use neither language nor nonlanguage communication systems. Children with hearing impairment and language disorders may evidence difficult behavioral problems, in part due to their frustration over their inability to communicate. Clinical studies of children with aphasia are under way (Tuchman, Rapin, & Shinnar, 1991).

PRAGMATICS

"Pragmatics is that component of communication that transcends language in terms of its isolated words and grammatical structure" (Milton, Prutting, & Binder, 1984). "Pragmatics refers to a system or rules that clarify the use of language in terms of situational or social content" (Sohlberg & Mateer, 1989). Pragmatics is heavily cultural laden. Pragmatics may be viewed as a distinct component of language, or it may be viewed as an umbrella function overlying all other aspects of language (Bates, 1979; Bloom & Lahey, 1978). The richness and complexity of a person's communication exists because of the contributions of both the right and left cerebral hemispheres. The right hemisphere is now known to play a major role in the prosody, attitude, emotions, and gestural behaviors involved in language and communicative behaviors. Ross and Mesulam (1979) argued that the right hemisphere is dominant for organizing the affective-prosodic component of language and gestural behavior.

Pragmatics is a young area of speech and language pathology. Tracking its development in childhood has not yet been extensively reported. It is known that before children begin to talk they use prosodic (detailed in the following material) features to express themselves. They learn from family and other caretakers how to alter pitch, loudness, tone, inflection, and duration to achieve a desired effect. Thus the quality of the child's cry may be different to indicate different needs. Around 6 months of age, the infant will begin to experiment with inflections heard in other voices. By listening to prosodic features in the language of others, the child learns their meaning. Children imitate rhythm and pacing of vocalization, which results in different dialects (Schuster & Ashburn, 1986). Recently it has been found that the parietal, occipital, and temporal lobes undergo marked development between ages 1 and 7.5 years (Allison, 1992). During this time children perfect their ability to form images. Parietal occipital development is enhanced during the ages of 11 and 13 years, and the temporal lobes mature further between ages 13 and 17 years (Allison, 1992). Pragmatics has not been specifically examined in aged persons as yet, but retrieval of visual-spatial memories is known to decrease more than retrieval of language-related memories after age 70.

Prosodia

Prosodia, referring "to the melody, pause, intonation, stresses and accents applied to the articulatory line," is the most studied aspect of pragmatics to date (Ross, 1985). Prosodia imparts affective tone, introduces subtle grades of meaning, and varies emphasis in spoken language (Bolton, & Dashiell, 1984). Prosodia is primarily responsible for the richness and complexity of communication with its many familial and cultural nuances. Some researchers claim that prosodia, not linguistics, forms the fundamental building blocks for language (Crystal, 1969, 1975; Lewis, 1936; Monrad-Krohn, 1963).

Prosodia was studied first by Monrad-Krohn (1947a). From this research Monrad-Krohn theorized that prosodia has four components: intrinsic, intellectual, emotional, and inarticulate prosodia. "Intrinsic prosodia serves specific linguistic purposes and gives rise to dialectical and idiosyncratic differences in speech quality" (Ross, 1985). Examples of intrinsic prosodia are as follows:

1. Stress differences on segments of word to clarify whether a noun or a verb (e.g., the noun *com bin'* or the verb *com' bin*)
2. Differences in pause structure of a sentence to clarify potentially ambiguous or unclear statements: the boy and girl with the dog (said with no pauses and meaning the dog was with both children) versus the boy (pause) and the girl with the dog (the four words said together) and meaning the dog was with the girl only
3. Changing pitch of voice to indicate a question rather than a declarative statement: "Not true?" (high-pitched ending), "Not true." (low-pitched ending)

Intellectual prosodia conveys the speaker's attitude about the information being communicated (e.g., "He is smart." with *is* stressed, reflects the speaker's acknowledgment that the person possesses the characteristic). Stress placed on "smart" may convey that although the person is smart, the use of the quality may not meet the speaker's approval.

Emotional prosodia contributes emotion to speech and has a large cultural component. Inarticulate prosody is the use of paralinguistic elements such as sighs, grunts, and groans.

The first studies of the right brain's role in the emotional aspects of communication took place in the 1970s. Zuriff (1974), Blumstein and Cooper (1974), and Van Lancker (1980) found that the left ear (right hemisphere) is better at understanding the intonational aspects of speech and the right ear (left hemisphere) is better at linguistic aspects of speech. Ross and Mesulam (1979) found that persons with right hemisphere damage could not insert affective and attitudinal variation into speech and gestural behavior. Affected persons cannot put any emotion into their voices and actions and are aware of this. They speak in monotone and do not use gestures. The listener cannot tell the difference between a flat commanding statement (e.g., "Get the door.") indicating a command and a pleasant request (e.g., "Get the door?"). Heilman, Scholes, and Watson (1975) found that right hemisphere damage disrupted comprehension of the affective components of language. Tucker, Watson, and Heilman (1977) demonstrated that persons with right hemisphere damage could not insert intonation on request or by imitation. Right hemisphere brain injury has been found to very seriously impair affective components of prosody and gestures (Heilman et al., 1975; Ross, 1981; Ross, Harney, de La Coste-Utamsing, & Purdy, 1981; Ross, Holzapfel, & Freeman, 1983; Ross & Mesulam, 1979; Tucker et al., 1977; Borod, 1992; Cancelliere & Kertesz, 1990). The linguistic (i.e., intrinsic) component of prosodia can be impaired by either right hemisphere brain injury or left hemisphere brain injury (Blumstein & Goodglass, 1972; Danly, Cooper, & Shapiro, 1983; Danly & Shapiro, 1982; Heilman, Bowers, Speedie, & Cosletter, 1983; Weintraub et al., 1981). Cancelliere and Kertesz (1990) found the basal ganglia most frequently involved in aprosodia syndromes, followed by anterior temporal lobe and insular involvement.

Kinesics (Gestures)

Kinesics is the study of limb, body, and facial movements associated with nonverbal communication (Critchley, 1970). When kinesic activity has a semantic purpose—that is, conveys a specific meaning—it often is referred to as pantomime. Pantomime conveys specific semantic information. When movements convey an emotional and attitudinal component, they often are referred to as gestures. Gestures are movements used to color, emphasize, and embellish speech and are highly reflective of one's cultural background (Ross, 1985).

Both the right and left hemispheres appear to contribute to kinesic comprehension and production, but the specific neuroanatomy/neurophysiology involved is not yet well understood. Disturbances in performance and comprehension of pantomime were found in persons with left hemisphere injury along with aphasia (Dent, 1990; Gainotti & Lemmo, 1976) (Goodglass & Kaplan, 1963). The pantomime comprehension deficit has been attributed to an inability to comprehend symbols. The deficit in execution of pantomime was found to best correlate with the presence of ideomotor apraxia (Goodglass & Kaplan, 1983). Ciconi, Wapner, Foldi, Zuriff, and Gardner (1979) found that persons with Broca's aphasia used more pantomime, whereas persons with Wernicke's aphasia used more gestures. Ross and Mesulam (1979) correlated loss of kinesic activity with right-sided brain injury. Injury to the right frontal inferior area resulted in complete loss of spontaneous gestural activity without the presence of apraxia.

The development of kinesic comprehension and production has not yet been explicated. It is known that at 9 months of age an infant gives attention to gestures. The expressions of meaning through body movement, or kinesics, are learned through observation initially within the confines of the family and other caretakers. Children learn meanings associated with certain body movements or gestures and how to use movement to accompany language or to substitute for language. One of the earliest gestures learned is that of the hand wave to indicate good-bye, and later, hello. The child also learns that a shoulder shrug can indicate "I don't know." (Schuster & Ashburn, 1986). The effects of aging in kinesics has not been specifically addressed.

Facial Recognition and Facial Expression

Facial recognition (prosopagnosia), a right-sided temporal function, is an inability to recognize previously known faces including one's own and to learn new ones (Milner, 1968). Actually the deficit is not limited to faces but extends to individuals in groups. Minor distinguishing features cannot be recognized.

Facial expressions convey mood and emotional state. They set the stage for the dynamics of communication. The right hemisphere is crucially concerned in the appreciation and production of emotional messages via facial expression (Code, 1987).

The development of facial recognition begins in the first months of life within the family and progresses as the temporal, parietal, and occipital lobes develop in childhood. The development of facial expression, comprehension, and production has not been specifically examined. Facial recognition has been found to decline after 70 years of age (Benton, Eslinger, & Damasio, 1981).

Pragmatic Deficits

Monrad-Krohn (1947c) defined dysprosody as a change in voice quality giving a different accent because of inability to properly stress segments and words. This definition limits dysprosody to a disorder of intrinsic prosodia. Aprosodia for Monrad-Krohn referred to a general lack of prosodia such as found in a person with parkinsonism because of akinesia and masked facies. Mesulam (1990) defined aprosodias as encoding and decoding disorders of affective behavior. Hyperprosodia is the excessive use of prosodia such as often found in persons with mania or persons with Broca's aphasia, who may be able to use few words effectively to communicate.

The anatomic/functional organization of prosodic deficits has been examined (Larsen, Skinhoj, & Lassen, 1978; Ross, 1981; Ross, et al., 1983). Based on their research, Ross et al. described an anatomic/functional classification model for the aprosodias that mirrors the organization for language presented early (Fig. 25-3). Table 25-4 summarizes the characteristics of these aprosodias.

A motor aprosodia is characterized by flat monotone speech with loss of spontaneous gesturing. Repetition of affective prosodia (e.g., repeating "I am having company for dinner." said in a happy voice) is severely compromised. However, comprehension of affective prosodia and visual comprehension of emotional gesturing are intact. Motor aprosodia is associated with right frontal and anteroinferior parietal damage and occasionally with subcortical right-sided basal ganglia and internal capsule damage. Accompanying clinical findings include moderate to severe left-sided hemiplegia, variable left-sided sensory loss, and transient dysarthria and anosognosia (e.g., inability to recognize the neurologic deficits being experienced). Under extreme emo-

tional conditions, persons with motor aprosodia often are able to laugh or cry in a fleeting all-or-none fashion, resembling the pathologic affect found in pseudobulbar palsy.

In sensory aprosodias there is severely impaired auditory comprehension of affective prosody, visual comprehension of emotional gesturing, and repetition of affective prosodia. Affective prosodia in speech and active gesturing, however, are intact. In fact the person may appear somewhat euphoric and overly happy even when talking about serious topics Sensory aprosodias is associated with right-sided posterotemporal and posteroinferior parietal injury. Sensory aprosodias may be accompanied by moderate deficits in left-sided vibration sense, position sense, and stereognosis as well as a dense left-sided hemianopia.

The person with global aprosodia has severely compromised comprehension and repetition of affective prosodia, severely compromised visual comprehension of emotional gesturing, and an inability to display affect through prosodia and gestures. The person exhibits a very flattened affect. Global aprosodia is associated with a large right-sided perisylvian injury involving the frontal, parietal, and temporal lobes and occasionally with deep right-sided intracerebral hemorrhage. Global aprosodia is accompanied typically by severe left-sided hemiplegia, left-sided hemisensory loss, and left-sided hemianopia.

Descriptions of transcortical motor aprosodia, transcortical sensory aprosodia, and mixed transcortical aprosodia are based on limited data and so must be discussed with caution. Transcortical motor aprosodia appears to manifest as aprosodic-gestural speech with preserved repetition and

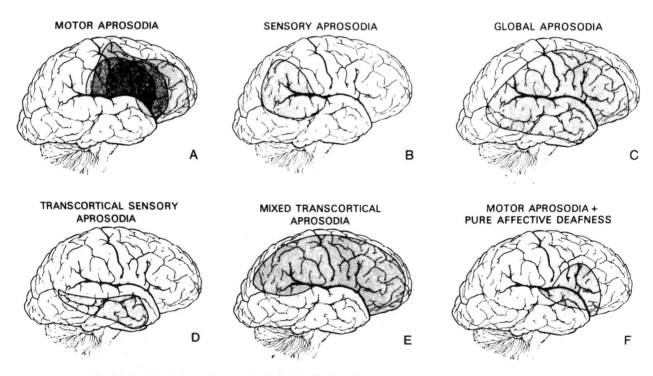

Fig. 25-3 Right lateral brain templates showing the distribution of infarctions seen on computed tomographic (CT) scans in 8 of 10 clients with various aprosodias. (From *Principles of Behavioral Neurology* by M-M Mesulam, 1985, Philadelphia, F.A. Davis. Copyright 1985 by F.A. Davis. Reprinted with permission.)

Table 25-4   The aprosodias

Aprosodias	Spontaneous affective prosody and gesturing	Affective prosodic repetition	Affective prosodic comprehension	Comprehension of emotional gesturing
Motor	Poor	Poor	Good	Good
Sensory	Good	Poor	Poor	Poor
Global	Poor	Poor	Poor	Poor
Conduction	Good	Poor	Good	Good
Transcortical motor	Poor	Good	Poor	Good
Transcortical sensory	Good	Good	Poor	Poor
Mixed transcortical	Poor	Good	Poor	Poor
Anomic	Good	Good	Good	Poor

From *Principles of Behavioral Neurology* (p. 246) by M.-M. Mesulam, 1985, Philadelphia: F.A. Davis. Copyright 1985 by F.A. Davis. Reprinted by permission.

comprehension of affective prosodia and emotional gesturing. Left-sided hemiparesis without sensory loss may be present. A right-sided basal ganglion injury is thought to produce such an aprosodia. Transcortical sensory aprosodia appears to manifest as a severely impaired comprehension of affective prosodia, while emotional gesturing, spontaneous affective prosodia and its repetition are intact. A right-sided anteroinferior temporal lobe injury is believed to account for this aprosodia. Mixed transcortical aprosodia is believed to manifest as absent gesturing and spontaneous affective prosodia, impaired but present repetition of affective prosodia, and poor comprehension of affective prosodia and emotional gesturing. The lesion is thought to be in the right suprasylvian region and a small portion of the posteroinferior temporal lobe. Severe left-sided hemiplegia and hemisensory loss also is present.

Pure affective deafness plus motor aprosodia is thought to be characterized by a flattened voice devoid of affective variation, blunted gesturing, poor comprehension, and repetition of affective prosodia but intact comprehension of emotional gesturing (i.e., visual comprehension is intact). But again data are limited. This aprosodia is accompanied by severe left-sided hemiplegia without sensory loss or aphasia. The right-sided inferior frontal, anterior insular, and anteroinferior temporal area is believed to be the location of the injury.

Developmental affective-prosodic deficits have been reported recently in children with congenital or very early right hemisphere injury; acquired motor-type aprosodia following acute right-sided focal brain injury have been documented in school-aged children (Basso, Farabola, Grassi, & Laiacona, 1990; Bell, Davis, Morgan-Fisher, & Ross, 1990).

Other pragmatic deficits discussed in the literature are inappropriate reactions to humor and misinterpretation of metaphors (Buck & Duffy, 1980; Thompkins & Mateer, 1985; Van Lancker, 1980). These deficits may arise with right hemisphere injury.

HIGH-LEVEL LANGUAGE SKILLS

Language is a cognitive system, and at the same time many cognitive functions mediated by the left hemisphere are language dependent. Human beings use language when performing cognitive activities. For example, the left hemisphere transfers memory and permanently stores memory in a language format. We form language concepts using symbolic representations and move from literal interpretations to abstract principles and meanings. Human beings think in symbols—that is, we think in words referred to as internal speech. Therefore distinguishing linguistic incompetence from cognitive disorders may be difficult, and dysfunction in any of the cognitive systems may seriously impact communication.

According to Groher (1977) confused language may result from disorientation in time and space, faulty short-term memory, poor thinking, mistaken reasoning, poor understanding of the environment, and inappropriate behavior. Aphasia may resolve into a more confused language profile (Groher, 1977; Weinstein & Keller, 1963). Development of cognitive functions and dysfunctions in cognitive systems are discussed in Chapter 26.

Dysfunction in any attentional system—arousal, selective attention, or vigilance (concentration)—produces altered communication patterns. Without arousal—that is, without awakeness or consciousness, mediated by the ascending reticular activating system of the brainstem—communication is tremendously restricted. There is no language and only inarticulate prosody (the most primitive nonverbal output). Reception of communication is limited and at a primary sensory level at best.

The selective attention system facilitates the orienting to specific information of interest. Selective orienting of attention may be either overt—that is, movement of the head, eyes, and body to the point of interest or covert—that is, mental shifting of attention to the source of interest. Recent evidence supports that the thalami mediate selective attention. The right-sided parietal area also has been demonstrated to mediate at least some aspects of selective attention, and with injury a unilateral neglect syndrome develops. When this syndrome is present, the person cannot orient to any sensory stimuli coming from the contralateral left side. This dysfunction will influence any communication embedded in that spatial, tactile, auditory, or visual information cannot be focused on. Pragmatics is impaired.

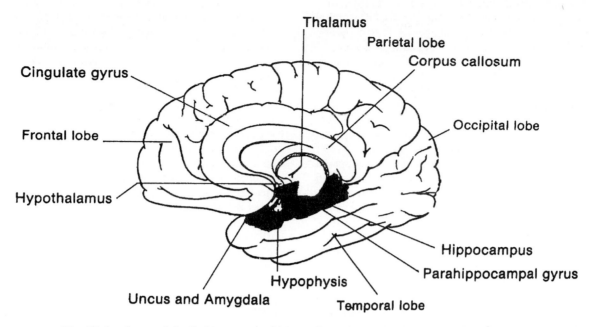

Fig. 25-4   Areas of the limbic system which mediate recent memory are shaded. (From "The Neurophysiologic Basis of Learning: Attention and Memory. Implications for SCI nurses" by B.J. Boss, 1993, *SCI Nursing*, 10, 125. Copyright 1993 by American Association of Spinal Cord Injury Nurses (AASCIN). Reprinted with permission.)

Since 1-month-old infants give some evidence of beginning selective attention and 2-month-old infants attend to objects and evidence some response to nearby voices and everyday noises, lack of visual selection attention after 6 weeks raises the question of the presence of a visual impairment. Likewise a dissociation between visual motor behavior and motor behavior during the first 6 months of life may suggest a visual impairment. Failure to "listen" or to pay attention to auditory stimulation in the environment is seen in children with autism. In any of these situations, communication is affected at the time as well as in the future.

The vigilance system provides the ability to sustain attention—that is, concentration over time. The prefrontal areas mediate vigilance. A more complex form of vigilance, called tracking, is the ability to maintain focus despite the presence of competing stimuli or the need to engage in alternating tasks (Boss, 1991). The person with a vigilance defect is inattentive or distractible. Concentration on the communication, in all of its fullness and complexity, is not possible; the person does not receive and register the communication: they do not hear, see, or feel the communication. The inattentive behavior is difficult for other persons to deal with and communicate around.

Vigilance develops as the prefrontal areas mature during the first 6 years of life. Continued maturation of these areas occurs at about 7.5 years of age. Vigilance does not decline with aging.

Memory is the encoding, consolidation, and retrieval of information. The recent memory system transfers short-term memories into permanent (i.e., long-term) memory stores. The encoding and consolidation of information (i.e., recent memory) is mediated by the hippocampi, amygdalae, and probably adjacent temporal lobe and diencephalic areas (Fig. 25-4). The left hippocampus and related temporal areas encode and consolidate language-related memories; the right hippocampus and related temporal areas encode and consolidate nonlanguage auditory and visual-spatial memory stores. The amygdalae are believed to participate in transferring the affective component of the experience into a permanent memory store. The recent memory system appears to be functional shortly after birth (Allison, 1992). The hippocampi develop quite early and have reached 40% of maturation by birth, 50% by 1 month and are fully mature by 15 months of age (Allison, 1992). The person with a recent memory deficit cannot learn any new information and is disoriented to all new persons, all new places, time, and current situation. Affected individuals do not remember what they have been told, what they have read, or what they have experienced. The individual's communication appears confused and not very meaningful, although syntax and semantics may be intact. The person appears forgetful. Recent memory decreases with aging but not sufficiently to impair cognitive functioning.

The remote memory system stores long-term memories. These long-term memories are believed to be sorted within the association areas of the parietal, temporal, and occipital lobes. The left hemisphere association areas store memories related to language, mathematics, and abstractions in language format; the right hemisphere association areas store nonlanguage sounds such as music, spatial relationships, and visual experiences. During the time that parietal, occipital, and temporal lobes undergo marked development between ages 1 and 7.5 years (Allison, 1992), children perfect their ability to form images, use words, and place things in serial order. By about age 10 years, children begin to perform simple operational functions such as weight determination and logical-mathematic reasoning. Parietal occipital development is enhanced during the ages of 11 to 13 years; the temporal lobes mature further between ages 13 and 17 years (Allison, 1992). Dysfunction in the remote memory system of the left hemisphere association areas may produce a loss of comprehension of verbal and/or written language—that is, an aphasia. Some of the deficits that may be produced by dysfunction in the remote memory system of the right hemisphere association areas are aprosody, loss of facial recognition, loss of facial expression, and loss of comprehension of gestures and pantomime. Visual-spatial memory retrieval is more impaired in normal aging than language-related memory retrieval.

Concept formation mandates an ability to analyze relationships between objects and their properties (Boss, 1991). The cortical association areas are believed to contribute to concept formation. The left hemisphere mediates formation of language concepts; the right hemisphere mediates formation of visual-spatial concepts. Concept formation is fundamental to language development. The ability to form concepts develops throughout childhood as was previously described under the remote memory system. Even before 6 years of age, children begin to develop tactics for problem-solving. The continuing development of the visual and auditory regions of the cortex permits children from 10 to 13 years of age to perform formal operations such as calculations and to perceive new meaning in familiar objects. The continued development of the visual-auditory, visual-spatial, and somatic systems in the early teenage years permit the adolescent to review formal operations, find flaws with them, and create new operations (Allison, 1992).

Due to developmental level, young children cannot draw relationships; therefore their communication uses concrete, literal interpretations. There is no richness and fullness to the communication. The communication of an individual unable to form and use concepts resembles the communication of a young child and requires persons trying to communicate with the individual to use concrete, literal language as well.

Aged persons appear to form language concepts and to use abstract concepts as readily as younger persons. However, aged persons form visual-spatial concepts and abstract less readily.

The executive system is a system of programming, verification, and correction mediated by the prefrontal areas (Boss, 1984a). Executive functions include the following:

1. Motivation, also called anticipation
2. Goal selection or goal formulation
3. Planning
4. Programming, which includes initiating, maintaining, and discontinuing actions
5. Self-monitoring
6. Use of feedback—that is, self-correction

The executive system develops in early childhood until 6 years of age. At about 7.5 years of age, the prefrontal areas again undergo accelerated development for a few years. The prefrontal areas finish their maturation between the ages of 17 and 21 years (Allison, 1992). Executive system dysfunction influences communication by impairing the programming of communicative activities and impairing

verification of the adequacy of the communication and correction of the inadequacy. One of the striking communication deficits in persons with diffuse traumatic brain injury is their loss of motivation to initiate communication. The apathy blocks their ability to communicate and hinders, if not totally discourages, other persons who may be trying to communicate with them. With an inability to goal form or goal select, the person is unable to communicate goals since they do not exist; therefore the persons appears indecisive. Communication is one-way with the other person acting as goal former and decision-maker. The person's communication evidences little if any planning and more reflects ill-conceived needs, wants, and desires that cannot be realized. Often the person acts without any preliminary communication of intentions. Because these individuals lack ability to self-monitor, they cannot recognize their communication deficits and cannot understand what the problem is with the other person. Feedback from others cannot be used, nor can these individuals use self-feedback. This makes rehabilitation extremely difficult and places most of the change on the other persons in the communication rather than on the affected person. In a child perseveration is a landmark sign of autism in the absence of a history of neurologic insult.

SPEECH

Speech is a highly coordinated, sequential pattern of muscular contractions of the respiratory, larynx, pharynx, palate, tongue, and lip musculature (Adams & Victor, 1989). This results in verbal output. Speech development is considered part of language development and was discussed under linguistics. Speech does not decline with normal aging.

Dysarthria

Dysarthria has been defined as a defect in articulation. Anarthria has been defined as the complete loss of articulation. However, speech problems that arise in dysarthrias are not exclusively articulatory but include respiratory deficits, phonation problems, and resonation difficulties. Loss of control of the vocal tract muscles produces phonation deficits that distort consonant and vowel sound production, which distorts the language (Ackermann & Ziegler, 1991a).

Dysarthrias are caused by central or peripheral nervous system motor disorders which produce weakness or paralysis, incoordination, or alteration in the muscle tone of the speech musculature. Different forms of dysarthria have specific characteristics. Adams and Victor (1989) described five types of dysarthria: lower motor neuron (flaccid), spastic and rigid, ataxic, hypokinetic, and hyperkinetic. Darley (1975) and Darley et al. (1969a, 1969b) described a sixth type of dysarthria, mixed.

Flaccid dysarthria, the most common type of dysarthria according to Basso (1987), is caused by paresis or paralysis of the muscles used for articulation. The neurologic damage is located in the motor nuclei of the lower brainstem or in cranial nerves VII (the facial nerve), IX (the glossopharyngeal nerve), X (the vagus nerve), and XII (the hypoglossal nerve). With this dysarthria there is a marked hypernasality (nasal speech) due to palatal immobility. Speech sounds are thick and slurred but feeble. Indistinctness of speech results from paresis or paralysis of the tongue musculature. Consonant production is imprecise, especially with vibratory consonants such as "r." With severe paresis or complete paralysis of all three cranial nerves, no lingual or labial consonants can be pronounced. Inspiration is audible. The voice is breathy. Persons with myasthenia gravis evidence flaccid dysarthria.

With hypokinetic dysarthria there is a slowness of articulatory movements. The range, direction, and force of muscle contraction are limited, making speech muffled and indistinct. There is monopitch and monoloudness. Clusters of prosodic insufficiencies are present. Persons with parkinsonism or Wilson's disease may evidence this dysarthria.

Hyperkinetic dysarthria is also caused by extrapyramidal system dysfunction. Hyperkinetic dysarthria is characterized by movements that are irregular, random, unpatterned, and rapid. Patterns of articulation are highly varied. There are sudden variations in loudness. Rhythmic hypernasality is present. Speech is described by Adams and Victor (1989) as "hiccup speech," a speech pattern evidencing abrupt breaks in flow due to the superimposed abnormal movements. Persons with Huntington's chorea evidence this type of dysarthria (Ackermann & Ziegler, 1991).

Spastic dysarthria is caused by the loss of inhibitory cortical influxes on the brainstem reflexes due to damage within the corticobulbar system. This is called a spastic bulbar palsy or pseudobulbar palsy. In spastic dysarthria there is a diffuse reduction, weakening, or loss of motor speech movement activity. Speech usually is slow with short utterances. Articulation is very imprecise. Pitch is low. Voice is harsh and strained-strangled. An acute brainstem trauma or stroke producing bilateral injury may initially produce complete flaccid anarthria, but if there is some improvement with time, the person may exhibit slow, thick, and indistinct speech.

Ataxic dysarthria results from a cerebellar dysfunction. Ataxic dysarthria is characterized by errors in timing, speed, range, and force of vocal tract muscles. This results in dysrhythmia of speech manifested by explosive and intermittent speech. Some words and syllables are spoken with too great a force, and other words and syllables are not audible because the person's breath is gone (Murdoch, Chenery, Strokes, & Hardcastle, 1991). Syllable repetition may be present. Phoneme and interval prolongation produce an unnatural separation of the syllables of words called scanning speech. There is imprecision in enunciation. Speech in monotonous. The rate of speech is slow. Respiratory and speech patterns are not coordinated. Persons with multiple sclerosis may evidence ataxic dysarthria as may an intoxicated person.

In mixed dysarthria there are two or more of the previously described types of dysarthria present in the same person. Two or more different neurologic systems have sustained injury. Persons with amyotrophic lateral sclerosis (ALS) may have combined flaccid and spastic mixed dysarthria (Ansel & Kent, 1992; Kent et al., 1991, 1992; Kertesz & McCabe, 1977).

PATTERNS OF RECOVERY AND FACTORS INFLUENCING RECOVERY

There is a strong tendency for some degree of spontaneous recovery from aphasia. At times recovery is early, rapid, and extensive. Early recovery—that is, in 1 to 2 weeks—is

due to improvement in anoxia, edema, cellular infiltration, and intracranial pressure. The most dramatic language recovery is seen in the first 2 or 3 weeks following a cerebrovascular accident (Kohlmeyer, 1976). Striking language recovery may still be found in the first 3 months, but there is a considerable decrease in language recovery after 6 months (Basso, Capitani, & Vignolo, 1979; Culton, 1969; Kertesz & McCabe, 1977; Sarno & Levita, 1981; Vignolo, 1964). Spontaneous recovery follows the path of a return of old knowledge and in no way resembles relearning of a child. In comparison studies it was found that comprehension recovers more quickly and more completely than expression (Hanson & Cicciarelli, 1978; Kenin & Swisher, 1972; Kertesz & McCabe, 1977; Lomas & Kertesz, 1978; Porch, 1967). In a longitudinal study, Basso et al. (1982) found that comprehension improved more and with greater speed than expression in both treatment and untreated groups. Oral language improved more than written language, but language training centered on oral remediation improved written language in addition.

Consistent data across studies have emerged related to the influence of handedness, etiology, and severity on recovery from aphasia. Left-handed and right-handed persons with a family history of left-handedness recover language more often than right-handed persons, but Basso et al. recently have offered data challenging this belief (Basso et al., 1990; Gloning, Gloning, Haub, & Quatemberr, 1969; Luria, 1970; Subirana, 1958). Persons with posttraumatic aphasia improve more often than do persons with dysphasia following a stroke (Basso et al., 1979; Burfield & Zangwell, 1946; Kertesz & McCabe, 1977; Luria, 1970; Marks, Taylor, & Rusk, 1957). Persons with focal damage are more likely to demonstrate overt speech and language disturbances, with anomic aphasia the most commonly occurring disturbance (Heilman, Safran, & Geschwind, 1971; Sarno, 1980a; Tucker et al., 1977). Persons with severe aphasias recover less language than persons with milder aphasias (Basso et al., 1979; Kertesz & McCabe, 1977; Sands, Sarno, & Shankweiler, 1969).

The empiric data are contradictory regarding the influence of age and type of deficit on recovery. Influence of age on recovery is debated. The research findings are inconsistent. Culton (1971) and Sarno (1980) found age to have no effect on recovery. Marshall, Thompkins, and Phillips (1982) found older persons recovered less language than did younger persons. Recently growing evidence has led pediatric experts to assert that cognitive skills, including language undergoing rapid development, usually are more impaired with neurologic insult. Children 4 months to 5 years of age are more prone to have overall language impairment. Children 6 to 9 years of age, following head injury, have been found to show much more impairment of written language skills. Injury in teenagers threatens their ability to extrapolate from concrete to basic abstraction, leaving them with only literal meaning.

Basso et al. (1975, 1979) found no difference in recovery between fluent and nonfluent aphasias. Burfield and Zangwell (1946), Messerli, Tissot, and Rodriguez (1976) and Kertesz and McCabe (1977) found the prognosis better for persons with Broca's aphasias, whereas Vignolo (1964) found the prognosis better in persons with Wernicke's aphasias. The problem of classification of aphasias and association of a classification system with severity has created difficulty in studying this area. Comprehension recovers more quickly and to a greater extent than expression in aphasic persons (Prins, Snow, & Wagenaar 1978).

Inconsistent data have been found regarding the prognostic value of intelligence and sex. Intelligence was found to be a factor in recovery from aphasia by Darley (1975) but Basso (1987) could demonstrate no correlation between intelligence and recovery of verbal comprehension. Basso et al. (1979) found no difference between men and women on 6-month recovery of comprehension, but 6-month recovery of oral expression was significantly better in women. Pizzamiglio, Mammucari, and Razzano (1985) found that at 6 months or less no difference existed between males and females on naming, but comprehension was better recovered on three of four tasks by women. Kertesz and Benke (1989) argue their data dispute gender differences in intrahemispheric cerebral organization.

The effects of therapy on recovery are highly debated. Several types of efficacy studies have been conducted and include (1) nonexperimental no control studies (Burfield & Zangwell, 1946; Marks et al., 1957; Sands et al., 1969); (2) studies with control for time (time series design) (Danly & Shapiro, 1982); (3) control group studies; and (4) comparison of different treatments (Loughrey, 1992). Vingolo (1964), Sarno, Silverman, and Sands (1970) and Levita (1978) found no difference with or without speech therapy, whereas Hagen (1973) and Basso et al. (1975, 1979) found the treatment group had greater improvement. Meikle et al. (1979) found no difference in recovery using therapist versus volunteers. Wertz et al. (1981), in a multicenter study, found greater improvement with individual versus group therapy sessions. Lincoln, Pickersgill, Hankey, and Hilton (1982) and David, Enderby, and Bainton (1982) found all clients improved regardless of treatment. Basso et al. (1979) found that the time lapse between onset of dysphasia and client evaluation correlated with degree of improvement. Generally the findings could be summarized as inconclusive, although Johnson and Pring (1990) argue that the benefit of speech therapy is documented by recent experimental studies.

Little research has been conducted on the influence of education, social milieu, general health, and occupational status on recovery from aphasia, although these factors generally are considered prognostic (Keenan & Brassell, 1974; Marshall et al., 1982; Sarno et al., 1970; Smith, 1971).

Patterns of recovery from pragmatic deficits are not well described. Clinical experts are of the opinion that persons recover more gestural ability than verbal prosody. In global prosody clinical experts believe that affective-prosodic comprehension and gesturing improve over time. Spontaneous affective prosody usually remains severely compromised.

Patterns of recovery from dysarthria are somewhat unclear. Some dysarthrias progressively worsen because of the progressive nature of the disease producing the dysarthria (e.g., ALS). If essential functions such as respiration are compromised by the disease process, prognosis is said to be poor. Recovery from dysarthria is not good. Enderby and Crow (1990) found that persons with severe dysarthria remain severely dysarthric, but improvement was seen at 18 months, 24 months, and 30 months in three of four persons. Small gains continued to 48 months following speech therapy initiation.

Related to pragmatics, cognitive systems, and speech, empiric evidence of the factors influencing recovery are lacking.

ASSESSMENT OF COMMUNICATION

Nurses and other health-related professionals as well as families and significant others ignore or dismiss language and speech errors because that is appropriate social behavior. It would be rude to focus on the deficit. Nurses mistakenly may view this deficit as solely within the arena of the speech/language pathologist and beyond the assessment skills of the nurse. Unfortunately such attitudes may mean that the deficit is never carefully and thoroughly evaluated and appropriate therapeutic interventions are not instituted. The informality possible with the nurse and the continuous intimate contact with the nurse makes nursing contribution to the assessment valuable. The best assessment takes place by observing clients in natural communication situations conversing with a partner who may be the nurse.

A comprehensive nursing assessment concerning communication includes information on health history, developmental level of the client, previous cognitive and communication abilities, and present communication abilities. A comprehensive evaluation of communication function would include assessment of language, cognition, pragmatics, and speech. An aphasia battery particularly is not sufficient for the diagnosis and description of language impairments associated with diffuse brain injury such as in closed head injury because it does not address cognitive factors and pragmatic skills (Levin, Grossman, & Kelly, 1976; Sarno & Levita, 1981; Sohlberg & Mateer, 1989; Thompson, 1975). This assessment also is used to identify areas of competence that may help the person cope with the communication deficits.

Before beginning, the assessment and its purpose need to be explained to the client. Describe what is to be done and describe why. Acknowledge the difficulty for the client. During the assessment observe for fatigue, pain, and undue frustration. Stagger the assessment as needed.

An aphasia assessment includes evaluation of spontaneous speech, comprehension of verbal language, comprehension of written language, ability to name, ability to repeat, and ability to write. The nurse observes the following:

Spontaneous speech
+ Is client fluent or nonfluent?
+ Is the speech hesitant and slow?
+ Are there misused words, grammatic errors, word substitutions, or neologisms?
+ What is client's response to his or her own speech?

Comprehension of the spoken word
+ Ask client to follow simple midline (truncal) commands (e.g., "Stand up," "Sit down").
+ Request client to follow simple extremity commands (e.g., "Point to the floor," "Point to the door").
+ Increase the complexity of the commands by joining

two or more requests together (e.g., "Stand up and walk to the bed"). Be careful not to give nonverbal cues.

Comprehension of written language

◆ Ask client to read out loud.

◆ Request that client follow a written command (e.g., write out "Point to the chair").

◆ If reading is impaired, determine client's ability to recognize letters and words.

Ability to name objects

◆ Request client to name objects in the room.

Ability to repeat

◆ Ask client to repeat what is said (e.g., "It is a cloudy day.").

Ability to write

◆ Request client write a spontaneous thought in a sentence (e.g., "Write in a sentence what you are thinking."). If this does not work, be more structured (e.g., "Write a sentence about your breakfast this morning.").

◆ Ask client to write what is dictated (e.g., "It is a sunny, warm day.") (Boss, 1984b).

Table 25-5 represents a detailed bedside aphasia testing outline.

Pragmatic assessment is not well established (Sohlberg & Mateer, 1989). A screening assessment includes evaluation of prosody, gestures, pantomime, facial recognition, and facial expression. The nurse observes the following:

Spontaneous use of affective prosody and gesturing during conversation

◆ Is there affective prosodia in client's voice, especially to emotionally loaded questions? (e.g., "How do you feel?")

◆ Does client convey emotional or attitudinal information appropriate to the situation?

Ability to repeat, through imitation, linguistically neutral sentences with affective prosodia

◆ Select a declarative sentence with no emotional words in it (e.g., "It is cloudy.").

◆ Ask client to repeat the sentence with same affective tone used by the examiner: happy, sad, tearful, angry, surprised, or disinterested voice.

Ability to auditorily comprehend affective prosodia

◆ Select a declarative sentence with no emotional words in it (e.g., "It is cold.").

◆ Standing behind client so he or she cannot see gestures and facial expression, ask client to identify the affect voiced by the examiner in saying the sentence.

Table 25-5 Outline for the long form for the examination of an aphasic client

Background information	Handedness, level of education, language history (e.g., native language, delayed speech, stuttering)
Spontaneous speech	Listen to client during a conversation and note the following: fluency, rhythm and melody, articulation, phrase length, paraphasia, and word content

Comprehension	Test client's comprehension by the following:
	  Commands: although client may comprehend, she may be apraxic, therefore also test with
	    Questions that can be answered with yes/no responses
	    Pointing (pointing to the ceiling)

Repetition	Ask client to repeat grammatic phrases (e.g., "no ifs, and, or buts"), numbers, and words

Naming	Test client's ability to name an article presented visually; test with objects, pictures of objects, colors, hospital-related items, and actions
	If client has difficulty with visual naming, try alternate afferent pathways (i.e., tactile, auditory, olfactory, taste)
	If client fails in naming, see if he will correct with the following tests:
	  Phonetic cueing (e.g., if one holds up a pencil and client cannot name it, give her a "p" sound)
	  Multiple choice questions (e.g., give him a list of names that includes the correct name and see if he can choose it)
	  Sentence completion (e.g., "Summer is hot and winter is .")

Series speech	Ask client to name the days of the week in order or to count sequentially

Reading skills	Listen to client read aloud; assess reading comprehension by asking client to respond to the following:
	  Commands
	  Matching words to pictures
	  Yes/no
	  Multiple-choice questions
	To test spelling, say a word and have client spell it; spell a word aloud and have client say it or point to object

Writing skills	Test writing in response to command (i.e., "Write a sentence about the weather today."), to dictation (i.e., "Write this."), or as an exercise in copying

Table 25-6   The pragmatic protocol

Name: _____   Date: _____
Communicative   Communicative
Setting   Partner's
Observed: _____   Relationship: _____

Communicative act	Appropriate	Inappropriate	No opportunity to observe	Examples and comments
VERBAL ASPECTS				
Speech acts				
Speech act pair analysis				
Variety of speech acts				
Topics				
Selection				
Introduction				
Maintenance				
Changes				
Turn taking				
Initiation				
Response				
Repair/revision				
Pause times				
Interruption/overlaps				
Feedback to speakers				
Adjacency				
Contingency				
Quantity/conciseness				
Lexical selection/use across speech acts				
Specificity/accuracy				
Cohesions				
Stylistic variations				
Varying of communicative style				
PARALINGUISTIC ASPECTS				
Intelligibility and prosodics				
Intelligibility				
Vocal intensity				
Vocal quality				
Prosody				
Fluency				
NONVERBAL ASPECTS				
Kinesics and proxemics				
Physical proximity				
Physical contacts				
Body posture				
Foot/leg and hand/arm movements				
Gestures				
Facial expression				
Eye gaze				

From "A Clinical Appraisal of the Pragmatic Aspects of Language" by C. Prutting and D. Kirchner, 1987, *Journal of Speech and Hearing Disorders, 52,* pp. 105-117. Copyright 1987 by AASP. Reprinted by permission.

Ability to visually comprehend gestures

✦ The examiner conveys an affected state by using gestures of face and limbs (e.g., "It is hot.") said neutrally but with facial expression indicating happiness, sadness, or anger.

✦ Ask client to identify emotion or describe emotion.

In addition the nurse asks about the client's internal emotional state (e.g., "How does this news make you feel?" "Tell me how you feel inside."). It is important to remember that clients with motor aprosodia will not display depression but remain able to experience depression.

An example of a more comprehensive pragmatic profile inventory is given in Table 25-6.

The cognitive assessments that must accompany language, pragmatic and speech assessment include evaluation of arousal, selective attention, concentration, recent memory, remote memory, concept formation, and executive functions. The nurse observes the following:

Arousal

✦ Is client awake?

Selective attention

✦ Is client able to focus his or her attention?

✦ Does client focus on external stimuli? If so, to what does client respond?

✦ Does client search his or her environment?

✦ What overt orienting behaviors are evidenced?

Vigilance

✦ Is client distractible or inattentive?

✦ Is client able to attend to and respond to questions?

✦ Does client require redirection?

✦ Can client maintain attention with the presence of competing stimuli?

Recent memory

✦ Is client oriented? Confused? If not, to what is client disoriented: self, person, place, time, situation? What confuses client?

✦ Is client able to learn new information? Language-related memory? Nonlanguage-related memory? If so, to what degree? Is emotional memory affected?

Remote memory

✦ Is client able to recall (retrieve) previously learned information? Language-related memory? Nonlanguage-related memory? If so, to what degree?

Concept formation

✦ Does client misinterpret information (illusion)?

✦ Is client able to abstract? Categorize? Sort? Identify similarities and differences?

✦ Is client able to interpret the current situation? Does client exhibit concrete thinking?

Executive functions

✦ Motivation

Does client lack motivation? Initiative? Does client initiate communication?

Does client exhibit a flat affect? Appear emotionless? Is client able to appreciate his or her communication deficits?

Does client lack social graces in conversation?

✦ Goal formulation or selection

Is client able to form or set communication goals?

Is client able to make decisions about communication?

✦ Planning

Is client able to make plans for achieving communication?

Is client's communication impulsive? Does client think through his or her communications?

✦ Programming

Is client able to initiate, maintain, and/or terminate communication activities? Does client know where to begin? Is client able to carry out a communication sequence?

Is client slow to shift or alter his or her communication responses?

Is speech perseveration present?

✦ Self-monitoring

Is client able to self-monitor his communication?

Does client recognize communication omissions and errors in his communication? Does client recognize mistakes in speech? Does client exhibit careless speech?

Does client overestimate his communication ability and performance?

✦ Use of feedback

Is client able to change communication based on feedback?

Is client able to use communication cues? (Boss, 1991)

High-level language tests reflecting sensitivity to abstract language such as thematic pictures, synonyms, antonyms, metaphors, verbal power, and speed (e.g., word fluency) exist. The neuropsychologist is the resource person to consult for further information on such tests.

A dysarthria assessment includes evaluation of articulation, respiration, phonation, resonation, and prosody. The nurse

1. Listens to client during normal conversation or while client reads aloud and notes the speech pattern. With a dysarthria the same speech sounds are equally affected consistently; self-correction is minimal and articulation errors are consistent throughout repeated testing.

2. Asks client to repeat test phrases or to rapidly repeat lingual (la-la-la-la), labial (me-me-me-me), or guttural (k-k-k-k-k) sounds.

3. Assesses movement of pharynx, tongue, face, and lips. The motor function of facial, vagus, and hypoglossal nerves are tested. (See box on p. 558 for details.)

4. Notes muscle tone of facial, palatal, and tongue muscles. Are there signs of spasticity, rigidity, or flaccidity?

5. Identifies any other factors that may contribute to a speech problem (e.g., drooling, ill-fitting dentures) (Boss, 1984b).

When a speech disorder is present, the rehabilitation nurse additionally assesses the client for other health problem often associated with a speech problem including eating difficulties (Chapter 17), inability to cough (see Chapter 18), and skin integrity problems (see Chapter 15) due to drooling (Boss, 1984b).

The nurse documents the findings of these assessments in the client record. Serial assessments are performed to evaluate and document changes over time so that the treat-

ASSESSMENT OF LOWER CRANIAL NERVES

FACIAL NERVE

+ Observe client's face for symmetry and form. Are naso-labial folds equal? Is expression mobile, stiff, or excessive? Have client puff out his or her cheeks or whistle. Have client smile to differentiate emotional from voluntary facial weakness.
+ Inspect for adventitious movements, fatigability, or automatic associated movements.
+ Test deep tendon reflexes by gentle tapping with reflex hammer.

GLOSSOPHARYNGEAL AND VAGUS NERVES

+ Test palatal movement. Does palate elevate in midline? Do pharyngeal walls approximate on saying "ah"?
+ Test swallowing. Is there nasal regurgitation or choking on swallowing? Does larynx elevate on swallowing?
+ Does client's voice have a nasal quality? Test laryngeal function.
+ Is client's voice hoarse? Can client say "a, e, i, o, u"?
+ Test reflexes (cough, gag). When there is an obvious deficit, testing gag is foolish and perhaps dangerous.

HYPOGLOSSAL NERVE

+ Inspect client's tongue at rest for symmetry, size, shape, and presence of fasciculations.
+ Is client able to protrude his or her tongue in midline as well as against cheeks? If there is paresis, tongue will protrude toward the weak side.
+ Test rhythmic movement and coordination by repetitive protrusion as well as by test phrases (e.g., "Round the rugged rock the ragged rascal ran.").

From "Dysphasia, Dyspraxia, and Dysarthria: Distinguishing Features, Part II" by B.J. Boss, 1984, *Journal of Neurosurgical Nursing 16,* p. 213. Copyright 1984 by AANN. Reprinted by permission.

NURSING DIAGNOSES RELATED TO COMMUNICATION DEFICITS

Impaired communication: Verbal (NANDA)
Impaired communication: written, emotional, and gestural
Potential for injury related to impaired communication
Sensory/perceptual alteration
Self-care deficit related to impaired communication
Anxiety
Altered family process
Social isolation

EXAMPLES OF TESTS FOR ASSESSING COMMUNICATION

DYSPHASIA TESTS

Boston Diagnostic Aphasia Examination (Goodglass & Kaplan, 1983)
Minnesota Test for the Differential Diagnosis of Aphasia (Schuell, 1965)
Porch Index of Communicative Ability (Porch, 1967)
Western Aphasia Battery (Kertesz, 1989)

For Children
Denver Developmental Screening Test (DDST)
Denver Prescreening Questionnaire (PDQ)

PRAGMATIC DEFICIT TESTS

Communication Performance Scale (Erlich & Spies, 1985)
Adapted from the pragmatic protocol to assist clinical judgment of client's progress following communication interventions to provide empiric documentation of change: 13 pragmatic behaviors rated on a 1-5 scale

Facial Recognition Test

Interactional Checklist for Augmentative Communication (INCH) (Bolton & Dashiell, 1984)
Observational protocol to assess pragmatic ability when communication is augmented: three components to protocol, strategies (skills client uses in a communication exchange); modes (means by which messages are transmitted—linguistics, paralinguistics, kinesic, proxemic and chronemic modes); and contexts (the particular communication partners and situations—e.g., relationship between sender and receiver, level of competence receiver has)

Pragmatic Protocol (Prutting & Kirchner, 1983)
Screening tool designed to assess how client uses language; 32 pragmatic behaviors in 4 categories: utterance act, propositional act, perlocutionary act, and illocutionary act

Profile of Nonverbal Sensitivity (PONS)
Evaluates ability to comprehend facial expressions, limb and body movements, and intonational qualities of the voice

DYSARTHRIA

Frenchay Dysarthria Assessment

For Children
Denver Articulation Screening Examination (DASE)

ment plan may be modified appropriately. Relevant nursing diagnoses are listed in the box on p. 558.

Magazines and books are excellent resources for pictures that can be used in assessing language, speech, pragmatics, and cognition. A list of some available standardized tests for aphasia, pragmatic deficits, and dysarthrias are given in the box on p. 558.

Comprehensive assessment provides a method for translating information gleaned through observation into treatment goals and establishing objectives such as the following:

- ✦ Assist client in achieving optimum communication
- ✦ Establish a functional means of communication
- ✦ Establish an environment conducive to communication
- ✦ Prevent injury
- ✦ Preserve client's self-esteem
- ✦ Promote social interaction
- ✦ Assist client in returning to social roles
- ✦ Provide communication opportunities
- ✦ Educate client and family regarding the communication deficit(s)

- ✦ Assist client and family in establishing effective support systems

Specific therapeutic goals for dysarthria are (1) to improve articulation and (2) to improve respiration, phonation, and resonance, which will make speech more intelligible.

REHABILITATION NURSING INTERVENTIONS

Rehabilitation nursing interventions for the client with a communication deficit depend on the client's unique needs. The members of the rehabilitation team, in addition to the nurse, who most frequently work with the client experiencing a communication deficit are the speech/language pathologist, physical therapist, occupational therapist, audiologist, dentist, social worker, psychologist, nutritionist, clergy member, and the primary physician or physiatrist (see the following box). A primary nursing role in this team is communicating to all members of the team information about the whole client, so that everyone on the team knows the client's underlying disease(s), physical/cognitive/psychological/social communicative limitations, coping and adaptation styles, and any current changes in the client. Nursing interventions are designed to provide a therapeu-

---

THE REHABILITATION TEAM FOR A CLIENT WITH A COMMUNICATION DEFICIT

Physiatrist	Provides a comprehensive approach to client experiencing functional limitations
Speech/language pathologist	Evaluates client's ability to understand verbal and written communications, to gesture, to speak spontaneously and on instruction, and to evaluate communication; implements appropriate treatment protocol for communication problem; also may evaluate swallowing and implement treatment protocol
Physical and occupational therapist	Plan physical therapies, taking into consideration client's communication problems, and use these therapies in conjunction with facilitation techniques to promote communication
Audiologist	Assesses hearing, selects hearing aid if needed, and teaches client to use the device
Social worker	Assists client or family with social and financial concerns related to healthcare costs, dependent family members, and postdischarge needs; provides counseling and assists client and family to grieve, cope, manage stress, and rebuild their lives
Psychologist	Provides counseling and assists client and family with complex adaptation and coping problems
Dentist	May be needed if dentures do not fit properly or teeth are in poor repair
Nutritionist/dietitian	Provides nutritional assessment and assists with providing special meals and supplements based on client needs
Clergy	Assists with meeting spiritual needs of client and family

tic, supportive environment for the client to facilitate actual communication and in order to educate the client and family.

Therapeutic Environment

The rehabilitation nurse plays a primary role in creating an environment that makes attempts at communication easier and less stressful. Specific interventions to promote the existence of a therapeutic environment are given in the following box.

In the acute rehabilitation setting, when a room is shared, the client with a problem in communication output—that is, a Broca's aphasia, motor aprosody, or dysarthria—benefits most from having a roommate who can understand the communication problem being experienced by the client. The environment most supportive of the client with a comprehension problem is one that does not cause excessive auditory or visual stimulation. The roommate of a client with Wernicke's aphasia who is talkative should not be troubled by spontaneous, frequent, meaningless verbalizations.

Impaired communication may seriously compromise the client's safety. Careful assessment with each client having a communication deficit for any special precautions needed to ensure safety is appropriate. Ways to call for help either in the acute rehabilitation setting or at home need to be established and the client taught how to use them. The client needs to be informed about environmental hazards despite the communication deficit by pictures, pantomime, or whatever it takes. Two examples to illustrate the safety hazards are given in the following box.

Supportive Behaviors

All rehabilitation team members who interact with the client need to monitor themselves for postures, behaviors, tone of voice, and facial expressions. All these communications need to be positive and supportive. Also team members need to behave as if communications are understood when in the presence of the client and need to assume that misunderstanding because of the communication deficit may readily occur. Misunderstanding is assessed for continuously and corrective actions are taken immediately.

◆

CREATING A THERAPEUTIC ENVIRONMENT

With any communication deficit
◆ Maintain a calm, relaxed, and unhurried environment.
◆ Maintain an uncluttered environment with equipment placed in least distracting areas.
◆ Maintain a routine in the schedule of activities.
◆ Avoid isolation.
◆ Recognize anxiety-provoking stimuli and eliminate stressors.
◆ Institute anxiety-reducing measures, as appropriate.

When output of communication is impaired while comprehension is relatively preserved
◆ Help client to communicate. Create an environment where communicating is a pleasant experience. Praise client for trying to communicate even when the results are far from perfect
◆ Stimulate communication during routine nursing care activities
◆ Provide client with frequent opportunities to experience communication: to hear speech; to practice listening to family and social conversation; to read; to practice interpretation of emotion, gestures, and pantomime, as appropriate. Radio and television may be used to some degree.
◆ Encourage client to participate in group activities for social value and communication stimulation.

When a comprehension deficit is present
◆ Avoid continuous noise and interaction.
◆ Avoid fatigue.
◆ Set limits on amount of praise given.
◆ Limit frequency and length of time that communication is stimulated.
◆ Limit frequency and length of group activities.
◆ If activity or interaction is confusing or stressful, discontinue the activity or interaction (Boss, 1984b).

◆

EXAMPLES OF SAFETY HAZARDS EXPERIENCED WITH CLIENTS WITH A COMMUNICATION DEFICIT

CASE STUDY 1

Mr. Jones, a 65-year-old man with a history of a myocardial infarction, had Broca's aphasia as a result of a stroke that occurred 6 weeks earlier. While ambulating in the hospital corridor, he experienced a severe episode of left-sided chest pain that radiated down his left arm. He became weak, fell to the floor, and remained there rubbing his arm. Initially the staff thought he had injured his arm in the fall. No one understood why he looked so apprehensive and pale. On taking his vital signs, the nurse discovered he was hypotensive and experiencing significant cardiac dysrhythmia. Fortunately, because the vital signs were taken, early treatment for the cardiac condition was initiated.

CASE STUDY 2

Mrs. Brown experienced Broca's aphasia as a result of an automobile accident. She continually rubbed her right eye but never verbally complained (she could not). She frequently was restless and often appeared uncomfortable, but no one could determine the cause. Sometimes when the eye became red, a wrist restraint was applied to stop her from irritating the eye by rubbing. The eye became severely inflamed so an ophthalmologist was consulted. Examination revealed that a piece of glass had become embedded in the eye at the time of the accident. Unfortunately the prolonged irritation left Mrs. Brown's cornea scarred.

Embarrassment about the inability to communicate in a meaningful way can discourage the client from interacting with others and participating in treatment. The nurse, other rehabilitation team members, and family can help reduce embarrassment by demonstrating acceptance and interest. Supportive behaviors are listed in the following box.

As the client physically recovers from the nervous system injury that produced the communication deficit, social interactions are encouraged. Initially interactions involve rehabilitation team members with whom the client regularly interacts, family, and close friends. Interaction involving one or two people usually is best because this makes it easier for the client to focus. Visitors or other clients need to be instructed regarding appropriate communication techniques. The nurse monitors visits to ensure that the encounters are pleasant and not too long.

When a client returns home, resumption of a "normal" social life often is difficult. Frustration and embarrassment about one's communication may result in a loss of interest in socializing: the stress itself is fatiguing.

Old friends often feel uncomfortable in initiating interactions because the interests once shared can no longer be pursued. Friends also may be frustrated by their inability to communicate effectively or to help the client communicate more effectively. They may be frightened by the changes seen in their friend (Broida, 1979). The nurse and the family can teach the client's friends ways to communicate. Friends, like family, need to be encouraged to visit and received recognition for the support offered. They too need a chance to verbalize their fears and frustrations.

Self-help organizations such as the American Heart Association Stroke Clubs, the National Head Injury Association chapters, and the National Alzheimer's and Related Disorders Association chapters help fulfill social, support, and education needs. These organizations not only are helpful to the client experiencing the communication deficit but to spouses and family members as well. These organizations may be particularly valuable when the client and/or family have few support systems. These organizations can serve as a source of new friends who understand, share good ideas regarding mutual problems, and are seeking new friends themselves.

Facilitation Techniques to Improve Communication

All members of the rehabilitation team need to be knowledgeable about communication processes and facilitation

---

SUPPORTIVE BEHAVIORS

✦ Evidence genuine concern for client.

✦ Recognize frustration and difficulty client is experiencing. Be patient and accepting of his or her anger and depression.

✦ Treat client as an adult even during times when his or her behavior may regress. Involve client in decision-making regarding his or her care and activities.

✦ Attempt to anticipate client's needs and validate specific needs with client. Be observant and sensitive.

✦ Encourage client in all of his or her communication efforts. Praise even the smallest gain.

✦ Help client develop constructive and positive outlook. Emphasize things that client can do. Build up his or her confidence. Reassure client that everyone has difficulty at times with self-expression.

✦ Do not be overly helpful. Allow client to take pride in being able to provide self-care as much as possible.

✦ Encourage client to be as independent as he or she wishes regardless of the communication deficit.

✦ Be honest with client regarding prognosis and difficulties in regaining communication abilities.

✦ Limit communication goals to those that can be accomplished. Emphasize short-term goals.

✦ Avoid placing demands on client that cannot be met.

✦ Do not force client to communicate or to see persons when he or she does not wish to.

✦ Do not remind client that once the client communicated well.

✦ If client laughs or cries uncontrollably, attempt to change subject or activity. If crying or laughing continues, remove client from situation.

✦ Begin language/speech therapy when client is interested and psychologically ready.

When comprehension and cognition are intact

✦ Do not behave or permit other persons to behave as if client does not understand or has lost some of his or her cognitive abilities.

When comprehension is impaired

✦ Do not discuss client in the client's presence without direct attempts to communicate this information to client as well.

✦ Accept paraphasia, "jargon speech," cursing, and other such output nonjudgmentally but attempt to inform client that you do not understand his or her communication.

✦ Use touch, tone of voice, and other nonverbal behaviors to communicate calmness, reassurance, and trustworthiness when language comprehension is impaired. When prosodic comprehension is impaired, put all emotions and gestural intentions into verbal language, and say what you mean.

✦ Carry out all activities in a calm, unhurried manner (Boss, 1984b).

techniques used to promote effective communication in clients with communication deficits. Often experimentation with various techniques is necessary to determine what works best for a particular client. Behaviors the rehabilitation nurse can use to facilitate communication are present in the following box.

◆ **Rehabilitation approaches**

The many widely different language interventions may be categorized into four main approaches. These approaches

have sometimes arisen in different countries under the influence of different psychological theory, but they are not necessarily mutually exclusive. Specific treatment applications depend on what theories are accepted by the therapist. Some treatments have a clear research base. Others are derived more from the theory but are without empiric evidence of efficacy.

The classical (or stimulation) approach encompasses many different intervention techniques, but all techniques are based on two assumptions. The first assumption is that

---

◆ BEHAVIORS TO FACILITATE COMMUNICATION

- ◆ Use spontaneous communication topics that are of interest to client or of immediate importance to him or her.
- ◆ Frequent but short communications are more beneficial.
- ◆ Postpone communication if client is fatigued or upset.
- ◆ Encourage use of gestures and other forms of communication when client's verbalizations are misunderstood.

When communication output is disturbed, but comprehension is intact
- ◆ Allow client to communicate for himself or herself. Provide opportunity for client to speak first, and provide the necessary time to communicate.
- ◆ Encourage all attempts to verbalize by acknowledging attempts and efforts. Encourage automatic speech or imitation (e.g., prayers, social responses such as "Hello."). Encourage singing if client enjoys singing.
- ◆ Use self-talk (i.e., speaking about the activity as nurse performs it).
- ◆ Use parallel talk (i.e., describing aloud the activity client is carrying out with nurse).
- ◆ Use expansion, which adds substance to the statement (e.g., adding to statement "drink of water," "You want a drink of water.").
- ◆ Attend very carefully to communications.
- ◆ With dysarthria, encourage client to say one word at a time with all sounds in each word produced and consonants emphasized. Encourage client to increase volume of voice.
- ◆ React with physical actions or verbalizations to convey your understanding of verbalizations.
- ◆ Assume some responsibility for misunderstanding communications.
- ◆ Do not interrupt while client is trying to communicate unless client becomes frustrated. Only then interpret or supply words.
- ◆ Encourage use of shorter phrases, single words, or slower verbalization if client is distressed or fatigued or if verbalizations are misunderstood (Piotrowski, 1978).
- ◆ Allow mistakes. Only occasionally correct client, if clearly appropriate. Do not insist that each word be pronounced perfectly.
- ◆ If client is having trouble with a word, use cueing (i.e., pronouncing the initial syllable of word), have client repeat the word after you, give an open-ended sentence to fill in the blank or try writing down word for client to read (Norman & Baratz, 1979).
- ◆ Request statements be repeated or rephrased if not understood.
- ◆ Serve as a good communication model to imitate when client is having difficulty.

When even a slight comprehension deficit is present (as with any aphasia or aprosodia)
- ◆ Provide a quiet environment for communication on a one-to-one basis at least initially. Turn televisions and radios off. Remove unnecessary items and equipment from client's visual field.
- ◆ Gain client's attention first. Get client to look at communication partner. Redirect client back to communication partner, if client becomes distracted (Norman & Baratz, 1979).
- ◆ Speak slowly and distinctly, using natural pauses. Use short simple instructions and/or explanations. Use gestures and pantomime along with verbalizations.
- ◆ Use simple, direct questions that are answerable with one word or short phrases. Use gestures and pantomime with verbal questions.
- ◆ Reinforce appropriate responses.
- ◆ Tell client when you do not understand him or her. Ask simple questions and systematically point and gesture until the point is uncovered.
- ◆ Do not raise your voice if client fails to understand or misunderstands. Signal client that there was a miscommunication and reword the communication. Try to use strong gestures and facial expressions. Do not become annoyed (Boss, 1984b).

aphasia is a central language deficit. An overall language pattern pervades all different language modalities, thus types of aphasia reflect only different levels of language dissolution. Aphasias are quantitatively different. The breakdown is in the one single central language mechanism (Basso, 1987; Schuell, Jenkins, & Jimenez-Pabon, 1964; Wepman, 1957). This assumption heavily influences rehabilitation because under this assumption improvement is simultaneous across all modalities. There is no need to focus on each modality using different techniques. For example, Schuell et al. (1964) recommended using intense auditory stimulation only controlling the amount of stimulation for the severity of the language disorder (i.e., less stimulation with dense dysphasia). Most therapists focus on oral language. Wepman (1957) uses the same exercises for comprehension and expression.

The second assumption is that "aphasia is characterized by reduced efficiency in gaining access to language knowledge" (Basso, 1987). Aphasia is a restriction of language availability, therefore therapy addresses levels of language availability (e.g., informative content versus automatic language and focuses on improving accessing strategies).

The second approach, called the Soviet approach, is built on Luria's theory that "any functional system may be deranged by lesions in diverse parts of the cortex, but the quality of the impediment is dependent on the localization of the lesion" (Basso et al., 1979; Luria, 1970, 1973; Beyn, Skokhor-Trotskaya, 1966). Recovery occurs through reorganization of the functional system under treatment in such a way that transfers affected function to a new structure. The defective link is replaced with a new one so that the function can reestablish itself. Intrasystem reorganization may take place at a more primitive (low) level or at a more intentional level. Therapy is directed at helping the person understand the nature of the impediment and to learn to do intentionally things that were previously automatic. There is conscious analysis of speech and thought processes, a step-by-step reconstruction of a functional language operation, which is exemplified in the substitute skills model therapies. External operations for each of the different links composing the function must then be progressively internalized. There are two fundamental rehabilitation rules: (1) the deficit must be rigorously differentiated, so there must be an accurate qualitative analysis of the deficit and (2) each deficit calls for its own rehabilitation program.

The operant conditioning approach is based in Skinner's (1972) principles of operant conditioning. The consequences (reinforcement) are manipulated. Baseline data are collected. Criteria for success are defined. Then the steps within the treatment program are implemented (Goldfarb, 1981). Examples of a behavioral approach are presented in the literature (Brookshire, 1969; Holland, 1970; Holland & Harris, 1968; Holland & Sonderman, 1974; Holland, 1977). Basso (1987) argued that this approach is a methodologic approach, not a content approach, but is a useful tool in systematically implementing any rehabilitation program.

The final approach is called a psycholinguistic approach. Linguistic criteria are the focus. Although the approach is not well established, examples of the psycholinguistic approach in the literature are Jakobson (1964), Chomsky (1978), and the substitute symbols systems including

Weigl's (1961) deblocking technique, Sparks' melodic intonation therapy (MIT) (Sarno et al., 1970; Sparks, Helm, & Albert, 1974) and its variant melodic rhythm therapy (TMR) (Van Eeckout, Honrado, Bhatt, & Deblais, 1983), the visual communication program (Gardner, Zuriff, Berry, & Baker, 1976), and visual action therapy (VAT) (Helm-Estabrooks, Fitzpatrick, & Barres, 1982). Amerind sign language (Skelly, Schinsky, Smith, & Fust, 1974) also has been used with some reported success, especially with severe Broca's aphasia. This approach has had a major impact on the diagnosis and classification.

Regardless of the approach used, therapeutic efforts generally are tailored on an individual basis. Generally therapies concentrate on improving spoken language. Impaired auditory language comprehension often is directly approached by exercises in listening to words and sentences. In severe cases lip-reading or reliance on writing may be used. Alexia and agraphia commonly are treated with traditional classroom work and then homework assignments. Children usually are taught language by traditional educational methods. The communication problems most resistant to direct therapeutic approaches and substitute skills models are profound anomia, severe agrammatism, severe alexia, profound impairment of word retrieval and language comprehension via both speech and writing, and severe impairment initiating or formulating an utterance (e.g., transcortical motor aphasia) (Goodglass, 1987).

◆ General therapeutic considerations

Some general principles that may help guide rehabilitation nurses as they attempt to facilitate the client's communication include the following:

1. It is common to distinguish between comprehension of communication and production of communication and reeducate each separately.
2. Because comprehension is believed to be easier than production, target it first (Basso, 1987; Basso et al., 1982; Schuell et al., 1964).
3. Language in context is easier to deal with than words or phrases isolated from immediate experience. Nurses have ample opportunity to provide language exchange in context.
4. Improvement brought about by retraining in one modality may be accompanied by corresponding improvement in untrained skills.
5. With sufficient repeated practice, it is possible either to restore functional efficiency to a defective capacity or bring an alternative route to a level of voluntary and eventual automatic skill (Goodglass, 1987). Interact with client while giving care and during activities as well as in practice sessions. Use facilitation techniques given in the previous Box.

With regard to pragmatics, treatment protocols are in the very early stages of development. There are some trial remediation programs mostly with head-injured clients. Some therapists have used a group approach (Ehrlich & Spies, 1985; Sohlberg & Mateer, 1989). Sohlberg and Mateer (1989) use a modular format to address four behaviors: nonverbal communication, communication in context, message repair, and cohesiveness of the narrative. The module is introduced by describing and demonstrating target behaviors to be learned. Then a role play is videotaped followed by review by the group. Participants are helped to look at specific behaviors that increase success or failure and identify ways to modify the communication behavior. Other therapists use an individual approach targeting particular communication behaviors that are deficient in individual clients. The therapist attempts to address the communication behaviors in a broad range of naturalistic communication environments. Family members receive descriptions of communication goals and suggestions for providing appropriate

feedback. Opportunity is provided to practice appropriate behaviors and to modify existing problem areas as well as to establish new, effective modes of communication.

With regard to dysarthria, rehabilitation nurses need to understand the specific treatments prescribed and the methods for applying the treatments during nurse-client interactions. Dysarthria therapy has three approaches:

1. Medical care of underlying neurologic disorder to prevent further deterioration
2. Prosthetic and/or surgical management

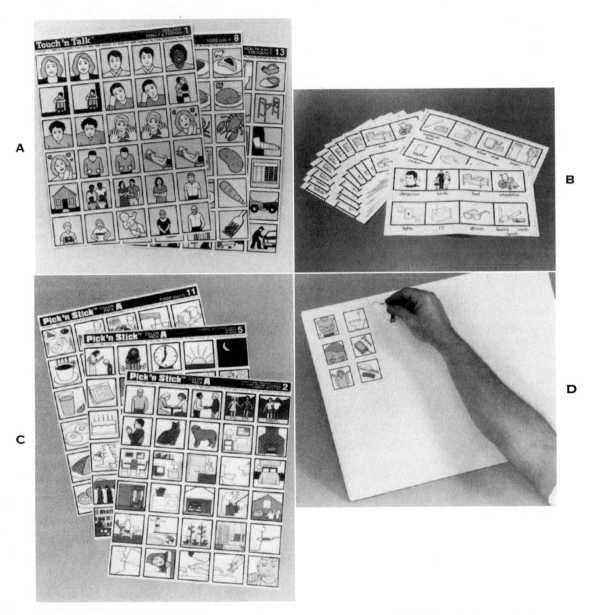

Fig. 25-5   Many assistive devices for improving communication with clients who have aphasia can be made at home. Some clients may have computers and software packages available. Easy to use and excellent commercial products include the following items. **A,** Touch 'N Talk picture board. **B,** Identification picture board. **C,** Pick 'N Stick Identification stickers. **D,** Picture stickers. (Reprinted by permission of Bissell Healthcare Corporation/Fred Sammons, Inc.)

3. Therapeutic approach of speech pathologist, which is usually behavioral in nature with some instrumental aids when such aids are available

The speech therapy approach is basically symptomatic and supportive or compensatory. To improve articulation, the speech pathologist determines the reason for the articulatory errors and designs and implements a hierarchy of exercises starting with sounds that sometimes are correct and ending with those sounds impaired most seriously. To improve resonance, which will reduce hypernasality, the palatal muscles (palatin vault) are strengthened using exercises such as sucking and blowing and by producing oral and nasal sounds alternately (e.g., "pa, ma, pa, ma"). To improve phonation, laryngeal valve exercises may be used (e.g., production of "i-i-i" or rapid pitch changes). To strengthen the respiratory muscles, clients may use incentive spirometry, counting aloud during expiration, and increasing loudness rapidly and dramatically. Exercises to help prevent air waste may be prescribed (e.g., "pa-pa-pa" to improve bilabial air control and "ta-ta′ta" for linguoalveolar air control).

The nurse needs knowledge about the use of prosthetic devices and alternate forms of communication used by the client. Some common strategies used when interacting with the person who is dysarthric are given in the previous Box.

Clients with aphasia, pragmatic deficits, and cognitive impairments need time to process incoming information. If the nurse has trouble eliciting a response from the client, the nurse's own communication needs to be examined.

◆ Alternate forms of communication

Some persons with only speech problems, such as dysarthria involving only speech, can communicate in writing. Other persons because of speech and arm motor problems cannot put out verbal or written language but can use communication boards, a spelling board, or cards that use printed words or require spelling out words, sentences, and so on. Typewriters, computers, and voice simulators address the same communication problems.

When aphasia is present, the communication boards, notebooks, or cards must use pictures of objects, persons, needs, actions, faces expressing moods, and so on. A computer-aided visual communication system (Fig. 25-5) has been developed for clients with aphasia.

Client and Family Education

Both the client and family need to understand the cause of the communication deficit, the purpose of language/speech therapy, and have a realistic view of the potential for recovery. All rehabilitation team members need to have knowledge of what the client and family have been told and by whom. Information on prognosis for recovery initially may be presented by the primary physician, physiatrist, or speech/language pathologist. Realistic hope for recovery of communication ability by the client and family is supported, but the client and family are informed that full recovery is not common.

The family is taught the importance of creating an environment that is physically and emotionally supportive and how to create that environment (see the box at right). Facilitation techniques found to promote more effective communication are taught to all persons who interact with the client.

Two references especially useful in assisting family members to cope with the problems of aphasia are the booklet entitled "Aphasia and the Family," available on request for a small fee from the American Heart Association and the article "An Open Letter to the Family of an Adult Patient with Aphasia," published in *Rehabilitation Literature*, volume 23, May 1962. This material can serve as reference material to give families.

Referrals

The nurse assumes a key role in the referral of clients to various health disciplines within rehabilitation institutions and the community. Close and often long-term interactions with the client provide the opportunity for identifying obvious and subtle problems. The nurse's findings need to be carefully and completely documented in the client's record.

◆

EDUCATION OF CLIENT, FAMILY AND FRIENDS

CLIENT TEACHING

In conjunction with other rehabilitation team members
- ◆ Teach client about the communication deficit.
- ◆ Help client learn how to help himself or herself and how to help other persons learn to assist him or her to communicate through supportive behaviors and behaviors that enhance communication.
- ◆ Teach client how to manage the environment.

FAMILY AND FRIENDS TEACHING

In conjunction with other rehabilitation team members
- ◆ Teach family and friends about the communication deficit.
- ◆ Provide explanations about behavioral changes that language and prosodia comprehension deficits often produce. Reassure family and friends about the etiology for these changes.
- ◆ Encourage family members and friends to continue normal home activities whenever possible and to encourage client to participate in appropriate activities. Help them guard against overprotectiveness.
- ◆ Help family and friends include client in making decisions related to family and mutual affairs but at the same time avoid excessive involvement with small, insignificant, day-to-day difficulties.
- ◆ Help family and friends learn how to help client communicate and how to help other persons facilitate client's communication through supportive behaviors and behaviors to facilitate communication.
- ◆ Provide family and friends with information on environmental management.
- ◆ Help family and friends to function as an outside monitor of communication effectiveness. (Boss, 1984a)

Nurses can assume a major role in seeing that information regarding communication techniques used with the client are communicated to other healthcare professionals and that techniques they have found useful are noted and shared both in the acute care facility and in the community setting.

Growing numbers of clients are receiving speech/language therapy on an outpatient basis in clinics and private practice settings. Likewise more and more community health agencies and home health organizations are beginning to offer speech/language therapy services. Because of prohibitive costs for continued therapy, some speech/language pathologists have designed programs that the family can use with the client. They see the client only for reevaluation and adjustment of the therapy program. The nurse may need to be involved in finding such resources for clients and encouraging the development of such programs.

Outcome criteria for the client experiencing a communication deficit are determined individually based on the client and situation. Potential outcome criteria are presented in the following box.

SUMMARY

New technologies have just opened the way to study communication systems in normal children and adults and in children and adults who have sustained neurologic insult. With these studies may come a true understanding of language, pragmatic, cognitive, and speech systems. These technologies also open the way to examine the effectiveness of language, speech, and pragmatic therapies in both children and adults. Much of the current controversy and debate will be put to rest with such research.

Rehabilitation nurses traditionally have remained on the sidelines in the area of communication rehabilitation, but increasing demand for cost containment, cross-trained rehabilitation specialists, early return to the community, and home-based healthcare services may mandate that nurses play a larger role in treating communication deficits. This is not an unreasonable or unmeetable request.

OUTCOME CRITERIA FOR COMMUNICATION DEFICITS

- ✦ Client participates in all activities planned to improve communication:
    - Participates in speech therapy sessions and periodic evaluation
    - Interacts and communicates with health team members, family, and friends
    - Explains, demonstrates, or recognizes speech therapy methods and communication techniques designed to improve communication
    - Explains and appropriately uses alternate forms of communication
- ✦ Client is in control of anxiety and frustration permitting him to
    - Participate in speech therapies
    - Effectively express anxieties and frustrations via verbalizations or gestures
    - Communicate needs to others
- ✦ Client functions safely and independently including searching for and accepting assistance of others as needed
- ✦ Client establishes a defined method of communication
- ✦ Client demonstrates ways to maximize his communication
- ✦ Client demonstrates attitude of self-worth as evidenced by
    - Spontaneous communication to others
    - Awareness and interest in other persons and environment
    - Expression of interest in appearance
- ✦ Client enjoys social interactions, as evidenced by
    - Identification of opportunities for social interaction
    - Participation in chosen activities
- ✦ Family provides effective support for client by
    - Identifying safety needs of client
    - Explaining cause of communication deficit
    - Explaining expected prognosis for recovery of communication
    - Providing realistic and honest support for client
    - Identifying importance of psychological support for themselves as well as client
    - Explaining and using facilitation techniques, methods for maximizing communication, and alternative methods of communication
    - Explaining importance of promoting maximum independence
    - Identifying methods for promoting maximum recovery

CASE STUDY

Mrs. Edwards, a 75-year-old widow, experienced an ischemic stroke involving the inferior trunk of the middle cerebral artery, causing dysfunction in the right temporooccipital areas 2 weeks ago. She was diagnosed concurrently with non-insulin-dependent diabetes mellitus and hypertension. She now has impaired comprehension of prosody, gestures, and pantomime with some loss of facial recognition. Because she has no sensory or motor impairment, she does not require inpatient hospitalization but will have outpatient cognitive rehabilitation with nursing providing home rehabilitation.

CARE PLAN

Create a therapeutic environment (Boss, 1984b).

1. Maintain a calm, relaxed, unhurried and uncluttered environment. Carry out all activities in a calm, unhurried manner.
2. Maintain a routine in schedule of activities.
3. Avoid isolation but avoid continuous noise and interaction as well as fatigue. Limit frequency and length of time that communication is stimulated. Limit frequency and length of group activities.
4. Recognize anxiety-provoking stimuli and eliminate stressors and institute anxiety-reducing measures, as appropriate. If the activity or interaction is confusing or stressful, discontinue activity or interaction.

Evidence supportive behaviors (Boss, 1984b).

1. Verbalize your caring about Mrs. Edwards.
2. Verbally recognize frustration and difficulty Mrs. Edwards is experiencing. Be patient and accepting of her anger and depression.
3. Treat Mrs. Edwards as an adult even during times when her behavior may regress. Involve Mrs. Edwards in decision-making regarding her care and activities.
4. Attempt to anticipate Mrs. Edwards's needs and validate specific needs with her. Be observant and sensitive.
5. Encourage Mrs. Edwards in all of her communication efforts. Praise even the smallest gain.
6. Help Mrs. Edwards develop a constructive and positive outlook. Emphasize things that Mrs. Edwards can do. Build up her confidence.
7. Be honest with Mrs. Edwards regarding prognosis and difficulties in regaining her comprehension of prosody, gestures, and facial recognition.
8. Limit communication goals to those that can be accomplished. Emphasize short-term goals.
9. Avoid placing demands on Mrs. Edwards that cannot be met.
10. Do not force Mrs. Edwards to communicate or to see persons when she does not wish to.
11. Do not remind Mrs. Edwards that she once comprehended prosody and gestures well.

Use techniques to facilitate communication (Boss, 1984b). Use conversations as therapy sessions for Mrs. Edwards to help her learn to communicate effectively in spite of the aprosody. During these therapy sessions

1. Use frequent but short communications initially. Postpone conversation session if Mrs. Edwards is fatigued or upset.
2. Provide a quiet environment and a one-to-one conversation initially. Turn televisions and radios off. Remove unnecessary items and equipment from Mrs. Edwards's visual fields.
3. Speak slowly and distinctly, using natural pauses. Use short simple topics of interest to Mrs. Edwards. Use simple, direct questions.
4. Accept literal interpretations of verbal communication and misinterpretations of communications. Inform Mrs. Edwards when you do not understand her emotional feelings and intent and ask simple questions about her emotions and feeling. Reinforce appropriate responses.
5. Put all emotions and gestural intentions into verbal language and say what you mean and feel.
6. Do not raise your voice if Mrs. Edwards fails to understand or misunderstands. Tell her that there was a miscommunication and reword the communication. Do not become annoyed.

Educate Mrs. Edwards, family, and friends (Boss, 1984b).

1. Teach Mrs. Edwards, family and friends about the communication deficit. Provide explanations about behavioral changes that prosody comprehension deficits often produce. Reassure family and friends about the etiology for these changes.
2. Help Mrs. Edwards learn how to help herself. Help family and friends learn how to help Mrs. Edwards comprehend prosody and gestures. Help Mrs. Edwards and family learn how to help other persons learn to assist her comprehend through supportive behaviors and behaviors that enhance her comprehension.
3. Teach Mrs. Edwards how to manage the environment. Provide family and friends with information on environmental management.
4. Help family and friends to function as an outside monitor of communication effectiveness.
5. Encourage family members and friends to continue normal home activities whenever possible and to encourage Mrs. Edwards to participate in appropriate activities.

REFERENCES

Ackermann, H., & Ziegler, W. (1991a). Articulatory deficits in parkinsonian dysarthria: An acoustic analysis. *Journal of Neurology, Neurosurgery and Psychiatry, 54,* 1093-1098.

Ackermann, H., & Ziegler, W. (1991b) Cerebellar voice tremor: an acoustic analysis. *Journal of Neurology, Neurosurgery and Psychiatry, 54,* 74-76.

Adams, R., & Victor, M. (1989). *Principles of Neurology* (4th ed.). New York: McGraw-Hill.

Allison, M. (1992). The effects of neurologic injury on the maturing brain. *Headlines, 3,* 2-6, 9-10.

Ansel, B.M., & Kent, R.D. (1992). Acoustic-phonetic contrasts and intelligibility in the dysarthria associated with mixed cerebral palsy. *Journal of Speech and Hearing Research, 35,* 296-308.

Basso, A. (1987). Approaches to neuropsychological rehabilitation: language disorders. In M. Meier, A.L. Benton, & L. Diller (Eds.), *Neuropsychological rehabilitation* (pp. 294-314). New York: Guilford Press.

Basso, A., Capitani, E., & Moraschini, S. (1982). Sex differences in recover from aphasia. *Cortex, 18,* 469-475.

Basso, A., Capitani, E., & Vignolo, L.A. (1979). Influence of rehabilitation on language skills in aphasic patients: A controlled study. *Archives of Neurology, 36,* 190-196.

Basso, A., Faglioni, P., & Vignolo, L.A. (1975). Etude controlce de la reeducation du langage dans l'aphasia: comparaison entre aphasiques traites et non-traites. *Revue Neurolgique, 131,* 607-614.

Basso, A., Farabola, M., Grassi, M.P., Laiacona, M., & Zanobio, M.E. (1990). Aphasia in left-handers. Comparison of aphasia profiles and language recovery in non-right-handed and matched right handed patients. *Brain and Language, 38,* 233-252.

Bates, E. (1975). *The emergence of symbols: Cognition and communication in infancy.* New York: Academic Press.

Bell, W.L., Davis, D.L., Morgan-Fisher, A., & Ross, E.D. (1990). Acquired aprosodia in children. *Journal of Child Neurology, 5,* 19-26.

Benson, D.F. (1979). *Aphasia, alexia and agraphia.* New York: Churchill Livingstone.

Benson, D.F., & Geschwind, N. (1985) Aphasia and related disorders: a clinical approach. In M.-M. Mesulam (Ed.), *Principles of behavioral neurology.* Philadelphia: F.A. Davis.

Benton, A.L., Eslinger, P.J., & Damasio, R. (1981). Normative observations on neuropsychological test performance in old age. *Journal of Clinical Neuropyschology, 3,* 33-42.

Beyn, E.S., & Shokhor-Trotskaya, M.K. (1966). The preventive method of speech rehabilitation in aphasia. *Cortex* 2, 96-108.

Bloom, L., & Lahey, M. (1978). *Language development and language disorders.* New York: John Wiley.

Blumstein, S., & Cooper, W. (1974). Hemispheric processing of intonation contours. *Cortex, 10,* 146-158.

Blumstein, S., & Goodglass, H. (1972). The perception of stress as a semantic cue in aphasia. *Journal of Speech and Hearing Research, 15,* 800-806.

Bolton, S.O., & Dashiell, S.E. (1984). *Interaction checklist for augmentative communication: An observational tool to assess interactive behavior.* Idyllwild, CA: Imaginart Communication Products.

Borod, J.C. (1992). Interhemispheric and intrahemispheric control of emotion: A focus on unilateral brain damage. *Journal of Consulting and Clinical Psychiatry, 60,* 339-348.

Boss, B.J. (1984a). Dysphasia, dyspraxia, and dysarthria: distinguishing features, part 1. *Journal of Neurosurgical Nursing, 16,* 151-160.

Boss, B.J. (1984b). Dysphasia, dyspraxia, and dysarthria: Distinguishing features, part 2. *Journal of Neurosurgical Nursing, 16,* 211-216.

Boss, B.J. (1991). Cognitive systems: Nursing Assessment and management in the critical care environment. *AACN Clinical Issues in Critical Care Nursing, 2,* 685-698.

Broca, P. (1965). Sur la faculte du langage articule, *Bulletin of Social Anthropology, 6,* 337-393.

Broida, H. (1979). *Coping with stroke: Communication breakdown within brain injured adults.* San Diego: College Hill Press.

Brookshire, R.H. (1969). Probability learning by aphasic subjects. *Journal of Speech and Hearing Research, 12,* 857-864.

Buck, R., & Duffy, R. (1980). Nonverbal communication of affect in brain damaged patients. *Cortex, 16,* 351-362.

Burfield, E., & Zangwell, O.L. (1946). Re-education in aphasia: A review of 70 cases. *Journal of Neurology, Neurosurgery and Pyschiatry, 9,* 75-79.

Cancelliere, A.E., & Kertesz, A. (1990). Lesion localization in acquired deficits of emotional expression and comprehension. *Brain and Cognition, 13,* 133-147.

Chomsky, N. (1978). *Syntactic structures.* The Hague: Mouton.

Ciconi, M., Wapner, W., Foldi, N., Zuriff, E., & Gardner, H. (1979). The relationship between gesture and language in aphasia communication. *Brain and Language, 8,* 324-349.

Code C. (1987). *Language, aphasia and the right hemisphere,* Chichester: John Wiley & Sons.

Critchley, M. (1970). *Aphasiology and other aspects of language.* London: Edward Arnold.

Crystal, D. (1969). *Prosodic systems and intonation in English.* Cambridge, England: Cambridge University Press.

Crystal, D. (1975). *The English tone of voice.* New York: St. Martin's.

Culton, G.L. (1969). Spontaneous recovery from aphasia. *Journal of Speech and Hearing Research, 12,* 825-832.

Culton, G.L. (1971). Reaction to age as a factor in chronic aphasia in stroke patients. *Journal of Speech and Hearing Disorders, 36,* 563-564.

Danly, M., Cooper, W.E., & Shapiro, B. (1983). Fundamental frequency, language processing, and linguistic structure in Wernicke's aphasia. *Brain and Language, 19,* 1-24.

Danly, M., & Shapiro, B. (1982). Speech prosody in Broca's aphasia. *Brain and Language, 16,* 171-190.

Darley, F.L. (1975). Treatment of acquired aphasia. In W.J. Friedlander (Ed.), *Advances in neurology* (Vol. 7) (pp. 111-145). New York: Raven Press.

Darley, F.L., Aronson, A.E., & Brown, J.R. (1969a). Clusters of deviant speech dimensions in the dysarthrias. *Journal of Speech and Hearing Research, 12,* 462-496.

Darley, F.L., Aronson, A.E., & Brown, J.R. (1969b). Differential diagnostic patterns of dysarthria. *Journal of Speech and Hearing Research, 12,* 246-269.

David, R., Enderby, P., & Bainton, D. (1982). Treatment of acquired aphasia: Speech therapists and volunteers compared. *Journal of Neurology, Neurosurgery and Psychiatry, 45,* 957-961.

Dent, C.H. (1990). An ecological approach to language development: An alternative functionalism. *Developmental Psychobiology, 23,* 679-703.

De Renzi, E., Motti, F., & Nichelli, P. (1980). Imitating gestures: A quantitative approach to ideomotor apraxia. *Archives of Neurology, 37,* 6-10.

Ehrlich, J., & Spies, A. (1985). Group treatment of communication skills for head trauma patients. *Cognitive Rehabilitation, 3,* 32-37.

Enderby, P., & Crow, E. (1990). Long-term recovery patterns of severe dysarthria following head injury. *British Journal of Disorders of Communication, 25,* 341-354.

Feldman, H.M., Holland, A.L., Kemp, S.S., & Janosky, J.E. (1992). Language development after unilateral brain injury, *Brain and Language, 42,* 89-102.

Gainotti, G., & Lemmo, M. (1976). Comprehension of symbolic gestures in aphasia. *Brain and Language, 3,* 451-360.

Gardner, H., Zuriff, E., Berry, T., & Baker, E: Visual communication in aphasia. *Neuropsychologia, 14,* 275-292.

Geschwind, N., & Levitsky, W. (1968). Human brain: left-right asymmetries in temporal speech region. *Science, 161,* 186-187.

Gloning, I., Gloning, K., Haub, C., and Quatemberr, R. (1968). Comparison of verbal behavior in right-handed and nonright-handed patients with anatomically verified lesion of one hemisphere. *Cortex, 5,* 43-52.

Goldfarb, R. (1981). Operant conditioning and programmed instruction in aphasia rehabilitation. In R. Chapey (Ed.), *Language intervention strategies in adult aphasia.* Baltimore: Williams & Wilkins.

Goodglass, H. (1980). Disorders of naming following brain injury. *American Scientist, 68,* 647-655.

Goodglass, H. (1987). Neurolinguistic principles and aphasia therapy. In M. Meier, A. Benton, & L. Diller (Eds.), *Neuropsychological rehabilitation* (pp. 315-326). New York: Guilford Press.

Goodglass, H., & Kaplan, E. (1963). Disturbance of gesture and pantomime in aphasia. *Brain, 86,* 703-720.

Goodglass, H., & Kaplan, E. (1983). *The assessment of aphasia and related disorders* (2nd ed.). Philadelphia: Lea & Febiger.

Green, H., & Howes, D. (1977). Conduction aphasia. In H. Whitaker & H.A. Whitaker (Eds.), *Studies in neurolinguistics* (Vol. 3), New York: Academic Press.

Groher, M. (1977). Language and memory disorders following closed head trauma. *Journal of Speech and Hearing Research, 20,* 212-223.

Grossi, D., Trojano, L., Chiacchio, L., Soricelli, A., Mansi, L., Postiglione, A., & Salvatore, M. (1991). Mixed transcortical aphasia: clinical features and neuroanatomical correlates: A possible role of right hemisphere. *European Neurology, 31,* 204-211.

Hagen, C. (1973). Communication abilities in hemiplegia: Effect of speech therapy. *Archives of Physical Medicine and Rehabilitation, 54,* 454-463.

Hanson, W.R., & Cicciarelli, A.W. (1978). The time, amount and pattern of language improvement in adult aphasics. *British Journal of Disorders of Communication, 13,* 59-63.

Harkness, S. (1990). A cultural model for the acquisition of language: Implications for the innateness debate. *Developmental Psychobiology, 23,* 727-740.

Heilman, K.M., Bowers, D., Speedie, L., & Cosletter, H.B. (1983). The comprehension of emotional and nonemotional prosody. *Neurology, 33*(Suppl. 2), 241.

Heilman, K.M., Safran, A., & Geschwind, N. (1971). Closed head trauma and aphasia, *Journal of Neurology, Neurosurgery and Psychiatry, 34,* 265-269.

Heilman, K.M., Scholes, R., & Watson, R.T. (1975). Auditory affective agnosia: disturbed comprehension of affective speech, *Journal of Neurology, Neurosurgery and Psychiatry, 38,* 69-72.

Helm-Estabrooks, N., Fitzpatrick, P., & Barresi, B. (1982). Visual action therapy for global aphasias. *Journal of Speech and Hearing Disorders, 47,* 385-389.

Hill, B.P., & Singer, L.T. (1990). Speech and language development after infant tracheostomy. *Journal of Speech and Hearing Disorders, 55,* 15-20.

Holland, A.L. (1970). Case studies in aphasia rehabilitation, using programmed instruction. *Journal of Speech and Hearing Disorders, 35,* 377-390.

Holland, A.L. (1977). Practical considerations in aphasia rehabilitation. In M. Sullivan & M.S. Kommeara (Eds.), *Rationale for adult aphasic therapy.* Omaha: University of Nebraska Medical Center.

Holland, A., & Harris, B. (1968). Aphasia rehabilitation using programmed instruction: An intensive case history. In H. Sloane & B. Mac Auley (Eds), *Operant procedures in remedial speech and language training.* Boston: Houghton Mifflin.

Holland, A., & Sonderman, J. (1974). Effect of a program based on the token test for teaching comprehension skills to aphasics. *Journal of Speech and Hearing Research, 17,* 589-598.

Jakobson, R. (1964). Towards a linguistic typology of aphasia impairments. In A.V.S. DeReuck & M. O'Connor (Eds.), *Disorders of language* (pp. 21-46). Boston: Little, Brown.

Johnson, J.A., & Pring, T.R. (1990). Speech therapy and Parkinson's disease: A review and further data. *British Journal of Disorders of Communication, 25,* 183-194.

Kean, M.L. (1977). The linguistic interpretation of aphasic syndromes. In E. Walker (Ed.), *Explorations in the biology of language.* Montgomery, VT: Bradford.

Kean, M.L. (1985). *Agrammatism.* San Diego: Academic Press.

Keenan, J., & Brassell, E. (1974). A study of factors related to prognosis for individual aphasic patients. *Journal of Speech and Hearing Disorders, 39,* 257-269.

Kenin, M., & Swisher, L.P. (1972). A study of pattern of recovery in aphasia. *Cortex, 8,* 56-68.

Kent, J.F., Kent, R.D., Rosenbeck, J.C., Weismer, G., Martin, R., Sufit, R., & Brooks, B.R. (1992). Quantitative description of the dysarthria in women with amyotrophic lateral sclerosis. *Journal of Speech and Hearing Research, 35,* 723-733.

Kent, R.D., Sufit, R.L., Rosenbeck, J.C., Kent, J.F., Weismer, G., Martin, R.E., & Brooks, B.R. (1991). Speech deterioration in amyotrophic lateral sclerosis: A case study. *Journal of Speech and Hearing Research, 34,* 1269-1275.

Kertesz, A. (1979). *Aphasia and associated disorders: Taxonomy, localization, and recovery.* New York: Grune & Stratton.

Kertesz, A., & Benke, T. (1989). Sex equality in intrahemispheric language organization. *Brain and Language, 37,* 401-408.

Kertesz, A., & McCabe, P. (1977). Recovery patterns and prognosis in aphasia. *Brain, 100,* 1-18.

Kohlmeyer, K. (1976). Aphasia due to focal disorders of cerebral circulation: Some aspects of localization and of spontaneous recovery. In Y. Lebrum & R. Hoops (Eds.), *Recovery in aphasics.* Amsterdam: Swets & Zeitlinger.

Larsen, B., Skinhoj, E., & Lassen, N.A. (1978). Variations in regional cortical blood flow in the right and left hemispheres during automatic speech. *Brain, 101,* 193-209.

Levin, H., Grossman, R., & Kelly, P. (1976). Aphasia disorder in patients with closed head injury. *Journal of Neurology, Neurosurgery and Psychiatry, 39,* 1062-1070.

Levita, E. (1978). Effects of speech therapy on aphasics' responses to the functional communication profile. *Perceptual and Motor Skills, 47,* 151-154.

Lewis, A. (1936). *Infant speech: A study of the beginnings of language.* New York: Harcourt, Brace & World.

Lincoln, N.B., Pickersgill, M.J., Hankey, A.I., & Hilton, C.R. (1982). An evaluation of operant training and speech therapy in the language rehabilitation of moderate aphasics. *Behavioral Psychotherapy, 10,* 162-178.

Locke, J.L. (1990). Structure and stimulation in the otogeny of spoken language. *Developmental Psychobiology, 23,* 621-643.

Locke, J.L. (1992). Thirty years of research on developmental neurolinguistics. *Pediatric Neurology, 8,* 245-250.

Locke, J.L., & Pearson, D.M. (1990). Linguistic significance of babbling: Evidence from a tracheostomized infant. *Journal of Child Language, 17,* 1-16.

Lomas, J., & Kertesz, A. (1978). Patterns of spontaneous recovery in aphasic groups: a study of adult stroke patients. *Brain and Language, 5,* 388-401.

Loughrey, L. (1992). The effects of two teaching techniques on recognition and use of function words by aphasic stroke patients. *Rehabilitation Nursing, 17,* 134-137.

Luria, A.R. (1970). *Traumatic aphasia: Its syndromes, psychology and treatment.* La Hauge: Mouton.

Luria, A.R. (1973). *The working brain, an introduction to neuropsychology.* Harmondsworth: Penguin.

Mancall, E.L. (Ed.). (1981). *Alpers and Mancall's essentials of the neurologic examination* (2nd ed.). Philadelphia: F.A. Davis.

Marie, P. (1906). Revision de la question de l'aphasie: la troisieme circonvolution frontale gauche ne joue aucun role special dans la fonction du language. *Seminars in Medicine, 26,* 241-247.

Marks, M., Taylor, M.L., & Rusk, H.A. (1957). Rehabilitation of the aphasic patient: A survey of three years experience in a rehabilitation setting. *Neurology, 7,* 837-843.

Marshall, R.C., Tompkins, C.A., & Phillips, D.S. (1982). Improvement in treated aphasia: examination of selected prognostic factors. *Folia Phoniatric, 34,* 305-315.

Meikle, M., Wechsler, E., Tupper, A.M., Benenson, M., Butler, J., Mulhall, D., & Stern, G. (1979). Comparative trial of volunteer and professional treatments of dysphasia after stroke. *British Medical Journal, 2,* 87-89.

Messerli, P., Tissot, R., & Rodriguez, J. (1976). Recovery from aphasia: some factors of prognosis. In Y. Lebrun & R. Hoops (Eds.), *Recovery in aphasia.* Amsterdam: Swets & Zeitlinger.

Mesulam, M-M. (1990). Large-scale neurocognitive networks and distributed processing for attention, language, and memory. *Annals of Neurology, 28,* 597-613.

Miceli, G., Mazzuchi, A., Menn, L., & Goodglass, H. (1983). Contrasting cases of Italian agrammatic aphasia without comprehension disorder. *Brain and Language, 19,* 65-97.

Milner, B. (1968). Visual recognition and recall after right temporal lobe excision in man. *Neuropsychologia, 6,* 191-209.

Milton, S.B., Prutting, C.A., & Binder, G. (1984). Appraisal of communicative competence in head injured adults. In R.H. Brookshire (Ed.), *Proceedings from the clinical aphasiology conference.* Minneapolis: BRK Publishers.

Monrad-Krohn, G.H. (1947a). Dysprosody or altered "melody of language," *Brain, 70,* 405-415.

Monrad-Krohn, G.H. (1947b). The prosodic quality of speech and its disorders. *Acta Psychiatr Neurol, 22,* 255-269.

Monrad-Krohn, G.H. (1947c). Altered melody of language ("dysprosody") as an element of aphasia. *Acta Psychiatr Neurol, 46*(suppl), 204-212.

Monrad-Krohn, G.H. (1963). The third element of speech: prosody and its disorders. In L. Halpern (Ed.), *Problems of dynamic neurology.* Jerusalem: Hebrew University Press.

Murdoch, B.E., Chenery, J.H., Strokes, P.D., & Hardcastle, W.J. (1991). Respiratory kinematics in speakers with cerebellar disease. *Journal of Speech and Hearing Research, 34,* 768-780.

Norman, B., & Baratz, R. (1979). Understanding aphasia. *American Journal of Nursing, 79,* 2135-2138.

Piotrowski, M. (1978). Aphasia: Providing better nursing care. *Nursing Clinics of North America, 13,* 543-554.

Pizzamiglio, L., Mammucari, A., & Razzano, C. (1985). Evidence of sex differences in brain organization from recovery in aphasia. *Brain and Language, 25,* 213-222.

Porch, B. (1967). *Proch index of communicative ability.* Palo Alto, CA: Consulting Psychologists.

Prins, R.S., Snow, C.E., & Wagenaar E: (1978). Recovery from aphasia: spontaneous speech versus language comprehension. *Brain and Language, 6,* 192-211.

Prutting, C., & Kirchner, D. (1983). Applied pragmatics. In T. Gallagher & C. Prutting (Eds.), *Pragmatic assessment and intervention issues in language.* San Diego: College-Hill Press.

Ross, E.D. (1981). The aprosodias: Functional-anatomic organization of the affective components of language in the right hemisphere. *Archives of Neurology, 38,* 561-569.

Ross, E.D. (1985). Modulation of affect and nonverbal communication by the right hemisphere. In M-M. Mesulam (Ed.), *Principles of behavioral neurology* (pp. 239-257). Philadelphia: F.A. Davis.

Ross, E.D., Anderson, B., & Morgan-Fisher, A. (1989). Crossed aprosodia in strongly dextral patients. *Archives of Neurology, 46,* 206-209.

Ross, E.D., Harney, J.H., deLaCoste-Utamsing, C., & Purdy, P. (1981). How the brain integrates affective and propositional language into a unified brain function. Hypothesis based on clinicoanatomic evidence. *Archives of Neurology, 38,* 745-748.

Ross, E.D., Holzapfel, D., & Freeman, F. (1983). Assessment of affective behavior in brain damaged patients using quantitative acoustical-phonetic and gestural measurements. *Neurology, 33*(Suppl. 2), 219-220.

Ross, E.D., & Mesulam, M-M. (1979). Dominant language functions of the right hemisphere? Prosody and emotional gesturing. *Archives of Neurology, 36,* 144-148.

Saffran, E.M., Schwartz, M.F., & Marin, O.S.M. (1980). The word-order problem in agrammatism II: Production. *Brain and Language, 10,* 263-280.

Sands, E., Sarno, M.T., & Shankweiler, D. (1969). Long-term assessment of language function in aphasia due to stroke. *Archives of Physical Medicine and Rehabilitation, 50,* 203-207.

Sarno, M.T. (1980a). Language rehabilitation outcome in the elderly aphasic patient. In L.K. Obler & M.L. Albert (Eds.), *Language and communication in the elderly: clinical therapeutic and experimental issues.* Lexington: D.C. Heath.

Sarno, M.T. (1980b). The nature of verbal impairment after closed head injury. *Journal of Nervous and Mental Disease, 168,* 685-692.

Sarno, M.T. (1981). *Acquired aphasia.* New York: Academic Press.

Sarno, M.T., & Levita, E. (1971). Natural course of recovery in severe aphasia. *Archives of Physical Medicine and Rehabilitation, 52,* 175-179.

Sarno, M.T., & Levita, E. (1981). Some observations on the nature of recovery in global aphasia. *Brain and Language, 13,* 1-13.

Sarno, M.T., Silverman, M., & Sands, E. (1970). Speech therapy and language recovery in severe aphasia. *Journal of Speech and Hearing Research, 13,* 607-623.

Schuell, H. (1965). *Differential diagnosis of aphasia with the Minnesota test.* Minneapolis: University of Minnesota Press.

Schuell, H., Jenkins, J.J., & Jimenez-Pabon, E. (1964). *Aphasia in adults—diagnosis, prognosis and treatment.* New York: Harper & Row.

Schuster, C.S., & Ashburn, S.S. (1986). *The process of human development: A holistic life-span approach* (2nd ed.). Boston: Little, Brown.

Skelly, M., Schinsky, L., Smith, R., & Fust, R. (1964). American Indian sign (AMERIND) as a facilitator of verbalization for the oral verbal apraxic, *Journal of Speech and Hearing Disorders, 39,* 445-456.

Skinner, B.F. (1957). *Verbal behavior.* New York: Appleton-Century-Crofts.

Skinner, B.F. (1972). *Cumulative records: a selection of papers.* New York: Appleton-Century-Crofts.

Smith, A. (1971). Objective indices of severity of chronic aphasia in stroke patients. *Journal of Speech and Hearing Disorders, 26,* 167-207.

Sohlberg, M.M., & Mateer, C.A. (1989). *Introduction to cognitive rehabilitation: theory and practice.* New York: Guilford Press.

Sparks, R., Helm, N., & Albert, M.L. (1974). Aphasia rehabilitation resulting from melodic intonation therapy. *Cortex, 10,* 303-316.

Subirana, A. (1958). The prognosis in aphasia in relation to the factor of cerebral dominance and handedness. *Brain, 81,* 415-425.

Thompkins, C., & Mateer, C.A. (1985). Right hemisphere appreciation of prosodic and linguistic indication of implicit attitude. *Brain and Language, 24,* 185-203.

Thompson, I.V. (1975). Evaluation and outcoming of aphasia in patients with severe closed head trauma. *Journal of Neurology, Neurosurgery and Psychiatry, 38,* 713-718.

Tuchman, R.F., Rapin, I., & Shinnar, S. (1991). Autistic and dysphasic children. I: clinical characteristics, *Pediatrics, 88,* 1211-1218.

Tucker, D.M., Watson, R.T., & Heilman, K.M. (1977). Discrimination and evocation of affectively intoned speech in patients with right parietal disease. *Neurology, 27,* 947-958.

Van Eeckhout, P., Honrado, C., Bhatt, P., & Deblais, J.C. (1983). De la T.M.R. et de sa pratique. *Reeducation Orthophonique, 21,* 305-316.

Van Lancker, D. (1980). Cerebral lateralization of pitch cues in the linguistic signal. *International Journal of Human Communication, 13,* 201.

Van Lancker, D., Canter, G.J., & Terbeek, D. (1981). Disambiguation of dystrophic sentences: Acoustic and phonetic cues. *Journal of Speech and Hearing Research, 24,* 330-335.

Velletri-Glass, A., Gazzaniga, M., & Premack, D. (1973). Artificial language training in global aphasics, *Neuropsychologica, 11,* 95-103.

Vignolo, L.A. (1964). Evolution of aphasia and language rehabilitation: A retrospective exploratory study. *Cortex, 1,* 344-367.

Weigl, E. (1961). The phenomenon of temporary deblocking in aphasia. *Zeitschrift fur Phonetik, Spruchwissen-schaft, und Kommunikationsforschung, 14,* 337-364.

Weinstein, D., & Keller, W. (1963). Linguistic patterns of misnaming in brain injury. *Neuropsychologia, 1,* 79-90.

Weintraub, S., Mesulam, M-M., & Kramer, L. (1981). Disturbances in prosody. *Archives of Neurology, 38,* 742-744.

Wepman, J. (1957). *Recovery from aphasia.* New York: Ronald.

Wertz, R.T., Collins, M.J., Weiss, D., Kurtzke, J.F., et al. (1981). Veterans Administration cooperative study on aphasia: a comparison of individual and group treatment. *Journal of Speech and Hearing Research, 24,* 580-594.

Wexler, K. (1990). Innateness and maturation in linguistic development. *Development Psychobiology, 23,* 645-660.

Whaley, L.F., & Wong, D.L. (1987). *Nursing care of infants and children* (3rd ed.), St. Louis, Mosby–Year Book.

Whaley, L.F., & Wong, D.L. (1991). *Nursing care of infants and children* (4th ed.), St. Louis: Mosby–Year Book.

Zukow, P.G. (1990). Socio-perceptual bases for the emergence of language: An alternative to innatist approaches, *Developmental Psychobiology, 23,* 705-726.

Zuriff, E.B. (1974). Auditory lateralization: prosodic and syntactical factors. *Brain and Language, 1,* 391-404.

Zuriff, E.B., Caramazza, A., & Myerson, R. (1972). Grammatical judgments of agrammatic aphasics. *Neuropsychologia, 10,* 405-417.

SUGGESTED READING

Alexander, M.P., Benson, D.F., & Stuss, D.T. (1989). Frontal lobes and language. *Brain and Language, 37,* 656-691.

Ball, M.J., Davies, E., Duckworth, M., & Middlehurst, R. (1991). Assessing the assessments: A comparison of two clinical pragmatic profiles. *Journal of Communication Disorders, 24,* 367-379.

Buckwalter, K.C., Cusack, D., Sidles, E., Wadle, K., & Beaver, M. (1989). Increasing communication ability in aphasic/dysarthria patients. *Western Journal of Nursing Research, 11,* 736-747.

Caramazza, A., & Hillis, A.E. (1991). Lexical organization of nouns and verbs in the brain. *Nature, 349,* 788-790.

Halpern, H., Darley, F., & Brown, J.R. (1973). Differential language and neurologic characteristics in cerebral involvement. *Journal of Speech and Hearing Disorders, 38,* 162-173.

Kolh, H. (1985, March). *Telegraphic speech and ellipsis.* Paper presented at Conference on Grammatical Processing in Aphasia: Cross-linguistic Studies. Royaumont, France.

Lesser, R. (1978). *Linguistic investigations of aphasia.* London: Edward Arnold.

Lund, N., & Duchan, J. (1993). *Assessing children's language in naturalistic contexts.* Englewood Cliffs, NJ: Prentice-Hall.

Prigatano, G. (1985). *Neuropsychological rehabilitation after brain injury.* Baltimore: Johns Hopkins University Press.

Steele, R.D., Weinrich, M., Wertz, R.T., Kleczewska, M.K., & Carlson, G.S. (1989). Computer-based visual communication in aphasia. *Neuropsychologia, 27,* 409-426.

Von Stockert, T. (1974). Aphasia sine aphasia. *Brain and Language, 1,* 277-283.

Wapner, W., Hamby, S., & Garner, H. (1981). The role of the right hemisphere in the apprehension of complex linguistic materials. *Brain and Language, 14,* 15-33.

Wepman, J., & Jones, L.V. (1964). Five aphasias: a commentary on aphasia as a regressive linguistic phenomenon. In D. Rioch & E.A. Weinstein (Eds.), *Disorders of communication.* Baltimore: Williams & Wilkins.

26

Cognition and Behavioral Patterns

Cindy Gatens, MN, RN, CRRN
A. René Hébert, MS, RN, CRRN

INTRODUCTION

Rehabilitation nurses encounter clients who have experienced cognitive alterations following injury or illness in all rehabilitation settings. The underlying assumptions for rehabilitation interventions with clients who have impaired or altered cognition include an individual's ability to remember and the capacity to learn new information, learning directed self-care; returning to a previous lifestyle; and maintaining independence despite specific deficits in cognitive functioning. The brain is able to recover variably from such injuries and deficits and is able to acquire compensatory capacities to replace deficits that are irrecoverable; the extent of recovery depends significantly on the individual's participation and response to specific therapeutic remediations or training interventions (Kottke & Lehmann, 1990). The expected outcome is coping effectively with the demands of daily living. Although some individuals appear to recover fully, many never return to their preinjury or predisease cognitive status. Rehabilitation nurses collaborate with the client, family, team, and community to facilitate the restoration of cognitive function, to ensure recovery or adjustment, and to capitalize on specific cognitive strengths, as well as manage deficits.

BRAIN FUNCTION

The nervous system is most central to our functioning as human beings. The body receives information, and the brain integrates the information to determine a response from the body. The brain is the command center for the nervous system. The brain controls or influences most organs and cell functions, either directly through nerves or indirectly through hormones.

Reticular Activating System

The brain is divided into various parts. The reticular formation of the brain lies within the central core of the brainstem. It is a system of neurons and their axons, which extend from the brainstem and thalamus to the cerebral cortex. Fibers project diffusely from the reticular core to all areas of the cerebral cortex. This reticular core plus the projections are known as the reticular activating system (RAS), which also is discussed in Chapters 23 and 24. The RAS is responsible for arousal, alertness, sleep, wakefulness, and basic orientation, and alerts the cerebral hemispheres to in-

coming stimuli. If injury occurs to this area, loss of arousal or coma may occur. Cerebral thrombosis, traumatic brain injury (TBI), intracerebral lesions, intracerebral hemorrhage, hydrocephalus, and a variety of metabolic disorders can affect consciousness, leading to confusion and decreased attention when information received from the reticular core is disrupted.

Brain stem

The RAS works in harmony with the brain stem reflexes, which are responsible for controlling circulation and breathing. The midbrain area, plus the pons and the medulla oblongata, comprise the portion of the brain called the brain stem, which serves as a conduction pathway between the spinal cord and other parts of the brain. The brain stem stores cell bodies for most cranial nerves, and each part is responsible for specific reflex centers. Nerve cell nuclei in the midbrain control various visual, auditory, and postural reflexes. The pons area is responsible for the nerve centers that control respiratory rhythm. Since the critical nerve centers for cardiac, respiratory, and vasomotor functions are located in the medulla, any injury to the brain stem may result in death.

Cerebellum

The cerebellum is located behind the brain stem. The purpose of the cerebellum is to coordinate voluntary movement, maintain trunk stability, and maintain equilibrium. Cerebellar function is essential for normal execution of movement. It regulates the rate, force, range, and direction of movement by innervation of opposing muscle groups and cerebellar function. It coordinates all visual, auditory, tactile, and proprioceptive impulses with muscle activity to maintain balance and equilibrium. As a result of an intact cerebellum, a person is able to walk steadily, maintain posture while standing and sitting, and alternate movements with the hands.

The effects of injury to the cerebellum depend on the exact location. Injury to the cerebellum will not cause paralysis but may produce tremors, incoordination of voluntary movement, and ataxic gait as well as decreased muscle tone, mild weakness, or disequilibrium. As a result a person may experience a variety of difficulties with ambulating, dressing, eating, hygiene, work, and recreation. The most common display of cerebellar dysfunction is alcohol intoxication.

Basal Ganglia

Also essential for the execution of voluntary movements is the basal ganglia system, a series of paired structures located in the cerebrum and midbrain, on either side of the thalamus. The basal ganglia include the caudate, putamen, globus pallidus, claustrum, subthalamic nucleus, and substantia nigra. This system regulates the initiation, execution, and completion of voluntary movement and automatic movements associated with skeletal muscle activity—most commonly, swinging of the arms while walking, swallowing saliva, and blinking. Parkinson's disease symptoms reflect disturbances in the basal ganglia system.

Cerebrum

The cerebrum, the largest part of the brain, is made up of two matched hemispheres separated by a longitudinal fissure. The corpus callosum, a band of nerve fibers, connects the two cerebral hemispheres and allows sharing of information between them. The cerebral hemispheres perform motor, sensory, and cognitive functions in specialized areas of the hemispheres. Each hemisphere contains four major lobes (Fig. 26-1) named for the skull bones that lie over them: frontal, parietal, temporal, and occipital.

Frontal Lobes

The frontal lobes appear to be particularly important in the components related to judgment, attention span, abstraction, sequencing thoughts, transference of knowledge from one situation to another, social inhibition, intellectual function, storage of sensory information, and motor activity. Within this lobe is an area called Broca's area. Broca's area is almost always dominant on the left side of the frontal lobe and is responsible for formation of words.

The frontal lobe and the limbic system interact to produce an individual's affective behavior and distinctive personality. The limbic system includes the thalamus, hypothalamus, and hippocampus, and has projections into the RAS and the cortex. The limbic system, located anterior to the brain stem, controls appetite, temperature, water balance, pituitary secretions, emotions, affect (rage, fear, instinct, self-preservation), and autonomic functions. Damage to or malfunction of a person's limbic system may affect a person's sexual behavior, emotional responses, motivation, and biologic rhythms. Figure 26-2 shows a lateral view of the brain.

Parietal Lobes

The parietal lobes receive and interpret sensory impulses from the skin, muscles, joints, and tendons on the opposite side of the body. Sensations interpreted in this lobe include pain, heat, cold, pressure, size, shape, texture recognition of objects, right/left differences, and body part awareness. The right side is usually dominant for perception.

Temporal Lobes and Occipital Lobe

The temporal lobes control hearing, olfaction, and taste. In addition, the temporal lobe of the dominant hemisphere (left side) receives and interprets sounds as words (Wernicke's area). Furthermore, this lobe integrates auditory and

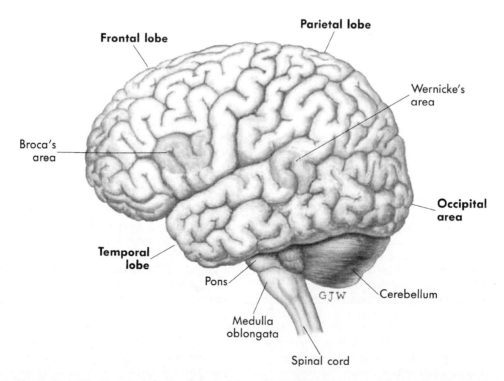

Fig. 26-1 Lateral view of the brain. (From *Neurological Disorders* by E. Chipps, N. Clanin, and V. Campbell, 1992, St. Louis: Mosby–Year Book. Copyright 1992 by Mosby–Year Book. Reprinted by permission.)

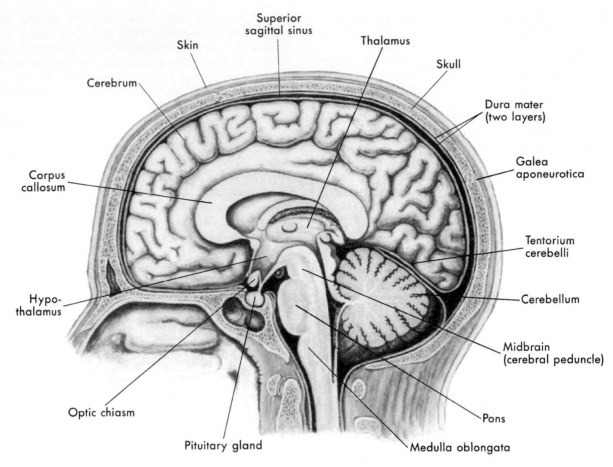

Fig. 26-2 Meningeal layers of the brain. (From *Neurological Disorders* by E. Chipps, N. Clanin, and V. Campbell, 1992, St. Louis: Mosby–Year-Book. Copyright 1992 by Mosby–Year Book. Reprinted by permission.)

visual sensations into an organized thought process, then holds information for short-term memory. The occipital lobe is responsible for the understanding of visual images in both eyes.

The hemispheres participate differently in various kinds of cognitive activity. The left hemisphere appears to be more active in cognitive activities that involve sequences of events, understanding the order of events, communication skills, mathematic sequences, and analytic skills. In contrast, the right hemisphere appears to specialize in situations in which the whole is evaluated, rather than the parts. Spatial and pattern perception and artistic forms of intelligence such as paintings, music, and three-dimensional objects also appear to be predominantly right hemisphere functions. From birth, one hemisphere (usually the left) develops more highly than the other and becomes dominant.

No one area of the brain is the primary section for cognition. Thinking makes up the total of cognitive activities in the brain. It involves remembering, planning, foresight, judgment, abstraction, problem-solving, and scholastic achievement. Functional cognition includes the ability to feel, emote, respond appropriately with joy and sorrow, and have acceptable behaviors. The brain functions as a whole, with lesions of specific areas of the hemispheres producing

characteristic dysfunctions. The location and nature of the insult or disease bear a direct relationship to the physical or cognitive impairments incurred. The thinking that is required to live in society requires the integration of cognitive activities from both hemispheres (Mitchell, Cammermeyer, O'Luna, & Woods, 1984).

CHILDREN AND COGNITION
Childhood Head Injury

Causes of cognitive impairments or alterations vary with age, severity, geographic location, and even season of the year. Children under 1 year sustain brain injuries commonly as a result of abuse. For older children the leading causes of cognitive impairments are falls, recreational activities, motor vehicle accidents (MVAs), assaults, and firearm accidents. Falls account for the largest number of head injuries in children (closed head injury [CHI]), whereas MVAs account for the largest number of severe injuries (Nelson, 1992). A 2-year retrospective descriptive study revealed that males between birth and under 15 years of age were 1.5 times more likely to sustain head injury than were females. The highest incidence of CHI in the population studied was during the first year and around age 6 years. Transportation-related causes accounted for most of the injuries, and falls were second. Seventy percent of CHI occurred between 2 and 6 AM and between 6 and 10 PM, with fewer CHI during winter than any other season (Henry, Hauber, & Rice, 1992).

Children's rehabilitation process needs differ from an adult program of cognitive rehabilitation. An adult with a cognitive deficit has to relearn what was once known. Children engage in some relearning, but because they are developing rapidly, much of what they encounter will be original learning. For example, a child who has cognitive deficits at age 6 years will learn to write (new learning) for the first time while dealing with the effects of a head injury. New motor function along with cognitive, emotional, social, sexual, and academic development can be affected when a child has a head injury.

Cognitive deficits may complicate the developmental process immensely. Depending on a child's age and stage, different developmental areas are affected (Russo, 1990).

Cognitive Development

Piaget emphasized the importance of early physical experience and motor activity in cognitive and intellectual development. Piaget's theory centers around the concept that motor actions, manipulation of objects, and physical exploration of the environment are the sources from which mental operations and intelligence emerge. According to Piaget's States of Description of Intellectual Development, one stage must be attained before transition to the next stage occurs. Each stage describes a way of thinking that determines how a child will experience and respond to activities in their environment (Ginsburg & Opper, 1988).

The stages of intellectual development (ages are approximate), are as follows:

1. Sensorimotor stage (birth to 2 years)
2. Preoperational stage (2 to 7 years)
   Preconceptual thought (2 to 4 years)
   Intuitive thought (4 to 7 years)
3. Concrete operational thought (7 to 11 years)
4. Formal operational thought (11 to 15 years) (Cox, Hinz, Lubno, Newfield, Ridenour, & Sridaromonp, 1989).

Cognitive development is a process that occurs as children grow, mature, and interact with their environment. All knowledge derives from actions the child performs within his environment. The development of spatial concepts begins in infancy. As the child moves, the opportunity to group objects in space and to visualize objects from different points of view are enhanced. As movement experiences continue and the brain matures, children develop an awareness of their body in space. Later, children learn to predict movement, which fosters the learning of academic skills (Rothman, 1989).

In the past a normal, healthy child who suffered a head injury causing cognitive deficits did not receive rehabilitation due to the classical belief that children's bodies and nervous systems would compensate for damage received by different parts of the brain taking over for the damaged parts. However, this belief no longer is accepted. Children's bodies compensate physically better than an adult's body, but cognitively a child's recovery is similar to that of an adult. Therefore children need rehabilitation to speed their recovery and to help their families cope with serious re-

sidual problems or subtle changes in cognition that have not yet resolved. Boyer and Edwards (1991) reported on a study of 220 children and adolescents who had experienced TBI. They measured progress over a 3-year period after injury in the areas of mobility, activities of daily living, education, and cognitive function. According to the study, physical recovery was most rapid in the first year, and cognitive and language gains occurred later, even up to 3 years after injury. Even for those children who were admitted in an unconscious state up to 62 days after injury, there was good potential for recovery. Overall, 14% returned to regular education, whereas 25% remained unable to return to any educational program. The majority of the subjects demonstrated cognitive deficits including perceptual, motor, memory, attention problems, and impulsiveness. Once children with cognitive deficits reach adolescence, there is a tendency for them to develop personality and behavior problems due to cognitive deficits and difficulties in adjusting to residual disabilities. This study confirms that children and adolescents have potential for continued recovery for at least 3 years after injury.

Another study by Jaffe et al. (1992) compared children with TBI with children without injury, individually matched for age, gender, school grade, behavior, and academic performance. Intellectual, neuropsychological, and academic assessments were done 3 weeks after full orientation was achieved. The impairments identified in this study reported that moderately and severely brain-injured children were at risk for problems in the acquisition of academic skills and higher cognitive abilities. Ideally rehabilitation programs for a child with cognitive deficits are provided by a team specializing in pediatrics. Understanding the implications of changes or alterations in pediatric cognitive development is a precursor to understanding normal growth and development. Commonly used tests for screening in children include the following:

1. Denver II Developmental Screening Test (DDST)
2. Pediatric Evaluation of Disability Inventory (PEDI)
3. Bayley Scales of Infant Development
4. Vineland Adaptive Behavior Scales (VABS)

Rehabilitation goals for the child with altered cognition promote age-appropriate growth and maturation. A child's altered cognition impacts the entire family. Education is a key to empowering and enabling family members to become actively participating members of the rehabilitation team. Family and caregiver roles are discussed further in Chapter 13.

AGING AND COGNITION
Cognitive Changes with Aging

Throughout life a person's body is challenged continuously by internal and external stimuli. Aging and/or diseases associated with aging result in altered brain function and can impact the individual, family and community; the financial burden can be overwhelming.

Research findings vary in regard to cognitive changes associated with normal aging. Short-term memory—the process used to acquire and retain information—declines during the aging process. Currently it is believed that older adults may have difficulty with recalling recent material correctly. Results from a metaanalysis study (Bashore, Osman, & Heffley, 1989) support that a generalized proportional decline in mental processing speed among older adults affects all elements of mentation equally; the exception being sensorimotor processes, which show few if any changes.

In addition to short-term memory decline, abilities that involve abstract reasoning, learning of new complex information, and learning of basic information may be impaired with age (DeBoskey, Hecht, & Calub, 1991). Timed cognitive performance tasks, associative memory, logical reasoning, and abstract thinking gradually decline throughout life. Overall, the more complex the mental task, the greater the effects of aging (DeLisa, Curric, Gans, Gatens, Leonard, & McPhee, 1988).

Johansson, Zarit, and Berg (1992) studied 324 people between 84 and 90 years of age over a 2-year interval, finding a small decline in mean scores from five cognitive tests. Their findings show that the average older adult does not regress in all abilities simultaneously. Abilities that require an adult to respond quickly and abilities that involve abstract reasoning decline earlier, whereas abilities acquired through education and those used in daily life decline later.

Cognitive decline in older adults may be related to a decrease in the cerebral reserve. Numerous postmortem studies indicate that brain weight and size are reduced in the older adult. Early studies of the aging brain found cerebral blood flow insufficiency and nerve cell loss as primary causes for memory loss (Maloney & Bartz, 1982). Health and lifestyle are as important as chronologic age in determining when change occurs.

The average healthy adult will maintain the ability to learn and retain adequate memory during normal aging. Long-term memory (storage of long-held knowledge) seems to change little with age. A person's motor skills and language habits also remain intact throughout normal aging. The processes of immediate memory of names and numbers, semantic memory of the context of a meaningful paragraph, remote memory to retrieve information from long-term storage, and retrieval of overlearned material do not seem to decline with age (DeBoskey et al., 1991).

Adults and Traumatic Brain Injury

Older adults may experience various multiple alterations or impairments in cognition following stroke, secondary to illness or drugs, as well as to MVAs or falls. Falls are serious, often preventable problems for older adults. Commonly contributing factors of falls resulting in TBI include postural hypotension, arrhythmias, seizures, medication side effects, alcohol, dementia, visual impairment, altered gait mechanics, and impaired balance or coordination (Goodman & Englander, 1992).

MVAs and pedestrian accidents are the next most common causes of TBI in older adults. Contributing factors for this type of injury are alcohol, previous TBI, and dementia.

A retrospective study (Englander, 1988) found that length of stay in rehabilitation was shorter for older adults (29 days) versus younger adults (45 days) for similar types of TBI. Also, older adults had longer periods of posttraumatic amnesia (PTA) (72% more than 28 days) than did younger persons (33% more than 28 days). As a result of earlier discharge and longer periods of PTA, older people with TBI were more disabled than younger adults on discharge. Davis and Acton (1988) compared discharge outcomes between young adults (under age 25) and older adults (over 50 years). Findings revealed that 85% of the older adult TBI group eventually went home; however, only 50% went directly home from acute rehabilitation. In comparison, 96% of the young adult group returned home directly after acute rehabilitation services. Those in the older adult TBI group who lived with family or friends before injury were more likely to have complete recovery than those living alone or in institutions.

Once an older adult is admitted into rehabilitation, the intensity of the therapy program is tailored to the individual's tolerance. Before rehabilitation, almost all clients have been on bed rest for several days and are deconditioned, presenting greater risks for older adults. An aware rehabilitation team anticipates pacing progress initially in older adults. Long-term outcomes for older adults who suffer from impaired or altered cognition are related to cognitive status, behavioral status, and social situation. When an individual outlives a caregiver/significant other, placement in an extended care facility is common.

NEUROBEHAVIORAL PROCESSES

Intact cognitive function reflects the highly integrated functions of many parts of the cerebral hemispheres, cortex, and subcortical structures. Cognitive function has many components. The most crucial components of cognitive functions involved in carrying out daily living activities are as follows:

- ✦ Orientation
- ✦ Memory
- ✦ Attention
- ✦ Judgment/reasoning
- ✦ Problem-solving
- ✦ Intellectual functioning skills
- ✦ Organization
- ✦ Initiation
- ✦ Sequence
- ✦ Motivation

Orientation refers to the ability to understand self and the relationship of self to the environment: person, place, and time. Those individuals who experience disorientation lack the very basic skills needed to participate in society (Rosenthal, Griffith, Bond, & Miller, 1990).

The ability to remember, or *memory,* is crucial to all other aspects of cognitive function. Memory is a complex process of placing information in memory banks, keeping it there, and producing it when needed. Memory is divided into immediate recall, short-term memory, and long-term memory. Immediate recall, or incidental recall, is the memory ability to recall information from the moment of reception and up to 1 minute after its reception. Short-term memory is the ability to reproduce or recall information from 1 minute to 1 hour after its reception. Long-term memory is the ability to store and retrieve information for more than 1 hour. Long-term memory is practically limitless. Short-term memory appears to be a necessary step in the storage of long-term memories. No specific brain location is associated with long-term memory; it appears that storage of such memory involves the brain as a whole (Mitchell et al., 1984).

Attention refers to the ability to respond to relevant information and to screen out information that is not important (DeBoskey et al., 1991). The three components of attention include alertness, effort or maintenance, and selection. Alertness is the degree of generalized readiness of the central nervous system to receive information. Effort or maintenance is the amount of attention needed for a task. Concentration, persistence, and the ability to maintain focus over long periods of time are examples of effort. Selection is the ability to choose the information while suppressing irrelevant stimuli. Attention is required for information to be coded and stored (Rosenthal et al., 1990).

Judgment/reasoning is the ability to determine what the consequences of a given action may be and the ability to act in a safe and appropriate manner.

Problem-solving is the ability to define and analyze a problem, choose and execute a strategy, and evaluate the results.

Intellectual functioning/thinking comprises remembering, planning, foresight, judgment, abstraction, and the ability to transfer information from one situation to another. Problem-solving is one form of thinking ability. Scholastic achievement is another.

Organization is the ability to establish a consistent relationship between objects, events, or features.

Initiation is the ability to start actions independently, continue, and carry them through to completion.

Sequencing is the ability to perform the steps of a task from start to finish.

Motivation refers to inner forces that regulate behavior in order to satisfy needs and achieve goals. Multiple factors influence a person's motivation to participate in self-care and rehabilitation.

To function as a fully functioning person, the quality and quantity of cognition must be intact. Being independent requires consciousness, mentation, and the ability to integrate cognitive and motor functioning.

PATHOPHYSIOLOGY OF DEFICITS IN COGNITION
Traumatic Brain Injury

TBI and CHI often are used interchangeably in literature and practice. An operational definition is "a structural injury of varying severity, resulting in direct mechanical injury or contusion of the brain cortex and a stretch-shearing, or diffuse axonal injury, of the underlying axons composing the hemispheric white matter and deeper structures" (Berroll, 1992). General physiologic effects that commonly are seen in moderate to severe head injuries include cerebral edema, increased intracranial pressure, sensorimotor deficits, and cognitive deficits (Chipps, Clanin, & Campbell, 1992).

Brain damage is categorized as "focal" or "diffuse" depending on the mechanism or how the damage occurred. Focal damage is discrete damage relatively localized in either hemisphere to produce a specific deficit pattern. Focal damage may result from falls, gunshot wounds, intracranial hemorrhage (including stroke), multiple sclerosis (MS), or brain tumors.

CHI, anoxia, and Alzheimer's disease produce a more diffuse damage to the brain. The primary mechanisms of injury in CHI are coup and contrecoup; coup being the injury to brain tissue at the site of the blow to the skull. With contrecoup the injury is to brain tissue on the opposite side of the brain from the impact, which is caused by the brain literally rebounding inside the skull. These are high acceleration injuries, often secondary to MVAs. Although focal lesions may occur in specific regions of the brain, more often the damage is diffuse and involves both hemispheres. Brain damage from anoxia and Alzheimer's disease produce more widespread deficits (Andrews, 1992). Two terms commonly used in conjunction with TBI are PTA and retrograde amnesia. PTA is the period of time between injury and recovery of continuous memory. Retrograde amnesia refers to the memory loss of the period before injury (Rosenthal et al., 1990).

Mild Traumatic Brain Injury

Much confusion exists over the "correct" definition of mild TBI (MTBI), although current literature reveals that MTBI can result in either little or no sequelae or alternately insignificant and long-lasting disability.

The Head Injury Interdisciplinary Special Interest Group of the American Congress of Rehabilitation Medicine (ACRM) proposed a common definition for MTBI as follows: "A patient with Mild Traumatic Brain Injury is a person who has had a traumatically induced physiological disruption of brain function, as manifested by at least one of the following:

1. Any period of loss of consciousness
2. Any loss of memory for events immediately before or after the accident
3. Any alteration in mental state at the time of the accident (e.g., feeling dazed, disoriented, or confused)
4. Focal neurologic deficit(s) which may or may not be transient, but where severity of the injury does not exceed the following:
   Loss of consciousness of approximately 30 minutes or less
   After 30 minutes, a Glasgow Coma Scale of 13 to 15 (see the following box)
   PTA not greater than 24 hours" (Evans, 1992)

Incidence of MTBI greatly outnumbers the incidence of severe TBI, spinal cord injury, and cerebrovascular accident (CVA) combined. Persons with MTBI can exhibit persistent emotional, cognitive, behavioral, and physical symptoms, alone or in combination, which may produce a functional disability. The symptoms generally fall into one of the following three categories and provide additional evidence that an MTBI has occurred:

1. Physical symptoms of brain injury (e.g., nausea, vomiting, dizziness, headache, blurred vision, sleep disturbance, fatigue, lethargy, or other sensory loss) that cannot be accounted for by peripheral injury or other causes
2. Cognitive deficits (e.g., involving attention, concentration, perception, memory, speech/language, or higher-level executive functions) that cannot be accounted for completely by emotional state or other causes
3. Behavioral change(s) and/or alterations in degree of emotional responsivity such as irritability, quickness

---

GLASGOW COMA SCALE

EYE OPENING

Spontaneous	E 4
To speech	3
To pain	2
Nil	1

BEST MOTOR RESPONSE

Obeys	M 6
Localizes	5
Withdraws	4
Abnormal flexion	3
Extension response	2
Nil	1

VERBAL RESPONSE

Orientated	V 5
Confused conversation	4
Inappropriate words	3
Incomprehensible sounds	2
Nil	1

Coma score (E + M + V) − 3 to 15

From *Management of Head Injuries* by B. Jennetti & G. Teasdale, 1981, Philadelphia, F.A. Davis. Copyright 1981 by F.A. Davis. Reprinted with permission.

---

to anger, disinhibition, or emotional lability that cannot be accounted for by a psychological reaction to physical or emotional stress or other causes (American Congress of Rehabilitation Medicine [ACRM] 1991)

Anoxia/Hypoxic Brain Injury

Anoxic brain injury (ABI) refers to injury to the brain caused by inadequate oxygen supply. The terms "anoxia" and "hypoxia" often are used interchangeably. Although the terms can be used to refer to the oxygen supply of the lungs or bloodstream, it is the lack of oxygen availability at the brain tissue level that causes ABI.

There are three principle mechanisms of brain anoxia:

+ Decreased oxygen moving from the lungs to the bloodstream
+ Decreased circulation of blood to the brain
+ Insufficient amount or ability of red blood cells to delivery oxygen to the brain

Frequently ABI occurs secondary to cardiac arrest. When oxygen supply to the brain is interrupted for an estimated period of time, brain cells die and serious ABI can occur. Although cardiopulmonary resuscitation restores some circulation, it is difficult to estimate the duration and severity of compromise of oxygen supply to the brain. Other causes of ABI include trauma, choking on food, lightning injuries, near-drowning, drug overdose, and perioperative complications (Long, 1989).

Secondary hypoxic damage also can occur after the initial brain insult. Arterial hypoxemia is present in more than a third of severely head-injured persons when they arrive at a major hospital after injury. When arterial Po_2 falls, a desaturation of arterial blood begins to occur, with a consequent fall in the volume of oxygen carried per unit volume of blood. Under normal circumstances this fall in oxygen content would be compensated for by a brisk cerebral vasodilation. In the damaged brain, however, a compensatory boost in blood flow does not occur or occurs to a lesser extent. Thus there is a reduction in oxygen reaching the brain cells in the most severely injured parts of the brain. Causes can range from airway obstruction secondary to blood, foreign bodies, poor positioning, aspiration of gastric stomach contents, and chest injury resulting in pneumothorax, hemothorax, or pulmonary contusion (Rosenthal et al., 1990).

Depending on the severity of the ABI, certain "generic" symptoms may be characteristic as follows:

Mild ABI

+ Decreased attention/concentration
+ Memory impairment (amnesia)
+ Decreased balance
+ Agitation/restlessness

Severe ABI

+ Decreased attention/concentration
+ Memory impairment (amnesia)
+ Agitation (may be persistent)
+ Soft, mumbled speech
+ Dysphagia
+ Balance/coordination difficulty
+ Seizures
+ Spasticity (may be monoclonus—sudden muscle jerking caused by movement)

Most severe ABI

+ Inability to communicate consistently
+ Not fully comatose
    Able to open eyes
    Inconsistent response to the environment

Other symptoms secondary to anoxia/hypoxia are receptive and/or expressive aphasia, apraxia (difficulty performing requested tasks despite adequate comprehension, strength, and coordination), and visual agnosia (inability to recognize something despite seeing it adequately).

Certain parts of the brain are especially sensitive to a lack of oxygen. Symptoms specific to brain regions/lobes occur depending on the severity of the anoxia. For example, anoxia/hypoxia to certain cells in the temporal lobe produces memory difficulty, whereas anoxia/hypoxia to cells in the cerebellum produces balance difficulties. If the oxygen shortage is prolonged and severe, numerous brain cells are damaged and the effects can be severe.

The brain areas affected after ABI differ from those affected by TBI; thus symptoms and course of recovery differ. For instance, anoxia injuries occur posteriorly, whereas TBI frequently causes damage to frontal/temporal areas of the brain; ABI causes loss of brain cells, whereas TBI leads to hemorrhage or bruising and edema.

It is very difficult to predict the course of recovery after an anoxic/hypoxic event, since most persons are comatose immediately after an anoxic event, but there are indicators for estimating severity or extent of impairment. One indicator for predicting outcome is pupillary response to light reflex. The duration of time a client requires to follow commands or speak is predictive of the course of recovery. Clients with ABI almost always regain communication abilities within the first 1 or 2 months when continuous recovery is occurring. On the other hand, clients with TBI sometimes show dramatic improvement after several months of unresponsiveness. Others demonstrate initial rapid improvements followed by a decrease in responsiveness, usually between the second and tenth days after anoxia; the reason for this is unknown.

Youth is an asset for recovery in ABI. With mild ABI many older persons become able to return to independent living. For all age groups difficulty in cognition indicates problems with attention, concentration, and memory that can severely limit a person's safety and ability to function independently in society. (Long, 1989).

Multiple Sclerosis

Charcot (1877) first discussed intellectual, emotional, and memory problems in people with MS. In a number of studies since Charcot's observation, broad estimates are that 30% to 50% of persons with MS experience some type of cognitive dysfunction; however, the degree of cognitive impairment has been difficult to define because estimates are dependent on the population studied and the method by which impairment is defined. McIntosh-Michaelis et al. (1991) studied a community-based population of people with MS and described neuropsychological test results. Cognitive impairment was found in 46%, memory impairment in 34%, and failure on tests of frontal lobe function in 33%. Memory impairment was more common in those who had MS for 10 years or more. The use of standardized neuropsychometric batteries in assessing cognitive deficits in MS has revealed even higher estimates of prevalence than studies using briefer bedside screening procedures (Strothcamp, 1991). Screening procedures such as person, place, and time orientation, and questions about family or current events may not indicate deficits. Requesting a history from the person or listening to a life description may reveal that subtle problems exist, thus defining the need for psychometric evaluation. Cognitive symptoms seen in MS can present in three major forms: relapsing and remitting, relapsing and progressive, or chronic progressive (Strothcamp, 1991).

Cognitive deficits commonly seen in MS include difficulty in learning new materials, deficits in verbal and nonverbal memory (may occur at very early stages), difficulty with information retrieval, and deficits in attention and concentration. Clients complain of fogginess, disorientation, or a sense of confusion, especially when fatigued. Sullivan, Edgley, and Dehoux (1990) surveyed 1180 individuals with MS to examine the degree to which they perceived themselves as experiencing cognitive difficulties. A substantive proportion of these individuals perceived that they had cognitive difficulties. Concerns have been raised about the validity of self-report measures of cognitive functioning. Self-report measures of cognitive problems can be useful in identifying cognitive functions not easily addressed by neuropsychological tests, and also can be helpful in pointing out

areas of activities of daily living that can be disrupted by deficits in cognition. Self-report measures are more individualized in regard to disruption in one's life activities because a person's environment is considered in relation to expression of problems.

Rao, Leo, Ellington, Navertz, Bernardin, & Unverzagt (1991) conducted neuropsychological testing on 100 clients with MS and classified them as either cognitively intact or cognitively impaired. After a neurologic examination, clients completed questionnaires on moral and social functioning, had an in-home occupational therapy evaluation, and were rated by a close relative or friend regarding personality characteristics. There were no significant differences between the two groups on measures of physical disability and illness duration. Those clients who were cognitively impaired were less likely to be working, involved in fewer social activities, reported more sexual dysfunction, and had more trouble performing routine tasks than did cognitively intact individuals. These findings suggest that cognitive dysfunction is a major factor in determining quality of life.

Cerebrovascular Accident

A CVA can be defined as an infarction of the brain, causing disruption of brain function due to ischemia or hemorrhage. Stroke is a term for any sudden-onset focal neurologic deficit. Generally the terms are used synonymously. A stroke can be caused by many different events including aneurysm, vascular malformation, emboli, cardiac failure, and hypertension. Rehabilitation following a stroke must take into account the severity of the initial event, the area of the brain affected, the resultant pathophysiology, and the deficits encountered. There are significant differences between the cognitive abilities of persons with left-sided hemiplegia (right hemispheric damage) and right-sided hemiplegia (left hemispheric damage).

✦ Left-Sided Hemiplegia

Persons with left-sided hemiplegia often experience visuomotor perceptual impairment, loss of visual memory, and left-sided neglect. But since this person still may be verbally fluent, the deficit may not be readily apparent. Impulsivity, disorganization in performance of activities of daily living, and lack of insight are all critical elements in safety. Lack of insight and judgment and inability to follow through are huge roadblocks to learning.

✦ Right-Sided Hemiplegia

Clients with right-sided hemiplegia have problems with effective communication. Vocabulary and auditory retention span are reduced. Since the right hemispheric functions of visuomotor perception and visuomotor memory should be intact, these should be utilized in teaching and learning. Early diagnosis of the specific communication problem should aid in the focus of how to plan a rehabilitation program such as limiting words and utilizing visual demonstration and imitation.

Alzheimer's Disease

Alzheimer's disease is a progressive, irreversible neurologic disorder resulting from significant destruction of brain tissue. Research has not yet confirmed what causes the disease but degeneration of specific nerve cells, presence of neuritic plaques, and neurofibrillary tangles pathologically confirm Alzheimer's disease. An autopsy conducted after the patient dies is the procedure used for confirming the actual diagnosis of Alzheimer's disease (Burns & Buckwalter, 1988).

The disease is characterized by progressive cognitive decline. Little is known about the typical rate of decline or the factors that influence the decline. Teri, Hughes, and Larson's (1990) descriptive and exploratory study investigated 106 clients with Alzheimer's disease and assessed them at 1 to 5 points in time, spanning 3 years. At each observation point in time the Mini–Mental State Examination (MMSE) (see Chapter 31) was administered. Baseline information regarding behavioral disturbances (presence/absence of hallucinations, depression, incontinence, wandering, agitation), health status (presence/absence of neurologic, cardiovascular, and other diseases), and descriptive information (gender, age of onset, duration of deficits) was obtained in the first part of the study. A two-stage random effects regression model was used. The data were used in assessing the effect of these behavioral, health, and descriptive measures on the rate of decline. The researchers found that the rate of cognitive decline in Alzheimer's disease is quite variable. Individuals with various health and behavioral problems declined at a rate between 1.4 and 5 times faster than those without such problems. Alcohol abuse, additional neurologic disease, and agitation were significantly related to the rate of decline, whereas the overall number of behavioral and health problems did not significantly affect the rate of decline.

Approximately 10% of persons between the ages of 65 and 75 years and 25% of those over 85 are reported to have some form of dementia (Evans, Funckenstein, Albert, Scherr, Cook, Chown, Hebert, Hennekens, & Taylor, 1989). Sixty percent of the elderly with dementia are reported to have Alzheimer's disease. As the number of older Americans increases from 11.3% in 1980 to 21.6% by the year 2040, the number of cases of Alzheimer's disease is expected to quintuple. The progression of Alzheimer's disease varies, the final stage being reached in some persons in 1 year and in others in 5 to 10 years. Which thought processes will be lost first and which are maintained longest are very unpredictable. Eventually there is complete memory loss, disorientation, and ultimately death. Alzheimer's disease reduces an individual's remaining life expectancy by at least half. Death usually results from the physical deterioration that accompanies the profound cognitive changes rather than the brain pathology itself.

Although "benign forgetfulness" is a familiar characteristic of the aged, the true hallmark of Alzheimer's disease is memory loss for recent events. Memory impairment becomes so severe that the individual is unable to carry on a conversation, follow a line of thought, or recognize familiar persons, places, or objects. The inability to remember, concentrate, calculate, discriminate, and make decisions leads to anxiety, irritation, agitation, withdrawal, and depression. Decreasing control over motor function and decreasing physical strength are the final behavioral alterations that result in institutional placement for people with Alzheimer's disease (Burns & Buckwalter, 1988).

NEUROBEHAVIORAL DEFICITS

The effects of altered cognition can range from minor annoyances to profound disruption of every aspect of living. Most people with cognition impairments from any source may exhibit a broad range of behaviors. These behaviors are apt to be most evident in situations in which the brain is being asked to process multiple stimuli or to respond to new situations. The source or cause of the behavior may be different depending on the type of insult, injury, or disease that the individual has experienced, but the techniques of management often are similar. The following are behaviors that often accompany altered cognition:

+ Disorientation/confusion
+ Apathy
+ Lack of initiation
+ Attention span deficits
+ Impaired judgment
+ Poor problem-solving skills
+ Impulsivity
+ Depression
+ Perseveration
+ Emotional lability
+ Agitation
+ Lack of insight

Disorientation/confusion can be a result of attentional problems, fluctuating states of alertness, and memory problems. An individual often appears incoherent. As a result of the loss in sense of direction, getting lost may be a real problem. The disoriented or confused individual most often will not know where he is, what time it is, or be unable to recall minute-to-minute, hour-to-hour, or day-to-day events in life. As a result the individual is unable to understand his current situation in light of what has happened or will occur in the future.

Apathy presents a bland affect, general lethargy, and low motivation. This behavior may be a result of an individual's frustration over what seems to be an impossible task or confusion. In response to this behavior, the individual may refuse to participate in daily self-care tasks, lose interest, and refuse to get out of bed or participate in rehabilitation.

Lack of initiation is when an individual is motivated to perform an activity but cannot determine how to carry it out. Lack of initiative may be evident when an individual does not experience self-starting and self-directed behavior. This often is mistaken as apathy, but it is important to differentiate the two behaviors.

Those exhibiting *attention span deficits* may be highly distractible by either internal or external events, go off on tangents when a single thought occurs to them, move quickly from one idea to another, and fail to attend for any period of time.

Individuals with *impaired judgment* may misinterpret the actions and intentions of others, may be unable to handle multiple pieces of information simultaneously, and may have an inaccurate perception of strengths and weaknesses. These poor self-monitoring skills can lead to problems with safety and ultimately functional independence.

Those individuals who have difficulty with the high-level skill of *problem-solving* generally have difficulty planning and organizing their thoughts and behaviors, formulating alternative solutions, and comprehending the potential consequences of their choices.

Lack of insight results in denial. These individuals may lack motivation for rehabilitation because they do not have internal feedback about their capabilities. They may blame others for their frustrations.

Impulsivity is the tendency to act without thought of consequences. Impulsive individuals may appear to act quickly, make continuous and unrelenting demands, and grab and reach for everyone and everything.

Depression is sadness that may be evident in social withdrawal, crying, self-degrading comments, anxiety, and irritability.

Perseveration is an individual's reflexive repetition of certain behaviors, either verbalizations or actions. There often is a consistent theme to perseveration, such as "I want to go home" or washing one extremity repeatedly during a bath.

Some individuals demonstrate episodes of *confabulation* where they compensate for memory and other deficits by inventing details to meet their needs. Although it is not done purposefully, it often reflects a person's inability to find other explanations for what is occurring to them. It may serve a purpose for the person, such as anxiety reduction.

Emotional *lability* is the inability to control emotions. It generally is evidenced in easily triggered bouts of crying or laughing even though the individual is not sad or happy. An exaggerated emotion may occur suddenly and then disappear suddenly.

For individuals to function within the social and cultural norms of society, they must be aware of behavioral norms and the feelings and needs of others. Lack of inhibition, or *disinhibition,* is the inability to control verbalizations or behaviors in a socially appropriate way.

Agitation can be generally defined as excesses of behavior. It often is characterized by restlessness, inability to focus or maintain attention, and irritability and may escalate to combativeness.

The cumulative effects of these emotional and behavioral changes often cause problems with personal and social relationships that can lead to increasing isolation for individuals and their families. Since the primary goal of rehabilitation is a return to family and community, simple containment or toleration of inappropriate behaviors within rehabilitation is not enough. The community will not tolerate such behavior. The plan for management should include elimination of socially unacceptable behavior and restoration of self-regulated and socially acceptable responses to environmental demands. The basic premise is to acknowledge an individual's limitation, but assume that with structure and guidance a person can gain control over behavior. It is essential that we teach family members about an individual's cognitive impairment and resulting behavior changes so they can deal with the behaviors appropriately.

ASSESSMENT

The basic function of the neuropsychological assessment is to provide a valid description of the client's mental status, covering both cognitive processes and affective state. Among the major cognitive processes that need to be assessed are attention-concentration, speed of information processing, decision-making, and communication skills. It is equally important that the presence of depression, agitation, and emotional lability be evaluated because these affective disturbances are prime determinants of a patient's ability to participate in rehabilitation.

I. PREINJURY NURSING ASSESSMENT
  A. Data before disease/injury/alteration in thought processes
    1. Medical history in regard to thought processes
    2. Past cognitive and behavioral functioning
      a. Ask family/friends to describe individual's preinjury behaviors and intellectual functioning
      b. Ask family/friends about individual's preinjury recreation, socialization, and occupation
      c. Assess child's level of development preinjury by talking with parents and pediatrician
    3. History of medications/alcohol/substance abuse
    4. History of activities of daily living
    5. History of sleep-wake pattern

CHILDREN'S COMA SCALE (MODIFIED GLASGOW COMA SCALE, RECOMMENDED FOR AGE 3 AND YOUNGER)

EYE OPENING	SCORE
Spontaneous	4
Reaction to speech	3
Reaction to pain	2
No response	1

BEST MOTOR RESPONSE

Spontaneous (obeys verbal command)	6
Localizes pain	5
Withdraws in response to pain	4
Abnormal flexion in response to pain (decorticate posture)	3
Abnormal extension in response to pain (decerebrate posture)	2
No response	1

BEST VERBAL RESPONSE

Smiles, oriented to sound, follows objects, interacts		5
Crying	*Interacts*	
Consolable	Inappropriate	4
Inconsistently consolable	Moaning	3
Inconsolable	Irritable, restless	2
No response	No response	1

Courtesy of Yoon Hahn, M.D. with the help of pediatricians and a neonatologist at Children's Memorial Hospital, Chicago, Illinois

II. POSTINJURY NURSING ASSESSMENT
  A. Data immediately after injury/onset of disease/alteration in thought processes
    1. Assess level of consciousness/cognition/behavior
      a. Glasgow Coma Scale (acute care tool) (see box, p. 578)
        1. Orientation
        2. Pupillary response
        3. Motor capability
      b. Children's Coma Scale (see box, p. 581)
      c. Rancho Los Amigos Levels of Cognitive Function Scale (see box below)
        1. Sequence of recovery from coma
        2. Tracking of behaviors
    2. Assess body systems
    3. Identify onset of symptoms/etiology of impairment
      a. Gradual onset
      b. Sudden onset
    4. Review medications: identify those that could alter thought processes
    5. Monitor for seizures
    6. Observe physical status/motor functioning
    7. Assess level of communication
      a. Verbal
      b. Nonverbal
    8. Assess sensory and perceptual function
      a. Apply tactile stimulation to skin and monitor response
      b. Assess level of responsiveness
      c. Assess visual-spatial alterations
III. ASSESSMENT CONCURRENT WITH REHABILITATION
  A. Data collected throughout rehabilitation process by nurses and members of rehabilitation team
    1. General orientation to person, place, and time
    2. Common bedside assessment for memory
      a. Recall for immediate memory (0 to 60 seconds)
      b. Short-term memory (1 minute to 1 hour)
      c. Long-term memory (greater than 1 hour)
    3. Assess attention span/concentration deficits
    4. Monitor judgment/intellectual functioning and thought content
      a. Examine ability to follow a sequence of commands
      b. Assess ability to problem-solve
        1. Follow simple assignments and instructions
        2. Solve problems and choose alternatives
      c. Assess ability to utilize self-monitoring skills and remain safe
      d. Monitor for phobias, perseveration of thought, or delusions
    5. Assess for changes in behavior
    6. Note changes in medications
    7. Observe patterns of seizures
    8. Monitor vital signs and test values
    9. Observe progression of physical status/motor control
    10. Note patterns of communication/language skills
    11. Monitor changes in sensory and perceptual functioning
    12. Assess ability to perform activities of daily living
    13. Observe motivation and cooperation with rehabilitation program
    14. Note sleep-wake cycles
    15. Assess community and social support systems
    16. Assess tests of orientation, mental clarity, and memory

---

RANCHO LOS AMIGOS LEVELS OF COGNITIVE FUNCTION SCALE: ADAPTED VERSION, 1979

  I. No response to pain, touch, sound, or sight
  II. Generalized reflex response to stimulation/pain
  III. Localized response: blinks to strong light, turns toward/away from sound, responds to physical discomfort, gives inconsistent response to commands
  IV. Confused-Agitated: alert; very active, aggressive, or bizarre behaviors; performs motor activities but behavior is nonpurposeful; extremely short attention span
  V. Confused-Nonagitated: gross attention to environment, highly distractible, requires continual redirection, difficulty learning new tasks, agitated by too much stimulation
  VI. Confused-Appropriate: inconsistent orientation to time and place, retention span/recent memory impaired, begins to recall past, consistently follows simple directions, goal-directed behavior with assistance
  VII. Automatic-Appropriate: performs daily routine in highly familiar environment in nonconfused but automatic robot-like manner, skills noticeably deteriorate in unfamiliar surroundings, lack of realistic planning for own future
  VIII. Purposeful-Appropriate

IV. ASSESSMENT TOOLS
  A. Assess test of orientation, mental clarity, and memory
    1. Common bedside examination
      a. MMSE (Mini–Mental State Examination) measures orientation, attention, short-term memory, ability to register new information, and recall (Chipps et al., 1992),
    2. Common neuropsychological tests
      a. GOAT (Galveston Orientation and Amnesia Test) measures cognition, PTA, and memory functioning (Rosenthal et al., 1990)
      b. Halstead Reitan Battery (HRB) measures problem-solving, attention, vigilance, abstraction, motor speed, and incidental memory. WMS-R (Wechsler Memory Scale–Revised) measures verbal, nonverbal, and memory functioning (Rosenthal et al., 1990)
      c. Luria-Nebraska Neuropsychological Battery (LNNB) measures simple and complex abilities in each sensory area (Bondy, 1994)

Cognitive impairments can impact how well an individual will function in rehabilitation and in society. Neuropsychological assessment tests have been developed to quantitate the severity of cognitive deficits by identifying brain-behavior relationships. For many the deficits are transient, and for some the cognitive deficits are permanent. In either situation a neuropsychological assessment test is used to clarify the nature and type of cognitive deficits. Vast numbers of neuropsychological tests are available. They derive from many scientific and clinical traditions. As a result of diversity in tests, a single index or measure cannot capture the pattern of cognitive strengths and weaknesses. Comprehensive neuropsychological assessment should be done with overlapping tests to survey cognitive functions. Comprehensive sampling permits the analysis of patterns of cognitive performance within an individual client. Once specific deficits are identified and quantified, a plan of individual care can be planned and implemented

NURSING DIAGNOSES

A number of nursing diagnoses can be formulated for the person with impairment in cognition. The following nursing diagnoses from the North American Nursing Diagnosis Association are related to cognition:

  1. *Altered thought processes:* state in which an individual experiences a disruption in cognitive operations and activities.

     Since "thought" is not a concrete entity, it often is conceptualized for the sake of assessment as a set of cognitive processes. Damage to the brain from neurologic disease or trauma can cause alterations in these cognitive processes. Changes may occur in memory, attention span, judgment, intellectual functioning/learning, language/comprehension, problem-solving, motivation, and social interactions.

  2. *Sensory/perceptual alterations* (visual, auditory, kinesthetic, gustatory, tactile, olfactory): state in which an individual experiences a change in the amount or patterning of incoming stimuli accompanied by a diminished, exaggerated, distorted, or impaired response to such stimuli.

     As nursing diagnoses, altered thought processes and sensory/perceptual alterations are both higher-order cognitive processes. A change in either process is likely to produce a change in the other.

  3. *Potential for injury:* state in which an individual is at risk for injury as a result of environmental conditions interacting with the individual's adaptive and defensive resources.

     Safety is a concern in the early phase of recovery of cognitive deficits due to confusion, agitation, and in the later phases due to wandering and poor judgment.

  4. *Self-care deficit:* state in which an individual experiences an impaired ability to perform or complete bathing/hygiene, dressing/grooming, feeding, and toileting.

     This impaired ability to perform self-care can be temporary or permanent and can occur as a result of decreased motor and/or cognitive function.

  5. *Knowledge deficit:* state in which specific information is lacking. It has been defined as an inability to state or explain information or demonstrate a required skill related to trauma/disease management procedures, practices, or self-care health management.

     Knowledge is the lowest level of cognitive learning such as in recalling or remembering information. The process of applying and synthesizing information in problem-solving is a higher level of learning.

  6. *Altered growth and development:* state in which an individual demonstrates deviations in norms from his or her age group.

     There are key aspects of cognitive development at the end of each of three age ranges: early childhood (2 to 5 years), middle childhood (6 to 11 years), and adolescence (12 to 18 years). Neurologic trauma and diseases affecting cognition can have a varied impact on individuals at any age (Rosenthal et al., 1990).

  7. *Altered sexuality patterns:* state in which an individual expresses concerns regarding his or her sexuality. This may occur due to actual or perceived difficulties, limitations, or changes in sexual behavior.

     With clients who have experienced alterations in cognition, both the client and family can be affected by altered sexuality patterns.

  8. *Altered parenting:* state in which the ability of the nurturing figure(s) to create an environment that promotes the optimum growth and development of another human being is at risk of being altered or is altered.

     A parent with an alteration in cognition may be unable to meet the physical/emotional needs of his or her child.

  9. *Altered role performance:* disruption in the way an individual perceives his or her role performance. Problems associated with role functioning include

role insufficiency, role distance, interrole conflict, intrarole conflict, and role failure.

10. *Impaired adjustment:* state in which an individual is unable to modify his or her lifestyle or behavior in a manner consistent with a change in health status.

   The individual with impaired adjustment experiences difficulty handling responsibilities and fulfilling personal needs and goals. A person with deficits in cognition may have difficulty in dealing with the losses and lifestyle changes associated with changed health status.

11. *Self-esteem disturbance:* state in which negative self-evaluation and feelings about self develop in response to a loss or change in an individual who previously had a positive self-evaluation.

   Self-esteem is the valuative component part of self-concept. How a person develops self-esteem depends on the number of repetitive positive experiences in interactions with significant others in the environment. It is the cumulative result of success or failure in these experiences over time. A person with deficits in cognition may recognize these deficits and be less confident.

12. *Social isolation:* state in which the individual has a need or desire for contact with others but is unable to make that contact because of physiologic, biologic, or sociocultural factors. It is a negative state of aloneness. Individuals cannot exist apart from relationships with other people.

   A neurologic disease or disabling injury may bring limitations and barriers to forming relationships for both an individual with a disability and his or her family.

13. *Ineffective family coping:* ineffective, insufficient, or compromised support, comfort, assistance, or encouragement, usually by a supportive primary person (family member, close friend). The client may need this to manage or master adaptive tasks related to his or her health challenge.

   When a family's usual patterns of functioning are disrupted, such as when a family member has experienced major trauma or neurologic disease with hospitalization, role changes, and prolonged disability, coping abilities are compromised.

14. *Altered family processes:* state in which a family who normally functions effectively experiences dysfunction.

   Relationship problems secondary to all the changes that may occur within the family unit with disease or disability are common (Thompson, McFarland, Hirsch, Tucker, & Bowers, 1989).

REHABILITATION INTERVENTIONS

In order for individuals to return as independent members of the community, they need skills that are essential for community living. Cognitive recovery usually occurs based on physiologic recovery after brain damage with restitution and substitution of function (Horn & Cope, 1989). Treatment interventions attempt to impact attention span, memory, language, reasoning, and visual-spatial skills depending on the deficits.

Coma Programs

Many terms have been used in describing programs to improve the level of responsiveness in comatose patients. "Coma arousal therapy," "sensory stimulation," or "coma rehabilitation" are examples. The conceptual proposal is that using a battery of stimuli to provide input via the senses can increase survival and hasten recovery (Horn & Cope, 1989). The effectiveness of coma stimulation is still unproven and thus controversial. The process utilizes periodic introduction of controlled stimuli including familiar strong odors (coffee, chocolate); familiar strong tastes (chocolate, salt, sugar); familiar sounds (family member's voice, favorite music); tactile stimulation with different fabric textures; and sometimes visual stimulation with large, colored cards (Chipps et al., 1992).

Disorientation/Confusion

Intact mentation requires an awareness of one's self. The recall of events, faces, times, situations, and sensations all influence the ability to learn and solve problems. It is imperative that in caring for a person with disorientation that the rehabilitation team works together in providing the individual with a consistent, predictable daily routine.

All clients who are confused should have a calendar in their room and a schedule with them all times—for example, on the arm of the wheelchair or in a shirt pocket. At the beginning of each contact with a client, each team member should review the client's name, team member's name, date, location, and name of the rehabilitation facility. All team members should encourage the person to look at calendars, clocks, name badges, and building signage to reinforce this information. After orienting the client, the staff should explain what is going to happen, using the language and terms at the client's level of understanding. This will increase the client's awareness. Activities are broken down into steps. For example, at end of each contact the client's schedule is used to elicit the next activity; then before leaving, the staff member reorients the person again to signal the activity is ending.

A structured environment is essential to maintaining a client in a constant physical environment. The room, personal belongings, nursing call light, and therapy sessions should remain as unchanged as possible. Consistency can be promoted when a client sees the same personnel daily and follows an established routine of care.

Currently it is not possible to repair or exchange nerve cells. However, with time and effort, memory skill can return by maximizing the use of remaining capacities.

Memory Loss/Attention Deficits

There are two major approaches for dealing with cognitive impairment. The first is individual cognitive retraining, which directly treats primary impairments (e.g., memory) through practice or instruction in compensatory strategies. Compensation strategies are as follows:

1. Teach clients memory mnemonics strategies and use memory aids and devices. Examples to promote memory recall are daily log book, activity board, maps, schedules, or lists.
2. Allow clients more time for encoding information.

Generally the more time spent on encoding, the better the chance of recall.

3. Provide repetition of information and make either verbal or visual associations that will promote remembering the information.
4. Teach clients to organize information in a logical way. For instance, when dressing, teach person to plan event in sequence of bathing, hygiene, underclothes, clothes).
5. Assist clients to anticipate situations when they will need to retrieve information.
6. Provide clients with a consistent, systematic way to remember or retrieve information.

If a daily log book and schedules are being used as memory aids, be sure that every team member and family/friends are all using the same method. The client will learn through repetition to rely on the daily log book for recent past events and the schedule sheet for upcoming activities (Deelman, Saan, & Van Zomeren, 1990).

Many persons with memory impairments can understand nonverbal cues better than verbal suggestions. It is important that the team members try to model calm, cool, and friendly behavior. Calm demeanor will reduce the person's fear and anxiety. The second component of cognitive retraining is the use of reality orientation groups. These sessions are held in a group setting one to three times a day and are led by team professionals. The group sessions should follow a consistent day-to-day format. The primary group goals are to promote orientation, self-esteem, socially appropriate behaviors, and group interactions. Each client's performance should be documented to monitor progress toward orientation.

Clients in the confused-disoriented stage often suffer from attention deficits. The most common form of attention disorder seen in a rehabilitation setting is a short attention span combined with distractibility. It is important to determine the client's attention span before scheduling therapies so as to not expect too much from the individual (Wood, 1990). When communicating with an individual who has a decreased attention span and altered cognitive status, it is important that the message be short, simple, and basic. The client also needs an environment free from noise and other distractions. Time, ranging from seconds to minutes, is needed to process information and to produce a response. Clients with attention deficits may have difficulties with the most basic, automatic activities. If instructed to get dressed in the morning, a client with attention deficits and no physical deficits may not be able to initiate or complete the task. Instead the client should be instructed in sequencing (identifying the components of getting ready in the morning). For example, instruct the client to turn the shower on, test the water, get into the shower, bath self, turn water off, dry self, then get out of the shower, and so on. For each component of the task, cue the client and allow sufficient time to complete it before providing the next cue. Allow disengagement from one task or stimulus before proceeding to another. It is very important that reinforcement and consistency be given when working with a client who has an attention deficit so as to decrease confusion and anxiety. When working with the client, omit interaction, conversation, and distractions for this may cause him to forget his task. As the client progresses, provide him with fewer cues.

In addition to attention span and memory, judgment, knowing, understanding, learning, and perceiving are all components of cognition. Cognitive rehabilitation is not an immediate treatment, such as surgery or medication. It usually involves a variety of strategies carefully matched to the needs of the client. There is no specific treatment that works for all clients with cognitive deficits.

Since clients with impairment in cognition have much difficulty with new learning and generalizing learning to new situations or new behaviors, it is important that treatment focus on skills that can be utilized in solving problems of everyday living. Teach the client to pair new learning with something familiar. For example, if the client is having difficulties remembering to brush her teeth, then have her family bring in her familiar toothbrush, toothpaste, mouthwash, favorite towel, and so on. Label specific items so the client has visual cues to guide her. On the outside of drawers, label items placed within each drawer. By labeling items and having the client utilize familiar items, performance in self-care activities should improve.

Inappropriate Social Behaviors

As a client progresses, incorporate self-monitoring skills. Before assisting a client with a task, have the client identify the steps needed to complete the task. For example, before transferring a client into a wheelchair, have the client state the necessary steps. This will help the client anticipate what will be occurring. In addition to reinforcing self-monitoring skills for tasks, promote self-monitoring of behaviors. Typically the person with cognitive impairments demonstrates inappropriate social behaviors and is unaware of these behaviors. When a client is demonstrating inappropriate behaviors such as perseveration, outbursts, and/or inappropriate conversation it is important to encourage the client to identify the behavior. If the client is unable to identify the behavior or inappropriateness of the situation, then the healthcare professional must define it. Once identified, the healthcare professional must retrain the client. One intervention may be to videotape the client when acting inappropriately and play it back for the individual to provide feedback. Role play can be an effective tool in retraining. It is important that the team provide a consistent, age-appropriate plan in dealing with inappropriate behaviors.

Comprehension Deficits

When dealing with clients who have comprehension difficulties, it is important that the healthcare professional clarify what the client is saying. Strongly encourage the client to ask for clarification. Assess for nonverbal and verbal behaviors that would indicate the degree of understanding. Initially when speaking with the client, do so in one-on-one conversation and not in informal conversations with other clients, family, and staff. Reading is the highest level of comprehensive skills. Provide discussions about events, current news, and items found in print. For example, the client may have the newspaper opened to the sports section as if trying to read it. Acknowledge the interest in sports and provide discussion about the newspaper article.

Reasoning/Problem-Solving Deficits

Another common deficit seen among persons with cognitive impairments is difficulty with reasoning/problem-solving due to lack of understanding of the problem, impulsive behaviors, and poor organization skills. Generally the steps of problem-solving include problem analysis, choosing alternatives based on past experience or knowledge, selection of a solution, execution, and evaluation. Clients with cognitive impairments often have difficulties in deciding vocational choices, social situations, day-to-day living decisions, and personal finances. The client's lack of awareness of a problem and potential alternatives to the problem are the major blocks in recovery of this cognitive skill.

In treating clients with problem-solving skills, the healthcare professionals and family can begin with simple problems that can be controlled. Card games, tic-tac-toe, simple board games, and meal selection are simple choices. Complexity of these tasks should be increased gradually. Computer games, difficult board games, and planning the day's events may be beneficial. Also, develop a problem-solving training program to allow clients to practice responses to common problem situations. Encourage the client to verbally rehearse and say alternative choices out loud before implementing the choice. Provide the client with choices/alternatives throughout each day. Provide positive reinforcement when the client makes an appropriate choice. As the client progresses, gradually introduce common problems that the client might be faced with in the community. Community outings are particularly helpful in testing problem-solving skills in real-life settings.

Computers can be helpful in treating cognitive impairments because a single stimulus can be presented. According to Lynch (1992) several variables should be considered when selecting software for computer-assisted cognitive retraining:

1. How well does client follow instructions?
2. How does client manage the keyboard?
3. How well does client manage other input devices?
4. Are there any problems with vision or hearing?
5. How difficult does client find the software?

All computer software programs should be selected and monitored by professionals on the team.

Many of the computerized treatment programs encourage clients to work through programs for attention training, memory functioning, and intellectual training. It has been found that clients generally improve on the tasks in the computer programs, but the evidence doesn't support that such achievements lead to improvements in real-life tasks requiring attention, memory, and perception (Deelman, Saan, & Van Zomeren, 1990). If computer-assisted cognitive retraining is used, it should not be utilized as a substitute for therapy with the healthcare professional.

Fatigue

Fatigue, lack of motivation, lack of initiative, depression, and deconditioning can limit participation in the recovery process. The client may tire more quickly after each activity. Even activities that normally are relaxing, like taking a shower, can tire a client. In managing fatigue, it is important that activities are monitored and frequent rest periods are provided, especially after strenuous activities.

In situations that show lack of motivation and initiative, clients have difficulty with planning and goal setting. They do not know how to begin, perform a task, or plan the activity, so consequently do nothing. Furthermore, the clients' fear of failure can generate an unmotivated response. In treating clients who are unmotivated, all team members need to involve the clients in goal setting. If the problem is interfering with the therapy program, a contract may need to be established with positive reinforcement behaviors (e.g., if the client participates in all therapies, he will be allowed time off unit with friends in the evening). It is important that the client receive praise/support for participating in task/therapy. Fatigue is discussed further in Chapter 23.

Inability to Initiate

Since initiation is the most challenging part of participation, provide a client with supervision, support, and assistance to begin an activity. For example, if the client is refusing therapy, an option may be to allow the client to choose someone (like a family member) to attend the first 5 minutes with him. If a client asks for assistance, work with the client together in completing the task. Break the task into smaller components. Do not ask the client "Do you want to . . ." for this gives the opportunity to say no. Instead give the client a choice between two activities. Let clients know that they can choose or you will make the choice.

Agitation

During the early stages of recovery from coma, agitation may result from severely compromised cognitive abilities. With many persons difficulties with orientation, memory, attention, judgment, problem-solving, and motivation compound the problem and provide a challenge for the rehabilitation team members working with persons who have brain injury and related behavior problems. Agitated or aggressive persons may be uncooperative, verbally abusive, and physically threatening. Impulsiveness and lack of self-control can cause self-injury or injury to others. Agitated behaviors can occur in the acute care setting, in rehabilitation, or in the community.

In the early recovery period, when clients are emerging from coma, environmental awareness is limited and clients are confused. Clients at Rancho Level III are emerging from coma. They begin to focus visually and track movement; appear alert; exhibit spontaneous, purposeful movement; follow one-step commands inconsistently; and may attempt to communicate (Connell, Borg, Cavaliero, Ross, & Watchmaker, 1992). The management techniques utilized in caring for clients with disorientation are useful in managing agitation outbursts at Rancho Level IV.

Other options for management include nursing actions to control environmental noise and safety. Due to their confusion, the clients are unable to participate actively in the program. Minimize stimulation that may precipitate agitation. Create a safe environment by covering the floor/walls with mattresses or padding. Clients then are allowed to lie on the floor and move around the room. Special beds such as the modified Craig bed or a net bed allow for safe client movement without restraint. Perform in-room or on-unit therapy to minimize movement and distraction since this can increase confusion and disorientation. Schedule a seclusion room, also padded, where the client can stay during an agitated episode.

It is important that surveillance be maintained whenever a person is secluded or isolated. A video camera can be used in the room to monitors all activities and allows continual observation by nursing staff who are outside the room. Physical restraints that provide the least amount of restriction may be necessary to prevent a client from self injury, pulling at tubes, or falling from the bed or wheelchair (Patterson & Sargent, 1990). Padded mitts, wrist restraints, locking bed belts, and lap restraints for the wheelchair could all be useful in preventing injury. Another option for arranging a safe environment is one-to-one monitoring. A staff member or sitter is assigned to be with the client at all times to provide structure, continuity, and continual monitoring. Depending on the actual clinical environment and available resources, management strategies may vary from institution to institution.

Pharmacologic management may be needed temporarily in a person who is recovering from coma but should be used only as necessary to ensure physical safety. When medications are used, it is important to monitor the side effects of sedation and interference with cognitive processes (Rosenthal et al., 1990).

As a person with brain injury becomes more neurologically stable with a higher cognitive level (Rancho Level V), there are other potential interventions that may be helpful in controlling agitation. At this level clients may be more predictable in terms of what causes them to act out. They can become irritable quickly and even combative with apparently little provocation. Flashes of irritability may occur when a client is attempting a task that is difficult. Frustration may occur, and the individual may strike out at someone or become verbally abusive since the ability to inhibit these impulses is disrupted. Agitation usually is not directed at the person who is verbally or physically abused. It is the client's inability to deal with surrounding circumstances or stimuli in an effective manner that produces the agitation.

In the early stages of an outburst, attempt to redirect the person's attention away from the cause of frustration. Elicit the person's attention in a calm manner, present an alternative idea or task, and help guide thinking about a new area. Implement further de-escalation techniques such as attempt to reduce stimulation and noise in the environment and decrease or remove the cause of the behavior, making the person as comfortable as possible. Use gentle talking and reassurance. Since the client may be restless and want to move about during this phase, restraints predictably increase frustration and aggression. Permit as much freedom of movement within a controlled area as possible, allowing the clients to walk until they become tired and less irritable. On the other hand, tired clients are more likely to be frustrated. Structure the person's time as much as possible, allowing time for rest periods. Model calm behavior with calm, relaxed facial expressions. When family members and

staff become upset, they fuel aggressive outbursts from clients. Agitated clients often react to aggressive nonverbal cues from staff more than to what a staff member is saying. Lack of training in behavior management may prevent staff from dealing with aggressive behavior with a confident approach. Many rehabilitation centers provide educational sessions designed to teach how to safely manage aggressive behaviors from clients. The educational component helps staff identify persons at risk for aggressive behavior, discusses de-escalation techniques, and important considerations in maintaining a safe environment. A practice session demonstrates how to physically contain clients who are out of control and dangerous to self or others. Role playing potential situations can help staff gain confidence and trust in their colleagues in dealing with potentially violent situations (Herbel, Schermerhorn, & Howard, 1990). The program also increases the awareness of the staff in maintaining themselves in a safe environment. Suggestions such as staff working in groups of two, avoid leaning over or bending down near a client, maintaining a calm approach, and positioning themselves in a room to allow easy escape are all ideas to incorporate in all plans of care where there is potential for violence. In all cases it is important that staff remain calm and not overreact.

Once the client has sustained memory and attention span and can participate actively in the program, a plan of behavior modification may be helpful in decreasing maladaptive and inappropriate behaviors. Behavior modification is an attempt to modify automatic or behavioral responses by manipulating reinforcement (Wood & Cope, 1989). The person must have the capacity to acquire new information and skills to retain this information. Once it has been determined that a client may benefit from behavior modification, the method of behavior modification and a specific plan must be identified.

Behavior modification can affect two types of behavior. It can affect behavior excesses: irritating behaviors such as physical and verbal aggression, alcohol and drug abuse, and impulsivity. It also can affect behavioral deficits such as social skill deficits, memory loss, and communication deficits (Burke & Wesolowski, 1988).

Behavioral deficits can interfere with participation in and cooperation with therapies, and lack of active participation in self-care can reduce the potential progress that could be achieved as a result of rehabilitation.

Numerous behavioral approaches are utilized in managing behavioral problems associated with brain injury (Wood & Cope, 1989). But the most common approaches used in working with clients in rehabilitation focus on influencing the behavior of an individual during interaction in a social environment. There are basically seven steps in the development of a behavior modification program. It is important that all team members including family are aware of the plan and how to implement it.

1. *Identify target behaviors.* This is the most important step in the program. Define them in an objective definable manner, so that all staff can identify the exact behaviors to be decreased. An example might be a client exhibiting a tantrum—that is, sitting in the wheelchair and shaking arms and legs wildly and screaming.

2. *Identify causes and consequences surrounding the behavior.* This may identify the environmental influences that may cause a behavior to occur. These are events or consequences that follow behavior and either strengthen or weaken that behavior. The consequences that result in an increase or strengthening of a behavior are called reinforcers. Consequences that cause a behavior to decrease or weaken are called punishers.

3. *Identify frequency of behavior.* Each instance of the behavior is recorded in a consistent manner.

4. *Identify new behaviors.* New, alternative desired behaviors must be identified. Since behavior modification is founded on learning theory, the premise is one of teaching new behaviors.

5. *Identify events or consequences that increase or strengthen the desired behaviors (positive reinforcers).* There are two types of reinforcers: learned and unlearned. Unlearned reinforcers do not depend on previous conditioning for their reinforcing power (e.g., food or pleasurable activities). Learned reinforcers have no initial effect on influencing behaviors. Examples are tokens, money, or praise. To make these reinforcing, they must be paired with unlearned reinforcers. For example, 100 tokens may be earned and exchanged for a pleasurable activity.

6. *Determine a schedule of reinforcement.* It is important to give the client an opportunity to perform the appropriate behavior. It may be more achievable if the behavior is broken down into several steps (e.g., the second step is to put his legs into the pants . . .). You would continue with additional steps until the person is able to zip the pants. By breaking the behavior down into simple steps, the person can experience success and receive reinforcement for each step that is learned.

7. *Implement/assess/evaluate and make changes in the program based on outcome.* You must determine whether the program had the desired result. If not, why not? Changes can be made to make it a positive outcome.

Another form of behavior modification program utilizes a seclusion or "time-out" room. Use of the time-out room means providing time out from positive reinforcements to eliminate inappropriate behaviors. The object is to ensure that an inappropriate behavior is followed by no positive reinforcement. There are a number of ways to take away positive reinforcement. Many behaviors can be ignored (verbally and nonverbally) on the spot. But the attention that an inappropriate behavior brings from fellow clients and families may necessitate removal from the situation. A seclusion or time-out room can meet this need. The hope is that implementing behavior management techniques early in rehabilitation will help clients gain control over behavior and prevent chronic behavioral problems that may prohibit a person from reintegrating back into the home and community. The theoretic base for social learning theory is discussed briefly in Chapter 1.

TEAM ROLES

All team members can make a unique contribution to promoting cognitive rehabilitation. The overall goal of the rehabilitation team is to help clients return to their previous lives at home, community, school, and/or workplace, even when there are residual cognitive and/or functional limitations.

Rehabilitation Nurse

In addition to the already mentioned nursing intervention, the nursing goals for a client with cognitive impairment include 24-hour assessment and supervision and the prevention of complications (in relation to safety, nutrition, elimination, coping, sexuality, and mobility). The nurses reinforce and complement the interventions of the rest of the rehabilitation interdisciplinary team.

Occupational Therapist

The occupational therapy goal for a client with cognitive impairment is to enhance performance in daily living. Commonly occupational therapists utilize two approaches: remediated and compensatory mechanisms. Remedial techniques emphasize improvement of impaired skills and mental strategies by using interventions such as computers and practicing activities of daily living. The compensatory approach emphasizes the task itself by using interventions that alter the environment or the use of memory aids (Poole, Dunn, Schell, Tiernan, & Barnhart, 1991).

Physical Therapist

The physical therapist must take into consideration a client's cognitive, emotional, and social consequences when designing and implementing a treatment program. The goal of a physical therapist when working with a person who has cognitive impairment is to influence the cognitive recovery process while addressing the physical management issues.

Clinical Neuropsychologist

The clinical neuropsychologist and psychologists assess and treat problems of cognition, behavior, and emotional adjustment associated with the disability. The assessment component is diverse and covers varying degrees of cognitive, perceptual, motor, personality, emotional, and functional abilities. Psychologists assess and treat problem areas. Intervention strategies include structured cognitive remediation, biofeedback, behavior modification, and other psychotherapies (Fletcher, Banja, Jann, & Wolf, 1992).

Social Worker

The social worker facilitates discharge planning for the person with cognitive impairment. Many times, these clients require 24-hour supervision and care. The social worker works with the person's support system and community resources in developing living arrangements that will provide a safe, therapeutic environment. Also, the social worker provides counseling and support to both the client and family.

Speech/Language Pathologist

The speech/language pathologist provides planned interventions that promote cognitive recovery. For clients who have cognitive problems without obvious speech deficits, speech/language pathologists will focus therapy on developing verbal reasoning, conversational speech, appropriate body language, and sustained eye contact as well as improvement of attention/concentration and higher-level cognitive functions.

Therapeutic Recreational Therapist

The therapeutic recreational therapist provides a person with cognitive impairment with recreational and leisure activities adjusted to any limitations. The goal is to resocialize the persons, promote appropriate social skills, and help in structuring time.

Physician

The physician, typically one who specializes in physical medicine and rehabilitation, establishes a medical diagnosis, prognosis, and prescribes medical management. If physical or chemical restraints are needed to manage a client's behavior, the physician will be required to order them. Also, the physician guides the treatment team in working collaboratively in a treatment plan.

Family

It is important that all the team members work together to obtain maximum cognitive recovery. However, the most important team members secondary to the client are family. The family who understands the team's approach and is involved in and supports the treatment plan will enhance the recovery process. The keys to getting the family involved are education and open communication throughout the continuum from admission through reintegration back to the community. Family coping is discussed further in Chapter 13.

COMMUNITY REINTEGRATION

The rate of improvement for persons with cognitive deficits is unpredictable. Many times individuals are discharged before full cognition recovery. Studies conducted with persons after mild, moderate, and severe brain injury revealed that cognitive and behavioral skills require longer time periods than physical skill to achieve optimal level (Rosenthal et al., 1990).

Throughout the acute rehabilitation phase, the rehabilitation team members must prepare the client and family for discharge. Unless the individual returns to full age-appropriate cognition, a post–acute rehabilitation plan is needed. Many factors must be identified before making a decision about a program: severity of deficits, support systems, functional abilities, financial status, and program availability.

In choosing a post–acute rehabilitation plan, the individual's current needs and future needs must be considered. A community re-entry plan includes planning for the person to live and receive treatment and training in a community setting other than a hospital or rehabilitation center (Rosenthal et al., 1990).

There is sparse information in the literature on the successes and outcomes of persons with cognitive deficits once they have left the acute rehabilitation facilities. But program options are available to help address the long-term care needs of those with cognitive deficits and their families. These programs should be as individualized as possible to promote functional life skills in the home or alternate care options utilizing resources in the community.

RESIDENTIAL PROGRAMS

One community re-entry option for the person with cognitive impairment is a residential program. A residential program provides supervision and care while the persons (referred to as residents) live within the facility. Residential programs are designed to simulate a home environment within a small community. Residents gradually take an increasing responsibility for their own care, meal preparation, laundry, and other basic living skills. It simulates a home environment and is designed as a small community. The individual is a resident of the facility only for the duration of treatment.

DAY TREATMENT PROGRAMS

Many individuals do not go to residential rehabilitation programs because there are very few of them, and it most likely they would be required to live away from their home and family. Another option (and the most common choice) is a rehabilitation day treatment program. A day treatment program allows a client to receive needed therapies, plus counseling and vocational rehabilitation, on a regular basis throughout the week. During the evening, night, and weekends the person is under the supervision and care of someone in their home. The day treatment program is an integrated program that differs from traditional outpatient therapies. A day treatment program intends to reintegrate an individual into daily living and the community.

An important step in cognitive recovery is getting a person back to gainful employment. Since this phase in recovery can span months or years, many persons return to work gradually with continuous monitoring and support.

DAY CARE PROGRAMS

Not everyone who has cognitive impairment will improve to the point of being able to live independently and maintain employment. Families are left to provide constant daily care and supervision, which can cause frustration and burnout. A possible option for managing this type of situation is a day care program. Day care programs are designed to provide cognitive, educational, and resocialization opportunities during set hours and days of the week, usually Monday through Friday. This option relieves the family from having to be with the client constantly, so they can pursue their own employment, and provides the family much needed respite (Deutsch & Fralish, 1991).

CASE MANAGEMENT

In the past the process of advancing the individual with cognitive impairment through the hospital stay and into the community was coordinated and planned by a variety of discharge planners. As a result discharge planning tended to be fragmented and inconsistent; often it was omitted. As a result a client's potential for recovery in a timely, cost-effective manner was hampered. In response, the concept of case management has emerged, prompting coordination of services by rehabilitation nurses. "The rehabilitation nurse case manager uses a goal-oriented approach emphasizing both quality and cost-effectiveness" (McCourt,

1993). External case managers coordinate and synthesize a client's plan of care throughout the client's disability (acute care through re-entry community). Internal case managers employed within a facility work with external case managers and coordinate a client's care so that the client is discharged in a timely and cost-effective manner from their facility. Chapter 8 provides detailed discussion of case management.

A study was conducted (Sargent & Patterson, 1993) to investigate the effectiveness of case management for a post–acute home-based head injury rehabilitation program. The case manager's role in this study was to provide support and coordination of a TBI post–acute home program. All seven clients who participated in the research over a 3-month interval made progress using the case management process. One of the major advantages of this type of treatment program is that the case manager and rehabilitation professional have the chance to develop skills with a client in the environment in which the skill will be used. Issues such as socialization, sexuality, and substance abuse are important to address and perhaps can best be accomplished by those who are working with the client and family in their own home and community.

In summary, in order for a person with a cognitive impairment to make continuous progress, the post–acute rehabilitation program must achieve salience between meeting the client's and family's needs on a daily basis and resolving a way for this individual to participate in society and contribute as possible.

To measure the success of a program, certain outcome criteria should be identified and measured. They may include the following:

1. Client improves memory for orientation and information.
2. Client demonstrates developmentally appropriate cognitive and problem-solving skills.
3. Client compensates for memory loss through use of aids and/or cues.
4. Client demonstrates ability to self-monitor and self-correct inappropriate behavior.
5. Client initiates and completes activities when appropriate structure is provided.
6. Client returns to preinjury environment, social interactions, and activities.
7. Client copes effectively with demands of daily living.

SUMMARY

Working with children and adults who have impairments in cognition requires a nurse to possess knowledge about the structure and function of the brain and the cognitive skills that allow individuals to live and function in society. An assessment of the neuropsychological status of the client who has experienced injury to the brain secondary to trauma, injury, or neurologic disease enables the interdisciplinary rehabilitation team to formulate an individualized plan of care related to cognitive and behavioral deficits.

Nursing interventions complement the interventions of the rehabilitation interdisciplinary team. Educating family members and the client about the disease or injury and the plan of care increases the chance of effective adjustment in dealing with temporary and/or permanent lifestyle changes related to cognition and behaviors.

CASE STUDY

Tina is a 19-year-old who sustained a TBI secondary to an MVA. Traumatic injuries included rib fractures, multiple abrasions, and left-sided frontal/temporal hemorrhagic contusions. After 2 weeks in the neurology intensive care unit, she was transferred to a neurology/trauma unit.

When admitted to the neurology/trauma unit, she was comatose and unresponsive (Rancho Level I: Unresponsive). She received physical and occupational therapies that provided verbal and tactile stimulation, passive range of motion, and splints to prevent contractures. After 1.5 weeks she began to move and make soft verbal sounds (Rancho Level II: Generalized Reflex Response).

During week 3 Tina became more alert. She was able to track movement with her eyes, make sounds in response to stimulation, turn her head toward noise, and squeeze her hand on command (Rancho Level III: Localized Response). At this point she was transferred to a TBI unit for rehabilitation.

By week 4 Tina moved into Rancho Level IV: Confused-Agitated. When awake, she pulled on all her indwelling devices (percutaneous endoscopic gastrostomy, tracheostomy, indwelling catheter), threw her legs over the bed rails attempting to get out of the bed, became combative, and screamed. Maintaining her safety was the rehabilitation team's first priority. A

bed sensor device was applied to her bed to alert staff of her attempts to climb out of bed. A locking bed belt restraint was applied to secure her from falling out of the bed and the reclining wheelchair. A behavior management attendant or sitter maintained one-to-one supervision with her during peak agitation periods. When appropriate, mitten restraints were applied. During week 5 her indwelling catheter was discontinued, and she was placed on a toileting program every 3 hours while awake. Her tracheostomy was discontinued. She began to eat a pureed diet with supervision and was gradually weaned from tube feedings. As a result of not having indwelling devices, she was placed in a protected bed environment and the bed restraint was discontinued.

By week 6 Tina entered into Rancho Level V: Confused-Nonagitated. Tina was speaking now but not everything she said made sense or was appropriate. She was able to participate in self-care activities but her attention span was limited. She could follow simple commands but she wouldn't initiate activity. She was distracted easily and suffered from severe memory impairments. After a splint was placed on her right leg, she could stand and walk with a walker.

During week 8 she entered into Rancho Level VI: Confused-Appropriate. Tina's biggest problem was her inappropriate be-

Continued.

CASE STUDY—cont'd

---

havior. Her outbursts of physical aggression, kicking and hitting, and verbal abuse escalated dramatically. Her behaviors prevented her from participating in her rehabilitation program. She constantly threatened to leave the hospital.

GOAL SETTING

The rehabilitation goal was to achieve behavioral control to allow Tina to participate in her recovery. Tina's only goal is to "go home." The family, parents, and younger sister are frightened by Tina's outbursts and seldom come to visit. The rehabilitation team decided to implement a behavior modification program with active participation of Tina's family.

INTERVENTIONS

The participants involved in developing the plan need to be identified. This may include appropriate rehabilitation team members, client, and family. Before initiating the plan, the family was educated on the behavior modification plan and asked to participate. It was decided that the family would take Tina out on short passes in the evening if she demonstrated appropriate behaviors. Very short-term goals were identified and feedback had to be immediate.

For the first 48 hours, everyone on the team and family observed Tina to clearly identify "target behaviors." Whenever Tina demonstrated an outburst, verbal or physical, it was documented on a tracking flowsheet. The time, activity before the outburst, and description of the behavior were documented. The target behaviors were identified as verbal and physical outbursts. After 48 hours of assessing the target behaviors, the team met and reviewed the findings to determine the causes surrounding the behaviors. It was identified that Tina acted inappropriately during the following situations:

1. When more than one person was interacting with her
2. When therapy schedules were changed
3. During late afternoon and mealtimes

The team limited the number of persons in contact with her by placing a sign at the nurse's station limiting visitors/staff to no more than one person at a time. This included nursing, team members, family, and friends.

The decision was made to do therapies on the unit. Interactions were to be short, simple, and basic. All other environmental stimuli (TV, radio) were to be turned off during interactions.

Also, it was agreed that her schedule would not be changed. If therapy could not be given at the scheduled time, it was canceled rather than rescheduled. Tina's schedule was placed in large print on her wall where she could read it. She also had her schedule taped to the arm of her wheelchair.

Since Tina's outbursts were greatest between 3 and 6 PM, she was scheduled to have quiet time in her room with no therapies, limited nursing contact, and no family or friends at that time. Tina would also eat meals in her room, free from distractions.

After identifying the target behaviors and a plan to minimize causative factors, the behavior plan was developed. Since Tina's primary goal was to go home, it was decided that the positive reinforcement for appropriate behavior would be evening passes with her family. As a result of her short-term memory impairment, impulsive and explosive outbursts, it was decided that she would be given 6 tokens each morning with an explanation by the psychologist of the behavior modification plan. The plan included that

1. Tina would receive 6 tokens at 8 AM.
2. If Tina demonstrated any type of physically or verbally inappropriate behavior, she would be given one warning to correct the behavior. She would be told how to correct the behavior such as the following:
   If hitting/kicking, she would be told to "stop" and "sit still."
   It was suggested that when she felt angry she could throw soft bean bags (kept in a bag on the back of wheelchair) onto the floor.
   If verbally abusive, she would be told to "stop" and "count numbers" and to start counting.
3. If after cueing, she resumed appropriate behavior, her positive behaviors would be acknowledged and praised and she would be reminded that she would keep her tokens and spend time on an evening pass.
4. If her inappropriate behaviors did not subside, then team/family would immediately place her in "time out" (quiet room free of all distractions) until inappropriate behaviors were gone. When removing Tina from quiet room, the purpose for "time out" would be explained, one token removed, and then Tina would resume her schedule.
5. At 6 PM her evening primary nurse would count the number of tokens left for that day. The plan was as follows:
   6 tokens left = 2 hour pass with family
   5 tokens left = 1.5 hour pass with family
   4 tokens left = 1 hour pass with family
   3 tokens left = ½ hour pass with family
   2 tokens left = 15 minutes outside building
   1 token left = 15 minutes off unit with family (canteen area)

Data should be collected/documented throughout the program in order to determine the program's effectiveness. A collaborative effort involving all rehabilitation team members, the client, and family throughout the process is essential. Changes may need to be made based on Tina's response and the outcome.

REFERENCES

American Congress of Rehabilitation. (1991). *Medicine: Definition of mild traumatic brain injury.* Chicago: Author.

Andrews, B.T. (1992). Initial management of head injury. *Physical Medicine and Rehabilitation Clinics of North America, 3,* 249-258.

Bashore, T.R., Osman, A., & Heffley, E.F. (1989). Mental slowing in elderly persons: A cognitive psychophysiological analysis. *Psychology and Aging, 4,* 235-244.

Berrol, S. (guest Ed.). (1992). [Special issue]. Traumatic brain injury. *Physical Medicine and Rehabilitation: Clinics of North America, 3*(2).

Bondy, K.N. (1994). Assessing cognitive function: A guide to neuropsychological testing. *Rehabilitation Nursing, 19,* 24-30, 36.

Boyer, M.G., & Edwards, P. (1991). Outcome 1 to 3 years after severe traumatic brain injury in children and adolescents. *Injury: the British Journal of Accident Surgery, 22,* 315-320.

Burke, W.H., & Wesolowski, M.D. (1988). Applied behavior analysis in head injury rehabilitation. *Rehabilitation Nursing, 13,* 186-188.

Burns, E.M., & Buckwalter, K.C. (1988). Pathophysiology and etiology of Alzheimer's disease. *Nursing Clinics of North America, 23,* 11-29.

Charcot, J. (1877). *Lectures on the diseases of the nervous system.* London: New Sydenham Society.

Chipps, E., Clanin, N., & Campbell, V. (1992). *Neurologic disorders,* St. Louis: Mosby-Year Book.

Connell, K, Borg, M.B., Cavaliero, L., Ross, I., & Watchmaker, A. (1992). From coma to discharge the story of a roller coaster recovery. *Nursing '92,* 44-50.

Cox, H.C., Hinz, M., Lubno, M., Newfield, S., Ridenour, N., & Sridaromont, K. (1989). *Clinical Applications of Nursing Diagnosis: Adult, Child, Women's Health, Mental Health, and Home Health.* Baltimore: Williams & Wilkins.

Davis, C.S., & Acton, P. (1988). Treatment of the elderly brain-injured patient: Experience in a traumatic brain injury unit. *Journal of the American Geriatric Society, 36,* 225-229.

DeBoskey, D.S., Hecht, J., & Calub, C. (1991). *Educating families of the head injured: A guide to medical, cognitive, and social issues.* Gaithersburg, MD: Aspen.

Deelman, B.G., Saan, R.J., Van Zomeren, A.H., (Eds.) (1990). Traumatic brain injury: Clinical, social, and rehabilitation aspects (pp. 104-143, 145-168). Amsterdam: Swets and Zeitlinger B.V.

DeLisa, J., Currie, D., Gans, B., Gatens, P., Leonard, J., & McPhee, M. (1988). *Rehabilitation medicine; Principles and practice.* Philadelphia: J.B. Lippincott Company.

Deutsch, P.M., & Fralish K.B. (Eds.). (1991.) *Innovations in head injury rehabilitation.* New York: Matthew Bender and Co.

Englander, J. (1988). Head injury after 50; How is it different? NHIF Seventh Annual Symposium. 1988.

Evans, D.A., Funckenstein, H.H., Albert, M.S., Scherr, P.A., Cook, N.R., Chown, M.J., Hebert, L.E., Hennekens, C.H., & Taylor, J.O. (1989). Prevalence of Alzheimer's disease in a community population of older persons: Higher than previously reported. *JAMA, 262,* 2551-2556.

Evans, R.W. (1992). Mild traumatic brain injury. *Physical Medicine and Rehabilitation Clinics of North America, 3,* 427-439.

Fletcher, E.F., Banja, J.D., Jann, B.B., & Wolf, S.L. (1992). *Rehabilitation medicine: Contemporary clinical perspectives.* Philadelphia: Lea & Febiger.

Ginsburg, H.P., & Opper, S. (1988). *Piaget's Theory of Intellectual Development, 3rd ed.* Englewood Cliffs, NJ: Prentice Hall.

Goodman, H., & Englander, J. (1992). Traumatic brain injury in elderly individuals. *Physical Medicine and Rehabilitation Clinics of North America, 3,* 441-459.

Henry, P.C., Hauber, R.P., & Rice, M. (1992). Factors associated with closed head injury in a pediatric population. *Journal of Neuroscience Nursing, 24,* 311-316.

Herbel, K., Schermerhorn, L., & Howard, J. (1990). Management of agitated head-injured patients: A survey of current techniques. *Rehabilitation Nursing, 15,* 66-69.

Horn, L.J., & Cope, D.N. (Eds.). Traumatic Brain Injury. (1989). *Physical Medicine and Rehabilitation: State of the Art Reviews, 3*(1).

Jaffe, K.M., Fay, G.C., Polissar, N.L., Martin, K.M., Shurtleff, H., Rivara, J.B., & Winn, H.R. (1992). Severity of pediatric traumatic brain injury and early neurobehavioral outcome: A cohort study. *Archives of Physical Medicine and Rehabilitation, 73,* 540-547.

Johansson, B., Zarit, S.H., & Berg, S. (1992). Changes in cognitive functioning of the oldest old. *Journal of Gerontology and Psychological Sciences, 47,* 75-80.

Kottke, F., & Lehmann, J. (1990). *Krusen's handbook of physical medicine and rehabilitation.* Philadelphia: W.B. Saunders Company.

Long, D.F. (1989). *What is anoxic brain injury?* National Head Injury Foundation, Washington D.C.

Lynch, W.J. (1992). Selecting patients and software for computer-assisted cognitive retraining: Key patient variables to consider. Part 2. *Journal of Head Trauma Rehabilitation, 7,* 106-108.

Maloney, J.P., & Bartz, C. (1982). Aging and memory loss. *Journal of Gerontological Nursing, 8,* 402-404.

McCourt, A.R. (Ed.). (1993). Cognitive-perceptual pattern. In *The specialty practice of rehabilitation nursing: A core curriculum* (3rd ed., pp. 130-146). Skokie, IL: Rehabilitation Nursing Foundation.

McIntosh-Michaelis, S.A.M., Roberts, M.H., Wilkinson, S.M., Diamond, I.D., McLellan, D.L., Martin, J.P., & Spackman, A.J. (1991). The prevalence of cognitive impairment in a community survey of multiple sclerosis. *British Journal of Clinical Psychology, 30,* 333-348.

Mitchell, P.W., Cammermeyer, M., O'Luna, J., & Woods, N.F. (1984). *Neurological assessment for nursing practice.* Reston, VA: Reston Publishing, Prentice-Hall.

Nelson, V.S. (1992). Pediatric head injury. *Physical Medicine and Rehabilitation Clinics of North America, 3,* 461-474.

Patterson, T.S., & Sargent, M. (1990). Behavioral management of the agitated head trauma client. *Rehabilitation Nursing, 15,* 248-249, 253.

Poole, J., Dunn, W., Schell, B., Tiernan, K., & Barnhart, J.M. (1991). Statement: Occupational therapy services management of persons with cognitive impairments. *The American Journal of Occupational Therapy, 45,* 1067-1068.

Rao, S.M., Leo, G.J., Ellington, L., Nauertz, T., Bernardin, L., & Unverzagt, F. (1991). Cognitive dysfunction in multiple sclerosis. *Neurology, 41,* 692-696.

Rosenthal, M., Griffith, E., Bond, M., & Miller, J.D. (1990). *Rehabilitation of the adult and child with traumatic brain injury.* Philadelphia: F.A. Davis Co.

Rothman, J. (1989). Early physical experience and cognitive development. *Clinical Management, 9,* 20-22.

Russo, D.C. (1990). Specialized rehab needs for head injured children. *Continuing Care, February,* 28-32.

Sargent, M., & Patterson, T.S. (1993). Postacute, home-based head injury rehabilitation: An outcome study. *Rehabilitation Nursing, 18,* 380-383, 387.

Saul, R. (1993). Neurobehavioral disorders following traumatic brain injury: Part I. Neurobehavioral sequelae in the early stages of recovery; Part II. Late neurobehavioral sequelae. *Physical Medicine and Rehabilitation: State of the Art, 7,* 581-592, 593-602.

Strothcamp J. (1991). Multiple sclerosis and its effect on cognition. *Rehabilitation Institute of San Antonio (RIOSA), 3*(2),9-15.

Sullivan, M.J.L., Edgley, K., & Dehoux, E. (1990). A survey of multiple sclerosis, Perceived cognitive problems and compensatory strategy use (Part I). *Canadian Journal of Rehabilitation, 4,* 99-105.

Teri, L., Hughes, J.P. & Larson, E.B. (1990). Cognitive deterioration in Alzheimer's disease: Behavioral and health factors. *Journal of Gerontology: Psychological Sciences, 45,* 58-63.

Thompson, J.M., McFarland, G.K., Hirsch, J.E., Tucker, S.M., & Bowers, A.C. (1989). *Mosby's manual of clinical nursing* (2nd ed.). St. Louis: Mosby–Year Book.

Wood, R.L. (1990). Rehabilitating the behavior disordered brain injured patient. In B.G. Deelman, R.J. Saan, & A.H. van Zomeren, (Eds.), *Traumatic brain injury: Clinical, social and rehabilitation aspects* (pp. 101-119). Amsterdam: Swets and Zeitlinger B.V.

Wood, R.L., & Cope, D.N. (1989). Behavioral problems and treatment after head injury. *Physical Medicine and Rehabilitation: State of the Art Reviews, 3,* 123-142.

SUGGESTED READINGS

Antai-Otong, (1993). Cognitive and affective assessment of the geriatric patient. *Medical Surgical Nursing, 2,* 70-74.

Ben-Yishay, Y., & Diller, L. (1993). Cognitive remediation in traumatic brain injury: Update and issues. *Archives of Physical Medicine and Rehabilitation, 74,* 204-213.

Bergman, G., & Thomas, R. (1990). Nursing Care. (Eds.) *Reviews in Physical Medicine and Rehabilitation, 4,* 517-526.

Cook, E.A., & Thigpen, R. (1993). Identification and management of cognitive and perceptual deficits in the rehabilitation patient. *Rehabilitation Nursing, 18,* 310-313.

Cronwall, D., Wrightson, P., & Waddell, P. (1990). *Head injury: The facts, a guide for families and caregivers,* Oxford: Oxford University Press.

Greenwood, R.J., & McMillan, T.M. (1993). Models of rehabilitation programs for the brain-injured adult: Current provision, efficacy, and good practice. *Clinical Rehabilitation, 7,* 248-255.

Helwick, L. (1994). Stimulation programs for coma patients. *Critical Care Nurse, 14,* 47-52.

Jacobs, H.E. (1993). *Behavior analysis guidelines and brain injury rehabilitation; People, principles and programs.* Gaithersburg, MD: Aspen.

Kaplan, C.P., & Corrigan, J.D. (1994). The relationship between cognition and functional independence in adults with traumatic brain injury. *Archives of Physical Medicine & Rehabilitaiton, 75,* 643-647.

Kay, T. (1993). Neuropsychological treatment of mild traumatic brain injury. *Journal of Head Trauma Rehabilitation, 8,* 74-85.

Le, N., Venti, C.R., & Levin, E.R. (1994). Initial assessment of patient cognition in a rehabilitation hospital. *Rehabilitation Nursing, 19,* 293-297.

Lynch, W.J. (1994). Software Update. . . Cognitive rehabilitation (CR) software. *Journal of Head Trauma Rehabilitation, 9,* 105-108.

Radomski, M.V. (March, 1994). Cognitive rehabilitation: Advancing the stature of occupational therapy. *American Journal of Occupational Therapy, 48,* 271-273.

Saul, R. (1993). Neurobehavioral disorders following traumatic brain injury: Part I. Neurobehavioral sequelae in the early stages of recovery; Part II. Late neurobehavioral sequelae. *Physical Medicine and Rehabilitation: State of the Art, 7,* 581-592, 593-602.

Seidel, G.K., Millis, S.R., Lichtenberg, P.A., & Dijkers, M. (1994). Predicting bowel and bladder continence from cognitive status in geriatric rehabilitation patients. *Archives of Physical Medicine & Rehabilitation, 75,* 590-593.

Yeaw, E.M.J. (1993). Identification of confusion among the elderly in an acute care setting. *Clinical Nurse Specialist, 7,* 192-197.

27

Sexuality Education and Counseling

Susan B. Greco, MSN, RN, CRRN

INTRODUCTION

Humans are sexual beings. The answer to the first question following ultrasonography, "Is it a boy or girl?" has a profound effect on a life from infancy to old age. Sexuality is a vital part of being that is a key component of rehabilitation nursing practice. The concept of human sexuality encompasses how one thinks, feels, and acts as a sexual being; needs and drives; expression of maleness or femaleness; gender roles; interactions with others; identity; and body development and function (National Guidelines Task Force, 1991). Who and what we are is incorporated with our sexuality; it is difficult to separate persons from their sexuality. Expressing sexuality through intimate involvement with another is a major developmental task of adolescence and young adulthood and may be lifelong.

The word sexuality refers to all aspects of being sexual including biologic, physical, psychosocial, and behavioral dimensions. Biologic factors largely control sexual development from conception to birth, the ability to reproduce after puberty, and certain sex differences in behavior; and produce physical responses such as those of sex organs or increased pulse rate. The physical side of sexuality affects sexual desire and sexual functioning, and may affect sexual satisfaction. The psychosocial dimension, the sense of gender identity, is shaped by information and attitudes transmitted by parents, peers, teachers, and society. Since sexual behavior is a product of biologic and psychosocial forces, it sheds light on why and how people act, not only what they do (Malek & Brower, 1984). Ultimately sexuality is construct of one's body image and self-concept.

Maslow (1954) identified the sexual drive as a basic human need that must be satisfied before higher needs could emerge. The ability to function as a sexual being depends on an individual's culture, life stage and status, physical and emotional well-being, and available opportunities. Sexuality has played a profound role in human lives throughout history. Essential to reproducing the species, sex influences day-to-day existence and impacts society as a whole. Sex is something we do; it implies the act of intercourse and all the behaviors that surround this act (Selekman & McIlvain-Simpson, 1991).

The positive nonreproductive purposes of sex include the following:

+ Strengthening of pair bonding
+ Fostering intimacy between partners
+ Providing pleasure
+ Bolstering self-esteem
+ Reducing tension and anxiety
+ Demonstrating one's masculinity or femininity (Reinisch, 1990)

The World Health Organization (1975) defined sexual health as "an integration of somatic, emotional, intellectual, and social aspects of sexual being, in ways that are positive, enriching, and that enhance personality, communication, and love." Included in this definition are three basic tenets: (1) the ability of a person to enjoy sexual and reproductive behavior in accordance with personal and social ethics; (2) freedom from fear, guilt, shame, and false information—which impair a sexual relationship and inhibit sexual response; and (3) freedom from organic disease and disabilities that present barriers to sexual and reproductive functions.

Culture defines what is usual and acceptable sexuality and sexual performance in a society, as well as variations of sexual pleasuring. In some cultures women are the sexual initiators, men in others. Sexual positions, presence or absence of kissing, desired duration of intercourse, sexual stimulation, sexual frequency, and intercourse during certain times in the female cycle are governed by cultural norms and prohibitions. Common threads among cultures forbid incest and advocate privacy during sexual relations (Woods, 1988b).

THE NURSE'S ROLE IN SEXUAL EDUCATION/COUNSELING

Personal sexual health is not guaranteed due to altered physiologic responses, psychosocial responses, and behavioral responses. Our social construction for persons with disabilities is as asexual beings, although sexuality is an essential core of their lives. Rehabilitation nurses work with clients who frequently do not experience sexual health; however, sexuality remains a difficult topic for rehabilitation team members. Thus a client encounters attitudes based on misinformation about sexual implications from a disease or disability, misconceptions about the sexual partner's expectations, unrealistic goals for sexual performance, and lack of open communication about the topic from those most available to promote sexual readjustment (Ducharme & Gill, 1990).

Physical disability may limit a person's opportunities for

sexual interaction and alter ability to perform and respond to sexual acts. An individual may compensate for these changes and achieve sexual health. The rehabilitation nurse must be willing to overcome the veil of silence that may surround sexuality and sexual function to help clients reach optimum function after disability. To achieve that goal, nurses must be knowledgeable about sexuality and sexual function, comfortable with their own sexuality, comfortable in discussing sexual function with clients, accept a client's need to know apart from sexual preferences and practices, and accept not discussing sexuality when a client so chooses. How can the nurse be prepared for this role?

Preparation for sexual counseling begins with self-education. To counsel others, the nurse becomes knowledgeable about the following:

✦ Human sexual response
✦ Variety of sexual behaviors existing in society
✦ Prevalence of sexual behaviors
✦ Types of sexual dysfunction
✦ Relationship of age, life events, pathologies, behavior problems, or pharmaceutic agents with sexual function
✦ Professional responsibility for holistic care

Comprehensive Sexuality Education

According to the Sex Information and Education Council of the United States, comprehensive sexuality education should address facts, data, and information; feelings, values, and attitudes; and the skills to communicate effectively and to make responsible decisions (Haffner, 1990). The goals of sexuality education are to

1. Provide information about human growth and development, human reproduction, anatomy, physiology, masturbation, family life, pregnancy, childbirth, parenthood, sexual response, sexual orientation, contraception, abortion, sexual abuse, sexually transmitted diseases (STDs), including the human immunodeficiency virus and acquired immunodeficiency syndrome (HIV/AIDS).
2. Develop values. As a result of sexuality education, people may question, explore, and assess attitudes, values, and insights about human sexuality. Understanding family, religious, and cultural values helps clarify personal values, increases self-esteem, provides insight about relationships with members of both genders, and defines personal responsibility to others.
3. Develop interpersonal skills. Participating in sexuality education can help people develop skills in communication, decision-making, assertiveness, peer refusal skills, and the ability to create satisfying relationships.
4. Develop responsibility. Providing sexuality education helps to develop a concept of responsibility extending to sexual relationships. Informed, responsible people are able to consider abstinence, resist pressure to become prematurely involved in sexual intercourse, properly use contraception, take other measures to prevent sexually related health problems such as teenage pregnancy and STDs, and resist sexual exploitation or abuse (Haffner, 1990).

Nurse Counselor Role

A nurse counselor becomes aware of a personal value system, including biases and beliefs about appropriate and inappropriate sexual behavior; all rehabilitation team members ideally understand their own sexuality. Nurses are never to negate their own beliefs, but while acknowledging the validity of their beliefs should be aware of what they can or cannot acceptably teach and refer clients to other health professionals if conflicts interfere with counseling or education. All persons providing counseling or education have limitations and at times refer to others who are qualified or able to provide the counsel or education the client desires or needs.

The individual is of primary importance in sex education or counseling. When providing sexual counsel, avoid generalizing either from the individual to an entire group or from group data to individuals within the group (Johnson & Kempton, 1981). Certainly there is a place for group classes, especially in rehabilitation and for sharing basic information; however, each client's needs are worth private discussion. Timing is important. For instance, a nurse may help a client restore body image by listening to expressions of grief and anger, then when ready, introducing clients to others who have developed effective coping skills with similar situations.

Holistic care for persons with disabilities means the rehabilitation nurse intervenes when problems of sexual function are discovered, observed, or expressed. Professionals need to be able to communicate with their clients on the client's level, using language the client understands, and be able to discuss sexuality with ease and confidence. Communication skills include active listening, techniques to elicit feelings, strategies for showing acceptance, goal setting, and problem-solving. Qualities of compassion, a sense of humor, patience, perceptiveness, ingenuity, and flexibility are strengths in counseling relationships.

Effective counseling begins with a willing available listener who spends quality time to listen to a client express needs as a sexual being. Empathetic listening and active listening are foundational techniques for counseling, guiding a client through problem-solving toward being comfortable in discussing sexuality, and eliciting specific needs relative to self and family members (Kerfoot & Buckwalter, 1985).

Counseling the Sexual Partner

Counseling the sexual partner involves giving information about how to react to changes in body image, being prepared for what can happen during sexual intercourse, and understanding the effects of medications and certain disabilities on sexual function—all of which can help alleviate the partner's anxiety about engaging in sexual acts (Kroll & Klein, 1991). Both the client and partner may need help in dispelling myths and misconceptions about alternate sexual options. The nurse can act as a validator to confirm that a particular sexual practice is acceptable and will not be harmful. Responses to clients must be appropriate to their sexual lifestyles and needs. The client and partner must make the final decisions concerning the guidelines they can comfortably function within.

The use of past successful coping strategies often will

help a client and partner place events in proper perspective. Nurses and family members can assist a client in identifying strengths and previous successes. The client and partner who can reframe the situation knowing that things have changed, but are not necessarily worse than before, may adjust better with alterations in sexual ability (Kroll & Klein, 1991).

All too often in Western culture, humor is lacking and sexual acts are taken too seriously. Humor can be used, according to Kerfoot and Buckwalter, "to release anxiety, to help clients anticipate potentially embarrassing moments, and can teach the client to help people laugh with him or her as a way of releasing tension associated with changes in sexual functioning" (Kroll & Klein, 1991).

Effective counselors anticipate a client's reactions to surgeries, procedures, or disabilities by supplying information before events and alleviating threats to self-esteem or perceived loss of control. A nurse who counsels clients benefits from experience with numbers of clients with similar disabilities, knowledge of the comprehensive health assessment, and competency in interventions for individuals with various developmental levels, and cultural, religious, and ethnic values.

The PLISSIT model developed by Annon (1976) is useful in helping nurses evaluate their role in sexual counseling. Each health professional is involved in counseling at a level of comfort. The acronym PLISSIT defines possible involvement levels: permission, limited information, specific suggestions, and intensive therapy. As comfort and experience increase, a nurse may employ more complex levels but may refer at any time.

✦ Permission

Permission is given to the client by the nurse to discuss concerns and problems related to sexuality; permission to be a sexual being. For instance, when a client is asked questions concerning sexuality during an admission assessment, the nurse leaves the door open for any questions or discussion by the client. The nurse may give permission through reassurance that the current sexual practices of the client are appropriate and healthy and that worrying about sexual function is common; or permission may be to experiment with new forms of sexual expression.

✦ Limited information

Clients should not leave the rehabilitation setting without limited information concerning how their illness or accident has or has not affected their sexual function. This should be part of the basic information given to each client. It should answer the questions they have concerning their current sexual function.

✦ Specific suggestions

Specific suggestions may be offered by the nurse to address specific concerns. For example, clients with total hip replacements should receive specific suggestions as to positions that would allow for sexual function while not causing hip flexion greater than 90 degrees or external rotation at the hip. Specific suggestions involve direct problem-oriented strategies or referral for specific medical interventions. The suggestions may help clients to rethink the prob-

lem and make changes to alleviate the concern. It may be helpful to have clients practice using the suggestions, perhaps on day passes at home, and to evaluate progress and problems.

✦ Intensive therapy

This is a referral mechanism used to meet the needs of a client whose problems cannot be solved using the preceding three levels. This level of intervention is required by only a few clients but is appropriate for persons with significant psychosocial sexual dysfunctions (Annon, 1976).

Rehabilitation nurses who are uncomfortable with any of these levels should refer the client to team members who are skillful and knowledgeable in specific areas for counseling and education. Team members who may be skilled in sexual counseling include the clinical nurse specialist, psychologist, social worker, rehabilitation counselor, therapy staff, gynecologist, physiatrist, urologist, and sex therapist.

Team Approach to Counseling

In the realm of rehabilitation, the sexual concerns of a client with a disability and the partner can best be managed by an integrated rehabilitation team approach. The nurse's team role functions follow the PLISSIT model discussed previously. The team approach offers the client opportunity for individual or group counseling and the resources of a number of healthcare professionals. Peer counseling may be another avenue in adjustment to a disability. Didactic and informational sessions led by members of the interdisciplinary team, although not sufficient for a behavioral change or resolution of sexual problems, provide a forum for discussion (Girts, 1990).

Many rehabilitation facilities have initiated sexual education programs by first educating members of the designated sexual counseling team by more experienced members, through reading printed information, and by attending seminars. Planned, structured opportunities allow healthcare professionals to desensitize themselves to hearing sexual terms and concepts, evaluate values and cultural practices through role play and small-group discussion, and consider personal feelings and beliefs about sexual behavior for themselves and others. Before they can comfortably assess, intervene, and evaluate problems related to sexual function, rehabilitation team members review information about normal sexual anatomy and physiology and changes associated with various physical disabilities.

Sexuality Across the Life-span

Although sexual counseling is primarily directed toward adults and older persons, sexual counseling is not an adults-only activity. When children and adolescents require sexuality information and counseling, parents are involved in setting up individualized or group sexual education programs for their children. Understandably parents may be anxious concerning sexual education for their children. More often parents will allow sexual education that does not teach only "how to do it" but rather emphasizes sex roles, understanding the body, and socialization skills. The sexual education program should not sexually stimulate the children or motivate them into undesirable behavior. Parents may leave or refuse at any point. Research findings indicate that students who understand their sexuality and the responsibilities that go with it are less likely to encounter sexual troubles than students who are uninformed. However, responsible presenters of sexual education programs do not impose their moral standards or values on their students. Parents have legal and ethical rights to retain primary responsibility for transmitting values and building morality with their children (Johnson & Kempton, 1981).

Rehabilitation nurses and case managers who work with pediatric and adolescent clients may become the providers of sexual education if parents are unable or unwilling to provide this information. In group homes where young persons with chronic, disabling, or developmental delays live, staff may become the providers of sexual information as imparted through daily contacts, as part of the fabric of daily life, as well as formal classes.

Sexual education programs for youth and adolescents include information on responsible sexual behavior such as social skills, how to avoid being sexually exploited, appropriate body exposure, privacy of sexual behavior, responsibility of sexual behavior including abstinence, and how to prevent pregnancy (Johnson & Kempton, 1981). A majority of children with disabilities will experience sexual maturation so they need to be prepared for the changes that will occur in their bodies when sexual maturation begins (Muscari, 1987).

The following information could be shared with parents of children with disabilities to enhance sexual education:

1. Parents should demonstrate acceptance of the child's body.
2. The first experience with love and socialization will be provided by parents and siblings.
3. Social relationships with siblings and friends should be encouraged.
4. Children need to understand the difference between private and public behavior.
5. Children need to learn the role behaviors of the same-sex parent in daily interactions (Selekman & McIlvain-Simpson, 1991).
6. Sexuality information is presented related to a child's age.

Table 27-1 illustrates age-related sexuality education for children.

PHYSIOLOGY OF SEXUAL RESPONSE

For rehabilitation professionals desiring to impart sexual information and counsel to their clients, one appropriate place to start is through learning the physiologic aspects of sexual response. Sexual response is a very complex neuronal phenomenon that involves all divisions of the nervous system, including those governing endocrine activity. To have normal sexual function, the system must be completely connected and able to maintain its homeostatic balance. Psychological desire also must be present for successful sexual performance.

Autonomic and Peripheral Nervous System

Male and female sex organs receive both sympathetic and parasympathetic innervation. In males sympathetic fibers originate from the intermediolateral columns of the spinal cord from T10 to L2 and from the inferior mesenteric ganglion. These fibers merge to form the hypogastric plexus, which provides efferent and afferent innervation to the testes, prostate, seminal vesicles, and vas deferens. Parasympathetic innervation is via the pelvic nerves that are formed

Table 27-1   Sexual information for children and adolescents

Ages 5-8 years	Ages 8-11 years	Ages 12-18 years
Correct name of body parts and their functions	Females should be taught about menses and males about nocturnal emissions	Health maintenance (i.e., regular breast examinations and testicular examinations, both self-examinations and physician examinations)
Differences and similarities between girls and boys	Signs and variability of puberty	
Elements of reproduction and pregnancy	Sexuality as part of the total self	
Qualities of good relationships (friendship, love, communication, respect)	Information on reproduction and pregnancy	Sexuality as part of the total self to include communication, dating, love, and intimacy
Decision-making skills and the fact that all decisions have consequences	Importance of values in decision-making	
	Communication within family unit about sexuality	Masturbation should be practiced privately
Beginnings of social responsibility, values, and morals	Masturbation	Importance of values in guiding one's behavior
Masturbation can be pleasurable but should be done in private	Abstinence from sexual intercourse	How alcohol and drug use influence decision-making
Avoiding and reporting sexual exploitation	Avoiding and reporting sexual abuse	Sexual intercourse and other ways to express sexuality
	Sexually transmitted diseases including HIV/AIDS	Birth control and the responsibilities of childbearing
		Reproduction and pregnancy
		Role of condoms in disease prevention: pros and cons

From "Sexuality Education for Children and Youth with Disabilities" in *News Digest*, 1992, Washington, DC: National Information Center for Children and Youth with Disabilities. Reprinted as desired.

by the preganglionic fibers originating in the intermediolateral nuclei of the sacral spinal cord between S2 and S4. These fibers innervate the penis, prostate, seminal vesicles, and vas deferens. Figure 27-1 provides an illustration of the autonomic nervous system. An afferent parasympathetic system also exists that enters the spinal cord at the posterior roots of S2 to S4 (Horn & Zasler, 1990). The pudendal nerve, a mixed motor and sensory nerve, supplies motor innervation to the pelvic floor from S2 to S4, and the sensory dermatomes are supplied from S2 to S5. This is true

in both sexes. Distally the pudendal nerve becomes the dorsal nerve of the penis or the nerve of the clitoris.

Functionally, in the neurologically intact male, erections can begin through both reflexogenic and psychogenic pathways (Fig. 27-2). Reflexogenic erections are mediated primarily via the autonomic sacral parasympathetics, S2 to S4, and can occur independent of conscious awareness and without brain input. The stimuli to which psychogenic erections are activated come from the brain in the form of mental images or nontactile sensory stimulation including

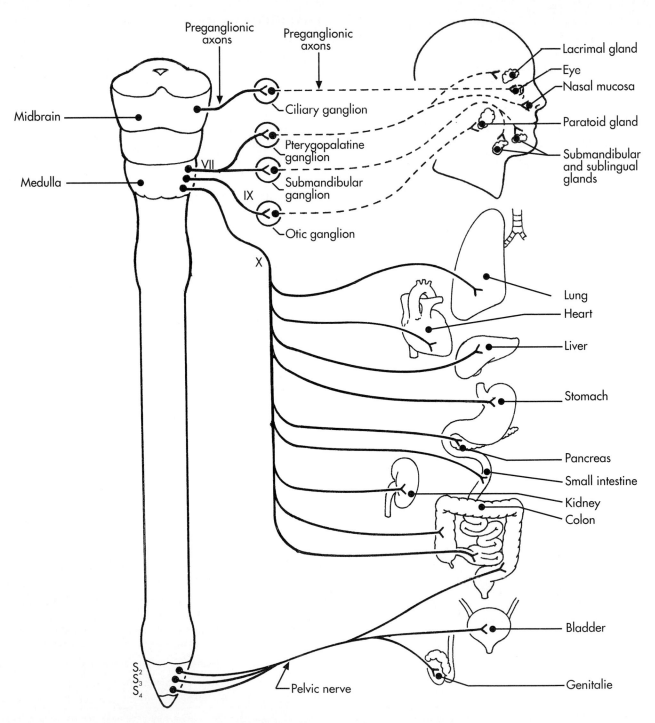

Fig. 27-1 The autonomic nervous system.

Fig. 27-2 Reflexogenic erections and psychogenic pathways in male reproductive organs. (From Woods, NF: *Human Sexuality in Health and Illness*, 3rd ed. by N.F. Woods, 1984, St. Louis: Mosby–Year Book. Copyright 1984 by Mosby–Year Book. Reprinted by permission.)

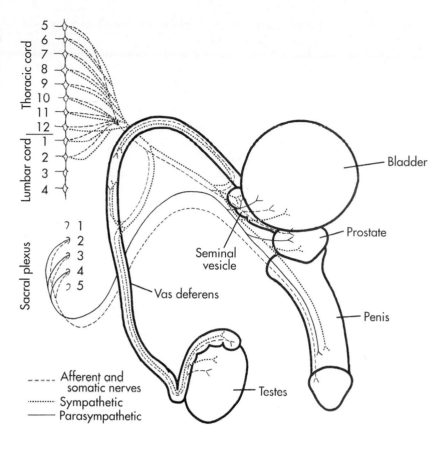

Fig. 27-3 **A,** Psychogenic erection: messages from the brain are blocked at the level of the lesion but may bypass the lesion via the autonomic nervous system. **B,** Reflexogenic erection: sensory nerve (1) relays message to the spinal cord and synapses with the nerve that carries information to the genitals (2) and produces erection. (From *Human Sexuality in Health and Illness* by N.F. Woods, 1984, St. Louis: Mosby–Year Book. Copyright 1984 by Mosby–Year Book. Reprinted by permission.)

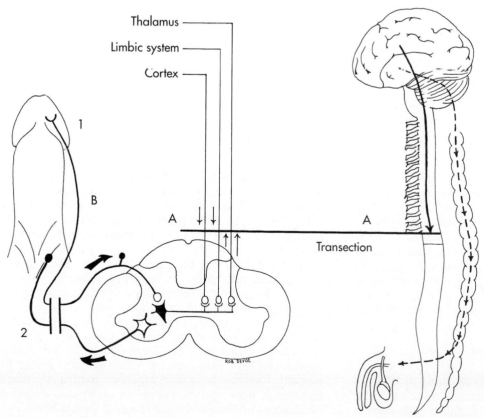

Table 27-2   Spinal cord injury: Level of injury and genital response—complete injuries

Level of injury	Male		Female
T11 and above	Reflex erectile function because sacral cord is intact. No psychogenic erection since sympathetic pathways have been interrupted. Ejaculation is rare.	No sensation	Reproductive function is not affected. Tumescence and vaginal lubrication occur. Orgasm is rare.
T12 and S1	Psychogenic and reflexogenic erections tend to be of poor quality and short duration. Orgasmic and ejaculatory sensations are lost, though seminal fluid discharge may occur. Female response is similar.	No sensation	Reproductive function is not affected.
Sacral injuries	Penile tumescence may occur secondary to sympathetic psychogenic activity; however, erections tend to be inadequate for intercourse. Ejaculation may occur.	No sensation	Reproductive function is not affected. Psychogenic stimulation does not appear to affect the vulva or vagina.

Adapted from "Neuroanatomy and Neurophysiology of Sexual Function," R.J. Horn and N.D. Zasler, 1990, *Journal of Head Trauma Rehabilitation, 5,* pp. 1-13. Copyright 1990 by Aspen. Reprinted by permission.

sights, sounds, tastes, and smells. The stimuli for psychogenic erections travel through the thoracolumbar sympathetics, T10 to L2, to the sex organs (Fig. 27-3).

Semen arriving at the prostatic urethra is dependent on intact hypogastric sympathetic nerve function, whereas true ejaculation results from pudendal nerve activity and the contraction of the pelvic floor muscles. Diseases affecting the peripheral or autonomic nervous system can impair erectile capacity, and almost any pathologic process involving the spinal cord may lead to erectile dysfunction. True ejaculation is rare in males with spinal cord injuries and is especially uncommon with complete quadriplegia (Horn & Zasler, 1990). Table 27-2 displays relationships between level of injury and genital response in males and females following complete spinal cord injury.

In females the sympathetic nerve supply is mixed and is carried by the preganglionic splanchnic nerves and the postganglionic fibers to the ovarian plexus. The parasympathetic nerve supply is through the pelvic nerves via the hypogastric and uterine plexus. The uterus and ovaries receive only sympathetic innervation, whereas the vagina, clitoris, and fallopian tubes receive mixed autonomic innervation. The pudendal nerve acts similarly in females as males (Fig. 27-4).

In females clitoral swelling and vaginal secretions are triggered by parasympathetic activity. Contraction of the vaginal sphincter and pelvic floor occur with stimulation of the somatic pudendal nerves. The autonomic nervous system does not seem to play as critical a role in fertility in females as it does in males. Fertility is a reality for most women with spinal cord injury who were fecund before injury.

Brain Structures and Their Effects on Sexuality

The brainstem plays a role in sexual function to maintain arousal and alertness. Without the brainstem's reticular activating system preparing people to process information,

any behavior would lose its driving force. Libido and potency may require specific activation within certain limbic and cortical structures, initiated by externally or internally generated stimuli. The brainstem also carries motor and sensory messages via the spinal tracts, which allow participation in sexual activity.

An intact thalamus probably plays a role in erection, and lesions in the thalamus have been associated with hypersexuality. Limbic and paralimbic structures play an intrinsic role in sexuality, especially the hippocampus (which may help produce erection), amygdala (associated with hypersexuality), septal complex (associated with erection and a pleasurable sexual sensation), and several hypothalamic nuclei (where damage can result in disturbances in sexual behavior). Temporal lobe epilepsy has been associated with disturbances in sexual function (Horne & Zasler, 1990).

Other higher brain centers affect sexual function. Damage to the frontal cortex may produce disinhibited, sexually inappropriate behavior that may be verbal and devoid of any true sexual arousal or more rarely may lead to increased promiscuity with full arousal. There may be erection or emission difficulties. Injury to the dorsolateral convexities of the frontal lobe produces a more apathetic and akinetic effect. Initiation is impaired, although erection and copulation are possible if the client is led step by step. Frontal injury may affect attention and impair the ability to fantasize.

Problems in the left brain hemisphere can affect sexual function. Language problems, as with aphasias, may impede an individual's ability to comprehend verbal requests or follow directions for sexual activity. Apraxia could impede motor planning for sexual performance. The right hemisphere is more active during orgasm; damage may produce impulsivity, denial, and occasionally euphoria. Visual/perceptual problems may interfere with a person's ability to properly align the body with a partner and hamper interpretation of nonverbal cues or ability to express emotional components of communication (Horn & Zasler, 1990).

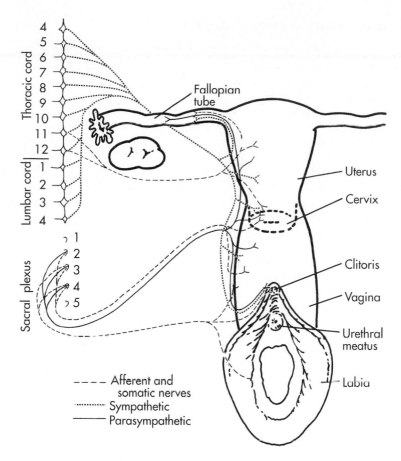

Fig. 27-4 Neurologic bases of female sexual response. (From *Human Sexuality in Health and Illness* by N.F. Woods, 1984, St. Louis: Mosby–Year Book. Copyright 1984 by Mosby–Year Book. Reprinted by permission.)

Influence of Hormones on Sexual Function

Hormones influence sexual activity from the womb throughout a person's lifetime. Damage to brain structures through brain injury or stroke can impact those structures, which regulate the body's hormone balance. This can be seen as secondary hypogonadism or as damage to the pituitary. In the 20% of persons who develop temporal lobe epilepsy following brain injury, 40% to 58% of males are impotent or hyposexual, and up to 40% of females have menstrual abnormalities with reproductive endocrine dysfunction (Horn & Zasler, 1990).

The most important hormone in sexual function is testosterone. Present in both males and females, this hormone is the principal biologic determinant of the sex drive in both men and women. Deficiencies may cause a drop in sexual desire, and excessive testosterone may heighten sexual interest. Too little testosterone may trouble men in obtaining or maintaining erections; except in the area of sexual desire, effects on females are unclear (Masters, Johnson, & Kolodny, 1986).

Estrogens are manufactured by the ovaries and testes. In women estrogen is important for maintaining vaginal elasticity, lubrication, and condition of the vaginal lining, in addition to preserving the texture of the breasts. Excessive es-

trogen in males can reduce libido, affect erection, and enlarge the breasts.

The hypothalamus, through gonadotropin-releasing hormone, controls secretion of two hormones made in the pituitary gland that act on the ovaries and testes. Luteinizing hormone stimulates the testes to manufacture testosterone and the ovary to ovulate. Follicle-stimulating hormone promotes production of sperm cells in the testes and prepares the ovary for ovulation.

There is not a direct relationship between hormones and sexual behavior, although deficient testosterone reduces sexual interest in both sexes. Low hormone levels do not cause loss of sexual ability in all persons, nor do hormone levels predict sexual behavior or interest of a particular person (Reinisch, 1990).

SEXUAL MATURATION

Puberty, the process that leads children from childhood to sexual and reproductive maturity, is marked by various physical, psychological, and social changes occurring on a highly individualized schedule. The process of puberty begins before birth and unfolds throughout childhood as various hormones effect changes in the brain and body. The same hormonal changes that stimulate physical develop-

Table 27-3 Reproductive and sexual changes during puberty

Males		Females	
Between ages 9 and 15	First external changes: testicles grow, scrotal skin becomes red and coarser, few straight pubic hairs appear, nipple areola grow and darken. Muscle mass develops, and height increases.	Between ages 9 and 15	Areola, then breast sizes increase to rounded shape; sparse pubic hair becomes darker and coarser; growth in height, body fat rounds body contours; normal vaginal discharge, active sweat and oil glands, and acne; vagina lengthens, external reproductive organs and genitals grow.
Between ages 11-16	Penis, testicles, and scrotum continue growth; pubic hair becomes coarser, curled, and spreads over area between the legs; growth in height, shoulders broaden and hips narrow; larnyx enlarges, deepening the voice; sparse facial and underarm hair appears.	Between ages 10 and 16	Breasts mound, areola and nipples grow; pubic hair grows to a triangular shape, axillary hair appears; menarche occurs as internal organs mature, enabling fertility; height growth slows.
Between ages 11-17	Penis circumference, length (more slowly), and testicle size increase; adult pubic hair texture; facial and underarm hair grow, may begin shaving and develop acne; matured internal reproductive organs produce the first ejaculation of semen and sperm; gynecomastia in 50% of males for 1-2 years.	Between ages 12 and 19	Adult breast size and shape, pubic hair covers mons and spreads to top of thighs, slight voice deepening, and regular menses; some body shape changes occur into the early twenties.
Between ages 14-18	Near adult height and reproductive shape and size; pubic hair to thighs and toward abdomen; chest hair, facial hair, and shaving. For some, increases in height, body hair, and muscle growth and strength continue into the early twenties.		

ment bring about normal sexual changes such as intensified sexual feelings and fantasies, more frequent spontaneous erections, increased vaginal lubrication, and tendency toward masturbation (Reinisch, 1990).

Tanner's (1962) classic grouping visually documented physical changes of puberty into measures of developmental stages for each sex. The typical physical stages for both sexes are described in Table 27-3.

For males the first changes of puberty are internal as testicles begin to mature and produce increased amounts of testosterone, in turn causing growth of the prostate gland and other internal organs related to male reproduction.

Females begin to develop sexually at an earlier age, with changes appearing in different order, beginning sometime between ages 8 and 11. Internal changes are initiated by hormones particularly estrogen.

Reproductive and Sexual Changes with Aging

Sexual changes occur with aging as maturation continues. In males primarily testosterone declines with age,

which may alter libido and create fewer viable sperm. As muscle tone decreases, the testes become more flaccid, and the diameter of the testicular tubules that store and transport sperm become increasingly narrow, predisposing benign prostatic hypertrophy. Contractions of the prostate may weaken, reducing the volume and viscosity of the seminal fluid and decreasing the force of ejaculation; the refractory period after ejaculation increases to intervals of 12 to 24 hours. Longer, more intense, direct stimulation precedes erection, which then can be maintained for longer periods and may contribute to partner satisfaction. Mulligan and Moss (1991) questioned male veterans, ages 30 to 99, concerning sexuality and found sexual interest lessened but remained as men aged. Vaginal intercourse was the uniformly preferred sexual contact regardless of age, availability of a partner, or current sexual activity level. All forms of sexual activity—kissing, petting, oral sex, partner masturbation, self-masturbation, as well as intercourse—were less prevalent among these older persons (Mulligan & Moss, 1991).

In females hormonal regulation is affected by aging, beginning with lowered estrogen levels during menopause, resulting in gradual atrophy of the uterus and vagina and concurrent reduced firmness and size of related genital tissues. The vaginal mucosa thins and the canal shortens; lubrication decreases as the Bartholin's glands decline in number and activity. The vagina may become friable, resulting in painful intercourse for some. The sexual response may change as well with the excitement level developing more slowly, the plateau stage lasting longer, and orgasm taking longer. These longer times may enhance a woman's sexual experience both physically and emotionally (Weg, 1978).

Normal Sexual Response

Regardless of age sexual response follows a natural progression. Masters, Johnson, Kolodny (1986) observed human sexual activity and described the changes during sexual responses in four categories: (1) excitement, (2) plateau, (3) orgasm, and (4) resolution.

The stages vary from time to time for an individual and between people. The physiologic processes of sexual response are not simply mechanical movements but are part of psychosexual involvement and identity of the whole person. Two basic physiologic reactions occur during human sexual response. The first is vasocongestion, an increased amount of blood concentrated in body tissues, in the genitals, and female breasts. The second is increased neuromuscular tension or myotonia, a buildup of energy in the nerves and muscles that occurs throughout the body, not only genitalia, in response to sexual arousal. Table 27-4 lists the four phases according to male, female, and both male and female responses.

Return to the unaroused state is called resolution. This phase coincides with a refractory period in males as loss of erection occurs and genital blood flow returns to baseline. A hyperventilated breathing pattern may be present just after orgasm, accompanied by a rapid pulse ranging from 100 to 160 beats/minute and rise in blood pressure, but all recede gradually as the entire body relaxes (Masters et al., 1986). If there has been considerable excitement but orgasm has not occurred, resolution takes longer. A lingering sensation of pelvic heaviness or aching is due to continued vasocongestion, which may create some discomfort. Generally relief occurs during sleep or by masturbation.

Table 27-4   Stages of Human Sexual Responses

Both male and female	Female	Male
EXCITEMENT STAGE I		
Increased muscle tension	Clitoris swells	Penis becomes erect
Increased pulse rate	Labia majora flatten and separate	Scrotum rises
Increased blood pressure	Vaginal lubrication	Testes swell and move to body
Sex flush	Breasts enlarge	
Nipple erection	Uterus elevates and expands	
PLATEAU STAGE II (TIME VARIES GREATLY)		
Muscle tension increases	Clitoris withdraws	Testes grow 2-3 times usual size
Pulse rate 100-160 beats/minute	Vaginal vasocongestion or orgasmic	Glans color deepens, head diameter
Fast breathing	platform narrows	grows
Sex flush	Vaginal opening expands inner two thirds	Cowper's secretion
	Uterus elevated	
	Breast areola swell	
	Vivid coloration of labia minora from	
	bright red to deep wine	
ORGASM STAGE III (LASTS A FEW SECONDS)		
Rhythmic muscle contractions, then	Clitoris retracts	Penis, urethra, and muscles at base of
intense physical sensations, then	Uterus contracts with outer third vagina	penis
relaxation	and anal sphincter	Ejaculation of initial spurts of semen;
Sex flush after pulse increases	Vaginal contractions or pelvic	bladder neck closes, gradually tapers
Blood pressure increases	throbbing—may have multiple orgasms	off
Respirations fast		
RELAXATION STAGE IV (LASTS A FEW MINUTES TO HOURS)		
Muscles relax	Clitoris descends	Loss of erection
Normal pulse	Labia, vagina, breasts, and uterus return	Scrotum and testes lower and return to
Normal blood pressure	to usual size and place	usual size and place
Nipple erection reduces		
Sex flush subsides		

Adapted from Masters and Johnson on Sex and Human Loving by W.H. Masters, V.E. Johnson, & R.C. Kolodny, 1986, Boston, Little, Brown. Reprinted with permission.

RELATIONSHIP FACTORS THAT MAY AFFECT SEXUALITY

Relationship factors affect the quality of sexual relationships and responses in males and females. With a strong relationship many obstacles can be overcome to achieve a satisfactory sexual relationship. Conversely a disability may further stress a marginal relationship, leading to separation of the couple. Sometimes a disability allows partners to focus on factors known to maintain relationships such as love, communication, maintaining trust, intimacy, affection, romance, timing, sensory stimulation, fantasy, and self-concept.

Love

"Love is patient, love is kind. It does not envy, it does not boast, it is not proud. It is not rude, it is not self-seeking, it is not easily angered, it keeps no record of wrongs. Love does not delight in evil but rejoices with the truth. It always protects, always trusts, always hopes, always perseveres. Love never fails" (1 Cor. 13:4-8a [Holy Bible]).

Because sexual desire and love may be both passionate and all-consuming, it is essential to distinguish the substance behind the intense feelings. Sexual desire is narrowly focused and rather easily discharged, whereas love is a more complex and constant emotion with respect for the loved one a primary concern. To maintain love or help it grow, marriage partners invest emotions, energy, and ongoing "giving" in communications, physical warmth, shared interests, and shared responsibilities through hard work and creativity (Masters et al., 1986).

The passion of romantic love fades quickly, whereas companionable love based on sharing, affection, trust, involvement, and togetherness is steadier and may include a satisfying sex life. It is characteristic of marriage and long-term relationships in working, raising children, having hobbies, and relaxing with friends (Masters et al., 1986).

Communication

Effective communication is a cornerstone of interpersonal and sexual intimacy that differs from communicating with others. Partners in a committed, intimate, and caring relationship have a safety net of trust and support wherein each one knows there is no deliberate hurt. Talking about feelings and experiences, simply holding one another, and sharing improve a sexual relationship and improve mutual understanding as well.

Communication is especially important in relationships where a partner has impaired or altered functions. With sensory loss, partners share what feels pleasurable, conveys no feeling, or is painful. Potential bowel or bladder incontinence is discussed before it is experienced. Partners tell one another when they experience fatigue, discomfort, or frustration. Communication adds stability and satisfaction.

Intimacy Built on Trust

Trust is necessary for sharing intimacy and develops over time as partners learn to rely on each other's word, commitment to value and honor one another, and to work on mutual problem-solving. Love is a choice to build security into a relationship (Smalley & Trent, 1988). Intimacy is an exchange of feelings, thoughts, and actions marked by mutual acceptance, commitment, tenderness, trust, caring, and sharing—which result in commitment through crises, boredom, and fatigue as well as through joy, prosperity, and excitement.

Affection

The expression of tenderness may be spoken by physical contact or other direct behavior. Consistent, gentle touching is one of the most powerful messages of security, emotional bonding, and romance—and may be more important than sexual activity for some. Meaningful touch occurs throughout a day with hugs, hand holding, back rubs, a kiss on the cheek, or a pat. Eye contact also is a form of intimate touch (Smalley & Trent, 1989). However, never hearing words of affection can be troubling and can lead to questions concerning whether partners really care. Persons with impairments may participate fully in intimacy, communication, meaningful touch, affection, and eye contact—which are the most important parts of the sexual relationship for many partners.

Romance

Romantic experiences help set the stage for a positive sexual experience and demonstrate the value of each one to the other—for instance, taking a walk, holding hands, talking in front of a warm fire, or spending a weekend away for two. Taking time for romance affords a chance for preparation, relaxation, and enjoyment; it sets the stage as limited only by one's imagination, privacy, and safety. Mirrors, for example, enhance visual enjoyment when a partner has impaired sensation; water beds simulate motion when a partner has immobility.

✦ Timing/mood

Preferred times of day or night when both partners feel rested, relaxed, and ready for sexual activities vary with couples. Some illnesses or injuries affect timing—for example, those with arthritis have improved function after morning stiffness has subsided. Those with spinal injury may schedule sexual activity after their bowel program to decrease the risk of incontinence.

✦ Sensory stimulation/fantasy

The greatest sense organ and central coordinating center for sexual activity is the brain. Sexual desire begins in the brain fueled by sensory input of sights, sounds, tastes, smells, or touches. Thus for some persons fantasy can be a powerful producer of sexual desire as well as a way to express sexual desire. Sexual fantasies can enhance both the psychological and physiologic sides of sexual response in several ways: countering boredom, focusing thoughts and feelings, boosting self-image, and imagining the partner who suits all needs (Masters et al., 1986).

Stimulation of the senses can enhance the psychological desire for sexual activity. Certain odors are relaxing and lead to sexual arousal in one individual, while repelling another. Some persons emit natural body scents or pheromones during arousal that are sensed by their partner. Pleasant environmental odors, incense or cologne for two, may enhance the sexual experience. Chapter 16 contains additional information on the senses.

Arousing touch includes massage with body oils, creams, or lotion; light touch to sensitive areas, kissing, or licking.

Heat or cold applications, rubbing, textures of material, or vibrators enhance sexual arousal through touch. Some individuals with sensory impairment report enhanced sexual feelings, almost orgasmic, from touch in areas of intact sensation (Woods, 1979). Chapter 24 has more content about sensation and perception.

Masters and Johnson's (1986) technique of "sensate focus" is recommended by some sex counselors. In this technique partners explore parts of each other's body without leading to intercourse or orgasm. The exploration concentrates on touching all areas of the body and telling the partner what feels good and what does not (Masters et al., 1986).

Sight is a powerful sensory tool enabling some individuals with disabilities to have a more positive sexual experience when they are positioned to see what is occurring. A lighted room and strategically placed mirrors allow the brain to enjoy what the eye can see, although the body may not be able to feel.

ALTERATIONS IN SEXUAL FUNCTION

Individuals with chronic disease or disability who are significantly inconvenienced because of sensory limitations or disorders involving one or more of the following body systems—neurologic, musculoskeletal, respiratory, cardiovascular, or digestive—are considered to have altered sexual function whether or not the sex organs are affected (Shrey, Kiefer, & Anthony, 1979). For example, fatigue with arthritis or positioning for lower extremity spasticity causes both partners to make adjustments. A shared concern is fear that engaging in sexual activity may accelerate the disease process or adversely affect the client. The following section discusses functional problems that may affect sexuality as a complication of a disease or disability.

Physiologic Alterations
✦ Impaired physical mobility

A freely movable body is an asset in expressing oneself as a sexual being. Impaired mobility impacts positions available for intercourse, especially when large joints or paralysis are involved. When the hands are involved, an individual may have difficulty in communicating using touch or caressing. Impaired mobility may limit the ability to transfer to a bed or couch, dress or undress, manage personal hygiene, insert or apply birth control devices, and perform the thrusting motion inherent in intercourse. Hypertonic muscles have the most effect on positioning, whereas apraxia and ataxia may limit the initiation of the motion or coordination of the motion. Balance also can have an effect on selection of positions. All of the preceding impact the safety of assuming certain positions.

✦ Increased or decreased sensation

When sensation is altered, the pleasure derived from stimulation no longer may be perceived in some erogenous zones of the body. In spinal injury the higher the level of the lesion, the less skin surface is available for stimulation. Following stroke some individuals experience decreased sensory function and touch to the hemiparetic side is not felt; others become hypersensitive on their hemiparetic side and experience any touch to this area as intense pain. Clients with brain injury may have increased or decreased sensory input, and some are very defensive concerning areas of the body that are hypersensitive.

✦ Pain

Pain contributes to sexual dysfunction in a number of chronic diseases, and constant pain creates real barriers to sexual desire and performance. Pain may limit positions or performance of movements required for sexual activities; when chronic, pain may lead to depression further dulling desire. Pain has been identified as a greater barrier to sexual intimacy than disabling characteristics (Conine & Evans, 1982).

✦ Bowel and/or bladder incontinence

Incontinence can result from neurologic, muscular, or urologic or intestinal damage, but the real challenges are social consequences and detrimental effects on sexual function. Both men and women worry about offensive odors and bowel and/or bladder incontinence during sexual activities, which can inhibit enjoyment. Women with incontinence may have more bowel accidents than men because the steady stretch from the penis inside the vagina may activate bowel reflexes that relax the anus and initiate emptying (Zejdlik, 1992). Preparation for sexual activity includes emptying the bowel and bladder, padding the bed, and adding scents in the environment and on the person. When the role transition from sexual partner to manager of bowel and bladder continence inhibits sexual desire, the caregiver role is best delegated to another person, if the pair choose.

✦ Fatigue

Brain injury, stroke, rheumatic disease, and multiple sclerosis all have fatigue as side effects. Fatigue may result from crises of disability and the accompanying depression. Persons whose daily living activities require a great expenditure of energy may have little energy left to engage in sexual activity. Chapter 23 provides additional discussion of fatigue.

✦ Changes in libido

Lesions in the thalamus, limbic system, or bitemporal injury have been associated with hypersexuality; disinhibited sexual behavior is associated with involvement of the paralimbic and neocortical frontotemporal areas. Although not scientifically defined, hypersexuality characteristics include (1) insatiable sexual activity that may interfere with other everyday functioning, (2) impersonal sexuality having no emotional intimacy, and (3) unsatisfying sex despite frequent orgasms (Masters et al., 1986). Hypersexuality can cause difficulties for clients and their partners. Following brain injury, hyposexuality is more common than hypersexuality. Decreased sex drive can be due to many factors including organic affective disorders, reactive depression, cognitive dysfunction, stress, and anxiety. Clients who have experienced stroke report decreased sexual interest (Renshaw, 1978).

✦ Genital sexual dysfunction

Erectile dysfunction, or impotence, is the inability to have or maintain an erection firm enough for coitus at least 25% of the time. Typically partial erections occur, but they are not firm enough for vaginal insertion. Diabetes and alcoholism are two prominent organic contributors to erectile dysfunction; others include neurologic damage, particularly spinal cord injury, and multiple sclerosis; infection or injury to the sex organs, hormone deficiencies, and circulatory problems.

Premature ejaculation is possibly the most common sexual dysfunction in the general U.S. population, with an estimated 15% to 20% of men having moderate difficulty controlling rapid ejaculation. Premature ejaculation rarely results from organic causes. In complete upper motor neuron spinal injury, ejaculation and orgasm are absent, reflex erection may be present, and should ejaculation occur, it often is retrograde ejaculation. For those with incomplete spinal injury, intercourse is possible for four out of five (Masters et al., 1986).

Female genital dysfunction may involve libido, excitement (vaginal lubrication), and orgasm. Any severe chronic illness may impair female orgasmic response: diabetes, alcoholism, neurologic disturbances, hormone deficiencies, and pelvic disorders such as infections, trauma, or scarring from surgery to name a few (Reinisch, 1990).

Both sexes can experience painful intercourse due to psychosocial or physical difficulties. For men infections, inflammations of the penis, foreskin, testes, urethra, or prostate are the most likely organic causes. Any condition in women that results in poor vaginal lubrication can produce discomfort during intercourse including medications, diabetes, spinal injury, vaginal infections, and estrogen deficiencies (Masters et al., 1986).

✦ Fertility

Men experience decreased fertility following spinal cord injury. Sperm counts may be lower than before injury and true ejaculation is rare, especially with higher cervical injury making fertility somewhat of a mechanical problem. Loss of temperature regulation by the testes and the tendency to retrograde ejaculation also impact infertility (Woods, 1984).

For females ovulation may occur before the menstrual cycle resumes, about 6 months following spinal cord injury, and fertility returns to preinjury levels. Fertility counseling is recommended early in rehabilitation care. Lack of knowledge about birth control is common among all persons, but a woman with a disability may face added physical and psychosocial problems from an unplanned pregnancy.

✦ Endocrine dysfunction

Fertility also may be altered in persons who have experienced brain injury. When damage affects the endocrine system, hormonal imbalance may decrease fertility. In sexually mature males decreased serum testosterone level is evident initially as a decrease in libido and later as impotence. Typical male sexual characteristics may decline, testes atrophy, and facial hair decrease, along with the inability to ejaculate after a brain injury. With prolactin overproduction, males may develop breast tissue and females may start producing milk (Horn & Zasler, 1990).

Acquired dysfunction of ovarian endocrine function will lead to female menstrual irregularities and more androgens, resulting in symptoms of hirsutism, acne, and obesity. Some women may develop polycystic ovaries and hypogonadotrophic hypogonadism.

Alcohol, even amounts below legal levels of intoxication, can inhibit arousal, reduce erectile capacity, and slow or eliminate ejaculation in healthy males. Alcohol weakens male masturbatory effectiveness and decreases the intensity and pleasure of male orgasm. In females alcohol has a similar negative impact on sexual arousal, vaginal blood volume, and orgasm. Alcohol has a physically inhibiting effect, yet most believe it increases their sexual responsiveness, in part because its disinhibiting effect makes it possible for sexual desire to emerge (Masters et al., 1986).

Long-term alcohol use can lead to significant physical changes that in turn affect sexuality. In males alcohol temporarily lowers testosterone levels and sperm counts. Regular or prolonged alcohol use leads to permanent sterility, testicular atrophy, and gynecomastia when estrogen increases. Alcohol use is known to have devastating effects on the fetus and is not to be ingested during pregnancy.

✦ Effects of medication

Analgesic drugs used in treating pain that depress the central nervous system may have an effect on sexual function similar to alcohol. Addictive narcotic drugs produce erectile dysfunction, retarded ejaculation, and low sexual interest in males and low sexual interest and orgasmic dysfunction in females. Many clients with neurologic involvement take medication to manage health problems or control symptoms caused by neurologic damage but find it also affects sexual function. Diazepam (Valium) is taken to decrease the hypertonic response of spasticity, but it also can reduce sexual desire and contribute to problems with ejaculation or orgasm. Lioresal (baclofen) use leads to problems with erection or ejaculation (see the box below).

Since hypertension is the major risk factor for stroke, many stroke clients may be taking antihypertensives (Reinisch, 1990). Tranquilizers reduce sexual desire; diazepam and alprazolam (Xanax) cause difficulty with ejaculation and orgasm. Carbamazepine and phenytoin may be used for clients who have sustained a head injury if they have posttraumatic seizure disorder. Some medications used

---

✦

SEXUAL PROBLEMS RESULTING FROM MEDICATION

Ejaculation problems: Diazepam (Valium), methyldopa (Aldomet), ranitidine (Zantac), phenytoin, baclofen (Lioresal), cimetidine (Tagamet), carbamazepine

Priapism: Hydralazine (Apresoline), prazosin (Minipress), labetalol (Trandate)

Gynecomastia: Methyldopa (Aldomet), hydrochlorothiazide and spironolactone (Aldactazide), Raudixin, Rauzide, reserpine (Serpasil), spironolactone.

Menstrual changes: Hydrochlorothiazide and spironolactone (Aldactazide), spironolactone (Weiss, 1991; Sullivan Lukoff, 1990).

Tranquilizers: Reduce desire and sexual function

Antihistamines: Produce drowsiness, reduced body fluids

to reduce excess body fluid cause men problems with reduced sexual desire and erection and women problems with reduced vaginal lubrication, causing intercourse to be painful (Reinisch, 1990).

Psychosocial Alterations

Psychosocial alterations that occur with disability and chronic illness—social isolation, partnership issues, and issues of self-esteem—may impact sexuality to the same extent as physical problems.

✦ Social isolation

Social isolation is a major barrier for persons with brain injury and their families (Davis & Schneider, 1990). During the time needed for recovery, friends move ahead in school or continue with work, leaving the person socially isolated, making it difficult to meet individuals of the opposite sex. When relationships are established, their own and others' reactions to disease or disability may be another barrier to communicating willingness to engage in sexual activity. Persons who have visible disabilities or use adaptive equipment may feel a need to make others feel at ease.

Researchers reported on 105 persons less than 60 years old who had experienced stroke: 60% said their sexual desire was the same or greater than before the stroke, 43% had decreased frequency of coitus, 22% had increased coitus, and 35% gave incomplete information. Most of the 105 stroke clients reported the same subjective sexual desire as previously but reported fewer sexual opportunities due to their partner's fear or abhorrence. Negative attitudes, however, may reflect a client's own feeling about self rather than that of the partner's (Renshaw, 1978).

✦ Self-concept

Self-concept includes all the beliefs people hold in regard to themselves; beliefs concerning the ideal self, the value of self or self-esteem, and internal feelings about body parts and body image. External factors such as cosmetics, clothes, and jewelry also express one's self-concept as shaped by environmental and genetic factors. Throughout the life-span, persons develop positive or negative views of self as they interact with others. The person with a disability may be forced to abdicate social roles for extensive periods. The ability to adjust to changes associated with chronic or disabling conditions varies among individuals, but almost always, there is some loss of body image and self-concept (Hirsch, Seager, Seldor, King, & Staas, 1990). Persons who held a positive body image before disability tended to cope with body changes more effectively than individuals who viewed themselves negatively before disability. Independence in self-care and social roles eliminates barriers and promotes positive self-concept.

✦ Partnership issues

Disability affects an individual and the entire family, notably the partner. When a spouse becomes disabled, the partner senses loss of the spouse's contribution to the relationship, particularly when disease or accident impairs a person's cognitive function. Crewe (1992) reports imbalance in relationships may occur after spinal cord injury. When one partner serves dual caregiver and provider roles, the burdens can lead to burnout and imbalance in the relationship. Too often a partner becomes preoccupied with tasks or financially unable to continue participation in activities that bring zest to life. Communication and problem-solving skills to bridge the strains of financial, health, and physical needs are vital issues for couples dealing with disability. Married women who experience spinal cord injury are vulnerable, with six out of seven eventually divorced (Smith, 1990).

A survey of 407 people selected from the National Spinal Cord Injury data bank 9 years after their injuries revealed 68% remained married as compared with 75% of the general population. Additionally divorce rates doubled for persons with spinal cord injury who married twice or more when compared with people who married for the first time (Divorce Trends in Spinal Cord Injury, 1990). Other research findings note that those who marry postinjury are happier with their sex lives, living arrangements, and social lives. The mitigating factor in this research may have been the survey sample that contained 79% employed persons (Smith, 1990).

Physical, psychological, cognitive, and behavioral alterations that affect sexuality also have profound effects on a homosexual relationship. Clients who are homosexual require information and counseling about sexual functioning. Each counselor must decide whether to provide education or refer to another professional for counsel.

Cognitive and Behavioral Alterations

To successfully participate in sexual activity, cognitive function must be intact. Cognitive impairments or alterations occur with brain injury, stroke, multiple sclerosis, Parkinson's disease, and other neurologic diseases. For example, attention, memory, executive function, communication, mood, and social perceptiveness are higher center skills and behaviors that affect sexual function or sexuality.

Deficits in attention can affect sexual function since one must be able to attend to task for the required period of time and not be distracted. In sexual activity a doorbell or ringing telephone can break attention and concentration, but with persistence partners can refocus their attention. Inattention disrupts the ability to concentrate and focus on the partner, fantasize, focus on sexual play, or maintain erection by psychogenic means. Memory can affect the frequency and rhythm of sexual activity—that is, persons remember the last encounter as part of their schedule as a couple and sexual preferences or dislikes.

Egocentricity—one partner focusing only on self and his or her own needs—detracts from a sexual relationship. Equally contributing persons, each focused on the other, create balance in a sexual relationship.

Executive function impairments affect the quality of reasoning, planning, organizing, and judgment. Sexual function is a high-level social skill that requires planning, preparation, and anticipation. In a sexual scenario this translates to understanding nonverbal as well as spoken signals, knowing what is expected of each partner, anticipating what comes next, and selecting the best approach—which all are difficult for those with impaired executive function.

Social perceptiveness—truly understanding the message of the other person and comprehending how one is being perceived—also may be altered by brain injury, causing other relationship problems. If an individual lacks the social skills to express personal feelings and to show love through actions, words, and nonverbal communication the entire intimate relationship, not only sexual relations, is threatened.

Intimacy is maintained and enhanced by effective communication: sharing hopes, dreams, values, and our most important needs. To communicate at this level requires high-level communication skills. With altered communication, such as experienced by persons following stroke or brain injury, a signal system may serve the couple to initiate sexual intimacy by one of the partners when a couple cannot communicate verbally. Sexual activity is a means of expressing love for one another and sharing intimate moments although the words cannot be retrieved. Depression, often following chronic or disabling conditions, can adversely affect libido and sexual performance. These work together in a cycle in which depression leads to decreases in sexual activity, which in turn may contribute to depression. Mood disturbances such as depression may decrease libido or alternatively if the mood disturbance is euphoria, increase libido. In either case sexual function may be altered.

Disinhibition differs greatly from depression as a cause of sexual dysfunction. Sexual function has its own set of social and cultural rules that vary greatly in practice among couples. Disinhibition can change the nature of the sexual encounter for some spouses. This may take the form of verbal interaction only or it may carry over into sexual relations, becoming a sexual turnoff for some partners. For some clients who are without a partner, sexual disinhibition can cause problems in the community, unless the person relearns that sexual activity is to be participated in only when in private.

Irritability is a potential behavior that occurs more frequently in persons with brain injury, stroke, or neurologic diseases. An irritable person does not necessarily make the best partner for sex since an incorrect perception of a partner's behavior elicits an irritable response, disrupting the sexual encounter. When assessing individuals for sexual function, a holistic approach to the person considers impaired or altered sexual function and sexuality in relation to the relationship as well as work, home maintenance, and recreation.

Assessment of Sexual Function

Sexuality and sexual response may not be a priority early in a client's rehabilitation process; later sexual function may become a major consideration for the client and the partner. A client may initiate discussion; sexuality is a major concern. Health professionals have responsibility not only to address the topic but to provide education and counsel to clients. As rehabilitation is a process that transcends disciplines, so is assessment of sexual function. Assessment data are collected from different disciplines. The nurse integrates data from nursing assessment with information from other team members to provide sexual education or counseling as a therapeutic intervention. The sexual assessment includes obtaining a sexual history, identifying physical and psychosocial strengths and limitations, determining the client's sexual values, and assisting with performing diagnostic tests.

The following list guides preparation for assessment:

- ✦ Assess information needs
- ✦ Individualize teaching and counseling
- ✦ Select the site
- ✦ Establish trust and rapport
- ✦ Assure confidentiality and privacy
- ✦ Legitimize sexuality
- ✦ Ask about cultural or ethnic needs
- ✦ Evaluate language and understanding
- ✦ Proceed logically with information
- ✦ Allow time and encourage questions
- ✦ Convey sexual health as part of personal health
- ✦ Validate and empower client
- ✦ Reassess for feedback

Clients are informed as the interview begins that they can refuse to answer any questions. Refusal may be due to sociocultural factors such as sex as a taboo topic, or age and gender may be barriers that dissuade clients from answering questions. Never cause a client or partner to come into conflict with their moral or ethical views. A referral to someone from the same religious or cultural background may be in order.

Questions proceed from less to more sensitive areas. A life cycle chronology provides a logical unfolding of events, as well as a progression from less to more threatening topics. The impact of any questions can be softened by making a general statement, then proceeding with the question. For instance, the nurse can make a general statement about masturbation as a normal form of sexual release, then ask the client's opinion about this practice. Or ask about the ideal rather than the real to facilitate communication such as, "Statistically people of your age have intercourse three times a week. In an average week how often do you have intercourse?" Once the nurse is familiar with interviewing techniques she can proceed to the sexual history (Woods, 1984).

✦ Sexual history

The purpose of the sexual history is to identify problems and misconceptions, as well as areas requiring education and counseling regarding sexual issues (see the box on p. 609).

✦ Physical examination

The physician, physician's assistant, or nurse practitioner (or nurses in some settings) conducts the physical examination. The information will guide content of sexual education and counseling.

External genitalia. In males inspect the penis for size and shape, presence of a foreskin and proper foreskin retraction; assess size and consistency of testicles. Small atrophic testicles may be due to primary or secondary hypogonadism.

In females inspect the external genitalia. A nurse practitioner or gynecologist may perform a bimanual examination, inspect the vaginal walls for atrophic changes and assess intravaginal tone, and complete a breast examination.

Neurologic assessment of the genital area: inspect rectal sphincter tone; normal sphincter tone indicates both the lumbar and sacral segments of the spinal cord are intact al-

---

SEXUAL HISTORY FORM

Name _____ Age _____
Marital/partnership status (includes quality, duration)
_____

Occupation _____ Highest education _____
Religion _____ Interests/hobbies _____
_____

MEDICAL HISTORY

Psychological/psychiatric problems _____
Behavioral/emotional problems _____
Renal insufficiency _____
Diabetes _____
Neurologic conditions _____
Hereditary disorders _____
Hypertension _____
Endocrine disorders _____
Sexually transmitted diseases _____

CURRENT MEDICATIONS

Antihypertensives _____
Antipsychotics _____
Antihistamines _____
Alcohol _____
Analgesics _____
Narcotics _____
Recreational drugs _____

PREMORBID SEXUAL FUNCTION

Description of sexual activities preferred _____
Frequency of sexual activity _____
Partner who generally initiates sexual activity _____
Sexual preferences of the client _____

SPECIFIC CONCERNS OF THE COUPLE

Fertility _____
Birth control _____
Importance of sex in the relationship _____

Physical issues that impact sexual function
Transfers _____
Ability to dress/undress _____
Hemiplegia/hemiparesis _____
Paraplegia/quadriplegia _____
Range-of-motion limitations _____
Hypertonicity _____
Hypotonicity _____
Endurance _____
Balance _____
Presence of sensation versus being hypersensitive ____
Presence of pain and location _____
Presence of bowel and/or bladder incontinence _____
Presence of genitourinary or gastrointestinal collection devices and their position
_____

Difficulty with vision, hearing, oral motor control
_____

General and genital hygiene and cleanliness _____

SEXUAL RESPONSE ISSUES

Female
  Menstrual history _____
  Sexual interest _____
  Frequency of sexual interaction _____
  Vaginal lubrication _____
  Sensation present _____
  Orgasmic capacity _____
  Fertility _____
Male
  Sexual interest _____
  Presence of morning erections _____
  Presence of erections with manual stimulation _____
  Process for ejaculation _____
  Sensation present _____
  Type of ejaculation and volume _____
  Fertility _____

---

lowing strong reflex erections in the male. Ask the client to contract the rectal sphincter voluntarily; ability to do this implies preservation of efferent motor fibers in the pyramidal tract system essential for ejaculation.

If pain and temperature are present in the saddle area, S2-4, sensory awareness of orgasm is present. Sensation from the testes enters the spinal cord at the T9 level. If squeezing the testicle elicits a pain response, then psychogenic erections can likely occur since the pathway for these is through T11-12 spinal nerves via the sympathetic nervous system (Fig. 27-2).

Assess the bulbocavernosus reflex manually by compressing the penis while palpating the perineum or anus for a reflex contraction. This reflex is present in approximately 70% of neurologically intact males. In females press on the clitoris to contract the rectal sphincter. In both males and females, contraction of the anal sphincter is a positive response and indicates an intact reflex arc, which allows for reflex erections in males. Use a pinprick to the anus to elicit contraction of the anal sphincter; the anal wink reflex indicates an intact sacral reflex arc and potential for strong reflex erections (Zasler & Horn, 1990).

Because the urinary tract and genital organs share much innervation, tests of bladder function (e.g., urodynamics) help in estimating the neurologic integrity of the genital system. Through urodynamic testing physicians can determine a person's reflex versus areflexic neurologic status and sphincter dyssynergia. Regarding sexual function, if reflexes are present then reflex erections are possible; if not, then psychogenic erections may be possible.

Efferent neurologic pathways can be assessed by nocturnal penile tumescence testing, which is a measure of penile erection during sleep, generally conducted in a sleep laboratory or at home. The test provides a reliable report of all nighttime penile activity for frequency, quality, duration, and amplitude of any nighttime erections. If erections occur during sleep, the clinician has some information about the motor and autonomic efferents involved in penile erection.

Another method that may be used to evaluate erection potential is intracavernosal injection of pharmacologic agents. The medication, papaverine or phentolamine, causes vasodilation when injected into the corpus cavernosum of the penis, leading to erection when all physical components of erection are present. Failure of the injection to produce erection suggests the vascular system to the penis is not intact and functioning, leading to impotence.

Other tests that are conducted in only a few rehabilitation centers are penile biothesiometry (skin vibration sensitivity) and dorsal somatosensory-evoked potential testing. Biothesiometry provides information on the sensory afferents through measuring the vibration perception threshold of the penis. A small electromagnetic test probe is placed on the penis and allowed to vibrate gently. Vibration testing evaluates only the function of the sensory nerves. Sensory nerve deficits are found in persons with diabetes or those with a history of alcohol abuse. Somatosensory-evoked potential testing allows specific localization of the anatomic lesion in peripheral, sacral, or suprasacral nerves. Impaired dorsal nerve activity adversely affects the ability to sustain penile erection (Zasler & Horn, 1990).

Penile arteriography and/or corpus cavernosography (radiographs taken of the penis after a special dye has been injected) can determine which blood vessels are involved. The arteries also can be evaluated by Doppler analysis, which uses ultrasonography to evaluate blood flow (Leslie, 1990). Diagnostic testing in females is not as sophisticated or available as with males. Changes in vaginal hemodynamics can be measured through photoplethysmography and heat electrode techniques. This technology can be incorporated in biofeedback programs to address orgasmic or arousal problems (Reinisch, 1990).

NURSING DIAGNOSES

Nursing diagnoses related to sexual function that are accepted by the North American Nursing Diagnosis Association include the following:

1. *Sexual Dysfunction, altered sexuality patterns:* lack of or compromised ability to respond to those activities or behaviors associated with stimulation of the erogenous zones. Sexual dysfunction describes perceived problems in achieving sexual satisfaction and includes clients with limitations on sexual expression imposed by disease or therapy. Planning is directed toward designing interventions to meet sexual adjustment goals that are realistic and attainable. The related factors that may contribute to this nursing diagnosis are accident or injury; altered body structure or function; motor/sensory deficits; knowledge deficit regarding sexual function and effects of disability; values/cultural conflict; lack of privacy; role changes; body image disturbance; unresolved relationship or sexuality issues before disability; pain or discomfort; medication side effects; dyspnea; and reduced activity tolerance (Mumma, 1987).

2. *Body image disturbance, personal identity distur-bance, self-esteem disturbance:* lowered self-concept possibly caused by impaired motor or sensory function, pain, fatigue, disfigurement, loss of control, loss of independence, social isolation, or depression. Body image disturbance is closely related to self-esteem disturbance and describes negative feelings or perceptions about characteristics, functions, or limits of the body or body parts. Planning is directed toward facilitating the process of adequate sexual adjustment while focusing on improving body image through attention to personal hygiene, dress, and mannerisms; assisting the client to resume social roles and change prevailing attitudes regarding male and female sexual roles; reestablishing personal identity; and improving self-esteem as former activities and roles are resumed in the usual or adapted ways. Related factors that might contribute to this nursing diagnosis include loss of a significant other; unrealistic self-expectations; repeated negative interpersonal experiences with significant others; separation from support systems while hospitalized; inability to adjust to and integrate body changes; and knowledge deficit regarding activities of daily living and potential abilities (Mumma, 1987).

3. *Social Isolation:* lack of or limited ability for social interaction because of impaired motor or sensory function or self-imposed isolation. This condition may result from voluntary or therapeutic isolation. Planning should focus on the identification of acceptable social interactions, recreational opportunities, and transportation options. Related factors for this nursing diagnosis include physical disability; cognitive impairment; emotional handicap to include depression or extreme anxiety; fear of embarrassment, rejection, discovery, environmental hazards; incontinence; body-image disturbance; disfigurement; sensory losses of sight or hearing; loss of usual means of transportation; loss of employment; insufficient community resources, or sociocultural dissonance (Mumma, 1987).

4. *Knowledge deficits:* lack of knowledge regarding alternative ways to achieve sexual functioning or lack of knowledge regarding birth control. The client may not be aware of alternatives to traditional sexual activities, and the disabling condition may result in motor or sensory impairments that interfere with the ability to perform sexual activities in the usual manner. The client may not be aware of ability or lack of ability to produce children. Planning should be directed toward teaching the client about options to facilitate satisfaction of sexual drives and birth control methods. Related factors for this nursing diagnosis include onset of disability; low readiness for reception of information; lack of interest or motivation to learn; cognitive limitations; psychomotor limitations; uncompensated memory loss; inability to use materials or information resources due to, for example, cultural or language barriers; change in health status; and new or complex treatment program (Mumma, 1987).

PLANS OF CARE

A plan of care is individualized, proactive, based on the assessment, and developed with the client and partner to synchronize the team with them toward the person's highest functional level. The plan of care includes nursing diagnosis, goals, interventions, time frames for completion, and evaluation of the goals and interventions. Much of the care plan related to sexual function focuses on education and/or counseling of the client and the partner, incorporating techniques for everyday functioning taught and practiced in the therapy departments and the nursing units. For example, transfers from the wheelchair to the bed are not considered sexual activity but may be preparations for sexual activity.

Goals

Realistic goals, mutually established with the client and partner, may include the following:

+ Maintenance or restoration of function as a sexual being
+ Sexual adjustment
+ Being knowledgeable concerning sexual options, compensation strategies, alternative positions, and devices
+ Decreased pain and potential for medical complications, if applicable, during sexual activity
+ Management strategies for bowel and/or bladder incontinence (practiced by those persons with incontinence or appliances)
+ Maintenance or restoration of positive self-concept, including improving body image
+ Being knowledgeable concerning fertility and birth control
+ Enabling client/partner to seek professionals who can provide sex therapy, further sex counseling, devices, birth control methods, and/or fertility information or services
+ Being knowledgeable concerning prevention of STDs

REHABILITATION NURSING INTERVENTIONS
Education for Client and Partner

The role of the rehabilitation professional in sexual counseling is twofold: educator and counselor. Through sexual education the rehabilitation nurse suggests interventions and provides information to a client and partner (or to a client through the course of daily interactions) about sexual options, positions for sexual activities, management or relief of pain, management of bowel and bladder function, psychosocial aspects of human sexuality, effects of medications on sexual function, prevention of STDs, and birth control methods. A session on human sexuality scheduled for regular client education programs is one method of reaching groups of individuals who have experienced alterations in sexual function and effectively coped or who need support. These groups are similar to support groups available in many communities for males experiencing impotence. Groups can be composed of clients who are at similar stages in the adjustment process or persons with similar diagnoses who may anticipate similar sexual problems; generally groups are composed of persons of the same sex. The groups focus on education and strategies to manage the problems encountered.

Compensation Strategies for Sexual Dysfunction

Clients may learn strategies for compensating for sexual dysfunction in all areas of deficit but especially for sexual activities that can be satisfying when intercourse is not an option. Most physical disabilities do not reduce interest in sex or the capacity for sexual functioning, although certain impairments make intercourse difficult or impossible. Many people with disabilities report difficulty with finding sexual partners, leaving masturbation to orgasm a common sexual activity for individuals. Masturbation is self-stimulation of the genitals to the point of orgasm, which is not physically harmful and provides relief of sexual tension for clients with normal sensation or limited loss of sensory function. In some disease processes such as myocardial infarction, masturbation may be advised as the first step back to sexual activity (Watts, 1979). One report suggests men who are not disabled, are married, and are regularly active with a partner (94%) masturbate; 60% to 80% of women were estimated to masturbate as well (Reinisch, 1990).

Manual sexual stimulation from a partner and orogenital sexual stimulation are options for some. Two types of orogenital activity are possible, depending on the sex of the person receiving the stimulation. Cunnilingus—stimulation of the female genitals by a partner's mouth or tongue—is very pleasurable for some women. A word of caution concerning cunnilingus is never to blow air forcibly into the vagina, as air embolism may result, leading to death of the woman and/or fetus if a woman is pregnant. Fellatio—stimulation of the male genitals by a partner's mouth or tongue—can provide pleasurable sensations and orgasm with or without ingestion of the ejaculated semen by the partner. A client with loss of sensation may perform manual or orogenital sexual stimulation on the partner and gain a sense of fulfillment from pleasing another person. Though generally common in the United States, some persons find the idea of orogenital sex incomprehensible or taboo for discussion (Reinisch, 1990). Discern the client's and/or the partner's feelings before presenting this as an option.

Erectile dysfunction can be compensated for by using various strategies. When a male is unable to have or sustain an erection, the partner may choose to use the "stuffing technique." The female positions the soft penis into the vagina, contracts the vaginal (pubococcygeal) muscles, and holds the penis in the vagina (Griffith & Trieschmann, 1983). In the dominant position the woman may perform a rotary or circular motion, which is useful when a partner is impotent, regardless of underlying pathophysiology.

Vacuum entrapment systems or pumps are external devices that can produce or maintain erection (Fig. 27-5). The man lubricates the flaccid penis and places it into a clear acrylic tube that is held tightly against the body. Then he uses the pump device to produce a vacuum in the acrylic tube, which forces blood into the penis. When the penis is rigid, a rubber ring is moved from the end of the tube onto the penis, around the base, to hold the blood in the penis. The tube then is removed, and the erection can be maintained for the length of time the rubber band can stay in place, which is 30 minutes. At orgasm the rubber ring can prevent ejaculation in some persons; some individuals report pain or numbness. There is the potential for damage to the penile shaft, to internal penile tissue, and for infection or irritation to the urinary tract. These devices should be used under a physician's supervision; the physician will provide counseling for both the client and partner and check for problems at frequent intervals.

There have been recent studies of small groups of persons who report success with a slightly different type of vacuum device that has a flexible tube for the penis and looks somewhat like a thick condom. This device is kept on the penis during intercourse (Reinisch, 1990).

Pharmacologic impotence management techniques include enteral agents that can be prescribed by a physician including dopamine agonists such as L-dopa and yohimbine. Yohimbine reduces the activity of certain nerves that naturally inhibit erectile function and may increase sexual desire; 20% to 25% of individuals experience improvement in impotence. Testosterone injections can help increase libido and even improve erectile function in persons with borderline low serum testosterone levels (Zasler & Horn, 1990). Those with a history of prostate cancer, or heart, kidney, or liver disease should not receive testosterone therapy. If testosterone levels are not low, there is no benefit to testosterone injections.

Physicians can prescribe medications for intracavernosal injection. Medications include papaverine, phentolamine, and prostaglandin E_1 injected via syringe and needle into the corpus cavernosum of the penis to stimulate erection through vasodilatation. Since this is a relatively new treatment, the long-term side effects are unclear. One concern is cavernosal fibrosis, which may have the potential to adversely alter erectile ability. Papaverine has not been approved for use in intracavernosal injection by the Food and Drug Administration. These injections affect erection only; there is no increased ability to ejaculate or experience orgasm. Priapism (a persistent painful erection) occurs in about 5%. Should priapism continue longer than 4 hours, treatment is required to reverse the erection and prevent tissue damage to the penis (Williams, 1989). Over 30,000 men are successfully using some type of penile injection therapy as their preferred treatment for impotence (Leslie, 1990). Researchers are experimenting with new orally administered drugs that produce erection without the risk of priapism.

Penile implants are an option for some males who are impotent as a result of spinal cord injury, diabetes, arterial ischemia, extensive pelvic surgery, or long-term use of certain drugs such as anti-hypertensives. Implantation may diminish the ability to achieve partial erection, but presurgical sperm count and sensations during intercourse will remain as before surgery. Penile implants or prostheses can be inflatable or noninflatable. Inflatable prostheses are close to natural functioning, being self-contained with a reservoir and tubing connected to two silicone cylinders placed in the erectile areas of the penis (Zasler, 1989) (Fig. 27-6). Disadvantages include a complicated mechanical system, extensive surgery requiring 5 hospital days, hospitalization for replacement of malfunctioning parts, training to operate, and manual dexterity on the part of the man or his partner (Leslie, 1990).

Noninflatable implants are either semirigid or hinged-malleable. The semirigid implant is a rodlike silicone form that is inserted into the penis. After surgery the penis is always erect but can be pushed down and concealed by clothing. The hinged-malleable implant has interlocking springs that lock into place when the penis is pulled straight outward and then pressed toward the body to lock into rigid position (Fig. 27-7). Afterward the process is reversed, and the springs unlock to allow for a more natural penis position in clothing. Both of these prostheses require a 3-day hospital stay to recover from surgery, but with fewer mechanical parts, these tend to have less replacement and be more maintenance free (Leslie, 1990).

Thousands of both types of penile implants have been used since the 1970s with 95% of users reporting general satisfaction. Concerns are that the penis is shortened surgically, and there is decreased penile sensitivity and loss of any existing natural erection. Implants may be reserved until other treatment options are exhausted and the involved parties are fully informed. Clients who cannot tolerate, or do not wish, penile implant surgery may select an artificial penis, a device strapped onto the groin that simulates natural erection. Others use a vibrator to intensify stimuli in the

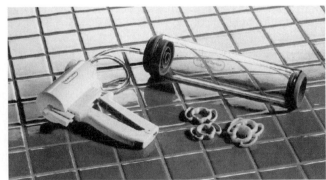
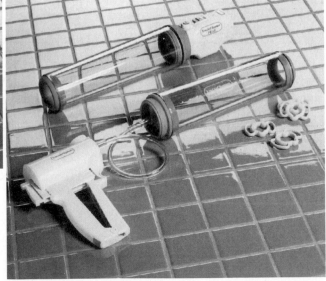

Fig. 27-5   **A,** ErecAid Hand-Pump System. **B,** ErecAid-Plus Battery-Operated System. (Courtesy of Osbon Medical Systems, Augusta, GA.)

genital area, thereby facilitating erection or masturbation. Because rough handling damages genital tissues and structures, a vibrator is used gently with a water-soluble lubricant. People are advised to stop use immediately on discomfort or irritation. Vibrator stimulation may enhance sexual function for some; however, clinicians report clients may become dependent on intense stimuli and find it more difficult to achieve orgasm from less stimulating touch.

About 5% of all persons with impotency may be candidates for some form of penile vascular surgery, microscopic reconstruction of the arterial blood supply, or removal of veins that drain blood from the penis too rapidly. Surgery is successful for 60% to 65% of candidates (Leslie, 1990). For males who are having problems with premature ejaculation, the "squeeze" technique delays ejaculation. A man must become aware when to signal withdrawal of stimula-

tion before ejaculation. Then either the man or his partner compresses the penis behind the glans or at the base, thereby inhibiting the ejaculatory reflex so intercourse can be resumed (Masters et al., 1986).

Some clients will accept and try some of the previously described approaches to sexual activity, whereas others will have concerns or prohibitive sociocultural beliefs. Sexual function is an individual choice, and the persons receiving education choose which activities they wish to learn about or practice based on their willingness to experiment or unwillingness to try new approaches.

Compensation for Motor Dysfunction and Positioning

Those who experience hypertonicity are persons with central nervous system injury including spinal cord injury above T12 or L1, multiple sclerosis, stroke, cerebral palsy,

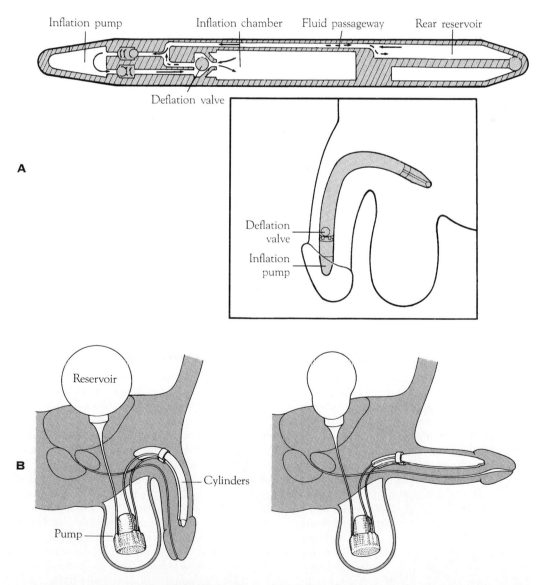

Fig. 27-6 **A,** One-piece inflatable penile prosthesis. **B,** Scott inflatable penile prosthesis. (From Mosby's Clinical Nursing, 3rd ed. by J.M. Thompson, 1993, St. Louis: Mosby–Year Book. Copyright 1993 by Mosby–Year Book. Reprinted by permission.)

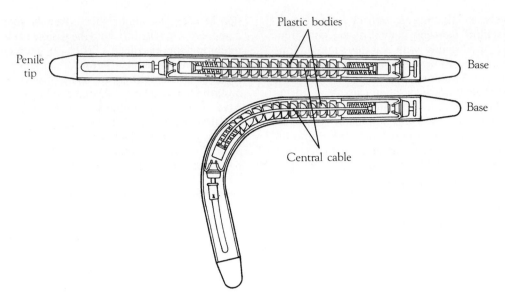

Fig. 27-7 One-piece prosthesis with a central cable that shortens the plastic bodies to produce erection. (From *Genitourinary Disorders* by M.L. Gray, 1992, St. Louis: Mosby–Year Book. Copyright 1992 by Mosby–Year Book. Reprinted by permission.)

spina bifida, or brain injury. Individuals who experience hypertonicity may have difficulty attaining and remaining in any position. Involuntary movements may be a source of embarrassment, as well as a matter of inconvenience, or impose a safety hazard during sexual activity. Medication may relieve or reduce the spasticity but reduce libido (Nygaard, Bartscht, & Cole, 1990). Steady stretching on a hypertonic muscle and avoiding jerking movements may relieve an isolated spasm, but it also may interfere with sexual activity. For persons with hemiplegia, position the affected side downward to allow free movement of the unaffected side.

Those persons who have hypotonicity use careful positioning as the best defense against subluxation at involved joints. Pillows or other supports prevent further stretching of ligaments, and joints are supported in proper alignment at all times.

A partner's inability to move the lower body places the responsibility for motor movement on the other partner. Water beds help, but may be difficult to get into and out of and can be hazardous to persons with limited head control while lying prone. A person with apraxia, motor planning dysfunction, may not be able to initiate the thrusting motor movement but may be able to assume the movement once the activity is initiated by the partner. One person initiates and simulates the motion. The partner must be willing to assume the dominant role in motor movement, which may be difficult for some females. Clients with ataxia, uncoordinated muscle movement, may need guidance and a position that provides stability to perform the motor components of coitus. Motor perseveration may interfere with moving from one activity to another; the partner may need to verbally or physically redirect the activity. In all cases of motor dysfunction, information benefits client and partner in their sexual activity.

A nurse may encourage clients to experiment with positions that are comfortable and appropriate for them and that enhance comfort and facilitate sexual activities. Information about alternate positions, as well as encouragement to experiment, often are welcomed by the individual and partner. Clients who have difficulty with bed mobility may need equipment such as side rails or bed loops for ease and safety in changing positions (Robunault, 1978). Loss of range of motion in the joints, particularly the hips, may limit movements during sexual activity and restrict their favorite positions. Pillows are positioners; those shaped like an armchair back can be beneficial in allowing the person with high spinal injury to see what is transpiring. Some persons are more comfortable in a recliner chair or other chair than in bed. Consider helping clients and their partners select positions that will place the least stress on involved parts of the client's body, thus managing pain or potential harm, and allowing the most sexual pleasure.

Precautions During Positioning

Some precautions are sensible in sexual positioning for clients who have been immobile for long periods of time or who do not bear weight on lower extremities. The weight of the partner on osteoporetic bones may be enough to cause fractures; others with recent orthopedic injuries with concomitant neurologic injuries may require bracing for bone stabilization. Until the physician decides it will be safe to remove a brace, the person wears it in bed during sexual activity. Generally a client may remove a brace when in bed but not during sexual activity. A brace also can determine positions as undue pressure should not be applied to the braced area of the body. Those persons with heterotropic ossification may have limited joint motion and painful joint areas and would benefit from positioning that would allow the most functional mobility while reducing pain.

Specific disabilities may preclude certain positions. For example, clients who have cardiac problems should avoid positions that place undue stress on the arms for sustained

---

CLIENT GUIDELINES FOR SEXUAL INTER-COURSE AFTER MYOCARDIAL INFARCTION

Familiar surroundings are important in diminishing psychological stress.

A comfortable temperature, neither too cold or hot, can decrease heart stress.

Prepare gradually for the increased activity of intercourse through foreplay; this helps to gradually prepare the heart.

Positions should be comfortable, relaxing, and permit unrestricted breathing. Usual positions are most comfortable.

Orogenital sex and masturbation cause no undue strain, so may be used for sexual expression if desired.

Intercourse is best performed when the couple is rested, so morning is an ideal time for couples at home.

Eating a heavy meal or drinking alcohol should be followed by rest of 3 hours' duration before sexual activity.

Take medications, such as nitroglycerin, before intercourse if required to prevent chest pain.

Sex with a new partner may incre-ase stress to the heart. (Seidl, Bullough, Scherer, Rhodes, Haughey, & Brown, 1991; Tardif, 1989).

---

periods. In this circumstance the client may find the supine position less stressful physically as long as breathing is not restricted. Often the side-by-side position and face-to-face position create less worry about compromising cardiac function. Sexual activity for the cardiac client should be resumed based on the physician's recommendation but is generally a few weeks after heart surgery and 3 to 8 weeks after myocardial infarction (Relf, 1991). Refer to the box above for guidelines for sexual intercourse following myocardial infarction. Chapter 19 discusses activity measures following myocardial infarction.

In the individual with spinal cord injury, especially complete injury at the T6 level or above, sexual activity may elicit autonomic dysreflexia or hyperreflexia, especially in certain positions that provide greater stimuli below the level of injury. Should symptoms of dysreflexia occur, the couple is taught to cease sexual activity so that the symptoms can subside. The client assumes an upright position, has blood pressure monitored, and takes prescribed medications. Medications such as mecamylamine hydrochloride (Inversine) may prevent dysreflexia symptoms but on the other hand may reduce desire and lead to erection problems.

Avoiding complications and providing a comfortable sexual activity are goals in experimenting with positions. Persons with rheumatic disease, for example, select positions that place the least stress on the involved joints. Those with loss of joint motion limit movement during sexual activity, and the client and partner may need to experiment with several positions before finding one that permits comfort and flexibility. About 70% of persons with arthritic hip joint problems reported sexual difficulties (Reinisch, 1990).

For females with arthritis affecting the hip joint, the spoon position where the male and female are side-lying, with the man behind the woman for rear entry into the vagina by the penis, is recommended. For men with hip problems the first recommendation is a position in which the couple lies side by side facing each other and the woman wraps her upper leg around the upper hip of her partner, or both legs around his hips. In another position the man lies supine while the woman sits astride his hips with her knees, lower legs, and feet on either side of his body if her legs are limber and knees support her. She can put her hands on the bed to control her weight on his pelvis (Reinisch, 1990). Pillows all around help support the weight and cushion painful joints.

Those with multiple sclerosis who experience fatigue and spasticity consider scheduling and positioning that is the most comfortable and least tiring (Valleroy & Kraft, 1984). Persons with spinal cord injury may need encouragement to experiment with various positions. Usually the person with spinal cord injury assumes the bottom position due to motor dysfunction and lack of movement. Pillows placed under the hips of the female make this a comfortable position for her, but she may experiment with the prone or side-lying positions.

Persons with disabilities may use variations of the four basic positions, all of which provide access for genital-to-genital contact, cunnilingus, and fellatio. The advantages and disadvantages of these positions are described in the following material.

1. Face-to-face, man above, or missionary position, allows partners to engage in continued kissing and hand touching of the body. The male controls movement in this position, which permits deep penile penetration. Pillows placed under the woman's back and buttocks allow deeper penetration, which may help impregnation because the semen is pooled at the top of the vagina. This position may be difficult if the man is overweight or the woman is pregnant. There are at least four disadvantages to this position: (1) the woman may feel "pinned" underneath the weight of her partner, making it more difficult to engage in pelvic movement; (2) the woman has little control over the depth of penetration; (3) the man may find it tiring to support his weight on his elbows and knees; and (4) the man may have less control over ejaculation than in other positions.

2. Face-to-face, woman above position allows for increased control by the female both from a psychological and mechanical viewpoint. Both partners may engage in kissing and touching of the body. Woman on top positions often are suggested for women who have difficulty experiencing orgasm during intercourse. They allow the woman more freedom to adjust her body to increase stimulation on whichever areas she finds most pleasurable. They also permit her more control over the depth of penetration and the rhythm of thrusting, other factors important in achieving orgasm. Some men do not feel comfortable emotionally with the control exercised by the woman in this position.

3. Face-to-face, side-lying position provides for freedom

of movement for both partners. It allows for kissing, touching, and exploration. Since neither partner is supporting the weight of the other, it can be less tiring and more relaxing over an extended period of time. Pillows may be used to support various areas such as the back and legs and to provide for increased comfort and decreased strain on muscles and joints. Penetration in the side-lying position is not as deep as in those positions where the male or female is on top.

4. Rear entry position is possible from a side-lying or sitting position or when the woman is kneeling or lying prone. Hand stimulation is possible for both partners, and penetration into the vagina may be regulated. Variations in this position are possible because multiple approaches using pillows as supports can be used. Persons who feel that face-to-face contact is important during intercourse may not find these positions acceptable (Reinisch, 1990).

Compensation for Sensory Dysfunction

Persons who have lost sensation to the genital area are those who experienced spinal cord injuries that are complete or affect sensation; persons with diabetes or multiple sclerosis; and a small number who may have heightened or diminished sensation on the affected side of their body following stroke. Persons with spinal cord injury report a wide variety of sexual sensations ranging from anesthesia to orgasm, and some report heightened pleasurable sensation that is similar to orgasm in other areas of the body during sexual activity. These include intact areas generally considered erogenous zones like the breasts, ears, eyes, neck, lower abdomen, groin, inner thighs, and the back above the level of the spinal cord lesion (Woods, 1984).

Sensory stimulation may enhance sexual enjoyment. Seeing the activity may enhance pleasure for those persons with decreased genital sensation, especially for males. Lighting the room, placing mirrors, and positioning for visualization may enhance sexual pleasure. The senses may promote fantasy; pleasant sounds, certain music, or the noises and words uttered during sexual activity may increase sexual desire or release. Touch as a sense is a major contributor to sexual pleasure, especially to intact areas of sensation. Rubbing or caressing using various textured items or lotions heightens touch. Smell is a sense probably not used as much as it could be to enhance sexual pleasure. Pleasant smells in the environment, on the person, and from sexual activity can be a powerful precursor to sexual pleasure. The taste of the partner is unique, and the special taste during sexual excitement may bring sexual pleasure to some persons.

Sensory amplification involves thinking about a physical stimulus very intensely and mentally amplifying that sensation to an intense degree. This technique can in some instances facilitate psychogenic orgasm.

Pain Control During Sexual Activity

Pain and sexual activity usually are associated with rheumatic diseases and joint replacement surgery. Many activities taught to clients by rehabilitation team members can be useful in providing pain control during sexual activity. Malek and Brower (1984) suggest several techniques to al-

---

◆ PAIN MANAGEMENT

Malek and Brower's (1984) techniques to alleviate or control pain during sexual activity for persons with rheumatoid arthritis

◆ Practice muscle relaxation techniques and mental imagery to promote comfort and tranquility

◆ Practice range-of-motion exercises without resistance to promote comfortable movement

◆ Apply moist heat to painful joints 10-15 minutes before sexual activity to reduce swelling and promote increased range of motion

◆ Rest after completion of bathing and grooming activities

◆ Position pillows under affected, painful limbs for support; always remember to remove these pillows after sexual activity to prevent contractures

◆ Schedule pain medications and arrange for sexual activities around the period of maximum drug effectiveness, when possible

◆ Explore alternative styles of sexual expression to convey caring, concern, and love

OTHER SUGGESTIONS TO REDUCE PAIN INCLUDE THE FOLLOWING:

◆ A warm water bed, an electric blanket over the client, or a bed warmer under the sheets to ease pain or stiffness, or a moist heating pad for a particularly painful joint

◆ Precede sex by a warm bath or massage, and mild exercise

◆ Some persons' pain may be relieved better by using cold applications rather than heat, especially for inflamed joints

◆ Frequent sexual activity may reduce pain of arthritis by stimulating adrenal glands to increase production of body's own natural antiinflammatory and pain-reducing corticosteroids (Reinisch, 1990)

---

leviate the pain of rheumatoid arthritis when engaging in sexual activities (see the box above). They stress avoiding fatigue and engaging in anticipatory planning and activity management. Their suggestions would be helpful to clients with other conditions involving painful muscles, and joints.

Often couples develop techniques to inform the partner that a particular activity or position is painful. With the "hand riding" technique, the person with pain places a hand on the partner's hand, signaling should distress occur. When intercourse is painful for either person, a thorough medical examination may identify organic causes and suggest corrections. Without a physical cause, referral to a certified sex therapist may be appropriate, as psychosocial conditions can contribute to painful intercourse (Reinisch, 1990).

Women, particularly postmenopausal women or those with spinal cord injuries, may experience discomfort during intercourse because of decreased vaginal lubrication. As a woman's estrogen level decreases, she is more likely to experience vaginal dryness, atrophy of the vagina and external genitalia, thinning of the vaginal lining, and a tendency to vaginal and urinary tract infections. Treatment for postmenopausal women includes use of vaginal lubrication, hormone replacement therapy, and preventing or treating infections. Only water-soluble lubricants that can be removed easily are used. These include K-Y Jelly, Lubrin inserts, Replens, and Astroglide. Oil-based lubricants are not recommended as they increase risk of infection, particularly for females, and rapidly destroy the effectiveness of rubber condoms, diaphragms, and cervical caps.

Bowel and/or Bladder Management

Persons with bowel and/or bladder incontinence are anxious about the possibility of urinating or defecating during sexual activity. Because the autonomic nervous system regulates sexual function and influences bowel and bladder control, activation of one set of neurons can activate the others. A partner is advised when potential for incontinence exists to prevent embarrassment and in preparation. Use protection for bed covers, rinse items in white vinegar with washing to eliminate any urine odor, and use incense or cologne to mask odor if no one is sensitive or allergic. Prepare by emptying the bladder and limiting liquid intake; schedule sexual activity soon after completing an established bowel program.

A man with an indwelling urinary catheter tapes it in place with nonstick tape near the base of the penis or sheathes it in a condom. Apply lubricant to smooth the presence of the catheter or tape. Women tape an indwelling catheter to the abdomen or remove it before sexual activity and replace it afterward. Suprapubic or ileoloop appliances need not be removed but are taped to the abdomen. Urinary flow to any catheter cannot be obstructed for long periods without increasing the risk for urinary tract infection.

Medication Management

Medications and other ingested substances can effect sexual performance. It is possible that medication taken for the treatment of hypertension, heart disease, anxiety or stress, depression, psychiatric illness, sleeplessness, convulsions, gastrointestinal disorders, or arthritis may affect sexual functioning. Symptoms of sexual dysfunction may not develop immediately after taking a medication; the onset may be later in the course of drug therapy. If sexual dysfunction develops, the client is advised to discuss the effects with a physician, who can try a different dosage or an alternative drug. Clients who go against medical advice by experimenting with dosages or deleting medications without the consent and advice of the physician may jeopardize their health. A woman who intends or suspects pregnancy is referred to her physician, so medications can be evaluated to aid in prevention of birth defects (Reinisch, 1990).

Fertility, Infertility, and Birth Control

Fertility and infertility are both major issues for persons of childbearing years who have experienced an accident or illness. Some form of birth control or permanent sterilization are options if they do not desire to become pregnant. Birth control information shared with all fertile clients and partners is an essential element in education. Often society

and the client mistakenly assume that disability results in infertility and no precautions are needed. Clients who have the ability to impregnate or become pregnant need to know correct information before sexual activity to avoid future physical, social, emotional, vocational, and spiritual problems for themselves and partners.

Instruction includes information on sexual anatomy, the physiology of contraception, and birth control devices or methods. A contraceptive method is chosen based on accurate information about failure rates, reversibility, safety, and personal health status. The nurse obtains feedback from the couple about previous birth control practices (before injury or illness) and preparation to meet future birth control needs. Referral to a gynecologist or urologist may be required for the birth control method of the couple's choice.

Table 27-5 and the following material provide a brief discussion of birth control methods, including effectiveness, availability, and advantages and disadvantages for certain disability groups.

✦ Oral contraceptives (the pill)

The pill does not protect from STDs and may reduce the effectiveness of antibiotics (ampicillin and tetracycline). Antibiotics also can reduce the effectiveness of the pill, as can anticonvulsants (phenytoin and primidone). This is important information for some of our adolescent patients who may take antibiotics for acne or head injury patients who take anticonvulsants as a preventative or treatment after head injury.

PREGNANCY

Women with chronic illnesses or traumatic injuries generally maintain their fertility, keeping childbearing an option. Although women with chronic illness or traumatic injury, including rheumatic disease and spinal cord or head injury, can give birth to healthy infants, supervision by a trained physician is advisable since there are risks during pregnancy, labor, and delivery for mother and infant.

Medication management is addressed before pregnancy or as early as possible. Baclofen for spasticity is tapered gradually to prevent seizures from sudden withdrawal. Anticonvulsant drugs, such as phenytoin or carbamazepine, are evaluated and managed carefully. A mother receiving antiseizure medication has double the risk (4% to 6% versus 2% to 3%) of bearing an infant with special needs; however, risk of falls during grand mal seizures resulting in injury to mother and fetus are greater. Diazepam raises the potential for fetal cleft palate and infant withdrawal after birth. Nonsteroidal antiinflammatory drugs are withdrawn in the client with rheumatic disease. As with all pregnant women, the use of alcohol and smoking is discouraged.

Complications of concern for a pregnant woman with spinal cord injury include urinary tract infections, anemia, pressure sores, sepsis, unattended birth, and autonomic hyperreflexia (Comaar, 1966). Interventions may vary with physicians but typically include prevention. For example, prophylactic antibiotics for urinary tract infection; monitoring weight gain that may inhibit movement and transfers; and skin inspection twice daily for preventing pressure ulcers; strict adherence to skin integrity principles, especially during labor and delivery. Should a pressure ulcer develop,

Table 27-5 Birth control methods

Method	Effects	Advantage	Disadvantages	Contraindications
Oral contraceptives: hormone pills taken 1 daily for 21 days, none for 7 days or placebo; then restart cycle on 5th day of menses.	Alter hormone patterns to supress ovulation; cervical mucosa and endometrium resist sperm. Note: Those with history of blood clots such as following SCI, multiple trauma, stroke, or coronary artery disease or those who have hypertension, diabetes, gallbladder disease, or irregular menses are not candidates for "the pill."	2%-3% fail due to irregular use. Reduced: PMS, cramps, fibrocystic breast disease, ovarian cysts. Highly reversible, convenient.	No STD protection, less effective with antibiotic therapy. Minor side effects usually decrease. Major concern: thromboembolus problems.	Teach client to report severe abdominal or chest pain; visual or speech changes; leg cramps or pain, headache, dizziness, weakness, or numbness; shortness of breath. Refer to physician.
Norplant: matchstick-like tubes inserted in arm above elbow in 15 minutes with local anesthetic.	Levonorgestrel is released steadily into bloodstream in small amounts; no estrogen; inhibits ovulation, thickens cervical mucosa to inhibit sperm motility.	Less than 1% failure. Minimal side effects, effective in 24 hours after implant and for 5 years; then new insert. Reversible. Continual protection over time without action.	No research regarding persons with disability; longer menses, but lighter.	Breast cancer, liver disease, uterine bleeding problems, breast-feeding or pregnant women.
IUDs inserted into uterus. Only 2 in USA: ParaGard (Copper T380A) and Progestasert, which is replaced annually.	Exact action unclear; prevent implantation of ovum.	5% fail with ParaGard; 2% with Progestasert. Reversible.	Check monthly for string placement; device must stay in place. With impaired hand function, partner may have to check; with decreased sensation in saddle area, pain or bleeding may be missed. No STD protection.	Not recommended for those exposed to multiple partners; at risk for PID or STDs.
Barriers: sperm trapped or prevented entry to cervix, or chemical spermicide. Condoms placed over penis before preejaculatory fluid. Female condom (Reality) under tests.	Only latex protects from HIV and hepatitis B. Oil-based lubricants destroy latex. Spermicide may be used with condom or applied if condom fails. Use new condom for each encounter, discard after use.	10% failure due to improper use or product failure; 2%-3% when used properly. Inexpensive, reversible, no prescription.	Must be used each time. Male is responsible. For person with impaired hand or range of function, partner must apply.	
Diaphragm: dome-shaped latex spread with spermicide cream or jelly; placed in vagina to cover and surround cervix.	Inserted before contact and remaining for 6 hours after intercourse; blocks sperm entry through cervix, spermicide destroys sperm. Sized and prescribed by physician or nurse practitioner; weight gain or loss, and childbirth may change size needed.	As low as 2% failure when correctly sized, placed, and used. 10%-19% failure in other studies.	Poor size may lead to pain or irritation, even infections. Menstrual use may lead to toxic shock; allergies to latex or spermicides.	With reduced flexibility, hand function, balance, or sensation, partner may have to insert diaphragm; if dislodged, may not be perceived by woman.

Method	Description	Effectiveness	Use/Instructions	Considerations for impairment
Spermicide foams, jellies, creams, dissolving tablets, or suppositories.	Active chemical attacks sperm and base forms mechanical barrier. With added nonoxynol-9 or octoxynol, protects against many STDs. Renew application for each encounter.	18%-21% failure when used alone; more effective in combination. No prescription; safe and inexpensive.	Cream, foam, jells must be inserted within 30 minutes of intercourse; tablet and suppository 10-15 minutes ahead. Douche may wash away spermicide.	Proper placement may be difficult for those limited hand function, balance, or flexibility.
Sponge: soft, round polyurethane sponge fits with dimpled end over cervix; loop on other side for removal.	Spermicide activated when moistened with water before insertion. For second encounter, retain sponge but reapply spermicide.	10%-20% failure rate. No prescription; protects against some STDs and PID.	Leave in place 8 hours after intercourse; remove and discard. Not used with menses or 3-6 weeks postpartum to avoid toxic shock syndrome.	Proper insertion needed and may require partner to insert and remove if woman has impairment.
Withdrawal (coitus interruptus).	Penis is moved from genital area and/or withdrawn from vagina before ejaculation.	23% failure rate. Cooperation, communication, and timing.	Sperm may be present in preejaculatory fluid; enjoyment may be frustrated, or partner may miscalculate.	Person with impairment may lose control; woman must decide timing when partner has limited movement or sensation.
Natural methods: rhythm, fertility awareness methods: calendar, basal body temperature, or cervical mucus test. Abstinence during at-risk times as determined by tests. Training and combination of techniques and regular cycle help.	Calendar: track start and stop of menstrual cycle for 6 months. Abstain 10+ days midcycle. Basal temperature: Daily AM temperature of woman. Increase of 0.4-0.8° F within 24 hours of ovulation. Abstain 7 days before and 3 days after rise. Cervical mucus: observe cervical mucus for raw egg white status and stretches to ∠ inch strand between fingertips signals ovulation. Safe days are after ovulation until menses; days after menses when mucus negative.	Inexpensive, reversible, no chemicals or hormones. 2%-10% failure for those with regular cycles and proper use; 24% failure overall but 40% with mucus alone. Promotes woman's awareness of her own body. Home urine test kits detect LH used for both preventing and detecting pregnancy.	Requires training, commitment to testing, and abstinence. Both partners agree and participate. Ovum may be fertilized 1 day in a cycle, but sperm can reach ovum from semen deposited in vagina approximately 8 days before ovulation, plus the ovulation day. Thus abstinence before ovulation is necessary. No STD protection.	Persons must be cognitively able to calculate and responsible for adhering to schedules.
Permanent sterilization: vasectomy or tubal ligation. Surgical techniques.	Vasectomy: vas deferens cut to block sperm ejaculation. Tubal ligation: fallopian tubes surgically blocked, preventing ova from reaching uterus or fertilization in tubes.	Effective and popular for couples >30 years of age who have established families. Failure 160/100,000 for vasectomy and 276-326/100,000 for tubal ligation. Vasectomy simpler and safer.	Surgical techniques. Irreversible except in specific cases, then requires surgery with no guarantee.	Informed consent couple must understand permanency. May have ethical issue when used for vulnerable populations.

SCI, spinal cord injury; STD, sexually transmitted disease; IUDs, intrauterine devices; PID, pelvic inflammatory disease; HIV, human immunodeficiency virus; LH, luteinizing hormone.

the resulting nutritional catabolic state or anemia is treated aggressively to avoid inhibiting fetal growth. Attention to decreased gastrointestinal motility with pregnancy may prevent constipation and maintain bowel programs (Craig, 1990).

Vaginal checks for signs of premature labor begin at 26 weeks. If sensation is diminished, monitor contractions and educate the client with injury above the T10 level about increased vaginal discharge as a signal of undetected labor pain. Uterine contraction and cervical dilation travel via sympathetic nerves entering the spinal cord between T10 and L1. In later stages of labor, impulses from the perineum travel via the pudendal nerves, which enter the spinal cord at S2-S4; as a result those with lesions below T12 may have uterine sensation but perineal anesthesia. Labor pains are recognized in some women as abdominal spasms, leg spasms, difficulty in breathing, or back pain (Wanner, Rageth, & Zach, 1987). Episodic hypertension may be the first sign of uterine contractions since the uterus contracts during labor by intermuscular communication without a connected nerve supply (Nygaard et al., 1990). With lesions at the T10 to T11 level, poor uterine contractions may necessitate cesarean section; forceps may facilitate delivery when abdominal muscles are paralyzed.

Autonomic hyperreflexia may occur during labor and delivery in as many as two thirds of carefully observed pregnant women with spinal cord lesions at T6 or above (Nygaard et al., 1990). Suggestions for prevention of dysreflexia include topical anesthetic whenever procedures such as catheterizations, rectal manipulation, or vaginal examination might produce symptoms. Regional anesthesia, such as epidural or spinal block, can prevent or control autonomic dysreflexia during labor; similarly, epidural or spinal narcotics are preferable to anesthesia, which also inhibit the spinal reflexes that cause hyperreflexia (Baraka, 1985). The nurse assesses for noxious stimuli, a full bladder or bowel, and monitors blood pressure. Physicians may order medication for blood pressure control to include nifedipine, nitroglycerin, hydralazine, prazosin, or atropine. Upright positioning to decrease symptoms and assisted delivery to shorten labor may be indicated (Nygaard et al., 1990). Postpartum, observe for deep vein thrombosis and urinary tract infection.

Many conditions contribute to infertility: erectile or ejaculation dysfunction, decreased sperm count or motility, altered thermoregulation to the testicles from autonomic nervous system dysfunction, or hormonal irregularities in both sexes following brain injury. Until recently infertility in persons with disabilities was not treated aggressively. Currently several centers in the United States provide programs for couples who are infertile, have disabilities, and wish to bear children. Sperm may be collected using vibrators, rectal stimulation, or intrathecal injections, then washed and used for artificial insemination or in vitro fertilization. Couples who have had successful unprotected intercourse for 1 full year during the woman's most fertile time in each cycle without pregnancy benefit from fertility evaluation. If a health problem affects fertility for one partner, a fertility clinic is recommended. Fertility problems generally are equal between male and female partners. An accessible fertility clinic for persons with disabilities would be the choice for infertility management.

Prevention of Sexually Transmitted Diseases

STDs are near epidemic levels in the United States and are increasing in incidence. STDs can be uncomfortable or painful, inconvenient, embarrassing, anxiety producing, or fatal to a large percentage of those infected. They also can be persistent or leave residual damage as with *Chlamydia* and gonorrhea. The persistent herpesvirus has been found in up to 30% to 40% of single, sexually active people, and syphilis is at a 40-year high. Any symptoms of genital infection must be diagnosed immediately and treated to protect both the infected individuals and partners. All sexually active persons, especially those not in mutually exclusive relationships or who have changed partners, need to know the common symptoms of STDs and be tested during annual medical examinations. Early diagnosis and treatment may prevent some long-term complications.

Guidelines for safe sex include abstinence until marriage, monogamous sex, and marriage for life. Safer sex guidelines were developed (see the following box on p. 621) for all persons, although they were developed in response to the AIDS epidemic. The guidelines reduce risks when used properly and every time.

Psychosocial Factors
✦ Self-concept disturbance

Because self-concept is composed of self-ideal, self-image, and self-esteem it may be affected adversely by altered sexual abilities. Nurses enhance a client's self-concept throughout rehabilitation interventions. Successful bowel and bladder retaining, transfer training, and ADL training improve self-concept. Self-esteem thrives in a therapeutic environment where a trusting relationship is formed with caregivers who communicate acceptance and inclusion of a client as a worthwhile and unique human being apart from the disability. The sooner one returns to meaningful work and becomes a productive financial provider for the family, the greater the self-esteem and role balance. All factors that build self-concept contribute positively to the sexual relationship. On the other hand, self-concept may be affected by a decrease in sexual abilities and performance. Men who are anxious about sexual problems may voice concern about their ability to provide satisfaction for their partners. When role changes become necessary for sexual activities, the nurse provides support and encouragement, as well as education about compensation strategies or fertility clinics when appropriate.

✦ Social isolation

A client whose self-concept is threatened may avoid contact with others and become socially isolated. Involving the client in social interaction as early as possible, complimenting efforts to appear attractive, discussing individual sexual concerns, and accepting concerns matter-of-factly may help the client maintain or restore self-concept.

In a facility clients are encouraged to eat with others in the dining room, participate in groups in the therapy departments and on nursing units, participate in education pro-

---

SAFER SEX GUIDELINES

1. Delay sexual intercourse as long as possible. Abstinence is the only completely safe behavior.

2. Restrict the number of sexual partners you have. The fewer sexual partners you have in your lifetime, the smaller the chance of being exposed to an STD.

3. You are at lower risk for catching STDs when you are in a mutual sexually exclusive relationship. This means you and your partner have sex only with each other. If neither you nor your partner is infected with an STD, then you can safely engage in any sexual activity with each other that you choose.

4. Learn as much as possible about any new potential sexual partner, but don't accept answers at face value. Unfortunately research shows that people lie about things such as how many partners they have had. In one study 47% of men and 42% of women admitted telling dates that they had fewer partners than was really the case. Researchers suspect people are even more likely to lie about homosexual activity, sex with prostitutes, or the use of illegal drugs.

5. Do not assume that what people call themselves (heterosexual or homosexual) tells you anything about their actual sexual behavior. Studies of men from the general population show that more than 30% have had at least one sexual experience with another male since puberty. Three studies of homosexual men reported that between 62% and 79% had engaged in heterosexual intercourse. Four other studies found that 15% to 26% of homosexual men had been married. A recent study of lesbian women found that 74% had engaged in heterosexual intercourse at least once since age 18. Do not assume that a female partner is automatically in a low-risk group for STDs or that a male partner has never had sex with other men (Kinsey, 1990).

6. Avoid high-risk sexual behavior until you are certain your partner is not infected with an STD. The most risky behaviors are unprotected anal intercourse and unprotected vaginal intercourse (i.e., without using a condom and a spermicide containing nonoxynol-9 or octoxynol). Anal intercourse appears to be the sexual activity that most easily transmits the AIDS virus if it is present, perhaps because the anal and rectal tissues are more likely to be damaged, thereby providing easy access into the body (Reinisch, 1990). Also refrain from unprotected orogenital sex, fisting, or rimming unless you are certain neither you nor your partner is infected. Fisting even without the presence of infection can be harmful including rupture of the anal sphincter, perforation of the colon, various rectal infections, and tears in the mucous membranes of the anus or rectum. Perforation occurs when force is used against the natural curves and broad muscle supports of the pelvis. Pressure on the vagus nerve, which has receptors in the colon, can produce heart arrhythmias that could be fatal. Damage to the vagina and cervix is also a possible result of vaginal fisting (Reinisch, 1990).

7. Any activity that exposes a person to blood, semen, vaginal secretions, menstrual blood, urine, feces, or saliva should be considered high-risk behavior unless partners are in a mutually sexually exclusive relationship and neither is infected. The AIDS virus and other STD organisms can enter the mucous membranes of the mouth, vagina, or rectum through even microscopically small breaks anywhere on the skin.

8. If you decide to have penile-anal intercourse, using a condom and a spermicide with nonoxynol-9 or octoxynol as an ingredient can provide good protection against many STDs. Condoms don't provide protection when an infectious area is not covered. For example, a herpes sore on the scrotum would not be covered.

9. If you decide to engage in fellatio (oral sex on a penis), using a condom provides good protection if either of you is infected. Put the condom on before touching the penis with your mouth, lips, or tongue.

10. If you decide to engage in cunnilingus (oral sex on a vulva), placing a dental dam (or other latex) over the vulva provides good protection if either of you is infected. Dental dams are thin sheets of latex rubber used by dentists to isolate an infected area of the mouth during dental work. They may be available at a medical supply store (Reinisch, 1990).

11. Vibrators, dildos, or other items used for sexual stimulation should not be shared with another person until thoroughly washed with soap and water. Plenty of lubricant should be applied, and these items should be used gently to avoid irritating the skin or breaking vaginal or rectal tissues.

---

grams and in social skills groups and support groups. Peer groups and peer counselors may be helpful in overcoming social isolation. Some support groups have special meetings for survivors or former clients to help meet social needs. Volunteering in the community provides a social outlet as well as a service to others. Providing lists of community resources helps clients to meet persons with similar interests and may facilitate the return to work or school.

Social isolation reduces opportunity to meet that special someone with whom the client would desire to build a strong interpersonal or sexual relationship. Community resources include church singles ministries, special-interest groups, community education classes and programs, participative sports programs, and volunteer opportunities as places for meeting people. Concerning fostering relationships:

- ✦ Don't believe that no one will love you because you have a disability
- ✦ Don't build your life in search of romance; use activities to meet people
- ✦ Be a friend first

+ Keep up on current events
+ Be patient in your search for connection with others
+ Be open about your disability
+ Regardless of your disability, lovemaking is possible (National Information Center for Children and Youth with Disabilities, 1992)

+ Education concerning building and maintaining relationships

Information concerning building and maintaining relationships should be an essential component of the education provided to clients and their partners. Masters et al. (1986) give some pointers concerning communicating about sex (see the following box).

One area where men and women differ is communication. In general, researchers find (Smalley & Trent, 1988) men process and remember in conversation mainly through the left side of the brain. They then focus on the actual words said and process the literal words and factual data while missing the underlying emotions. Women, however, store nonverbal and emotional communication, perceiving the tone of voice as well as the emotional or pictorial messages. To reconcile the differences, the researchers recommend a technique of developing and presenting word pictures to aid each in better understanding the other. Word pictures or analogies bridge both sides of the brain and enable a couple to unlock the gateway to intimacy (Smalley & Trent, 1988). In communicating with a partner to assure understanding, build the message through use of analogy: "I'll love you until I've drained the Pacific Ocean by removing the water one bucket at a time." Relationships are nutured by the daily sharing of our feelings, needs, hopes, and dreams, and by being a good listener when our partner shares.

+ Trust and honor

Building trust and honor is a choice involving a lifelong commitment to stay together, understand each other's needs, develop the skills to meet those needs, and desire to resolve conflicts and promote harmony. Following an illness or injury partners choose to accept the one injured as the unique, complete person that is loved and to look for ways to comfort and nurture.

+ Affection and romance

Couples can be encouraged to express affection through meaningful touch during their loved one's hospitalization and are allowed the privacy to greet one another with a kiss or hug. Meaningful touch is one area opened to all disability groups, as most have some areas of intact sensation. Verbally conveying feelings is opened to all those who can communicate verbally or through sign language. Eight to ten meaningful touches a day keeps the fires of the relationship burning (Spica, 1989). Romance is a shared emotional experience of special times that focus on how valuable each is to the other, but couples may require careful planning and conversation to rediscover romance and to build romance into their daily lives. Encouragement is given to schedule intimate times together in spite of the pressures of life with a disability (Smalley & Trent, 1988).

Preparing for Home

Increasingly rehabilitation nurses are working in the community as consultants or providing direct services. A great deal of a client's adjustment to disability will occur after hospitalization. Rehabilitation nursing assessment and interventions during hospitalization are instrumental in identifying sexual problems requiring early intervention, discharge planning, and follow-up. Problems resolved during the hospitalization with staff intervention lay the groundwork for problem resolution at home.

Ideally rehabilitation facilities provide privacy for the client to be alone or with the spouse to experiment with techniques. Facility personnel and clients decide what they feel comfortable in providing and allowing. Some inpatient facilities allow sexual activity only for married couples to prevent lawsuits and protect those incompetent to make ratio-

---

COMMUNICATING ABOUT SEX

+ Talk with your partner about how and when it would be most comfortable to discuss sex. This will let your partner know you are interested in feedback about your sexual interaction.
+ Consider the possibility of using books or other media sources to initiate discussions. One disadvantage is that books do not always suit the personal style of the couple, so choose one that is not offensive.
+ Use "I" language as much as possible when talking about sex together and try to avoid putting blame on your partner for your own patterns of response (or lack thereof).
+ Remember that if your partner rejects a type of sexual activity that you think you might enjoy, he or she is not rejecting you as a person.
+ Be aware that sexual feelings and preferences change from time to time.
+ Don't neglect the nonverbal side of sexual communication, since these messages often speak louder than words.
+ Don't expect perfection.
   Talking about sex with your partner is not something to do once and then put aside. Like all forms of intimate communication, this topic benefits from the ongoing dialogue that permits a couple to learn about each other and resolve confusion or uncertainties over time (Masters et al., 1986).

nal decisions. Visiting for sexual purposes may be allowed only in certain areas where more privacy is allowed. All staff members should be required to knock on a client's closed door and wait for permission to enter as a common courtesy. Weekend passes while the client is still hospitalized can be helpful in providing opportunities to try out new sexual options in the privacy of their own surroundings. Time should be planned to discuss the weekend experiences with the client and spouse, if they desire.

Rehabilitation nurses also need to know the community and community-based nurses well enough to arrange appropriate referral sources for individuals who require continuing services as part of the team plan. Follow-up appointments with a member of the rehabilitation team may be scheduled to deal with sexual difficulties related to the disability.

Some clients and their partners will require intensive therapy. Two professional organizations, the Society for Sex Therapy and Research (New York) and the American Association of Sex Educators, Counselors, and Therapists (Washington, D.C.), publish national directories of qualified sex therapists. Local medical societies, psychological associations, and certified psychiatric or mental health nurses, mental health associations, and other nurses working in rehabilitation centers or as members of a sexual management team may be helpful in identifying qualified sex therapists in an area.

Evaluation

Evaluation is an essential part of the nursing process. As related to the nursing interventions of education or counseling, there are two methods to use in evaluation. One is demonstration of skills taught; the other is by having the information verbally repeated by the learner. Since sexual activity is a private matter, the only evaluation method that would be socially acceptable to most people is questioning and then evaluating the verbal responses. The nurse could ask which of the individualized goals have been achieved. The client and partner are free to decide if they wish to answer the questions. Relationship factors can be evaluated by observation of interactions of the client and partner. When teaching concerning use of devices to promote erection such as injections or the vacuum device, and birth control devices, return demonstration for use of the device should be required before use to assure correct placement or usage of the device. Ordinarily this would be done at the prescribing physician's office. The effectiveness of birth control methods can be evaluated by the absence of pregnancy and side effects.

CONCLUSION

The ability to function as a sexual being is a basic need of all persons. This need coexists with chronic illness or disability, where sexual concerns sometimes become a major focus. Since sexual concerns are tremendously complex, no simple behavioral or medical approach will suffice to assess or treat individual sexual problems. Ideally a sexual management team—whose members are comfortable with their own sexuality, knowledgeable about sexuality, and willing to commit a considerable amount of time—is required to plan and implement a team approach for the individual with sexual problems.

Rehabilitation nurses frequently deal with these problems at their level of comfort, refer to other team members if unable to address the problems expressed, and participate as members of the sexual management team. It is the responsibility of every rehabilitation nurse to give the client permission to discuss sexual concerns and then to deal with any expressed difficulties appropriately. Clients should leave rehabilitation settings knowledgeable concerning their sexual function, with their questions answered, prepared to manage their sexual function independently or direct their partner in the process.

CASE STUDY 1

Daniel Lacey is a 57-year-old Black male who experienced a left middle cerebral artery cerebrovascular accident 3 months ago. Currently he is ambulatory for community distances using a straight cane; his right arm (his dominant hand) is hypertonic and has minimal movement; sensation is diminished on the right side. He has predominately expressive aphasia and a right visual field cut. He is independent in self-care, in some home maintenance, and is bowel and bladder continent.

Mr. Lacey is unable to return to his previous job as a truck driver. The Laceys have been married for 30 years and have four grown children. He regularly attends a Baptist church. Church attendance and family visits are his primary outings. Mrs. Lacey works full time and feels she cannot quit her job, especially now that her husband is not working. The Laceys have a strong relationship and premorbidly had a good sexual relationship, especially after the children left home. Mrs. Lacey had a tubal ligation shortly after the birth of her last child. Their usual method of sexual expression is penile-vaginal intercourse.

During his rehabilitation stay Mr. Lacey attended a group class on sexuality, but due to his communication problem he did not verbally participate. Upon his follow-up visit at 3 months, his wife requested from the physiatrist, "Can we resume our sexual relationship or is that not possible?" The physiatrist assured her they can resume but felt they needed more education than he had time to give. The Laceys were referred to the case manager, a nurse, for further counseling.

The case manager identified the need for education concerning compensation strategies for sexual function as a primary need for this couple, especially as related to their communication problem and Mr. Lacey's motor and sensory deficits. She also noted a need to work with Mr. Lacey concerning issues of self-esteem related to the change in his role of provider.

The nurse did a thorough assessment and reviewed the physical examination completed by the physician. She noted that Mr. Lacey had normal rectal sphincter tone and control of external anal and bladder sphincters. He had normal sensation when his testicles were squeezed and his bulbocavernosus and anal wink reflexes were normal. Premorbidly Mr. Lacey had normal sexual function.

The nurse identified problems that could be encountered sexually by this couple. She developed the following nursing diagnoses:

1. Knowledge Deficit concerning how stroke affects sexual function; positioning for sexual function for a person with hemiparesis; compensation for sensory dysfunction and communication impairment
2. Self-concept Deficit related to recent change in lifestyle
   GOALS: Following the education provided by the case manager the Laceys will:
1. Be knowledgeable concerning basic information on the effects of the cerebrovascular accident on sexual function
2. Discuss information about sexual options, compensation strategies, and devices
3. Begin to participate in sexual activity at a level near their preillness level
4. Experience maintenance or restoration of a positive self-concept including improving body image

The case manager's plan of care included teaching the Laceys the following information:

1. Because of his normal sensation and voluntary motor control over bowel and bladder function, sexually Mr. Lacey's body should work like it did before his stroke. It may take some time, 6 to 7 weeks poststroke, to return to previous levels.
2. Participation in sexual activities would not increase Mr. Lacey's potential for another stroke or harm him.
3. Positions that may increase Mr. Lacey's ability to move and participate include side-lying with the right side on the bed to free his more mobile side for stroking or caressing his wife. Having his right side downward would also allow his wife to be in his intact field of vision. Positioning could include face to face or front to back. Another possible position is male on his back, female on top. For Mr. Lacey semisitting in a supported position would allow increased visualization. Mrs. Lacey would have to assume the motor movement in this position. To gradually work back into genital intercourse, dual partner stimulation may be initiated as a first step.
4. Other sexual activities that have been pleasurable should be encouraged such as kissing, touching sensitive body areas, caressing, licking, hugging, or oral sex, and so on.
5. To compensate for diminished sensation on the involved right side, the intact side of the body should be used for rubbing and pleasuring. The couple may wish to use sensate focus activities to redefine the pleasurable areas or activities. Leaving the light on may be helpful with decreased visual fields. Auditory and olfactory stimuli may be increased as compensation.
6. The communication problem is a major barrier to the sexual relationship. The couple may want to discuss, using yes/no communication, the development of a signal to use for interest in sexual activity and a signal for discomfort, should that occur during sexual activity. Some couples express that, with the decreased intimacy resulting from the communication deficit, sexual activity helps maintain the couple's oneness.
7. Working to build self-esteem involves every facet of life, not sexual function in isolation. Mrs. Lacey should allow her husband to be as independent as possible and to contribute as much as possible to family responsibilities and their relationship. Finding an effective method for communication through continued speech therapy would be helpful. The nurse suggests psychological counseling. Medication may be ordered by the physician. This may have the adverse effect of decreasing libido, so caution should be advised. To compensate for lost work status and social isolation, a volunteer position or return to work in a different capacity may be suggested.

Outcome several months later showed that Mr. and Mrs. Lacey increased their understanding of compensation strategies and returned closer to their premorbid rate of sexual activity over a period of time using the compensation strategies. They discovered the pleasurable sensory areas and used increased sensory stimulation. Their intimacy grew through sexual expression, as did Mr. Lacey's self-concept. Frustration with limited communication continues to be a problem, but speech therapy continues.

CASE STUDY 2

Pam Delaney is a 27-year-old white female who experienced a complete spinal cord injury at T10 in a motor vehicle accident. She has been married 4 years and has a 2-year-old son. Before the accident she was a speech/language pathologist; her husband Jim teaches history in the local high school. Pam is in an acute rehabilitation hospital. She attends daily group education classes on spinal injury. The team feels she will be independent with transfers, activities of daily living, and home management including child care upon discharge. She will wear a clam shell body brace for 3 months from the date of the accident. The rehabilitation nurse will teach an individualized education program to Pam and her husband on the subject of sexual function. Pam and Jim had a satisfying sexual relationship before the accident, and he has been supportive of her since.

The teaching plan includes the following nursing diagnoses:

1. Sexual dysfunction related to motor and sensory deficit, reduced activity tolerance, and body image disturbance
2. Knowledge deficit concerning the effects of T10 spinal cord injury on sexual dysfunction; positioning for sexual function; compensation for sensory loss; special precautions and birth control issues

GOALS: Following the education provided by the rehabilitation nurse the Delaneys will

1. Be knowledgeable concerning the effects of complete spinal cord injury at the T10 level on sexual function
2. Be knowledgeable concerning compensation for sensory loss, positioning and motion for sexual function, special precautions, and birth control
3. Begin to accept Pam's altered body image and experience beginning return of positive self-concept

The teaching plan included the following information regarding the overview of changes related to sexual function: Pam will have no sensation related to genital sexual function. She will have no ability to move the pelvic area of her lower body or to position her legs without use of her hands. Pam may not experience vaginal lubrication during sexual stimulation. She will experience the same level of fertility as before injury since there was no damage other than spinal cord injury. Brain function is intact and so is sensation above T10. Pam has good hand function and will eventually have good bed mobility skills as well as the ability to perform all activities of daily living including bowel and bladder programs.

Compensation strategies to be taught:

1. Compensation for sensory loss will include manual stimulation of the female to the intact areas of function including the breasts, face, ears, and eyes. Pam can supply manual stimulation to her husband in all areas. Increasing visual stimuli by having lights on may be helpful. Fragrance worn by both partners may be positively stimulating. Using fantasy for both partners may promote sensory appreciation.

2. Positions that will be suggested include face to face or front to back with the woman on the bottom, or side-lying. Pam should be cautioned to wear her back brace during sexual activity for as long as the physician recommends it for support. Also, both should be cautioned that osteoporosis makes her bones more prone to fractures, so the weight of her husband should be kept off her legs. They may participate in orogenital intercourse if they desire. Movement may be enhanced for Jim by use of a full-motion water bed.

3. Vaginal lubrication should be recommended if not sufficient for genital intercourse. This should be replaced every few minutes to prevent problems and must be water-soluble. A gynecologist may recommend an estrogen cream or vitamin E to enhance vaginal moisture.

4. Education concerning maintaining relationships should be provided to this couple. Information concerning the value of each to the relationship, honoring each other, and building romance and fun into their time together should be shared. Working together to build self-esteem should be encouraged.

5. To enhance self-esteem, Pam should consider a return to work at a later date. She also should practice child care from her wheelchair and assume that role as soon as feasible. She should be shown dressing and makeup techniques to enhance attractiveness in the wheelchair. Social skills training should be a part of the education. She should go home as soon as possible to help in maintaining relationships. Rehabilitation should continue on an outpatient basis.

6. Pam should be referred to her gynecologist for birth control advice and ordering. She should be instructed that she is fertile. The gynecologist also should be consulted for decisions concerning pregnancy in the future. Referrals should be made to other professionals as required.

EVALUATION: Pam and Jim state they understand the information presented. They accept the written information given. An appointment is made with the gynecologist. They are encouraged to call the nurse should they have questions or encounter problems after returning home. More information and counseling may be required at a later date, and appropriate referrals can be made through the outpatient program.

RESOURCES FOR FURTHER INFORMATION

AIDS Hotline 1-800-342-AIDS

American Association for Marriage and Family Therapy
1717 K Street NW, Suite 407
Washington, D.C. 20006

American Association of Sex Educators, Counselors, and
Therapists
11 Dupont Circle NW, Suite 220
Washington, D.C. 20036

American Fertility Society
2140 11th Avenue South, Suite 200
Birmingham, AL 35205-2800

Coalition on Sexuality and Disability
122 E 23rd Street
New York, NY 10010

Information Center for Individuals with Disabilities
20 Park Plaza, Room 330
Boston, MA 02116

National Center for Youth with Disabilities
University of Minnesota
Box 721
420 Delaware Street SE
Minneapolis, MN 55455
1-800-333-6293

National Head Injury Foundation
333 Turnpike Road
Southborough, MA 01772

Recovery of Male Potency (ROMP)
27211 Lahser Road, Suite 208
Southfield, MI 48034

Research and Training Center in Independent Living
University of Kansas
3111 Haworth Hall
Lawrence, KS 60045

SIECUS Sex Information and Education Council of the U.S.
33 Washington Place, Fifth Floor
New York, NY 10003

REFERENCES

Annon, J.S. (1976). The PLISSIT model: A proposed conceptual scheme for behavioral treatment of sexual problems. *Journal of Sex Education Therapy, 2,* 1-15.

Baraka, A. (1985). Epidural meperidine for control of autonomic hyperreflexia in a paraplegic parturient. *Anesthesiology, 62,* 688-690.

Comaar, A.E. (1966). Observation on menstruation and pregnancy among female spinal cord injury patients. *Paraplegia, 3,* 263-272.

Conine, T.A., & Evans, J.H. (1982). Sexual reactivation of chronically ill and disabled adults. *Journal of Allied Health, 11,* 261-270.

Crewe, N.M. (1992). Marital status adjustment to spinal cord injury. *Journal of the American Paraplegia Society, 15,* 14-18.

Craig, D.I. (1990). The adaptation to pregnancy of spinal cord injured women. *Rehabilitation Nursing, 15,* 6-9.

Davis, D.L., & Schneider, L.K. (1990). Ramifications of traumatic brain injury for sexuality. *Journal of Head Trauma Rehabilitation, 5,* 31-37.

Divorce trends in spinal cord injury: Worth taking the chance. (1990). *Spinal Network Extra, 41.*

Ducharme, S., & Gill, K.M. (1990). Sexual values, training, and professional roles. *Journal of Head Injury Rehabilitation, 5,* 38-45.

Girts, C. (1990). Nursing attitudes about sexuality needs of spinal cord injury patients. *Rehabilitation Nursing, 15,* 205-206.

Griffith, E.R., & Trieschmann, R.B. (1983). Sexual dysfunctions in the physically ill and disabled. In C.C. Nadelson & D.B. Marcotte (Eds.), *Treatment interventions in human sexuality* (pp. 241-277). New York: Plenum Press.

Haffner, D.W. (1990). *Sex education 2000: A call to action.* New York: Sex Information and Education Council of the U.S.

Hirsch, I.H., Seager, S.W., Seldor, J., King, L., Staas, W.E., Jr. (1990). Electroejaculatory stimulation of a quadriplegic man resulting in pregnancy. *Archives of Physical Medicine and Rehabilitation, 71,* 54-57.

Holy Bible, New International Version. (1983). Grand Rapids, MI: Zondervan Bible Publishers.

Horn, L.J., & Zasler, N.D. (1990). Neuroanatomy and neurophysiology of sexual function. *Journal of Head Trauma Rehabilitation, 5,* 1-13.

Johnson, W.R., & Kempton, W. (1981). *Sex education and counseling for special groups* (2nd ed.). Springfield, IL: Charles C Thomas.

Kerfoot, K.M., & Buckwalter, K.C. (1985). Sexual counseling. In G.M. Bulechek & J.C. McCloskey (Eds.), *Nursing interventions: Treatments for nursing diagnosis* (pp. 127-138). Philadelphia: W.B. Saunders Co.

Kroll, K., & Klein, E.L. (1991). *Enabling romance: A guide to love, sex, and relationships for the disabled (and the people who care about them).* New York: Crown.

Leslie, S.W. (1990). *Impotence: Current diagnosis and treatment.* Lorain, OH: Geddings Osbon, Sr. Foundation.

Malek, C.J., & Brower, S.A. (1984). Rheumatoid arthritis: how does it influence sexuality? *Rehabilitation Nursing, 9,* 26-28.

Maslow, A. (1954). *Motivation and personality.* New York: Harper and Row.

Masters, W.H., Johnson, V.E., & Kolodny, R.C. (1986). *Masters and Johnson on sex and human loving.* Boston: Little, Brown.

Mulligan, T., & Moss, C.R. (1991). Sexuality and aging in male veterans: A cross-sectional study of interest, ability, and activity. *Archives of Sexual Behavior, 20,* 17-25.

Mumma, C. (Ed.). (1987). *Rehabilitation nursing: Concepts and practice—A core curriculum.* (2nd ed.). Evanston, IL: Rehabilitation Nursing Foundation.

Muscari, M.E. (1987). Obtaining the adolescent sexual history. *Pediatric Nursing, 13,* 307-310.

National Guidelines Task Force. (1991). *Guidelines for comprehensive sexuality education: Kindergarten–12th grade.* New York: Sex Information and Education Council of the United States.

Nygaard, I., Bartscht, K.D., & Cole, S. (1990). Sexuality and reproduction in spinal cord injured women. *Obstetrical and Gynecological Survey, 45,* 727-732.

Reinisch, J.M. (1990). *The Kinsey institute new report on sex: What you must know to be sexually literate.* New York: St. Martin's.

Relf, M.V. (1991). Sexuality and the older bypass patient. *Geriatric Nursing, 12,* 294-296.

Renshaw, D. (1978). Stroke and Sex. In A. Comfort (Ed.), *Sexual consequences of disability* (pp. 121-131). Philadelphia: George F. Strickley.

Robunault, I.P. (1978). *Sex, society and the disabled.* New York: Harper and Row.

Seidl, A., Bullough, B., Haughey, B., Scherer, Y., Rhodes, M., & Brown, G. (1991). Understanding the effects of a myocardial infarction on sexual functioning: a basis for sexual counseling. *Rehabilitation Nursing, 16,* 255-264.

Selekman, J., & McIlvain-Simpson, G. (1991). Sex and sexuality for the adolescent with a chronic condition. *Pediatric Nursing, 17,* 535-538.

Sexuality education for children and youth with disabilities. (1992). Fostering relationships: Suggestions for young adults. *News Digest.* Washington DC: National Information Center for Children and Youth with Disabilities.

Shrey, D.E., Kiefer, J.S., & Anthony, W.A. (1979). Sexual adjustment counseling for persons with severe disabilities: A skill-based approach for rehabilitation professionals. *Journal of Rehabilitation, 45,* 28-33.

Spica, M.M. (1989). Sexual counseling standards for the spinal-cord injured. *Journal of Neuroscience Nursing, 21,* 56-60.

Smalley, G., & Trent, J. (1988). *The language of love.* Pomona, CA: Focus on the Family Publishing.

Smalley, G., & Trent, J. (1989). *Love is a decision.* Phoenix: Today's Family.

Smith, J. (1990). Joy rises, misery falls, communication works. *Spinal Network Extra, 40.*

Sullivan, G., & Lukoff, D. (1990). Sexual side effects of antipsychotic medication: evaluation and interventions. *Hospital and Community Psychiatry, 41,* 1238-1241.

Tanner, J.M. (1962). *Growth at adolescence* (2nd ed.). Oxford: Blackwell Scientific.

Tardif, G.S. (1989). Sexual activity after a myocardial infarction. *Archives of Physical Medicine and Rehabilitation, 70,* 763-766.

Valleroy, M.L., & Kraft, G.H. (1984). Sexual dysfunction in multiple sclerosis. *Archives of Physical Medicine and Rehabilitation, 65,* 125-128.

Wanner, M.B., Rageth, C.J., & Zach, G.A. (1987). Pregnancy and autonomic hyperreflexia in patients with spinal cord lesions. *Paraplegia, 25,* 482-490.

Watts, R.J. (1979). Dimensions of sexual health. *American Journal of Nursing, 79,* 1568-1572.

Weg, R.B. (1978). The physiology of sexuality in aging. In R.L. Solnick (Ed.). *Sexuality and aging.* Los Angeles: University of Southern California Press.

Weiss, R.J. (1991). Effects of antihypertensive agents on sexual function. *American Family Physician, 44,* 2075-2082.

Williams, L. (1989). Pharmacologic erection programs: A treatment option for erectile dysfunction. *Rehabilitation Nursing, 14,* 264-268.

Wilson, P.S., & Dibble, S.L. (1993). Rehabilitation nurses' knowledge of and attitudes toward sexuality. *Rehabilitation Nursing Research, 2,* 69-74.

Woods, N.F. (1984). *Human sexuality in health and illness* (3rd ed.). St. Louis: Mosby–Year Book.

Woods, N.F. (1988a). Alterations in human sexuality. In P.H. Mitchell, et al. (Eds.), *Neuroscience nursing* (pp. 471-481). Norwalk, CT: Appleton and Lange.

Woods, N.F. (1988b). Human sexuality: An overview. In P.H. Mitchell, et al. (Eds.), *Neuroscience nursing* (pp. 459-469). Norwalk, CT: Appleton and Lange.

World Health Organization. (1975). *Education and treatment in human sexuality: The training of health professionals* (WHO Technical Report Series No. 572). Geneva: World Health Organization.

Zasler, N.D. (1989). Managing erectile dysfunction with external devices. *Practical Diabetology, 8,* 1-9.

Zasler, N.D., & Horn, L.J. (1990). Rehabilitative management of sexual dysfunction. *Journal of Head Trauma Rehabilitation, 5,* 14-24.

Zejdlik, C.M. (1992). *Management of spinal cord injury* (2nd ed.). Monterey, CA: Wadsworth Health Sciences Division.

SUGGESTED READING

Antidepressant-related sexual dysfunction. (1993). *Nurses Drug Alert, 19,* 74.

Banja, J.D. & Banes, L. (1993). Moral sensitivity, sodomy laws, and TBI Rehabilitation. *Journal of Head Trauma Rehabilitation, 8,* 116-119.

Blackerby, W.F. (1990). A treatment model for sexuality disturbance following brain injury. *Journal of Head Trauma Rehabilitation, 5,* 73-82.

Boldrini, P. Basaglia, N., & Calanca, M.C. (1991). Sexual changes in hemiparetic patients. *Archives of Physical Medicine and Rehabilitation, 72,* 202-207.

Burgener, S. & Logan, G. Sexuality concerns of the post stroke patient. *Rehabilitation Nursing, 14,* 178-181, 195.

Burling, K., Tarvydas, V.M., & Make, D.R. (1994). Human sexuality and disability: A holistic interpretation for rehabilitation counseling. *Journal of Applied Rehabil Counseling, 25,* 10-17.

Chicano, L.A. (1989). Humanistic aspects of sexuality as related to spinal cord injury. *Journal of Neuroscience Nursing, 21,* 366-369.

Closson, J.B., Toerge, J.E., Ragnarsson, K.T., Parson, K.C., & Lammertse, D.P. (1991). Rehabilitation in spinal cord disorders. 3. Comprehensive management of spinal cord injury. *Archives of Physical Medicine and Rehabilitation, 72,* S298-S308.

Cole, T., & Cole, S. (1976). *A Guide for trainers: Sexuality and physical disability.* Minneapolis: University of Minnesota Medical School, Multi-Resource Center.

Cross, L.L., Meythaler, J.M., Tiul, S.M., & Cross, A.L. (1991). Pregnancy following spinal cord injury. *Western Journal of Medicine, 154,* 607-611.

Falvo, D.R. (1994). Risk: Sexually transmitted diseases. *Journal of Applied Rehabilitation Counseling, 25,* 43-49.

Griggs, W. (1981). Sexuality. In H. Martin, N.B. Holt, & D. Hicks (Eds.), *Comprehensive rehabilitation nursing* (pp. 85-99). New York: McGraw-Hill.

Herbst, S.H. (1981). Impairment as a result of cancer. In N. Martin, N.B. Holt, & P. Hicks (Eds.), *Comprehensive rehabilitation nursing* (pp. 569-571). New York: McGraw-Hill.

Katchadourian, H.A. (Ed.). (1979). *Human sexual behavior: A comparative developmental perspective.* Berkley: University of California Press.

Katzin, L. (1990). Chronic illness and sexuality. *American Journal of Nursing, 90,* 54-59.

Kennedy, S., & Over, R. (1990). Psychophysiological assessment of male sexual arousal following spinal cord injury. *Archives of Sexual Behavior, 19,* 15-27.

Medlar, T., & Medlar, J. (1990). Nursing management of sexuality issues. *Journal of Head Injury Rehabilitation, 5,* 46-51.

Nay, R. (1992). Sexuality and aged women in nursing homes. *Geriatric Nursing, 13,* 312-314.

Sipski, M.L. & Alexander, C.J. (1993). Sexual activities, response and satisfaction in women pre- and post-spinal cord injury. *Archives of Physical Medicine and Rehabilitation, 74,* 1025-1096.

Smedley, G. (1991). Addressing sexuality in the elderly. *Rehabilitation Nursing, 16,* 9-11.

Smith, M. (1993). Pediatric sexuality; promoting normal sexual development in children. *Nurse Practitioner, 18,* 37-38, 41-44.

Szasz, G. (1991). Sex and disability are not mutually exclusive: Evaluation and management. *Western Journal of Medicine, 154,* 560-563.

White, M.J., Rintali, D.H., Hart, K.A., & Fuhrer, M.J. (1994). A comparison of the sexual concerns of men and women with spinal cord injuries. *Rehabilitation Nursing Research, 3,* 55-61.

White, M.J., Rintali, D.H., Hart, K.A., Young, M.E., & Fuhrer, M.J. (1994). Sexual activities, concerns and interests of women with spinal cord injury living in the community. *American Journal of Physical Medicine and Rehabilitation, 75,* 276-278.

28

Spirituality: A Rehabilitation Perspective

Mary Ann E. Solimine, MLS, RN
Shirley P. Hoeman, PhD, RN, CRRN

INTRODUCTION

Rehabilitation nurses are observing and practical professionals who have been educated to assess, plan, and intervene to resolve a problem. Nursing is concerned with the whole person—the client—not the disability. Nonetheless, when this biopsychosocial approach and the nursing process are completed, the spiritual aspect of care often remains unattended. Spiritual distress has been designated as a nursing diagnosis, but nurses on the whole remain unsure about how to assess and intervene in spiritual areas. Not only do nurses feel unsure about matters related to spirituality, but as they deal with health issues amenable to nursing therapeutics, the physical aspects of client care tend to have higher priority and prominence. However, spirituality fits well with rehabilitation principles (Davis, 1994) concerned with care and wholeness of being, rather than cure alone.

A spiritual assessment extends beyond merely ascertaining religious affiliation, church attendance, or dietary restrictions during an initial assessment. A number of multidimensional religious commitment tools are available for measuring religious status based on a client's responses to questions about religious practices, beliefs, and attitudes. Religion is an organized system of worship in which belief and moral norms are held in common and formal ritual and observances practiced that can be an expression of a person's spirituality, but not its core. Information about religious affiliation is important for understanding beliefs and practices that may influence how a client responds to an illness and for guiding specific nursing interventions.

Religion and spirituality are not the same. When religious data are the only information gathered, a nurse forfeits opportunities for insight into a deeper part of a client's background. Inadvertently, a client may not activate a spiritual coping strategy in a healthcare environment because the kind and depth of information collected for planning care was limited to religious data. Whether consciously or unconsciously, many persons acknowledge their spiritual relationships or dependence on God only when facing illness or incapacity. "Nursing care which fails to recognize spiritual needs as a vital part of whole-person care, and does not allow these needs to emerge and be addressed, becomes disrespectful and unethical" (Pettigrew, 1990).

DEVELOPMENT OF CARING OVER TIME

Caring for the sick dates back to prehistoric times when wellness meant survival of the fittest to obtain resources and avoid environmental dangers. Even in primitive societies the impulse to care for the sick and for weaker members was expressed according to the religious practices. In early organized societies worship and purification ceremonies—whether with shaman, tribal elder, or priest—were difficult to distinguish from medical and nursing measures. Outside fundamental family caregiving the men and women who served in temples received their training at the clients' bedside but eventually acquired basic skills in caring for the sick and were called on to nurse others. In other societies shamanism, spiritists, curanderos, wise women and other varieties of traditional healers connected religion with magic, herbs, and healing.

In the early Christian era, the ideals of charity, service, self-sacrifice, and brotherhood espoused by the church inspired workers to tend the ill and needy in everyday life. Some of these deacons and deaconesses were appointed as the need arose and others served in atonement for their own sins. Many religious orders became dedicated to providing nursing care while guaranteeing the inner being was tended also. Although healing was promoted and pain minimized, these caregivers provided comfort, potions, and attempted healing but had few cures to offer. They tried to reconcile their clients to the suffering of this world and prepare their souls for the next one, contributing comfort to a client's peaceful death.

By the Industrial Revolution sick persons were segregated from others, as medical practitioners came to understand more about the relationship between crowded living conditions in tenement settlements and the spread of infectious diseases. Over time secular institutions joined religious groups as healthcare providers, with a growing focus in nursing practice on specialties and tasks. As a result the spiritually interactive aspects of nursing practice diminished. Forging ahead with new theories, medical advances, and treatments, nurses were caught up with giving state-of-the-art care. The federal government enacted legislation appropriating funds for Medicare; the increasingly scientific base for medical education and business interests stimulated technical advances. Social thought changed with the new technologies. Rather than palliative comfort, people have come to expect that diseased organs will be replaced and disability or death will be postponed. They demand modifications and interventions by outside forces, giving up control of their lives in exchange, often resembling people of "parts." In this scenario the art and mystery of healing vanish, nurses lose sight of the client, and the client loses a most powerful resource: an inner, enabling vigor.

Florence Nightingale had developed the concept of nursing as a secular, economic, and independent vocation—an art requiring intelligence and technical skill as well as devotion and moral purpose (Griffin & Griffin, 1973). Concerned with the dimensions of mind-body-spirit of those she served and the influence of their environment on their experiences, Nightingale entrusted nurses with the goal of smoothing away any hindrances that did not allow the healing nature from within the client to operate (Nightingale, 1970).

A resurgence of holism has redirected spirituality into research for scientific verification and validity. Today's rehabilitation nurse may continue to regard the profession as a vocational "calling" from which to access, diagnose, and intervene to help clients create healing based on an interaction with the environment and God. The professional nurse "assists an individual, family or community, to prevent or cope with the experience of illness and suffering, and, if necessary, find meaning in these experiences" (Donley, 1991).

SPIRITUALITY

We are all spiritual beings. Rather than being an isolated dimension, the spirit is the essence of a person; it is the breath (from its Latin root) pervading and integrating the system. Our spirituality is a reflection of this force; it is what gives the mind and body life and character, making the wholeness sound and giving it purpose and meaning. Terms often used for this unity of caring are "connectedness" or "interconnectedness," signifying unity of the artificially partitioned physical, psychological, and social self, or as the image of God, to fill the need as it arises.

Thus spirituality is an internal guidance system basic to human well-being—influencing life, behavior, and health regardless of a person's religious philosophy, beliefs, or practices (Fig. 28-1). With wisdom, understanding, belief, and love, spirituality has power to shape and give meaning to the pattern of a person's self-becoming, expressed in being, knowing, and doing (Burkhardt, 1989)—a creative and energetic spiritual perspective. Apart from a complex theory or religious requirement, when actions are guided by the belief that it is better to create harmony than disharmony, a person is practicing spirituality (Glenndinning, 1990). Sig-

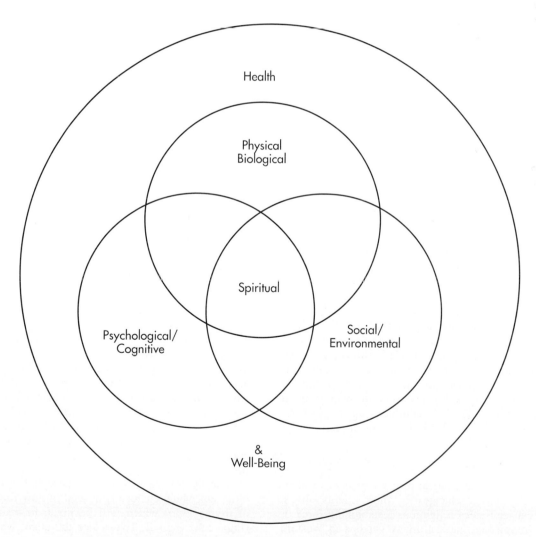

Fig. 28-1 A model for incorporating spirituality into holistic biopsychosocial health.

nificant others and total life events play major roles in spiritual growth (Haase, Britt, Coward, Leidy, & Penn, 1992).

Since being holy is no guarantee of good health, and sickness or trauma do not imply spiritual shortcomings, our physical bodies show imperfection by acting up or breaking down. Many persons believe otherwise. "Our understanding of the relationship between spirituality and healing is vastly incomplete. We shall have to be willing to stand in the unknown" (Dossey, 1993). In the case of a person's illness or disability, the spirit within will first act as a mediator for the individual to gain strength to overcome the disharmony that is experienced as disorganization, disruption, sadness, anger, guilt, anxiety, despair, or hopelessness. Next the spirit will aid in reorganization and finally resolution of the disability into the person's life, creating a general sense of wellness that unifies the person with others, nature, and a higher power or ultimate other: God.

Spirituality is encompassing, pervasively present in all dimensions and phases of life, seemingly beyond the concept of "well-being." However, spiritual well-being has been defined as "the affirmation of life in relationship with God, self, community and environment that nurtures and celebrates wholeness" (National Interfaith Coalition, 1975). Others suggest "spiritual integrity" (Labun, 1988) or spiritual "more-being" (Paterson & Zderad, 1976) to be accurate terms for an infusion of spirituality into one's life processes.

Spirituality can exist by degrees; the greater the degree of spirituality, the greater the influence on life and health. Although the inherent vital force, which is a person's spirit, does not weaken of itself, a person's reflection of spirituality may be affected by physical or environmental factors that influence the harmony of life, obscuring spirituality. In a physical analogy the body may suffer respiratory distress when a ventilatory problem causes misery or affects the mind, as with hypoxia. A variety or multiplicity of causes may have led to impaired ventilation, including pneumonia, chronic obstructive pulmonary disease, asthma, neoplasms, or diseases from the occupational environment. The etiology of "dis-spiriting" is similarly multiple and diverse, but spiritual needs are manifested through the physical symptoms of hurting, doubt, disquietude, or desperation and by psychosocial behaviors, body language, speech, and/or silence. Commonly a client will express feelings of boredom, tepidness, grief, or lack of comfort.

Clients may find relief when a nurse is able to assist them to enact or persevere in an affirmative relationship with their God. Encouraging clients to adhere to any personal resolution or practice of prayer or meditation may "inspirit" them at these times. "Spiriting" is the concept of finding meaning, peace, and/or joy from an inner strength and relationship with self, God, nature and others—one toward which nurses aim for themselves, as well as for their clients (Burkhardt, 1989).

Multidisciplinary Focus

Within the last decade, clinical psychologists have identified spiritually based changes in their clients' lives. Whether an earlier loss of religion as a stabilizing force or an upswing in spiritual interest, many persons in Western culture are recognizing now what has been evident in some other cultures: that everything seen is formed and sustained by what is not seen; that each one is an immortal spirit. Until recently the possibility of predicting a person's quality of life based on their satisfaction gained from religion was discounted; a person's needs for being, having, and relating were linked to a narrow definition of well-being. New structures based on the energy and values of the soul—the part always reaching for harmony, cooperation, sharing, and reverence for life—may displace the external power that now leads only to violence and destruction (Glenndinning, 1991). Although clients and professionals alike have not always perceived that life has a spiritual root, the hunger and search for intimacy and transcendency, personal friends, and a personal God to love and worship is not the latest fad but the oldest truth (Peterson, 1993).

Now medical sages are arguing calmly for holism. Chief among them is Dossey (1993), who makes clear his belief that illnesses and life-threatening diseases are changeable, depending on how the client perceives the meaning of the illness. Meaning is being, Dossey contends; therefore healing requires a "fundamental change in our own being" under the powers of the mind, through hope, prayer, and other expressions of "the secret helper and invisible power within."

In this Dossey would have the blessing of Osler, a physician who regarded life as a journey of the spirit, with the body as its conveyance. He ministered to this spirit through warm human contact, without the necessity for any shared theology but with shared belief. The concerned spirit of the physician reached out to the troubled spirit of the client, which was yearning for compassion and counseling, kindness and optimism—particularly when cure was impossible. Knowing his own limitations, Osler recognized the natural healing power latent in each client: faith. To the body of medical knowledge he added a soul (Wheeler, 1990).

A recent issue of *JAMA* (Cowl, 1991) devoted a section to religious essays, poetry, and features pertinent to clinical encounters. The idea of medical school as an arena for connecting health with spirituality has stimulated workshops for faculty in some schools where they learn to teach how to humanize client care and "heal lives rather than just treat diseases" (Siegel, 1986).

Pain and Suffering

Pain and suffering tend to be associated with hospitalization. Clients find themselves in unfamiliar, intimidating, and even frightening situations where pain and fatigue make them feel vulnerable and alienated, isolated from connecting relationships and out of control. When a client has a disability, negative feelings may exacerbate suffering. Above all, a person may come to fear not being heard so intensely that thoughts and fears are not voiced. A nurse is the professional who may be able to assure a client who is suffering that value and meaning enable some persons to come to grips with the real meaning and seriousness of their life.

"Earthly suffering, when it is accepted in love, is like a bitter nut which encloses the seed of new life, the treasure of divine glory which will be given to man in eternity" (Pope John Paul II, 1984). For the client who is a Christian, this "gospel of suffering" has two messages: the model of Christ and a promise that loving endurance of suffering will clear the way for the grace which transforms the human soul; to the caregiver it calls for compassion, action to relieve needless suffering, and reassurance to the client. The challenge to affirm life and love as a result of physical, mental, or spiritual suffering holds greater meaning than day-to-day "productive" work (Mahony, 1994). Values provide awareness and access to personal spirituality, but completing meaningless tasks closes access to spirituality and the result is depressed instinct and morals.

Clients from differing cultures or religious preferences other than Christian can be expected to choose their own explanations for suffering. Clients and families may believe that specific interventions and behaviors performed by certain individuals are necessary to alleviate pain and ward off suffering. Persons of many faiths consider suffering to be a punishment for wrongdoing or for failing to perform some action. Suffering, for others, may be the product of an event outside of their control or because someone or something has caused them to suffer. The extensive array of beliefs that individual clients may have about this universal experience cannot be listed, but a careful and complete assessment may lead a nurse to determine the unique nature underlying a particular client's suffering.

Prayer

Many sick or disabled persons have recognized that their ailment eventually became a gift because it taught them how to "let go and let God" (be God). It is important for these persons to be able to receive from God. Many persons are able to trade their weakness for God's strength and then they in turn begin "doing" for others, even if it is "doing without doing," by cooperating with the natural order in thoughts and prayers (Soeken & Carson, 1987). The very acts of worship they perform refocus their attention, distracting them, directing energy away from their pain, and replacing loneliness with the feeling of being in communion with God and those for whom they pray.

Not offering clients the opportunity to pray is tantamount to withholding medication. This spirit of prayerfulness is the interiorized sense of the sacred; the sense of being aligned with "something higher." Thus their praying is not directed somewhere out into the universe but inward to the spirit residing in the core of their being. An outward demonstration of feeling is not an indicator of prayer for a client who moves beyond formulas and ulterior wishes. However, some clients may require other persons, often a leader or designated spiritual person, to assist them, mediate for them, or conduct ceremonial acts as a part of their prayer. In a prayerful state a client may have "a sense in which a 'cure' can occur—the realization that physical illness (or trauma) no matter how painful or severe, is at some level of secondary importance in the total scheme of existence. One's authentic higher self is completely impervious to the ravages of any ailment whatsoever—utterly beyond the ravages of disease and death" (Dossey, 1993).

Children in rehabilitative care may be slow to enter into a relationship with those who are responsible for painful procedures and the invasion of their privacy. Although children do not always show appreciation, they value the times when a nurse is willing to listen when they question pain and suffering. Children need to feel free to express anger and bewilderment over what they may consider injustice or betrayal. When a child does express an intimate concern, a nurse can convey authentic hope beginning with a willingness to share their concerns. Offering platitudes or threatening divine retribution do little to increase trust and rapport with a child. Although it is difficult to confess a lack of understanding about why and to whom accidents and illness happen, children recognize honesty. A trusted nurse can help children appreciate their God's love for them. With this comes knowledge that they can be given strength to survive or to come to terms with their condition—and even to move forward—with the power of prayer and personal relationships.

Taking each day as it comes, children are able to respond to shared stories and experiences of others that affirm their perceptions and offer hope. Open and informal conversations with peers, teachers, clergy, or members of their church's youth group may provide good opportunities for a child to reflect on questions in the light of specific religious traditions. Different religions and belief systems will have their own ways of making contact with key persons, relating the stories, and performing ceremonies important to their children and families. Spiritual-based stories on tape could be used, after which instructions on how to "create your own TV show in your head about the story" would reinforce the message. Children have vivid imaginations, which can be put to use in positive ways. Relaxation, imaging, and centering techniques can be used with them, as well as innovative and imaginative games in support groups (Hendricks & Wills, 1975). Rituals can be ways of letting children know that they have a remembered place in their families and that their God will always be with them (Sommer, 1989).

Logotherapy

Logotherapy, or therapy through meaning, was conceptualized by Frankl after his experiences as a prisoner in concentration camps during World War II. Logotherapy suggests a model for overpowering suffering, thereby finding meaning in it. Thus Frankl's version of modern existential analysis teaches that

◆ Life has meaning under all circumstances, even the most miserable
◆ Humans have a will to meaning, which is their main motivation for living
◆ Persons have freedom to find meaning in what they do, what they experience, or at least in the stand they take in the face of a situation of unchangeable suffering (Frankl, 1984)

The object and challenge of logotherapy is to weave the slender threads of a broken life into a firm pattern of meaning and responsibility. It focuses on the future; on the meanings of the client to be fulfilled so that each person is confronted with and reoriented toward the meaning of his own life. Each one is questioned by life but only can answer to life for her own life and respond by being responsible. The five steps taken in logotherapy are as follows:

1. Self-discovery, leading to hidden values
2. Choice in action, experience, or attitude
3. Stressing the uniqueness of contribution of each person's suffering

4. Response-ability; how person responds according to personal values
5. Transcendence; meaningful spiritual acts (Stavros, 1994)

Logotherapists are a growing professional group who often have vested interest in their work. Although once considered for a career as a pitcher for a major league team, one individual who incurred tetraplegia following a diving accident found his meaning in life as a logotherapist. Psychoneuroimmunologists are professionals who have begun to study the connections and relationships among meaning and attitude, hope and prayer—expressions of the invisible spiritual power within—and the transformation of disease.

Nursing Imperative

Why are more nurses not engaged in providing spiritual care? Ask yourself—if you are among those who do not—why not? Then choose from among the following hypotheses about beliefs:

+ Belief that matters of spirituality do not concern nurses but rather psychologists or pastoral caregivers
+ Belief that nurses are so technologically oriented that they are not comfortable with spirituality
+ Belief that clients are uncomfortable discussing spiritual matters with a nurse; social restraint
+ Lack of education/experience having anything to do with issues spiritual; own shortcomings
+ Feeling that one's own beliefs/culture would contradict the clients' spiritual perspective
+ Feeling that one's own spiritual wellspring is depleted and would not be equal to the task; emotional risk; vulnerability
+ Lack of time to devote to what is perceived as an arduous endeavor

All or any part of these hypotheses may relate to a nurse-client encounter. Many nurses fear "meddling" in a client's spiritual life and correctly so. However, clients interviewed concerning spiritual needs have chosen nurses second to clergy as those with whom they wish to discuss spiritual matters. A nurse educates a client about the condition and rehabilitation techniques that may seem strange or frightening, addresses most physical needs without calling on a physician, and intervenes with many psychosocial or emotional responses without relying on a psychologist. A nurse advocates for a client and understands when a referral is needed, then selects the appropriate professional.

The foundation for religious belief is formed during the same developmental stage as the ability to trust. Thus a nurse may work with clients to create an environment and foster an atmosphere of trust wherein a client is encouraged to relax and be able to confide religious and spiritual needs. The professional must be as comfortable with the subject and setting as is the client. The pattern of how sexuality was treated in rehabilitation is a comparison. For many years sexuality was a topic seldom mentioned in rehabilitation and less often with the client. When the subject was introduced, professionals felt unqualified and "out of bounds" about the discussion, while clients wondered if their questions were inappropriate and at the same time experienced frustration because they were left without answers about their sexuality. Today sexuality is discussed freely, whereas spirituality remains a less approachable topic.

When a nurse-client relationship is bound by confidentiality and respect, spirituality becomes an acceptable topic. However, when a client believes illness or disability appears as a punishment for wrongdoing, especially perceived sexual transgressions, clerical intervention is needed. For example, those who value the ministry of confession are taught through grace to view God as a present friend rather than perceiving a punishing enemy. Some clients who continue to have serious adjustment problems of conscience may benefit from referral for psychological help.

In many instances what a client wants and expects is simple: someone to be there: to listen, acknowledge, touch, empathize, show concern, quietly reassure, patiently explain, allow crying or crying out, or to exercise nonjudgmental understanding (Ellis, 1980). This essence of nursing existed before technology and social thought steered nurses' attention in directions apart from their clients' spirituality. The nurse who chooses to become a spiritual resource cannot be personally depleted, either physically or spiritually. Regardless of spiritual background or personal beliefs, a nurse who fortifies others' personal spiritual perspective must find time apart to relax, imagine an uplifting scene, pray for guidance, and seek counsel when needed before becoming a resource. Sharing and demonstrating the benefits of personal renewal with a client may become mutual reinforcement for spiritual expression.

"Being there" is acknowledged as important by many clients. Also called "presencing," this is participation in an experience at the invitation (not demand) of the client. Presencing is recognized by a sense of meaningful self-giving when the client needs it most; it can be offered but never forced. "Revealed, directly and unmistakably, in a glance, a touch, a tone of voice" (Paterson & Zderad, 1976); "being there" implies closeness, openness, receptivity, readiness and availability, willingness to hear, and involvement. There is healing and being healed; no "saying or doing the right thing," only exposing oneself to feelings of awkwardness and discomfort, possibly to fear and pain, vulnerability meeting vulnerability in "safe silence." Each person has a reflexive, immediate impulse to fill silence with speech, and an excess of speech tends to occur with nervous or tense feelings. The person who is able to still the impulse may discover a subtle quieting of the mind, giving opportunity to experience a magnified awareness of inner wisdom, a "centering."

Achieving centering requires an individual to exclude extraneous, distracting thoughts and feelings. Instead the focus centers on the client without conflicting personal concerns intruding into the interaction. Once established in a relationship, presencing does not require large amounts of time. It may occur in sitting with a client in crisis when requested; with a smile, a passing glance, or a hug when leaving; with praise for trying something; or while sharing laughter or tears; and is known by really attentively "being there" as well as physically being there. The spiritual nature of presencing is the feature that continues to minister long afterward; "a remembered countenance still inspiriting" (Pettigrew, 1990).

ASSESSMENT

The initial spiritual assessment is conducted toward the end of history taking when there has been opportunity to assess psychosocial background and gain trust and rapport with the client. A client may express offense, feel threatened, or appear to be puzzled by a spiritual perspective during an assessment. Explain the importance of understanding each person's sources of strength in holistic care. Even when a client appears not to be concerned with spiritual needs, the ways in which a client responds and the content of answers to the questions will be valuable in providing care. Respect a client's right to object to any questions, decide not to answer, or maintain private information about beliefs and religious preferences.

Stoll's (1995) Spiritual History Guide can be incorporated into any general nursing history. Based on four areas of concern, the following questions may be arranged in any order to elicit data about spirituality from a client.

Sources of hope and strength (support system)
✦ Who is the most important person to you?
✦ To whom do you turn when you need help? Are they available?
✦ In what ways do they help?
✦ What is your source of strength and hope?

SPIRITUAL WELL-BEING SCALE

For each of the following statements *circle* the choice that best indicates the extent of your agreement or disagreement as it describes your personal experience:

SA = Strongly Agree   D = Disagree
MA = Moderately Agree   MD = Moderately Disagree
A = Agree   SD = Strongly Disagree

1. I don't find much satisfaction in private prayer with God   SA MA A D MD SD
2. I don't know who I am, where I came from, or where I'm going   SA MA A D MD SD
3. I believe that God loves me and cares about me   SA MA A D MD SD
4. I feel that life is a positive experience   SA MA A D MD SD
5. I believe that God is impersonal and not interested in my daily situations   SA MA A D MD SD
6. I feel unsettled about my future   SA MA A D MD SD
7. I have a personally meaningful relationship with God   SA MA A D MD SD
8. I feel very fulfilled and satisfied with life   SA MA A D MD SD
9. I don't get much personal strength and support from my God   SA MA A D MD SD
10. I feel a sense of well-being about the direction my life is headed in   SA MA A D MD SD
11. I believe that God is concerned about my problems   SA MA A D MD SD
12. I don't enjoy much about life   SA MA A D MD SD
13. I don't have a personally satisfying relationship with God   SA MA A D MD SD
14. I feel good about my future   SA MA A D MD SD
15. My relationship with God helps me not to feel lonely   SA MA A D MD SD
16. I feel that life is full of conflict and unhappiness   SA MA A D MD SD
17. I feel most fulfilled when I'm in close communion with God   SA MA A D MD SD
18. Life doesn't have much meaning   SA MA A D MD SD
19. My relation with God contributes to my sense of well-being   SA MA A D MD SD
20. I believe there is some real purpose for my life   SA MA A D MD SD

Note: Items are scored from 1 to 6, with a higher number representing more well-being. Reverse scoring for negatively worded items. Odd-numbered items assess religious well-being; even numbered items assess existential well-being.
Ellison, Craig W. *Address:* Alliance Theological Seminary/Nyack College, Nyack, New York 10960.
Title: Professor of Urban Studies and Counseling. *Degrees:* AB, The King's College; MA, PhD, Wayne State University. *Specializations:* Social-developmental psychology, urban psychology.
From "Spiritual well-being: Conceptualization and Measurement" by C.W. Ellison, 1982, *Journal of Psychology and Theology, 11,* p. 340. Copyright 1982 by C.W. Ellison and R.F. Paloutzian. Reprinted by permission.

✦ What helps you most when you feel afraid or need special help?

Concept of God/deity

✦ Is religion or God significant to you? If yes, can you describe how?
✦ Is prayer helpful to you? What happens when you pray?
✦ Does God/deity function in your personal life? If yes, can you describe how?
✦ How would you describe your God or what you worship? (Draper, 1965)

Relation between spiritual beliefs and health

✦ What has bothered you most about being sick (or in what is happening to you)?
✦ What do you think is going to happen to you?
✦ Has being sick (or what has happened to you) made any difference in your feelings about God or the practice of your faith?
✦ Is there anything that is especially frightening or meaningful to you now?

Religious practices

✦ Do you feel your faith (or religion) is helpful to you? If yes, would you tell me how?
✦ Are there any religious practices that are important to you?
✦ Has being sick made any difference in your practice of praying? Your religious practices?
✦ What religious books or symbols are helpful to you? (Stoll, 1995).

To this might be added

✦ Is there anything I can do to help you in your practice of faith?

Additional Modes of Spiritual Assessment

The Spiritual Well-Being Scale is another assessment tool for eliciting spiritual data (Ellison, 1982) (see the box on p. 633).

The North American Nursing Diagnosis Association (NANDA), approved Spiritual Distress (distress of the human spirit) as a nursing diagnosis during their fifth national conference. It is included herein as an assessment framework useful in rehabilitation nursing practice (Kim, McFarland, & McLane, 1993) (see the following box).

In another view, Table 28-1 contains descriptors of four spiritual needs that a client may have and lists the signs that indicate a client may have spiritual problems. These are comparable to the nursing diagnosis of Spiritual Distress and assess spiritual health or spiritual more-being. Adapted for rehabilitation, the information in the tables could be used to construct an assessment checklist. Ultimately the information about a client's spirituality could be integrated with other data to formulate a nursing diagnosis and care plan and to verify that a client's values are reflected in rehabilitation goals (Highfield & Cason, 1983).

A nurse may advocate to incorporate a spirituality assessment component into the client history. Whatever questions are used for an assessment, they must be validated as relevant, sensitive, and reflective of the fundamental values of respect, understanding, caring, and fairness—both for client and interviewer. Nurses working in a facility or a community agency would benefit from an inservice or continu-

---

◆

SPIRITUAL DISTRESS (DISTRESS OF THE HUMAN SPIRIT)

Disruption in the life principle that pervades a person's entire being and that integrates and transcends one's biological and psychosocial nature

RELATED FACTORS

Separation from religious and cultural ties
Challenged belief and value system (e.g., result of moral or ethical implications of therapy or result of intense suffering)

DEFINING CHARACTERISTICS

Expresses concern with meaning of life and death and/or belief systems
Anger toward God (as defined by the person)
Questions meaning of suffering
Verbalizes inner conflict about beliefs
Verbalizes concern about relationship with deity
Questions meaning of own existence
Inability to choose or chooses not to participate in usual religious practices
Seeks spiritual assistance
Questions moral and ethical implications of therapeutic regimen
Displacement of anger toward religious representatives
Description of nightmares or sleep disturbances
Alteration in behavior or mood evidenced by anger, crying, withdrawal, preoccupation, anxiety, hostility, apathy, etc.
Regards illness as punishment
Does not experience that God is forgiving
Inability to accept self
Engages in self-blame
Denies responsibilities for problems
Description of somatic complaints

From *Pocket Guide to Nursing Diagnosis,* 2nd ed. by M.J. Kim, G.K. McFarland, and A.M. McLane, 1987, St. Louis: Mosby–Year Book. Copyright 1987 by Mosby–Year Book. Reprinted by permission.

---

ing education program about spirituality before instituting any change. A community assessment to determine the various patterns of beliefs held by clients in a community will assist nurses in identifying specific information they need to learn about their clients.

Local or traditional helpers who are involved in healing, spirituality, holistic health, or related activities may be consulted. Some of these lay healers may be available to provide practical information that would prevent unintended errors or forestall awkward situations based on assumptions. Eventually the change could result in increased awareness, expanded education about an area of practice, and improved community relations; it could also offer encouragement for other nurses. Whether formal or ongoing during nursing care, assessment questions elicit information about how the

Table 28-1 Spiritual barometer

Need	Behavior or condition
SIGNS OF SPIRITUAL PROBLEMS*	
Need for meaning and purpose in life	Expresses that he has no reason to live
	Questions the meaning in suffering, disability, and death
	Expresses despair
	Exhibits emotional detachment from self and peers
	Jokes about life after death
Need to receive love	Worries about how the rest of his family will manage after his death
	Expresses feelings of a loss of faith in God
	Expresses fear of dependence
	Does not discuss feelings about disability with significant others
	Does not call on others for help when he needs it
	Expresses fear of tests and diagnosis
	Expresses feeling lack of supportive others
	Behaves as he "should" by conforming to the behavior of a "good" client or person
	Refuses to cooperate with health-care regimen
	Expresses guilt feelings
	Confesses thoughts and feelings about which he is ashamed
	Expresses anger with self/others
	Expresses ambivalent feelings toward God
	Expresses despondency during illness/hospitalization
	Expresses resentment toward God
	Expresses loss of self-value due to decreasing physical capacity
	Expresses fear of God's anger
Need to give love	Worries about financial status of family during hospitalization/separation from family
	Worries about separation from others through death
Need for hope and creativity	Expresses fear of loss of control
	Is unable to pursue creative outlets due to high level of physical disability
	Expresses boredom during illness and hospitalization
	Exhibits overly dependent behaviors
	Expresses anxiety about inability to pursue career, marriage, and parenting because of illness
	Expresses fear of therapy
	Denies the reality of his condition
SIGNS OF SPIRITUAL HEALTH (MORE-BEING)	
Need for meaning and purpose in life	Expresses that he has lived in accordance with his value system in the past
	Expresses desire to participate in religious rituals
	Lives in accordance with his value system at present
	Expresses contentment with his life
	Expresses hope in the future
Need to receive love	Expresses hope in life after death
	Expresses confidence in the health-care team
	Expresses feelings of being loved by others/God
	Expresses feelings of forgiveness by others/God
	Expresses desire to perform religious rituals leading to salvation
	Trusts others/God with the outcome of a situation in which he feels he has no control
Need to give love	Expresses love for others through actions
	Seeks the good of others
Need for hope and creativity	Asks for information about his condition realistically
	Talks about his condition realistically
	Sets realistic personal health goals
	Uses time during illness/hospitalization constructively
	Values his inner self more than his physical self

*Now would be nursing diagnosis of Spiritual Distress

From "Spiritual Needs of Patients: Are They Recognized?" by M.F. Highfield and C. Cason, 1983, *Cancer Nursing, 6.* Reprinted by permission.

◆

BELIEF INDICATORS

NEED	AFFECT
Achievement/purpose	Use of money, talents, time
Love/belonging/dependence	Source of solace
Self-worth	Esteem of self/God/others
Security/wholeness	Source of help
Sensory stimulation	Religious practices (Ellis, 1980)

client's spiritual beliefs affect his needs (see the box on this page).

In the course of a spiritual assessment, a client may manifest spiritual needs, recall an internal guidance system, feel less inhibited, spontaneously acknowledge problems, and confide in the nurse. A client may express spiritual needs subjectively during seemingly routine conversational exchanges, as interactions during daily care. Being prepared to assess the subtle expression of spiritual needs allows a nurse an opportunity to interject questions about a client's spiritual integrity and intervene to strengthen it. This is one step in understanding and predicting how a client may respond to disability or participate in therapy.

Table 28-2   Spiritual distress (distress of the human spirit)

Related factors: Challenged belief in God; separated from formal religious and family support*
  Richard J. Fehring and Audrey M. McLane

Client goals/expected outcomes	Nursing interventions/scientific rationale
IMPROVE SPIRITUAL WELL-BEING AS EVIDENCED BY THE FOLLOWING:	
Achieves high score (80-120) on Spiritual Well-Being Scale of Paloutzian and Ellison	Provide models of persons who have overcome difficulties, using examples from literature, Bible, personal experiences, and so on
Makes positive statements about self and life	Encourage/accept verbalization of feelings of anger
Articulates and is comfortable with belief system	Teach cognitive strategies (e.g., combating distorted thinking and values clarification) *(clarification of values will help client develop short- and long-term goals for spiritual growth)*
	Provide referral to spiritual counselor
	Monitor spiritual distress with Spiritual Well-Being Scale of Paloutzian and Ellison
	Provide daily prayer/meditation booklet congruent with reading level and expressed religious/denominational preference
	Use imagery/prayer/music to heal past life hurts
	Discuss importance of trying new religious exercises more than one time *(spiritual well-being/distress may differ from day to day; spiritual exercise may not be effective the first time)*
DEVELOP SUPPORT SYSTEM WITH FRIENDS/CHURCH MEMBERS AS EVIDENCED BY THE FOLLOWING:	
Initiates ongoing relationship with another individual	Encourage participation in adult prayer, social, and athletic groups
Feels someone cares about her	Use role playing to prepare client for new relationships
Participates in group activities (alcohol support group, prayer group, and so on)	
PARTICIPATE IN ALCOHOL REHABILITATION PROGRAM AS EVIDENCED BY THE FOLLOWING:	
Enters and adheres to alcohol rehabilitation program	Refer and advocate client's entrance into inpatient alcohol and drug treatment program *(advocacy will help gain entrance into inpatient program, especially if client has failed in previous outpatient treatment programs)*
FIND A JOB AND/OR ENGAGE IN VOLUNTEER ACTIVITY AS EVIDENCED BY THE FOLLOWING:	
Obtains job counseling	Refer to social worker/vocational counselor
Participates in volunteer program	Explore volunteer opportunities
Attends basic reading program	Enroll in basic reading program *(ongoing social support of case workers and learning basic reading skills will help client gain self-esteem, establish new goals, and obtain employment)*
Articulates goals in life	

*For a homeless person who believes in God and abuses drugs and alcohol.

A client's spiritual resources, as well as needs or distress, can be built into an individualized care plan when they are identified and validated. Other cues are observed directly, such as the presence of religious books or objects, facial expressions and gestures, or a humorous reference to God or religion as if to provoke a response (Ellis, 1980). Careful assessment eliminates false assumptions about client behaviors; all observations are validated before any interventions are planned.

Two prototypes demonstrating clinical decision-making with spirituality are included in this chapter. Both have been developed using the nursing diagnosis of Spiritual Distress. The first prototype contains a plan for a homeless person who abuses alcohol, which may be closer to a feasible approach during physical rehabilitation (Table 28-2). The second case study contains a client's situation in depth and provides multiple nursing interventions.

The spiritual aspects of healthcare have been influential in rehabilitation. Many rehabilitation facilities have regularly planned events and contact with clergymen and other religious persons. Major rehabilitation organizations have scheduled sessions, established special-interest groups, and published articles dealing with spirituality or pastoral care and rehabilitation.

For example, at a regional meeting of the Association of Rehabilitation Nurses (ARN), Nicosia presented his "healing paradigm," which was designed for an interdisciplinary approach in rehabilitation settings. The paradigm displayed in the following box "provides a way to devise care plans, encourage client involvement, and measure the effectiveness of treatment in all its forms" (Nicosia, 1994).

During a medical crisis the immediate concern is with the person's physical entity; some thought is given to psychological needs, but even when the emergency is resolved, spirituality remains unattended. Shortened stays in acute care settings do not allow delving below presentation of self unless the client projects distress unmistakable as a spiritual crisis. In rehabilitation or home care, nurses attuned to enabling a client to optimize functional potential may overlook the influence of spiritual attitude on all that has and is happening for a client.

Spiritually focused intervention will vary with religious groups, cultures, beliefs, and practices of both nurses and clients. Resource guides, such as those listed in reference books or articles, can be maintained on file and updated with new or additional information as it is learned about a group. However, not all persons uniformly adhere to the beliefs and practices of their culture or ethnic group; few persons practice all commonly known rituals, and most practice variations. Those who have become acculturated into Western medical practices and the mainstream of the United States may not employ any culturally specific practices apart from personal idiosyncracies or choices.

On the other hand, when threatened with illness or disability, persons may return to their origins and participate in cultural or religious practices more faithfully than when unthreatened. Di Meo's (1991) guide to religious practices or an outline of beliefs that can affect therapy, culled from 32 religious denominations throughout the United States (Nursing Update, 1979) are examples of resources that can be used and supplemented with data about religions in a cachement area. Apart from specialized knowledge of a person's background, clients have some universal needs that are eased by arranging for privacy during prayer, meditation, or spiritual reading; by allowing opportunity to offer a blessing before meals; by observing for indications that a client wishes to discuss spiritual anxieties; by scheduling for pastoral visitors; and by assuring access to religious services (Ellis, 1980).

In a practical vein a client may respond to activities such as keeping a journal, entering personal thoughts in a notebook, or speaking into a tape recorder. A client is able to review past thoughts and look for meaningful patterns in behavior. At times, contact with a person of the same cul-

---

HEALING PARADIGM

RESULTS	ELEMENTS	NURSE ASSISTS
Meaning and purpose	Open to discussion	Problems bearable
Self-esteem	Approach client; decision-making	Self-awareness; sense of worth
Interpersonal relationships	Encourage group activities	Connect with others
Ability to make choices	Decision-making	Control over life
Acceptance of circumstances	Knowledge/choices	No denial
Future orientation	Perceive goals and realize them	Courage to hope/independence
Sense of accomplishment	Reinforce and affirm contributions	Achieve recognition as self
Religious significance	Knowledge and support	Community worship (Nicosia, 1994)

ture who has a similar situation may be helpful; at other times this approach may create conflict or confusion. Some clients may find help from a prayer card or spiritual poetry, inspirations, or essays; or from audiotapes of inspirational music or relaxation sounds for meditation; or from opportunities for prayer. Appropriate humor may ease tension as the Yiddish proverb that says: "Soap is to the body as laughter is to the soul." Art or music therapy, bibliotherapy, or role playing can have spiritual themes.

Some facilities have initiated ecumenical prayer groups (Clifford & Gruca, 1987). The idea is that clients who already share through rehabilitation therapies and goals are able to form a group whose members would foster self-esteem, mutual support, prayer, and "deepen their hopes and make use of the present moment" (Durkin, 1992). Few opportunities allow persons with disabilities to meet and connect in a spiritual way. Brochures or articles about spiritually oriented camps, retreats, or religious or self-help groups may indicate sessions for persons with a particular illness or disability.

For example, Christian Overcomers Camp is a camp, Handicapped Encounter Christ is a retreat, and Joni and Friends is a religious group, which offers a variety of services based on the ministry of a young woman athlete who incurred traumatic quadriplegia. As an interest in spirituality becomes apparent, members of the team who feel so inclined may volunteer for training to specialize in spirituality therapy, or spiritual leaders and pastoral workers may be invited to join the team. However, at no time are professionals required to abdicate their own beliefs, make statements, or to practice behaviors that are inconsistent or in opposition to their faith or spiritual beliefs.

Meditation

Meditation as a means of achieving relaxation has been experienced in Eastern and Western cultures throughout the ages. Rather than searching for quiet, meditation is finding the quiet within. Meditation techniques include yoga, Zen, transcendental meditation, and hypnosis. Those who practice regular meditation twice a day have shown themselves to be in better health, have sharper minds, and live longer than their contemporaries (Di Meo, 1991). A quiet environment, an object to dwell on, a passive attitude allowing thoughts to pass through, and a comfortable position are the requirements for mediation.

Meditation occurs in Christian, Judaic, and Eastern religious literature as an inward exercise, a prayer from the heart centered on divine things and in true contact with the immovable, central core of being. Participants repeat and meditate only on thoughts and words chosen from their religion or belief system. In many spiritual meditations a person (1) prepares specific acts or petitions; (2) considers basic truths or petitions for grace; and (3) comes to conclusions that may involve resolution to make changes, such as to do something in the service of God.

At any time in the exercise of meditation, the client can engage in thoughts of the topic chosen the previous evening, or in conversation with God, returning to the simple breathing formula from time to time. Throughout the busy day, from awakening on, recalling the meditation will reinforce the technique until the client is able to create an atmosphere of prayer. Thus a client who began meditation after breakfast and continued into therapy sessions also could make a prayer offering of the work of therapy.

Practicing the technique of breathing and gazing downward while mentally saying the chosen word or prayer ensures a client is never far away from immediate personal contact with the infinite and intimate spiritual presence within. This breath of spirit can then flow out carrying the holy words, prayer lines, Bible phrase, Hebrew word, or whatever the client has chosen. Some clients may use a technique in which they focus on an image that embodies their sense of the divine. In the Kundalini form of meditation, there is a short "seven breath" meditation that can be done in a minute or two, wherever one is and whatever one is doing (Selby & Selig, 1992).

The "centering" used by many nurses who practice the principles of therapeutic touch has been likened to the senses attained through meditation. Although therapeutic touch is not associated with meditation techniques or mental effort, it depends on the universal healing power being channeled through the nurse as a conduit to provide comfort or healing. Those who desire that a time be set aside for a meditation period may need assistance from a nurse to find a secluded place in a rehabilitation facility or a "Do Not Disturb" sign on the door to their room. A guide to assisting clients with meditation as a means of managing stress is included in Chapter 13.

Imagery and Visualization

Imagery requires focused concentration using imagination and all the senses as a client attempts to dismiss anxiety and reach to spiritual resources within. Use of imagery techniques has been thought to influence the peripheral and autonomic nervous systems by reducing stressful symptoms and speeding recovery from illness. Many people choose images related to God (or an inner guide) and creation as their resources. A nurse who is interested in helping clients access their inner healing resources first becomes familiar with types of imagery (receptive, active, concrete, symbolic process end-of-state, and general healing) and studies ways to guide clients on their healing journey (Dossey, 1991).

Begin by guiding a client to identify the problem or goal for imagery, then to a relaxed state. When relaxed a client can begin to visualize images of the stressor; to create imagery of internal and external healing resources; and then to envision the goal. A commercial audiotape of relaxation exercises, or a self-made one with a personalized script, may enable a client to create wordless pictures in a compassionate imagery or to construct wordless but deliberate thoughts toward a goal.

Serenity

Trauma, major illness, and increasing age give way to a search for inner peace, or serenity, during troubled times. Serenity "gives one a healthy mastery of emotions, decreases stress, and leads to improved relationships with others and especially with God, through prayer; zest for living, acceptance of one's self as worthy, increased compassion and self-possession during trying times, and trust in a higher power" (Dossey, 1991). A serene person is caring, active, involved and responsible, not passive or detached.

Under an exterior equanimity, tranquility, and acceptance lies quiet inner-directed action.

The nurse who desires personal serenity is attuned to assess a client's serenity. Rehabilitation nurses may ask themselves, "What is the effect of a nurse's level of serenity on a client's health?" (Roberts & Messenger, 1993). Nurses could do no better for clients than to acquire for themselves the serenity which is deemed to be so efficacious. Characteristics of a serene person that may be detected during an assessment interview include a client's awareness of an "inner haven," detachment, belonging, giving, trust, acceptance, problem-solving, presentness, forgiveness, and a view of the future. Behaviors such as anxiety, anger, lack of faith, impatience, and unhealthy lifestyle behaviors are among those found in the nonserene.

Interrelationships among a client's view of an "inner haven," means of cognitive restructuring, and physical well-being must be considered when planning interventions. Before planning and setting goals, learn what the client may be doing already, what is possible in the present environment, and how to implement an integrated, holistic approach involving members of an interdisciplinary team. An individual who is able to achieve serenity may have a strategy for coping with chronic or recurring diseases, addictive behaviors, and other comorbid conditions that may accompany disabilities. Alcoholics Anonymous, in its quest for serenity for its members, has made famous the simple serenity prayer:

God grant me the serenity to accept the things I cannot change, courage to change the things I can, and wisdom to know the difference (Niebuhr, 1943)

ONCOLOGY REHABILITATION

With improved outcome for many clients, cancer has gained a place among chronic and disabling diseases, as well as being associated with terminal conditions. Furthermore, a client with a disability may have a dual diagnosis of a cancer. Clients who are expected to improve following diagnosis and treatment of cancer are appearing for therapeutic and preventive interventions and adaptive equipment or assistive devices available in rehabilitation settings. Clients seeking oncology rehabilitation include persons who have breast or bone reconstruction, grafts, amputations, surgical removal of portions of muscle or tissue (e.g., enterostoma or ostomies), sectioning or removal of functional parts such as the larynx, or altered sensory function, chronic pain, and so on.

Oncology rehabilitation may be categorized as preventive, restorative, supportive, and palliative. Dietz (1981) prefers the term "readaptation" because of a general reluctance, on the part of the public and health professionals alike, to view rehabilitation as relevant to clients with cancer. Dietz has defined the term as "accommodation to personal needs for physical, psychological, financial, and vocational survival; the initial goals as the elimination, reduction or alleviation of disability; and the ultimate goal as the reestablishment of clients as functional individuals in their environments." A nursing definition of cancer rehabilitation is less dogmatic: "a dynamic, ongoing, health-oriented process designed to promote maximum levels of functioning and independence in individuals with cancer-related health problems" (Watson, 1992).

In dealing with oncology in rehabilitation, the nurse and other team members, client, and family comprise a sociocultural, psychoemotional, holistically interactive unit dedicated to identifying and mobilizing a client's internal and external coping resources. Rehabilitation outcome improves when a client has an active support system, including professional support for timely referrals to counseling and acute care services. A nurse may function as a short-term adjustment counselor: promoting effective coping behaviors and a constructive attitude toward participation in a program of rehabilitation; keeping client and family informed and educated; and advocating for client needs, including referrals.

The spiritual nature of oncology rehabilitation nursing practice exists in empathetic listening, sensitivity to a client's needs and potential, managing a client's anxiety and maintaining hope, offering opportunity to vent emotions, or assisting with time and atmosphere for spiritual presencing. The client, informed of a malignancy, experiences system disorganization as evidenced by confusion, anger and frustration, and impersonalized feelings. A client may exhibit altered self-esteem and body image; impaired sexual adjustment, emotional insecurity, or reduced task motivation; changes in behavior leading to dependency; or regress to immature behavior, among other responses.

The team is challenged to assist the client to find a meaning and purpose according to the person's belief system. Many persons believe that God will impart direction amidst crisis and within the limitations imposed by the client's condition. Clients who experience changes in body image due to treatment or surgical intervention benefit from being able to focus on values of spiritual growth apart from their outward appearance. A client who centered personal worth on physical appearance or abilities may be at risk for psychosocial breakdown when body image is altered. This person may find former levels of self-confidence, self-esteem, assertiveness, trust, and hope, as well as interpersonal relationships, have been threatened or destroyed.

A client benefits from a sense of being in control of life following the invasive procedures associated with many cancer treatment regimens. These tend to erode strength and endurance, tax coping abilities, and invade personal space and privacy, leaving a person with feelings of powerlessness. A nurse advocating for client empowerment may assess potential and actual disabilities and ways to prevent or manage them so as to reduce the extent to which they interfere with activities of daily living and independent function; perform nursing therapeutics and teach self-care skills; have an understanding of the disease trajectory in view of the prognosis and data all physicians and other healers have given the client; assess needs in re-entering community life and meeting individual goals after discharge; offer resources for cosmetic or assistive devices, support groups, and long-term counseling; and assure a client is able to incorporate personal preferences, lifestyle choices, and cultural ways into all decisions concerning personal care and plans for the future.

A great deal of oncology research is under way that can be expected to produce findings about ways to combat cancer. At this time nurses can target interventions that improve a client's comfort, strength, well-being, and attitude. Nutritional planning and supplements; pain management and control, if relief is not possible; attention to detail such as skin integrity to protect from further disabilities or complications; use of technologic advances in care and for maximum functional abilities; promoting effective coping behaviors; and establishing the spiritual presence will enable a client to live with the highest possible quality of life.

Support groups for clients, family members, and friends are active in most community settings, and client-to-client volunteer networks are available. The American Cancer Society offers information and education programs that are advertised in local telephone directory listings. A client may learn all or any of the methods of in-spiriting discussed previously to be useful during the rehabilitation program and continue them throughout life in the community. Clients with an oncology diagnosis deal with some degree of uncertainty and other issues that may be managed through spiritual means, regardless of outcome.

Hope

Recent developments toward understanding disease etiology, improving treatment methods, validating research findings, and instituting interdisciplinary teamwork with oncology rehabilitation have stimulated services and programs for clients and their families. With more choices from effective interventions and treatments able to be blended with rehabilitation techniques, team members are optimistic themselves and thus better able to help clients generate models of hope. Indeed, oncology rehabilitation nursing imparts a philosophy of hope. Hope may transcend all time.

Hope, by definition, is future-oriented, necessary for sustaining life, involved in achieving goals, and embodying interpersonal relationships—the ultimate of these existing between a person and the perception of the Almighty. The opposite of hope is hopelessness, often accompanied by helplessness, which itself is preceded by loss of control of one's own life and independence. Clients who feel hopeless are not demanding or noisy; rather they present themselves as passive and depressed, wreaking further adversity on their quality of life.

Acknowledging a client's seeming hopelessness, offering to discuss problems, and assisting in constructive ways may begin a supportive nurse-client relationship from which to foster hope. Strategies include teaching coping behaviors, aiding in goal identification, reframing a view of health problems as opportunities for adaptation and physical and spiritual growth.

Clients who have cancer tend to set goals that are general rather than specific, open-ended rather than at set times, and focused on adapting to altered functional status. These goals may reflect their expectations and avoid disappointment. However, when goals are unrealistic or not embraced by a client, trust and rapport with the nurse will erode. At times a nurse may be able to reinforce a client's satisfaction with small gains; a client may become motivated to work toward higher expectations. Goals must be mutually agreed upon, attainable, realistic, and appropriate for the client's lifestyle. The resulting optimism leads to an integral, though constantly modified, part of the client's existence—

hope—the hope that is kept alive by an eternal hope in God and is a sign of spiritual integrity.

Loss and Change

The loss of a limb to cancer forces an individual to confront real limitations in life and to reevaluate goals and hopes. The functional reality of limb loss is different for each client and is experienced by sifting through each one's separate impressions, which are unlike anyone else's and dependent on many factors. While letting go of various things during life is something everyone goes through, it is a big step every time it happens. The crisis of amputation requires letting go of more than the limb itself; it is comprised of a myriad of smaller stages spread out over time. There are some ways to make losses easier:

+ Take time to say good-bye
+ Reach out to others
+ Accept change
+ Learn to trust in God
+ Make happiness a habit
+ Live your life well (Idowu, 1993)

To these we might add: pray constantly. Increased demanding and fault-finding, withdrawal, and low ability to control frustration that may occur perplex both the client and the family. Labile emotions may be anticipated during acute crisis that may occur for approximately 6 to 8 weeks and are one part of guidance counseling to be discussed with client and family.

It may require months, even years, for a client to become accustomed to an altered body image and for the associated problems to be resolved. An independent person with a positive and stable sense of self can come to accept personal limitations and those of others. After the person with an amputation begins to adjust to personal emotional shock, the primary concern shifts to the effect of loss on loved ones, a spouse's love and acceptance, and children's understanding and comfort; these responses are as important as personal adjustment. Practical problem-solving predictably would address changes in family roles, functional abilities and independence, and a client's fears for a place in the community—be it loss of work, change of career, return to school or training, or maintaining a home (Dise-Lewis, 1988).

At first, original goals in life appear meaningless. Ideally, spiritual maturity results in actively planning approaches to modify goals. Small goals, easily attained with the least amount of frustration, are documented, even videotaped for reinforcing playback. The entire process of educating the person with a new amputation uses language that is relevant, sensitive, and easily understood in repeated small doses. A fearful person, expecting to fail, may have spiritual distress, suffering from feeling a loss of God's love as a self-punishment for real or imagined "crimes."

Fearful on one hand, this client may become angry and revolt against religion. The client may resist choosing a prosthesis out of a belief that it is undeserved or will be impossible to use. The rehabilitation nurse who understands the need and creates a safe atmosphere for emotional and spiritual expression enables a client to know it is acceptable to experience and communicate feelings. During such times a caring and sensitive team will provide privacy and protect the client's dignity.

When clients agree, the rehabilitation nurse may arrange opportunities for them to share their amputation crisis experience. For example, persons may room together, have common free time, and participate in special-interest or support group activities for clients who have experienced amputations. In one institution, members of a self-help group for persons with amputations meet regularly in the evening, hold picnics, participate in education programs for health professionals, and help conduct summer camps for adolescents and young children who have amputation experiences. While the physical aspects of edema, pain, wound healing, phantom pain, and others are very real concerns, the spiritual and psychosocial aspects are the more challenging for the rehabilitation nurse. One method may not work; try another. Do not let a client become a "spiritual dropout."

Rehabilitation nurses have encountered clients who have stubborn persistence of hope and courage and those who are devoid of hopes and dreams. In either case, nurses know to be more sensitive, more compassionate, and more caring to those committed to their care (Leffall, 1994)—for "someday after mastering the wind, the waves, the tides and gravity, we shall harness for God the energies of love and then for the second time in the history of the world man shall have discovered fire" (Teilhard deChardin, 1984). The practical rehabilitation nurse can exemplify that same love and fire when helping clients to presence and become in-spirited.

Table 28-3   Client Goals & Nursing Interventions

Client goals/expected outcomes	Nursing interventions/outcome evaluation
Determine substance and design in own existence, illness, and distress *Self-esteem* *Sense of accomplishment*	Be available to listen; employ readings that depict people who found significance in difficult circumstances; teach meditation, imagery, and centering; help to view problems in perspective and to find how to use them to grow *Self-awareness* *Connect with others* *Volunteer activities*
Feel sense of pardon and diminished connotation of guilt by healing former offenses *Discussion of guilt feelings* *Forgiving oneself and accepting God's love and forgiveness*	"Be there" when client wishes to share feelings; suggest use of tape machine to record thoughts of hurt and guilt; in-spirit with centering and prayer techniques to ask God to forgive and replace guilt with love *Feel God's love and extend it to others* *Share guilt of past*
Feel that God will sustain client and alleviate misery *Receive serenity* *Embrace affliction*	Give assurance of nurse's willingness to be present when client is in distress; suggest imaging and prayer—offer self and touch during praying *Feeling that God will help* *Comfort and peace* *No denial*
Recognize and understand principles and values *Clarification of same*	Request client list what is important (goals and tasks) *Asks God for advice*
Feel less helpless and lonely as pertains to disassociation from religion *Involvement in rituals*	Have client discuss background; provide with others who have coped; share prayer and rituals; refer to spiritual advisor *Seeks religious resources* *Finds comfort and community in rituals*
Expand affinity with God *Feel closeness*	Be available; teach relaxation techniques; mention need to find God in self, environment, and others; refer to requested clergy *Seeks spiritual counsel* *Enjoys prayer and meditation*

◆

CASE STUDY

Mrs. G. is a 28-year-old female who was diagnosed with os-teosarcoma of the left radius, with subsequent above-elbow amputation. She is married and the mother of a 3-year-old daughter. A right-handed sports enthusiast, she is active in swimming, golf, and tennis. Her husband visits regularly. Her parents are deceased, but she has a very supportive sister and her in-laws are, in her words, "sympathetic and helpful." Mrs. G. had mild edema of the left arm on admission to the rehabilitation center but has made no complaints about pain, although she was observed biting into her lower lip several times. Since admission, she has been very quiet and does not initiate conversation with other clients.

One morning, upon awakening, she was seen to have tears on her cheeks by an aide whom she berated for "spying." Several times Mrs. G. has found fault with her food tray. She attends therapy sessions but takes little interest in care of her residual limb and participates as little as possible in therapy activities. The prosthetist says Mrs. G. displays no interest in fittings and refuses to make any choices.

On the nursing unit, Mrs. G. does not display any pictures of her husband or daughter in her room because "she cries each time she sees their pictures." When family members visit, Mrs. G. does not talk about her disability or her job. Her husband appears bewildered by the recent events and is overly cheerful and talkative when visiting. Informally, the nurses have ascertained that Mrs. G. is saddened and perhaps feeling angry about the loss of her arm and the impact on her having a productive place in society.

No spiritual integrity assessment form is established in the institution. However, religious data indicate the client's religion to be "R.C." and "N.P." ("nonpracticing"). Mr. G. is Protestant, but their daughter was baptized Catholic. Mrs. G. displays articles among her possessions, such as a rosary in her drawer and a guardian angel pin on her shirt, that suggest some affinity for her religion. She refused to have a priest visit her. The evening nurse recognizes several signs including inattention to basic tasks, impersonalized feelings, emotional detachment, rejection of the prosthesis, and excessive weeping that suggest Mrs. G. may be experiencing spiritual distress.

NURSING DIAGNOSIS: SPIRITUAL DISTRESS

The nurse plans to interview Mrs. G. in greater depth concerning spirituality, using questions from a spiritual history guide (Stoll, 1995), or Ellison and Paloutzian's Spiritual Well-Being Scale (box, p. 633) as a model. The nurse may begin by requesting Mrs. G. to answer the questions because she is concerned that everything is not well and is offering her help or she may ask questions to elicit data while performing routine care. The responses will allow a nurse to confirm the diagnosis and plan an effective intervention strategy.

After many conversations with Mrs. G., she agrees to meet with a woman who is a member of the social and support group for persons with amputation. The two women talk for some time, and Mrs. G. agrees to attend a meeting "some time later

on." The nurse has been teaching meditation techniques to Mrs. G. and assists her with relaxation before meditation. On one occasion the nurse prayed silently with Mrs. G., then offered her a book of spiritual readings from the library. A few evenings later Mrs. G. called the nurse to her bedside, then tearfully thrust her journal at the nurse. "Read this in private because I can't tell you my 'secret' aloud," Mrs. G. cried.

The nurse discovers that Mrs. G. has written her "secret" in the form of a confession. At age 15 years Mrs. G. had an abortion. She writes that she now is certain that God has punished her for this by removing her left hand and arm because this was the hand on which she wore her wedding ring. She believes God did this to remind her that she is unworthy of her husband or child because of the abortion. The amputation will be a reminder to her whenever she glances down to where her ring once was.

The nurse returns to Mrs. G. in her room and invites her to join in centering and praying, especially to ask God to forgive her and to substitute love for her feelings of guilt. A few days after the nurse spoke with Mrs. G. about an all-loving God, Mrs. G. asks to see a priest for reconciliation, and the nurse facilitates the visit. The nurse discusses other community services as referral options with Mrs. G. They agree that a counselor from Project Rachel, which is part of the Catholic Community Service located in every diocese, would be an acceptable resource. Making use of the spiritual readings and tapes, the nurse encourages Mrs. G. to continue practicing imagery and meditation.

Mr. G. is relieved and happy to have his wife talking and being cheerful but is puzzled about the behavior change. After discussing the entire event with his wife, Mr. G. brings her wedding ring to the rehabilitation center. With some small ceremony, he slips the ring on Mrs. G.'s ring finger of her right hand while repeating his wedding vows.

Mrs. G. began to cooperate with her therapy programs and self-care activities. Soon thereafter the nurse observes Mrs. G. as she is visiting with a client newly admitted to the rehabilitation center following a lower limb amputation. She is offering the newcomer a handmade prayer card and laughingly pointing to her daughter's computer-imprinted picture on her sweatshirt. Mrs. G. is fond of saying she carries her daughter everywhere, even without using her arm. Mrs. G. still has bouts of weeping but relaxes, meditates, prays, and after a visit from an empathetic fellow teacher, makes plans to return to teaching school in the fall.

DOCUMENTING SPIRITUAL DISTRESS IN A CARE PLAN

Table 28-3 illustrates how the nurse documented goals and outcome evaluation in the care plan concerning Mrs. G.'s nursing diagnosis of Spiritual Distress. The spirituality care plan has client-related factors of separation from formal religion, sense of being remote from God, sense of guilt and shame, and low self-esteem.

REFERENCES

Burkhardt, M.A. (1989). Spirituality: An analysis of the concept. *Holistic Nursing Practice, 3*, 69-77.

Clifford, M., & Gruca, C. (1987). Facilitating spiritual care in the rehabilitation setting. *Rehabilitation Nursing, 12*, 331-333.

Cowl, C.T. (Ed.). (1991). Religion in the clinical encounter. (Pulse section). *JAMA, 266(21)*, 3062-3067.

Davis, M.C. (1994). The rehabilitation nurse's role in spiritual care. *Rehabilitation Nursing, 19*, 298-301.

Dietz, J.H., Jr. (1981). *Rehabilitation oncology.* Melbourne, FL: Krieger.

Di Meo, E. (1991). Rx for spiritual distress. *Rehabilitation Nursing, 54*, 22-24.

Dise-Lewis, J.E. (1988). Psychological adaptation to limb loss. In D.J. Atkins & R.H. Meier (Eds.), *Comprehensive management of the upper-limb amputee* (pp. 165-172). New York: Springer-Verlag.

Donley, R. (1991). Spiritual dimensions of health care. *Nursing and Health Care, 12*, 178-183.

Dossey, B. (1991). Awakening the inner healer. *American Journal Nursing, 91*, 31-34.

Dossey, L. (1993). *Healing words: The power of prayer and the practice of medicine.* San Francisco: Harper & Row.

Draper, E., et al. (1965). On the diagnostic value of religious ideation. *Archives of General Psychology, 13*, 202-207.

Durkin, M.B. (1992). A community of caring: patients in a rehabilitation unit experience holistic healing through a spiritual support group. *Health Progress, 73*, 48-53, 70.

Ellis, D. (1980). Whatever happened to the spiritual dimension? *Canadian Nurse, 76*, 42-43.

Ellison, C.W. (1982). Spiritual well-being; Conceptualization and measurement. *Journal of Psychology and Theology, 11*, 330-340.

Frankl, V.E. (1983). *Man's search for meaning.* New York: Washington Square Press.

Glenndinning, C. (1990). *When technology wounds: the human consequences of progress.* New York: Morrow Publishers.

Griffin, G.J., & Griffin, J.K. (1973). *History and trends of professional nursing.* St. Louis: Mosby–Year Book.

Haase, J.E., Britt, T., Coward, D.D., Leidy, N.K., & Penn P.E. (1992). Simultaneous concept analysis of spiritual perspective, hope, acceptance and self-transcendence. *Image, 24*, 141-147.

Hendricks, G., & Wills, R. (1975). *The centering book: Awareness activities for children, parents and teachers.* Englewood Cliffs, NJ: Prentice-Hall.

Highfield, M.F., & Cason, C. (1983). Spiritual needs of patients: Are they recognized? *Cancer Nursing, 6*, 187-192.

Idowu, F. (1993). Let go and live. *America, 169*, 20-21.

Kim, M.J., McFarland, G.K., & McLane, A.M. (1993). *Pocket guide to nursing diagnoses* (5th ed.). St. Louis: Mosby–Year Book.

Labun, E. (1988). Spiritual care: An element in nursing care planning. *Journal of Advanced Nursing, 13*, 314-320.

Leffall, L.D., JR. (1994). Medical ethics in today's society. *Bulletin of the American College of Surgeons, 79*, 6-11.

Mahony, R. (1994). "Gospel of suffering" teaches important message. *Catholic Advocate, 44*, 19.

National Interfaith Coalition on Aging. (1975). *Spiritual well-being: A definition.* Athens, GA: Author.

Niebuhr, R. (1943). *Serenity prayer.* Heath, MA: Written for service in the Congregational Church.

Nicosia, J. (1994). Healing the human spirit: The healing paradigm. *Journal of Religion Disability Rehabilitation, 1*, 65-74.

Nightingale, F. (1970). Notes on nursing. (Facsimile reprint of 1860 ed.) Princeton, NJ: Brandon Systems Press.

Nursing Update. (1979). Beliefs that can affect therapy. *Pediatric Nursing, 5*, 298-301.

Paterson, J.G., & Zderad, L.T. (1976). *Humanistic nursing.* New York: John Wiley and Sons.

Peterson, E.H. (1993). The spirit quest. *Christianity Today, 37*, 27-30.

Pettigrew, J. (1990). Intensive nursing care: The ministry of presence. *Critical Care Nursing Clinics of North America, 2*, 503-508.

Pope John Paul II. (1984, February 1). Apostolici letter Salvifici Doloris: On the Christian meaning of human suffering. Washington, DC: U.S. Catholic Conference.

Roberts, K.T., & Messenger, T.C. (1993). Helping older adults find serenity. Are there potential nursing interventions that may help older adults reach a serene state? *Geriatric Nursing, 14*, 317-322.

Selby, J., & Selig, Z.J. (1992). *Kundalini awakening: A gentle guide to chakra activation and spiritual growth.* New York: Bantam Books.

Siegel, B. (1986). *Love, medicine and miracles.* New York: Harper & Row, Publishers.

Soeken, K.L., & Carson, V.J. (1987). Responding to the spiritual needs of the chronically ill. *Nursing Clinics of North America, 22*, 603-611.

Sommer, D.R. (1989). The spiritual needs of dying children. *Issues in Comprehensive Pediatric Nursing, 12*, 225-233.

Stavros, M. (1994). Logotherapy: Bringing meaning out of suffering. *SCI Psychosocial Processes, 7*, 22-26.

Stoll, R. (1995). Personal communication. Messiah College, PA.

Teilhard deChardin, P. (1984). *On love and happiness.* San Francisco: Harper & Row Publishers, Inc.

Watson, P.G. (1992). The optimal functioning plan: A key element in cancer rehabilitation. *Cancer Nursing, 15*, 254-263.

Wheeler, H.B. (1990). Shattuck lecture—healing and heroism. *New England Journal of Medicine, 322*, 1540-1548.

V

SPECIAL POPULATIONS AND REHABILITATION NURSING

29

Restorative Rehabilitation with Burn Injuries

Angela Moy, MSN, RN, CRRN

INTRODUCTION

It has been estimated that 1% of the population of the United States, or 2 million persons, will receive a burn injury each year; 6000 of these will prove fatal. One million persons, half of those with burns, will have injuries severe enough to restrict daily activities in the home, school, and workplace and frequently will seek rehabilitation services.

This chapter discusses what rehabilitation offers these clients, information about burn injuries, rehabilitation nursing assessment and interventions, and the impact of rehabilitation nursing care on outcome for the client who has an injury from burns. As with other clients, a key rehabilitation nursing function is to educate clients to be able to direct their own care, facilitating and encouraging them to do so. This advocacy begins with establishing trust and rapport from the time a client is admitted to service and maintaining a positive relationship throughout rehabilitation.

Incidence Across the Life-span

Children (2 to 4 years old) and young adults (17 to 25 years), especially males, comprise the age groups with greater numbers of injuries from burns. In fact, burn injuries rank second only to motor vehicle accidents as a cause of death during childhood. On the other end of the life-span, elderly persons experience high mortality and morbidity rates from burns. Older persons may not detect danger when preexisting problems such as altered or impaired judgment, decreased coordination and tactile sensation, or impaired vision and smell inhibit their awareness. Fifty percent of burns involve the upper extremities. As a result long-term impairments of arm, hand, and upper torso function may be painful; limit manual activities; alter a client's movement, facial expression, or overall appearance; and lead to psychosocial problems with body image.

CHANGES IN BURN CARE

The survival rate after burn injury has increased significantly over the past two decades. For instance, in 1964 a young person (10 to 30 years old) with a second- to third-degree burn covering 50% of total body surface areas had a 50% chance of survival; by 1984 the same person would have had a 90% survival rate. These dramatic improvements in mortality rates have been attributed in part to the expansion of approximately 200 specialized burn centers throughout the United States (Helms, 1992). A national survey of burn rehabilitation services in the United States revealed substantial improvements in comprehensiveness and ser-

vices over the past decade. Minimum guidelines for burn rehabilitation care are proposed as a next step (Cromes & Helms, 1992).

Traditionally clients were admitted to a burn unit directly from the emergency room and then received acute care, treatment, and therapy. Once discharged to home, they relied on outpatient care for follow-up treatment and evaluation. However, ongoing advances in burn care technology, health system changes, and demonstrated cost-effectiveness of comprehensive rehabilitation services have produced a trend toward inpatient rather than outpatient care for these clients, in contrast to most other health services.

Inpatient rehabilitation offers continual medical services, wound care programs, rehabilitation nursing and therapies, and treatment modalities for conditioning, strengthening, and improving functional mobility. However, the pendulum may have swung too far in the direction of inpatient treatment without sufficient attention to rehabilitation services for clients postdischarge and community follow-up. In a Delphi study, nurses who were burn specialists identified preparing clients and families, as well as community health nurses, to perform posthospitalization care as a priority need for nursing interventions and research (Bayley et al., 1992).

Community-based interventions support research findings that clients who have burn injuries require long-term psychosocial support and vocational benefits. However, many disability benefits are available only when a client's condition is carefully and precisely documented (Salisbury, 1992).

Types of Burns

Burn management decisions are based in part on an understanding of the type of burn injury. For example, some burn injuries, sun exposures for instance, will manifest symptoms rapidly within 12 to 24 hours, whereas others, such as electrical burns, though possibly superficial in appearance, may cause deeper tissue or organ damage that may not become apparent until days later.

Seventy percent of burns result from thermal injury either from dry heat (flame) or moist heat (hot liquid). Thermal injury results in marked changes in the vascular and metabolic responses of the body, leaving clients at risk for infection due to loss of skin integrity and postburn immunosuppression. Thus effective management of the client sustaining a major thermal injury requires understanding the interaction of changes occurring on the vascular, metabolic, and physiologic levels (Winkler, DiMola, & Wooten, 1993).

These issues are addressed critically in the acute care setting, but it is essential for nurses to acknowledge these interactive changes during rehabilitation and to continue supportive care for all three levels to achieve a successful outcome. By recognizing that the recovery process at a cellular level is continuous up to 1 year, rehabilitation nurses can anticipate that complications such as heterotopic ossification, contractures, or hypertrophic scarring may emerge over time; they can be prepared to make early assessments and interventions.

Six percent of burns occur as a result of electrical injury. Electrical injury varies with type of circuit, voltage, amperage, resistance, pathway, and duration. Lightning, representing 3% of electrical injury, kills more people in the United States every year than any other natural disaster (Winkler et al., 1993). Following electrical injury, clients require massive fluid resuscitation, complicated multisystem stabilization, cardiac evaluation, fasciotomy, and possibly amputation. Rehabilitation interventions for clients who have electrical injuries include pain control, nutritional support,

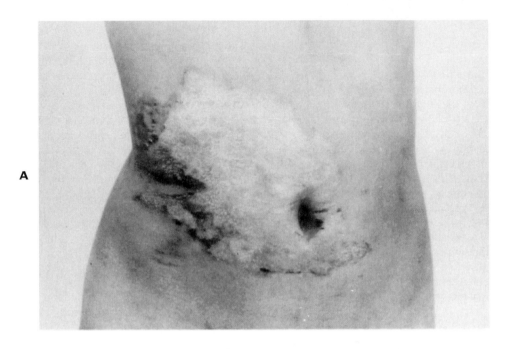

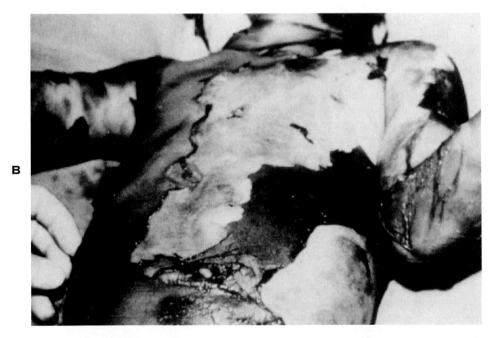

Fig. 29-1   **A,** Partial-thickness burn to the abdomen. **B,** Full-thickness burn to the chest, flank, and arms. (From *AACN's Clinical Reference for Critical Care,* 3rd ed. by Kinney, Packa, & Dunbar (Eds.), 1993, St. Louis: Mosby–Year Book. Copyright 1993 by Mosby–Year Book. Reprinted by permission.)

wound care, and with amputation, preparation of a residual limb for prosthetic fitting.

Four percent of burns are due to chemical injury. A chemical burn can result when tissue contact is made with a chemical whose inherent structure is capable of causing necrosis. The severity of damage can range from local to systemic according to several factors: chemical strength of the agent, quantity of the agent, manner and duration of skin contact, penetration, and mechanism of action. Burns caused by chemical agents usually are progressive; the chemical "burn" process often continues after contact. Initial damage to the skin is caused by the heat of the chemical reaction, with subsequent changes occurring as the chemical reacts with the protein in the skin. Tissue damage will continue until the chemical is inactivated by a neutralizing agent or diluted with water. Treatment and management options include topical agents, surgical excision, and immediate grafting (Winkler et al., 1993).

Depth of Burn Injury

Burn depth traditionally was ranked and numbered as first, second, or third degree based on visual appearances and signs and symptoms of tissue damage. The current rating terminology for burns is partial thickness or full thickness, terms that are more anatomically descriptive. With a partial-thickness burn, tissue damage and destruction does not invade the deep dermal layer, and tissue may regenerate. With a full-thickness burn, all skin layers are destroyed and subcutaneous tissues, muscle, and bone may be damaged. Full-thickness burn wounds require skin grafting to replace destroyed tissues (Fig. 29-1) (Bayley, 1990; Cromes & Helms, 1993).

Superficial or shallow partial-thickness burn depths may be noted when injury involves the epidermis and the dermis but excludes the dermal appendages. These injury sites are erythematous but can be blanched with fingertip pressure and then observed to refill, indicating that damaged tissue remains viable and will regenerate. Deep partial-thickness wounds involve the epidermis and most of the dermis.

PATHOPHYSIOLOGY

When burn injury occurs, a complex chain of events may be happening locally in the skin itself or systemically in other organ systems. The initial response to burn injury can be life-threatening; stabilizing multisystems, replacing fluids and electrolytes, and preventing infection are crucial.

Local Effects

The initial physiologic response to partial- and/or full-thickness burn injury is capillary vasoconstriction. Soon after, vasodilation occurs and plasma is released to the injury site. Within 24 hours increased clotting may occur, which will decrease or eliminate blood flow; without proper blood supply, further cellular death will occur. Because of this dynamic process, the exact depth of a burn injury may not be apparent for 3 to 5 days. During this process massive fluid loss from open wounds and evaporation will occur, resulting in heat loss and elevated metabolism. Furthermore, when skin integrity is compromised, the body is no longer protected from bacteria and local sepsis will occur rapidly

as bacteria enter the wound. If the infection is not monitored closely and treated carefully, tissue will be destroyed; depth of burn injury deepens as a partial-thickness burn converts to full thickness. Life-threatening systemic involvement also may occur.

In partial-thickness burns sensory nerve fibers are damaged but not destroyed, and clients experience severe pain. In full-thickness injury, however, nerve endings are destroyed and there is little pain. Commonly both partial- and full-thickness injuries occur and clients experience pain (Cromes & Helms, 1993).

Systemic Effects

Burn shock may occur as a result of hypovolemia. As fluid escapes to surrounding tissue, edema progresses until fluid pressure impairs range of motion (ROM) and blood flow to other tissues. Cellular death, damage to peripheral nerves, and sensory and/or motor loss to unscathed areas of the body may occur. The respiratory system is affected either by facial/neck edema following burn injury or by hyperventilation and increased oxygen consumption from smoke inhalation, possibly requiring emergent intubation. Other systemic effects involve the gastrointestinal and renal systems. Because of the hemodynamic changes that occur with postburn crises, renal insufficiency as well as gastric dilation and gastrointestinal ileus are concerns. Additionally a suppressed immune system creates an ongoing risk of infection (Bayley, 1990; Cromes & Helms, 1993; Winkler et al., 1993).

Wound Healing

In partial-thickness burns, the epidermal cells lining the hair follicles and sweat glands remain intact. Healing occurs as these cells migrate from the wound margin and join any small intact pieces of epithelium to form new epithelium, which will cover the burn wound in 14 to 21 days, depending on the depth of injury. This newly formed epithelium is extremely delicate and must be shielded until capable of performing temperature regulation functions and protecting the body from infection.

Deeper full-thickness burns heal with a different process, beginning with phagocytosis by white blood cells to clear the wound area of debris and bacteria. Fibroblasts secrete collagen at the same time as marginal epithelial cells migrate from the wound periphery and injured venule buds form capillary networks to restore circulation. This process creates granulation tissue that is reddened, highly vascular, warm to touch, and hypersensitive.

Hypertrophic scarring may occur in nongrafted partial-thickness and full-thickness burns. The collagen that is deposited during the healing process is not uniformly laid down and takes on an abnormal configuration, which contributes to severe contractures and cosmetic deformity. Concurrently the surrounding epithelium continues to encroach from the margins inward, altogether forming a closed wound with elevated scars (Cromes & Helms, 1993; Winkler et al., 1993).

Phases of Injury and Goals

The three phases of burn care are the emergent or resuscitative phase, the acute phase, and the rehabilitative phase.

The emergent stage involves critical care, often instituted in the emergency room or on site, at the place of the injury. The acute phase encompasses the period from burn injury until the client is considered stable and until all full-thickness burns are covered with skin (2 days to 2 weeks) (Winkler et al., 1993). Whereas the goals of the emergent and acute phase are multisystem stabilization, wound care, infection control, and restorative care are emphasized during rehabilitation. As a client progresses through the three phases of burn injury, the daily responsibility of burn care gradually moves from the burn team to the client. It is the role of the rehabilitation nurse to facilitate this transition and transfer of control, thus facilitating client empowerment.

The therapeutic management of burn rehabilitation begins with a coordinated interdisciplinary team approach necessary to develop the comprehensive treatment plan required for a client who has a burn injury, beginning with admission and continuing throughout recovery. Initial goals set during acute care are directed toward preserving joint mobility, strength, endurance, and controlling edema, with some attention to promoting independent self-care and educating clients and families about burn recovery. Subsequent goals expand with objectives to prevent further disability and complications, such as disfigurement related to scar contracture. The goals of rehabilitation are directed toward minimizing scar contracture formation; increasing flexibility, strength, and endurance; and promoting independence in normal daily activities. Long-term goals for clients are to improve physical skills for returning to work or school and for community reintegration.

ASSESSMENT, INTERVENTION, AND OUTCOMES

The rehabilitative aspects of care and management with a client who has a burn injury are discussed in this section of the chapter. Specific areas of concern or potential problems for clients with burn injuries are discussed using the nursing process as a guide and emphasizing the need for consistent long-term follow-up.

The Burn-Specific Health Scale (BSHS) is an 80-item questionnaire designed to quantify problems that may occur for persons who have sustained burn injuries. The eight subscales are mobility and self-care, hand function, role activities, body image, affective, family and friends, sexuality, and general health concerns (Blades, Mellis, & Munster, 1982). The questionnaire has been standardized, but reliability and content validity have not been tested. One study using the BSHS found clients had a wide range of rehabilitation goals, which were aligned with problems they experienced (Blalock, Bunker, Moore, Foreman, & Walsh, 1992).

In the emergent and acute phase of burn management, assessment is constant to ensure the stabilization of a client's medical condition and to detect significant alterations in hemodynamic status and circulatory compromise. Likewise, assessment during the rehabilitative phase is ongoing, but the focus shifts to detecting changes, supporting and promoting healing of various systems, and preventing complications related to physical or physiologic processes and those that may hinder functional abilities over time. Rehabilitation nurses assess each client's psychosocial changes and adjustments following burn injuries, providing interventions or referrals as needed.

Nutritional Assessment and Interventions

Assessment of a client's nutritional status following burn injury includes evaluation of protein and catabolic needs. Elevated metabolism occurs with burn injury due to stress, fluid loss, fever, infection, immobility, and hypercatabolism. Individual nutritional requirements vary with the extent and depth of injury, client age, and preburn nutritional status. Catabolic needs nearly double from 1700 to 3000 kcal to 3000 to 5000 kcal, and protein requirements triple from 0.8g/kg to 2 to 4 g/kg during the recovery period following burn injury.

Although precise mineral requirements remain undetermined, research-based guidelines are under way. As a rule vitamins and minerals are supplemented at two times the recommended daily allowance. In addition, oral iron replacement may be used to supplement any anemic state, and vitamin C, up to 1 g daily, may be given to facilitate wound healing and prevent infection. Zinc supplementation may be given to enhance hepatic protein synthesis and improve wound healing, since deficiencies in this mineral may occur with impaired cellular immunity and anorexia, as well as with altered taste and smell (Carvajal & Parks, 1987; LeMaster, 1983).

The duration of the catabolic phase post–burn injury continues for 30 to 40 days; however, the anabolic phase may last up to a year. Thus assessment of the digestive system is essential. Clients are advanced to a regular diet with high-protein supplements as soon as possible. Because constipation and fecal impaction are common complications during the recovery period, foods and beverages high in roughage are encouraged to aid in elimination.

Integumentary Assessment and Wound Management

Assessment of the integumentary system goes beyond evaluation of injury sites. By the time the client has reached the rehabilitative phase, escharotomies, debridements, and grafting procedures have been completed. Thus a client may enter rehabilitation with a wound that is covered but with extremely fragile skin. The goals of wound care during rehabilitative recovery focus on attending to healed areas and donor sites, preventing infection, protecting new skin from further trauma, and preparing skin for compression. An understanding of the physiologic alterations of skin resulting from burn injury, along with its impact on lifestyle, underlies all interventions and ongoing management.

Wound care consists of dressing changes, cleansing of wounds, and debridement of dead tissue on a daily basis. Often hydrotherapy treatments accompany wound care procedures by providing gentle debridement with decreased pain (Fig. 29-2). Hydrotherapy tub sessions should be limited to 20 minutes to prevent a client from becoming chilled. Wounds are gently patted dry before application of topical agents. Wound cleansing agents may be either sterile water or saline solution with a mild bacterial cleansing agent (diluted povidone-iodine [Betadine] or chlorhexidine [Hibiclens]) (Bayley, 1990; Canter, 1991).

The purpose of applying topical ointment is to control burn wound sepsis by reducing the number of bacteria

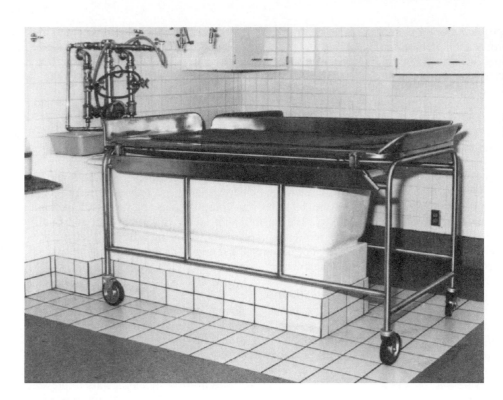

Fig. 29-2 Shower table used for daily hydrotherapy, debridement, and hygiene. (From *AACN's Clinical Reference for Critical Care,* 3rd ed. by Kinney, Packa, & Dunbar (Eds.), 1993, St. Louis: Mosby–Year Book. Copyright 1993 by Mosby–Year Book. Reprinted by permission.)

present in the wound. Before a new layer of topical agent or cream is applied to a wound, all residue from previous applications, as well as serous exudate, must be removed. Sterile technique with gloves is used to apply a new layer, then the wound must be covered with a sterile dressing (Poh-Fitzpatrick, 1992).

No single topical agent has been demonstrated to be universally effective for burn care. Alternative agents may be used concurrently on different burn sites as the wound and its bacterial flora change (LeMaster, 1983; Winkler et al., 1993). The most popular topical agent in use is silver sulfadiazine 1%, a water-based cream effective against gram-positive, gram-negative, and *Candida* organisms. Other agents commonly used include mafenide acetate (Sulfamylon), povidone-iodine, silver nitrate 5%, and cerium nitrate 1.74%. Over-the-counter topical agents may include bacitracin with polymyxin B and neomycin sulfate (Poh-Fitzpatrick, 1992). Recently occlusive, semiocclusive, hydrocolloid, and hydrogel products have been shown to offer a clinically significant improvement in wound care. Comparison studies have shown these various products (versus topical agents) are more cost-effective and result in better wound healing, repigmentation, less pain, and fewer dressing changes (Wyatt, McGowan, & Najarian, 1990).

Long-Term and Community-Based Wound Management

Persons who have had a burn injury may retain impairments for a long time following hospitalization. Many of these impairments are difficult to assess and document. For example, heat/cold intolerance, decreased strength and coordination, photosensitivity, or changes in sweating, and psychosocial problems may complicate rehabilitation outcome (Salisbury, 1992).

For example, a burn injury that extends to the dermis also will destroy hair follicles and sebaceous and sweat glands which arise from this skin layer. Also lost are the abilities for these structures to regenerate. Scar tissue may take up to 2 years to mature; thus the skin is continually changing, healing, and evolving during this posthospitalization phase. As a result the client must deal with skin that is thinner, less pliable, drier, more sensitive to temperature changes, and more prone to blistering and itching.

✦ **Dryness.** Topical emollients supply external moisture and lubrication to the newly healed skin. Lotions that contain both water (for absorption) and lipid (to retard evaporation) are recommended. In general, it is best to avoid creams, lanolins, and cocoa butter with nonessential or poorly characterized ingredients such as fragrance, exotic plant oils, or extracts, which only will mimic adequate lubrication. These nonessential ingredients can cause irritation or contact sensitization. As a supplement, a room humidifier may help to reduce epidermal dehydration.

✦ **Photosensitivity.** Avoiding sunlight exposure for 6 months or longer after a burn injury is recommended to prevent sunburn and permanent hyperpigmentation. Return of melanin pigments to newly healed skin or grafts varies, depending on the extent of injury. Commonsense measures include use of a hat and appropriate clothing, timing of outdoor activities for early morning or late afternoon, and application of sunscreen to newly formed skin. A product with a sun protection factor (SPF) rating of at least 15 should be used when sunlight exposure cannot be avoided. Sunscreens labeled "water resistant" will retain their protective ability for 40 minutes of sweating or swimming, whereas those labeled "waterproof" will retain their effectiveness for up to 80 minutes of activity. New sunscreen products are being developed each season.

✦ **Pruritus.** Pruritus is a significant problem during the recovery period. If not treated and controlled, the itching can destroy fragile grafts and healing donor sites. Strategies of daily hygiene, conscientious lubrication, appropriate thermal protection, alternatives to scratching, and antipruritic medications must be incorporated into the client's lifestyle if successful management is to be achieved. Itching of healing burn areas and new skin can be a severe discomfort. The use of systemic antihistamines in conjunction with topical antipruritic agents may ease some symptoms. An emollient lotion containing menthol (¼% to ½%) and camphor (½% to 2%) feels cool to the skin and may provide temporary relief while countering dryness. Refrigerated lotions as cold applications may be soothing for some persons. Topical anesthetics (e.g., pramoxine hydrochloride 1%) are available in ointments, creams, and lotions; however, topical benzocaine preparations are not recommended due to potential allergic sensitization (Poh-Fitzpatrick, 1992).

✦ **Lifestyle.** Assessment of each client's lifestyle, preferences, and habits as they were lived before injury is essential in developing an effective and realistic plan of care. Clients who learn and practice new strategies to care for their "now new body" will experience improved outcomes. Simple but regular strategies of daily hygiene, vigilant lubrication, avoidance of strong sun exposure and temperature changes, appropriate thermal protection, and antipru-

ritic measures are incorporated as much as possible into lifestyle and preferences. Although these strategies may be intrusive for some, they are necessary for effective long-term skin care management (Hegel, Ayllon, VanderPlate, & Spiro-Hawkins, 1986).

Self-Care

Self-initiated programs give clients the psychological benefit of actively participating in their own rehabilitation and promote the habits of a daily routine, which must be conscientiously adhered to after discharge. Active participation in wound care, hygiene, and self-exercise programs are crucial to prevent complications and increase functional ability. The rehabilitation nurse educates client and family and reinforces modifications for the client's lifelong lifestyle, not only for the duration of the rehabilitation wound management program.

✦ Mobility

Assessment of a client's mobility status is an ongoing process since functional recovery may be a long and laborious process and usually involves interdisciplinary assessments and interventions. Positioning, exercise, compression, and splinting are basic burn rehabilitation treatment procedures. The purposes of these modalities are to prevent loss of function and promotion of functional independence.

Fig. 29-3 **A,** Supine positioning of the burn client to prevent contracture formation. (Courtesy Shriners Burns Institute, Galveston, Texas. From *AACN's Clinical Reference for Critical Care,* 3rd ed. by Kinney, Packa, & Dunbar (Eds.), 1993, St. Louis: Mosby–Year Book. Copyright 1993 by Mosby–Year Book. Reprinted by permission.)

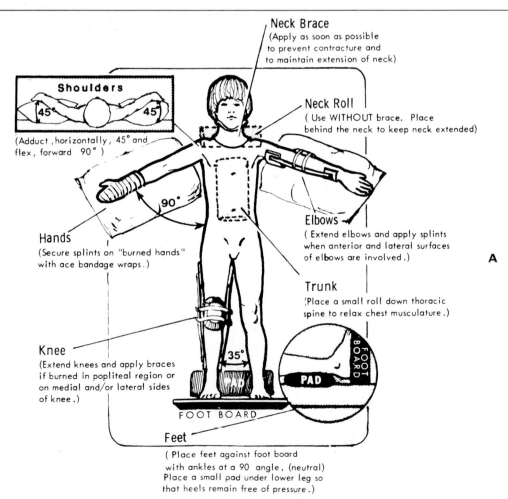

Neck Brace
(Apply as soon as possible to prevent contracture and to maintain extension of neck)

Shoulders
45°   45°
(Adduct, horizontally, 45° and flex, forward 90°)

Neck Roll
(Use WITHOUT brace. Place behind the neck to keep neck extended)

90°

Hands
(Secure splints on "burned hands" with ace bandage wraps.)

Elbows
(Extend elbows and apply splints when anterior and lateral surfaces of elbows are involved.)

Trunk
(Place a small roll down thoracic spine to relax chest musculature.)

Knee
(Extend knees and apply braces if burned in popliteal region or on medial and/or lateral sides of knee.)

35°

PAD

FOOT BOARD

PAD

A

Feet
(Place feet against foot board with ankles at a 90 angle. (neutral) Place a small pad under lower leg so that heels remain free of pressure.)

With advances in splinting and other modalities, most clients can expect to approximate their preinjury level of function. Assistive devices or adapted equipment may be needed to ensure function. Reconstructive surgery may be necessary for a client to regain function when scar contractures have formed.

✦ **Positioning.** Proper positioning begins at onset of injury and is evaluated regularly throughout rehabilitation. During the acute phase of injury, proper positioning minimizes edema, provides safe and proper joint alignment, and maintains tendon balance between overstretching and promoting contracture formation. During the rehabilitative phase of recovery, the goal is to continue effective positioning to prevent contractures (LeMaster, 1983). Since clients are encouraged to become ambulatory as soon as possible, using an assistive device if needed, proper positioning is part of learning upright sitting and standing posture. Whether a client's wound management dictates total body or partial positioning, various burn injury sites require special attention to prevent complications of pressure necrosis, dependent edema, or flexion contractures. Common factors that may affect positioning are edema, donor sites, graft areas, and respiratory function.

Figure 29-3 illustrates how position devices of cloth rolls, foam wedges, straps, foot boards, and slings may be used to assist with proper positioning. Burns involving the head, face, or neck require individualized positioning according to the area burned. Pillows are not recommended because their use may lead to secondary conditions, such as neck flexion contractures and pressure to the ears. The supine position, using a small foam pad instead of a pillow, is recommended for severely burned clients. As general rules, knees, hips, elbows, and interphalangeal joints are placed extended in neutral alignments. Ankles and feet are dorsiflexed at a 90-degree angle, wrists are dorsiflexed at 10 to 20 degrees, and a shoulder is placed in neutral alignment supported in a 90-degree abduction (Winkler et al., 1993).

Splints are one way to immobilize an area of the body and place it in a position that will preserve or restore function. However, a client must adhere to a schedule for wearing a splint, practice routine cleaning, and inspect the skin before and on removal of the splint to achieve desired outcomes (Leman, 1992).

✦ **Exercise.** Joint function may diminish as a result of bed rest, decreased protein, altered fluid and electrolytes, and poor circulation until ultimately contractures occur and heterotopic bone is formed. Full ROM joint exercises for all joints begins early in the wound management process and continues at regular daily intervals. Active and passive exercises may be combined, depending on a client's capabilities; however, joints are not moved beyond their free range unless prescribed by a physician and directed by a physical therapist.

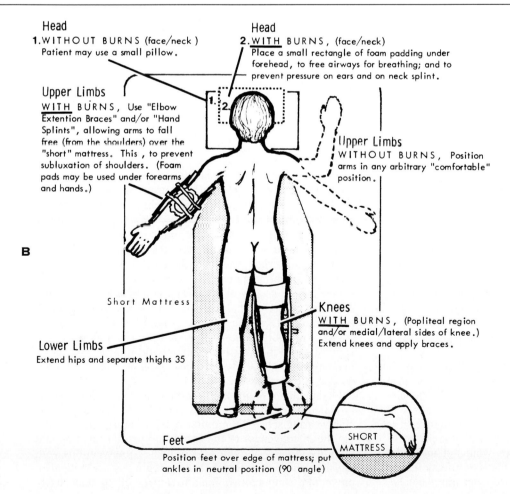

Head
1. WITHOUT BURNS (face/neck)
Patient may use a small pillow.

Head
2. WITH BURNS, (face/neck)
Place a small rectangle of foam padding under forehead, to free airways for breathing; and to prevent pressure on ears and on neck splint.

Upper Limbs
WITH BURNS, Use "Elbow Extention Braces" and/or "Hand Splints", allowing arms to fall free (from the shoulders) over the "short" mattress. This, to prevent subluxation of shoulders. (Foam pads may be used under forearms and hands.)

Upper Limbs
WITHOUT BURNS, Position arms in any arbitrary "comfortable" position.

Knees
WITH BURNS, (Popliteal region and/or medial/lateral sides of knee.) Extend knees and apply braces.

Short Mattress

Lower Limbs
Extend hips and separate thighs 35

Feet
Position feet over edge of mattress; put ankles in neutral position (90 angle)

SHORT MATTRESS

B

Fig. 29-3, cont'd. **B,** Prone positioning of the burn client to reduce contracture formation.

Successful outcomes of burn injury cannot be achieved when a client relies solely on the benefits of scheduled therapies. In home and community settings, rehabilitation nurses can assist community health nurses and other community resources to intervene with exercise modalities for stretching and increasing ROM, which are both creative and cost-effective. In the home, assistive devices such as splints, wedges, pulley systems, slings, shoes, or pillows may be effective in incorporating active and/or passive exercises into daily routines. As part of self-care a client is expected to follow through with these mobility skills during non-therapy hours, and family members are taught how to assist. A program or system established in the rehabilitation setting will be followed more consistently when it is appropriate and adaptable to the home environment. Ideally a client will understand, initiate, and incorporate these strategies into everyday routine.

Some clients may find it difficult to adhere to a prescribed exercise program due to pain, diminished endurance, low levels of motivation, other chronic or disabling conditions, or knowledge deficit. The rehabilitation nurse may be instrumental in educating a client and family about strategic ways to address issues such as anticipating and treating pain before exercise, developing and tolerating wearing schedules of compression garments and splints, coordinating wound management with other treatment regimens, and ensuring effective positioning of extremities and trunk. Successful adaptations of these necessary lifestyle changes can be achieved better when clients have incentives for high levels of motivation.

✦ **Compression.** A primary treatment for prevention and reduction of hypertrophic scarring is compression therapy. Once wounds are closed, custom-fitted garments are worn over affected areas. These garments ideally are worn 24 hours every day and are removed only for hygiene and skin care. These garments are worn for as long as 1 to 2 years or until scar tissue matures. Clearly this long-term treatment relies on interdisciplinary teamwork with a fully participating client and family for successful outcome (Leman, 1992; LeMaster, 1983; Winkler et al., 1993).

Preparation and toughening of the skin to tolerate the custom-fitted garment for such long duration is a primary goal of the interdisciplinary team. Pressure may be applied to burn areas gradually and through various methods. Products such as elastic wraps (ACE bandages), premade tubular elastic garments (Tubigrip) or tailor-made burn garments (Jobst) (Fig. 29-4) are designed to apply varying degrees of pressure to the scar tissue. Inserts of foam or silicone may be applied underneath the pressure garment to increase direct pressure to a specific area. The length of time a client is scheduled to wear a particular pressure application is increased gradually and as tolerated.

Whenever the compression garment, or other device, is removed, the nurse conducts a complete head to toe skin assessment. The nurse specifically pays attention to any pressure areas that may be developing and evaluates skin tolerance to compression treatment. With burn injuries it is not uncommon for blisters to develop on healed areas; these differ from pressure areas. Blisters are evaluated and noted but left intact unless accompanied by signs of infection. Any sign of infection is reported to the physician immediately.

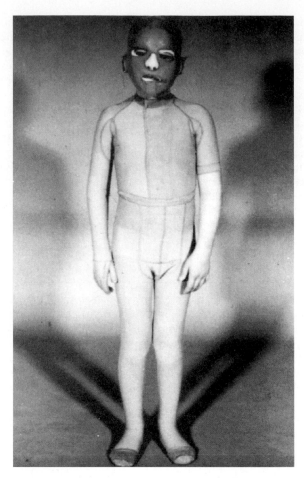

Fig. 29-4　Client in full Jobst garments. (From *AACN's Clinical Reference for Critical Care,* 3rd ed. by Kinney, Packa, & Dunbar (Eds.), 1993, St. Louis: Mosby–Year Book. Copyright 1993 by Mosby–Year Book. Reprinted by permission.)

✦ **Splinting.** Splints are created by occupational therapists. As assistive devices they may be used on various parts of the body for support, to promote mobility, and to enable a client to perform self-care activities. Splinting aids joint positioning and decreases scar contractures and hypertrophy. Splints are necessary to maintain the length of soft tissue joint structures; however, they are used cautiously to avoid prolonged immobilization and fibrosis of soft tissue. Static splints can be used over compression garments to maintain increases in motion that have been achieved with therapeutic exercise. Dynamic splints provide continuous gentle stretch when full motion is not achieved with exercise and activity. Once the skin has matured and joint ROM can be maintained with active exercise, splints are no longer needed (Leman, 1992).

Nursing interventions with splint treatment include assisting client and team with initiating and adhering to a tolerable wearing schedule, monitoring skin status, and evaluating the effectiveness of the splint regimen on function and mobility in daily activities. Coordinated interventions with physical and occupational therapy regimens are critical in preventing contractures. Team members, client, and family must coordinate treatments and devote attention to each phase of the treatment to achieve desired outcomes, which are to preserve function and minimize complications associated with burn injury.

Pain

Severe pain often accompanies partial-thickness burns due to damaged but not destroyed sensory nerve fibers. In contrast, little if any pain is associated with full-thickness injury because nerve endings are in large part destroyed.

Nurses are aware that each client is the authority on the pain he is experiencing. Chapter 24 contains principles for nursing assessment and management of pain and pain relief that apply to clients who have burn injuries. Thus the most valuable nursing intervention with clients who have pain is pain relief through administering prescribed medications (often narcotics), implementing comfort measures, and assisting clients to use alternative techniques. Relaxation techniques of imagery and distraction heighten the effects of analgesia for many clients. These are discussed in more detail in Chapter 13.

Coordinating therapy procedures, anticipating energy requirements for activities, planning for rest periods interspersed with therapies, and promoting time and guidance for self-help strategies contribute to minimizing pain; this in turn allows a client to participate in activities of daily living (ADL) (Blumenfield & Schoeps, 1992). A client who is involved in wound care and decision-making processes feels more empowered, thereby enhancing feelings of control related to pain management.

PSYCHOSOCIAL ADJUSTMENT AND FAMILY INVOLVEMENT

With few exceptions the psychological implications for a client who has a burn injury are extensive. Nurses may witness clients who exhibit a variety of responses and emotional reactions, depending on their phase of recovery. Initially a client may be delirious as a result of burn shock in combination with medications. Later, depression becomes a major factor as the realization of drastic changes in personal appearance, seemingly endless treatments, and functional implications for the future become more apparent. At some time fear of death is a major concern for many. Other fears commonly expressed by clients are fears of pain, suffering, disfigurement, prolonged hospitalization, and concerns about disruption in lifestyle (Blumenfield & Schoeps, 1992).

The nursing goals during these early phases are to decrease pain, ensure gentle physical care and handling, answer questions as completely as possible, and to begin to elicit client and family participation. There is some evidence that children who have burn injuries ultimately may experience less psychological impact than do their parents. However, findings from this study do not negate psychosocial adjustment problems for children.

Researchers conducted a study with an annual assessment of the psychological adjustment of 25 children aged 1 to 9 years who had a burn injury. Results were based on a child's behavior using testing and parent-teacher reports. As a group the children were found to have normal age behavior problems. However, parents expressed high levels of stress, difficulty relating to their child in a parenting role, and were socially isolated. Parents described their children as moody, demanding, and disappointing, but their relationships improved over time (Blakeney et al., 1993).

The stress of lifestyle changes and the constant demands of active participation in various preventive procedures can be extremely difficult for many persons. Coupled with body image concerns, functional limitations, and adapted lifestyle, and perhaps a changed vocation, the client re-enters society essentially as a changed person with a "now new body." Thus some type of grief response to changed body image usually occurs. These internal changes and adjustments are heightened by the multiple reminders of changes in appearance or ability that a client will encounter on re-entering society. Assertiveness training has helped many clients deal with social responses—ranging from avoidance, ridicule, stares, to excessive sympathy—which threaten a client's self-confidence.

The 1-year postinjury mark appears to be significant for persons who survive burn injuries. For many, emotional issues are resolved as physical function is restored and most extensive treatment such as compression is completed, and there has been time to adjust to social issues. These factors coincide with scar tissue maturation and improved sensation, which also may be occurring at approximately 1 year. Work and family roles may have been renegotiated by this time. Although prognosis for most adults is positive, Andreasen, Norris, and Hartford (1971) found a third of adult clients continued to experience emotional problems in areas of work, recreation, family, and interpersonal relationships as long as 1 to 1.5 years postinjury. Persons whose burn injuries involved the face or hands were found to have greater difficulty with community re-entry and adjustment, possibly due to the visible nature of their injuries. Juvenile delinquency, divorce, and depression have been documented when following clients with visible wounds at 1 year post–burn injury.

Family involvement is crucial during both initial and recovery periods. Tremendous sadness or guilt of being a survivor may accompany clients when a loved one was lost as a result of the burn injury event. The family is often the single most important continuing force in a client's life and the primary resource in redefining identity when the client re-enters the community. Allowing and encouraging regular family visits during all phases of recovery may accomplish the following three goals:

1. Providing a client opportunity to express emotions and encouraging expression of frustrations and concerns
2. Allowing family members to observe wound healing and adjust to changes in client's physical appearance and functioning
3. Aiding family in understanding a client's day-to-day struggles and offering insight into physical and emotional challenges during rehabilitation

The absence of family or significant other in the ongoing recovery process impedes a client's motivation and creates further stressors in the discharge process. Depending on the extent of the burn injury and physical functioning, family involvement and support may be a deciding factor in whether a client returns to live at home or in a skilled care facility.

Sexuality

Although the recovery period following a burn injury may require up to 5 years, a milestone is achieved when a client is able to look, touch, and care for the affected areas. Many times clients have disassociated themselves from the burn areas, perhaps for the first year. Rehabilitation nurses who conduct ongoing assessment will be attuned to a client's psychological readiness for redefining body image and self-esteem. Sexual functioning becomes a concern as other issues are resolved.

Andreasen et al. (1971) reported clients had few long-term problems in sexual functioning and more with sensuality. Unpleasant sensations may be due to hypersensitivity of immature scar tissue, irritable feelings from itching, blisters, or changes in heat and cold sensation, which affect normal pleasure response. Often significant others do not know how to deal with sexuality issues. For instance, they may fear causing injury to fragile healing skin sites, may experience frustration with role changes, or in some circumstances may be dealing with their own discomforts resulting from burn injuries incurred during the same event.

If sexual and social adjustment is to be successful, preparation for privacy, time, and supporting client and family needs for intimacy during all or any phases of recovery is planned. Information regarding sexual potential and emotional adjustment is provided along with specific sexual education on positioning, pleasuring, and alternative methods of sensuality in the reestablishment of intimacy. Questions of fertility may arise secondary to physical injury to genitalia or interruption of organ functioning (e.g., scrotal edema or amenorrhea). Chapter 27 presents a more complete discussion of sexuality and options for persons with chronic or disabling disorders.

Vocational Implications

Research findings indicate that most people who are employed at the time of their burn injury will return to work. The extent, etiology, and site of burn injury influence a person's return-to-work status. Functional limitations resulting from burn injuries may temporarily or permanently determine the ability to return to work. Related factors include stamina and endurance; tolerance to standing, walking, or sitting; and degree of hand grip and upper extremity strength. A comprehensive medical evaluation by a vocational specialist is required before a client is cleared to resume occupational roles. Sequelae issues such as personal fears of reinjury, concern about peer reaction, and a client's confidence level about resuming a work role may hinder success regardless of medical status (Cheng & Rogers, 1989). Vocational issues are a major correlate of long-term

psychosocial or emotional problems. When clients hold positive perceptions about how their roles in family, work, social network, and other activities will be resumed, these attitudes indicate strengths toward effective coping and adjustment.

Strengths and Resources

All severe burn injuries, regardless of origin, can alter the function of many body systems. Although most systems will recover and resume normal functioning, some processes may be compromised and others will never regenerate. When a client is able to construct a realistic assessment of these functions, the nurse is able to assess the beginning of psychosocial and emotional recovery, just as wound healing marks the beginning of physical recovery.

Ongoing support from family members and the interdisciplinary team is critical during all phases of institutional care and on community re-entry. The rehabilitation nurse functions as advocate, educator, and facilitator to assist clients in realistic appraisal of their status, emphasizing ability rather than limitations or disability. During follow-up appointments, clients need guidance, encouragement, empowerment, and reassurance about emotional adjustments; rehabilitation nurses may use these opportunities to promote effective coping behaviors.

In the community clients and families benefit from association, awareness, and utilization of community-based services and resources. Examples include hospital- or center-based support groups, peer groups, volunteer or not-for-profit self-help groups established by persons who have themselves survived burn injuries (e.g., Phoenix Foundation or the Knapp Foundation), and national organizations (e.g., American Burn Association).

OUTCOMES AND RESTORATIVE NURSING PRACTICE

The transition from client with a burn injury to person who has survived a burn injury and re-entered the community is the ultimate outcome desired following a rehabilitation program. The client is educated, motivated, and empowered to become the director of her own care. The roles of rehabilitation are pivotal to achieving successful outcomes of burn rehabilitation. This is one practice area in the growing field of restorative nursing care. As medical advances continue and healthcare system changes occur, rehabilitation nurses can anticipate active practice roles in planning, implementing, and evaluating services for clients who require extensive, long-term restorative care for a wide variety of conditions, in addition to those persons with burn injuries.

CASE STUDY

Jose G. is 32-year-old male from Ecuador who sustained a 55% total body surface area flame burn as a result of a boiler explosion aboard ship. He was resuscitated and received acute care treatment in his native country before being transferred to a specialized burn unit in the United States, where he underwent split-thickness skin grafts, transfusions for anemia, and a gastric tube (G-tube) for nutritional support. The acute hospital course was complicated by superventricular tachycardia (SVT), wound infections, and urinary tract infections. With status post (S/P) ventilatory support for 1 week for adult respiratory distress syndrome, he was transferred to a rehabilitation unit for treatment of severe contractures of both upper extremities and ongoing burn care.

STATUS ON REHABILITATION ADMISSION:

Medical: mild anemia with iron replacement; IV fluids and digoxin for SVT; etidronate disodium (Didronel) for heterotopic bone formation in both (B) elbows; limited ROM mainly in (B) axilla, elbow, and wrist.

Nutrition: regular diet following S/P G-tube removal; low protein and albumin level. Admission weight: 104 lb.

Bowel and bladder: spontaneous and continent with occasional constipation.

Activity: poor endurance for therapies, as well as frequent complaints of pain and discomfort secondary to tightness and/or sleep disruption.

Skin: multiple superficial open areas with small amount of serous drainage and frequent complaints of pruritus. Graft sites completely healed, except on buttock, and hypertrophic scarring on right anterior chest and arm.

Communication: client is alert, oriented × 3 (person, place, and time). Primary language is Spanish; an interpreter is available during therapy hours. No neurologic injury due to explosion.

ADL: due to severe mobility restrictions, client is dependent for all ADL, including self-feeding.

Psychosocial: following high school, he was employed as a sailor aboard a cargo ship. Client is recently separated, with two children and his family living in Ecuador. His mother returned to Ecuador during his acute hospitalization with plans to return to the United States during rehabilitation.

In summary, Jose was ambulatory once in a standing position but was unable to pull up his pants, feed, or toilet himself. He was fatigued easily, thin, and felt isolated due to the language barrier. Jose had some newly healed skin but abnormal scarring and ectopic bone formation.

REHABILITATION MANAGEMENT PLAN

The primary goal of the interdisciplinary team was to establish a communication system to meet client needs and provide care. Since the injury was a work-related case, Workers' Compensation benefits were subsidizing the hospitalization and related costs. For example, an interpreter was available during therapy hours; short-term goals were that Jose be able to communicate basic needs via use of interpreter, communication board, or with gestures. His understanding of hospital routine, schedules, exercise programs, and treatment regimen was essential to facilitate decision-making, enhance participation, and encourage motivation.

Skin care was crucial not only for ongoing care of current wounds but also for long-term skin management. His participation in skin and wound issues was essential; inspecting open wounds and healed areas for signs of infection, performing daily hygiene, and applying frequent lubrication to counter dryness were a few of the routine treatments that Jose was not particularly interested in doing for himself. Premorbidly Jose had not been a daily bather and found this requirement uncomfortable and disruptive. Further, Jose disassociated himself from his wounds as evidenced during dressing changes: Jose would allow the nurses to care for his wounds and would not look at his newly healed skin during the procedure.

Since Jose needed to recognize physiologic changes and physical care of his new body, client education centered on pathophysiology of burns, the effect on normal skin, and need for long-term management. Goals were for Jose to participate in wound care, identify potential skin problems, and incorporate lifestyle changes into daily routine. Outcomes were to rebuild skin integrity and eventually to prevent or minimize hypertrophic scarring and to tolerate wearing a Jobst garment.

Due to his severe contractures, mobility became a major limitation for Jose. Long-term goals include independence with mobility skills with assistive device as appropriate, ability to perform or direct all aspects of ADL, and attain a functional ROM by following through with mobility skills learned in therapy. The nursing unit provided an unstructured home setting so that skills and techniques conducted at home were conquered first while on the unit. Therapeutic interventions are an exercise in futility when clients return home and fall into habits that may lead to complications. For Jose, correct and consistent use of assistive devices was critical to achieving functional independence.

Jose's therapy programs and exercise regimen included using a pulley system designed to increase ROM of (B) axilla. Though reluctant at first, Jose eventually contracted to participate in scheduling mutually agreed-upon times for wearing the device during therapy and nontherapy hours, as well as to increase wearing time and degree of flexion as tolerated. Pain and fatigue were considered when scheduling and weekly measures evaluated increase in range. Thus Jose maintained control over the exercise regimen and developed incentives for a self-directed exercise program.

Nutritionally Jose's visceral protein status was depleted, but he tolerated a general diet. Goals were to attain and maintain a normal weight and for Jose to be educated about selecting foods appropriate for a high-protein diet. During rehabilitation, Jose received a high-protein, high-calorie diet of 2000 kcal every day, and high-protein supplemental shakes added to each meal and at night. Jose was weighed weekly, and serum albumin levels were assessed every 2 weeks. Assisted by his interpreter and with dietary guidance, Jose selected high-protein foods from a preprinted hospital menu and learned to identify traditional Ecuadorian foods compatible with his recommended diet.

Jose's premorbid bowel pattern was used to establish a realistic program in which he actively participated to resolve constipation. He requested a simple plan of care during the interim period, but desired only dietary regulation as a long-term goal. The nurse educated him about fluids, activity, diet, and use of an oral bulk laxative and stool softener for regulation—followed by periodic evaluation.

Jose experienced persistent pruritus severe enough that he could not tolerate therapy some days or sleep through the night. For pruritic relief, Jose chose medication and fluids and was encouraged to practice good hygiene, frequent lubrication, and alternatives to scratching. He found incorporating these new

Continued.

CASE STUDY—cont'd

tasks into his daily routine intrusive. Although he understood the need for interventions, combining more than two methods was difficult for him to accomplish. During early hospitalization the nursing staff completed most treatments for Jose, but as he progressed, the nurses transferred control to Jose, who was expected to assume these responsibilities.

COMMUNITY RE-ENTRY

Due to the language barrier, it was difficult to assess Jose's self-image post–burn injury; also he was reluctant to express his feelings with the interpreter present. Nonverbally, the nursing staff assessed a self-distancing during wound care and initial avoidance of mirrors and windows. Thus a major milestone was reached when Jose began to visualize and touch affected areas during wound care. Jose was encouraged to continue to participate in wound care, dressing changes, and treatment programs. Over time, through nonverbal gestures and general self-care abilities, Jose demonstrated the important goal of incorporating burn areas into part of self, significant in the long recovery.

Many factors affected Jose's ability to cope effectively: hospitalization, disability, communication, and most of all cultural separation. Ironically, being away from his homeland had some positive factors. For instance, he was appreciative of all that the United States healthcare system had to offer to someone in his position. His anger about his disability, though present, was reactionally appropriate. The ability to participate in decision-making was a fairly new concept to Jose since he willingly wanted his healthcare providers to make decisions for him and to set his plan of care. By empowering Jose as decision-maker about care, the nurses encouraged positive coping behaviors and helped him to elevate his self-esteem.

Many questions about life in the community remained unanswered for Jose. Was he capable of returning home? Who would be his caregiver? Would the environment permit him to be functionally independent? If he stayed in the United States, where would he live? What follow-up plan of care would be practical for someone whose homeland was at a distance? Communication was obviously a key factor at this complicated juncture. By becoming knowledgeable about the options, client, mother, interpreter, and team members were able to weigh realistic and practical needs in perspective for the immediate postdischarge period and project future needs for the following 1 to 2 years. Realistically Jose was not independent with self-care. To continue with mobility skills, Jose needed ongoing follow-up care from the acute burn team, as well as outpatient therapy. Long-term goals included regaining function and mobility, then returning to Ecuador.

DISCHARGE STATUS

Medical: stable—continues with mild anemia, maintained by diet. SVT: stable with digoxin.

Mobility: continued on etidronate disodium for heterotopic ossification. Serial computed tomography scans will monitor for bone maturation with pending surgery as indicated. In the interim, a pulley system was fabricated for home use under supervision of outpatient therapist.

Nutrition: increase in protein and albumin levels noted to low normal range. Net gain of 5 lb before discharge.

Bladder and Bowel: discharged on oral program with constipation resolved.

Skin: superficial areas remained; continued dressing changes with over-the-counter topical ointment and gauze. Client independently directing schedule for fluids, hygiene, lubrication, and medications. Client was tolerating Jobst garment for 20 hours with a second custom garment to be fitted in outpatient department.

ADL: independent with adaptive equipment for showering and eating. Independently directs dressing changes. Minimal assistance for lower extremity dressing, waistband, and zippers. Minimal assistance for toileting, moderate assistance for upper extremity dressing, buttoning, and clothing management.

Discharge: client and his mother were set up at a nearby apartment to ease and facilitate regular visits to the outpatient therapy department. Jose would be able to walk to rehabilitation facility daily for therapy.

ONE YEAR POST–REHABILITATION DISCHARGE

Jose underwent ectopic bone removal approximately 16 months after receiving burn injuries from the boiler explosion. Jose's mother returned to Ecuador shortly after surgery. Jose's level of self-care ability improved to minimal assistance, and a caregiver assisted with AM and PM care approximately 5 hours daily. His increased weight necessitated a newly sized Jobst garment. Jose continues with outpatient therapy approximately three times weekly.

TWO YEARS POST–REHABILITATION DISCHARGE

Jose now is living independently. He has completed the rehabilitation program and met all established goals. Jose has returned to his native country where the government will continue assessment/evaluation of vocational opportunities in the Ecuadorian Navy.

REFERENCES

Andreasen, N.J.C., Norris, A.S., & Hartford, C.E. (1971). Incidence of long term psychiatric complications in severely burned adults. *Annals of Surgery, 174,* 785-793.

Bayley, E.W. (1990). Wound healing in the patient with burns. *Nursing Clinics of North America, 25,* 205-222.

Bayley, E.W., Carrougher, G.J., Marvin, J.A., Knighton, J., Rutan, R.L., & Weber, B.F. (1992). Research priorities for burn nursing: Rehabilitation, discharge planning, and follow-up care. *Journal of Burn Care Rehabilitation, 13,* 471-476.

Billmire, M.E. & Myers, P.A. (1985). Serious head injuries in infants: accident or abuse? *Pediatrics 75(2),* 340-342.

Blades, B., Mellis, N., & Munster, A.M. (1982). A burn specific health scale. *Journal of Trauma, 22,* 872-875.

Blakeney, P., Meyer, W., Moore, M.A., Murphy, L., Broemeling, L., Robson, M., & Herndon, D. (1993). Psychosocial sequelae of pediatric burns involving 80% or greater total body surface area. *Journal of Burn Care Rehabilitation, 14,* 684-689.

Blalock, S.J., Bunker, B.J., Moore, J.D., Foreman, N., & Walsh, J.F. (1992). The impact of burn injury: A preliminary investigation. *Journal of Burn Care Rehabilitation, 13,* 487-492.

Blumenfield, M., & Schoeps, M. (1992). Reintegrating the healed burned adult into society. *Clinics in Plastic Surgery, 19,* 599-605.

Canter, K.G. (1991). Conservative management of wounds. *Clinics in Podiatric Medicine and Surgery, 8,* 787-798.

Carvajal, H.F., & Parks, D.H. (1987). *Burns in children.* St. Louis: Mosby–Year Book.

Cheng, S., & Rogers, J.C. (1989). Changes in occupational role performance after a severe burn: A retrospective study. *The American Journal of Occupational Therapy, 43,* 17-24.

Cromes, G.F., & Helms, P.A. (1992). The status of burn rehabilitation services in the United States: Results of a national survey. *Journal of Burn Care Rehabilitation, 13,* 656-662.

Cromes, G.F., & Helms, P.A. (1993). Burn injuries. In M.G. Eisenberg, R.L. Glueckauf, & H.H. Zaretsky (Eds.), *Medical aspects of disability* (pp. 92-104). New York: Springer Publishing Co.

Hegel, M.T., Ayllon, T., VanderPlate, C., & Spiro-Hawkins, H. (1986). A Behavior procedure for increasing compliance with self exercise regimen in severely burn injured patients. *Restorative Therapy, 24,* 521-528.

Helms, P.A. (1992). Burn rehabilitation: Dimensions of the problem. *Clinics in Plastic Surgery, 19,* 551-559.

Leman, C.J. (1992). Splints and accessories following burn reconstruction. *Clinics in Plastic Surgery, 19,* 721-731.

LeMaster, J.E. (1983). Rehabilitation and burn care. In T.L. Wachtel, V. Kahn, & H.A. Frank (Eds.), *Current topics in burn care* (217-230). Rockville, MD: Aspen.

Poh-Fitzpatrick, M.B. (1992). Skin care of the healed burned patient. *Clinics in Plastic Surgery, 19,* 745-751.

Salisbury, R. (1992). Burn rehabilitation: Our unanswered challenge. The 1992 presidential address to the American Burn Association. *Journal of Burn Care Rehabilitation, 13,* 495-505.

Shapiro, K. (Ed.). (1983). *Pediatric head trauma.* Mount Kisco, NY: Futura Publishing Co.

Winkler, J.B., DiMola, M.A., & Wooten, J.A. (1993). Burns. In M.R. Kinney, D.R. Packa, & S.B. Dunbar (Eds.), *Clinical reference for critical-care nursing* (3rd ed., pp. 1195-1231). St. Louis: Mosby–Year Book.

Wyatt, D., McGowan, D.N., & Najarian, M.P. (1990). Comparison of a hydrocolloid dressing and silver sulfadiazine cream in the outpatient management of second degree burns. *Journal of Trauma, 30,* 857-865.

30

Pediatric Rehabilitation Nursing

Josephine Ricci-Balich, MSN, RNC, CRRN
Judith A. Behm, MSN, RN, CRRN

INTRODUCTION

Pediatric rehabilitation nursing is a specialty practice area that continues to grow within the field of rehabilitation. This chapter traces the evolution and the expanding scope of this specialty. Medical and societal trends that affect the field are identified. The unique role of the pediatric rehabilitation nurse is examined. A developmental framework is suggested as a conceptual model for practice, and the impact of disabilities across developmental stages is discussed. Public laws protecting the rights of children with disabilities are identified as are issues related to the transition into adulthood. Strategies for assessment are presented along with interventions based on nursing diagnoses commonly associated with selected chronic and disabling conditions. Evaluation and standardized outcome data are addressed.

This chapter is intended as a template of pediatric rehabilitation nursing. The nursing process and case histories are used to highlight selected chronic and disabling conditions of childhood and adolescence. Examples of pediatric rehabilitation are contained in other chapters of this book as part of the focus of life-span needs for rehabilitation nursing practice. Clearly an entire textbook would be necessary to adequately address the myriad issues of this specialty practice area. Content of this chapter provides an introduction to the unique and comprehensive nature of pediatric rehabilitation nursing.

THE EVOLUTION OF PEDIATRIC REHABILITATION

The field of pediatric rehabilitation has experienced marked development over the past century. In the late nineteenth and early twentieth centuries, "homes" and training schools were established for individuals with specific problems such as blindness and crippling conditions (Edwards, 1992). Near the turn of the century, the concept of a multidisciplinary approach emerged, as restorative and reconstructive procedures were incorporated into the care of persons with disabilities (Allan, 1958).

During the 1940s many new rehabilitation facilities were established, some of which specialized in the care of children (Allan, 1958). Congenital neurologic and orthopedic problems commonly were seen. More recently the scope of the field has broadened. In addition to congenital problems, chronic conditions and acquired disabilities, as well as developmental disabilities, have expanded the field.

Chronic disabling conditions have increased due to improved survival rates for illnesses and injuries that once were fatal. Today, 10% to 20% of American children have some form of chronic health condition, with almost 5% experiencing some limitation in usual daily activities (Perrin & MacLean, 1988).

Children with cerebral palsy (CP) are among the largest population requiring (re)habilitative services (Molnar, 1992). Among the multiple causes of CP (i.e., intrauterine infections, toxins, and delivery complications), prematurity is the most significant contributing factor (Astbury, Orgill, Bajuk, & Yu, 1990; Drillien, Thompson, & Burgoyne, 1980; Molnar, 1992). Figure 30-1 shows sites of origin for neuromuscular disorders. The number of children with spastic diplegia due to prematurity referred for diagnosis and treatment increased during the 1980s, while term infants with this diagnosis were seen rarely (Binder & Eng, 1989). The broad span of etiologies accounts in part for the number of associated problems seen in children with this condition: hearing, vision, and speech impairments; feeding problems and malnutrition; seizures; mental retardation; in addition to various motor impairments (Cioffi & Gaebler-Spira, 1990). Spasticity is a particularly difficult to manage complication. Figure 30-2 illustrates two children who have spasticity producing "scissoring." Infants of drug addicted mothers are another group of children requiring early and ongoing intervention.

The sequelae of hematology problems (leukemia, sickle cell anemia) and oncology problems (brain/spinal cord tumors, lymphomas) are being seen more frequently in rehabilitation settings. In the recent past limited survival rates precluded the need for such services. However, the positive effects of rehabilitation on functional outcome following treatment for primary brain tumors were described by Philip, Ayyanger, Vanderbilt, and Gaebler-Spira (1994).

The number of children who are human immunodeficiency virus (HIV) positive and those manifesting symptomatic HIV infection also is rising steadily. The first case of acquired immunodeficiency syndrome (AIDS) in the pediatric population was reported in 1982. From that time through March 1990, there were 2192 cases in children under 13 years reported to the Centers for Disease Control (CDC) (Caldwell & Rogers, 1991). As the incidence of the disease rises and as life expectancy of those infected improves, rehabilitation specialists will be treating clients with

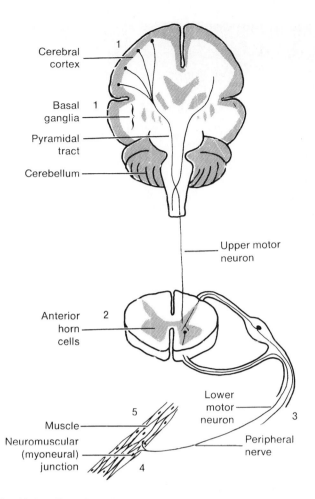

Fig. 30-1 Site of origin for neuromuscular disorders. *1*, Cerebral palsy; *2*, poliomyelitis, spinal muscular atrophy; *3*, mononeuropathies, polyneuropathies; *4*, myasthenia gravis, neurotoxic disorders; *5*, muscular dystrophies. (From *Nursing Care of Infants and Children*, 4th ed. by Whaley & Wong, 1991, St. Louis: Mosby–Year Book.)

a wide variety of resulting limitations. Traditionally rehabilitation nurses have emphasized education toward self-care and independence. However, modifications in the treatment approach may be necessary to accommodate the deconditioned state of the acutely ill child. In addition to the medical aspects of this disease, many psychosocial issues also must be considered. Support and guidance for terminally ill children and their families will require a shift in focus for the pediatric rehabilitation nurse. Chapter 22 contains additional information about pediatric AIDS.

Homelessness is an additional societal problem that influences chronic illness and disability in children and adolescents. In 1988 it was estimated that 3 million persons were homeless nationwide. Families with children represented 28% of the homeless population. An additional 200,000 were runaway adolescents. Health problems among these populations include underimmunization, malnutrition, high infant morbidity and mortality rates, lead poisoning, illicit drug use, and child abuse. In addition, chronic illness is twice as prevalent among the homeless. Homeless adolescents are at increased risk for sexually transmitted diseases and psychosocial problems as well (Alperstein & Arnstein, 1988).

Accidental and nonaccidental trauma contribute significantly to the increasing number of youngsters with disabilities. Traumatic brain injury is a major cause of disability in children. It is estimated that 200,000 children are hospitalized each year with head trauma. About 15,000 sustain some form of lifelong disability (Kraus, Fife, & Conroy, 1987). Falls are responsible for the majority of brain injuries, resulting in over 100,000 hospitalizations per year (Jaffe et al., 1992), followed by traffic-related accidents and blunt trauma (i.e., beatings or being struck by an object) (Di Scala, Osberg, Gans, Chin, & Grant, 1991).

The National Pediatric Trauma Registry (NPTR), established in 1985, provides educational and service information for families and professionals. The goal is to study the causes, circumstances, and consequences of injuries to children in the United States, with a view to the unique aspects of pediatric injuries from birth through age 19 years (NPTR, 1993).

Violence is reaching epidemic proportion in our society. From 1980 through 1989, 11,000 homicides were committed by high-school-aged youths. Firearms accounted for more than 65% of these fatalities (CDC, 1991a). In addition to the deaths, significant numbers of adolescents and children sustained long-term disability as a result of violence. Immediate access to potentially lethal weapons is a major contributing factor.

A 1990 survey revealed that about 20% of all students in grades 9 through 12 reportedly carried a weapon during the 30 days preceding the survey. Knives and razors were the most common weapons; however, 1 in 20 students reported carrying firearms. Handguns were the predominant type (CDC, 1991a).

Domestic violence is another significant contributor to childhood injury. Approximately 2 million children are seriously abused each year by their parents, guardians, or others. At least 1000 children die as a result of abuse (American Hospital Association [AHA], 1992), and the sequelae of countless other injuries are all too often witnessed in the rehabilitation setting. It is suggested that 65% to 80% of head injuries in children under 12 months of age may be due to nonaccidental trauma (abuse) (Billmire & Myers, 1985; Rivara, Kamitsuka, & Quan, 1988; Shapiro, 1983). Public awareness, education, primary prevention programs, and legislation (Spivack, Prothrow-Stith, & Hausman, 1988) are among the intervention strategies necessary to reduce violence-related deaths and injuries among our youth.

Location and Duration of Services

The location, type, and duration of rehabilitation services has changed markedly over the past few decades. At one time training schools provided treatment for specific populations such as the "deaf and blind." Later, a more collaborative multidisciplinary approach was espoused to treated a wider variety of chronic disabling conditions. Services were provided in hospitals and rehabilitation centers. Inpatient stays, once long and arduous, have been streamlined significantly. Hospitalizations for spinal cord injury, which

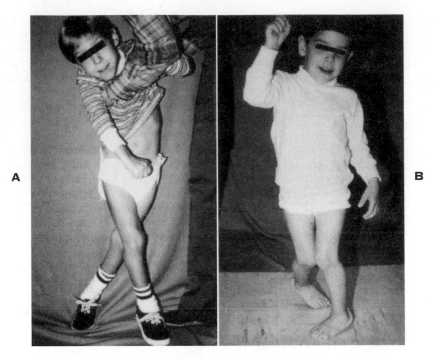

Fig. 30-2 Two children with adductor spasticity producing scissoring. **A,** Severe spasticity in nonambulatory child who has adduction deformity and severe scissoring. **B,** Ambulatory child with spastic diplegia whose legs scissor during walking. (From *Operative Pediatric Orthopaedics* by S.T. Canale & J.H. Beaty, 1991, St. Louis: Mosby–Year Book.)

once spanned 6 to 12 months, have now been reduced to 60 days in some cases.

Today the trend is clearly toward outpatient services, be it traditional outpatient therapy or more comprehensive outpatient day programs (i.e., brain injury recovery). This trend supports the philosophy of keeping children in their most natural environment: family and community. In addition, it is a cost-effective approach to rehabilitative care.

Services also may be received in home or school settings as an adjunct to facility-based therapy. The Education for All Handicapped Children's Act (Public Law 94-142) and its amendments (Public Law 99-457) ensure in-school therapy to the extent that is is needed to facilitate learning. Chapter 5 provides other discussion of these laws.

Many children require additional services; however, these often are secured at "out-of-pocket" expense to the parents. The increased demand for pediatric rehabilitation services has given rise to private, for-profit practices. These practices often are appealing due to more convenient locations, flexible service hours, and minimal waiting lists.

Uniqueness of the Pediatric Rehabilitation Nurse

Although rehabilitation services have been provided to children for quite some time, the field of pediatric rehabilitation nursing is relatively new (Selekman, 1991). In the mid-1980s the Pediatric Special-Interest Group (PSIG) was formed within the Association of Rehabilitation Nurses. The membership described the role of the pediatric rehabilitation nurse in a recent publication (PSIG, 1992).

Pediatric rehabilitation nurses are unique as they are both specialists and generalists: specialists by virtue of age of the client and generalists due to the broad diagnostic categories served. Infants, children, and adolescents with a variety of chronic disabling conditions receive specialized care from pediatric rehabilitation nurses in hospital, clinic, home, and school settings (PSIG, 1992).

Inherent in the specialized approach is the nurse's acceptance of a child with disability as first and foremost a child, and second as a child with special needs. A child must be viewed as an integral part of a family system, with the family and home as the central focus of the child's world. The family is primarily responsible for the child's development (DiCowden, 1990). The nurse along with other rehabilitation specialists assist the family in the child's development (habilitation) or recovery (rehabilitation) of skills needed to conduct activities of daily life. Rehabilitation nurses and other personnel who have contact with children with disabilities and their families share an important role and responsibility in shaping the child's future. It is during the earliest rehabilitation experience that the "seeds of empowerment of a fully functioning, integrated citizen with a disability are planted" (Bibb, 1990).

Developmental Framework

Developmental theory is fundamental to pediatric rehabilitation nursing. Children grow and develop in several realms: physical, cognitive, social, and emotional. Growth and development proceed in a sequential fashion for all children. It is the rate and level of achievement that vary. In the physical realm growth occurs in a cephalocaudal manner. Height, weight, and head circumference are important growth parameters. Children also must acquire the mobility and skills to eat, dress, toilet, and groom themselves in addition to negotiating their environment.

Cognitive development progresses from concrete to abstract thinking, which ultimately provides for learning and problem-solving (Piaget, 1952). In the social realm children develop a trusting relationship first with their parents or primary caregivers, their siblings, and ultimately with strangers (Erickson, 1963). They also learn socially appropriate behavior and culturally acceptable norms.

A positive body image and self-esteem are essential building blocks of healthy emotional development. A child's early experiences related to the disability can influence future adjustment to residual limitations, development of self-esteem and relationships, and career choices (Molnar, 1988). A parent's difficulty in adjusting to a child's disability could adversely affect the child's self-image. However, a consistent, nurturing, and stimulating environment can support healthy adjustment (Burkett, 1989; Selekman, 1991).

The pediatric rehabilitation nurse must tailor assessment skills to measure the physical, cognitive, and psychosocial parameters of growth and development. Appropriate communication skills, knowledge of developmentally appropriate play, and creative problem-solving are necessary elements for promoting developmental milestones (Selekman, 1991). In addition, major emphasis always should be placed on the child's abilities rather than limitations. An appreciation of cultural values and beliefs is key to successful education and treatment outcomes (Hoeman, 1989).

Clearly, special skills are needed to optimally care for children with disabilities, as "children are not small adults."

Nursing approaches vary depending on the developmental stage of the child (Fig. 30-3). The concepts developed for pediatric rehabilitation should be applicable across the spectrum of diagnostic categories. Therefore a developmental framework is the optimal approach to the myriad needs of children with disabilities and chronic illness (Carlson, Ricci, & Shade-Zeldow, 1990; DiCowden, 1990; Molnar, 1988; Selekman, 1991).

IMPACT OF DISABILITY

The following section discusses the impact of disability across developmental stages. Developmental tasks, coping processes, and strategies for intervention are highlighted. A summary is presented in Table 30-1.

Infancy

When a child is born with or acquires a chronic or disabling condition during infancy, the implications are far reaching. Parents often experience guilt and may grieve the loss of the child of their dreams (Solnit & Stark, 1962). Parent-infant bonding may be interrupted, separation anxiety may be exacerbated with multiple hospitalizations, marital discord, financial burden, and stress on siblings—which are additional problems all too commonly encountered (Carlson et al., 1990).

The infant may experience interruptions in timely and consistent nurturing, adequate nutrition, sensory stimulation, and freedom of movement—all of which facilitate physical well-being and the development of trust (Carlson et al., 1990; Perrin & Gerrity, 1984). Professionals can help parents to influence the infant's potential by offering clear, concise information regarding diagnosis, treatment, resources, and anticipatory guidance (Carlson et al., 1990).

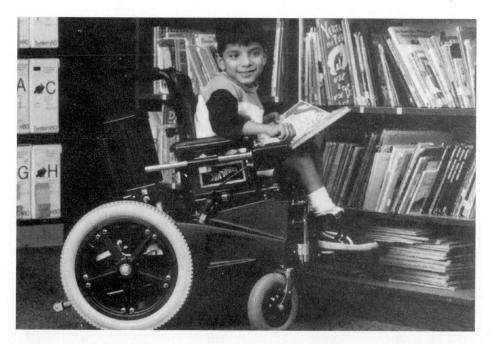

Fig. 30-3   Children are not miniature adults. They require care and equipment designed especially for their growth, development and disabling disorders. (From *Rehabilitation/Restorative Care in the Community* by S.P. Hoeman, 1990, St. Louis: Mosby–Year Book. Courtesy of Everest & Jennings, Inc.)

Table 30-1 Summary of psychosocial issues, coping process, and interventions

Stage	Developmental	Cognitive appraisal	Coping process		Strategic interventions
			Adaptive tasks	Coping skills	
Infancy	*Trust/mistrust* Achieve emotional stability Eye-hand coordination Sensory discrimination Motor skills Object permanence Eat solid foods	N/A	Integrating environmental experience	Motor activity (tension reduction and/or goal oriented) Crying, kicking	Consistency in nurturing Sensory stimulation Freedom to move Consistent caregiving Timely responses to needs Verbal soothing Clear information to parents
Toddlerhood	*Autonomy/shame and doubt* Self-control Language development Fantasy and play Elaboration of locomotion Sense of autonomy/asserting independence Functional communication Interpersonal control	Egocentrism (limited ability to imagine alternative viewpoint) Questioning through play Transductive reasoning	Mastery through fantasy and play Separation from parent Exploring environment Increasing communication skills Improved frustration tolerance	Repetitive activity and play (for mastery and anxiety reduction) Protest Fantasy Comfort Time-out Experimentation Restricting environment	Information giving to parents Teaching parents caregiving and limit-setting skills Encourage age-appropriate responses Acknowledge aggression as healthy response Set limits Provide safe tension-reduction outlets Encourage engaging activities Parental/sibling involvement during hospitalization Safe havens for parents and children Age-appropriate explanation
Early childhood	*Initiative/guilt* Exploration and mastery Independent activity	Rudimentary conscience Understands right and wrong (views conflict in these terms)	Independence Develop and identify role in family Maintain and protect body integrity	Routines Ritualized activities	Encourage play/fantasy to explore feelings about illness/treatment Concise, honest, age-appropriate information Support established routines Presence of parents to decrease anxiety

Middle childhood	*Industry/inferiority* Skill mastery Contending with feelings of inferiority Peer relationships Sensitivity to society expectations	Can perceive past/future Consideration of other points of view Questions beliefs Causal thinking Trial and error problem solving	Successful productivity Peer relationships Acceptance	Problem-solving Humor Withdrawal Aggression Control of behavior	Use models/diagrams in clarifying information Participation in self-direction of procedures Enhance opportunities to relate to others with similar difficulties Use humor in relationships Facilitate maintenance of family, peer relationships during illness Encourage responsibilities and chores
Adolescence	*Identity* Perception of self in eyes of others Testing autonomy Emotional independence Peer relationships Body awareness and comfort control Positive body image and self esteem Realistic future orientation	Higher order reasoning Propositional logic (formal operations) Strategic interventions Use of imaginary audience Interpretation of earlier experience	Reconstruction of experience (reframing, incorporating past) Integrating thinking of others Contending with self-consciousness Competition Transition to adult roles Successful integration of disability with identity Emotional stability Independence from parents Identify personal identity Sexuality Separation from peers	Repression, denial Intellectualization Conformity Behavioral control Motor activity Withdrawal	Understand perceptions of illness via listening Clarify misconceptions Encourage and support independence Involve in care as much as possible Respect need for privacy Encourage choice/decision making wherever possible Create opportunities for dialogue Facilitate peer support opportunities

From "Psychosocial Aspects of Disability in Children." by C.E. Carlson, J. Ricci, and Y. Shade-Zeldow, 1990, *Pediatrician, 17,* pp. 213-221. Reprinted by permission.

Families benefit from knowing and understanding their child's condition and trajectory of illness or condition. Illustrations, such as Figure 30-4, which diagram changes in the spine with meningocele and myelomeningocele, help families to visualize the condition. Chapter 13 discusses other ways of assisting children and their families with these conditions.

Toddlerhood

Egocentricity limits toddlers' ability to consider the world from any viewpoint other than their own. The toddler is a concrete thinker who affords life and function to all objects. Reasoning is transductive; therefore illness may be viewed by the child as a consequence of "bad" behavior (Pontious, 1982).

Play is the life work of children, occupying the majority of the day. It is the child's vehicle for exploration and learning. Play also helps children to master anxiety-provoking situations—for instance, catheterizing a doll during medical play.

Mobility, exploration, and separation from parents for short periods of time are normal activities that help toddlers to gain autonomy. Disability or chronic illness may disrupt these developmental processes. Strategies to minimize potential adverse responses to disability during this phase include parent/sibling involvement in healthcare regimens; stress management techniques (time-outs, physical comfort, reassurance); provision of a safe place for mobility and exploration; and age-appropriate explanations (Vipperman & Rager 1980). Parents also need information, caregiving skills, and guidance related to balancing encouragement and limit setting. At times parents may be reluctant to set appropriate limits for their challenged children; however, failure to do so may interfere with development of impulse control (Perrin & Gerrity, 1984).

Early Childhood/Preschool

The preoperational phase of cognitive development (Piaget, 1952) provides the preschool child with a basic understanding of rules of social behavior and a basic sense of right and wrong (Kohlberg, 1969). Fantasies are prominent, and maintenance of body integrity is of primary importance, as are routines and rituals at this stage of development. Magical thinking prevails, and illness still may be viewed as punishment for bad behavior. Body invasion and mutilation are key fears; thus treatments including burn dressings, bladder catheterization, and injections may be perceived as punitive or hostile (Carlson et al., 1990).

Improved understanding and coordination enable the child to take initiative in dressing, eating with utensils, and other self-care activities. The desire to move about is a strong motivating factor for this age group (Molnar, 1988). Disabilities that limit the child's ability to communicate, explore, and navigate the environment such as CP, spinal cord injury, and ventilator dependency may reduce the potential for achieving age-appropriate developmental tasks (Carlson et al., 1990).

Intervention strategies should focus on capabilities rather than disabilities. Feelings and perceptions about illness, treatment, and limitations can be explored through creative modalities such as imaginative play and art and music therapy. Routines and rituals should be supported and opportunities for successful mastery of situations provided. Concise, honest, age-appropriate explanations are important, as are parental and sibling involvement and support (Carlson et al., 1990).

Middle Childhood/School Age

The school-aged child has a greater understanding of the body, causation of illness, and treatment processes. Concerns exist about physical abilities such as control of the body and ability to master new experiences. However, there is a shift in emphasis to educational pursuit and psychosocial development. School is the workplace of the child (Perrin & Gerrity, 1984). The industrious child needs to learn, master, and produce even during illness (Carlson et al., 1990). To facilitate learning and mastery, voice or word communicators and switch-activated computers are available for school assignments and for playing action-oriented video games. This allows for a previously unattainable level of independence in a child with severe motor limitations (Molnar, 1988).

In addition to academic learning, the structure of a classroom and interactions with classmates provide an environ-

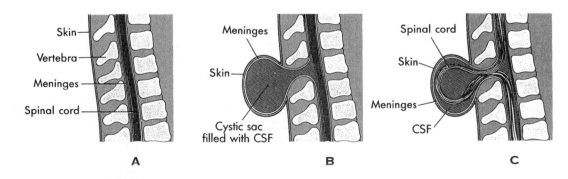

Fig. 30-4 Myelodysplagia is classified according to the pathophysiology of the lesion or defect of the spinal cord and surrounding structures. **A**, Normal spine; **B**, meningocele; **C**, myelomeningocele. (From *Primary Care of the Child with a Chronic Condition* by Jackson & Vessey [Eds.], 1992, St. Louis: Mosby–Year Book, Inc.)

ment for learning social skills. This is especially important for children with disabilities whose social experiences may otherwise be limited compared with those of their able-bodied peers (Molnar, 1988). Isolation, withdrawal, depression, and social dysfunction can result if the child is not well integrated into family, school, and community life. Therefore therapies and other health-related activities should be scheduled such that they do not interfere with education and peer relationships.

Health-related teaching can be facilitated with the use of diagrams and models. Clarification and correction of disability-related misconceptions is important. School-aged children are eager to participate in or direct self-care and therapeutic procedures. Peers with similar disabilities can provide support and serve as role models (Carlson et al., 1990).

Involvement in sports can enhance socialization, fun, exercise, and self-esteem. Assignment of a developmentally appropriate household chore can reduce parental tendency toward overprotection and promote a sense of responsibility and accomplishment for the child (Carlson et al., 1990; Vipperman & McCook-Rager, 1980).

Adolescence

Adolescence is a period marked by rapid growth, profound physiologic changes, development of higher-order reasoning abilities, an emerging personal identify, and a budding interest in the opposite sex (Molnar, 1988). It is a tumultuous time for adolescents as they strive to attain independence from their parents.

Although seeking a separate identity, the adolescent often travels the road of conformity to that end. The peer group is highly influential, and there is a strong need to be a part of the crowd. Body image is of critical concern. There is a preoccupation with physical characteristics, and "different" automatically implies "imperfect" (Perrin & Gerrity, 1984).

Whether the disability is congenital, as with limb deficiency, or acquired, such as traumatic amputation, the impact on psychosocial functioning can be great due to the many concerns of adolescence. The adolescent may have to adapt to separation from school and peers, changes in body image, discomfort, limitations in mobility, and involvement with the healthcare system. At a time when independence is a major developmental task, a condition that limits functioning and increases dependency on others can be extremely disruptive. Feelings of denial, anger, depression and fear—which normally are experienced during adolescence—may be exaggerated (Carlson et al., 1990).

Strategies for intervention at this developmental stage include careful listening, honest information giving, offering choices, and provision of privacy. Health-related misconceptions should be clarified. However, it is not uncommon for adolescents to be hesitant about sharing thoughts and feelings, particularly with adults. Therefore clinicians must be alert to subtle and overt cues (Carlson et al., 1990) that may indicate a desire to talk. Peer counselors may be helpful in providing support and encouragement.

Maintaining contact with friends is important, as is participation in school and other age-appropriate activities. Unfortunately, geographic integration in a regular classroom does not necessarily result in social integration. Isolation, poor self-image, and loneliness are problems faced by many adolescents with physical disabilities (Molnar, 1988). Those with visible physical disability, burn, or spinal cord injury, for example, often experience rejection by peers (Harper, Wacker, & Cobb, 1986). Individual or group counseling may provide an avenue for honest discussion, support, and encouragement.

Older Adolescence/Young Adulthood

The development of trust during infancy culminates with the establishment of intimate relationships in young adulthood. At this point in life, young adults have solidified their self-identity and career plans and have established or are working toward personal and financial independence.

Unfortunately social and physical barriers may impede or delay the accomplishment of the development tasks of this stage. Thus it is imperative that preparations for the fully functioning adult lifestyle begin at the person's point of entry into the (re)habilitation system. In addition, young adults must be well versed in their rights. Chapter 5 provides a detailed discussion of the Americans with Disabilities Act.

The passage into adulthood brings with it some unique concerns related to health maintenance. One issue is that of the transition from the pediatric to the adult rehabilitation team. Ideally the stage is set for this transition in the mid-to-late teenage years.

Sexuality is a concept that should be addressed throughout the life-span of an individual. However, specific issues may surface at this stage related to sexual functioning and fertility. Honest, accurate information and referral to specialists in the field are helpful intervention strategies. Chapter 27 provides detailed discussion of sexuality and sexual counseling.

PREVENTION

Prenatal intervention is one of the major defenses against children with congenital disabilities resulting from prematurity, low birth weight, and associated medical problems. A good prenatal diet; absence of smoking, alcohol, and recreational drugs; and adequate medical monitoring increase the chances of having a healthy infant. Inadequate amounts of folic acid are now cited as a contributing factor in the incidence of neural tube defects (CDC, 1991b). Teenage pregnancies, which often result in premature deliveries, contribute to a variety of problems for infants born at risk for special needs, including CP. Well child care, including immunizations, can prevent disabling illnesses such as measles encephalopathy, influenza, meningitis, and polio.

Although children with congenital disabilities make up a significant number of the disabled population under 21 years of age, many more are disabled as a result of trauma (Jaffe et al., 1992). Injury to children is the leading cause of acquired disabilities. The use of infant/child car seats, helmets, and other protective gear while bicycling or skating has helped to decrease residual disability related to traumatic brain injury and other physical injuries.

Educating both children and adults in all areas of safety and injury prevention is key to decreasing the incidence of trauma. Liller, Kent, and McDermott's (1991) survey of postpartum mothers revealed that although participants had some knowledge of prevention strategies, deficits were noted in prevention of burns, motor vehicle accidents, drownings, and falls. Greater than 50% of the mothers did not know the temperature of their hot water heater (recommended water temperature is 120° in the home) (Binder, 1992), and 22.4% did not use car safety seats with previous children (Liller et al., 1991).

Another cause of injury in children is child abuse. According to the CDC, abuse accounts for the majority of burned children under 2 years of age (Showers & Garrison, 1988). Lack of parental supervision resulting in unsafe play contributes to injuries as well. By increasing public awareness regarding child abuse and neglect as well as providing such services as hot lines, parenting classes, and mentor programs, health professionals are attempting to decrease the incidence of abused children. The increasing number of persons with substance abuse problems, however, is adversely affecting such efforts.

EARLY INTERVENTION AND THE LAWS

Changes are being made in our federal, state, and local laws as the public becomes more aware of the needs of children with chronical illness and disabilities, and as parents become more verbal regarding the challenges of caring for these children. In 1975 Public Law 94-142, Education for All Handicapped Children's Act, mandated that states provide children a free education in the least restrictive environment (Reynolds, 1986), allowing many children with disabilities to be "mainstreamed." Other amendments such as Public Law 99-457 and Public Law 90-538 provide early intervention programs for children below school age, including infants and toddlers. Early intervention includes several types of services: those that focus on the child's family; facilitate entry into service programs; and those that provide direct services to a child (Bird, Castellani, & Nemeth, 1990). The focus is now on access and full inclusion.

In 1990 then-President George Bush signed the amendment to the Education of Handicapped Act (EHA), naming it the Individuals with Disability Education Act (IDEA) to change the term "handicapped" to "disabled." Through this act the federal government provides financial assistance to state and local education agencies to meet special education needs. Part B of IDEA requires that each state have policies and procedures in place to guarantee that children between the ages of 3 and 21 years receive appropriate services in order to qualify for federal funds (Committee on Education and Labor, 1991).

Despite the increasing number of laws and incentives, parents of young children with disability or developmental delay still are struggling with limited programs and waiting lists. In 1980 there were an estimated 1.1 million children with disabilities whose mothers were in the workforce (Fewell, 1986). It is now estimated that this number has increased to over 1.5 million. Crowley (1990) also estimated that over 5 million children with chronic illness had mothers working outside the home. Because of limited early intervention programs, some parents have sought day care centers that accept children with milder disabilities; however, these also are difficult to find.

A survey of 70 day care centers revealed that over half the centers indicated a willingness to enroll children with disabilities; however, only 20% actually enrolled such children (Beck & Beck, 1982). Crowley (1990) found that many centers require children to be ambulatory and toilet trained, thus disqualifying many children with disabilities. Mainstream day care centers often lack staff who are adequately trained or experienced in the management of children with disabilities. Therefore they are reluctant to undertake this responsibility. Fewell (1986) outlines the necessary requirements for successful integration of children with disabilities into day care systems, including the following:

+ A higher ratio of staff to children
+ Staff training in management of children with special needs
+ Alteration in physical space to allow for increased equipment and mobility of wheelchairs
+ Appropriate equipment and learning materials
+ Availability of healthcare supports

By providing day care personnel with the appropriate resources and training, there is hope that a greater comfort level will be achieved in caring for this population, thus increasing enrollment. Increased enrollment provides opportunities for nurses to become involved in health education of child care providers and legislative activities, to serve as liaisons to the community, and to advocate with parents for increased services.

COORDINATION OF CARE SERVICES/CASE MANAGEMENT

Case management has quickly been acknowledged as a cost-effective method of coordinating services for persons with chronic disabling conditions requiring multiple healthcare services. Part H of the EHA amendment mandates the coordination of program services for infants and toddlers (birth to 3 years) by a case manager (Public Law 99-457). According to *Federal Register* Guidelines (1989), case management for children with disabilities is defined as an active and ongoing process of seeking and obtaining appropriate services for the benefit of infants and toddlers throughout their eligibility period. The role of case manager has been assumed by a variety of professionals, as well as by laypersons. In some models case managers are parents, a lead agency providing services, or a combination of health professionals (Gittler, 1988). According to a survey by Davis and Steele (1991), only 21% of families had a professional healthcare worker as a case manager. Some parents were acting in this role on their child's behalf. Many other families had no case manager identified.

Qualifications for a case manager include knowledge of infants and toddlers; the requirements of EHA part H; the nature and scope of services available in the state; early intervention programs; and payment sources (Public Law 99-457). The elements of case management involve health assessment, planning, procurement, delivery and coordination of services, and monitoring of all services provided (ANA, 1988). Chapter 8 provides case management information including a life care plan model. Pediatric rehabilitation nurses have traditionally cared for children and families from a holistic perspective, thereby uniquely qualifying them to function in the role of case manager. With greater numbers of children and families requiring these services, it is likely that nurses will increasingly assume case management responsibilities.

THE TECHNOLOGY-DEPENDENT CHILD

Another population of children that is increasing is the chronically ill and disabled requiring high-technology services in the home. The Office of Technology Assessment (OTA) has attempted to estimate the number of technology-dependent children, albeit with some difficulty (Teague et al., 1993). In 1987 it was estimated that there were between 10,000 and 68,000 children receiving care in their homes (OTA, 1987).

With the increase in children receiving these services comes a myriad of issues affecting the entire family. Blum (1986) states that there is an increase in marital stress, deprivation of leisure time, fatigue, and social isolation among these families. Financial difficulties also may cause additional burden. Inadequate respite care adds to the family's social isolation, fatigue, and limited leisure time. Any respite a parent receives usually comes from the family network rather than the community (Florian & Krulik, 1991). Assisting parents in locating respite services, either within the extended family network or community, can be an extremely valuable role for nurses and social services. Parents assisting parents through support groups or other activities also can facilitate the coping process.

There are many other opportunities for professional nurses to assist in minimizing a parent's stress as a result of caring for these children. Teague et al. (1993) noted that nurses were frequently identified by families as their most accessible professional resources. Visiting Nurse Associations (VNAs) and home health agencies have acknowledged the need for supportive services to manage high-tech equipment as well as to educate and support parents in learning these skills. Nurses also can work with families to help structure routine care delivery and therapy, thus increasing free time and reducing stress (Ray & Ritchie, 1993).

Education is a critical aspect of all children's lives. Involvement in a stable school setting can help to provide normalcy. By educating school personnel, nurses can contribute to the placement of technology-dependent children into the appropriate classroom setting.

TRANSITION TO ADULTHOOD

The transition from childhood to adolescence and adulthood is challenging for all children, but often it becomes a more difficult process for the child with a disability. First, the child with a disability may have been protected from family responsibilities and therefore may be lacking in basic skills such as performing household chores. Children and adults without disabilities often feel the need to protect and make decisions for the child with a disability. Thus an adolescent may not have had the opportunity to develop decision-making skills.

Second, mothers who may have developed a pattern of overprotection may ignore the child's age and ability to speak for herself. Mothers often continue to speak for their adolescents, such as during visits with nurse practitioners or physicians, further limiting opportunities for the adolescent to express feelings and concerns. A teen who is capable of communicating is allowed time alone with the physician or nurse to ask questions and voice concerns.

Socialization is another problem area for adolescents with disabilities. At a time in life when body image, peers, and sexual attraction are major developmental issues, adolescents may find themselves with limited friends and minimal opportunities for social interactions. Getting to school functions may be logistically difficult, which diminishes opportunities to be with peers. However, camps and clubs provide an atmosphere to meet others and for establishing friendships.

Other important milestones include the 3D's of "dating, driving, and dressing" according to Thompson (1990). Limited ability to perform any of these functions may create social isolation. It is important that the adolescent be given as much control and mobility as possible. Electric wheelchairs may provide a means by which to keep up with friends. However, a person whose physical appearance is altered or who may require assistive devices for mobility may be perceived as less attractive to members of the opposite sex (Thompson, 1990). Attention to overall appearance, cleanliness, and developmentally appropriate styles can boost the adolescent's self-esteem and increase attractiveness to others around them. Because body image is so important and control over one's body increases self-esteem and confidence, every attempt should be made to get youngsters out of diapers through intermittent catheterization programs and/or external devices as appropriate.

Many adolescents and young adults continue to be followed by their pediatrician because of difficulty finding a general physician willing or capable of providing care (Thompson, 1990). Health professionals can assist in the transition process by educating parents to allow teens to make informed decisions about their healthcare; addressing the adolescent as the "client" rather than the parent; assisting in accessing appropriate healthcare services; and educating the adolescent on self-care management to enhance independence.

Driver's evaluation and training programs are available through some vocational rehabilitation centers or departments. Assessments can be made of the cognitive and physical abilities required for safe-driving skills. If driving is not feasible, educating the adolescent/young adult in utilizing public transportation of all types can increase locus of control. Feeling in control of one's life is essential in establishing the independence and self-determination needed to function as an adult in society.

STRATEGIES FOR ASSESSMENT

Children with chronic illness or disability are assessed at regular intervals and at all points along the healthcare continuum: from preadmission through postdischarge follow-up. Assessments can occur in clinics, hospitals, rehabilitation facilities, and home and school settings. Assessment is a critical element in the nursing process, as it is the basis from which planning and evaluation of therapeutic interventions stem.

Holistic assessments encompass the physical, cognitive,

social, emotional, cultural, and spiritual aspects of a child's life. In addition, the child is assessed within the context of the family system. Privacy and dignity must be afforded the child/adolescent during the assessment process. Fear and anxiety can be allayed or minimized by providing honest, concise, and age-appropriate information to the child. Toys for younger children and other age-appropriate items such as puppets, anatomically correct dolls, diagrams, and books may also help to calm and elicit information from the child. Although parents/guardians usually are the primary historians, children/adolescents should never be overlooked or excluded from conversations regarding themselves. The nurse's behavior must convey the fact that the child is the central focus of the interaction and a valuable source of information. The box on pp. 671-675 is a sample data collection tool that can be used to guide nursing assessment of the child with rehabilitative needs across the continuum of healthcare settings.

The Denver Developmental Screening Test (DDST, 1969) is a standardized tool that can assist the practitioner in evaluating children in the following areas: gross motor, fine motor-adaptive, language, and personal-social. Skills in these areas are graded from 1 month through 6 years. The administration of the DDST is relatively simple, requiring minimal and easily accessible equipment. In addition, instructions are summarized on the back of the scoring sheet (Golden, 1983).

COMMON CHRONIC AND DISABLING CONDITIONS IN CHILDREN AND ADOLESCENTS

It is clearly beyond the scope of this chapter to provide a comprehensive review of all the diagnoses encountered in the field of pediatric rehabilitation. However, this section addresses some of the more common conditions with respect to nursing diagnoses and interventions.

I. CEREBRAL PALSY
   A. HIGH RISK FOR ALTERED NUTRITION: LESS THAN BODY REQUIREMENTS
      Interventions
      1. Prepare child and family for fluoroscopic swallowing study as needed to rule out aspiration and ensure safe oral feeding
      2. Collaborate with physician and speech therapist to establish a safe feeding regimen (adjust consistency of food and fluid to ensure safe consumption)
      3. Collaborate with occupational therapist to provide adaptive feeding utensils and techniques; collaborate with physical therapist to ensure proper seating and positioning
      4. Provide client/family education regarding feeding regimen and techniques
      5. Involve school nurse/personnel in feeding program to ensure community follow-through
      6. Educate client/family and school personnel in care and use of an enteral feeding tube as appropriate
      7. Monitor weight and plot on growth chart; assess skin turgor/mucous membranes and specific gravity to ensure adequate hydration

   B. IMPAIRED PHYSICAL MOBILITY RELATED TO SPASTICITY
      Interventions
      1. Passive/active range of motion (ROM) at least twice daily
      2. Encourage warm bath/shower and/or other relaxation techniques (guided imagery, deep breathing) to facilitate movements
      3. Ensure follow-through of physical and occupational therapy exercises in the rehabilitation, home and school settings
      4. Ensure that prescribed assistive devices are available and utilized
      5. Encourage self-care to child's maximum potential
      6. Educate client/family and school personnel in mobility requirements/restrictions
      7. Ensure appropriate seating and positioning in wheelchair; prone stander

   C. IMPAIRED COMMUNICATION
      Interventions
      1. Provide adequate time and a supportive environment for child to attempt to communicate
      2. Collaborate with speech therapist to establish a communication system (picture, word, alphabet board; computer; voice computer)
      3. Educate child, family, and school personnel regarding communication system to ensure consistency

   D. HIGH RISK FOR ALTERED BOWEL ELIMINATION: CONSTIPATION RELATED TO DECREASED FLUID AND BULK INTAKE; DECREASED MOBILITY
      Interventions
      1. Evaluate child's current bowel patterns
      2. Establish least invasive, most cost-effective bowel program focusing first on dietary and fluid measures, regular exercise/increased mobility, and scheduled toileting
      3. Use stool softeners and/or laxatives as an adjunct to dietary measures and exercise as necessary
      4. Determine that child can communicate need to use toilet; educate family and school personnel to ensure follow-through with established program
      5. Collaborate with physical therapist to ensure supported seating (commode chair) for relaxation of tone and facilitation of elimination

   E. HIGH RISK FOR IMPAIRED SKIN INTEGRITY RELATED TO SPASTICITY, FRICTION, AND MOISTURE
      Interventions
      1. Prevention is the primary intervention
      2. Skin checks at least twice daily (long-handled mirror can increase child's involvement and promote independence; special attention should be given to areas under braces and other orthoses)
      3. Ensure position changes to prevent prolonged pressure

Text Continued on p. 676.

PEDIATRIC ASSESSMENT GUIDE

Date _____

Client name _____   Date of birth _____

Historian _____   Sex _____

Client/parent/guardian goals _____

_____

_____

T _____   P _____   R _____   B/P _____   WT _____   HT _____

Head circumference (cm) _____(clients ≤5 yrs)   Arm span _____   (MM clients and SCI clients ≤5 yrs)

1. MEDICAL DIAGNOSIS (include date of onset, course, and other significant information) _____

_____

_____

2. SIGNIFICANT MEDICAL HISTORY

   A. Diabetes No/Yes _____

   B. Recent infection No/Yes _____

   C. Past surgeries No/Yes _____

   D. Allergies No/Yes _____

   E. Medications No/Yes _____

_____

_____

_____

   F. Immunizations

     DPT: (date) 1st _____ 2nd _____ 3rd _____ Booster _____

     OVP: (date) 1st _____ 2nd _____ 3rd _____ 4th _____

     Measles (date) _____

     Mumps (date) _____

     Rubella (date) _____

     Haemophilus influenza

     type B (date) _____

     Pneumovax (date) _____

     Tuberculosis test

        PPD (date) _____Result _____

        Tine (date) _____Result _____

     Hepatitis B (date) 1st ___ 2nd ___ 3rd _____

   G. **Childhood Disease History**

     Has your child had any of the following?

     If Yes, when?

     Chicken pox   No/Yes _____

     Measles   No/Yes _____

     Mumps   No/Yes _____

     Rubella   No/Yes _____

     Tetanus   No/Yes _____

     Pertussis (whooping cough)   No/Yes _____

     Rheumatic fever   No/Yes _____

     Tuberculosis   No/Yes _____

     CMV   No/Yes _____

     Rotovirus   No/Yes _____

     Hepatitis   No/Yes _____

     Has your child been in contact with any of these illnesses in the past 4 weeks? No/Yes

MM, myelomeningocele; SCI, spinal cord injured; DPT, diphtheria-pertussis-tetanus; OVP, oral poliovirus vaccine; PPD, purified protein derivative; H/O, history of; CMV, cytomegalovirus; BM, bowel movement; LMP, last menstrual period; ROM, range of motion; UE, upper extremity; LE, lower extremity. Adapted from **Inpatient Nursing Admission Form** (1991) and **Pediatric Nursing Admission Form Supplement,** Division of Nursing, Rehabilitation Institute of Chicago, Chicago, Illinois.

Continued.

PEDIATRIC ASSESSMENT GUIDE—cont'd

3. COGNITIVE/COMMUNICATIVE

  A. Mental status

      Alert Yes/No _____

      Orientation (circle) person place time

      Memory intact: short term Yes/No _____

                       long term Yes/No _____

      Loss of consciousness No/Yes _____

      Client responds to (circle) voice   pain   neither

      Client is "Yes/No" reliable (circle)   Yes   No

  B. Safety issues No/Yes _____

      Seizures No/Yes _____

      _____

  C. Communication: language spoken _____

      Spontaneous speech Yes/No _____

      Speech intelligible Yes/No _____

      Alternative communication system used No/Yes _____

      _____

      Was child speaking before onset of illness/disability

      No/Yes _____

  D. Visual problems No/Yes _____   Glasses No/Yes _____

      Hearing problems No/Yes _____

      Assistive device No/Yes _____

4. CARDIOVASCULAR

  H/O cardiac problems No/Yes _____

  H/O hypertension No/Yes _____

  Chest pain No/Yes _____

  Pulses palpable: brachial _____ radial _____ pedal _____

5. RESPIRATORY

  H/O respiratory problem (asthma) _____

  Current status (breath sounds) _____

  _____

  Tracheostomy No/Yes _____

  (size, type, fenestration, date last changed, corking

  program) _____

  Respiratory management (include oxygen, assistive cough,

  suctioning, incentive spirometer) _____

  _____

  _____

  _____

6. NUTRITION

  Type and texture of diet _____

  Route _____

  Enteral feedings No/Yes (type; amount of feeding) _____

  _____

  Type/size tube _____ Date last changed _____

  Problems sucking, chewing, pocketing food, swallowing

  No/Yes _____

  _____

  Dentition _____

  Likes _____

  Dislikes _____

◆

PEDIATRIC ASSESSMENT GUIDE—cont'd

Appetite: good _____ poor _____ fussy eater _____

Uses: cup _____ bottle _____ straw _____ pacifier _____

        fork _____ spoon _____

Special feeding techniques/equipment _____

_____

Indicate means of communicating: drink _____

water _____ milk _____ hunger _____

other _____

7. ELIMINATION

    A. Bowel: continent Yes/No _____

       Last bowel movement _____

       Premorbid pattern _____

       Current status (include bowel sounds) _____

       _____

       Indicate means of communicating need for toileting/BM

       _____

    B. Urinary: continent Yes/No _____

       Last void _____

       Management program _____

       Indwelling catheter No/Yes (type, size, date last changed)

       _____

       Intermittent catheterization program (include size, type of

       catheter; clean or sterile technique; level of

       independence) _____

       _____

       Indicate child's means of communicating need to void _____

       _____

       _____

8. GYNECOLOGIC

    A. Age at menarche _____ Date LMP _____

    B. Date last PAP smear _____

    C. Performs breast self-examination No/Yes _____ Date last done _____

       Level of independence _____

    GENITOURINARY

       Performs self-testicular examination Yes/No _____

       Frequency _____ Date last done _____

       Level of independence _____

9. INTEGUMENT

    A. Sensation (circle)   intact   impaired   absent

    B. Skin intact Yes/No _____

       (describe type lesion, location, grade/stage, measurements,

       treatment) _____

       _____

       PHOTO OPTIONAL

    C. Prevention program (describe turning, sitting tolerance)

       _____

       Special mattress/cushions used _____

       Method and frequency of pressure relief _____

       Method and frequency of skin checks _____

Continued.

◆

PEDIATRIC ASSESSMENT GUIDE—cont'd

10. ACTIVITY/MOBILITY
    A. Motor function (i.e., describe paraplegia; left-sided hemiparesis)

    _____

    _____

    B. Ambulatory Yes/No _____

       Assistive device(s) No/Yes _____

    C. Decrease in ROM No/Yes _____

    D. Contractures No/Yes _____

    E. Edema No/Yes _____

    F. Pain No/Yes _____

    G. Recent fracture No/Yes _____

11. REST/SLEEP
    A. Naps No/Yes _____

    B. Normal AM waking time _____

    C. Normal bedtime _____

    D. Does child sleep through the night Yes/No _____

    E. Child sleeps in (circle)   bed   crib

    F. Does child sleep alone Yes/No _____

    (if shares bed/room, with whom) _____

12. PSYCHOSOCIAL
    A. Family unit (with whom does child live; list names and ages of siblings) _____

       _____

       _____

    B. Primary caretaker _____

    C. Others that care for child (grandparents; neighbors; baby
       sitters) _____

    D. Pets _____

    E. Religious affiliation _____

    F. Any religious/cultural/traditional beliefs of which staff
       should be aware _____

    G. Leisure/play activities enjoyed by child _____

       _____

    H. Does child have special toy or comfort item No/Yes _____

       _____

       Was it brought with child today No/Yes _____

    I. Does child play well with other children Yes/No _____

       _____

    J. Does child attend school No/Yes _____ Grade _____

    K. Does child have any problems in school No/Yes _____

       _____

    L. Parent/guardian-child interaction _____

       _____

       _____

13. DEVELOPMENTAL
    A. Milestones: before illness/disability—was child
       Walking No/Yes _____ (age) _____
       Talking No/Yes _____ (age) _____
       Feeding self No/Yes _____ (age) _____
       Toilet trained No/Yes _____ (age) _____

    B. Fears
       Does child have any fears about which staff should be aware (dark; strangers; needles; animals; other) _____

       _____

PEDIATRIC ASSESSMENT GUIDE—cont'd

What behavior does child exhibit when frightened _____

How is your child comforted _____

14. SAFETY
   A. Birth to 4 years
      Do you have a car safety seat for your child Yes/No _____
      Do you consistently use safety seat Yes/No _____
   B. Four years and older
      Does your child wear a car safety belt Yes/No _____
   C. Does your child wear a helmet for bike riding; skating
      Yes/No _____
   D. History of tobacco use No/Yes _____
   E. History of alcohol use No/Yes _____
   F. History of drug use No/Yes _____

15. DISCHARGE PLANNING (FOR INPATIENT)
   Where will child be going at discharge _____
   Is residence accessible Yes/No _____
   Pediatrican _____
   School to which child will be returning _____

16. FUNCTIONAL LEVELS: ACTIVITIES OF DAILY LIVING
   [*Scale:* 5 = Independent; 4 = Minimal physical assistance (client does 75% or more); 3 = Moderate assistance (50% or more); 2 = Maximal assistance (25% to 50% or may direct); 1 = Dependent]
   Oral/facial _____   Eating _____
   Hygeine/bathing _____   Turning _____
   Dressing UE _____   Transfers _____
   Dressing LE _____   Toileting _____

17. NURSING DIAGNOSES
   _____
   _____
   _____
   _____
   _____
   _____
   _____
   _____

18. MUTUAL GOALS
   _____
   _____
   _____
   _____

19. EDUCATIONAL NEEDS (include assessment of learning style)
   _____
   _____
   _____
   _____
   _____

RN   SIGNATURE   _____

4. Establish bowel and bladder programs and collaborate with speech therapist to minimize drooling to decrease moisture

II. MYELOMENINGOCELE
   A. ALTERED PATTERN OF URINARY ELIMINATION: URINARY RETENTION
      Interventions
      1. Educate client/family and appropriate school personnel regarding bladder program (usually clean intermittent catheterization)
      2. Encourage child's progression toward maximal independence with bladder program
      3. Educate child/family regarding urinary tract health maintenance
         · Adequate fluid intake
         · Signs, symptoms, and steps to take for urinary tract infection
         · Prevention of bladder overdistention
         · Routine urologic evaluations as recommended by physician (generally every 6 to 12 months)
   B. HIGH RISK FOR ALTERED NUTRITION: MORE THAN BODY REQUIREMENTS RELATED TO DECREASED MOBILITY
      Interventions
      1. Educate client/family early on regarding healthful nutrition patterns
      2. Encourage child to participate in selection and preparation of healthy meals and snacks
      3. Encourage regular exercise and/or involvement in adapted sports/recreational activities
      4. Monitor weight and plot on growth chart
      5. Encourage and praise child regarding healthy nutritional choices and progress toward weight goal
   C. HIGH RISK FOR DISTURBANCE IN SELF-CONCEPT
      Interventions
      1. From earliest point of intervention with child, encourage family to focus on child's special qualities, uniqueness, and abilities rather than disabilities
      2. Encourage self-esteem by providing positive reinforcement and praising child
      3. Help parents to set reasonable expections for child
      4. Educate parents in importance of appropriate limit setting with child
      5. Encourage responsibility by assigning appropriate chores (ensure that expectations are within child's ability to master successfully)
      6. Ensure appropriate school placement
      7. Facilitate involvement with peer counselors and support groups as indicated
      8. Involve child in adapted sports/recreational programs
      9. Refer child and family to appropriate community resources (i.e., local chapter of Spina Bifida Association; YMCA)
   D. HIGH RISK FOR INJURY RELATED TO COGNITIVE AND PHYSICAL LIMITATIONS

Interventions
   1. Ensure safety awareness and problem-solving ability with respect to all aspects of care (i.e., bowel, bladder, skin, respiratory, wheelchair management)
   2. Educate client/family in safety related to areas such as
      · Lower extremity management (i.e., prevent burns, frostbite, pressure ulcers, trauma)
      · Community issues (i.e., traffic and playground safety, stranger danger; fire; poison prevention)
      · Personal (child sexual abuse prevention: child is in charge of own body, private versus nonprivate body parts, and child's right to say no)

III. BRAIN INJURY
   A. HIGH RISK FOR INEFFECTIVE FAMILY COPING
      Interventions
      1. Educate client/family regarding brain injury (i.e., location and sequelae of injury; potential physical and cognitive deficits; strategies for managing residual effects)
      2. Assist family to verbalize feelings related to situation (structured counseling sessions and/or spontaneous interactions through the course of daily activities)
      3. Assist family to implement established behavior program
      4. Refer client and family to head injury support groups
      5. Assist client/family to locate appropriate community resources (i.e., day care programs; respite services; attendant care)
   B. SLEEP PATTERN DISTURBANCE
      Interventions
      1. Log current sleep-wake patterns; determine child's premorbid sleep patterns
      2. Schedule therapies and other medical procedures during nonsleep, nonrest periods
      3. Establish appropriate rest periods and bed times
      4. Ensure that environment is conducive to uninterrupted sleep (i.e., decrease light, noise, and schedule medical and nursing procedures such that sleep is not disturbed)
      5. Ensure that nourishment and toileting needs are addressed before rest/sleep times
      6. Implement relaxation techniques before hour of sleep (i.e., warm bath or shower, deep breathing, guided imagery, soft music, child's favorite comfort item within reach [stuffed animal, blanket])
      7. Give medications as ordered to reverse or facilitate sleep cycle
   C. ALTERED THOUGHT PROCESS RELATED TO DECREASED ATTENTION SPAN; MEMORY LOSS; IMPULSIVITY; PROBLEM-SOLVING DEFICITS

Interventions
1. Provide concrete explanations to child regarding all interventions
2. Cue child to provide direction
3. Provide a low-stimuli environment to increase ability to attend to task
4. Develop a memory book to assist child with daily routine
5. Collaborate with psychologist to develop a behavior program
6. Praise and reward child for appropriate behaviors and redirect from inappropriate behaviors
7. Ensure proper school placement based on neuropsychological testing
8. Ensure that behavior programs are understood and implemented consistently by interdisciplinary team, family, and school personnel

IV. BURNS
  A. ALTERED COMFORT RELATED TO DRESSING CHANGES AND THERAPY PROCESS
     Interventions
     1. Explain rationale and importance of procedures to child (based on developmental age) and family
     2. Offer choices where they exist (i.e., "We can do your dressing change at 8 AM or 10 AM. Which would you prefer?")
     3. Provide analgesia as ordered before painful procedures (i.e., dressing changes, application of pressure garments, and therapy)
     4. Assess and document effectiveness of medication to ensure appropriate analgesia
     5. Implement relaxation techniques before painful procedures (i.e., deep breathing, guided imagery)
     6. Encourage client/family participation in dressing changes and/or therapy as much as possible
     7. Praise child for cooperation with procedures; never chastise child for crying or demonstrating fearful or pain-related behaviors; comfort child as appropriate
  B. ALTERED NUTRITION: LESS THAN BODY REQUIREMENTS
     Interventions
     1. Educate child/family on the important role of nutrition in burn healing and tissue repair
     2. Assist child to select preferred foods to ensure high-protein, high-calorie diet
     3. Supplement meals with high-protein, high-calorie snacks two to three times daily
     4. Monitor weights weekly; graph for visual assessment of progress toward goal
     5. Encourage family to bring preferred foods from home or pack preferred foods to send to school for lunch and snacks
     6. Encourage child to participate (as appropriate) in meal/snack preparation; this process also could incorporate upper extremity ROM exercises

  C. HIGH RISK FOR IMPAIRED SOCIAL INTERACTIONS
     Interventions
     1. Encourage child to communicate feelings regarding burn procedures and disfigurement (via verbalization, drawing, interactions with "burn puppets")
     2. Encourage child's participation in hospital socialization (i.e., child life and/or therapeutic recreation activities) and school functions
     3. Educate other children on hospital unit and/or in child's classroom around sequelae of burns and what to expect regarding appearance and experiences of affected child
     4. Refer child/family to burn support group and/or introduce peer counselor
     5. Assist child in identifying an area of interest on which child can focus, interact with peers, and achieve some mastery (Hoeman, 1992; Ricci-Balich, 1994)

OUTCOMES

Rehabilitation facilities, like most organizations, measure outcomes as a method of evaluating the effectiveness of their programs. Outcome measurement tools are used to identify the level at which a client is functioning on admission and discharge, thus enabling detection of improvement in functional categories or activities of daily living (ADL). These measures are being evaluated for use in home and community settings, as well. Some examples of areas that are rated include transferring, toileting, bathing, and cognitive functioning (i.e., communication, problem-solving, memory). The information is utilized by rehabilitation programs to assess their effectiveness and make necessary adjustments to improve client outcomes. Chapter 11 provides detailed information for all age groups.

Outcome measurement tools traditionally were developed by individual programs or facilities. However, it became apparent that there was a nationwide need for documenting the severity of disability and the outcomes of medical rehabilitation in a uniform language. The Uniform Data System (UDS) for Medical Rehabilitation was established to ensure uniformity in definitions and measures of disabilities and outcomes in rehabilitation. The Functional Independence Measure (FIM) tool was developed to assess 18 items relative to self-care, sphincter management, mobility, locomotion, communication, and social cognition on a seven-level scale.

The UDS serves as a central repository for client data and provides reports of comparable data for quality management to subscribing facilities. The process is dependent on reliable data collection and reporting by facilities and quality control of data received by the UDS. Raters are credentialed to ensure knowledge of FIM definitions and levels (UDS, 1991).

A Functional Independence Measure for Children (WeeFIM) was developed to reflect functional and criteria differences seen in children due to developmental age. The tool is used with children from 6 months to 16 years of age. Although very young children may score with a higher dependency factor at both admission and discharge due to de-

◆

FUNCTIONAL SKILLS CONTENT OF THE PEDIATRIC EVALUATION OF DISABILITY INVENTORY

SELF-CARE DOMAIN	MOBILITY DOMAIN	SOCIAL FUNCTION DOMAIN
Types of food textures	Floor locomotion	Comprehension of word meanings
Use of utensils	Chair/wheelchair transfers	Comprehension of sentence complexity
Use of drinking containers	Opening and closing doors	Functional use of expressive communication
Toothbrushing	In and out of car	Complexity of expressive communication
Hair brushing	Bed mobility	
Nose care	Stand/sit in tub or shower	Problem resolution
Hand washing	Method of indoor locomotion	Social interactive play
Washing body and face	Distance/speed indoors	Peer interactions
Pullover/front-opening garments	Pulls/carries objects	Self-information
Fasteners	Method of outdoor locomotion	Time orientation
Pants	Distance/speed outdoors	Household chores
Shoes/socks	Locomotion on outdoor surfaces	Self-protection
Toileting tasks	Scooting up and down stairs	Community function
Control of bladder function	Walking up and down stairs	
Control of bowel function		

From PEDI Research Group, New England Medical Center Hospitals, Boston, Massachusetts.

---

velopmental age, scores for older children can reflect gains in any or all areas measured. The WeeFIM can be used in both inpatient and outpatient settings, as well as in schools and community-based agencies.

The Pediatric Evaluation of Disability Inventory (PEDI) is a recently developed functional evaluation measurement tool (see the box above). The PEDI provides a comprehensive clinical assessment of key functional capabilities and performance in children between the ages of 6 months and 7 years. Older children whose functional abilities are not equivalent to chronologic norms, may be evaluated. The unique feature of the PEDI is the attempt to include social outcome measures, as well as those for ADL. The three domains attempt to measure what a child "does do" rather than what cannot be accomplished and the level of caregiver assistance required. A separate scale, the modifications scale, documents environmental modifications or adaptive equipment a child uses to perform ADL. The PEDI has been standardized on a sample of able-bodied children in the targeted age range (Feldman, Haley, & Coryell, 1990); other research to evaluate reliability and validity with specific populations, such as children with CP, is in progress. Rehabilitation professionals administer the PEDI in a clinical setting or by structured interview of parents, requiring approximately 45 minutes. Individual record booklets for maintaining a long-term profile and data entry software programs are available.

SUMMARY

The field of pediatric (re)habilitation continues to grow and evolve. Emerging populations (HIV/AIDS, drug-addicted infants, nonaccidental trauma, and the technologically dependent) present new challenges to the pediatric team. Chronic illness and disability affect children and their families at each developmental stage (Stein & Jessop, 1984). A developmental approach provides a useful framework for the pediatric rehabilitation nurse to address the physical, cognitive, and psychosocial needs of children with chronic disabling conditions.

Other issues that are critical to the field include strategies to promote health, prevent accidental and nonaccidental injuries, and provide early and ongoing intervention as indicated. Federal and state legislation has helped to ensure the rights of children and adults with disabilities. Although healthcare reform has not yet been clarified, universal coverage and health maintenance will certainly be beneficial for children. However, efforts toward cost containment undoubtedly will raise ethical questions, particularly related to high-tech procedures and ongoing care. Case management clearly will play an important role in quality and efficiency, as well as cost-effectiveness. The pediatric rehabilitation nurse is uniquely qualified to function in the role of case manager for children with disabilities. The nurse and other members of the pediatric rehabilitation team are influential in the development of children with chronic and disabling conditions as they mature into productive adults in our society.

CASE STUDY 1

Adam is a 6-year-old child with myelomeningocele who began first grade a few weeks before coming in for an outpatient evaluation. During this evaluation with the rehabilitation team, his mother reported to the nurse that Adam recently had expressed embarrassment about wearing diapers and had been teased by his peers. She was concerned that Adam was becoming more withdrawn and irritated. After completing the assessment, the following nursing diagnoses were identified:

1. Altered pattern of urinary elimination: urinary retention
2. Altered pattern of bowel elimination: neurogenic (areflexic bowel)
3. High risk for impaired skin integrity related to incontinence
4. Ineffective individual coping
5. Family coping-potential for growth

Short-term goals were to establish urinary and bowel continence through intermittent catheterization or external collecting device, and a regulated bowel program, and to promote effective coping for Adam and his family. Long-term goals included independence in bladder and bowel program and continued individual family coping.

In developing an educational plan, it is important to consider both the developmental age and any associated learning disabilities common in children with myelomeningocele.

Adam was encouraged to express his feelings about being different from his peers and about the teasing. His desire to get out of diapers was established and his participation in the plan was elicited. Since school-aged children are industrious and eager to master skills, Adam was given clear and concrete information regarding his urinary and gastrointestinal systems. Pictures and anatomically correct dolls were used to facilitate understanding of the body systems and the relationship between dietary measures and elimination.

Both Adam and his mother were taught how to perform the bladder and bowel programs. Adam was allowed to practice catheterization skills first on the model (doll), then on himself. Since he could not yet tell time, the catheterization schedule was linked to familiar events (when he awakened, after lunch and school, and before bedtime). A watch with an alarm helped to remind Adam of his schedule. The teacher and school nurse were involved to facilitate success of the program. He also was given the responsibility of recording his catheterization volumes on a chart (by coloring in the appropriate amount on a predrawn graduated cup). Adam's mother was responsible for supervision, coaching, and praising her son's efforts and achievements. She also maintained contact with the teacher, school nurse, and rehabilitation nurse. Both Adam and his mother were referred to the local Spina Bifida Association for support groups and family activities.

Over time, Adam gained more control over his body by participating in self-catheterization and bowel regulation. He achieved continence, which increased his self-esteem and allowed him to get out of diapers. Adam's mother and teacher reported that the child seemed happier and more confident, and that the teasing had ceased.

CASE STUDY 2

Anna is an 8-year-old child who was diagnosed with CP (spastic diplegia) at 2 years of age. She is the youngest of two children in her family. She attends an elementary school that has a separate classroom for children with orthopedic and cognitive disabilities.

Anna and her parents came to the pediatric rehabilitation clinic for a full evaluation and to address several specific concerns: bowel and bladder incontinence; limitations in communication with family and friends; and an ill-fitting wheelchair that she had outgrown. During the evaluation session, the nurse elicited more information from the parents regarding current bowel and bladder status and the impact of Anna's limited communication skills on toileting. Mild scoliosis also was identified on physical assessment.

During the session Anna's mother also expressed her concerns about her daughter being separated from able-bodied peers in school. Both she and Anna voiced the desire for mainstreaming at least part of the school day. Anna's parents also discussed the need for respite services, stating their difficulty in finding someone to care for Anna.

At the completion of the evaluation, the interdisciplinary team met with Anna and her parents to identify needs and to set mutual goals. The following were some of the goals:

1. Establish bowel and bladder continence and regularity
2. Control scoliosis with appropriate seating system and body jacket if necessary
3. Increase communication with augmentative system
4. Increase interactions with peers through inclusion in mainstream classroom, if appropriate, and other social situations
5. Locate appropriate respite services to allow child and parents some time away from each other

NURSING DIAGNOSES

1. Altered bowel elimination: incontinence and constipation
2. Altered urinary elimination: incontinence
3. Impaired communication
4. High risk for impaired mobility related to scoliosis
5. High risk for impaired social interactions

6. High risk for impaired skin integrity related to new body jacket and wheelchair

INTERVENTIONS

The nurse met with Anna and her mother to develop a bowel and bladder program. She collaborated with the physical therapist to identify a comfortable supportive seating device to be used for toileting needs and collaborated with the speech therapist to work on a means to communicate the need for toileting. School personnel were involved in the process to facilitate community follow-through and success of the program.

Since constipation was a problem identified by Anna's mother, education was focused on dietary, fluid, and mobility measures to enhance elimination. Some changes were suggested for Anna's diet and activity level. A toileting routine based on Anna's current elimination patterns was devised to establish continent voids and predictability of bowel elimination. The physical therapist recommended a commode chair, which provided support. She also instructed Anna's mother in transfer techniques and positioning to facilitate relaxation using a footrest.

The nurse instructed Anna and her parents on skin management and suggested a schedule to increase tolerance with the new body jacket and wheelchair. They also were instructed to report any skin compromise immediately, so that needed adjustments could be made promptly.

Social services and the neuropsychologist were involved to investigate the appropriateness of mainstreaming for Anna. Her parents also were provided information on the rights and entitlements that Anna could expect based on federal and state laws. They also were given information on resources for leisure and recreational activities to increase socialization in the community.

At the end of the session, a follow-up appointment was made to evaluate progress toward goals and implement changes as needed. Anna and her parents were encouraged to keep a record of successes and any problems that they may encounter with the established programs.

REFERENCES

Allan, W.S. (1958). *Rehabilitation: A community challenge*. New York, John Wiley & Sons.

Alperstein, G., & Arnstein E (1988). Homeless children—A challenge for pediatricians. *Pediatric Clinics of North America, 35*, 1413-1425.

American Hospital Association. (1992). *Something to think about . . .family violence: Report of the section for maternal and child health.*: Chicago, IL.

American Nurses' Association. (1988). *Nursing case management*. Kansas City, MO: Guturr.

Astbury, J., Orgill, A., Bajuk, B., & Yu, V. (1990). Neurodevelopmental outcome, growth and health of extremely low birthweight survivors: How can we tell? *Developmental Medicine and Child Neurology, 32*, 582-589.

Beck, H., & Beck, M. (1982). A survey by day care centers and their services for handicapped children. *Child Care Quarterly, 11*, 211-214.

Bibb, T. (1990). Planting seeds: Thoughts on pediatric rehabilitation. *Journal of Rehabilitation, 56(3)*, 11.

Binder, H., & Eng, G.D. (1989). Rehabilitation management of children with spastic diplegia cerebral palsy. *Archives of Physical Medicine and Rehabilitation, 70*, 482-489.

Binder, H. (1992). Rehabilitation of the burned child. In G. Molnar (Ed.), *Pediatric rehabilitation* (2nd ed.). Baltimore: Williams & Wilkins.

Bird, W., Castellani, P., & Nemeth, C. (1990). Access to early intervention services in New York State. *Journal of Disability Policy Studies, 1*, 65-84.

Blum, R. (Ed.). (1986). *Chronic illness and disabilities in childhood and adolescence*. Orlando: Grune & Stratton.

Burkett, K.W. (1989). Trends in pediatric rehabilitation. *Nursing Clinics of North America, 24*, 239-255.

Caldwell, M.B., & Rogers, M.F. (1991). Epidemiology of pediatric HIV infection. *Pediatric Clinics of North America, 38*, 1-16.

Carlson, C.E., Ricci, J., & Shade-Zeldow, Y. (1990). Psychosocial aspects of disability in children. *Pediatrician, 17*, 213-221.

Centers for Disease Control (1991a). Weapon carrying among high school students. United States, 1990. *MMWR, Oct 11, 1991, 40(40)*, 681-684.

Centers for Disease Control. (1991b). Use of folic acid for prevention of spina bifida and other neural tube defects—1983-1991. *MMWR, Aug 2, 1991, 40(30)*, 513-516.

Cioffi, M., & Gaebler-Spira, D. (1990). Selective posterior rhizotomy and the child with cerebral palsy. *Topics in Pediatrics, Lesson 10*, 1-14.

Committee on Education and Labor. U.S. House of Representatives. Report on the Individual with Disability Education Amendment of 1991.

Crowley, A. (1990). Integrating handicapped and chronically ill children into day care centers. *Journal of Pediatric Nursing, 16*, 39-44.

Davis, B.D., & Steele, S. (1991). Case management for young children with special health care needs. *Journal of Pediatric Nursing, 17*, 15-19.

Denver Developmental Screening Test (1969). Denver: John F. Kennedy Child Development Center, University of Colorado Medical Center.

DiCowden, M. (1990). Pediatric rehabilitation: Special patients, special needs. *Journal of Rehabilitation, 56(3)*, 13-17.

Di Scala, C., Osberg, J.S., Gans, B.M., Chin, L. J., & Grant, C.C. (1991). Children with traumatic head injury: Morbidity and post-acute treatment. *Archives Physical Medicine and Rehabilitation, 72*, 662-666.

Drillien, C.M., Thompson, A.J.M., & Burgoyne, K. (1980). Low birth weight children at early school age. A longitudinal study. *Developmental Medicine and Child Neurology, 22*, 26-47.

Edwards, P. (1992). The evolution of rehabilitation facilities for children. *Rehabilitation Nursing, 17*, 191-195.

Erickson, E.H. (1963). *Childhood and society (2nd ed.)*. New York: Norton.

U.S. Department of Education. *Federal Register.* (1989). *Department of Education Part III. Early intervention programs for infants and toddlers with handicaps, Final regulations, June 22, 1989. 54*, 119.

Feldman, A.B., Haley, S.M., & Coryell, J. (1990). Concurrent and construct validity of the pediatric evaluation of disability inventory. *Physical Therapy, 70*, 602-610.

Fewell, R. (1986). Child care and the handicapped child. In E. Grunzenhauger & O.B., Caldweel (Eds.), *Group for young children*. Skillman, NJ: Johnson & Johnson.

Florian, V., & Krulik, T. (1991). Loneliness and social support of mothers of chronically ill children. *Social Science Medicine, 32*, 1291-1296.

Golden, G. (1983). The assessment of normal and abnormal development. In C.W. Daeschner, Jr. (Ed.), *Pediatrics an approach to independent learning*. New York: John Wiley & Sons.

Gittler, J. (1988). *Community based case management*. Paper presented at U.S. Surgeon Generals Conference, Washington, DC.

Harper, D.C., Wacker, D.P., & Cobb, L.S. (1986). Children's social preferences toward peers with visible physical differences. *Journal of Pediatric Psychology, 11*, 323-342.

Hoeman, S.P. (1989). Cultural assessment in rehabilitation nursing practice. *Nursing clinics of North America, 24*, 277-289.

Hoeman, S.P. (1992). Pediatric rehabilitation nursing. In G. Molnar, (Ed.), *Pediatric rehabilitation* (2nd ed.), (pp. 202-219). Baltimore: Williams & Wilkins.

Jaffe, K.M., Fay, G.C., Polissar, N.L., Martin, K.M., Shurtleff, H., Rivara, J.B., & Winn, H.R. (1992). Severity of pediatric brain injury and early neurobehavioral outcome: A cohort study. *Archives of Physical Medicine and Rehabilitation, 73*, 540-547.

Kohlberg, L. (1969). Stage and sequence: The cognitive-developmental approach to socialization. In D.A. Goslin (Ed.), *Handbook of socialization theory and research*. Chicago: Rand McNally.

Kraus, J.F., Fife, D., & Conroy, C. (1987). Pediatric brain injuries. The nature, clinical course, and early outcome in a defined United States population. *Pediatrics, 79*, 501-507.

Liller, K.D., Kent, E., & McDermott, R.J. (1991). Postpartum patient's knowledge, risk perceptions and behaviors pertaining to childhood injuries. *Journal of Nurse-Midwifery, 36*, 355-360.

Molnar, G. E. (1988). A developmental perspective for the rehabilitation of children with physical disability. *Pediatric Annals, 17*, 766, 768-771, 773-776.

Molnar, G. (Ed). (1992). *Pediatric rehabilitation (2nd ed.)*. Baltimore: Williams and Wilkins.

National Pediatric Trauma Registry Fact Sheet Publications (NPTR). (1993). *RTC on rehabilitation and childhood trauma*. Boston: New England Medical Center and Tufts University School of Medicine.

Office of Technology Assessment (OTA) (1987). Technology dependent children: hospital versus home care. A technical memorandum. (OTA-TM-H-38). Washington, D.C., US Congress.

Pediatric Special Interest Group. (1992). *Pediatric Rehabilitation Nursing-Role Description*. Skokie, IL: Association of Rehabilitation Nurses.

Perrin, E.C., & Gerrity, P.S. (1984). Development of children with a chronic illness. *Pediatric Clinics of North America, 31*, 19-31.

Perrin, J.M. & MacLean, W.E. (1988). Children with chronic illness: The prevention of dysfunction. *Pediatric Clinics of North America, 35*, 1325-1337.

Philip, P., Ayyanger, R., Vanderbilt, J., & Gaebler-Spira, D. (1994). Rehabilitation outcome in children after treatment of primary brain tumor. *Archives of Physical Medicine and Rehabilitation, 75*, 36-39.

Piaget, J. (1952). *The origins of intelligence in children*. New York: International Universities Press.

Pontious, S. (1982). Practical Piaget: Helping children understand. *American Journal of Nursing, 82*, 114-117.

Ray, L.D., & Ritchie, J.A. (1993). Caring for chronically ill children at home. Factors that influence parent coping. *Journal of Pediatric Nursing, 8*, 217-225.

Reynolds, M. (1986). The educational needs of disabled children and youths. In R. Blum (Ed.), *Chronic illness and disabilities in childhood and adolescence* (pp. 75-96). Orlando, FL: Grune and Stratton.

Ricci-Balich, J. (1994) *Content from clinical practice guidelines at Rehabilitation Institute of Chicago*. Rehabilitation Institute of Chicago, IL.

Rivara, F.P., Kamitsuka, M.D., & Quan, L. (1988). Injuries to children younger than 1 year of age. *Pediatrics, 81,* 93-97.

Selekman, J. (1991). Pediatric rehabilitation: From concepts to practice. *Pediatric Nursing, 17,* 11-14.

Showers, J., & Garrison, K.M. (1988). Burn abuse: A four year study. *Journal of Trauma, 28,* 1581-1583.

Solnit, A., & Stark, M. (1962). Mourning and the birth of a defective child. *Psychoanalytical Study of Children, 17,* 523-536.

Spivak, H., Prothrow-Stith, D., & Hausman, A.J. (1988). Dying is no accident: Adolescents, violence, and intentional injury. *Pediatric Clinics of North American, 35,* 1339-1347.

Stein, R.E., & Jessop, D.J. (1984). General issues in the care of children with chronic physical conditions. *Pediatric Clinics of North America, 31,* 189-198.

Teague, B.R., Fleming, J.W., Castle, A., Kiernan, B.S., Lobo, M.L., Riggs, S., & Wolfe, J.G. (1993). "High tech" home care for children with chronic health conditions: a pilot study. *Journal of Pediatric Nursing, 8(4),* 226-232.

Thompson, C.E. (1990). Transition of the disabled adolescent to adulthood. *Pediatrician, 17,* 308-313.

Uniform Data System (UDS). (1991). *Uniform data system for medical rehabilitation.* (1991). Buffalo: State University of New York at Buffalo.

Vipperman, J.F., & McCook-Rager, P.M. (1980). Childhood coping: How nurses can help. *Pediatric Nursing, 6,* 11-18.

31

Geriatric Rehabilitation Nursing

Maria Brighton Radwanski, RN, MSN, CS, CRRN
Shirley P. Hoeman, PhD, RN, CRRN, CNAA, CCM

INTRODUCTION

Living longer in the United States presents an interesting paradox between retiring and enjoying the "golden years" and an 80% probability of acquiring one or more chronic, disabling conditions. Chronic illness and physiologic changes of aging increase the likelihood of physical limitations and disability disproportionately for older persons compared with younger adults. Furthermore, the number of older persons will triple by the end of the century in the United States as compared with the year 1900, while healthcare costs continue to rise. Members of this group consume a third of the country's healthcare resources; in another 50 years the figure will be 50%, including a 40% increased demand for hospital services (U.S. Bureau of the Census, 1990).

However, families continue to care for most older persons with disabling conditions; relatively few are in nursing homes. On the other hand, as many as 5 million older persons who are hospitalized annually would benefit from rehabilitation services. Whether in the acute stage of an illness or injury or in the community, rehabilitation services for the older person are built around maintaining functional abilities, assuring safety, promoting effective coping, preventing complications, and modifying the environment for maximum independence.

A key barrier to services is the misleading social construction of older persons into two distinct groups—those who are aging and those with disabilities—when in many instances they may be composed of the same persons. Another barrier is the medical model focus on cure for a population that relies heavily on care and assistive programs. Because the U.S. health system is in reality an illness care system, despite motions toward reform and cost benefits, the level and numbers of community-based services that would support self-care and rehabilitation interventions for older persons are fragmented and too few. Both barriers influence legislation, funding, and public policy against provisions for older persons, regardless of a person's function or severity of disability or impairment (Sheets, Wray, & Torres-Gil, 1993).

There are important differences in geriatric rehabilitation that require special attention from rehabilitation nurses. Beginning with recognition that chronic disease and age-related changes are irrevocable and often progressive, rehabilitation nurses promote the highest level of independent function possible across the continuum of care. Rehabilitation nursing expertise to assess; plan; offer early, rapid intervention; and identify factors that inhibit long-term management and protection of health, apart from disability, ultimately improves outcome (Brummel-Smith, 1990). Empowerment, independence, choosing and decision-making, dignity, self-esteem, and actualization often are ignored as values for older persons. In fact, the very nature of many programs and services limits older persons and fosters dependency (Hendricks & Leedham, 1991).

Demographics

Chronic disease and physical limitations that occur in the aging process make it difficult to discern whether a client's impaired functions result from preexisting limitations, as secondary symptoms or sequelae, or from an acquired condition or disability. Between 1983 and 1989 prevalence of chronic disease in persons over age 65 with a disability increased by 4 million persons, which represents roughly 40% of all persons with disabilities (Brummel-Smith, 1990). Numbers of persons with a disability who were over 85 years of age increased 27.9% over the same 6-year span. Advanced age also is related to incidence of chronic and disabling conditions: arthritis (49%), hypertension (37%), heart disease (30%), and orthopedic impairment (16%) (American Association of Retired Persons, 1990; Needham, 1993). Three fourths of persons older than 75 years have at least one limitation in their ability to perform activities of daily living (ADL) (U.S. Bureau of the Census, 1990).

HEALTHCARE FINANCES

In addition to carrying the largest burden of chronic illness, disability, and disease of any age group, older persons encounter multiple social, emotional, and financial disadvantages. Even when already designated as poor, elderly persons' poverty is 1.6% greater than for younger persons who are poor (Zarle, 1989). A familiar scenario is when postretirement income has not been sufficient to meet successive increases in healthcare costs coupled with injury or chronic disabling illness over a longer lifetime. Social Security, never meant to be the sole source of income for so many older persons, often is just that. In a related scenario, elderly widows who have never worked toward Social Security credits are living poorly without benefit of their de-

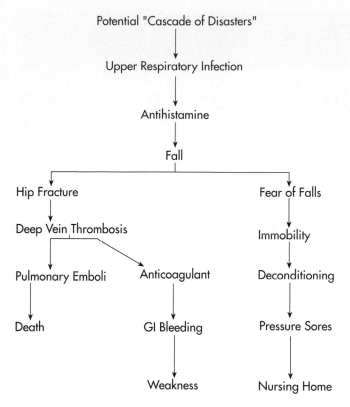

Fig. 31-1 Potential "cascade of disasters."

ceased spouse's vested pension income. Medicare provides scant coverage for treatment of chronic conditions or for health promotion. This trio of lowered income power, financial dependence with limitations in healthcare coverage, and chronic disabling conditions has a significant impact on health outcomes for older persons.

Clients who have experienced medical and functional difficulties before age 70 years are particularly frail. These frail elderly persons who develop a chronic, disabling condition become a particular challenge for rehabilitation nurses. At risk for complications, sequelae, and further disabilities that may lead to successive hospitalizations, their complex problems have been described as a potential "cascade of disasters" (Fig. 31-1) (Kemp, Brummel-Smith, & Ramsdell, 1990).

Similarly, community health nurses are familiar with frail elderly persons who have unmet basic needs, diminished social status with reduced opportunities for interaction and support, lowered self-esteem and sense of well-being, fewer choices for healthcare services, and decreased financial and physical access to appropriate healthcare products.

Upon assessment, frail elderly persons may have altered signs of a disorder accompanied by dulled or variant symptoms; thus skillful assessment is crucial to identify early signs warning of potential problems. Once hospitalized or with readmission, a client is guarded against developing disability or complications due to infection, immobility, impaired skin integrity, altered cognition, and preventable iatrogenic complications. Primary care needs of elderly clients cannot be ignored in lieu of attending to chronic, dis-

abling conditions. Maintaining general health status is another avenue of defense for these clients. Ideally rehabilitation nurses serve as clinical consultants to colleagues working with frail elderly clients in acute and community settings with goals of preventing complications through specialized assessment and attention to rehabilitation nursing principles. Key principles are those that promote the highest possible independent function and may influence long-term success (Brummel-Smith, 1990).

THEORETIC BASES OF AGING

A number of theories offer ideas about the aging process and views of social stereotypes about aging and elderly persons. Many have been questioned as discussed further in Chapter 1. The following Box summarizes commonly held theories and concepts about aging.

Variables Associated with Aging

The multiple physical, financial, social, and psychological variables associated with aging require a rehabilitation nurse to be astute about the uniqueness of this population. For instance, an older person may experience numerous mental and physical changes throughout a typical day. As a result symptoms often are expressed vaguely, and different caregivers may offer contradictory information about a client's behavior and status. Older persons may use different language or terms to describe or refer to conditions; some may not speak English well; others may be modest about discussing certain topics. Assuring that older persons have privacy and treating them with dignity and respect goes a long way toward building trust and rapport.

Data collection may occur at intervals over several days, take longer to collect, and be volunteered at a slower pace. Careful attention to what the client states as the problem, or how a chronic condition is described, will assist the rehabilitation nurse to make an accurate comprehensive assessment.

FUNCTIONAL ASSESSMENT

Functional assessment has become an essential component of rehabilitation nursing practice. Subjective assessment of health is the most significant predictor of functional status in the elderly adult, especially when clients return to live in the community. In a 4-year study of outcomes, persons (n = 2624) were assessed within 7 days of admission to 43 proprietary nursing homes after hip fracture and again at 1 month. Multivariant analysis of data revealed persons who had functional abilities and social supports were more likely to return home; those with physical or cognitive impairments and who used certain medications (cardiac, antidepressants, or narcotics) were at risk for dying (Kiel, Eichorn, Intrator, Silliman, & Mor, 1994).

The emphasis is on the person's physical and psychosocial abilities to perform life skills, rather than on the parameters of physical or mental health, because ability to perform these skills directly impacts independence and promotes mobility. In this regard, health problems and complications, including mental health, have been linked with lowered level of activity or inability to perform ADL. Maintaining function is a most important aspect of health to the older person because it impacts quality of life. Research

THEORIES OF AGING

Biologic theories	Describe cause-and-effect relationship between body system function and effect on individual over time.
Cross-link theory	Explains that chemical reactions within the body's DNA block cell division and affect normal function of the cell.
Immune theory	Implies that immune responses create an internal war within the aging body, which essentially destroys itself from an autoimmune response.
Free-radical theory	States lipofuscin occurs from fat-protein metabolism. In the aging body this chemical increases in amount and interferes with diffusion and intracellular transport.
Stress theory	Accounts for aging due to "wear and tear" of physiologic parts over time and load on psychosocial responses.
Programmed theory	States that aging occurs as a result of a genetically predetermined time clock that runs out, causing aging to occur in every individual.
Psychosocial theories	Indicate there are some interactions between aging adult and society, which result in changes in relationships.
Disengagement theory	Suggests a norm for society and aging person to withdraw from one another to allow society to continue its function without interference with youth.
Activity theory	Suggests society and aging adult continue to have an interdependent relationship, and although roles change for aging persons, they have continued importance. New roles and activities are expected in order to fulfill needs of the community.
Developmental theory (or continuity theory)	Implies that there are a wide variety of relationships between aging individual and society, which is influenced by individual's previous life roles and behaviors. Erickson's last developmental stage of Integrity versus Despair states that developmentally certain tasks are necessary for aging person to successfully adjust to the last years. Failure to achieve integrity results in despair, even death. These tasks include retirement, adjusting to loss and relocation, as well as maintaining generational ties. Other developmental tasks are to find new interests and hobbies while trying to find meaning to life and prepare for death.

findings indicate persons were significantly at risk for dying when they experienced loss of ability to manage money or make telephone calls accurately (cognitive decline) when they had a simultaneous decline in lower body functioning (Zadai, 1985).

Successful long-term or discharge planning takes into account a client's lifestyle, health beliefs, and practices before hospitalization. When a client seemingly is resistant to a care plan, ask questions to elicit details about the person's premorbid self-care practices, management of health and chronic illness, perceived functional impairment, and level of understanding, which may conflict with the care plan. The following box contains questions to assist nurses to obtain lifestyle information when interviewing an older client.

A number of functional evaluation instruments are avail-

♦

GERIATRIC ASSESSMENT STRATEGIES

Rehabilitation nurses are encouraged to incorporate the following questions into their interviews with clients who are older adults. Client responses to the questions, which address areas of particular pertinence and sensitivity for many older clients, predictably will provide information that would have been absent from a standard assessment. Specific strategies to elicit geriatric concerns will lead to more accurate and appropriate assessments, goals, and plans for care—thereby improving a client's trust and participation.

Don't ask if . . . ask how much
Present a potentially value-laden question in a neutral tone.
Example: Instead of "Do you drink alcohol?" ask: *"How many six-packs can you drink in a week?"*

Ask why, why, why
Persist with questioning to try to get to the root of a symptom, particularly if complaints are vague or confusing.
Example: *Why does the client have skin breakdown?*
   Because she has diarrhea.
Why does she have diarrhea?
   Because she has had it since surgery last year.
Why has she had it since surgery?
   Because she has been on a low-residue diet and anticholinergic drugs.

Ask specific questions about previous medication schedule practices at home
What medications have you been taking at home?
When did you take your medication?
What over-the-counter medications do you use from the drugstore?
How often do you skip your medication to make it last longer?
What medications do you share with someone else who has similar problems?
Have client bring medications from home. Observe client's dexterity, and ability to read medication labels. Older persons may share medications, use multiple or outdated prescriptions, use home remedies, or visit other healing practitioners without offering this information.

Ask specific questions about client's ability to perform functional skills at home
What trouble have you had managing your checkbook?
How often have you fallen within the past year?
Tell me what you usually eat each day for breakfast, lunch, dinner, and snacks?

Are there things you must ask family or others to do for you when they visit?
Ask who purchases, prepares, and stores food. Request clients to describe or demonstrate how they perform an activity or task. People devise innovative means for accomplishing their needs. Safety is one issue, but assistive devices or adaptive equipment may be other solutions to maintain independence.

Ask about health management practices
How many times did you visit the doctor last year?
Determine purpose of visits, number of physicians client visited, problems client was experiencing at each time.
What problems have you had in keeping the doctor's advice?
Do you visit or consult with other "doctors" or healers?
Do you have specific health practices that are important to you?
What does the health behavior or practice mean to you?
What will happen if you do not do this (behavior or treatment)?
What else do you do along with this action?
Evaluate folk practices, cultural beliefs and behaviors, personal patterns, and use of multiple lay and professional practitioners.

able to provide objective, reliable, and valid information to help members of the rehabilitation team to fully appreciate the functional status of each client. Chapter 11 provides information on functional evaluation. When evaluation scores are integrated with other observations, the nurse can work with the client and family to determine the meaning of impairments in their lives. For instance, a client's ability to understand, obtain, and self-administer medications is a practical functional ability that improves the likelihood of being able to live in one's own home in the community.

Principles associated with geriatric rehabilitation integrate chronic illness, the aging process, and functional abilities for the whole person (Zuckerman, Zetterburg, & Frankel, 1990). Risk factors related to disease, physical performance, cognitive impairment, and others may predispose a client to developing complications or further disability. During all levels of healthcare, not only during rehabilitation, preventive interventions and attention to maximizing functions improve outcomes and quality of living (Andrews, 1985). The case study (p. 697) highlights how and why rehabilitation nursing principles transfer across institutional lines and levels of intervention by tracing the path of a person with renal disease through the health system.

However, factors that may inhibit a client's full potential require repeated assessment before planned changes are incorporated into a person's routine. For instance, when retraining a client to learn ADL such as dressing or bathing, the nurse should include healthcare practices as part of the daily routine. Since many rehabilitation skills are taught using repetition, assure the environment remains nonthreatening and focus on skills a client will use on returning to the home environment. Although there are barriers in the community and obstacles in the home, the controlled environment of a rehabilitation facility can in itself place limits on a client's functional outcomes.

The following example illustrates a common obstacle to effective change in healthcare practices. A rehabilitation nurse is teaching a client who has insulin-dependent diabetes how to monitor her blood glucose levels in preparation for her to continue monitoring at home. A daughter shops for groceries but does not understand her mother's diabetic diet. The "cascade of disasters" (Fig. 31-1) occurs when the client becomes disoriented with hyperglycemia, forgets what she was taught about treating hyperglycemia with an extra insulin dose and monitoring blood glucose. The client quickly is readmitted to an acute care hospital for "noncompliance" in diabetic management. In contrast, an effective interdisciplinary rehabilitation plan would include both client and daughter, encourage them to plan a week's menu under a dietitian's supervision, and demonstrate knowledge and skills before the client's discharge to home. One rehabilitation nursing role function is to identify factors that may inhibit healthy lifestyles, which ultimately impact self-care and independence.

EFFECTS OF THE AGING PROCESS ON BODY FUNCTION

Some changes that occur due to aging processes may be difficult to distinguish from those that occur in response to disease (e.g., cardiopulmonary changes). The box on p. 688 displays a list of body system changes that may be due to chronic conditions or associated with aging. Vague and nonspecific symptoms, often poorly described by clients, may mask or mimic disease or chronic conditions. For example, cardiopulmonary system problems may underlie what initially are thought to be signs of renal disease. Conversely, symptoms of angina may appear only as numbness in the hands or lower arms without other classic signs.

Activity and Falls

Physical functioning in older adults is a key to maintaining cardiopulmonary fitness, muscle and bone mass, flexibility, independence, and quality of life as well as reducing body fat and perception of pain. However, only 39% of older adults exercise on a regular basis; many are afraid to exercise due to the ever-present fear of falling. In fact, this fear is well founded as falls are a leading cause of death in older adults, and many more persons live after a fall with compromised lifestyles or disabling conditions. Safety is a priority issue for older clients in a facility but especially a concern for those living at home. Ironically, chance of falling is increased with age and sedentary lifestyle changes in body weight, fat, and muscle distribution, which alter a person's center of gravity. This combination triggers a rapidly descending spiral trajectory as the older person's strength, flexibility, and cardiopulmonary function decrease (Daleiden, 1990).

Exercise and Cardiopulmonary Status

With aging, the heart has a reduced level of reflex tachycardia from physical activity and experiences orthostatic hypotension more frequently, but at the same time has a higher normal resting systolic blood pressure (160/90 mm Hg). The heart is more prone to arrhythmias because the sinus node is working with only 10% of the original pacing cells. The ventricles thicken, and more of the heart's work depends on atrial contraction. The lungs have a lower vital capacity from decreased elasticity of the chest wall. Those who lead a more sedentary lifestyle can expect to experience more cardiopulmonary compromise when compared with persons of the same age who regularly exercise. Although the maximal heart rate decreases with age, exercise improves oxygen uptake as the respiratory rate increases with activity to compensate for the decrease in lung function. Chapter 19 provides additional information about cardiac function, and Chapter 18 provides additional information about pulmonary function.

Therapeutic Activity

A preactivity assessment is important to identify the client's preexisting cardiopulmonary history and exercise tolerance before initiating the exercise program to anticipate any problems. Monitor vital signs (including lying and sitting): blood pressure, pulse, and respirations at rest and with initial trials of new activities. Vital sign and symptom assessment (see box, p. 689) is important when initiating new activity in older adults to assure cardiopulmonary tolerance to new activity stressors (Morgan, 1993). If symptoms are observed, activity is halted, and the client is reassessed after 5 minutes of rest (van Parys, 1987).

EFFECTS OF AGING PROCESS AND CHRONIC ILLNESS

Cardiopulmonary	Reduced work capacity, reduced reflex tachycardia, orthostatic hypotension, decreased pumping force of heart, higher resting systolic blood pressure, decreased lung vital capacity, increased risk of pulmonary infection, increased AV blocks and other arrhythmias, increased significance of risk factors for cardiopulmonary disease
Musculoskeletal changes	Decreased height; decreased stature and posture; decreased mobility; redistribution of body mass, fat, and bone minerals; muscle atrophy from disuse; slowed movement to accommodate for decreased range of motion, diminished strength, stiffening of joints
Skin changes	Thinner; paler; delayed healing time; less vascularity to skin and subcutaneous tissue; fewer sweat and sebaceous glands; dryer; less thermoregulatory control; nails more brittle; increased incidence of corns, calluses
Neurologic	Decreased cerebral blood flow, short-term memory; decreased balance and coordination; slowed reflexes and decreased response time
Sleep patterns	Longer to fall asleep, less REM sleep, more nighttime awakenings, quicker transitions between sleep cycles, frequent daytime and early evening "catnaps"
Bowel function	Less saliva, decreased gastric juices, less peristalsis, slower absorption
Genitourinary function	Hypertrophy of bladder wall, diverticula formation, decreased size and capacity, elevation in postvoid residual, change in sensation, vaginal hypertrophy resulting in urethral changes, female stress incontinence, prostatic enlargement
Liver function	Decreased size; decreased drug metabolism; and decreased protein synthesis
Renal	Decreased vascularity of nephrons, decreased glomerular filtration rate, decreased creatinine clearance, increased serum BUN and creatinine, decreased sodium conservation, slower adjustment to acid-base balance
Endocrine	Reduced insulin secretion and decreased glucose tolerance

AV, atrioventricular; REM, rapid eye movement; BUN, blood urea nitrogen.

Medications

Anticipate that older adults may need medication adjustment (e.g., antihypertensives) with the initiation of physical activity. Ask the client how the activity is being tolerated. With any activity, an individual with a sedentary lifestyle, a disabling condition, and/or cardiopulmonary compromise will expend more energy per unit of time. Regardless of physical limitations, allow clients to move at their own pace to achieve improved cardiopulmonary and musculoskeletal conditioning without symptoms of cardiopulmonary compromise (Fintarone & Evans, 1990). Evaluate safety techniques, environment; client's balance, alertness, and strength; time of day and energy level; current psychosocial attitude; and activity goals versus tolerance (Hamdorf, Withers, Penhall, & Plummer, 1993; Lampman, 1987; Simpsom, 1986).

PREPARATION FOR FUNCTIONAL INDEPENDENCE AFTER REHABILITATION

Rehabilitation nurse's assessment of the home environment before a client leaves the facility can provide the basis for an individualized plan to maximize the client's function in the home environment. Balance problems, limitations in mobility from age-related musculoskeletal changes and acquired disabilities, or sensory deficits, as well as cognitive impairments, may hinder a client's ability to live at home safely. Home accidents or illness leading to reinstitutionalization may impede the elderly person's functional abilities and eventually cause premature death.

A major goal is to prevent rehospitalization. Findings from research on functional changes in the elderly clearly link hospitalization with reduced functional abilities. Furthermore, although reduction in functional abilities is a consequence of aging, the capacity for improved function and community residency is possible for many older persons (Mor, Wilcox, Rakowski, & Hiris, 1994). Thus rehabilitation nursing interventions during a rehabilitation program optimize a client's cardiopulmonary and musculoskeletal function by encouraging the individual to engage in therapeutic activity essential to improve functional abilities and prevent complications. Many rehabilitation facilities have small apartments furnished and equipped to simulate a

---

VITAL SIGN PARAMETERS DURING PHYSICAL ACTIVITY

Evaluate and document vital signs before and 5 minutes after initiating new physical activity. Stop activity if any of the following are observed:

- ✦ Resting heart rate >100 beats/minute
- ✦ Exercise heart rate >35% above resting heart rate
- ✦ Exercise systolic blood pressure >25-30 mm Hg above resting blood pressure
- ✦ Decrease in systolic blood pressure >20 mm Hg
- ✦ Angina at rest or with activity
- ✦ Increased work of breathing including use of accessory muscles or substernal retraction
- ✦ Diaphoresis
- ✦ Dizziness/lightheadedness
- ✦ Excessive fatigue
- ✦ Pallor/cyanosis
- ✦ Onset of mental confusion or restlessness
- ✦ Inappropriate incoordination or change in coordination

---

home environment. Families and clients are able to test their skills and abilities privately but with the confidence of nursing backup in event of an emergency. Preparation for living at home begins with identifying each client's individual needs and preferences for personal care, then adapting the unit environment in the institution to closely resemble the environment on discharge, so a client can make the transition home safely and easily. In some instances older persons may not speak English. Without translation assistance information about daily activities and instructions will not be clear, and schedule changes may lead to confusion or misunderstanding. To assure continuity, the facility-based rehabilitation nurse places referrals and consults with community health nurses or community-based rehabilitation nurses and case managers.

Modifications to a person's home intrude on a very private part of life; some changes may reduce the aesthetic nature of the home. Explaining the reasons and the exact nature of changes in advance, involving the client and family in decision-making, being sensitive to their lifestyle and values, seeking the easiest and least expensive options possible to achieve necessary results, and helping them to envision how changes will create a safe environment for optimal independent function, while eliminating the risk for falls, are all ways to minimize the loss and stress of change (Tideiksaar, 1990). Provisions of the Americans with Disabilities Act (ADA) are pertinent to access for older persons and explained further in Chapter 5. Members of the interdisciplinary team may be able to make recommendations about ways to alter the client's home environment to assure safety while maintaining maximum independent function. Community health nurses in conjunction with the client, family, and members of the interdisciplinary team offer the most effective recommendations. Several special environmental needs common to safe function for older persons include adequate lighting, level and uncluttered floor

walkways, water temperature controls on bath fixtures, smoke detectors, furnace and electrical inspections including small appliances, access to telephone and ability to dial and communicate, emergency response system, food preparation and storage, and adaptive equipment maintenance and repair. Some persons require emergency backup systems for electricity in event of a power outage. A cordless telephone that can be transported while the client is using a walker or is in a wheelchair makes it easier to dial or answer the telephone but also may prevent injury from hurrying to answer the telephone. Chapter 9 details components of a home assessment.

Consider a Client's Home Environment and Lifestyle

The following questions help nurses to plan with clients and families for appropriate and relevant living at home while meeting rehabilitation goals:

- ✦ How far (how many feet) is client's bathroom from the usual daytime activity area?
- ✦ How far is client's bathroom from client's bedroom?
- ✦ Is client currently being wheelchair-propelled everywhere? (Should wheelchair use be discontinued in light of an approaching discharge date and inability to alter home environment?)
- ✦ Does client need to adjust before discharge to changes in environment or have appropriate changes been made at home to accommodate the new limitations? (An appropriate adjustment to the home would be to use a portable commode at the bedside or daytime activity area.)
- ✦ What type of bed will client be using? Is client dependent on head of hospital bed being elevated to get out of bed independently? (Client will never be able to get out of bed safely at home if current practice is continued until discharge. A potential alternative would be to remove head elevation controls from bed and assist client to learn to sit up from the supine position by rolling to her side and then push up with her arm or to use a rope ladder tied to the foot of the bed for client to hold onto and pull up.)

The rehabilitation nurse's understanding of these variables and effect on the functional outcome translate into therapeutic activity during care and treatment on the rehabilitation unit. The rehabilitation nurse encourages increased participation in all self-care activities while keeping in mind the need to balance therapeutic activity with energy conservation and rest. Creative therapeutic activities have been widely and enthusiastically received in rehabilitation facilities using seated exercise programmed to nostalgic music. Older adults feel safer working on increasing strength to arms and legs with low risk of falling and harming themselves. Quadriceps and gluteal sets, and upper body slow stretch activities promote needed conditioning and strengthening as well as improve walking gait and tolerance for distances. Side benefits are found in cardiovascular and respiratory conditioning.

OUTCOMES OF THERAPEUTIC ACTIVITY FOR PERSONS WITH SPECIFIC CONDITIONS

In clients with Parkinson's disease, activity and exercise enhance function by increasing the gait, grip strength, and fine motor coordination (Andrews, 1985; Korman & James, 1993). Unfortunately a therapeutic exercise program has little effect on changing the degree of rigidity and bradykinesia in the older person with Parkinson's disease. A high-carbohydrate and low-protein diet has been found to increase the efficacy of levodopa (Korman & James, 1993).

Many older persons who have undergone amputations of body parts also have existing cardiopulmonary conditions and other medical limitations. These persons experience great difficulty in the functional use of the prosthesis due to the cardiopulmonary stress from the weight of the prosthesis; even wheelchair mobility may be too stressful. With a lower extremity amputation, the condition of the remaining leg, such as peripheral vascular circulation, and premorbid functional level will impact prognosis for the person to walk with a prosthetic leg (St. George, 1993).

Soon after an amputation, clients have a tendency to develop maladaptive posturing habits that alter balance (Jackson-Wyatt, 1992). Typically clients hyperextend or flex the pelvis and lumbar areas, changing the center of gravity from midline to over the residual leg, resulting in altered balance and difficulty with gait training. Eventually adaptive pain syndromes may occur in various areas of the body (Jackson & Wyatt, 1992). A client requires consistent feedback from the rehabilitation nurse and interdisciplinary team members about postural maladaptation, each time these are observed, in order to prevent patterns of disabling behavior from developing.

Older clients with peripheral vascular disease are able to improve functional abilities through a therapeutic exercise program, as long as activity continues to the point when the client perceives fatigue or experiences intermittent claudication (Cifu, Means, Currie, & Gershkoff, 1993). Measurable gains in endurance and function for older persons with general deconditioning cannot be anticipated unless rest periods are interspersed with therapeutic activities; these clients simply do not have endurance and stamina.

As a rule, clients do better with short intervals of rest than with longer rest periods offered less frequently. Thus clients may be scheduled to lie in bed to rest for 20- to 30-minute periods spaced at intervals every 2 to 3 hours to allow two to three rest times throughout the activity portion of the day. The rehabilitation nurse and the team must consider individualized approaches to educating older adults regarding how to maintain a higher level of activity and adequate rest at home to prevent a return to a sedentary level of activity, in addition to ensuring the client's safety.

The person with an arthritic condition may alter posture and movement in response to pain. For instance, a client may hyperextend and flex the neck as a pain-blocking response—a maneuver that blocks cervical arteries as they pass through the vertebrae and produces cerebral ischemia, manifested as confusion and syncope episodes. The greatest rehabilitation outcomes are achieved through consistent interventions: ensuring adequate rest between therapeutic exercises, managing pain effectively, treating muscle spasms with graded activity, and teaching the client how to use movement principles to prevent further injury or complications (Cifu, Means, Currie, & Gershkoff, 1993).

Prolonged immobility may occur as an elderly person is stabilized following stroke. Immobility prolongs the time and level of intervention needed for functional training programs and adversely effects survival. Chapter 14 contains detailed information about complications of immobility and preventive nursing interventions. Exercise and activity increasingly are being initiated into the plan of care early on in the stroke program as a cost-effective form of preventive intervention. The results are to decrease the frequency of reflex sympathetic dystrophy-associated pain in shoulder-hand syndrome complications and the frequency and severity of contracture formation (St. George, 1993).

Shoulder-hand syndrome begins with pain in the shoulder, arm, and hand on the affected side of the body. Autonomic dysfunction emerges quickly, manifested by edema, pain, and altered sweating and skin color from altered circulation (Roth, 1988). Once skin and bone have atrophied, symptoms have progressed, until contracture occurs when pain and edema are resolved. Isolated shoulder pain occurs in up to 72% of persons who require extensive treatment time (2 months or longer) following stroke. In many cases isolated shoulder pain can be attributed a premorbid problem such as bursitis, prior trauma, or arthritis. Rehabilitation nurses are client advocates for assessing pain and discomfort, assuring pain management, and preventing chronic pain or distress. Nonsteroidal antiinflammatory agents (NSAIDs) commonly are used to manage these symptoms (Roth, 1988).

For either isolated shoulder pain or shoulder-hand syndrome, the affected arm requires protection early on and needs to be maintained within the joint space during range of motion and functional activities (Roth, 1988). This is best accomplished by supporting the arm on a lapboard or hemiboard attached to the arm of the wheelchair and with pillows under the elbow while in bed. Supports must be applied and positioned properly, monitored to assure they remain in place, and evaluated for therapeutic value. As a rule, slings and shoulder supports are not recommended as they may encourage synergistic spasticity within the scapulae and prohibit functional use of the affected extremity.

Spasticity and flexion-extension synergy begins as cortical shock resolves, approximately 2 to 3 weeks poststroke. Slow, sustained stretch of the affected side can prevent complications by eliminating synergy from primitive reflexes (St. George, 1993). Encourage clients to use the affected side as early as during acute levels of care and then in rehabilitation, as the limb has strong potential for function. This potential for function was demonstrated in a study of elderly persons who had hemiplegia following stroke. Clients in the experimental group allowed their affected arms to be restrained, while persons in the control group received no restraint. Clients were asked to move the affected arm by trying to remove the restraint, which subtly translated to self-taught movement. All clients in the experimental group used their affected arms, even though the arm was flaccid before the study (Taub et al., 1993).

Aging and Spinal Cord Injury

For the most part, spinal cord injuries are associated with older adolescents and young adults, usually as a result of trauma. However, over the past 10 years the mean age of persons treated following trauma has moved from 28 to 39

(Lazelek, 1994), which is attributed in part to the graying of America, prevention education programs, air bags, and increased seat belt use. Spinal cord compression as a result of degenerative disease and spinal cord abscesses are accounting for a larger number of older adult spinal cord injuries. It is often more difficult for the older adult who is frail and has reduced muscle strength to achieve the potential functional level.

As medical advances have made survival possible, rehabilitation nurses have prepared plans of care for the person who ages with a spinal cord injury. Less information is known commonly about quadriplegia and paraplegia that occur in older adults as a result of ischemia from spinal cord compression due to conditions such as tumors, spondylosis of the spine, or progressive neuromuscular complications; falls and accidents also increase the prevalence. Client outcomes are hampered by limitations of the aging process. For instance, musculoskeletal problems, including arthritis and general deconditioning, prohibit a client from achieving levels of rehabilitation outcome possible for younger clients. Restricted movement creates difficulties for preventing complications since many functional skills require a fair amount of upper body strength.

For example, independent management for pressure sore prevention by performing weight shifts while in the wheelchair or for bed mobility exercises may be difficult, even impossible, for an older person with cervical or lumbar spinal injuries to accomplish. Spinal cord injury creates limits in movement of respiratory muscles, which coupled with reduced mobility increases respiratory disease for older persons. This client's lifestyle, family situation, and psychosocial strengths and needs may dictate alternative or reduced expectations when setting functional goals.

Persons who incurred spinal cord injuries as youths and now are aged 65 years and older are experiencing onset of problems resulting from the physical wear and tear placed on their bodies. For instance, 70% have problems with their shoulders due to stress from upper extremity weight-bearing, including rotator cuff tears from transfers and wheelchair mobility, or crutch walking with lower-level injuries; pathologic fractures from changes in bone mineral density; and chronic pain in the lower back from the torquing of the back during transfers (Cifu, Means, Currie, & Gershkoff, 1993). Ambulation for persons with lower-level or incomplete injuries becomes less likely with aging as the person has decreased ability to handle the high energy demands.

As with the "cascade of disasters" (Fig. 31-1), decreased vital capacity has been attributed to problems with chronic gastric dilatation. Gastrointestinal function is a concern for the many adults with spinal cord injuries who have been maintaining a bowel management program twice a week, rather than more frequently. After years on a twice a week bowel program, a client may have chronic gastric dilatation, which adds difficulty to bowel emptying.

Continuing the "cascade of disasters," decreased vital capacity is associated with frequent respiratory infections and respiratory failure from increased respiratory weakness. Also these clients are more susceptible to pressure areas from the shearing forces during transfers, have decreased skin- and wound-healing time, and literally sit differently due to changes in the distribution of the body's fat and muscle. Obesity may occur with decreased activity even though a client maintains the same caloric intake. Personal attendants to assist with care, adjusting rest and activity levels and monitoring nutrition and medications, help clients to remain healthy.

Paced activities to improve strength are useful because cardiopulmonary improvement occurs at a lower threshold in elderly persons (i.e., with less activity) as compared with younger clients. When clients fail to improve or develop frequent cardiopulmonary symptoms, further assessment is needed to identify potential causes of cardiopulmonary compromise. Relatively low-cost assessment of work capacity and tolerance through the use of Holter monitoring, pulse oximetry testing with and without activity, and exercise endurance testing may identify why a client is unable to perform. The dosage of antihypertensive and diabetic medications in particular may need to be adjusted. Adding low-flow oxygen during activity will significantly improve the client's functional ability when tissue oxygen desaturation is identified.

With pulmonary disease, older clients receive the most benefit from rehabilitation when goals focus on maximizing existing respiratory abilities. Improving pulmonary function is not possible, but increased tolerance to activity and improved quality of life are possible when a client is taught to use techniques that conserve energy, pace activities, and enhance respiratory exercises, and to effectively use relaxation techniques (Zadai, 1985).

Sequelae of Early Life Disability in the Aging Adult

The child who experienced poliomyelitis in the 1950s now is middle- to geriatric-aged. More than 25% of these persons are experiencing post-polio syndrome with new residual effects after having reached a plateau in function for 25 years or more. Symptoms include excessive fatigue, progressive weakness, pain, functional deficits, and respiratory impairment (Macdonald, Gift, Bell, & Soeken, 1993). One theory is that muscle fibers that became overworked supplying energy for residual muscles after the onset of polio are tiring and aging early (Currie, Gershkoff, & Cifu, 1993). The cumulative effect of overuse and mechanical strain of compensating for weaker areas of the body has spawned new complications. Severity of new symptoms coincides with severity of the original disease symptoms but are worsened by recent stressor events such as bed rest due to illness, a fall, accident, or chronic illness.

Interventions for the person with post-polio syndrome are geared to reduce mechanical strain by supporting the weakened area and stabilizing joint movements. Chronic and acute pain management include moist heat applications or transcutaneous electrical nerve stimulation (TENS) to localized painful areas, posturing and biomechanics to avoid unnecessary strain, stress management techniques, alignment of balance of rest and activity with lifestyle, weight management, and supplemental oxygen or nighttime assistance with mechanical ventilation. Respiratory assistance may influence a client's overall sense of well-being and provide strength to perform functional activities independently during the day (Macdonald et al., 1993).

Cognitive Function

Cognitive function in the older person is an enigma for most healthcare professionals. Although acute and chronic cognitive impairment problems exist in the elderly, there is inadequate understanding, underdetection, and inadequate treatment and care (Neelon & Champagne, 1992). Confusion among the elderly fails to reach the attention of many healthcare professionals, perhaps because confusion as a normal aging response has become yet another medical myth. Indeed, confusion is a significant and highly prevalent health problem for persons who are acutely ill; prevalence is documented to be as high as 80% among hospitalized elderly adults (Evans, Kenny, & Rizzuto, 1993), often appearing as soon as the second day of hospitalization.

Environmental, sensory, and physiologic alterations may in themselves produce acute confusion. When confusion occurs fairly rapidly after a client is admitted to a facility, a combination of stressors related to hospitalization, medication, and associated physical illness must be ruled out. Some facilities permit a family member to stay with the client. An available family member recognized by the client may provide enough consistency in the environment to prevent or alleviate acute confusion. Later in hospitalization, confusion may have a variety of causes. For instance, electrolyte imbalances, hyperglycemia, hypoglycemia, dehydration, infection, fecal impaction, cardiopulmonary problems, nutrition, and drug use are frequent culprits leading to signs of cognitive impairment (Hadley Vermeersch, 1992; LeSage, 1991).

Acute confusion is a frightening state for clients and their families that shares some of the same symptoms as chronic cognitive impairment in dementias, such as in Alzheimer's disease (see the following box). Most professionals tend to rely on a client's alertness and orientation when assessing the confusional state. However, a more comprehensive assessment is required to determine the scope and characteristics of the confusional state (Champagne & Weise, 1992). Cognitive assessment encompasses perception, thinking ability, and memory, as well as alertness and orientation.

Assessment enables rehabilitation nurses to identify aspects of confusion specific to a client and interventions to prevent or reverse acute confusion that may be present (Champagne & Wiese, 1992). Acute confusion is treatable but when undiagnosed can continue indefinitely and progress to a more chronic confusional state. Cognitive dysfunction also inhibits the client's ability to perform personal care activities, inhibiting the functional outcomes of the rehabilitation program. Interventions must focus on preventing future problems, as well as addressing current problems that have caused the confusional state.

The Folstein Mini–Mental State Examination is used widely with well-established reliability and validity, but the instrument may not be specific enough for acute confusional states. The Folstein Mini-Mental State Examination assesses orientation, registration of information, attention and calculation, recall, and language. As with all the assessment tools, errors may occur due to medication use (Siebens, 1990), impaired verbal communication, sensory deficits, (Wilson, 1993), and cultural differences that may effect the outcome (Needham, 1993). Research results suggest that some alternatives in questions may be helpful in eliciting the information needed to identify deficits in cognition especially for long-term residents. (Feidler & Kilingbeil, 1990) (Table 31-1).

Delirium Versus Dementia

Delirium requires other management by first identifying potential causes, then aiming treatment toward underlying problems. Medications must be reconsidered; renal and hepatic changes in aging affect drug reabsorption; and excretion and toxicity may occur quickly. Medications that are problematic may be replaced with similarly acting drugs or eliminated whenever possible. Dehydration is another frequent culprit controlled by monitoring fluid intake, correcting imbalances in electrolyte values, and assuring adequate protein intake. Many of the newer antibiotics require clients to drink plenty of water, as much as 10 to 12 glasses a day, which many elderly persons do not like to do. Mobility, activity, socialization, and environmental cues with calendars, clocks, and adequate lighting (Gugel & Eisdorfer, 1986) are factors that may eliminate and prevent altered cognition for some. Reality orientation through group and individual therapy sessions will help the person to become more consistently oriented.

◆

CHARACTERISTICS OF CONFUSIONAL STATES

ACUTE CONFUSION (DELERIUM)	**CHRONIC CONFUSION (DEMENTIA)**
Acute onset; short duration	Long duration
Fluctuation in symptoms	Progressive symptoms
Short attention span	Short attention span
Reduced ability to shift attention	Personality changes and progressive behavioral problems
Impaired orientation (severity fluctuates)	Severe disorientation with confusion and mood fluctuations
Impaired short-term memory	Impaired long- and short-term memory
Distorted thinking	Impaired thinking and judgment
Distorted perception (delusions, hallucinations, or illusions)	Confabulates, unable to admit to memory deficits; impaired abstract thinking
Variable psychomotor behavior	Impairments interfere with social and functional abilities
Reversed sleep-wake cycles	Chronic confused sleep-wake cycles

Dementia is chronic confusion that does not respond to nursing interventions used for delirium. A number of physiologic and psychological causes for chronic dementia include brain tumors, hypothyroidism and hyperthyroidism, vitamin deficiencies, head trauma, degenerative neurologic diseases including Parkinson's disease, irreversible infectious diseases including acquired immunodeficiency syndrome (AIDS) and syphilis, and Alzheimer's disease. Confusion management in the elderly person with chronic confusion aims to balance doses of reality with meeting clients where they are. Thus reality orientation for persons who are chronically confused may increase the person's level of agitation.

A helpful alternative is reminiscence therapy (Needham, 1993), which places a focus on the reality that the person is currently engaged in through reliving past events. The nurse or therapist engages a client to review the important features of the life events being recalled and remembered. Instead of forcing a client to deal with present realities, the nurse engages the person in a discussion about the importance of the relationships and experiences from the past. For example, a client reminisces about her wedding day or the first time she waited for her children to come home from school. These exercises can be therapeutic and assist with meeting the person's developmental needs.

Restraints Versus Injury Prevention During the Rehabilitation Process

Clearly the use of chemical and physical restraints impede the rehabilitation process. The Omnibus Budget Reconciliation Act of 1987 (OBRA) provided landmark regulatory requirements for skilled nursing facilities. The act states all have "the right to be free from physical or mental abuse, corporal punishment, involuntary seclusion, and any physical or chemical restraints imposed for purposes of discipline or convenience and not required to treat the resident's medical symptoms" (OBRA, Section 1819(c)). Restraints have not been found to prevent many injuries; in fact, clients are at greater risk for complications associated with immobility, altered mental status, and loss of control or personal dignity (Quinn, 1994).

Exploring alternatives to restraint use has challenged personnel in all health facilities to identify multiple types of restraints, provide safe alternatives to restraints, and incorporate nursing interventions. The desired outcome is to provide a more therapeutic environment for older adults. For example, inadequate lighting and other unthoughtful difficulties in the older adult's environment alter perception and sensation, altering the older adult's awareness of time, place, and mentation. Higher levels of natural or artificial lighting are needed in order for older adults to see ad-

Table 31-1   Mini–mental state examination with rationale for the elderly

Assessment	Rationale
1. What is the date, season, day, month of the year?	Season, month, and year may be used if necessary to elicit client's orientation.
2. Question of location.	Suggest deleting this item because it has not tested as discriminating in research.
3. Tell client: "There are three items on a shopping list. (Name three objects that are associated independently.) You will be asked to recall them later."	Not as difficult to remember as compared with three disparate objects.
4. Tell client: "You buy a candy bar for 10 cents. You give the clerk a quarter. (Show client the quarter.) How much change should the clerk return to you?"	Erratic answers were around the number 10; found with spelling "world" and counting backward from 100 by 7's.
5. Ask client to repeat the three items from number three above.	
6. Ask client to repeat the following: "Cotton is grown in warm countries."	Phrase is propositional and is a reliable assessment of memory vs. "no ifs, ands, or buts," which could be repeated as rote return.
7. Instruct client to "Put (or mark) an 'X' on this paper, fold the paper, and give me the paper."	This is a more accurate three-step command as compared with, "Take this paper in your right hand, fold it in half, and put it on the floor." This is actually four steps.
8. Instruct client to write on this paper, "Put your hand on your head."	The command, "Close your eyes" was not discriminatory between two study groups.
9. Ask client to read the sentence, "We are going to paint the kitchen next week." Then ask client to write the sentence as read.	Telling a client to write a sentence was nondiscriminatory in the study group.
10. Instruct client to copy a design, a picture of a spoked wheel (example provided to client should be very round).	Copying a pentagon shape was not discriminatory between two groups.
11. Inform client: "You are late for an appointment with your doctor. What will you do?"	This is a newly added item intended to assess a client's multiprocess reasoning.

From "Cognitive-Screening Instruments for the Elderly" by I.G. Feidler & G. Klingbeil, 1990, *Topics in Geriatric Rehabilitation, 5,* 10-19. Reprinted with permission.

Table 31-2 Caring for persons at risk of falling

Risk factors	Nursing interventions
New admission or relocation	✦ Orient thoroughly to environment including use of call bell and bedside items ✦ Introduce to nursing staff and roommate(s) ✦ Provide agreed-upon place to store belongings and personal care items, dentures, prostheses, or assistive devices ✦ Encourage family involvement and visits ✦ Provide visible clock, calendar, familiar objects, family pictures, favorite pillow ✦ Use nightlight at bedside at night; keep surroundings well-lit during day ✦ Provide frequent observation by nursing staff, especially during night
History of falls and/or physical weakness	✦ Assess thoroughly for risk factors and causes ✦ Explore associated events (before, during, after fall) ✦ Use wheelchair, chair, bed alarm devices ✦ Provide antiskid mat at bedside ✦ Ensure easy access to bathroom and assure call bell is answered promptly; observe frequently ✦ Encourage timed voiding every 2 hours during daytime, every 4 hours during sleep ✦ Use bedside commode during hours of sleep for clients experiencing severe urgency, frequency, nighttime confusion, dizziness, unsteadiness at night ✦ Use comfortable chairs such as rockers, recliners instead of wheelchair when client is in bedroom or lounge ✦ Encourage mobility and activity ✦ Provide close supervision ✦ Encourage reconditioning exercises ✦ Encourage frequent, short rest intervals ✦ Provide nonrestrictive reminders to remain seated ✦ Use appropriate assistive devices
Altered mental status	✦ Provide visual cues to client to remind him to call for help ✦ Eliminate unnecessary noise ✦ Reduce visual stimulation ✦ Assign a room near nurses' station ✦ Provide adequate lighting ✦ Provide family education and encourage involvement ✦ Use companion or closer supervision ✦ Implement orientation exercises ✦ Consider medication, dehydration, or nutritional or electrolyte imbalances as potential causes
Altered psychosocial or emotional status	✦ Encourage decision-making ✦ Involve in establishing short-term goals or plan of action ✦ Perform psychosocial or psychiatric assessment and treatment as indicated ✦ Ask client and family to identify measures to aid in relaxation for inducing sleep (back rub, tea, music) ✦ When appropriate, gradually expand psychosocial environment
Visual impairment	✦ Assess vision ✦ Ensure eyeglasses are cleaned regularly ✦ Assess eyeglasses ✦ Encourage use of visual aids ✦ Provide adequate lighting ✦ Remove unnecessary furniture ✦ Avoid highly polished floors that produce glare ✦ Have unobstructed and nonskid floor surfaces ✦ Use colors to increase visibility (avoid blue/green combinations; use contrasting colors)

Adapted from *Reducing Restraints: Individual Approaches to Behavior: A Teaching Guide* by N. Strumf, J. Wagner, L. Evans, and J. Patterson, 1992, Huntington Valley, PA: Geriatric Research and Training Center. Copyright 1992 by University of Pennsylvania, School of Nursing. Adapted by permission.

Table 31-2 Caring for persons at risk of falling—cont'd.

Risk factors	Nursing interventions
Actual or potential incontinence	✦ Ensure easy access to bathroom and assure call bell is answered promptly ✦ Assess cause of incontinence ✦ Encourage timed voiding every 2 hours during daytime, every 4 hours during hours of sleep ✦ Use bedside commode during hours of sleep for clients experiencing severe urgency, frequency, nighttime confusion, dizziness, unsteadiness at night ✦ Have picture of toilet on bathroom door ✦ Encourage using easily manipulated clothing such as elastic waistbands
Postural hypotension	✦ Perform initial assessment of blood pressure lying, sitting, and standing ✦ Ensure adequate hydration (1500-2000 ml/24 hours unless restricted) ✦ Use elastic stockings ✦ Provide education regarding slow, gradual position changes
Medications	✦ Assess drug actions, interactions, side effects; include self-medication and over-the-counter products ✦ Assess drug substitutions or eliminations ✦ Consider changing medications that produce adverse side effects or discomfort ✦ Consider drug holidays with physician's order
Comfort	✦ Use relaxation measures identified as helpful by client and family ✦ Provide pain medication on a schedule if client is experiencing pain (or when suspected in client who is unable to communicate)

equately. "Sundowning" or simply giving thought to turning lights on before dark will prevent evening changes in mentation.

Falls are not random occurrences in the older adult. Common causes of falls in older adults include age-related physical changes and health problems (see box, p. 688), environmental factors, and other causes such as medication use and improper use of assistive devices. The elderly person must be identified for risks of falling and interventions initiated to prevent falls from occurring (Table 31-2). The most common locations for falls are bedrooms and bathrooms, for reasons such as trying to get to the bathroom and getting out of the bathtub.

Pain Management

"Few things we do for patients are more fundamental to the quality of life than relieving pain" (Dunwoody, 1987). However, pain is not always identified through nursing assessment or considered relevant enough in the care of older adults. The accuracy of pain perception frequently is devalued by the nurse. Physical signs vary, and client reports of pain are influenced by cultural and social norms, as well as communication and cognitive deficits, and may be confused with distress or anxiety. Pain assessment is identified most accurately by personal report. Pain is "whatever the experiencing person says it is, existing whenever he says it does" (McCaffery, 1979).

Assessment of pain is best accomplished by first determining the location of the pain. What precipitates pain; what typically relieves it? What is the severity of the pain? Severity of pain can be assessed easily using descriptor scales similar to those used with children. The vertical Visual Analogue Scale accurately and reliably depicts the escalating nature of pain, and the Faces Scale may be useful for persons with aphasia or slight confusion. Chapter 30 provides illustrations of Pain Assessment Scales. Pain Assessment Scale scores are used to reveal measures of the intensity of the pain experience at a given moment, assist the nurse with data to determine the most appropriate analgesic management, and evaluate the effectiveness of pain relief interventions.

Analgesic management has been established using standards set up by the World Health Organization (WHO, 1986) and the American Pain Society (1989). Analgesic management of acute, chronic, and neuropathic pain in older adults becomes a little more cumbersome due to age-related changes associated with drug metabolism.

Nonopioid analgesia works well in the treatment of mild to moderate pain intensity using acetaminophen, salicylate, or nonsteroidal antiinflammatory drugs NSAIDs. However, to obtain relief from pain that is constant, chronic acetaminophen use can cause problems with liver toxicity when exceeding more than 2500 mg/day. Administration of salicylate and NSAIDs requires special considerations in client pain management as gastric irritation and bleeding are frequent side effects except with choline magnesium trisalicylate (Trilisate).

Moderate to severe pain is best managed by combination therapy using nonopioid analgesics in addition to an appropriate opioid agent. Intramuscular routes are not recommended in any adult as the rate of absorption varies greatly and tissue necrosis is likely. Meperidine (Demerol) is of particular concern in the elderly as it will cause central nervous system neuroexcitation from intramuscular metabolism.

Neuroleptic agents such as phenytoin (Dilantin) and tricyclic antidepressants are helpful in potentiating the action of analgesics for mild to severe pain. In their own right, they are the preferred method of management for neuropathic pain that occurs as a result of neurologic injury or insult, tumors, or other causes. The client needs to be persistent with treatment as pain relief from these agents cannot be expected for at least 2 to 3 weeks after initiating their use. Some of the tricyclic antidepressants with anticholinergic side effects (such as amitriptyline) are best substituted with agents with lower anticholinergic side effects (such as fluoxetine hydrochloride) or the serotonin uptake inhibitors (such as paroxetine hydrochloride and sertraline hydrochloride), which also are effective in the management of neuropathic pain. Agency for Health Care Policy and Research (AHCPR) Clinical Practice Guidelines are available for rehabilitation nurses on the topic of pain management.

Teaching the Older Adult

Effectively teaching the older adult new skills in rehabilitation requires astuteness in assessment, communication skills, and ability to be flexible in approach. At the first level, assessing the client and family system's ability for new learning requires understanding of the client's traditionally preferred method for learning new information. Is the client a listener, reader, watcher, or a doer? Are there any age-related sensory changes that create challenges? Is the client's vision and hearing adequate to take in new information? Is this the best time of day for communication? For instance, older persons may experience diminished hearing acuity in early afternoon or when tired, as well as other subtle alterations in sensory functions not readily apparent. What does the client and family stand to lose by using this new information in practice? Is there a conflict with cultural practices, home remedy practices, or a shift in power or lifestyle for someone? What have the client and family's previous successes been with learning situations? What is the client and family's level of motivation? Is the client depressed, anxious, or confused? Can the client and family see any special benefits from learning the new information?

These questions are necessary to determine if there is readiness to learn new information and then use what is gained. "Noncompliance" is a loaded term often used by healthcare professionals to refer to behaviors when a client and family have not acted on plans or information taught to them. Most often the client and family have not incorporated the information into their routine because of misunderstood or deficient knowledge, functional inability or inadequate resources to carry out the recommendations, or lack of fit with lifestyle, preferences, or culture. Complexity of the treatment, cognitive dysfunction, and communication impairments are all barriers to compliance (Stilwell, 1988).

Older adults were "brought up" on a healthcare system that taught the clients to know little about their health status. Some of these traditional "customs" are attitudes that persist among healthcare providers today. For example, from acute care across the spectrum into long-term care, some health professionals continue to excuse family members from a client's bedside while treatments are performed. Then, when a discharge date is set, the client and family finally receive instruction about the treatment. The client and family passively learned the treatment was a "hands-off" item until directed by a nurse to learn "how" as a condition of discharge. How much easier and empowering for the client and family to participate in planning the treatment, observing and learning from the beginning with a gradual transition of skill and responsibility while the client was within the system.

Older adults and their caregivers respond well to information presented in layperson's terms that reflect understanding of what they really need to know. In other words, what value does the information have on the outcome of the client's care? The elderly adult and family need to see relevance in the information. If skills are required, what steps can be cut to make the skill as easy and as practical as possible for the home environment?

The rehabilitation nurse's nonverbal communication has tremendous impact on the learning experience. Take the example of teaching a female to self-catheterize. Does the nursing staff procrastinate teaching her for several days? (The client may think: "If they don't want to teach me, it must mean it's too hard for me to learn.") What impact does this have on the client's confidence in performing this skill? What merit does the client see in doing the procedure? She won't see much merit if she sees no personal gains. Could a personal motivator be dry skin and no urinary tract infections as per her history over the past 10 years? What merit would she see in "complying" with the catheterization schedule if she sees herself unable to leave home because she's only ever seen the procedure performed in bed? Tell her the expected outcomes from the beginning: she will learn first in bed to find the location of her meatus, identify how it feels, insert the catheter, and then she'll learn to do this on the toilet.

The older adult learns best when these needs are considered. As with all adult learners, adult learning principles need to be incorporated. Dialogue, consideration of the client's values and goals, and flexibility in approach reap the best outcomes. Finally, there is a need for repetition in order for older persons to incorporate new ideas into their lifestyle. Mutual goal setting and discharge planning initiated at admission drive this process, but clearly learning becomes part of daily activities when practiced routinely. There is no alternative: the rehabilitation nurse needs a clear insight into a client's needs early in the rehabilitation process. All staff involved in a client's care need to incorporate teaching the client and family the necessary skills early on to allow for sufficient practice and the beginning of new routines. Chapter 10 provides more information about client and family education.

LIFELONG, MULTISITE FOCUS OF REHABILITATION NURSING

As mentioned with the case study of a client with a renal impairment, many persons are living longer with multiple diagnoses, comorbidity, impairments, and altered functional status. These persons have chronic, disabling, or developmental conditions that generally will not be cured or resolved. They require comprehensive management that begins with onset or at admission to acute healthcare and continues through community re-entry and lifelong follow-up. Rehabilitation nursing process and management are key variables in improving outcome. When rehabilitation nurs-

CASE STUDY

A.M. is a 79-year-old widow who lives alone. Although childless, she has several very supportive friends. Her one-level ranch-style home has 13 steps to the front door, with a side hand rail extending from the street to the front door. For several months A.M. has experienced an altered gait unsteady enough to make walking difficult, but she denies any falling episodes. However, she does not go anywhere alone, depending on her friends to assist her with shopping and banking. She has performed household chores independently. She washes her clothes by hand in the sink as she has no access to a laundry.

During a routine visit to her primary physician, she reports the problems she has had with walking and notes that her urine has been chalk colored for some time. The physician admits her to the hospital for tests, which reveal acute and chronic renal failure, uremia, and anemia. After a 15-day hospitalization to begin dialysis, she is given a Tenckhoff shunt in the right side of her neck until a Dacron shunt is inserted in her arm.

A.M. is transferred to a rehabilitation hospital for acute rehabilitation. She is admitted with deconditioning. At admission she has difficulty walking, requiring moderate assistance for balance and use of a single-point cane. She requires moderate assistance with dressing and hygiene and displays signs of cognitive deficits. Her vital signs are stable, and she receives a 2-g sodium and potassium-restricted diet and fluids restricted to 1500 ml/day. Laboratory data obtained during her 3-day-a-week dialysis indicate elevated levels of potassium, sodium, phosphorus, BUN, and creatinine clearance. Results from the Folstein Mini–Mental State Examination suggest she has difficulty with short and intermediate recall and problem-solving.

A.M.'s goals on admission are to improve her strength so that she may return home and function independently with previous living arrangements. The rehabilitation nurse's goals are to evaluate the client's cognitive function concerning deficits related to renal failure, teach her about the disease process, prevent complications of renal failure by teaching and encouraging her about dietary, fluid, and medication management, and establish a bowel elimination program. The client's friends reveal that she has been consistently confused for several months before the hospitalization and express concern about her safety while at home.

The rehabilitation nurse notes that A.M. is experiencing difficulty learning her medication schedule. Therapists and other nursing staff report she has had difficulty reaching her rehabilitation goals of independence in ambulation and ADL. An interdisciplinary evaluation raises questions about her endurance. For instance, she experiences difficulty with endurance and complains of tiring easily during therapy; on the nursing unit she frequently asks nursing staff to lie down when she is not attending a therapy session. Her endurance appears to worsen during those days that precede her evening dialysis after therapy sessions are completed. A cardiopulmonary evaluation reveals that A.M. is desaturating during physical activity, with pulse oximetry dropping to 82% during ambulation. Oxygen is ordered at 2 L via nasal cannula during exertion.

During the interdisciplinary evaluation conference, team members express concern about safety and the level of assistance A.M. would require in order to return to her home. They argue that her confusion and inability to perform self-care activities will prevent her from living alone and file application for nursing home admission. A.M. is adamantly against this discharge plan and insists that she will not give up living in her home. She expresses mistrust of the social worker during discharge planning discussions.

Over the next 2 days, A.M. complains of shortness of breath, has a nonproductive cough, elevated temperature, apraxia with gait, and complains of pain under her rib cage with cough. She is noted to have increased confusion. Her legs are edematous, but her lung sounds are clear. Following a lung scan and chest radiograph, she is diagnosed with congestive heart failure (CHF), which is treated during hemodialysis. Over the next week A.M. is very weak after dialysis, prompting therapists to note a decline in her functional abilities. However, gradually her strength and mentation improve.

As a result of A.M.'s unwillingness to discuss and plan alternative living arrangements, the nurse and the social worker proceed with the plan for a discharge to home. A.M. begins an independent living program, gradually assuming responsibility for initiating ADL, performing her routine at the bedside on the nursing unit, and accepting responsibility for learning her medication schedule using a Mediset. Most of her medications require once-a-day dosing, and she receives one medication three times a day. The plan for medication administration at discharge will be for her to have medications prepoured weekly by a friend into the Mediset, and she will take the medications independently. She will receive Meals on Wheels, a home health aide will assist her with household chores, and she will receive occupational therapy and physical therapy two to three times a week once she is home. A.M. will take public transportation to and from the dialysis center three times a week. The dialysis is changed to daytime hours to accommodate public transportation.

Before discharge her weakness and confusion clear as a result of treatment of uremia and CHF. A.M. was successfully discharged home with visiting nurse services; she functions independently in self-care activities with a follow-up visit scheduled for 30 days after discharge. A.M. refused the home health services, and occupational and physical therapy services no longer are necessary. She continues to receive Meals on Wheels and takes public transportation to the dialysis center as scheduled. A.M. states she is pleased with her ability to continue to live independently and assures the nurse that she is doing very well at home.

The rehabilitation nurse prepares an inservice about the progressive effects of impaired renal function, which may affect every organ system in the body **(Fig. 31-2)**. A case study of A.M. is used to illustrate the multiple clinical manifestations that may occur with, mask, and exacerbate chronic uremia and how these manifestations may vary among clients.

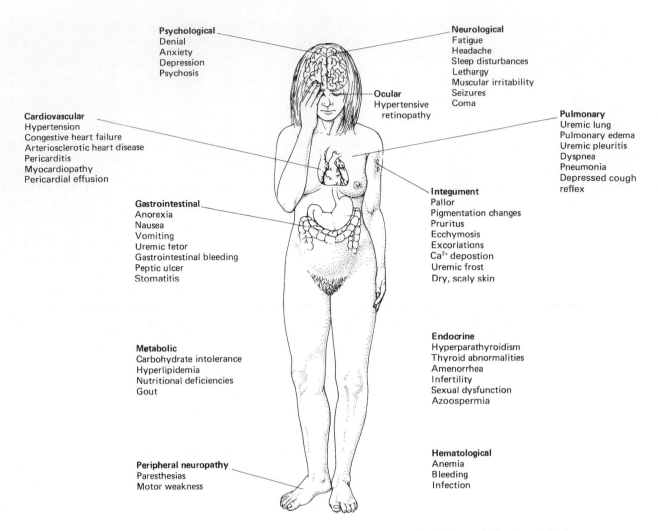

Psychological
Denial
Anxiety
Depression
Psychosis

Neurological
Fatigue
Headache
Sleep disturbances
Lethargy
Muscular irritability
Seizures
Coma

Ocular
Hypertensive
retinopathy

Cardiovascular
Hypertension
Congestive heart failure
Arteriosclerotic heart disease
Pericarditis
Myocardiopathy
Pericardial effusion

Pulmonary
Uremic lung
Pulmonary edema
Uremic pleuritis
Dyspnea
Pneumonia
Depressed cough
reflex

Gastrointestinal
Anorexia
Nausea
Vomiting
Uremic fetor
Gastrointestinal bleeding
Peptic ulcer
Stomatitis

Integument
Pallor
Pigmentation changes
Pruritus
Ecchymosis
Excoriations
Ca^{2+} depostion
Uremic frost
Dry, scaly skin

Metabolic
Carbohydrate intolerance
Hyperlipidemia
Nutritional deficiencies
Gout

Endocrine
Hyperparathyroidism
Thyroid abnormalities
Amenorrhea
Infertility
Sexual dysfunction
Azoospermia

Hematological
Anemia
Bleeding
Infection

Peripheral neuropathy
Paresthesias
Motor weakness

Fig. 31-2 Clinical manifestations of chronic uremia. (From *Medical Surgical Nursing,* 3rd ed. by S. Lewis and I. Collier, 1993, St. Louis: Mosby–Year Book. Copyright 1993 by Mosby–Year Book. Reprinted by permission.)

ing principles and techniques are instituted early and applied consistently during a client's plan of care, many threats to functional abilities and quality of life may be avoided or minimized. As hospital length of stay continues to be shortened, more clients have multiple diagnoses and problems, and acuity levels rise in rehabilitation and community settings, nurses must prepare themselves to attend to continuity in prevention of further complications or disability at all points of the healthcare system.

The nursing care guideline in Appendix 31-A is included to demonstrate how rehabilitation nurses may contribute to improving outcome for a client who has had a stroke, beginning with admission to a facility. It also contains information that will alert rehabilitation nurses to times and ways they may contribute, as well as receive nursing information, through nurse-to-nurse consultation with colleagues in acute care.

REFERENCES

American Association of Retired Persons. (1990). *A profile of older Americans.* Washington, DC: Department of Health and Human Services.

American Pain Society. (1989). *Principles of analgesic use in the treatment of acute pain and chronic cancer pain* (2nd ed.). Skokie, IL: American Pain Society.

Andrews, K. (1985). Rehabilitation of conditions associated with old age. *Internal Rehabilitation Medicine, 7,* 125-129.

Brummel-Smith, K. (1990). Introduction. In B. Kemp, K. Brummel-Smith, & J. Ramsdell (Eds.), *Geriatric rehabilitation* (pp. 3-22). Boston: Little, Brown.

Champagne, M., & Weise, R. (1992). Research on cognitive impairment: implications in practice. In S. Funk, E. Tornquist, M. Champagne, & R. Wiese (Eds.), *Key aspects of elder care* (pp. 340-6). New York: Springer.

Cifu, D.X., Means, K.M., Currie, D.M., & Gershkoff, A.M. (1993). Geriatric Rehabilitation. Diagnosis and management of acquired disabling disorders. Part 2. *Archives of Physical Medicine and Rehabilitation 74,* S406-S412.

Currie, D.M., Gershkoff, A.M., & Cifu, D.X. (1993). Mid- and late-life effects of early-life disabilities. Part 3. *Archives of Physical Medicine and Rehabilitation, 74,* S413-S416.

Daleiden, S. (1990). Prevention of falling: Rehabilitative or compensatory interventions? *Topics in Geriatric Rehabilitation, 5,* 44-53.

Dunwoody, C.J. (1987). Patient-controlled analgesia: Rationale, attributes, and essential factors. *Orthopedic Nursing, 6,* 31-36.

Evans, C.A., Kenny, P.T., & Rizzuto, C. (1993). Caring for the confused geriatric surgical patient. *Geriatric Nursing, 14,* 237-241.

Feidler, I.G., & Klingbeil, G. (1990). Cognitive-screening instruments for the elderly. *Topics in Geriatric Rehabilitation, 5,* 10-19.

Finatarone, M. & Evans, W. (1990). Exercise in the oldest old. *Topics in Geriatric Rehabilitation, 5,* 63-77.

Gugel, R.N., & Eisdorfer, S.E. (1986). Psychosocial interventions. *Topics in Geriatric Rehabilitation, 1,* 27-34.

Hadley Vermeersch, P. (1992). Clinical assessment of confusion. In S. Funk, E. Tournquist, M. Champagne, and R. Wiese (Eds.), *Key aspects of elder care* (pp. 251-261). New York: Springer.

Hamdorf, P.A., Withers, R.T., Penhall, R.K., & Plummer, J.L. (1993). A follow-up study on the effects of training on the fitness and habitual activity patterns of 60- to 70-year-old women. *Archives of Physical Medicine and Rehabilitation, 74,* 473-477.

Hendricks, J. & Leedham, C.A. (Eds.). (1991). *Dependency or empowerment? Toward a moral and political economy of aging.* Amityville, NY: Baywood.

Jackson-Wyatt, O. (1992). Age-related changes in amputee rehabilitation. *Topics in Geriatric Rehabilitation, 8,* 1-12.

Kemp, B., Brummel-Smith, K., & Ramsdell, J. (1990). *Geriatric rehabilitation,* Boston: Little, Brown.

Kiel, D.P., Eichorn, M.S., Intrator, O., Silliman, R.A., & Mor, V. (1994). The outcomes of patients newly admitted to nursing homes after hip fracture. *American Journal of Public Health, 84,* 1281-1286.

Korman, L., & James, J. (1993). Medical management of Parkinson's disease in the elderly. *Topics in Geriatric Rehabilitation, 8(4),* 1-13.

Lampman, R. (1987). Evaluating and prescribing exercise for elderly patients. *Geriatrics, 42,* 63-76.

Lazelek, U. (1994, May 31). LVH trauma unit treats fewer but older patients. *The Morning Call.* Bethlehem, PA.

LeSage, J. (1991). Polypharmacy in geriatric patients. *Nursing Clinics of North America, 26,* 273-290.

Macdonald, L.P., Gift, A.G., Bell, R.W., & Soeken, K.L. (1993). Respiratory muscle strength in patients with postpolio syndrome. *Rehabilitation Nursing Research, 2,* 55-60.

McCaffery, M. (1979). *Nursing management of the patient in pain* (2nd ed.). New York: J.B. Lippincott.

Mor, V., Wilcox, V., Rakowski, W., & Hiris, J. (1994). Functional transitions among the elderly: Patterns, predictors, and related hospital use. *American Journal of Public Health, 84,* 1274-1280.

Morgan, S. (1993). Effects of age on cardiovascular functioning. *Geriatric Nursing, 14,* 249-251.

Needham, J.F. (1993). *Gerontological nursing: A restorative approach.* Albany, NY: Delmar.

Neelon, V., & Champagne, M. (1992). Managing cognitive impairment: The Current bases for practice. In S. Funk, E. Torniquist, M. Champagne, & R. Wise (Eds.), *Key aspects of elder care: Managing falls, incontinence and cognitive impairment.* New York: Springer.

Quinn, C.A. (1994). The four A's of restraint reduction: Attitude, assessment, anticipation, avoidance. *Orthopaedic Nursing, 13,* 11-19.

Roth, E.J. (1988). The elderly stroke patient: Principles and practice of rehabilitation management. *Topics in Geriatric Rehabilitation, 3,* 27-61.

Sheets, D.J., Wray, L.A., & Torres-Gil, F.M. (1993). Geriatric rehabilitation: Linking aging, health, and disability policy. *Topics Geriatric Rehabilitation, 9,* 1-17.

Siebens, H. (1990). The adverse and therapeutic effects of medications on cognition of older adults. *Topics in Geriatric Rehabilitation, 5,* 20-25.

Simpson, W. (1986). Exercise: prescriptions for the elderly. *Geriatrics, 41,* 95-100.

St. George, C.L. (1993). Spasticity: Mechanisms and nursing care. *Nursing Clinics of North America, 20,* 819-827.

Stilwell, J.E. (1988). Common problems that threaten compliance in the elderly. *Topics in Geriatric Rehabilitation, 3,* 34-40.

Taub, E., Miller, N.E., Novack, T.A., Cook, E.W. III, Fleming, W.C., Nepomuceno, C.S., Connell, J.S., & Crago, J.E. (1993). Technique to improve motor deficit after stroke. *Archives of Physical Medicine and Rehabilitation, 74,* 347-354.

Tidelksaar, R. (1990). Environment adaptations to preserve balance and prevent falls. *Topics in Geriatric Rehabilitation, 5,* 78-84.

van Parys, E. (1987). Assessing the failing state of the heart. *Nursing 87, 17,* 42-50.

Wilson, L. (1993). Sensory perceptual alteration: diagnosis, prediction, and intervention in the hospitalized adult. *Nursing Clinics of North America, 28,* 747-764.

World Health Organization. (1986). *Cancer pain relief* (2nd ed.). Geneva: Author.

Zadai, C.C. (1985). Pulmonary physiology of aging: The role of rehabilitation. *Topics in Geriatric Rehabilitation, 1,* 49, 57.

Zarle, N.C. (1989). Continuity of care: Balancing care of elders between health care settings. *Nursing Clinics of North America, 24,* 697-705.

Zuckerman, J., Zetterburg, C., & Frankel, V. (1990). Principles of treatment of orthopedic injuries in the elderly. *Topics in Geriatric Rehabilitation, 6,* 1-17.

◆

Appendix 31-A   Nursing care guideline: Rehabilitation nursing focus in the acute care of a person over initial seven days following a stroke*

Usually clients who have had a stroke are admitted to the acute hospital via the emergency room. Clients with a diagnosis of stroke are a most heterogeneous population: symptoms may range from mild deficits to catastrophic loss of function. Assessment and intervention strategies are established according to the client's level of medical and neurologic instability and amount of stroke-related deficits. The first week following a stroke is the period when the risk of having another stroke or developing complications from the stroke is at its highest. The client's neurologic, cardiac, and respiratory status must be monitored closely. Although the acute phase is a period of risk, rehabilitation nursing interventions are incorporated into care from the time of hospital admission. Interdisciplinary planning and coordination of care is essential as the Diagnosis-Related Group (DRG) length of acute hospital stay for an uncomplicated stroke is currently 7.1 days.

I. Days 1 to 2
   A. Nursing Assessment
      The following nursing assessments are performed:
      ◆ Neurologic assessment
      Motor, sensory, and cognitive assessment
      Swallowing assessment including tongue strength and mobility, gag reflex, swallowing reflex, and ability to cough
      ◆ Cardiac and respiratory status
      Vital sign monitoring every 2 to 4 hours
      Electrocardiogram (ECG) monitoring
      Cardiac telemetry
      Monitoring of cardiac enzymes
      Respiratory rate and rhythm
      Breath sounds
      Ability to handle secretions
      Assessment and monitoring of laboratory studies
      ◆ Assessment and monitoring of volume status
      Intake and output measurement
      Daily weight
      ◆ Monitoring for presence of deep vein thrombosis (DVT): induration, warmth and pain at site of thrombosis
      ◆ Nutritional assessment
      Swallowing and eating ability
      Weight, height
      Diet history, dietary requirements
      Baseline laboratory measures of nutritional status
      ◆ Medical history: previous stroke, transient ischemic attack (TIA), hypertension, diabetes, cardiac or pulmonary disease, history of smoking, excessive alcohol intake
      ◆ Medication history, medication compliance
      ◆ Functional status before admission, living arrangements before admission
      ◆ Assessment of family and social support

      ◆ Beginning fall risk assessment: history of falls before admission
   B. Interventions
      ◆ Notify physician of any changes in neurologic, cardiac, or pulmonary status, or of any abnormal laboratory findings
      ◆ Maintain optimum pulmonary function
      Turn every 2 to 4 hours
      Encourage deep breathing and coughing to clear airway
      Chest physiotherapy as needed
      Oxygen therapy as needed
      ◆ Monitor blood pressure control within physician-designated parameters. In some cases the physician may determine that blood pressure is to be maintained at a higher level to assure cerebral perfusion. Antihypertensive medications may be held and blood pressure left untreated until it reaches a level of approximately 200/100 mm Hg.
      ◆ Monitor fluid status
      Intravenous (IV) fluids will most likely be given in the event of an ischemic event to keep blood volume high and assure cerebral perfusion, especially if the client is not able to maintain hydration. If there is a significant medical history of fluid regulation difficulty (CHF, pulmonary edema, renal failure, etc.), the client's fluid status is monitored carefully. In the event of a hemorrhagic stroke, with increased risk of increased intracranial pressure, IV fluids may be restricted.
      ◆ Client activity
      The client is typically on bed rest for the first 24 hours. Bed rest is maintained for the purposes of ruling out myocardial infarction and/or providing adequate cerebral perfusion. The client with a stroke involving the posterior circulation or the client with poor cerebral perfusion may need to remain in bed with the head of the bed flat. Otherwise, if the client is on bed rest, the head of the bed is elevated 30 degrees for aspiration precautions. The client is turned and repositioned every 2 hours with bony prominences and skin assessed with repositioning. Affected limbs should be positioned to protect joint mobility and prevent injury. The client is moved in bed carefully to prevent injury to paretic limbs; a pull sheet is used to prevent pulling on hemiparetic limbs. Range of joint motion is provided to involved limbs to promote movement and prevent joint contracture formation. Splints are used as needed; splints removed and skin inspected frequently. Bed mobility is encouraged by having client assist with turning and moving in bed. Fall prevention strategies are initiated: bed alarms, toileting schedule.
      ◆ Institute measures to prevent DVT
      The client is treated prophylactically for DVT prevention. If the client is receiving anticoagulant therapy with IV heparin, additional interventions are not necessary. If not, depending on the

stroke etiology, the client is placed on subcutaneous heparin, pneumatic antiembolus boots, or antiembolus stockings. If there is a question of the stroke being hemorrhagic, then subcutaneous heparin would not be the treatment of choice.

◆ Monitor anticoagulation

Clients often considered candidates for anticoagulation therapy include those with a history of atrial fibrillation; suspicion of a cerebral embolism of cardiac origin; or those with occluded or stenosed carotid arteries. Clients initially are placed on anticoagulation therapy with IV heparin, and when laboratory values reflect a therapeutic level of anticoagulation, are then switched to oral sodium warfarin (Coumadin). The amount of time that the client is maintained on oral anticoagulation therapy is dependent on the cause of stroke and the practice of the attending physician.

◆ Prepare client and family for evaluative procedures

The client and family need to be prepared for the variety of evaluative procedures that may occur in the first few days of hospital admission: computed tomography scan, magnetic resonance imaging, Holter monitor, echocardiography.

C. Consultation

Consultations to be made within the first 24 hours include

Social services

Physical and occupational therapy

Additional consultations to be made within the first 24 hours based on neurologic findings include

Swallowing therapy

Speech therapy

Nutrition

Neuropsychology

Interdisciplinary collaboration in establishing goals of care is initiated. Some factors that need to be considered include client's medical status and rehabilitation potential, availability of family/community supports, and availability of needed services and programs.

D. Client and Family Teaching

Client and family education about stroke begins on admission. Interdisciplinary team members collaborate and provide the family with initial information about stroke; the impact of stroke; the rationale for initial medical, nursing, and therapeutic interventions; evaluative procedures; and the experience of acute hospitalization. The family is provided with reading materials about stroke and invited to stroke education forums.

II. **Days 3 to 4**

A. Nursing Assessment

Assessment is ongoing and dependent on the severity and complications of the stroke

◆ Neurologic assessment

The results of assessments are compared with baseline and subsequent assessments. If indicated, more detailed language and perceptual assessments are initiated.

◆ Cardiac, respiratory assessment

As the client's activity level is increased, endurance should be monitored through frequent vital sign measurements and assessment of the client's appearance and complaints of fatigue.

◆ Functional assessment

After the first 24 to 48 hours, the client may be ready for increasing activity. It is at this time that the client can be evaluated further for increasing levels of functional ability: bed mobility, sitting balance, transfers ability, standing balance, and walking ability. Orthostatic hypotension is evaluated before getting the client out of bed. Self-care ability should be evaluated and includes bathing, grooming, feeding, dressing, and toileting.

◆ Swallowing and nutritional assessment

Swallowing is continually evaluated, especially if there is a question of the client's ability to swallow on the initial examination. The nutritional assessment continues: calorie counts are maintained and/or initiated if the client's intake is questionable. If the client is unable to eat or drink, it is time to address the need for an enteral feeding source such as nasogastric or gastrostomy tube.

◆ Bladder and bowel assessment

Urinary and fecal incontinence may be an outcome of stroke. Indwelling catheters should be removed as soon as possible. For continued urinary incontinence, review additional factors: history of incontinence, physical examination, urinalysis, functional ability, mental status, presence of urinary tract infection, gynecologic or prostatic problems. Obtain a 24-hour incontinence record. Identify type of bowel dysfunction and evaluate cause: immobility and inactivity, inadequate fluid or nutritional intake, infection, cognitive deficit, impaired mobility.

◆ Fall risk assessment

The client is assessed continually for falls and falling risk. If the client's activity is increased, the client's balance and stability while sitting and walking is evaluated. Mental status evaluation and perceptual evaluation are other factors to consider.

◆ Language assessment

Speech therapy should be consulted if there is any indication that the client is having difficulty with the production or comprehension of language; with reading, writing, or using gestures; or with the ability to move the lips, tongue, and mouth in a coordinated fashion to produce speech.

◆ Perceptual assessment

Occupational therapy will assist the nurse in identifying the presence of any perceptual deficits. Examples of some client cues: lack of acknowledgment of one side of the environment; inability to recognize function of object by shape and/or touch; denial of one side of the body; denial of illness.

B. Interventions

The level of nursing intervention is dependent on the severity of the client's stroke and resultant functional and cognitive deficits as well as medical condition. Many of these interventions are initiated in the acute care setting and continued in the rehabilitation setting or the home. Interdisciplinary collaboration is an integral aspect of planning interventions.

✦ Continue cardiac monitoring
  Cardiac telemetry most likely will be continued if arrhythmias are present, otherwise telemetry generally will be discontinued
  Continue to monitor pertinent laboratory results
✦ Continue respiratory monitoring
  Continue to monitor respiratory status
✦ Client activity
  The client should be out of bed, sitting in a chair, as soon as medically and neurologically possible. The client's level of activity is determined by cardiac and respiratory status and level of endurance. The initiation of rehabilitation therapies—physical therapy, occupational therapy, speech therapy, and swallowing therapy—should begin as soon as possible. The client is encouraged to participate in as many self-care activities as possible.
✦ Approaches to swallowing
  Identify needed changes in positioning: position of trunk, position of head
  Identify need for changes in food consistency, temperature, bolus size
  Identify environmental factors: need for decreased distractions, quiet and privacy during eating
✦ Approaches to urinary incontinence include
  Early removal of indwelling urinary catheter
  Determination of postvoid residuals through catheterization; if residual is greater than 100 ml, determine need for intermittent catheterization
  Place client on scheduled program of toileting, with schedule based on 24-hour incontinence record
  Protection of skin through cleansing and use of skin barriers
  When necessary, containment of urine through condom drainage system for men
✦ Approaches to bowel care
  Establishment of a bowel program based on previous bowel pattern
  High-fiber diet if possible
  Adequate fluid intake
  Elimination schedule
  Stool softener, suppository regimen, judicious use of laxatives
✦ Approaches to language disturbance
  Collaborate with speech therapist in planning communication strategies
  Keep communication with client simple
  Attempt to limit client's frustrations with limitations in communication ability

✦ Approaches to perceptual deficits
  Collaborate with occupational therapist and all members of interdisciplinary team in planning strategies of care
  Identify methods to promote client safety
  Identify environmental factors that may enhance perceptual ability
C. Client and Family Teaching
  Clients and families will need continued support and education. At this time teaching should center on assessing the family's ability to be involved in the client's care. Once the family's level of involvement is determined, learning needs can be better established. During this time of great stress, explanations may require frequent repetitions. Results of tests and procedures may be available and need to be shared with the client and/or family. Further investigation of the client's living situation and potential discharge plans should begin to be addressed. The social worker will be informed of the needs and involved in the planning. Discussion of the need for rehabilitation and the type of needed setting are initiated.

III. Days 4 to 7, Through Discharge
  A. Nursing Assessment
  The focus of nursing assessment is shifted toward assessment of rehabilitation needs and discharge planning. Client and family coping will be continually addressed as well. Nursing assessment should continue to include all of the previously discussed areas with particular emphasis on the neurologic and functional status; an ongoing assessment of the client's ability to swallow and nutritional status if a problem has been identified in these areas; cardiac telemetry will be discontinued if the client has remained stable hemodynamically—otherwise, it will continue until any problems have been addressed; monitoring of laboratory results will continue throughout the hospitalization, particularly if the client is receiving anticoagulant therapy or has an ongoing medical problem.
  B. Interventions
  The client's functional status and available family and community supports will determine the need for continued rehabilitation services. Discharge planning will be the major focus at this time. Members of the interdisciplinary team are actively involved in identification of need for continued rehabilitation and selection of the best type of facility or agency to provide needed services. Ideally a home assessment is made on site.
  C. Client and Family Teaching
  The client and family are involved with the rehabilitation efforts and discharge planning. Education should be ongoing as the client progresses toward discharge. Medication changes should be reviewed as they are made. Families are urged to continue participation in family education programs and review of materials about stroke. Families should be provided as much information as possible about rehabilitation programs and services. Staff need to

continually assess the client and family's understanding of the information provided. Follow-up appointments with physicians and therapists should be scheduled before discharge. Visiting nurse and discharge summaries should be prepared for discharge.

---

*Courtesy of Ann Connor, RN, MS, Stroke Nurse Specialist and Marion Phipps, MS, RN, CRRN, FAAN, Rehabilitation Nurse Specialist, Beth Israel Hospital, Boston, MA.

SUGGESTED READINGS

Asberg, K.H. (1989). Orthostatic tolerance training of stroke patients in general medical wards. *Scandinavian Journal of Rehabilitation Medicine, 21,* 179-185.

Axelsson, K., Asplund, K., Norberg, A., & Alafuzoff, I. (1988). Nutritional status in patients with acute stroke. *Acta Medica Scandinavia, 224,* 217-224.

Brody, E.M. (1985). Parent care as a normative family stress. *Gerontologist, 25,* 19-29.

Bronstein, K.S., Popovitch, J.M., & Stewart-Amidei, C. (1991). *Promoting stroke recovery: A research-based approach for nurses.* St Louis: Mosby–Year Book.

Chapron, D.J. (1993). Insights into the prevention of predictable complications of nonsteroidal antiinflammatory drugs in the elderly. *Topics in Geriatric Rehabilitation, 8,* 38-51.

DeVincenzo, D.K., & Watkins, S. (1987). Accidental falls in the rehabilitation setting. *Rehabilitation Nursing, 12,* 248-252.

Gross, J.C. (1990). Bladder dysfunction after stroke: It's not always inevitable. *Journal of Gerontological Nursing, 16,* 20-25.

Hamrin, E. (1982). Early activation in stroke: Does it make a difference? *Scandinavian Journal of Rehabilitation Medicine, 14,* 101-109.

Johnson, J.H., Searles, L.B., & McNamara, S. (1993). In-home geriatric rehabilitation: Improving strength and function. *Topics in Geriatric Rehabilitation, 8,* 51-64.

Lund, C., & Sheafor, M.L. (1985). Is your patient about to fall? *Journal of Gerontological Nursing, 11,* 37-41.

Matteson, M.A., & McConnell, E.S. (1988). *Gerontological nursing: Concepts and practice.* Philadelphia: W.B. Saunders.

Means, K.M., Currie, D.M., & Gershkoff, A.M. (1993). Geriatric rehabilitation: Assessment, preservation, and enhancement of fitness and function. Part 4. *Archives of Physical Medicine and Rehabilitation, 74,* S417-S420.

Mol, V., & Baker, C.A. (1991). Activity intolerance in the geriatric stroke patient. *Rehabilitation Nursing, 16,* 337-342.

Pasquearello, M. (1990). Developing, implementing, and evaluating a stroke recovery group. *Rehabilitation Nursing, 15,* 26-29.

Pressure ulcers in adults: Prediction and prevention: Clinical practice guideline (AHCPR Pub. No. 92-0050). Rockville, MD: US Department of Health and Human Services.

Rempusheski, V.F. (1989). The role of ethnicity in elder care. *Nursing Clinics of North America, 24,* 717-724.

Rogers, J.C. and Holm, M.B. (1991). Teaching older persons with depression. *Topics in Geriatric Rehabilitation, 6*(3).

Smith, E.L., DiFabio, R.D., & Gilligan, C. (1990). Exercise intervention and physiologic function in the elderly. *Topics in Geriatric Rehabilitation, 6,* 57-68.

Steiner, D., & Marcopulos, B. (1991). Depression in the elderly: characteristics and clinical management. *Nursing Clinics of North America, 26,* 585-600.

Urinary Incontinence in Adults: Clinical Practice Guidelines (AHCPR Pub. No. 92-0038). Rockville, MD: US Department of Health and Human Service.

US Bureau of the Census (1992). Report of the US Census for 1990. Washington, D.C.

Venn, M.R., Taft, L., Carpentier, B., & Appelbaugh, G. (1992). The influence of timing and suppository use on efficiency and effectiveness of bowel training after stroke. *Rehabilitation Nursing, 17,* 116-120.

Appendix: ARN Standards of Care and Standards of Professional Performance

Following are selections that are reprinted with the permission of the Association of Rehabilitation Nurses from Association of Rehabilitation Nurses, 1994, *Standards and Scope of Rehabilitation Nursing Practice,* 3d ed., Skokie, IL: Author. Copyright © 1994 by Association of Rehabilitation Nurses.

STANDARDS OF CARE

STANDARD I. ASSESSMENT
The Rehabilitation Nurse Collects Client Health Data.

1. The priority of data to be collected is determined by the client's immediate condition and/or needs.
2. Using appropriate assessment parameters, the rehabilitation nurse collects pertinent data about the client, including data in these areas:
   a. Adaptation, adjustment, and coping
   b. Perception of goals, of potential barriers to achieving goals, and of possible strategies to overcome barriers
   c. Cognitive and communicative status
   d. Economic resources
   e. Environmental factors (in places such as the workplace, home, and school)
   f. Family dynamics
   g. Functional ability (in areas such as self-care, elimination, and mobility)
   h. Knowledge about the nature of his or her own disability or chronic illness
   i. Level of impairment
   j. Physiological status, and
   k. Safety
3. Data collection involves, as appropriate, the client, significant others, and healthcare providers.
4. The data collection process is systematic and ongoing.
5. Relevant data are documented in a retrievable form.

STANDARD II. DIAGNOSIS
The Rehabilitation Nurse Analyzes the Assessment Data When Determining Diagnoses.

1. Diagnoses are derived from the assessment data.
2. Diagnoses are validated with, when possible, the client, significant others, and healthcare providers.
3. Diagnoses are documented in a manner that facilitates the determination of expected outcomes and of a plan of care.

STANDARD III. OUTCOME IDENTIFICATION
The Rehabilitation Nurse Identifies Expected Outcomes Individualized to the Client.

1. Outcomes are derived from the diagnoses and commonly deal with these areas:
   a. Adaptation, adjustment, and coping goals
   b. Learning goals for the client and significant others
   c. Functional goals
   d. Health management goals
   e. Self-advocacy goals, and
   f. Self-care goals
2. Outcomes are mutually formulated and prioritized with, when possible, the client, significant others, and healthcare providers.
3. Outcomes are documented as measurable goals.
4. Outcomes are realistic in relation to the client's present and potential functional, emotional, and developmental capabilities.
5. Outcomes are attainable in relation to the human, financial, equipment, and community resources available to the client.

STANDARD IV. PLANNING
The Rehabilitation Nurse Develops a Plan of Care that Prescribes Interventions to Attain Expected Outcomes.

1. The plan of care is individualized according to the client's condition, needs, and priorities.
2. The plan of care is developed with, when appropriate, the client, significant others, and healthcare providers.
3. The plan of care reflects current nursing practice.
4. The plan of care is documented.
5. The plan of care provides for continuity of care.
6. The plan of care and the interdisciplinary treatment plan are congruent and coordinated.
7. The plan of care is consistent with resources available to the client and significant others.
8. The plan of care promotes independence in functional, life care, and decision-making skills and progressively transfers that independence to the client and significant others.
9. The plan of care includes estimated time frames within which goals should be achieved.

STANDARD V. IMPLEMENTATION
The Rehabilitation Nurse Implements the Interventions Identified in the Plan of Care.

1. Interventions are consistent with the established plan of care, the interdisciplinary treatment plan, and available economic resources.
2. Interventions are implemented in a safe and appropriate manner.
3. Interventions are documented.
4. Interventions facilitate the independence of the client and significant others.
5. Interventions include the education of the client and significant others in regard to these areas:
   a. Adjustment to chronic illness or disability
   b. Management of behavior
   c. Community resources and re-entry
   d. Communication skills
   e. Decision-making
   f. The environment
   g. Functional and self-care skills
   h. Health maintenance and management
   i. Safety, and
   j. Self-advocacy

STANDARD VI. EVALUATION
The Rehabilitation Nurse Evaluates the Client's Progress Toward Attainment of Outcomes.

1. Evaluation is systematic and ongoing.
2. The client's and significant others' responses to interventions and progress toward outcomes are documented.
3. The effectiveness of interventions is evaluated in relation to achievement of outcomes.
4. Ongoing assessment data are used to revise, as needed, diagnoses, outcomes, and the plan of care.
5. Revisions in diagnoses, outcomes, and the plan of care are documented.
6. When appropriate, the client, significant others, and healthcare providers are involved in the evaluation and revision process.

STANDARDS OF PROFESSIONAL PERFORMANCE

STANDARD I. QUALITY OF CARE
The Rehabilitation Nurse Systematically Evaluates the Quality and Effectiveness of Rehabilitation Nursing Practice.

1. The rehabilitation nurse participates in quality-of-care activities as appropriate for his or her position, education, and practice environment. Such activities may include the following:
   a. Identifying aspects of care important for quality monitoring
   b. Identifying indicators used to monitor the quality and effectiveness of nursing care
   c. Collecting data to monitor the quality and effectiveness of nursing care
   d. Analyzing quality data to identify opportunities for improving care
   e. Formulating recommendations to improve nursing practice or client outcomes
   f. Implementing activities to enhance the quality of nursing practice
   g. Participating on interdisciplinary teams that evaluate clinical practice or health services, and/or
   h. Developing and revising policies and procedures to improve the quality of care
2. The rehabilitation nurse uses the results of quality-of-care activities to initiate changes in practice.
3. The rehabilitation nurse uses the results of quality-of-care activities to initiate changes throughout the healthcare delivery system, as appropriate.

STANDARD II. PERFORMANCE APPRAISAL
The Rehabilitation Nurse Evaluates His or Her Own Nursing Practice in Relation to Professional Practice Standards and Relevant Statutes and Regulations.

1. The rehabilitation nurse appraises his or her own performance on a regular basis, identifying areas of strength as well as areas for professional practice development.
2. The rehabilitation nurse seeks constructive feedback regarding his or her own practice.
3. The rehabilitation nurse includes in ongoing self-evaluations an appraisal of sensitivity to issues of cultural diversity, discrimination, language, prejudice, access, and civil rights that affect individuals with disability and chronic illness.
4. The rehabilitation nurse takes action to achieve goals identified during a performance appraisal.
5. The rehabilitation nurse participates in peer review as appropriate.

STANDARD III. EDUCATION
The Rehabilitation Nurse Acquires and Maintains Current Knowledge in Nursing Practice.

1. The rehabilitation nurse participates in ongoing educational activities related to clinical knowledge, professional and healthcare issues, and the functioning of the interdisciplinary team.
2. The rehabilitation nurse seeks experiences to maintain and improve clinical skills.
3. The rehabilitation nurse seeks knowledge and skills appropriate to the practice setting.
4. The rehabilitation nurse continually increases his or her knowledge of cultural, public policy, scientific, and social issues related to rehabilitation.
5. The rehabilitation nurse meets continuing education requirements for maintaining licensure, if such requirements exist, and for maintaining certification, if applicable.

STANDARD IV. COLLEGIALITY
The Rehabilitation Nurse Contributes to the Professional Development of Peers, Colleagues, and Others

1. The rehabilitation nurse shares knowledge and skills with colleagues and others.
2. The rehabilitation nurse provides peers with constructive feedback regarding their practice.
3. The rehabilitation nurse contributes to an environment

that is conducive to the clinical education of nursing students and other students, as applicable.

STANDARD V. ETHICS
The Rehabilitation Nurse's Decisions and Actions on Behalf of Clients are Determined in an Ethical Manner.

1. The rehabilitation nurse's practice is guided by *Code for Nurses with Interpretive Statements* (ANA, 1985) and by *Association of Rehabilitation Nurses Position Statement: Ethical Issues* (ARN, in press).
2. The rehabilitation nurse maintains a client's confidentiality.
3. The rehabilitation nurse acts as a client advocate.
4. The rehabilitation nurse delivers care in a nonjudgmental and nondiscriminatory manner that is sensitive to clients' diversity.
5. The rehabilitation nurse delivers care in a manner that preserves and protects clients' autonomy, dignity, and rights.
6. The rehabilitation nurse maintains an awareness of his or her beliefs and value systems and what effect they may have on care he or she provides to the client and client's significant others.
7. The rehabilitation nurse supports the client's right to make decisions that may not be congruent with the values of the rehabilitation team.
8. The rehabilitation nurse seeks available resources to help formulate ethical decisions.
9. The rehabilitation nurse promotes the provision of information and discussion that allows the client to participate fully in decision-making.
10. The rehabilitation nurse participates in decision making regarding allocation of resources.

STANDARD VI. COLLABORATION
The Rehabilitation Nurse Collaborates with the Client, Significant Others, and Healthcare Providers in Providing Client Care.

1. The rehabilitation nurse communicates with the client, significant others, and healthcare providers regarding the client's care and nursing's role in the provision of care.
2. The rehabilitation nurse obtains and communicates client data so that information from the nursing assessment is integrated into the interdisciplinary treatment plan.
3. The rehabilitation nurse includes the client and significant others in the collaborative work of the team whenever possible and appropriate.
4. The rehabilitation nurse collaborates with the team in establishing specific goals for the client.
5. The rehabilitation nurse makes referrals, including referrals to provide for continuity of care, as needed.
6. The rehabilitation nurse consults with healthcare providers for client care, as needed.

STANDARD VII. RESEARCH
The Rehabilitation Nurse Uses Research Findings in Practice.

1. The rehabilitation nurse uses interventions substantiated by research as appropriate to his or her position, education, and practice environment.

2. The rehabilitation nurse participates in research activities as appropriate for his or her position, education, and practice environment. Such activities may include the following:
   a. Identifying clinical problems suitable for research
   b. Identifying research questions that address the influence of societal discriminatory attitudes and/or barriers on the optimal independence of clients and their significant others
   c. Participating in data collection
   d. Participating in unit, organization, or community research committees or programs
   e. Sharing research activities with others
   f. Conducting research
   g. Critiquing research for its application to rehabilitation nursing practice, and/or
   h. Using research findings in the development of policies, procedures, and guidelines for client care.

STANDARD VIII. RESOURCE UTILIZATION
The Rehabilitation Nurse Considers Factors Related to Safety, Effectiveness, and Cost in Planning and Delivering Client Care.

1. The rehabilitation nurse evaluates factors related to safety, effectiveness, and cost when more than one practice option would result in the same expected client outcome.
2. The rehabilitation nurse assigns tasks or delegates care based on the needs of the client and the knowledge and skills of the provider the nurse selects.
3. The rehabilitation nurse assists the client and significant others in identifying and securing appropriate and available services to address health-related needs. Such services may include
   a. Community resources for housing and attendant care
   b. Healthcare and follow-up services
   c. Supplies, equipment, and repair services necessary for health maintenance, and/or
   d. Support groups and other emotional resources
4. The rehabilitation nurse considers financial resources when planning and delivering care.

DEFINITION OF TERMS

Assessment: "A systematic, dynamic process by which the nurse, through interaction with the client, significant others, and health care providers, collects and analyzes data about the client. Data may include the following dimensions: physical, psychological, sociocultural, spiritual, cognitive, functional abilities, development, economic, and life-style" (ANA, 1991a).

Client: "Recipient of nursing actions. When the client is an individual, the focus is on the health state, problems, or needs of a single person. When the client is a family or group, the focus is on the health state of the unit as a whole or the reciprocal effects of an individual's health state on the other members of the unit. When the client is a community, the focus is on personal and environmental health and the health risks of population groups.

Nursing actions toward clients may be directed to disease or injury prevention, health promotion, health restoration, or health maintenance" (ANA, 1991a).

Continuity of care: "An interdisciplinary process that includes clients and significant others in the development of a coordinated plan of care. This process facilitates the client's transition between settings, based on changing needs and available resources" (ANA, 1991a).

Criteria: "Relevant, measurable indicators of the standards of clinical nursing practice" (ANA, 1991a).

Diagnosis: "A clinical judgment about the client's response to actual or potential health conditions or needs. Diagnoses provide the basis for determination of a plan of care to achieve expected outcomes" (ANA, 1991a).

Evaluation: "The process of determining both the client's progress toward the attainment of expected outcomes and the effectiveness of nursing care" (ANA, 1991a).

Functional ability: "The ability to perform a variety of skills necessary for physical, cognitive, behavioral, and social activities.

Guidelines: "Describe a process of client care management which has the potential of improving the quality of clinical and consumer decision making. Guidelines are systematically developed statements based on available scientific evidence and expert opinion" (ANA, 1991a).

Healthcare providers: Individuals with special expertise who provide healthcare services or assistance to clients. They may include nurses, physicians, psychologists, social workers, nutritionists and dietitians, and various therapists. Providers also may include service organizations, vendors, and payers.

Implementation: "May include any or all of these activities: intervening, delegating, coordinating. The client, significant others, or health care providers may be designated to implement interventions within the plan of care" (ANA, 1991a).

Interdisciplinary treatment plan: A comprehensive, coordinated, individualized plan for each client that addresses the desired outcomes for the client for each service provided.

Nursing: "The diagnosis and treatment of human responses to actual or potential health problems" (ANA, 1980).

Nursing intervention: "Any direct treatment that a nurse performs on behalf of a client. Nursing interventions include nurse-initiated treatments and physician-initiated treatments" (McCloskey & Bulechek, 1992).

Outcomes: "Measurable, expected, client-focused goals" (ANA, 1991a).

Plan of care: "Comprehensive outline of care to be delivered to attain expected outcomes" (ANA, 1991a).

Rehabilitation setting: Any environment in which nurse-client interactions are grounded in the philosophy and concepts of rehabilitation nursing practice. Such environments could include rehabilitation centers, rehabilitation units, acute care units, ambulatory clinics, home health agencies, insurance companies, and long-term care facilities.

Significant others: "Family members and/or those significant to the client" (ANA, 1991a).

Standard: "Authoritative statement enunciated and promulgated by the profession by which the quality of practice, service, or education can be judged" (ANA, 1991a).

Standards of care: "Authoritative statements that describe a competent level of clinical nursing practice demonstrated through assessment, diagnosis, outcome identification, planning, implementation, and evaluation" (ANA, 1991a).

Standards of nursing practice: "Authoritative statements that describe a level of care or performance common to the profession of nursing by which the quality of nursing practice can be judged. Standards of clinical nursing practice include both standards of care and standards of professional performance" (ANA, 1991a).

Standards of professional performance: "Authoritative statements that describe a competent level of behavior in the professional role, including activities related to quality of care, performance appraisal, education, collegiality, ethics, collaboration, research, and resource utilization" (ANA, 1991a).

REFERENCES

American Nurses Association (ANA). (1980). *Nursing: A social policy statement.* Kansas City, MO: Author.

American Nurses Association. (1985). *Code for nurses with interpretive statements.* Washington, DC: Author.

American Nurses Association. (1991a). *Standards of clinical nursing practice.* Washington, DC: Author.

American Nurses Association. (1991b). Task force and nursing practice standards and guidelines: Working paper. *Journal of Nursing Quality Assurance, 5,* 1–17.

American Nurses Association & Association of Rehabilitation Nurses (ARN). (1977). *Standards of rehabilitation nursing practice.* Kansas City, MO: American Nurses Association.

American Nurses Association & Association of Rehabilitation Nurses. (1986). *Standards of rehabilitation nursing practice* (2nd ed.). Kansas City, MO: American Nurses Association.

American Nurses Association & Association of Rehabilitation Nurses. (1988). *Rehabilitation nursing: Scope of practice; process and outcome criteria for selected diagnoses.* Kansas City, MO: American Nurses Association.

Association of Rehabilitation Nurses. (in press). *Association of Rehabilitation Nurses position statement: Ethical issues.* Skokie, IL: Author.

McCloskey, J. C., & Bulechek, G. M. (1992). *Nursing intervention classification (NIC).* St. Louis: Mosby–Year Book.

National Institute of Child Health and Human Development (NICHHD). (1993). *Research plan for National Center for Medical Rehabilitation Research* (NICHHD Publication No. 93-3509). Bethesda, MD: Author.

INDEX

Illustrations are indicated by italics.

Notes